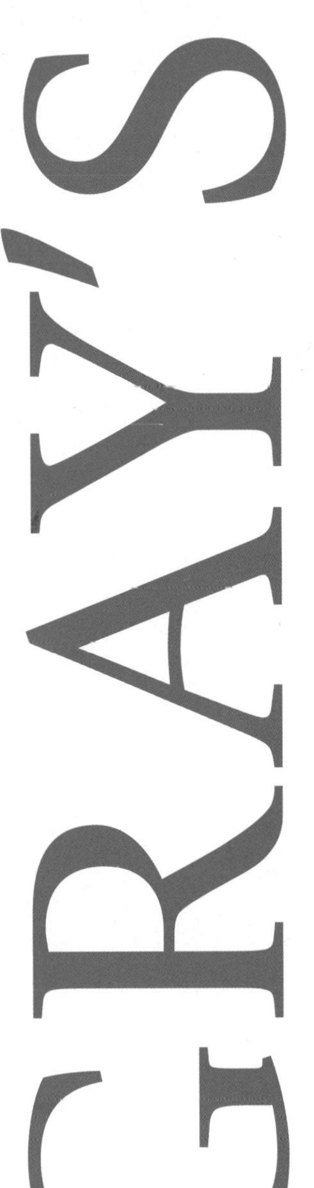

CLINICAL PHOTOGRA

DISSECTOR OF THE HUMAN BODY

Third Edition

Marios Loukas, MD, PhD
Dean School of Medicine,
Professor, Department of Anatomical Sciences
Professor Department of Pathology,
St. George's University, School of Medicine, Grenada, West Indies

Dean, College of Medical Sciences, Nicolaus Copernicus Superior School, Olsztyn, Poland

R. Shane Tubbs, PhD, MSc, PA-C
Professor
Director of Surgical Anatomy, Tulane University School of Medicine
Program Director of Anatomical Research, Clinical Neuroscience Research Center
Department of Neurosurgery,
Department of Neurology,
Tulane University School of Medicine
Department of Structural and Cellular Biology,
Department of Surgery, Tulane University School of Medicine;
Department of Neurosurgery and Ochsner Neuroscience Institute,
Ochsner Health System
New Orleans, Louisiana
University of Queensland
Brisbane, Australia
Department of Anatomical Sciences
St. George's University
Grenada, West Indies

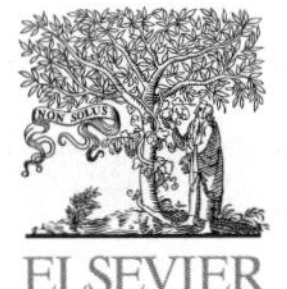

Elsevier
1600 John F. Kennedy Blvd.
Ste 1800
Philadelphia, PA 19103-2899

GRAY'S CLINICAL PHOTOGRAPHIC DISSECTOR OF THE HUMAN BODY, THIRD EDITION
ISBN: 978-0-443-10709-2

Publisher: Jeremy Bowes
Director, Content Development: Rebecca Gruliow
Publishing Services Manager: Deepthi Unni
Book Specialist: Kamatchi Madhavan
Design Direction: Amy Buxton

Printed in India

Last digit is the print number: 9 8 7 6 5 4 3 2 1

I would like to dedicate this book to my brilliant and wonderful wife, Joanna, who has been the bright star of my life. Her continuous support, dedication, love, and affection give me the energy and courage to fulfill all of our dreams.

ML

I would like to thank my wife, Susan, and son, Isaiah, for their support and patience during the writing of this book. All that I do, I do for them. I also want to dedicate this book in memory of my brother-in-law, Nelson Jones, whose intellect, engagement of others, and curiosity about life have been examples for me.

RST

Preface

Even in the modern era, the exploration of the human body through dissection remains an invaluable method for comprehending its complexities. The tactile engagement in dissection and the variations witnessed among specimens provide students with a profound understanding of the human structure, ultimately providing the basis to become a better physician. However, as time for anatomical education diminishes in many curricula, courses must adapt. In this context, anatomy courses utilizing cadaver dissection must make the most of the available time.

Traditionally, anatomy courses begin with students following guided dissection instructions, much like a recipe in a cookbook. These guides typically lack visual, step-by-step depictions of the dissection process, often resorting to schematic drawings that diverge from real anatomical structures. Recognizing this gap, we have assembled a collection of dissection photographs with accompanying descriptions and dissection tips and tricks. Our aim is to better support anatomy students by providing a visual representation of what they can anticipate uncovering during dissection, progressing from surface to depth. Moreover, the photographs within this book faithfully capture a realistic process of cadaveric dissection that every student will encounter in the anatomy laboratory. Deliberately, we refrain from portraying an immaculately dissected specimen, instead opting for a true-to-life representation. By enhancing their learning experience in this manner, we hope to enable students to maximize their efficiency and utilize their time effectively. In addition, in this edition, we follow the terminology of anatomical terms as outlined in the most recent edition of *Terminologia Anatomica,* 2nd edition (https://fipat.library.dal.ca/ta2/).

We hold the aspiration that both students and educators will derive satisfaction from exploring the intricacies of the human body with the assistance of *Gray's Clinical Photographic Dissector of the Human Body.* This approach aims to facilitate an efficient and productive learning experience, forming a solid foundation for comprehending the underlying mechanisms of diseases and clinical manifestations.

Marios Loukas
R. Shane Tubbs

Acknowledgments

This dissection book is the work not only of the authors but also of numerous scientific and clinical friends and colleagues who have been so generous with their knowledge and who have given significant feedback and help. This book would not have been possible were it not for the contributions of the colleagues and friends listed below.

The two main contributors, Nelson Davis, BSc, and Damion Richards, BSc, provided superb dissections and technical expertise for this project.

We thank the following faculty members of the Department of Anatomical Sciences, St. George's University, School of Medicine, Grenada, West Indies, for their incredible artistic talents and significant contribution throughout the book with numerous illustrations:

Sue Simon, MS, CMI
David Nahabedian, MSMI, CMI
Sarah Gluschitz, MA, CMI
Linden Pederson, MSMI
Claudia Cárceles Román, MA
Jack Nelson, BFA
Farihah Khan, BSc

The following individuals from the Department of Anatomical Sciences at St. George's University have been very helpful with their comments and criticisms:

Danny Burns, MD, PhD
Maira DuPlessis, MSc
Deon Forrester, MD
Rachel George, MD
Robert Hage, MD, PhD
Ahmed Mahgoub, MBBS
Kazzara Raeburn, MD
Ramesh Rao, MD
Deepak Sharma, MD
Tyan Mitchell, BSc

The following individuals from the Department of Pathology at St. George's University have also been very helpful with their comments and criticisms.

Ewarld Marshall, MD
Sasha Lake, MD

We are also grateful to the following members of St. George's University for their photographic and technical expertise and laboratory assistance:

Joanna Loukas (photography and design)
Rayn Jacobs (design)
Paulette Mitchell (laboratory technician)
Lillian Best (laboratory technician)
Reynard McDonald (laboratory technician)
Nicholas Phillip (laboratory technician)
Shiva Mathurin (laboratory technician)
Romeo Cox (laboratory technician)

Thanks also to *Ms. Yvonne James, Ms. Nafeza Baksh*, and *Ms. Tracy Shabazz* for their invaluable assistance.

A special thanks to our friends and partners in Elsevier for this project—*Jeremy Bowes, Rebecca Gruliow*, and *Madelene Hyde*.

We would like to acknowledge all our former and current students who have kept our thinking fresh and edgy with all their comments to improve the learning and teaching of anatomy.

The authors state that every effort was made to follow all local and international laws and ethical guidelines that pertain to the use of human cadaveric donors in anatomical education and research.[1] The authors extend their appreciation and gratitude to those who generously donated their bodies to science. Their contribution facilitated this anatomical educational project, enhancing students' learning and, ultimately, contributing to the improvement of patient care. Therefore these donors and their families deserve our utmost gratitude.[2]

[1]Iwanaga J, Singh V, Takeda S, et al. Standardized statement for the ethical use of human cadaveric tissues in anatomy research papers: recommendations from anatomical journal editors-in-chief. *Clin Anat.* 2022;35(4):526–528.

[2]Iwanaga J, Singh V, Ohtsuka A, et al. Acknowledging the use of human cadaveric tissues in research papers: recommendations from anatomical journal editors. *Clin Anat.* 2021;34(1):2–4.

Contents

Video Contents

The authors wish to express their profound gratitude to those remarkable individuals who selflessly donated their bodies to further the advancement of anatomical science. Their extraordinary gift has been the cornerstone of this project, enabling students and graduates to deepen their understanding and share invaluable knowledge with the next generation of medical professionals.

SECTION I

INTRODUCTION

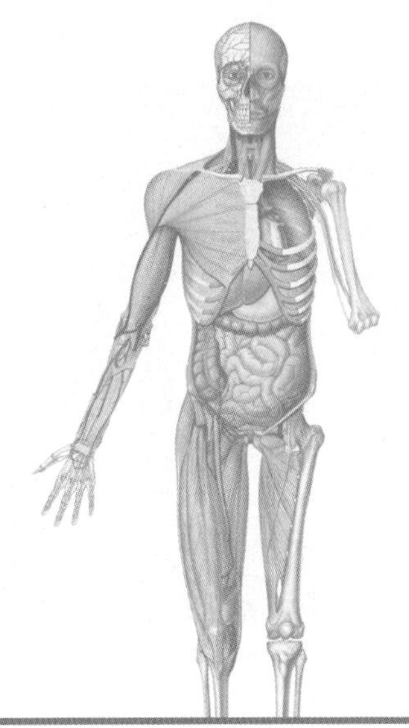

CHAPTER 1 DISSECTION LABORATORY MATERIALS, TOOLS, AND TECHNIQUES

Using appropriate dissection laboratory materials and tools is essential in making the dissection of a cadaver as rewarding as possible. Many experienced dissectors have their favorite tools. Obtaining the following materials and dissection tools allows dissectors to care for their cadaver donor while acquiring experience and knowledge of a successful dissection. Although not comprehensive, this list provides appropriate tools to dissect a cadaver donor in the anatomy teaching laboratory.

MATERIALS

Cadaver Materials

- Blocks
  Plastic or wooden blocks of different shapes and sizes (6–18 inches) can be used to position the cadaver (Fig. 1.1).
- Stands
  Removable stands that either bridge or attach to dissection tables are useful for holding dissection guides, texts, and atlases for dissection.
- Plastic sheets
  Plastic sheets can be used to cover the cadaver, which usually comes with a shroud and a cotton sheet. This helps maintain moisture within the cadaver, to prevent drying, and to allow dissection of appropriately hydrated tissues.
- Cotton sheets
  Surgical green or blue sheets covering a plastic sheet help preserve the cadaver and create a professional working environment.
- Spray bottle with wetting solution
  An individual plastic spray bottle (1 quart) at each cadaver station allows dissectors to maintain good-quality tissue (see Fig. 1.1). An alternative is a 2- to 3-gallon pressure spray unit shared among the dissection laboratory stations.
- Holding container
  The plastic 5- to 10-gallon container with a spigot stores cadaver hydration solution.
- Cadaver hydrating solution
  Several types of mixtures are available to hydrate and maintain cadaver tissue. The authors use a solution with 3000 mL of propylene glycol, 500 mL of ethyl alcohol, and 300 mL of fabric softener, in a 10-gallon holding unit, with the remainder filled with water.
- Cadaver bag
  The bag helps to maintain hydration of the cadaver (Fig. 1.2).

Dissector Materials

- Scrubs
  Comfortable clothing also can be worn with scrubs or under a lab coat.
- Disposable shoe covers
  Shoe covers protect shoes worn in the laboratory during dissection and can be disposed of on exiting the lab, ensuring cleanliness inside and outside the laboratory (Fig. 1.3). Closed-toed shoes should be worn in the dissecting laboratory.
- Goggles
  Protective safety goggles or glasses should be worn at all times during dissection (see Fig. 1.3).
- Face shields
  Shields can be worn when using bone saws or when excessive fluids are present (see Fig. 1.3).
- Gloves
  Gloves vary in the type of synthetic material used; powdered gloves and powder-free gloves are

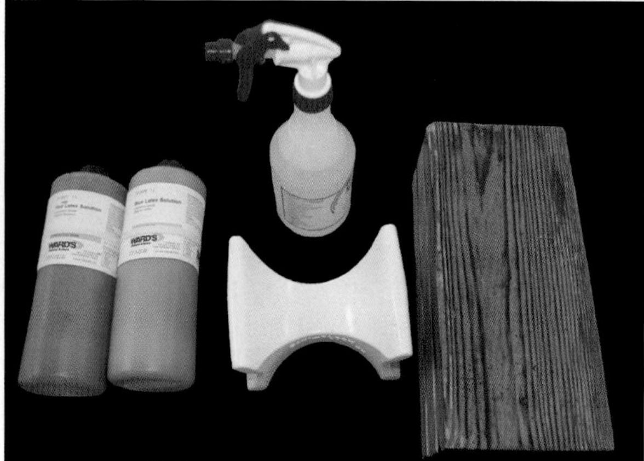

Fig. 1.1 *Red* and *blue* latex wrap (to keep cadaver moist); spray bottle; plastic and wooden blocks.

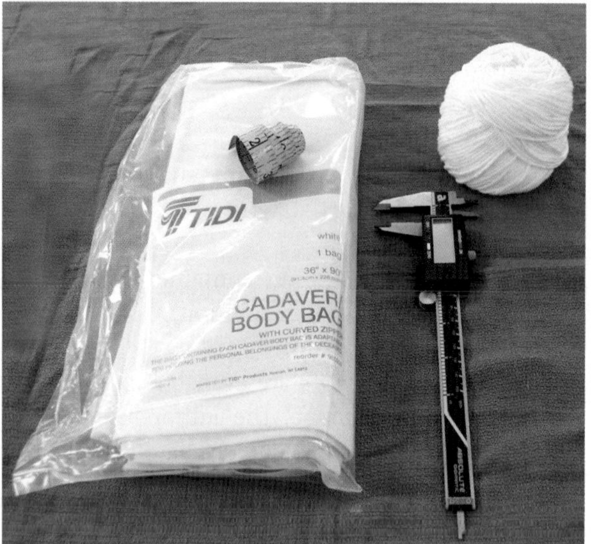

Fig. 1.2 Cadaver bag and cloth measuring tape; ball of string; digital calipers.

available (Fig. 1.4). Offer both types to protect dissectors with different skin sensitivities. *Double gloving* helps to prevent contact with cadaver embalming fluids, which may irritate sensitive skin.

- First-aid kit

  In a dissection laboratory, nicks and pricks are inevitable, so an up-to-date first-aid kit is essential. It should contain adhesive strips (e.g., Band-Aids), cleansing solutions (e.g., hydrogen peroxide), gauze rolls/pads, and eyewash solution. The phone number of the lab director and/or physician should be posted on a wall inside the lab so that users can contact them to answer any emergency issues that may arise if students are allowed to dissect during nonformal hours.

Dissection Tools

- Cloth/paper measuring tape

  A cloth or paper measuring tape can be invaluable when measuring distances from landmarks of surface anatomy (see Fig. 1.2).

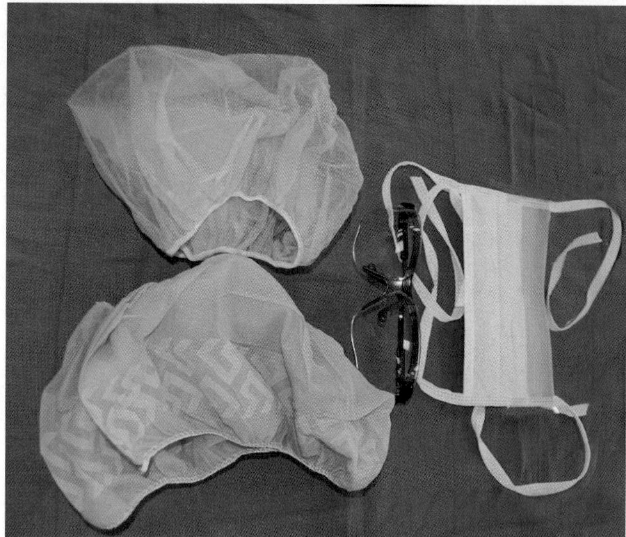

Fig. 1.3 Disposable hair and shoe covers; mask with eye shield; goggles.

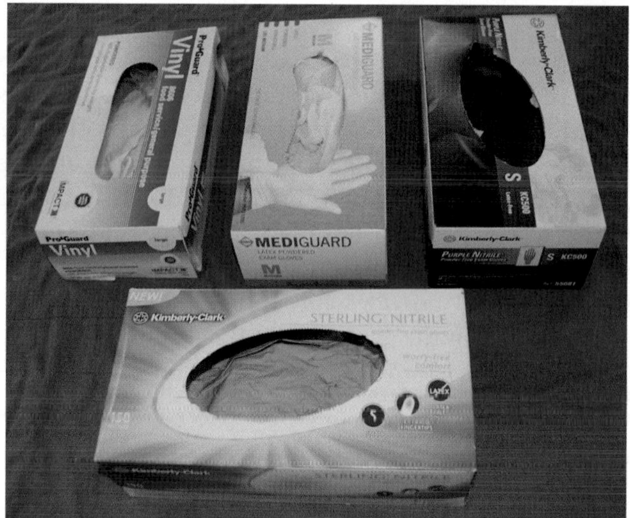

Fig. 1.4 Laboratory gloves differentiated by powder and powder free, latex and latex free.

- Skin marker

  Marking pens can be helpful tools for tracing out the incision before dissection. Markers can also be used to highlight surface anatomy (Fig. 1.5).

- Disposable scalpels

  Disposable scalpels have an advantage because the blade is already secured to the handle (see Fig. 1.5). Have a disposable sharps bin in the laboratory.

- Scalpel handles and blades

  Metal scalpel blades are relatively standardized. Many different blade shapes and sizes are available; however, dissectors should experiment to determine which best suits them and the targets to be dissected. The authors prefer larger blades for their students. Scalpels are used primarily to make skin incisions but also can be used to reflect the dermis and areas with dense connective tissue.

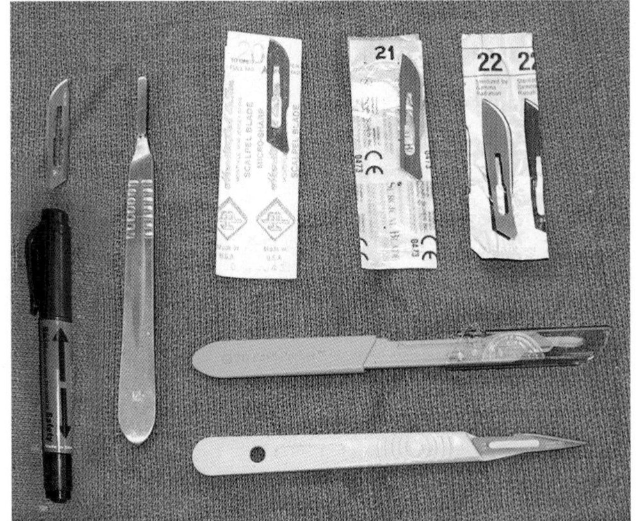

Fig. 1.5 Various scalpel blades and handles (metal and disposable scalpels). An example of a skin marker that can be used for outlining skin incisions is shown.

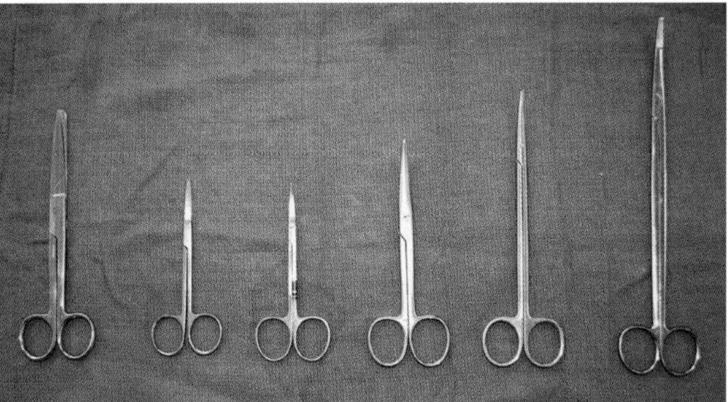

Fig. 1.6 Various scissors differentiated by length and blade type (straight or curved, pointed or blunted): 6-inch Deaver, straight fine scissors, curved fine scissors, 5-inch Mayo, 7-inch Metzenbaum, 9-inch Metzenbaum.

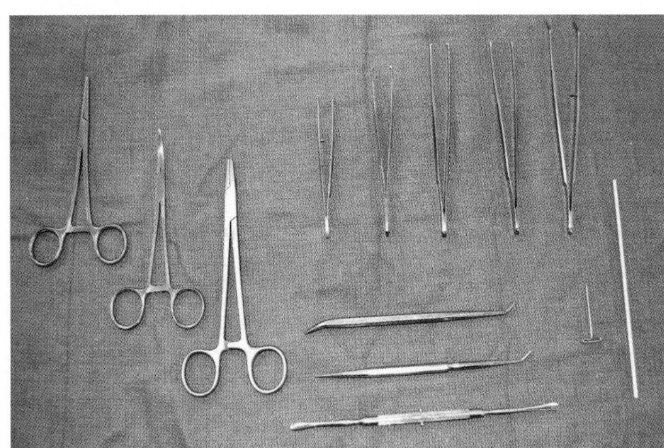

Fig. 1.7 *Left,* Hemostat or artery clamps (straight and curved). *Upper,* Needle holder; various forceps differentiated by length, toothed and nontoothed. *Lower,* Probes and dissectors. *Right,* T-pin and orange stick.

- Sharps bin or container

  For safety compliance, all dissection laboratories should have a sharps bin to dispose of scalpel blades, disposable scalpels, pins, and needles.
- Scissors

  Both 5- and 7-inch straight and curved scissors may be used. It is important that the scissors used for each dissection are appropriate in size (Fig. 1.6). Generally, head and neck dissections can be conducted with 5-inch scissors. The remainder of the body can be dissected with 7-inch scissors. The classic scissor dissection technique is a *reverse dissection.* Straight and curved scissors tend to be user specific.
- Hemostat clamps

  Corrugated and smooth, 5- and 7-inch hemostat clamps are available (Fig. 1.7). The corrugated type can be used to clamp onto the edge of skin incisions to aid in flap removal. Smooth clamps can be used to hold onto delicate structures during dissection. Hemostat clamps can be used when retracting tissue over relatively long dissection periods.
- Needle holders (drivers)

  The needle holder allows the user to secure and remove scalpel blades (see Fig. 1.7).
- Forceps

  Toothed and nontoothed forceps are either 5 inches or greater than 5 inches long. Toothed forceps enable the dissector to grip tissue without it sliding out of the hands. Nontoothed forceps allow the dissector to control delicate tissues during meticulous dissection without damaging the tissue (see Fig. 1.7).
- Spatula probe/pointer

  Instruments that have a probe or tip on one end and spatula on the other can be used to highlight dissected structures. The spatula can aid blunt dissection (see Fig. 1.7).
- T-pins

  T-pins (1½–2 inches) are useful in securing structures away from the desired dissection region. T-pins also can be used when setting up laboratory examinations (see Fig. 1.7).
- Chisel (osteotome)

  Narrow-blade and broad-blade chisels are important for performing osteotomies and can help dissect, for example, between the occipital condyles and various vertebrae (Fig. 1.8). Chisels can be used to break up a bone surface to view the soft tissue deep to it (e.g., anterior cranial fossa).
- Rubber mallet

  A mallet is used when striking the chisel to crack surface areas, such as when performing osteotomies (see Fig. 1.8).
- Electric Stryker™ saw

  Used when cutting bone, the Stryker saw has a safety mechanism that prevents the blade from cutting the user's skin and soft tissue.

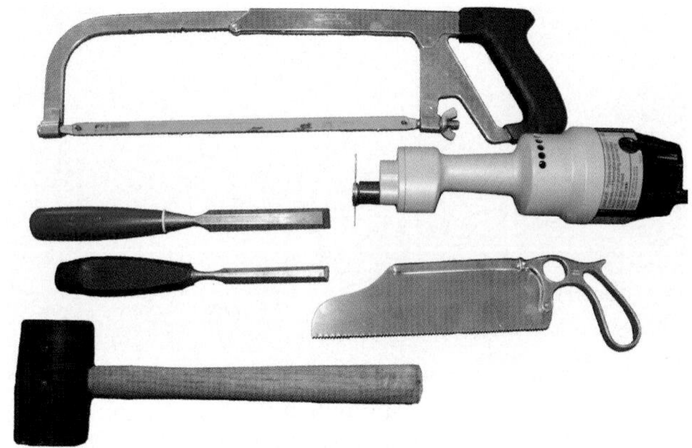

Fig. 1.8 Handsaws (long and short) for bone; electric Stryker bone saw; chisels (broad and narrow blades); rubber mallet.

- Handsaw

  A simple bone saw can be used to customize various dissections and amputations for plastination (see Fig. 1.8). A handsaw is important for hemipelvectomy dissections.

DISSECTION TECHNIQUES

Using the proper technique during dissection is important when developing good dissection skills. Initially, holding the instruments correctly and practicing the techniques may not feel natural. The authors believe that cadaver dissection techniques should reflect the techniques used during surgical procedures. Learning to hold forceps and scissors is fundamental during dissection. These techniques also can be used in the operating room and certain office settings during interventional procedures.

- Scalpel

  The technique for placing a blade onto a scalpel handle requires a hemostat to hold the blade and then place it onto the handle while holding the forceps (Figs. 1.9 and 1.10). When cutting with the blade, use the tip and the first centimeter of the blade. Direct the scalpel using smooth, sweeping motions (Fig. 1.11). Avoid "sawing" and "woodpecker" techniques. Dull blades that require "pushing" the scalpel are dangerous; therefore maintain a sharp blade at all times.

- Forceps

  Hold the forceps as you would hold a pencil, with a pincer grip. The classic mistake is holding the forceps in the palm of the hand as if grasping. Hold the forceps vertically and perpendicularly to the target tissue to allow a 360-degree window of use (Fig. 1.12).

- Scissors

  The appropriate technique when dissecting with scissors is called *reverse dissection* (Fig. 1.13). This requires the user to keep the scissor blades closed when entering into the tissue to be dissected, then opening the blades to create a splaying of the tissue. This results in natural separation of tissue structures and planes. Cut only tissue that is fully exposed so that the desired tissue can be preserved.

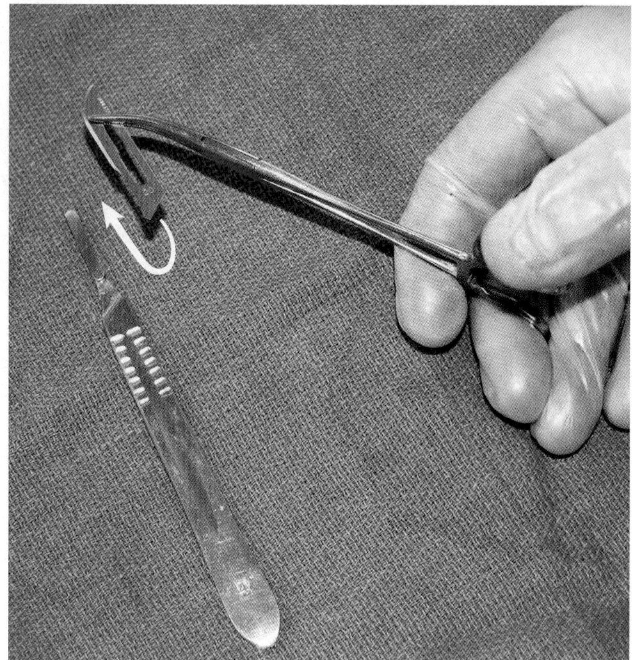

Fig. 1.9 Placing or replacing scalpel blades onto a scalpel handle. Use hemostat or needle holder to grip the scalpel blade. Line up the base angle of the blade with the tip-of-handle angle.

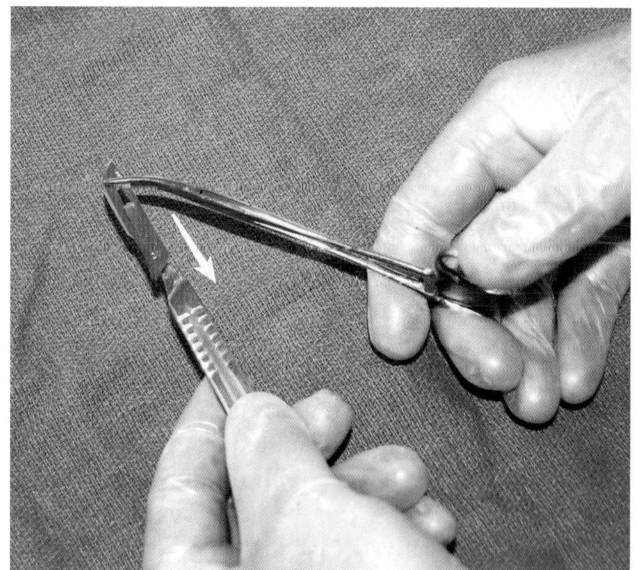

Fig. 1.10 Placing the blade onto the scalpel handle tip. Generally, a clicking sound confirms the blade is secured correctly.

- Buttonhole maneuver

  A buttonhole maneuver is helpful when dissecting a flap of dermis. Create a 2-cm parallel incision along

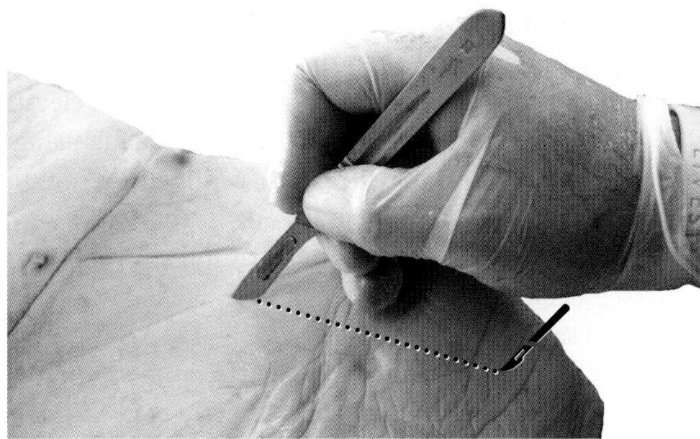

Fig. 1.11 Using the scalpel tip to create skin incisions. Note the grip of the scalpel provides side-to-side and back-to-front blade stability.

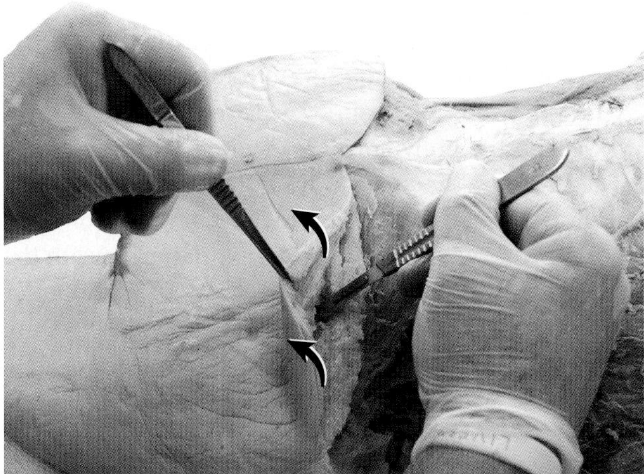

Fig. 1.12 Holding toothed forceps with a 360-degree view and using the scalpel tip between tissue layers while maintaining tension of superficial tissue layer.

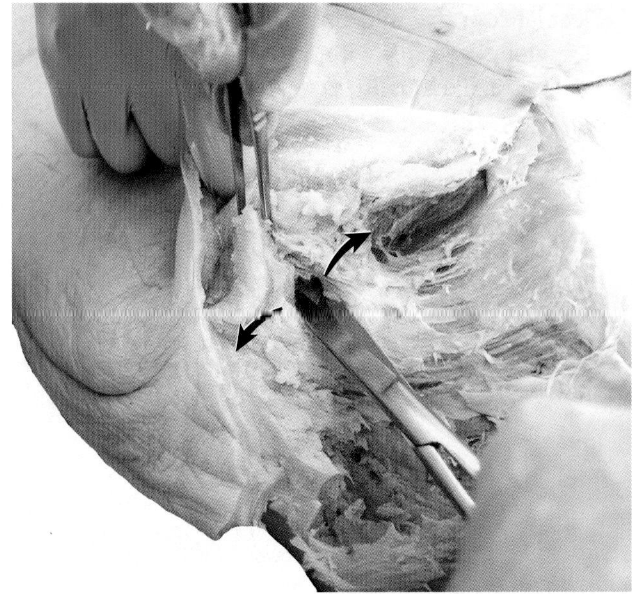

Fig. 1.13 Blunt dissection introduces the scissor tips into the tissue, and then reverse dissection opens the tissue planes.

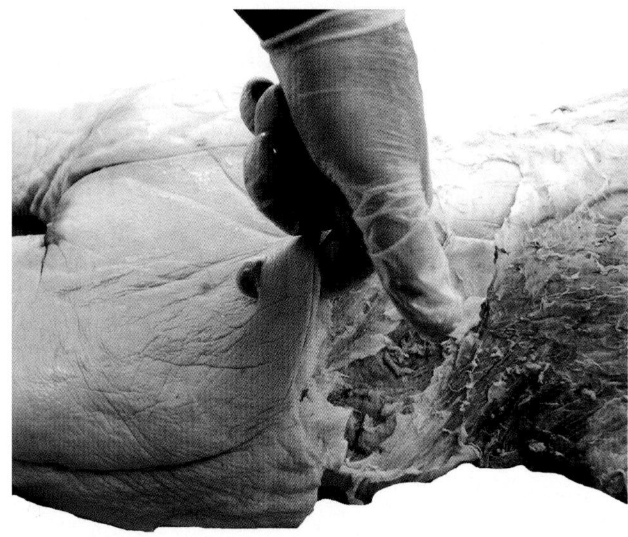

Fig. 1.14 The buttonhole maneuver is helpful when dissecting large skin flaps and provides appropriate tension to expedite dissection. Place your fingertip(s) into the parallel incision and retract with appropriate tension.

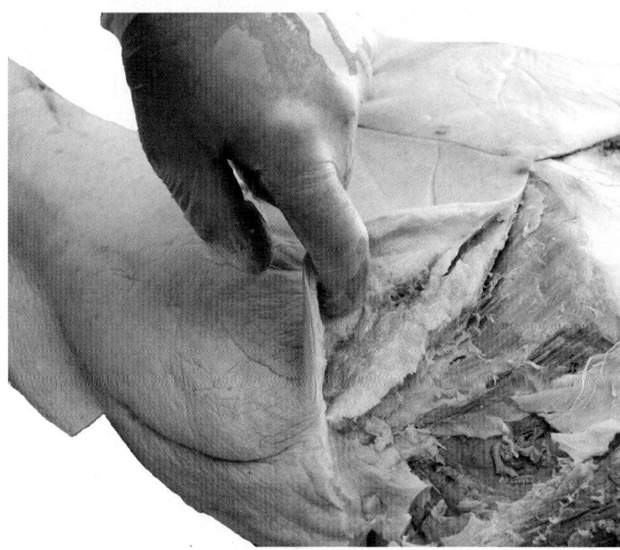

Fig. 1.15 The buttonhole maneuver for retraction of the skin allows adequate visualization of the underlying tissue for further dissection.

the original skin incision, 2 to 3 cm from the edge. Repeat this, generally near the corners of the skin flap. Place your index finger into the parallel incision, and retract the skin flap with appropriate tension that would allow either blunt dissection or a sharp edge to cut the apex of the flap (Figs. 1.14 and 1.15).

- Surface fracturing technique

The surface fracturing technique requires placing the broad blade of a chisel parallel to the bone and with as much of the blade along the bone. Strike the chisel head with a mallet using a technique that does *not* follow through once the head is struck. The objective is to direct the energy through the blade onto the bony surface, causing multiple fractured segments while protecting the soft tissue beneath the bone (e.g., fracturing anterior cranial fossa plate before superior orbit dissection) (Fig. 1.16).

- Direct fracturing technique
  The direct fracturing technique can be performed using a narrow-bladed chisel or by tilting a broad-bladed chisel so that a direct point touches the bone to be fractured. Strike the chisel head with the mallet as if driving a nail. This technique will fracture through a specific part of the outer layer of bone (Fig. 1.17).

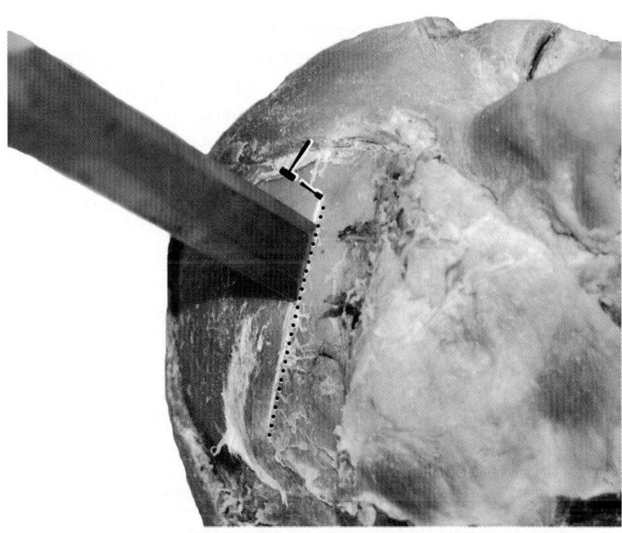

Fig. 1.16 Place chisel blade flat and parallel on the desired bone surface. The surface fracturing technique generally results in multiple fragments protecting the deep tissue.

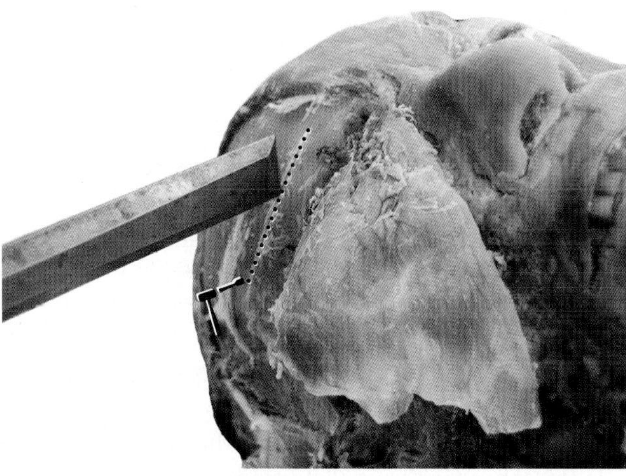

Fig. 1.17 Place chisel blade at an angle on the desired bone surface. The direct fracturing technique creates a specific fracture at the point of the chisel blade.

- Prying technique
  The prying technique requires placing the blade of a chisel into the gap created by a handsaw or electric saw. Once in the gap, rotate the chisel blade using a circular motion of the wrist while gripping the chisel to pry the two bony edges apart. Prying is especially useful when performing a craniotomy (see Chapter 23).
- Stryker saw
  The technique for using the electric bone saw is performed by placing the blade directly perpendicular to the bone. Place enough pressure onto the bony surface until the blade has gone through the thickness of the bone. Once through the bone, remove the blade and assess whether the prying technique is required.
- Stryker saw scoring
  The scoring technique requires using a Stryker electric saw blade to score the surface of the bone region to be removed. Often an "X" pattern of scoring can weaken the bony cortex. Once the scoring is completed, use the surface fracturing technique. This allows fracture of the cortex and removal of bony fragments without damaging soft tissue beneath the cortex (e.g., removing outer cortex of mandibular ramus; see Chapter 22).

SPECIALIZED MATERIALS TO HIGHLIGHT STRUCTURES

- Latex solutions
  Use latex solutions as an injection to highlight vessels, especially small vessels that may not be easily dissectible.
- Needle and syringe
  Multiple syringe sizes and needle sizes are used to inject latex or dye into spaces (Fig. 1.18). Injection of the globe (eyeball) with water also may be useful to obtain lifelike qualities.

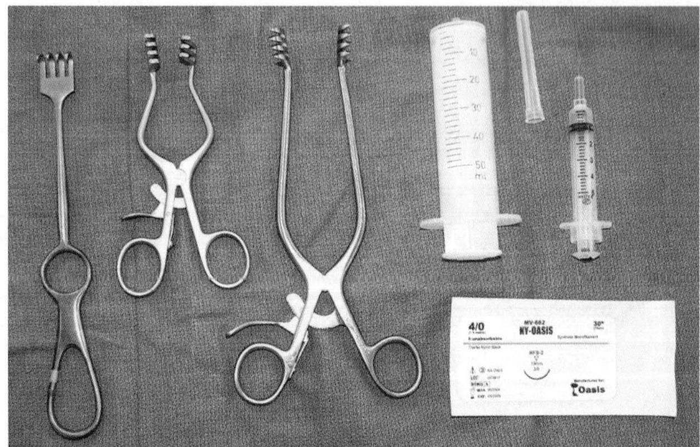

Fig. 1.18 *Left to right,* Handheld retractor (Volkmann); dynamic self-retaining retractors (Weitlaner); syringes (50 mL and 5 mL); suture material.

- Suture material
  Multiple sizes of suture material to reattach dissected structures can be useful when demonstrating superficial and deep structures after dissection (see Fig. 1.18).
- Retractors
  Types include (1) single-handled manual retractor for dynamic traction and (2) self-retractor used to retract two sides simultaneously, allowing the dissector to practice surgical procedures without needing others to retract structures manually (see Fig. 1.18).
- Food coloring
  Mix with a solution to inject into the body, to fill up potential spaces, and to highlight others.
- Electronic digital calipers
  Use to measure specific length, size, and shape of anatomic structures (see Fig. 1.2).
- Plastination
  The plastination technique preserves dissected regions or structures to be used as *prosected material*, with a life span of 6 months to 20 years, depending on technique, body part, and frequency of use.
- Rongeur and rib cutters
  These can be used to cut through small- to medium-sized bones and to customize cut ends of all bone sizes (Figs. 1.19 and 1.20).

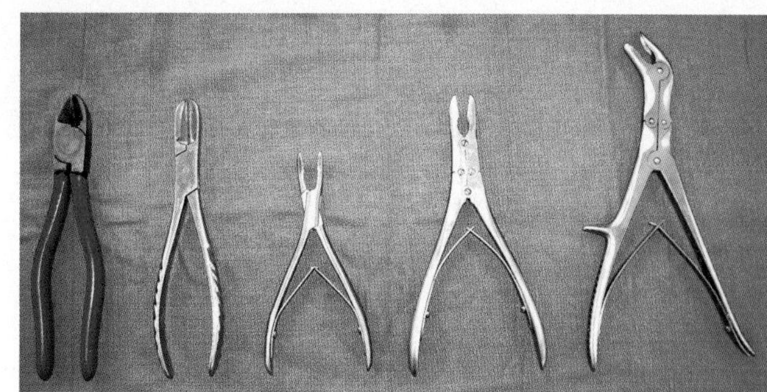

Fig. 1.19 *Left to right,* Metal wire cutters (2), bone cutter (Liston), 5-inch bone-cutter forceps, 7-inch bone-cutter rongeur (Stille).

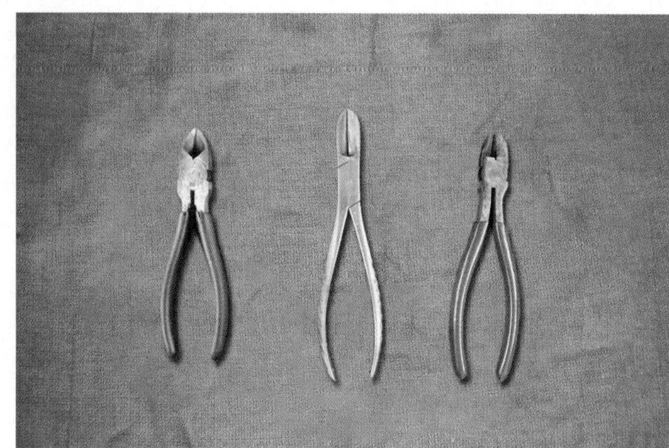

Fig. 1.20 *Left to right,* Rib cutters of several sizes.

SECTION II

BACK

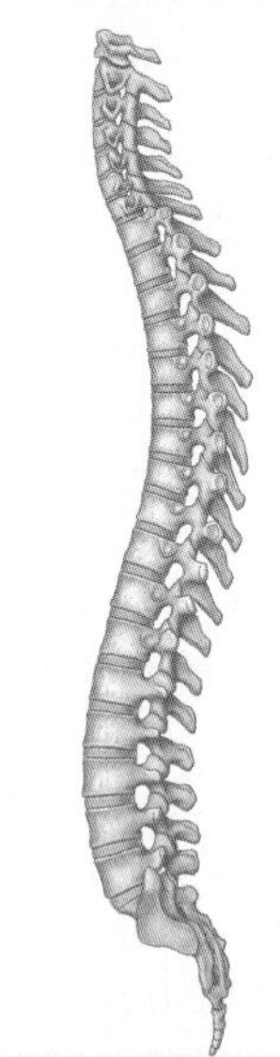

CHAPTER 2 MUSCLES OF THE BACK AND SCAPULA

BEFORE YOU BEGIN

Make sure that you have palpated the following anatomical landmarks on yourself and classmates:

- Superior nuchal line
- External occipital protuberance (inion)
- Mastoid process
- Spinous process of the 7th cervical vertebra (C7, vertebra prominens)
- Spinous processes of the thoracic and lumbar vertebrae, the sacrum, and the coccyx
- Medial and lateral parts of the clavicles
- Iliac crests
- Trapezius muscle
- Latissimus dorsi muscle
- Deltoid muscle
- Triceps brachii muscle
- Acromion

SKIN AND SUPERFICIAL FASCIA

- **Begin by palpating bony landmarks. With a skin marker, draw the following lines on the skin of the cadaver (Fig. 2.1):**
  1. From the external occipital protuberance, down the midline of the back to the sacrum.
  2. Laterally, from the external occipital protuberance to the mastoid process on each side of the cadaver.
  3. Laterally, from the spinous process of the vertebra prominens to the acromion of each shoulder.
  4. Superiorly from the sacrum, curving obliquely over the iliac crests to the midaxillary line on each side of the body, that is, to a point about halfway around the upper edge of each iliac crest.
- **Incise the skin along the lines just described, beginning at the point where the incisions for the midline and from the shoulders meet (Fig. 2.2).**
- **Retract the skin carefully (with toothed forceps), leaving the adipose tissue (superficial fascia) intact (see Fig. 2.2).**

DISSECTION TIP

Place absorptive cloths at the inferolateral spaces of the iliac crest. Excessive amounts of embalming fluid often accumulate at this location.

DISSECTION TIP

Make necessary "buttonholes" in the skin to facilitate the dissection (Fig. 2.3), as indicated in Chapter 1.

- **On one side of the body, the dissectors should first reflect only the skin, leaving the superficial fascia (tela subcutanea) in place.**
- **Start the separation of the superficial fascia from the underlying deep fascia in the midline by identifying a small part of the trapezius muscle.**
- **Carefully remove the superficial fascia from the surface of the muscle with your scalpel (Fig. 2.4).**

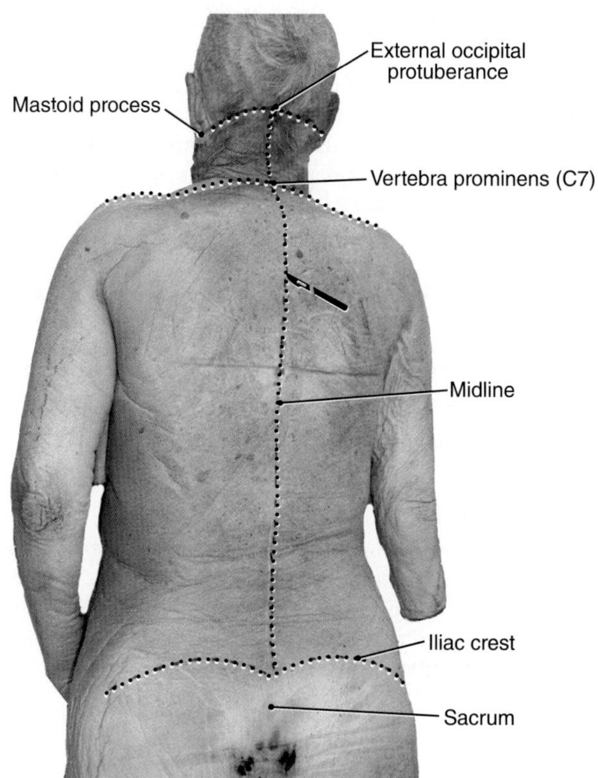

Fig. 2.1 Skin markings for incision lines: neck and back.

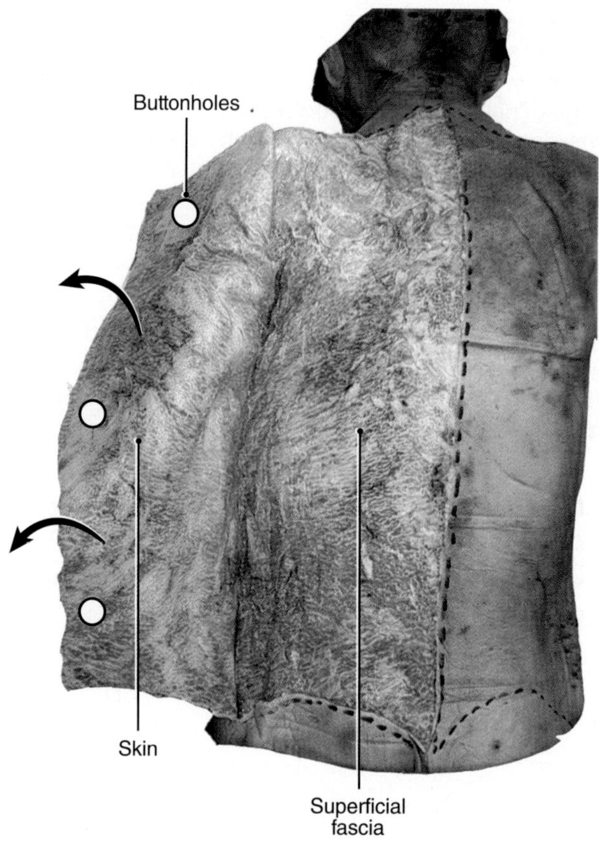

Fig. 2.3 Make "buttonholes" in the skin to facilitate its reflection from the underlying superficial fascia.

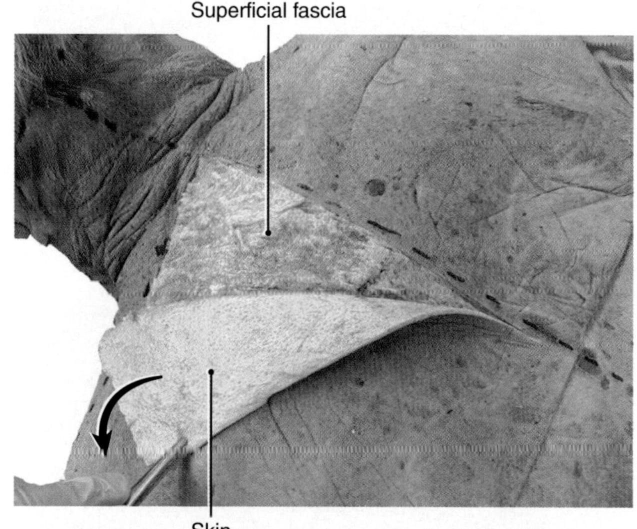

Fig. 2.2 Reflection of skin from the superficial fascia.

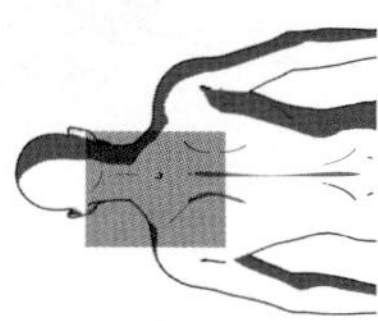

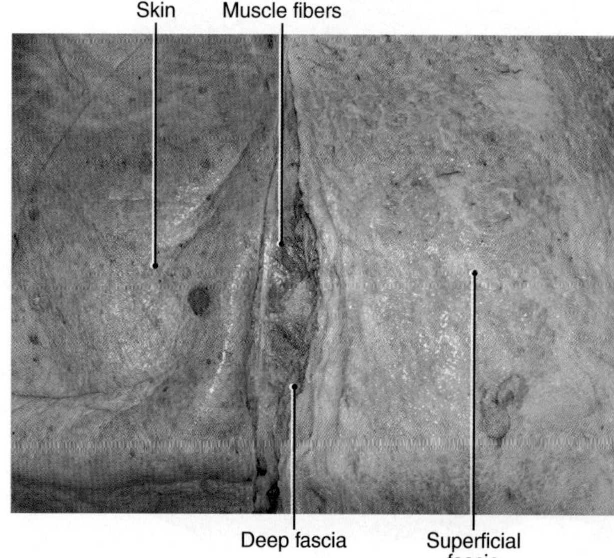

Fig. 2.4 Deep skin incisions showing deep fascia and muscle fibers.

DISSECTION **TIP**

As the superficial fascia is reflected, watch for the passage of neurovascular bundles from the deep fascia into the deep surface of the superficial fascia. Save short segments of several of these for later demonstration and review.

DISSECTION **TIP**

Take precautions to avoid cutting too deeply with the scalpel. In some cadavers, the superficial fascia is very thin, and more deeply situated structures can be cut and destroyed (Figs. 2.5 and 2.6).

- **Completely remove superficial fascia over the latissimus dorsi muscle.**
- **On the other side of the body, the skin and superficial fascia can be reflected together.**

DISSECTION **TIP**

Care must be taken in this latter approach to avoid damage to the underlying muscles, especially the trapezius and latissimus dorsi muscles and their aponeuroses. Identify these before the skin and fascia are reflected more than a few centimeters.

SUPERFICIAL MUSCLES OF THE BACK: PART 1

- **Remove enough deep fascia to clarify the borders of the two most superficial muscles of the back, the trapezius and latissimus dorsi (Fig. 2.7).**

ANATOMY **NOTE**

Note the diamond-shaped aponeurotic area of the trapezius at the upper middle thoracic region (see Fig. 2.7). The skin, superficial fascia, and deep fascia are relatively thin here. This is in contrast to the lateral lumbar region, where the amount of subcutaneous fat is increased (see Fig. 2.6).

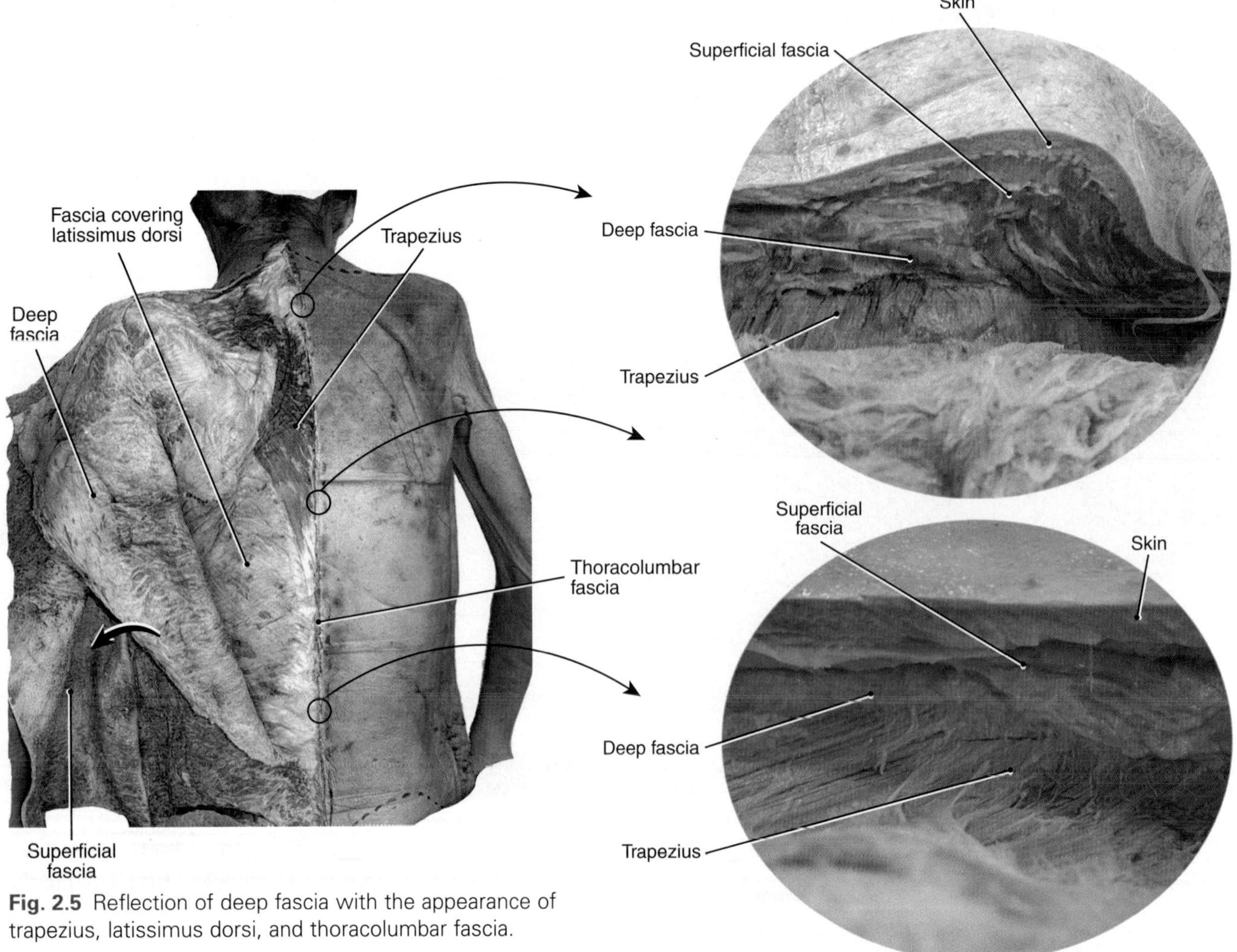

Fig. 2.5 Reflection of deep fascia with the appearance of trapezius, latissimus dorsi, and thoracolumbar fascia.

Fig. 2.6 Note possible differences in the thickness of the skin and fascia. Avoid cutting too deeply with the scalpel to prevent damage to superficial structures when exposing them.

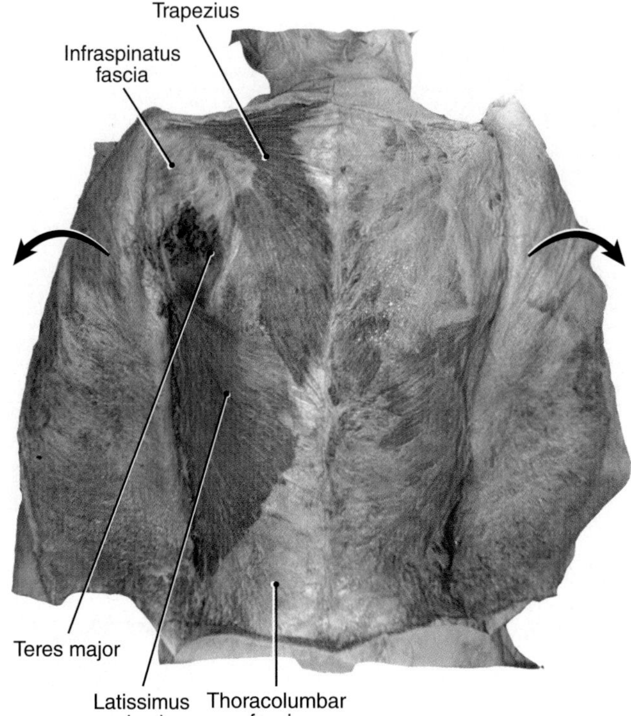

Fig. 2.7 Complete removal of superficial fascia over trapezius, latissimus dorsi, and posterior layer of thoracolumbar fascia on the left side of the cadaver. Deep fascia and some adipose tissue have been left intact on the right side.

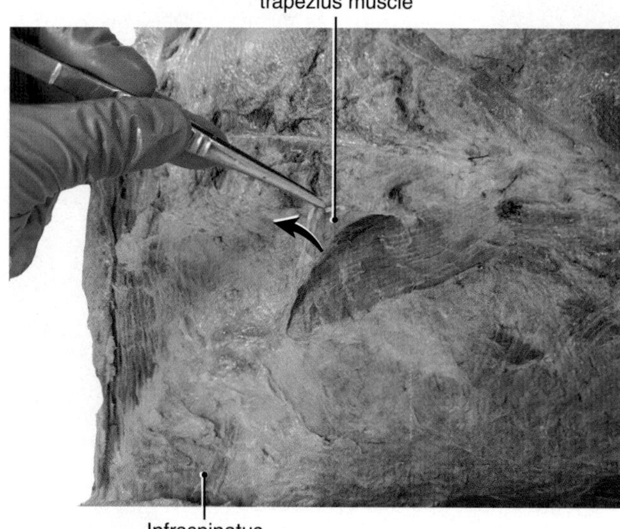

Fig. 2.8 Careful separation of deep fascia covering the trapezius muscle.

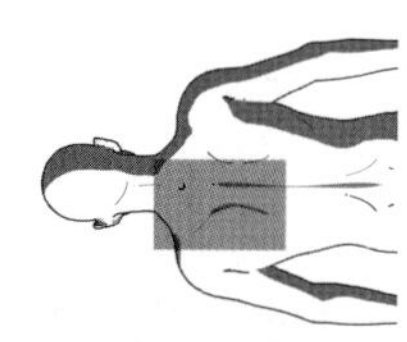

- **Identify the teres major muscle and the infraspinatus fascia (see Fig. 2.7).**

ANATOMY **NOTE**

This fascia covering the infraspinatus muscle is attached to the margins of the infraspinatus fossa and is continuous with the deltoid fascia along the posterior border of the muscle.

- **Carefully separate the deep fascia covering the trapezius muscle (Fig. 2.8).**
- **While cleaning away the fascia that overlies the most cranial portion of the trapezius (Figs. 2.9 and 2.10), look for the greater occipital nerve.**
- **This nerve usually can be found approximately 1 inch (2.5 cm) from the midline and 1 inch inferior to the superior nuchal line, as the nerve pierces the trapezius (Figs. 2.11 and 2.12).**
- **Also at this location, locate the occipital artery and preserve it as the trapezius is reflected (see Fig. 2.12).**

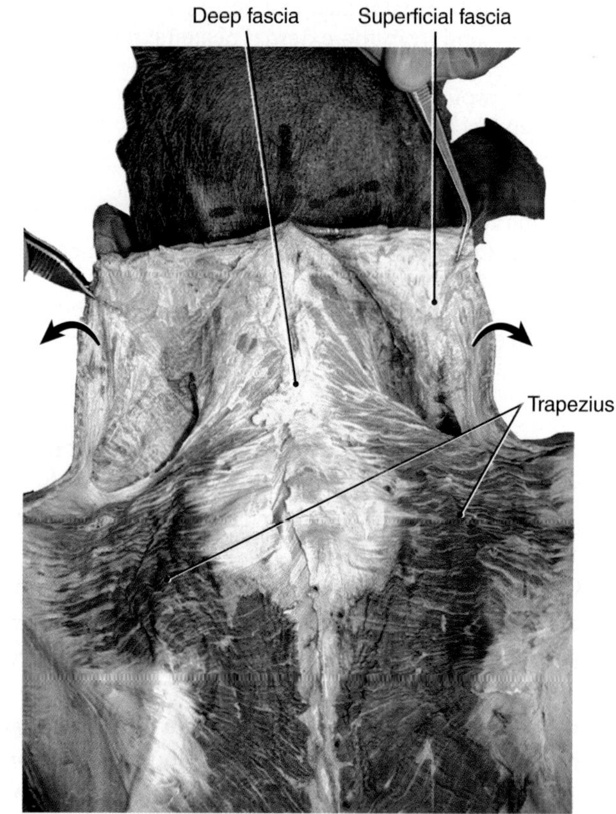

Fig. 2.9 Exposure of the trapezius with portions of deep fascia still covering its uppermost portions.

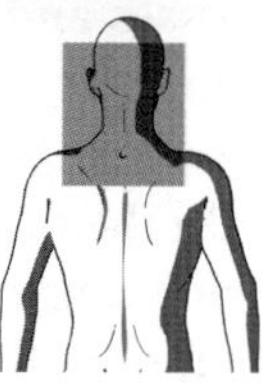

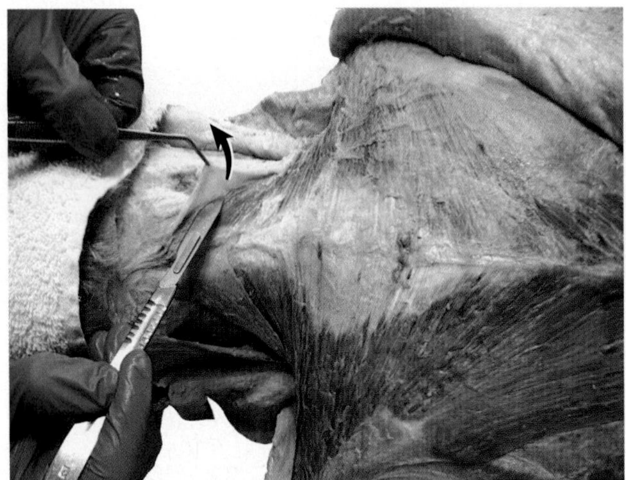

Fig. 2.10 Reflection of the deep fascia covering the upper portion of trapezius.

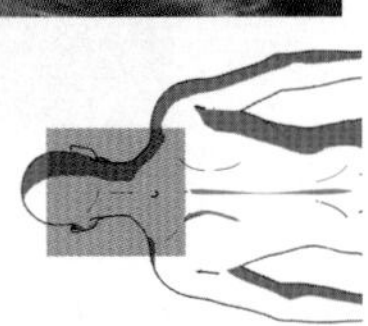

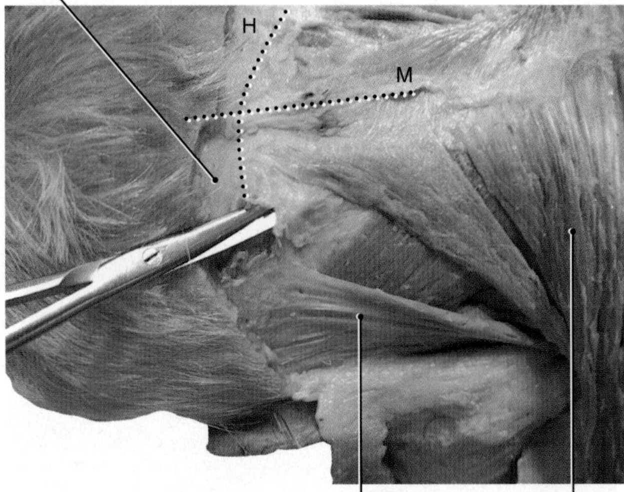

Fig. 2.11 After identifying the greater occipital nerve, separate and remove the deep fascia. *H,* Horizontal line; *M,* midline.

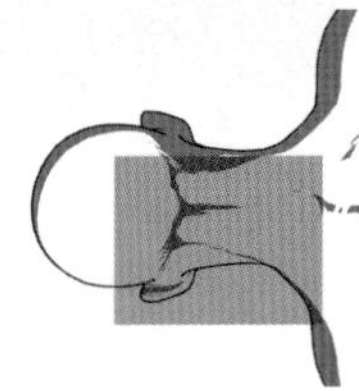

DISSECTION TIP

GREATER OCCIPITAL NERVE

To identify the greater occipital nerve, draw a horizontal imaginary line from the external occipital protuberance to the mastoid process. At 3 cm lateral to the external occipital protuberance on the imaginary line, remove the deep fascia to identify this nerve.

THIRD OCCIPITAL NERVE

Usually, the deep fascia over the trapezius muscle below the superior nuchal line is very thick and difficult to cut until the 7th cervical vertebra (C7) level. Pay special attention to the dissection process. Intermingled with the deep fascia over this area is the **third occipital nerve;** try to expose and save it (Fig. 2.13).

- **To detach the trapezius from its origin, first make a small vertical cut through the lower part of the trapezius at the 12th thoracic vertebra (T12) level as it attaches to the midline.**
- **Continue the incision to the external occipital protuberance. Define and loosen the trapezius with your fingers or with scissors before you proceed further upward along the midline (Fig. 2.14).**
- **Detach the trapezius from its origin on the superior nuchal line and the external occipital protuberance, and sever the fibers that arise from the spinous processes and associated ligaments of the cervical and thoracic vertebrae. Reflect the trapezius laterally toward its insertion onto the scapula (Fig. 2.15).**
- **On the deep surface of the trapezius, near the superior angle of the scapula, look for the nerve that supplies the trapezius, the spinal accessory nerve.**

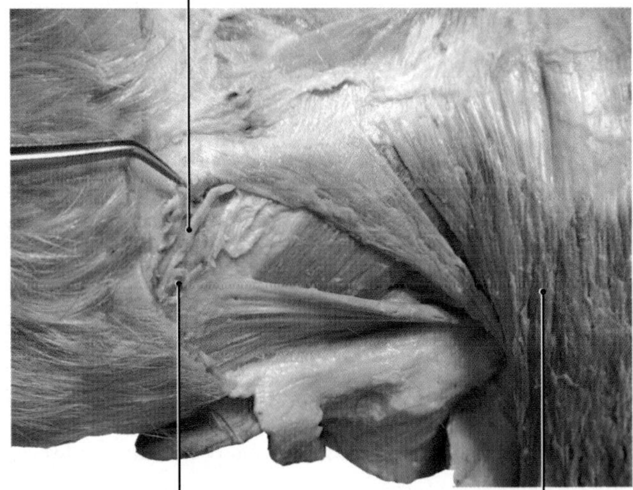

Fig. 2.12 Deep fascia is cut, and the greater occipital nerve and occipital artery are visible.

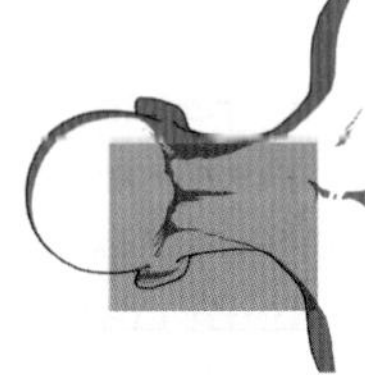

- **Note the artery that supplies the trapezius muscle, the ascending branch of the transverse cervical artery.**
- **Identify the levator scapulae, rhomboid minor and major muscles, and neurovascular bundle (Fig. 2.16).**
- **Clean the fascia from these muscles so that their fibers can be seen clearly.**

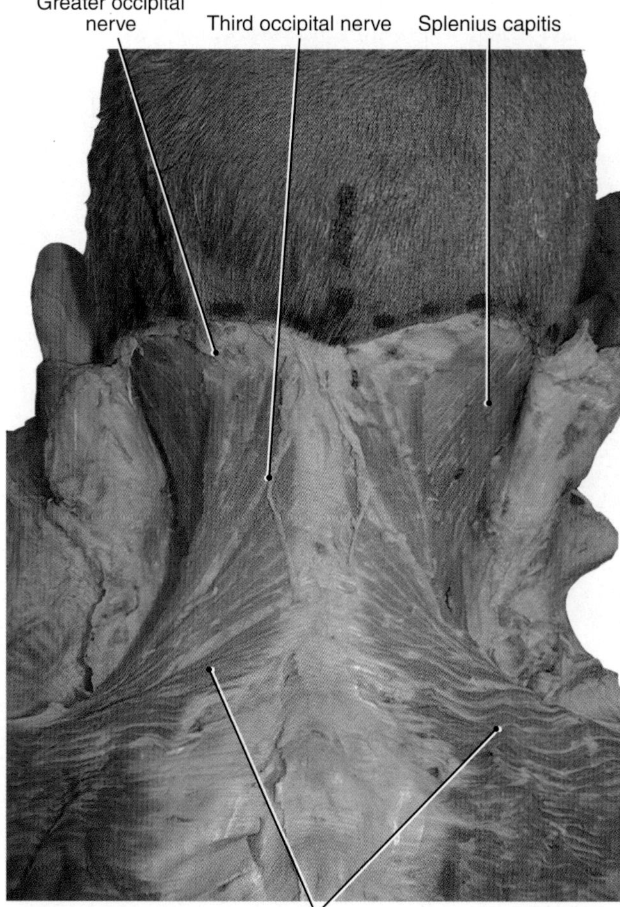

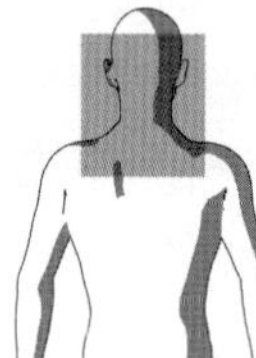

Fig. 2.13 Complete exposure and detachment of the superior part of the trapezius from the deep fascia. Observe the third occipital nerve.

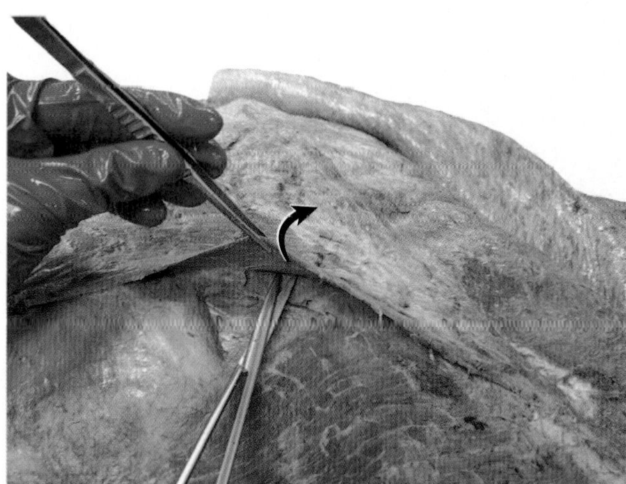

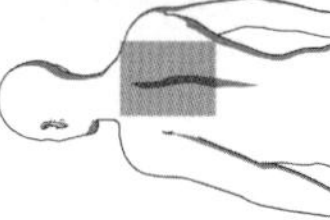

Fig. 2.14 Dissection of the lateral edge of the trapezius muscle facilitated by a separation technique using dissecting scissors.

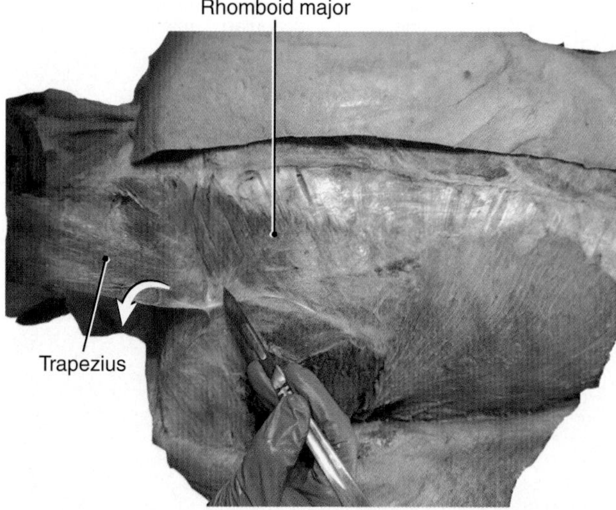

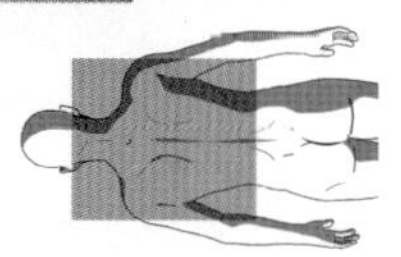

Fig. 2.15 Separation of the connective tissue on the deep surface of trapezius.

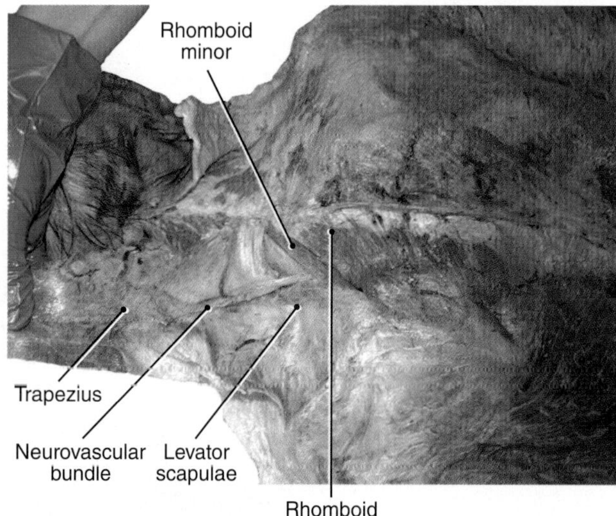

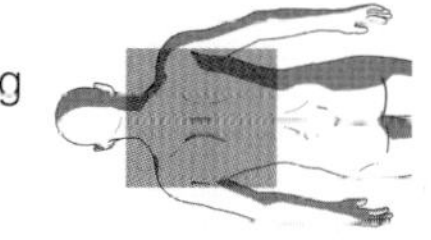

Fig. 2.16 Complete reflection of the trapezius and appearance of the underlying levator scapulae and rhomboid muscles, and neuromuscular bundle.

- **Gently retract the levator scapulae muscle medially. At the midpoint of the levator scapulae muscle, you will see the spinal accessory nerve exit and run on the internal surface of the trapezius muscle (Figs. 2.17 and 2.18).**
- **Carefully separate the neurovascular bundle to identify the spinal accessory nerve, ascending branch of the transverse cervical artery, and tributaries of the transverse cervical vein (Figs. 2.19 and 2.20).**

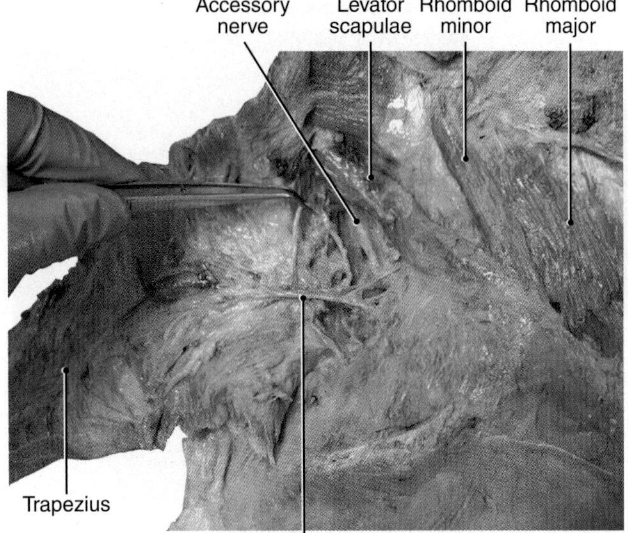

Fig. 2.17 Identification of spinal accessory nerve, emerging deep from the medial side at the midpoint of levator scapulae muscle.

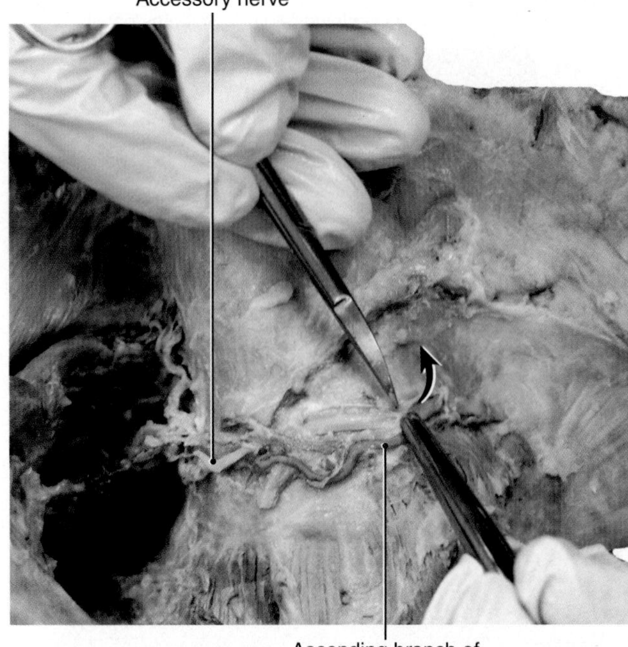

Fig. 2.18 Careful separation of neurovascular bundle to identify spinal accessory nerve, ascending branch of transverse cervical artery, and tributaries of transverse cervical vein.

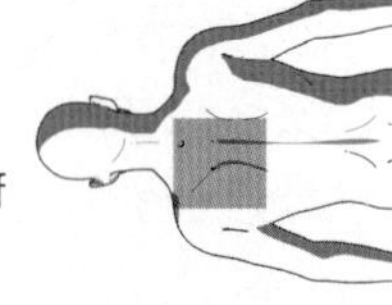

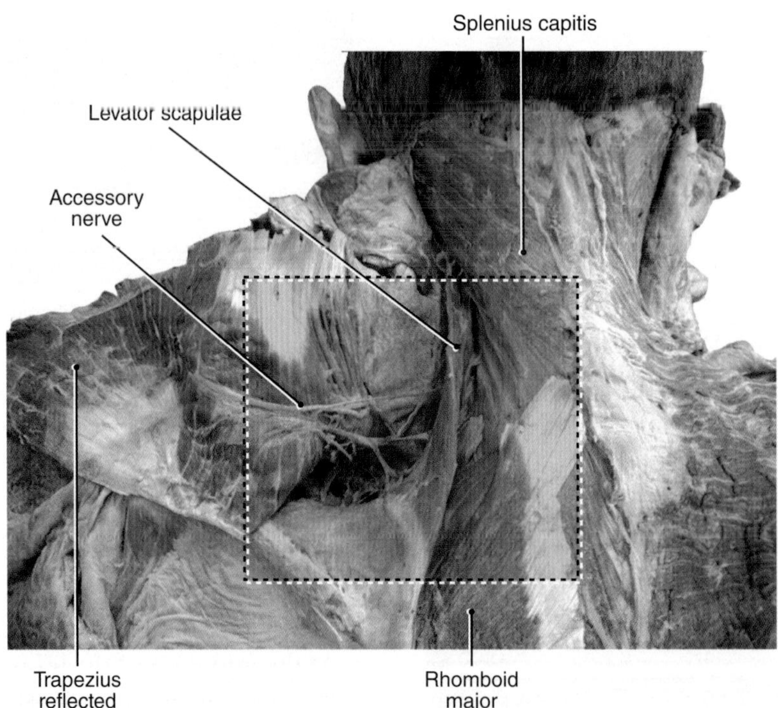

Fig. 2.19 After careful dissection of connective tissue, the trapezius muscle is reflected and the spinal accessory nerve is identified.

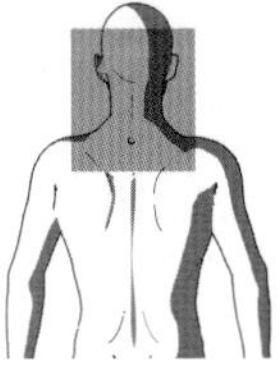

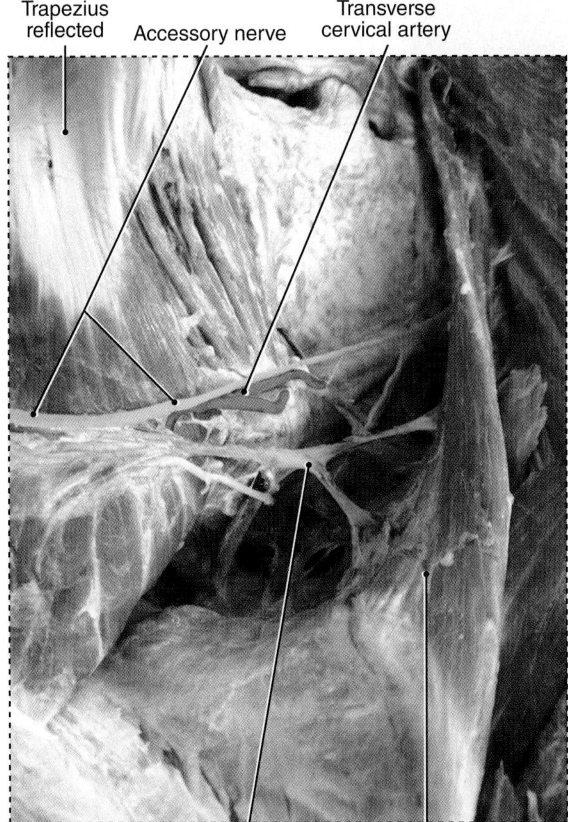

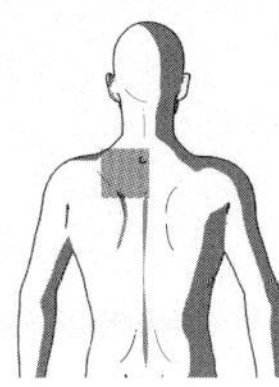

Fig. 2.20 Trapezius muscle is reflected, and the spinal accessory nerve is identified.

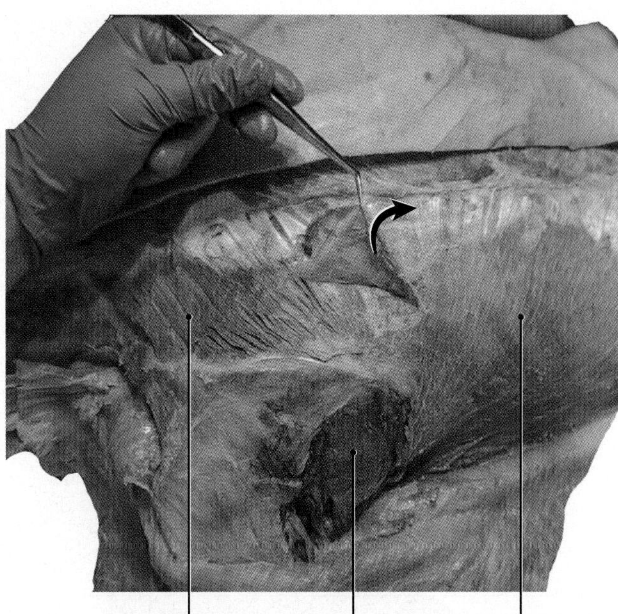

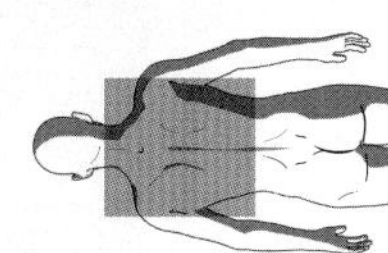

Fig. 2.21 Carefully expose the deep fascia over the rhomboid major and minor muscles.

- **Carefully expose the deep fascia over the rhomboid major and minor muscles. In some specimens the line of cleavage between the rhomboid muscles may be unclear (Figs. 2.21 and 2.22).**
- **Reflect the rhomboid muscles laterally toward their insertion onto the medial border of the scapula (Fig. 2.23 and Plate 2.1).**
- **Deep to the rhomboids, identify the serratus posterior superior muscle, which inserts onto the ribs rather than onto the scapula. (This fact will assist you in its identification.)**
- **On the deep surface of the rhomboids, try to identify the dorsal scapular nerve and dorsal scapular artery (Fig. 2.24).**

ANATOMY **NOTE**

The dorsal scapular nerve innervates the rhomboid and levator scapulae muscles (in addition to branches from C3 and C4). The dorsal scapular nerve arises from C5, one of the two nerves that arise directly from the anterior (ventral) rami of the brachial plexus.

ANATOMY **NOTE**

In about 50% of the specimens, the dorsal scapular artery is absent, and the deep branch of the transverse cervical artery replaces it. The dorsal scapular artery typically arises from the third part of the subclavian artery and runs posteriorly usually through the brachial plexus.

MUSCLES OF THE SCAPULA

ANATOMY **NOTE**

The infraspinatus fascia is attached to the scapula around the boundaries of the attachments of the infraspinatus, teres minor and major, long head of triceps brachii, and deltoid muscles.

- **Clean the teres major muscle (Fig. 2.25).**
- **Identify the teres minor and deltoid muscles and the long head of triceps brachii (Fig. 2.26).**

ANATOMY **NOTE**

The fibers of the teres minor muscle run more or less parallel to the fibers of the teres major and are medial to the long head of the triceps brachii and deltoid muscles (see Fig. 2.25).

- **Beginning superiorly, reflect the infraspinatus fascia to expose the long head of triceps and deltoid muscles (Figs. 2.27 and 2.28).**

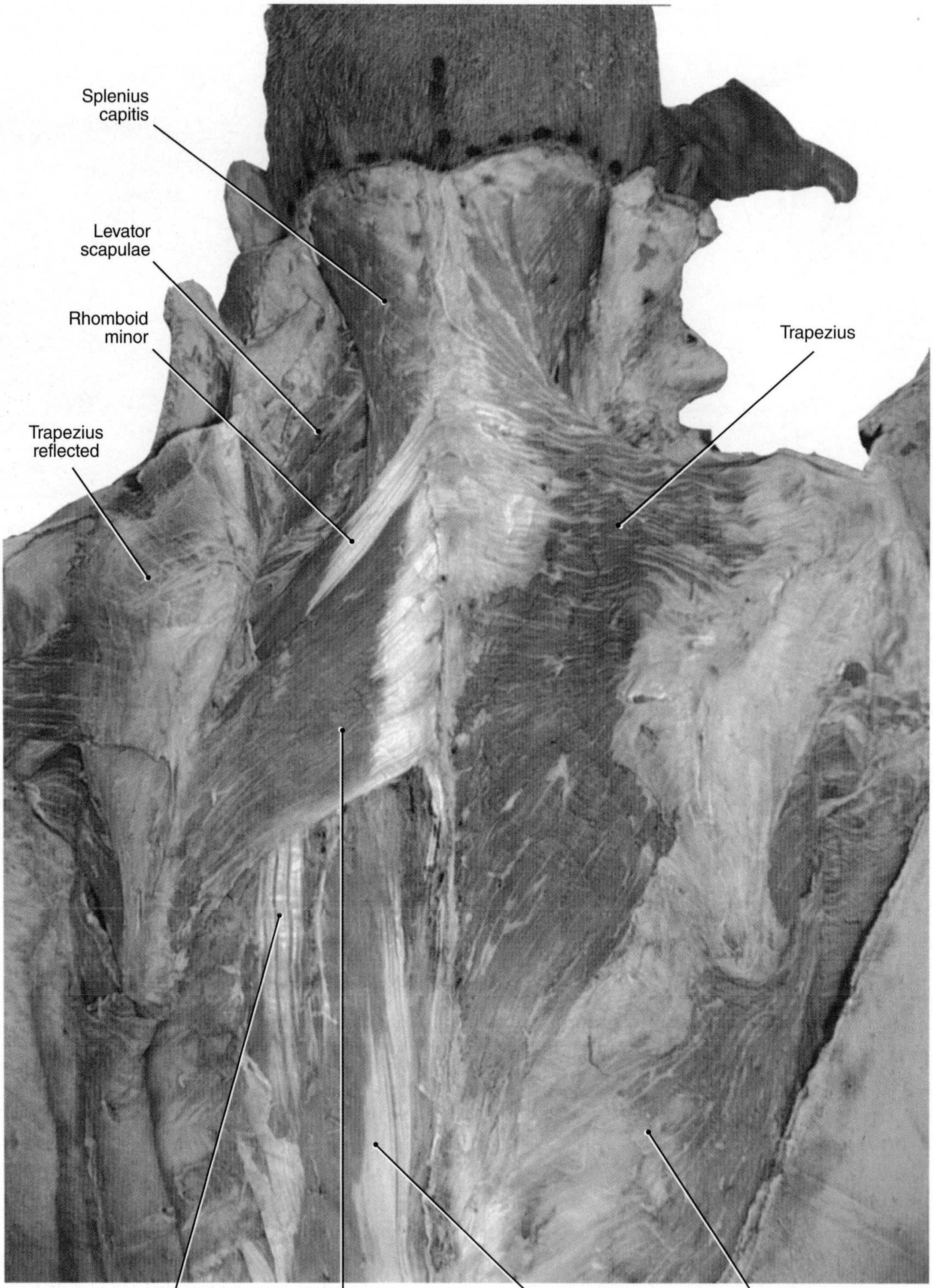

Fig. 2.22 Trapezius and latissimus dorsi muscles are reflected exposing the intermediate group of the extrinsic muscles of the back.

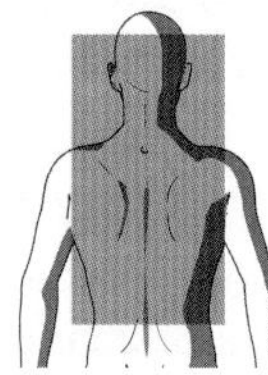

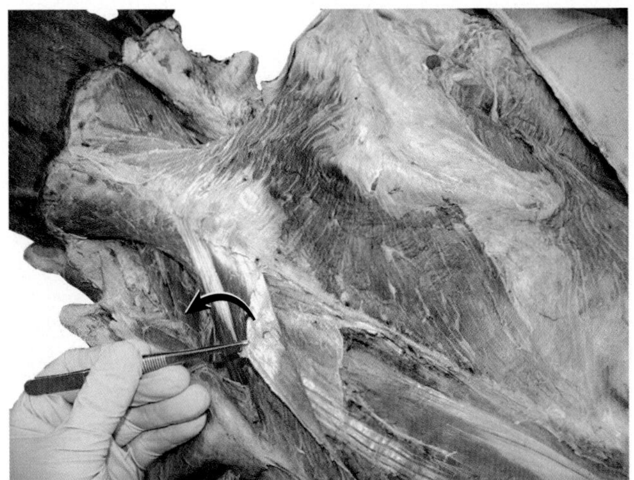

Fig. 2.23 After the trapezius is exposed, reflect the rhomboid major and minor muscles to expose the serratus posterior superior.

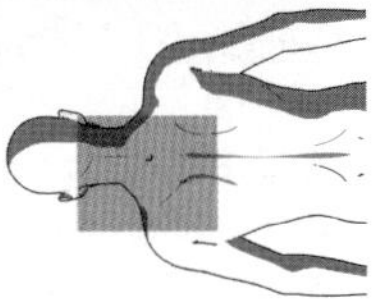

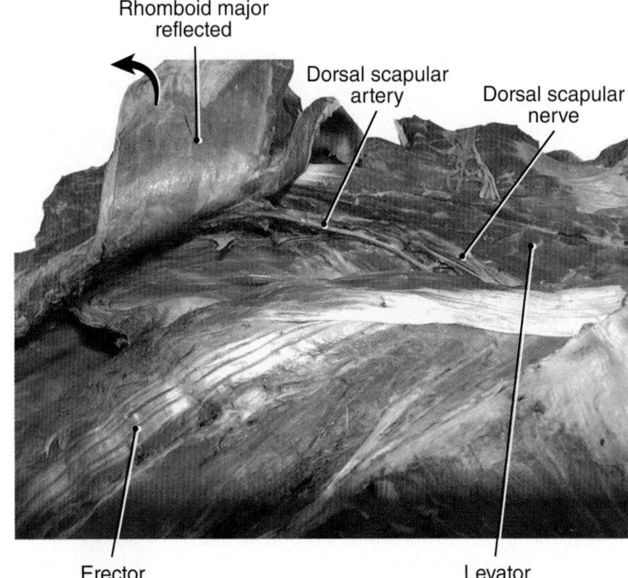

Fig. 2.24 View of deep surface of scapula illustrating dorsal scapular artery and nerve running at the medial border of scapula.

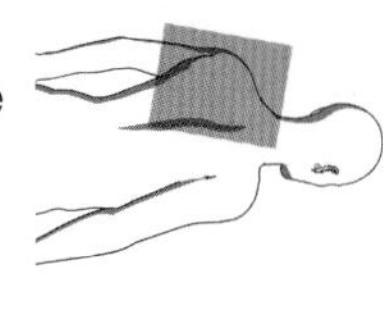

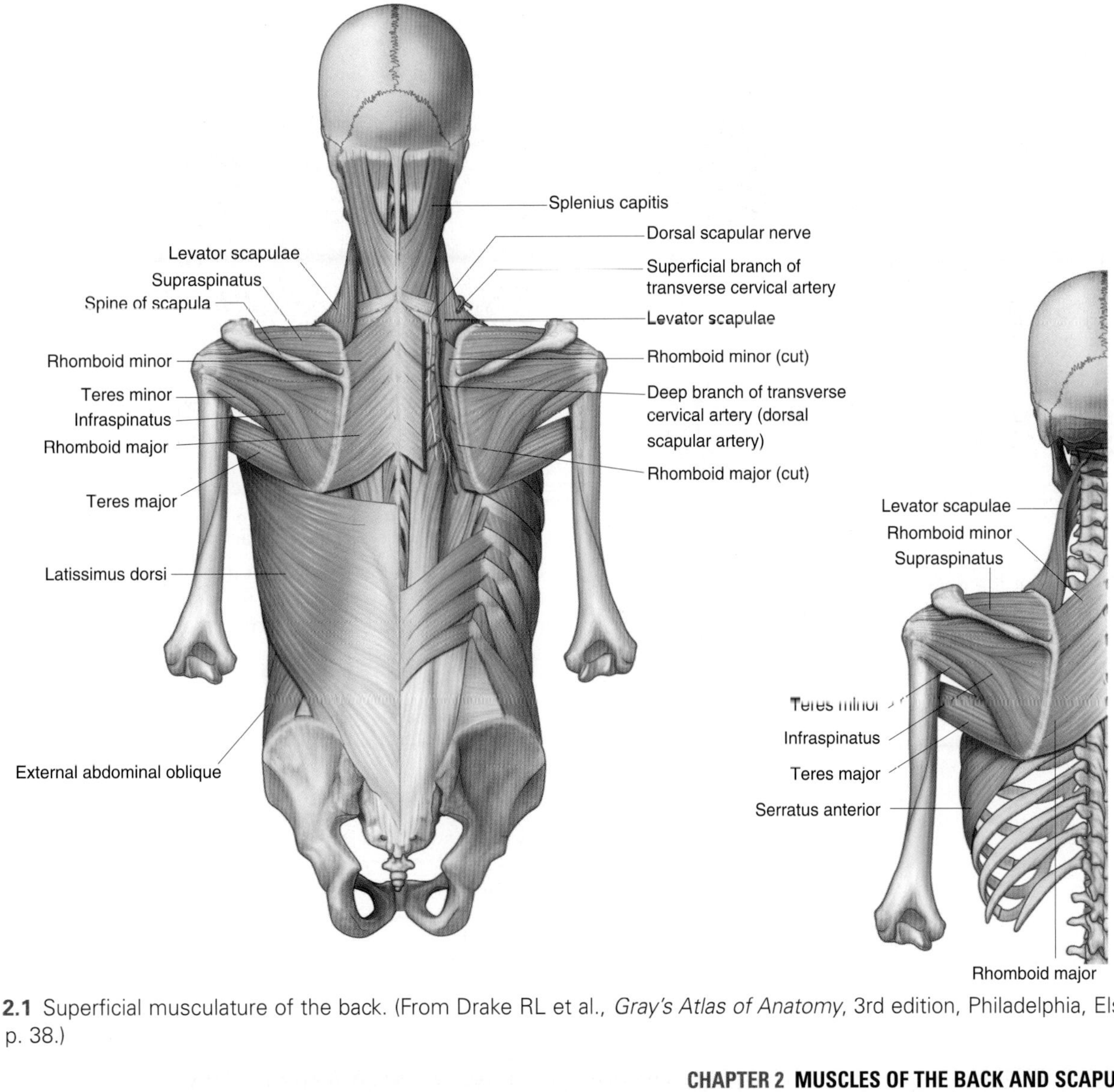

Splenius capitis
Dorsal scapular nerve
Superficial branch of transverse cervical artery
Levator scapulae
Rhomboid minor (cut)
Deep branch of transverse cervical artery (dorsal scapular artery)
Rhomboid major (cut)
Levator scapulae
Supraspinatus
Spine of scapula
Rhomboid minor
Teres minor
Infraspinatus
Rhomboid major
Teres major
Latissimus dorsi
External abdominal oblique
Levator scapulae
Rhomboid minor
Supraspinatus
Teres minor
Infraspinatus
Teres major
Serratus anterior
Rhomboid major

Plate 2.1 Superficial musculature of the back. (From Drake RL et al., *Gray's Atlas of Anatomy*, 3rd edition, Philadelphia, Elsevier, 2021, p. 38.)

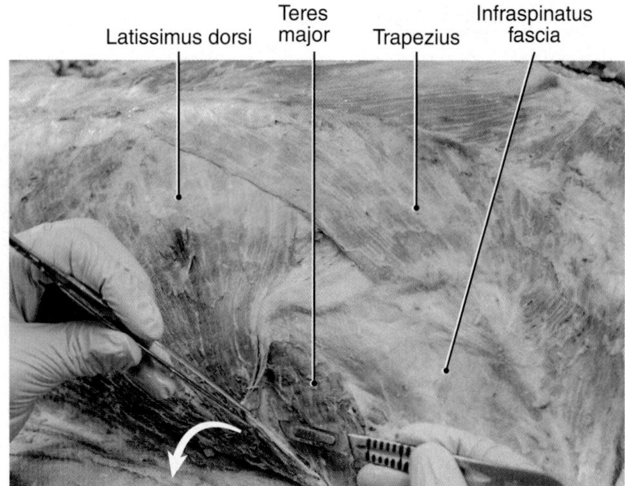

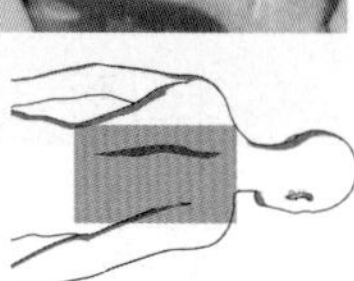

Fig. 2.25 Careful separation of the teres major muscle from the upper border of the latissimus dorsi muscle.

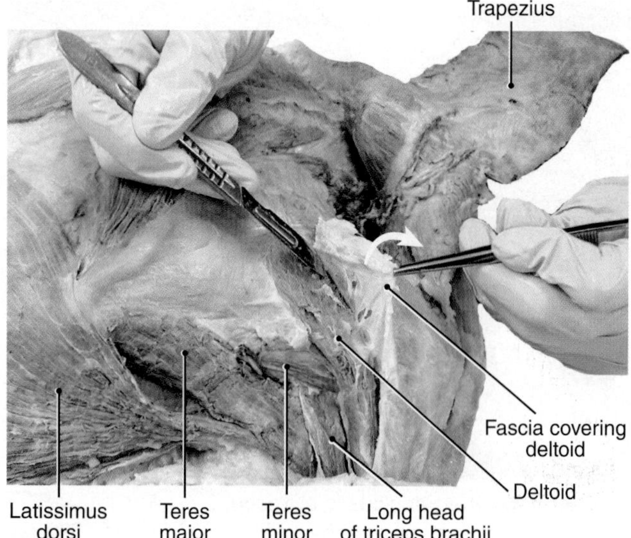

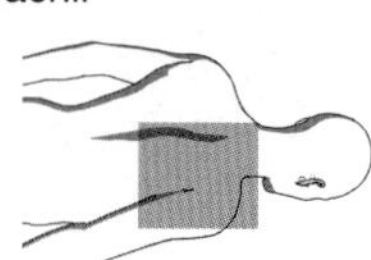

Fig. 2.27 With the scalpel, carefully detach deep fascia covering the posterior fibers of the deltoid muscle.

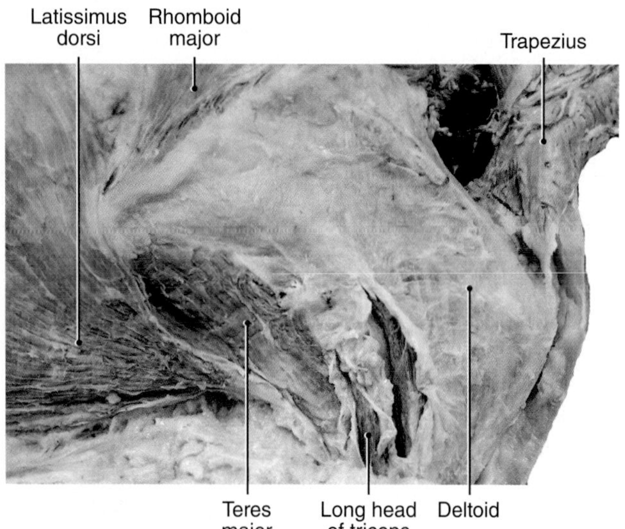

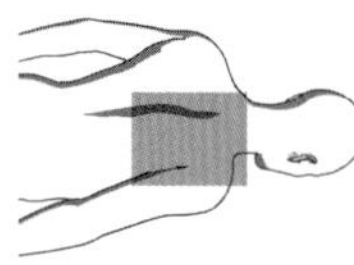

Fig. 2.26 View of the posterior scapular region. The long head of triceps brachii and deltoid muscles are exposed after careful separation from infraspinatus fascia.

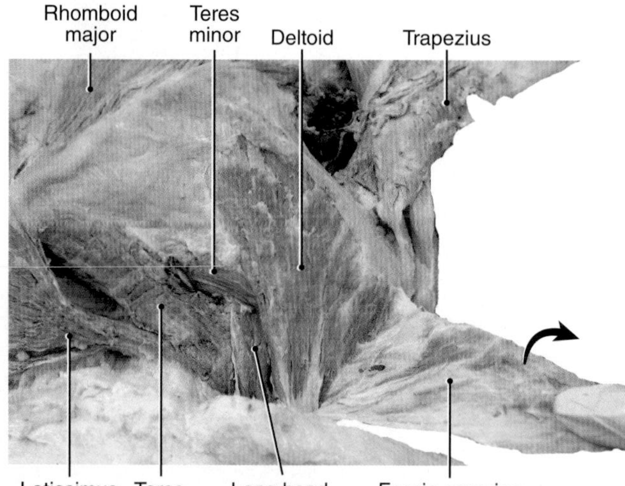

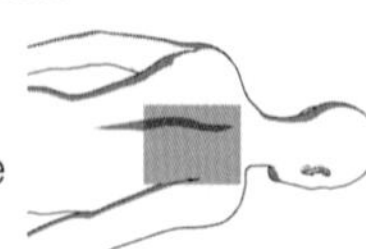

Fig. 2.28 Deep fascia covering the deltoid muscle is reflected, exposing the deltoid muscle with its attachments onto the spine of the scapula.

- Insert your index finger under the deltoid muscle (Fig. 2.29).
- Using toothed forceps, scalpel, and scissors, reflect the posterior border of the deltoid laterally, separating it at its attachment on the spine of the scapula and acromion (Fig. 2.30).

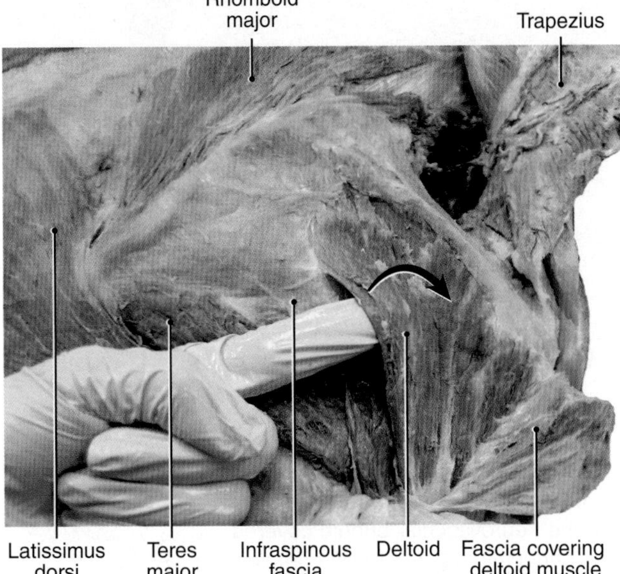

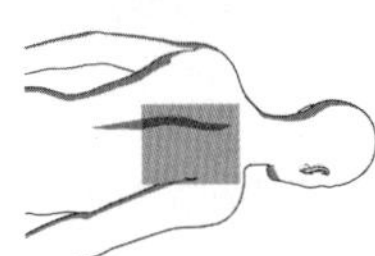

Fig. 2.29 Insert your index finger under the deltoid muscle, and with a scalpel, detach its attachments to the scapula.

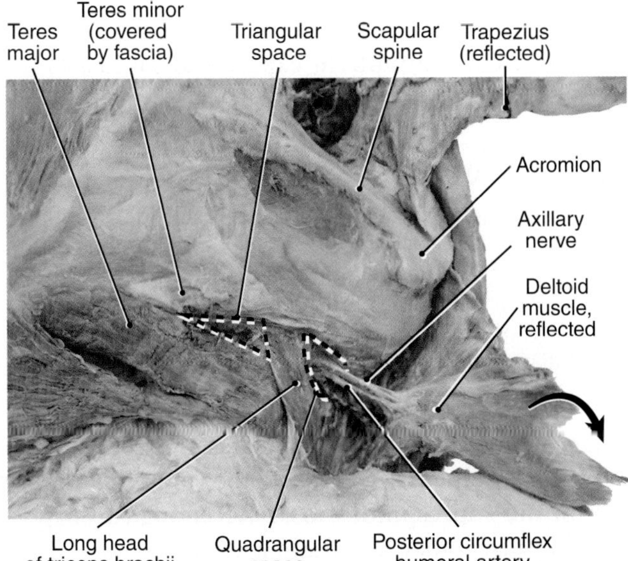

Fig. 2.30 View of the internal surface of reflected deltoid muscle with the posterior circumflex humeral artery and axillary nerve exposed. Note the quadrangular and triangular spaces.

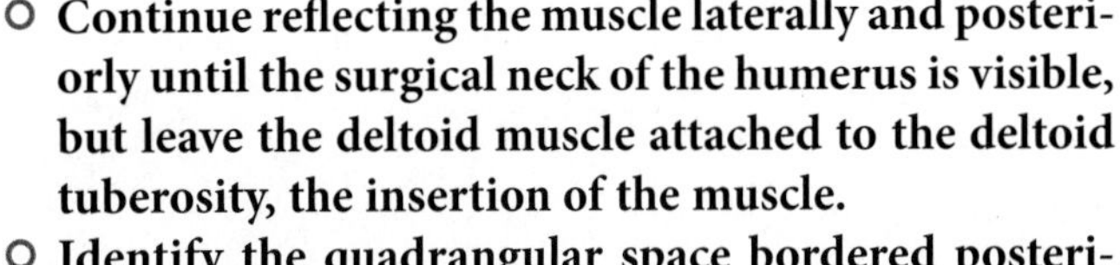

- Continue reflecting the muscle laterally and posteriorly until the surgical neck of the humerus is visible, but leave the deltoid muscle attached to the deltoid tuberosity, the insertion of the muscle.
- Identify the quadrangular space bordered posteriorly by the teres major and minor muscles, long head of triceps brachii, and surgical neck of the humerus (see Fig. 2.30).
- Identify the axillary nerve as it appears posterior to the surgical neck of the humerus (see Fig. 2.30). The nerve is accompanied by the posterior circumflex humeral artery, a branch of the third portion of the axillary artery. The axillary nerve and posterior circumflex humeral artery appear in the field by emerging through the quadrangular space.
- Thoroughly clean the axillary nerve and the posterior circumflex humeral vessels at their entrance into the deltoid muscle behind the surgical neck of the humerus. Protect these as you clean connective tissue away from the muscles that help form the boundaries of the quadrangular space.

DISSECTION **TIP**

The axillary nerve typically branches off into several smaller branches and is usually superior to the posterior circumflex humeral artery.

- Identify the triangular space between the teres minor, teres major, and the long head of the triceps brachii (see Fig. 2.30).
- Identify the scapular circumflex artery within the triangular space.

ANATOMY **NOTE**

This artery originates from the subscapular artery, one of the three branches of the third part of the axillary artery. The scapular circumflex artery branches to the overlying skin of the triangular space before turning around the lateral border of the scapula and passing deep to the infraspinatus muscle.

DISSECTION **TIP**

The scapular circumflex artery typically is located at the midpoint of the lateral border of the scapula (see Fig. 2.33).

ANATOMY **NOTE**

The infraspinatus and supraspinatus fasciae are attached to the scapula around the boundaries of the attachments of the infraspinatus and supraspinatus muscles, respectively.

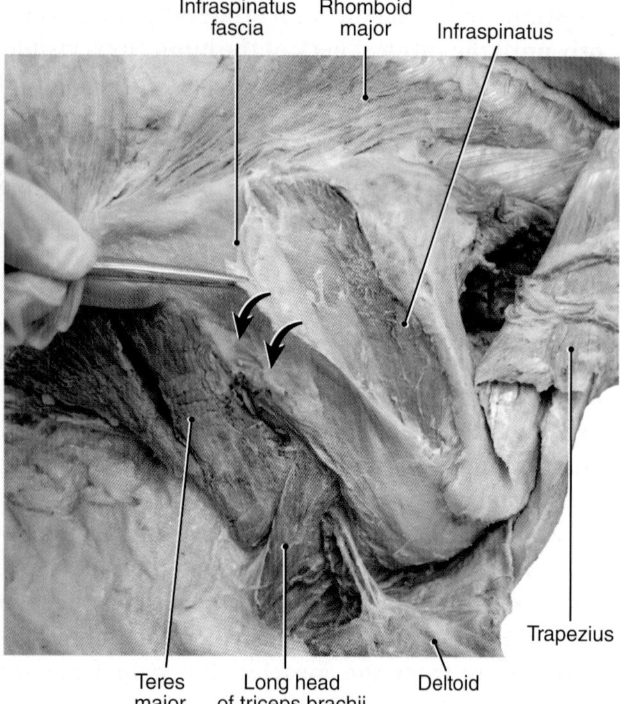

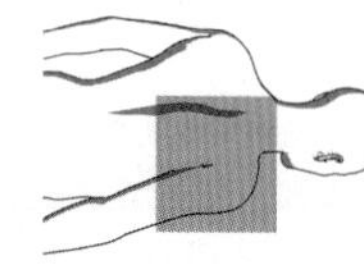

Fig. 2.31 With a scalpel, carefully detach the deep fascia (infraspinatus fascia) covering the infraspinatus muscle.

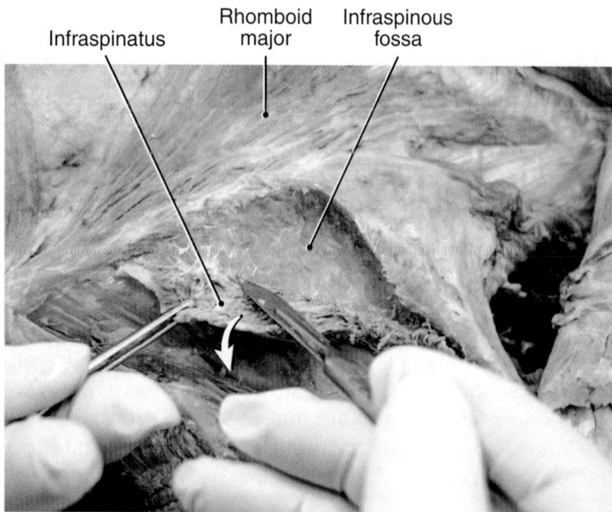

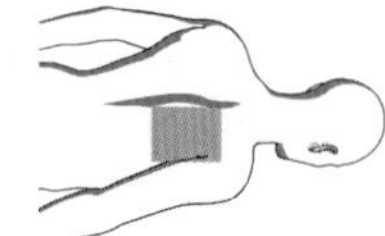

Fig. 2.32 With a scalpel, carefully detach the infraspinatus muscle from the infraspinous fossa.

- **Identify the medial border of the infraspinatus muscle.**
- **With a scalpel, carefully detach the deep fascia (infraspinatus fascia) covering the infraspinatus muscle (Fig. 2.31).**
- **Carefully detach the infraspinatus muscle from the infraspinous fossa (Fig. 2.32).**

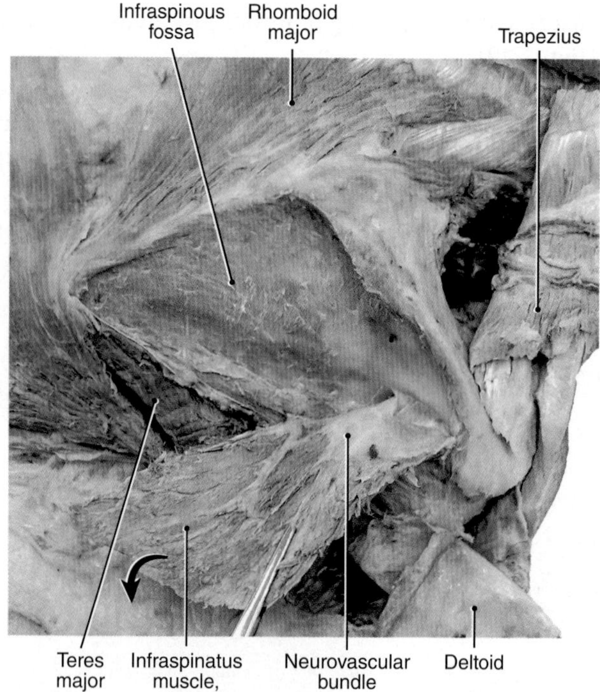

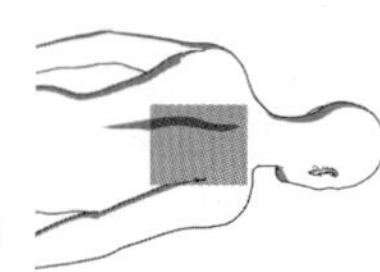

Fig. 2.33 View of infraspinous fossa with infraspinatus muscle reflected. Note the neurovascular bundle covered with connective tissue, which contains the suprascapular artery, vein, and nerve.

- **Reflect the infraspinatus muscle laterally from the infraspinous fossa toward its humeral insertion (Fig. 2.33). Note the neurovascular bundle covered with connective tissue, which contains the suprascapular artery, vein, and nerve.**
- **Carefully separate the connective tissue over the neurovascular bundle to expose the suprascapular artery, nerve, and vein (Fig. 2.34).**

ANATOMY **NOTE**

The suprascapular artery has a rich anastomosis with the scapular circumflex artery. This arrangement allows the formation of a collateral arterial supply between the subclavian artery and the third part of the axillary artery in the event of occlusion of the more proximal portions of the axillary artery.

- **Identify and clean the supraspinatus muscle (Fig. 2.35).**
- **Beginning medially, reflect the muscle laterally from the supraspinous fossa far enough to expose the suprascapular nerve and artery.**
- **Identify the suprascapular artery and trace it from its origin to its crossing of the superior transverse scapular ligament to enter the supraspinous fossa, deep to the supraspinatus muscle (Fig. 2.36). Note the passage of the suprascapular nerve and vessels around the scapular notch, where they enter the infraspinatus muscle (Plate 2.2).**

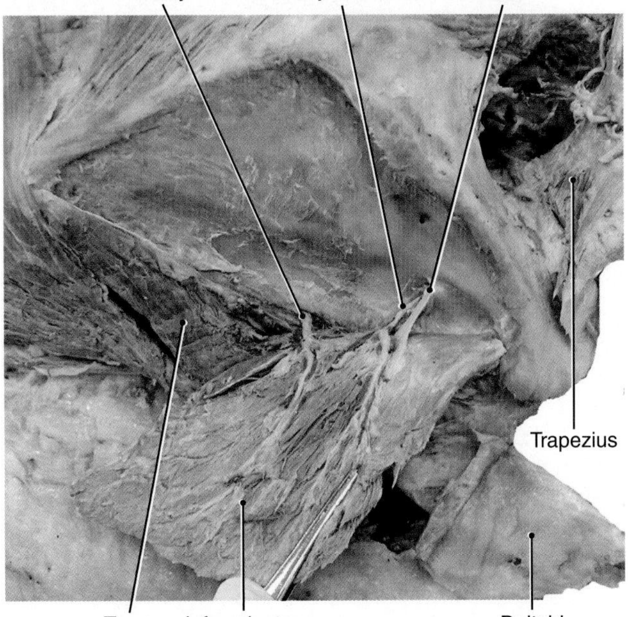

Circumflex scapular artery
Suprascapular artery and vein
Suprascapular nerve
Trapezius
Teres major
Infraspinatus reflected
Deltoid (reflected)

Fig. 2.34 Connective tissue is dissected away, exposing the suprascapular artery, vein, and nerve, as well as the scapular circumflex artery.

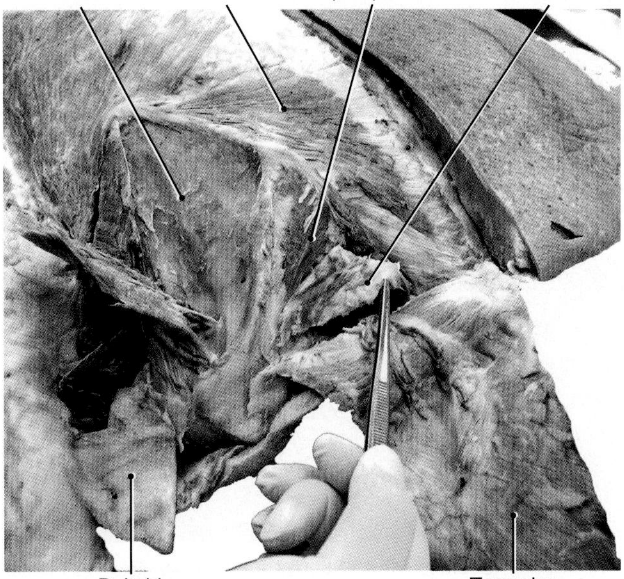

Infraspinatus fossa
Rhomboid major
Supraspinatus
Supraspinatus fascia
Deltoid
Trapezius

Fig. 2.35 Supraspinatus fascia is reflected, and the supraspinatus muscle exposed.

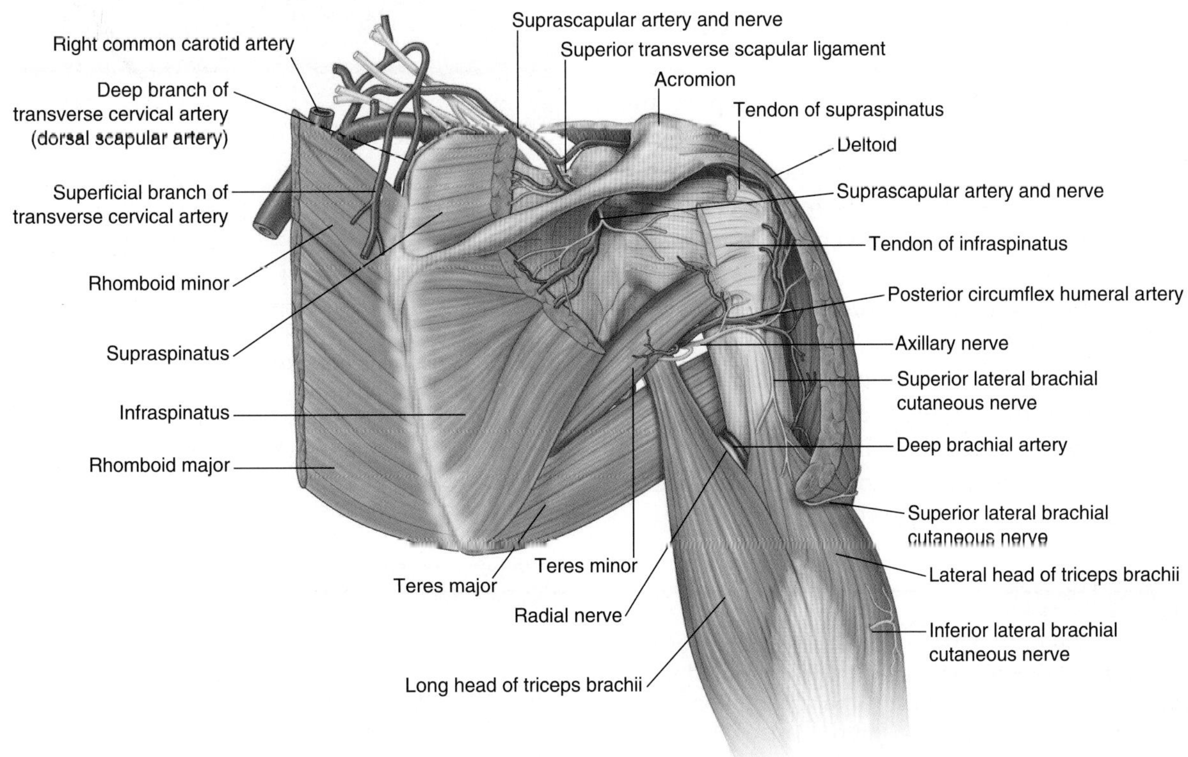

Plate 2.2 Collateral arterial supply between the subclavian artery and the third part of the axillary artery through anastomoses of the circumflex scapular artery and the suprascapular artery. (From Drake RL et al., *Gray's Atlas of Anatomy*, 3rd edition, Philadelphia, Elsevier, 2021, p. 402.)

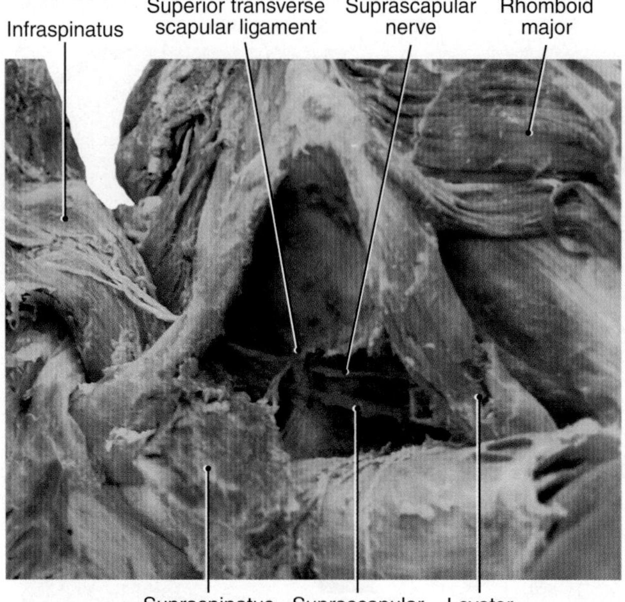

Fig. 2.36 View of the internal surface of the supraspinous fossa. Notice the suprascapular artery passing over the superior transverse scapular ligament and suprascapular nerve underneath it.

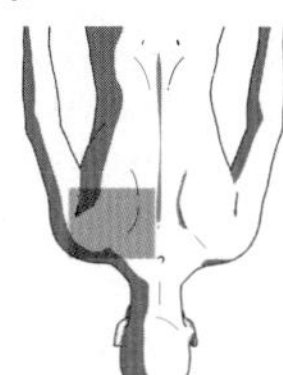

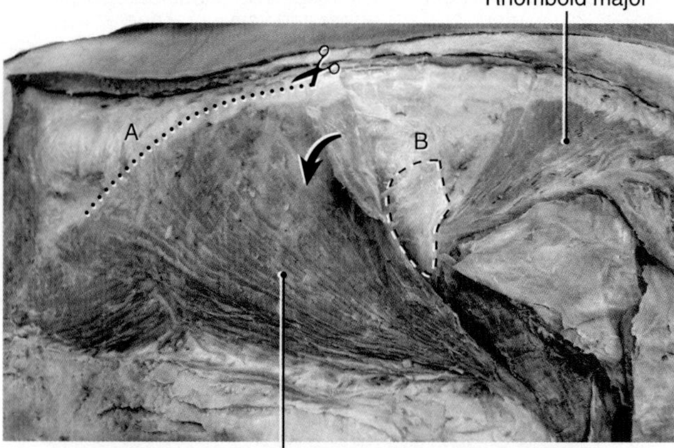

Fig. 2.37 *Dotted line A* shows location of incision through the aponeurosis of latissimus dorsi muscle. *Dotted line B* shows area of connective/adipose tissue covering serratus anterior muscle.

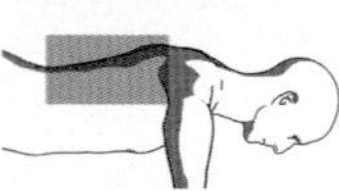

SUPERFICIAL MUSCLES OF THE BACK: PART 2

- **Completely remove the deep fascia to expose the latissimus dorsi muscle.**
- **Make an incision through the aponeurosis of the latissimus dorsi muscle about ½ inches (1.25 cm) from the midline of the back and cut its attachments to the crest of the ilium.**
- **Reflect the latissimus dorsi muscle superiorly and laterally (Fig. 2.37).**
- **Reflection of the trapezius and latissimus dorsi muscles exposes underlying the intermediate group of the extrinsic muscles of the back.**
- **Identify the serratus anterior and the serratus posterior inferior muscles (Fig. 2.38).**

DISSECTION TIP

If you do not exercise care, you will reflect the serratus posterior inferior muscle with the latissimus dorsi. The key to their separation lies in the recognition that although the serratus posterior inferior arises in common with part of the latissimus dorsi, the serratus inserts onto the lower ribs. These fibers can be observed as they diverge from those of the latissimus to pass to their insertion (Fig. 2.39).

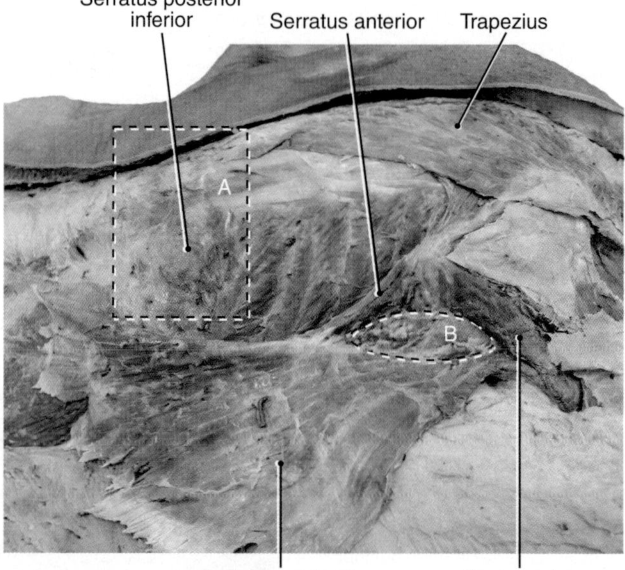

Fig. 2.38 Latissimus dorsi muscle is reflected, and *dotted outline A* shows the serratus posterior inferior muscle. Connective/adipose tissue of Fig. 2.33 is removed and serratus anterior muscle exposed. *Dotted line B* shows the second area of connective/adipose tissue between serratus anterior and latissimus dorsi muscles.

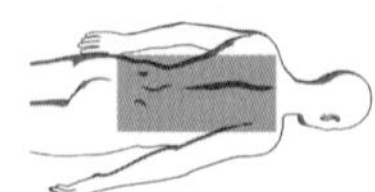

- **Pay special attention when removing the connective adipose tissue between the latissimus dorsi, serratus anterior, and teres major muscles so as not to injure the thoracodorsal artery and vein (Figs. 2.40 and 2.41).**
- **Cut the origin of the serratus posterior inferior muscle and reflect it toward its insertion.**

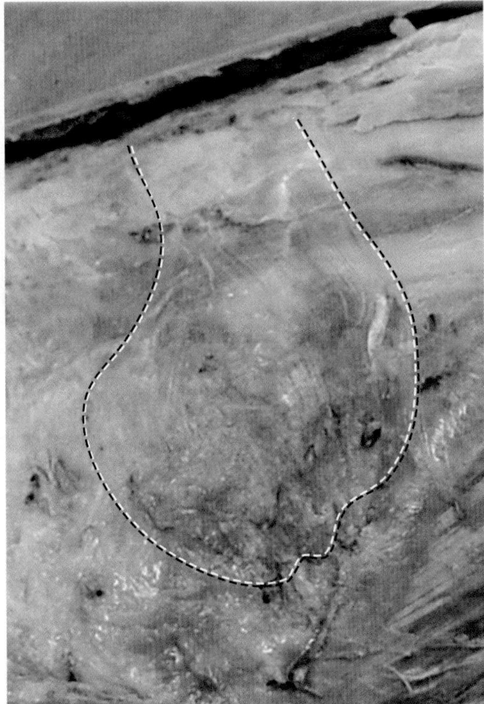

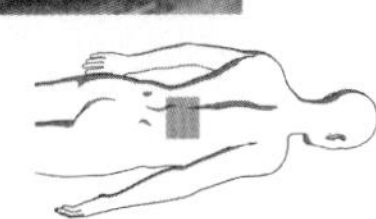

Fig. 2.39 *Dotted line* shows borders of serratus posterior inferior muscle.

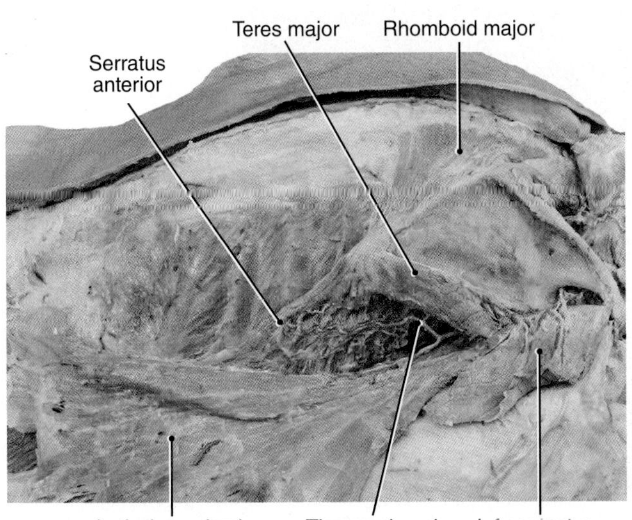

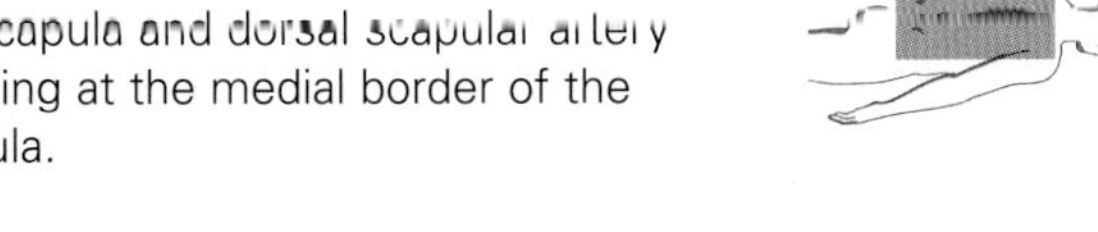

Fig. 2.40 View of the internal surface of the scapula and dorsal scapular artery traveling at the medial border of the scapula.

- **Make a longitudinal incision through the lumbar part of the thoracolumbar fascia near the midline. Then, by cutting its attachments to the underlying musculature, reflect this thick fascia/aponeurosis combination laterally far enough to expose the erector spinae muscle layer (Figs. 2.42 and 2.43).**

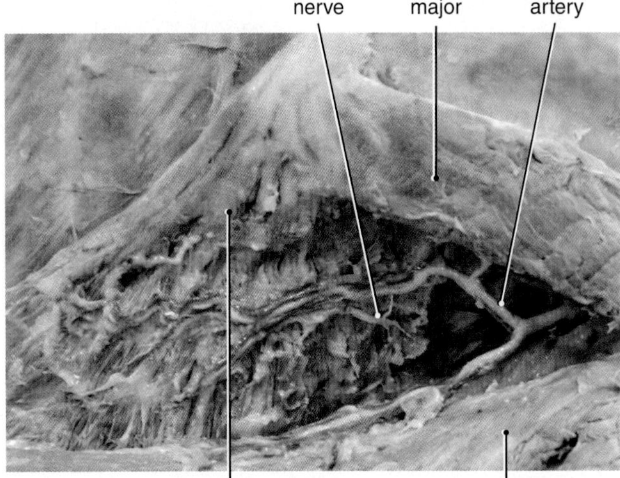

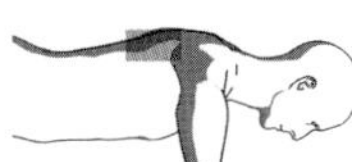

Fig. 2.41 Close-up view of space between teres major, serratus anterior, and latissimus dorsi muscles (area *B* in Fig. 2.38). Note the thoracodorsal artery and long thoracic nerve supplying the serratus anterior muscle.

DISSECTION **TIP**

The reflection of the thoracolumbar fascia is performed in the lumbar region only. For the thoracic region, it is unnecessary because the fascia is much thinner there. In this specimen, the fascia in the thoracic region was thick enough to be reflected (see Fig. 2.42).

- **Identify and separate the three longitudinally oriented columns of the erector spinae muscle: the spinalis, longissimus, and iliocostalis (Fig. 2.44).**

ANATOMY **NOTE**

The spinalis is the more medial muscle; the longissimus is the longest muscle, extending to the neck, and the iliocostalis is the most lateral of the three muscles, attaching the iliac crest to the ribs.

DEEP MUSCLES OF THE BACK

- **To expose the deeper musculature, remove a block of the erector spinae muscle several inches long from the lower thoracic and upper lumbar region and identify the transversospinalis musculature (Figs. 2.45 and 2.46). The transversospinalis muscles include the semispinalis, multifidus, and rotatores.**

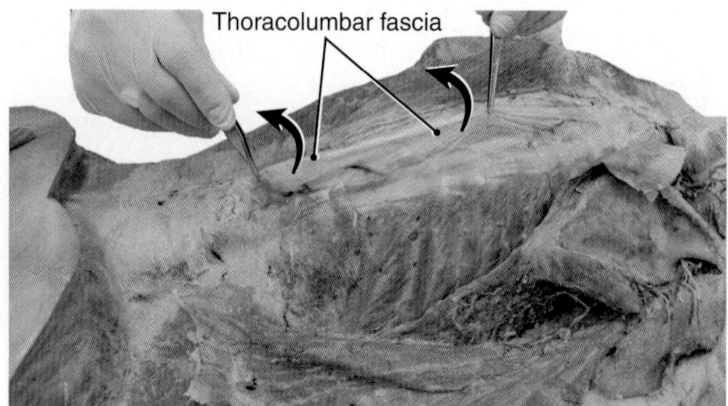

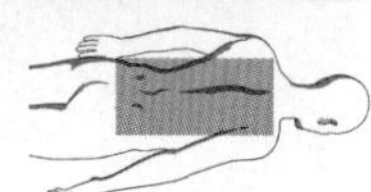

Fig. 2.42 Reflection of thoracolumbar fascia.

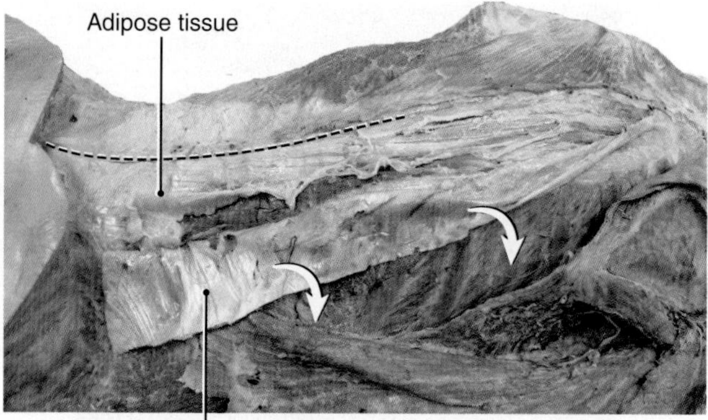

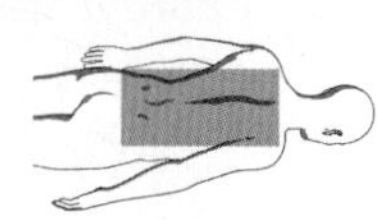

Fig. 2.43 Thoracolumbar fascia is reflected, and erector spinae muscle is exposed. Note adipose tissue overlying erector spinae. *Dotted line* represents longitudinal incision of thoracolumbar fascia from the midline.

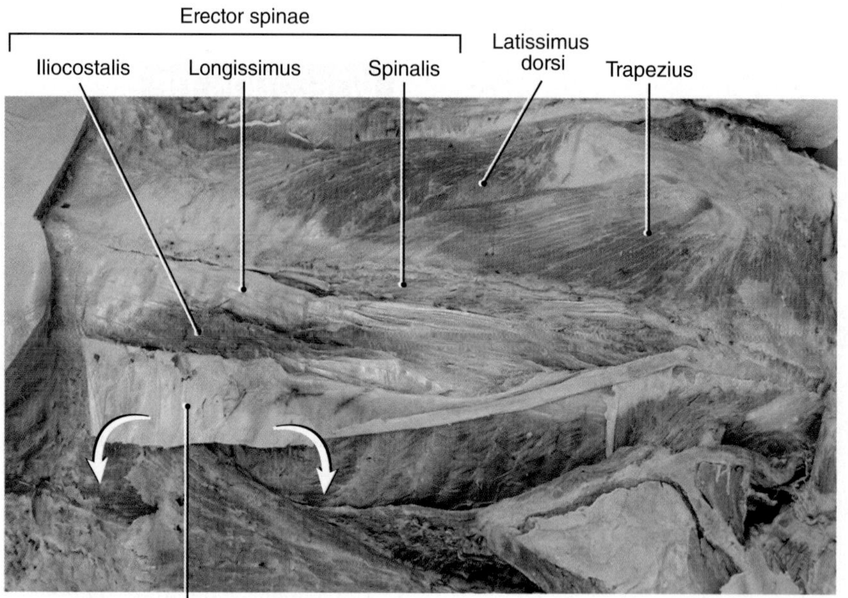

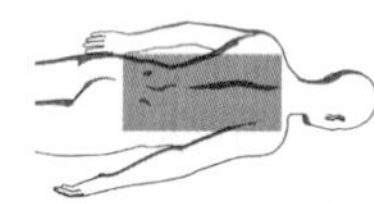

Fig. 2.44 The thoracolumbar fascia is reflected, and the erector spinae muscle is exposed.

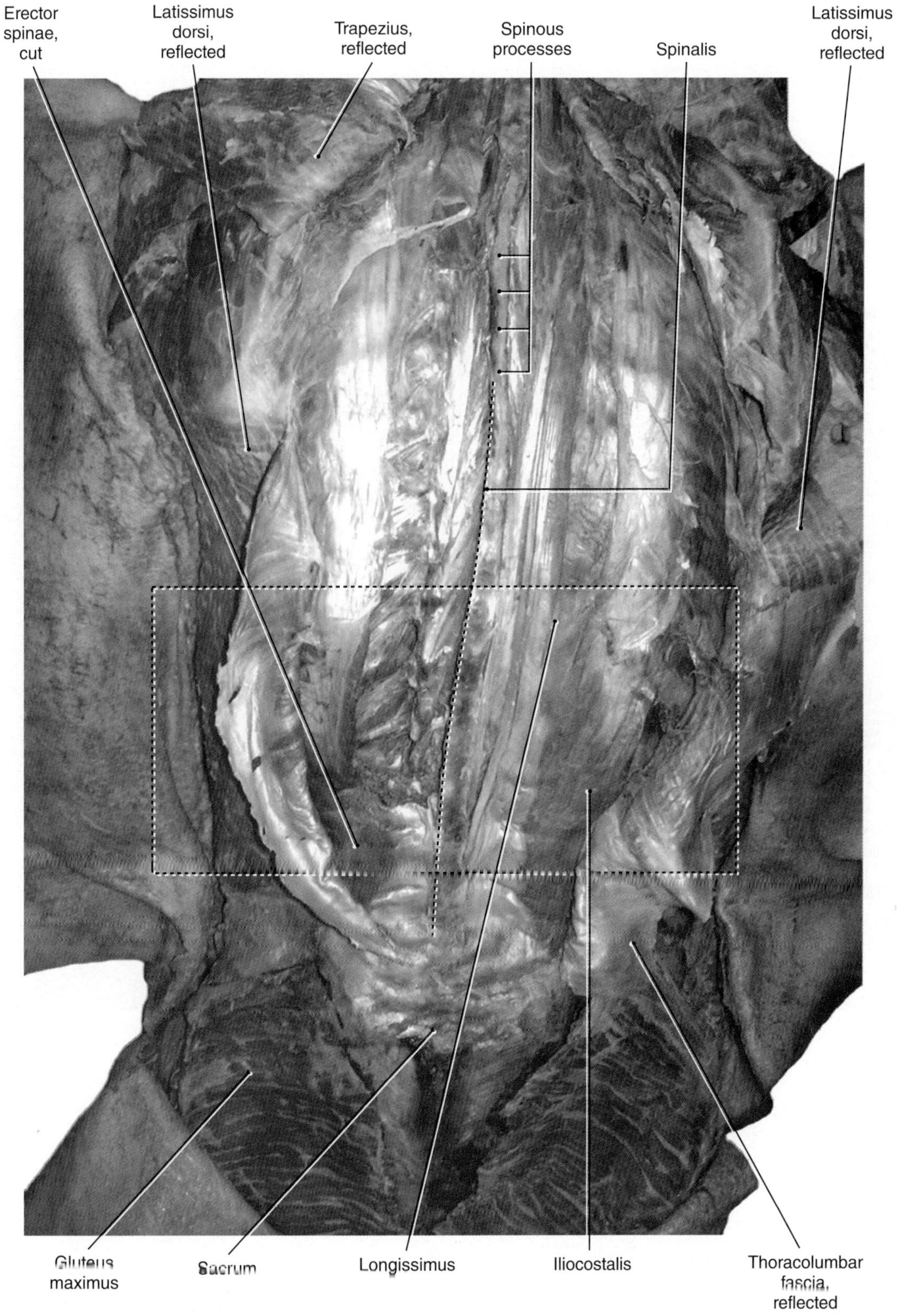

Erector spinae, cut
Latissimus dorsi, reflected
Trapezius, reflected
Spinous processes
Spinalis
Latissimus dorsi, reflected
Gluteus maximus
Sacrum
Longissimus
Iliocostalis
Thoracolumbar fascia, reflected

Fig. 2.45 The posterior lamina of the thoracolumbar fascia is reflected laterally, and the erector spinae muscle (spinalis, longissimus, and iliocostalis) is exposed on the right. On the left, the erector spinae muscle is cut to expose the deeper muscles of the back.

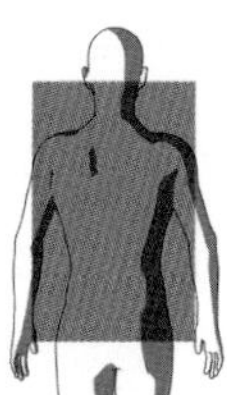

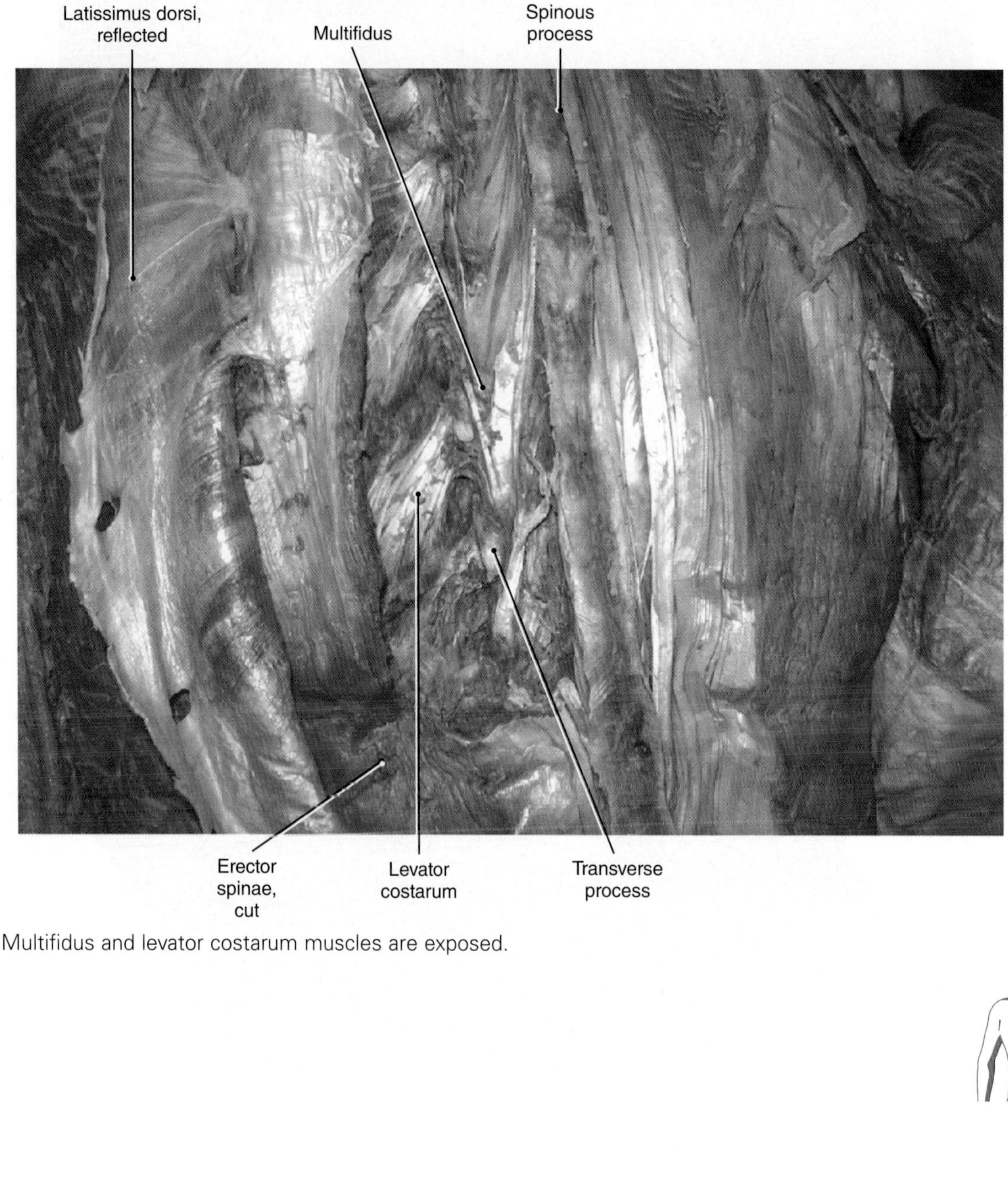

Latissimus dorsi, reflected
Multifidus
Spinous process
Erector spinae, cut
Levator costarum
Transverse process

Fig. 2.46 Multifidus and levator costarum muscles are exposed.

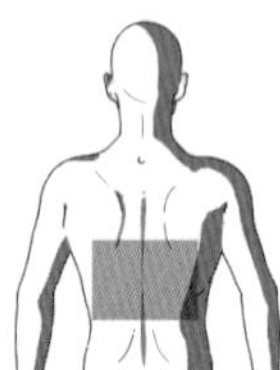

LABORATORY IDENTIFICATION CHECKLIST

OSTEOLOGY
- ☐ Skull and vertebrae
- ☐ Superior nuchal line
- ☐ External occipital protuberance
- ☐ Mastoid process
- ☐ Vertebra prominens (C7)
- ☐ Spinous processes of thoracic and lumbar vertebrae, sacrum, and coccyx

CLAVICLE
- ☐ Medial and lateral ends, body, and curvatures

SCAPULA
- ☐ Acromion
- ☐ Spine of scapula
- ☐ Medial or vertebral border
- ☐ Superior border
- ☐ Scapular notch
- ☐ Inferior angle
- ☐ Superior angle
- ☐ Lateral or axillary border
- ☐ Coracoid process

OTHER
- ☐ Iliac crests

MUSCLES
- ☐ Trapezius
- ☐ Latissimus dorsi
- ☐ Serratus posterior inferior
- ☐ Serratus posterior superior
- ☐ Levator scapulae
- ☐ Rhomboid minor
- ☐ Rhomboid major
- ☐ Deltoid
- ☐ Triceps brachii, long head
- ☐ Supraspinatus
- ☐ Infraspinatus
- ☐ Teres major
- ☐ Teres minor
- ☐ Transversospinalis
  - ☐ Semispinalis
  - ☐ Multifidus
  - ☐ Rotatores
- ☐ Semispinalis
- ☐ Splenius capitis
- ☐ Erector spinae
  - ☐ Spinalis
  - ☐ Longissimus
  - ☐ Iliocostalis

NERVES
- ☐ Greater occipital
- ☐ Spinal accessory
- ☐ Dorsal scapular
- ☐ Suprascapular
- ☐ Axillary

FASCIAE
- ☐ Thoracolumbar
- ☐ Supraspinatus/infraspinatus

LIGAMENT
- ☐ Superior transverse scapular

ARTERIES
- ☐ Occipital
- ☐ Suprascapular
- ☐ Scapular circumflex
- ☐ Transverse cervical
- ☐ Dorsal scapular
- ☐ Posterior circumflex humeral

VEIN
- ☐ Transverse cervical

SUBOCCIPITAL TRIANGLE

- Make a midline skin incision from the spinous process of the 7th cervical vertebra (C7) to the external occipital protuberance (Fig. 3.1).
- At the level of the external occipital protuberance, make a horizontal skin incision connecting the right and left mastoid processes.
- Reflect the skin and the subcutaneous adipose tissue as one layer.
- Beneath the subcutaneous tissue, a connective tissue layer covers the upper portion of the trapezius muscle (Fig. 3.2); dissect away this layer and expose the trapezius (Fig. 3.3).
- While cleaning out the fascia that overlies the most cephalic portion of the trapezius muscle (see Fig. 2.10), look for the greater occipital nerve (Fig. 3.4).
- Also at this location, locate the occipital artery and preserve it as the trapezius is reflected.

ANATOMY NOTE

The greater occipital nerve usually can be found about 1 inch (2.5 cm) from the midline of the neck and 1 inch inferior to the superior nuchal line, as this nerve pierces the trapezius muscle (see Figs. 2.11 and 2.12).

DISSECTION TIP

Usually, the deep fascia over the trapezius muscle, below the superior nuchal line, is thick and difficult to cut until the C7 level. About 1 cm lateral to the midline, the third occipital nerve (medial branch of posterior ramus of C3 spinal nerve) is seen along the nuchal ligament (ligamentum nuchae) intermingled with the deep fascia over this area (see Figs. 3.3 and 3.4). Generally, the third occipital nerve is very small and often is cut during routine dissections.

- Identify the greater occipital nerve and the third occipital nerve, and preserve them after reflecting the trapezius away from its cranial and cervical attachments. Carefully reflect the trapezius muscle from its cranial and cervical attachments (Figs. 3.5–3.7).

DISSECTION TIP

The trapezius is thin at its cephalic and cervical attachments (see Fig. 3.6). Be careful during its reflection. While reflecting the trapezius up from its distal end, keep the scalpel blade facing downward toward the vertebrae, not upward, in order to prevent damage to the muscle.

- The small amount of connective tissue between the trapezius and splenius capitis muscles can be removed.
- At the lateral border of the splenius capitis, identify the lesser occipital nerve (see Fig. 3.7).
- Identify the splenius capitis and splenius cervicis muscles; divide them at their origins from the spines of the cervical and upper thoracic vertebrae and reflect them laterally, exposing the semispinalis capitis muscle (Figs. 3.8–3.10).
- Cut the attachment of the semispinalis capitis muscle from the skull and the nuchal ligament to reveal the suboccipital triangle. Preserve the greater occipital and lesser occipital nerves as the semispinalis capitis muscle is reflected.

DISSECTION TIP

Make one small cut on the semispinalis capitis muscle medial to the greater and lesser occipital nerves (Fig. 3.11). In this way, the semispinalis capitis muscle easily can be reflected laterally without disturbing the course of the nerves (Fig. 3.12).

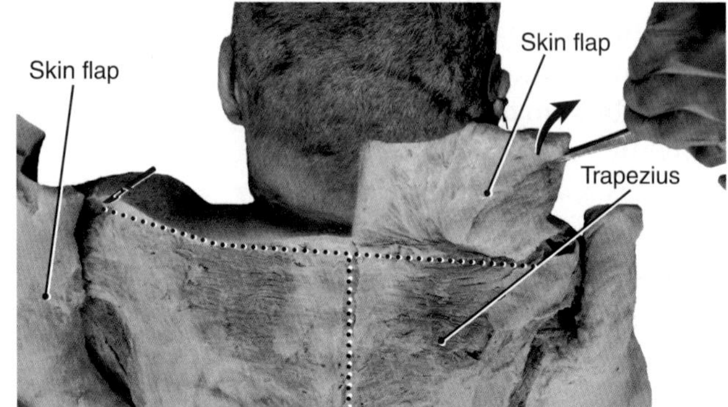

Fig. 3.1 Once the overlying skin is reflected, the deeper lying trapezius muscle is seen.

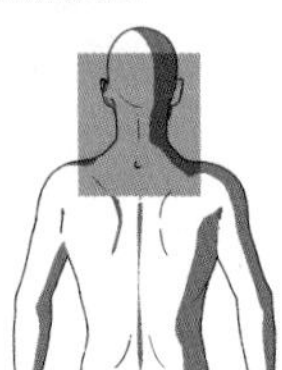

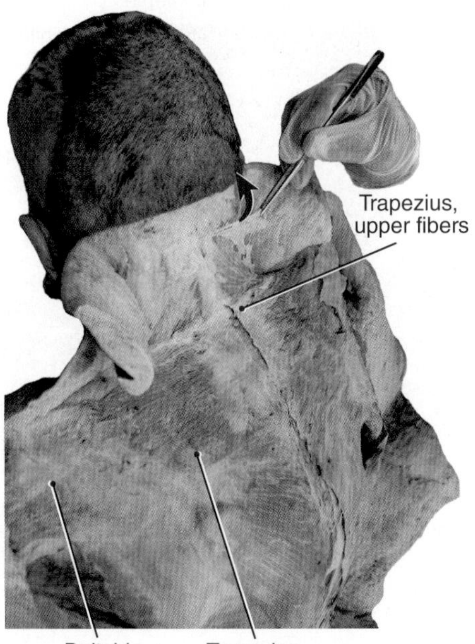

Fig. 3.2 Reflected skin and fascia revealing upper, middle, and lower fibers of the trapezius muscle.

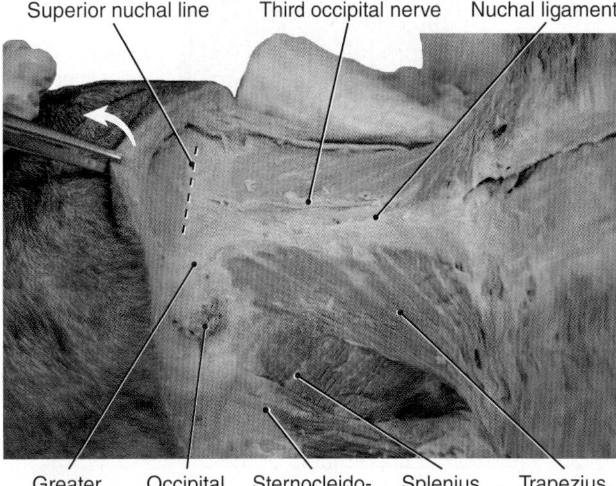

Fig. 3.4 Structures superficial to suboccipital triangle: nuchal ligament, trapezius (upper fibers), splenius capitis, sternocleidomastoid, third occipital nerve, and occipital artery.

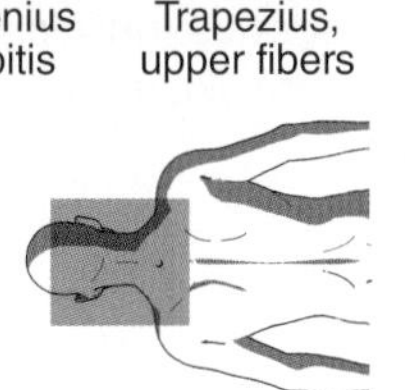

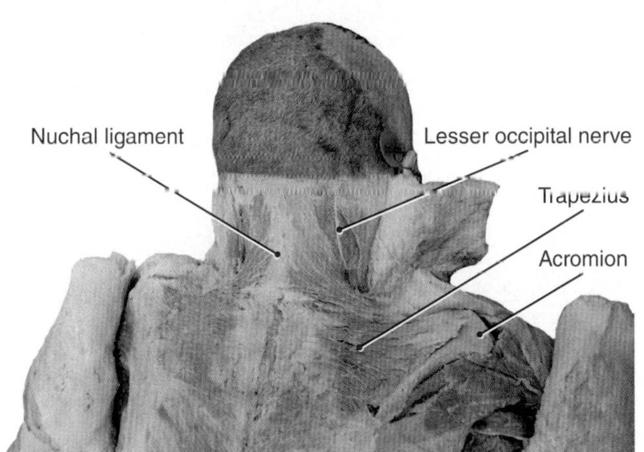

Fig. 3.3 Superficial upper back and suboccipital regions: upper, middle, and lower fibers of the trapezius muscle and nuchal ligament (ligamentum nuchae).

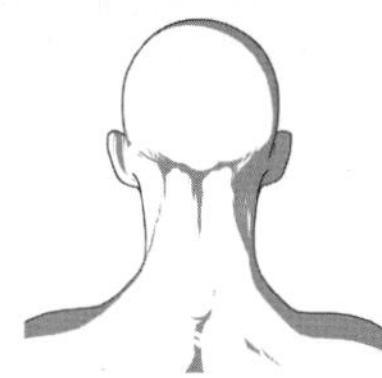

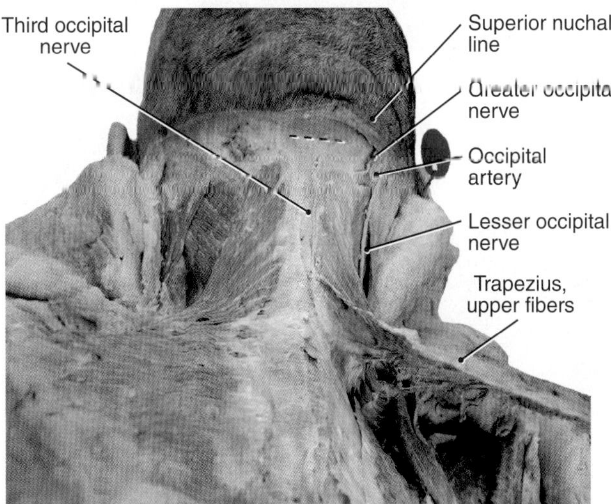

Fig. 3.5 Initial reflection of the trapezius muscle.

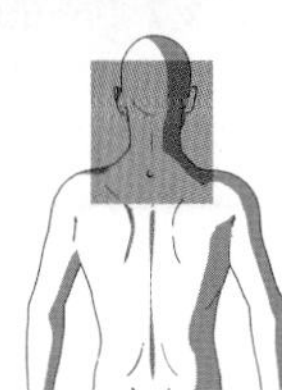

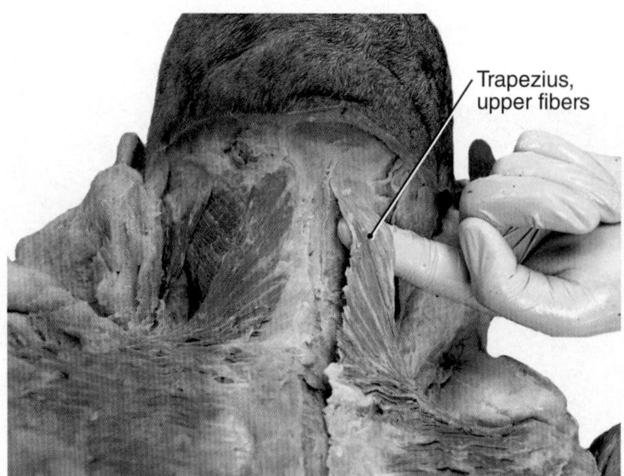

Fig. 3.6 Elevation of upper fibers of the trapezius muscle reflected away from the nuchal ligament.

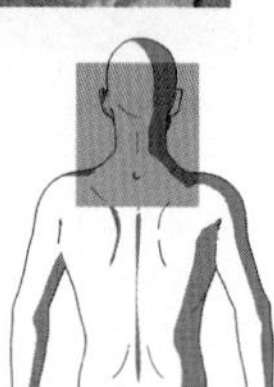

Fig. 3.8 Insert the scissors deep to the splenius capitis muscle at the midline and continue the incision inferiorly along the nuchal ligament.

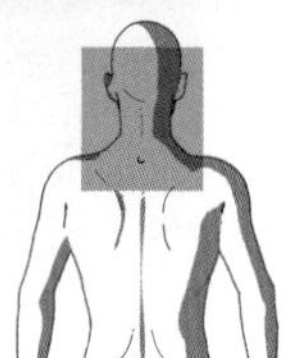

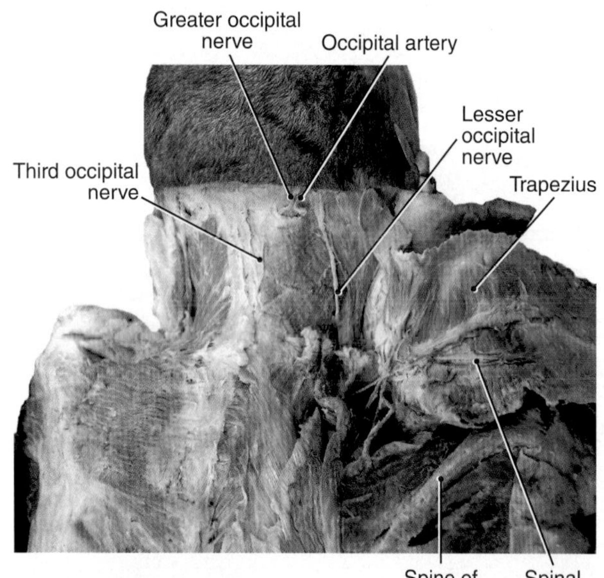

Fig. 3.7 Posterolateral view of the superficial suboccipital region with reflected trapezius muscle and its associated neurovascular bundle seen on its undersurface.

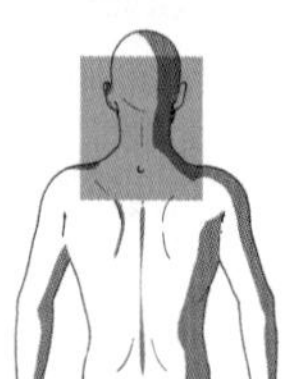

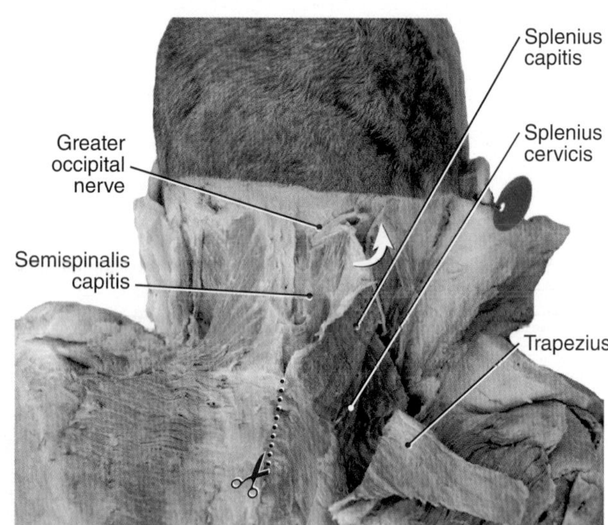

Fig. 3.9 Reflect the splenius capitis laterally, and then continue incision toward first thoracic vertebra (T1) level.

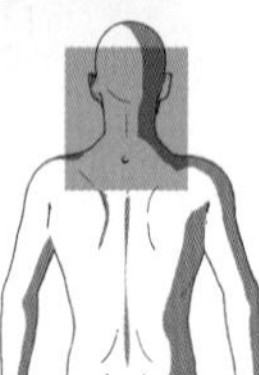

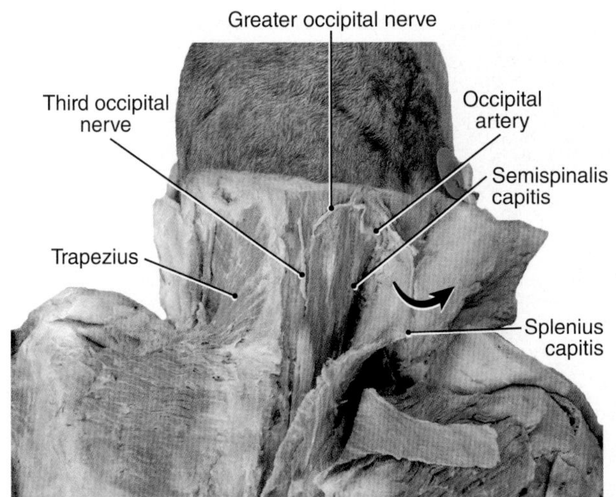

Fig. 3.10 Complete reflection of the splenius capitis muscle laterally.

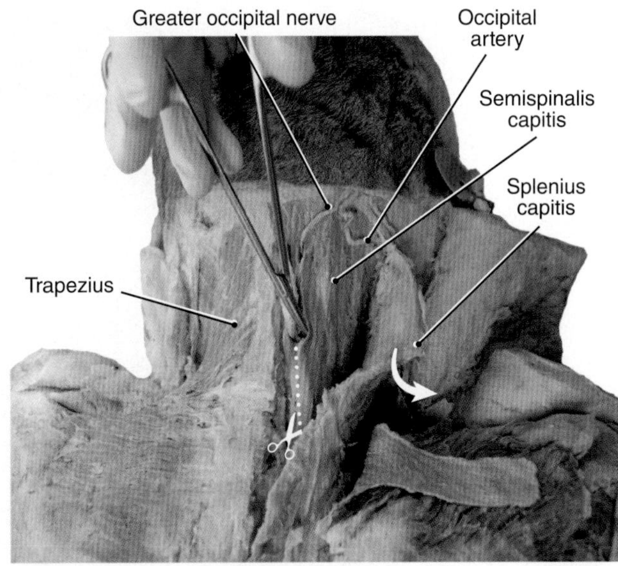

Fig. 3.11 Make an incision into the semispinalis capitis muscle near the midline down to approximately the T1 level. Preserve the greater and third occipital nerves.

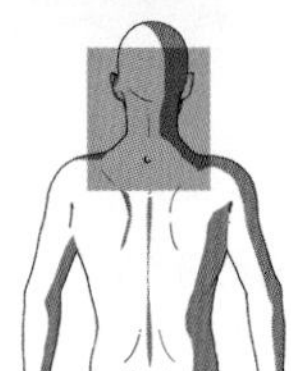

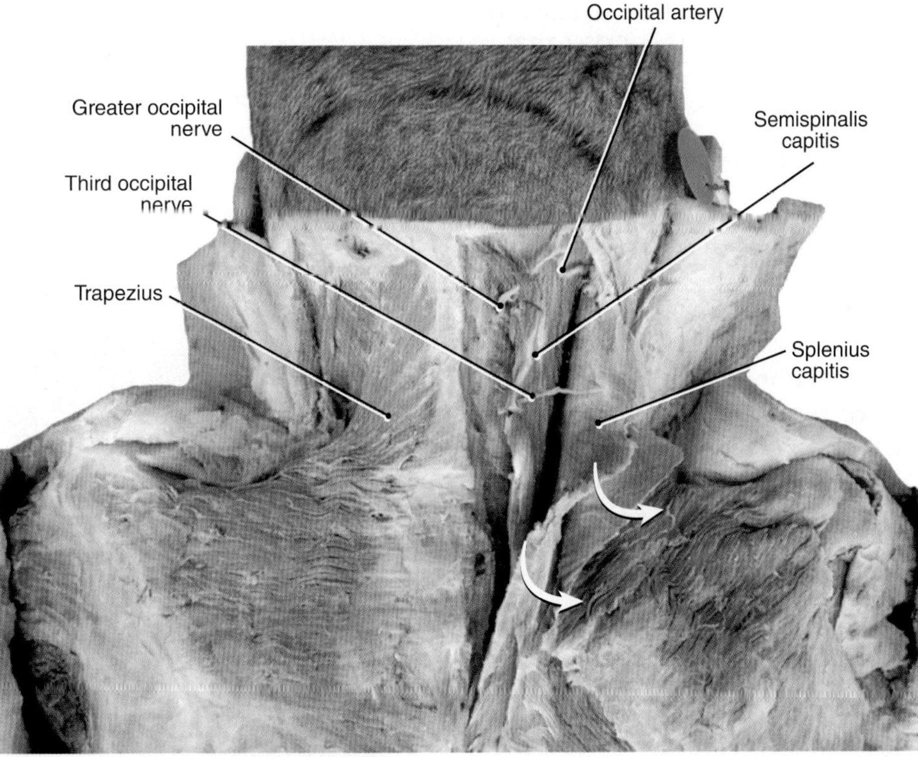

Fig. 3.12 Reflected trapezius, splenius capitis, and semispinalis capitis muscles.

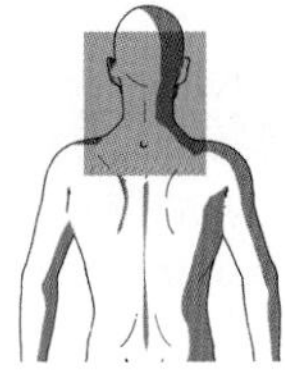

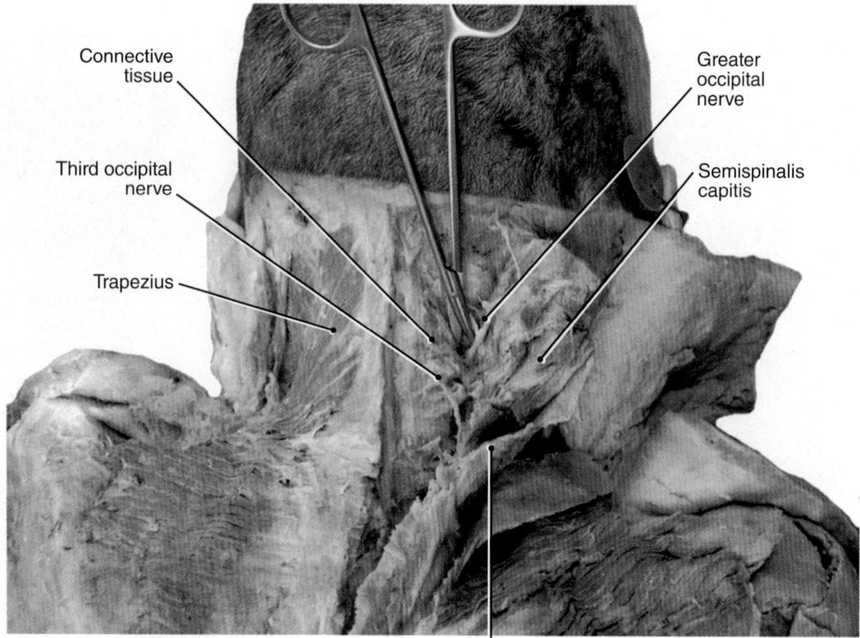

Fig. 3.13 Remove fat and connective tissues from around the greater and third occipital nerves. Use the separation technique with your scissors.

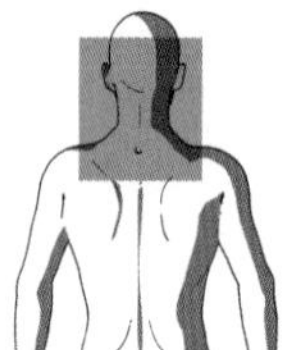

- **Trace the occipital nerves down through the underlying fat and connective tissue, clearing away the connective tissue using the "separating scissors technique" (Fig. 3.13).**

DISSECTION **TIP**

Even after the semispinalis capitis muscle is reflected, generally the boundaries or contents of the suboccipital triangle are not immediately apparent and are hidden by overlying connective tissue. Remove these tissues carefully (Figs. 3.14 and 3.15).

- **Place the tip of your finger into the suboccipital triangle to locate the posterior arch of the atlas.**
- **After removal of the connective tissue, identify the muscles that form the sides of the suboccipital triangle: inferior capitis oblique, superior capitis oblique, and rectus capitis posterior major (Fig. 3.16 and Plate 3.1).**

ANATOMY **NOTE**

The rectus capitis posterior major is found superficial to the rectus capitis posterior minor. Although the rectus capitis posterior minor is considered a "suboccipital" muscle, it does not contribute to the margins of the suboccipital triangle.

DISSECTION **TIP**

Use fine scissors and take your time to expose and clearly demonstrate the vertebral artery. Besides the connective tissue over the vertebral artery, a rich venous plexus is also present. Clean away the connective tissue and venous plexus. You will see only the posterior wall of the vertebral artery.

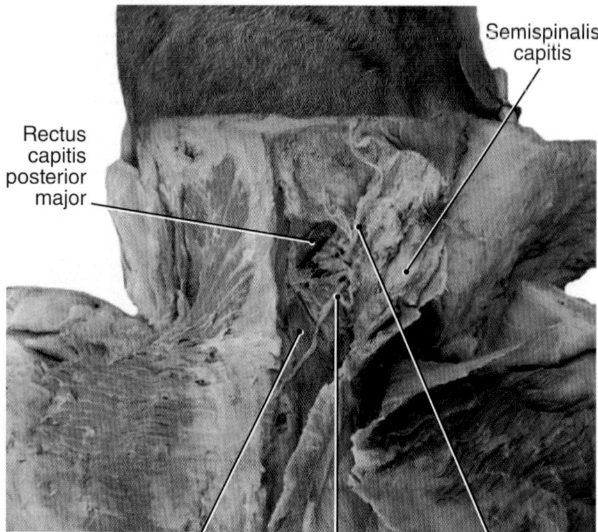

Fig. 3.14 Dissection of suboccipital triangle demonstrating the rectus capitis posterior major muscle and greater and third occipital nerves. Remove all fat and connective tissue.

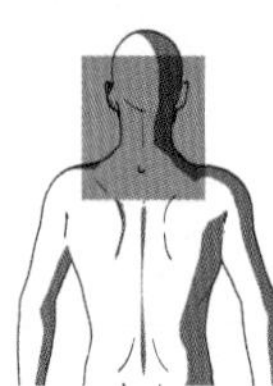

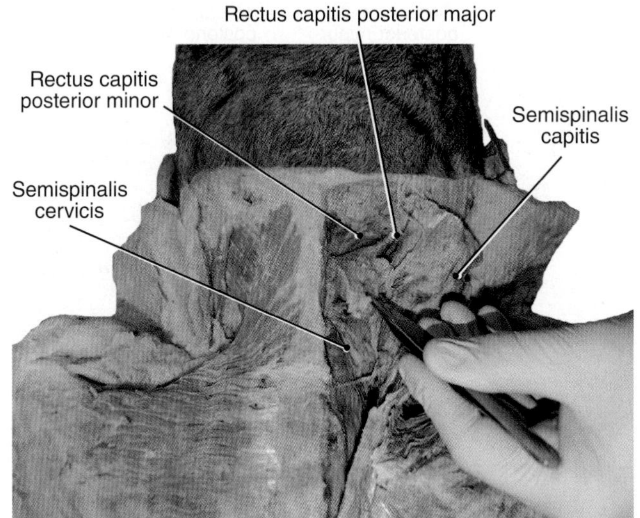

Fig. 3.15 Dissection of the suboccipital triangle revealing surrounding muscles, including the rectus capitis posterior major and minor and semispinalis capitis muscles.

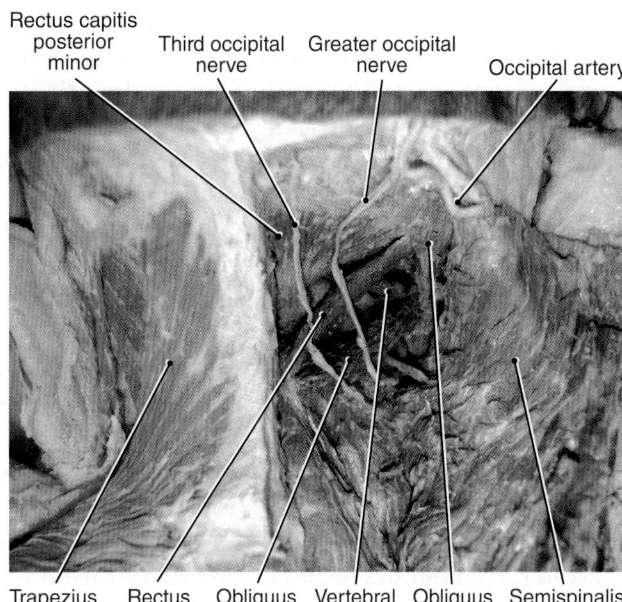

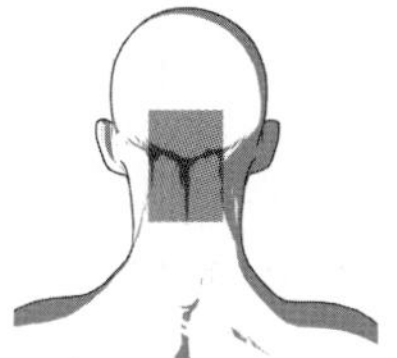

Fig. 3.16 Dissection of the suboccipital triangle highlighting its borders and contents.

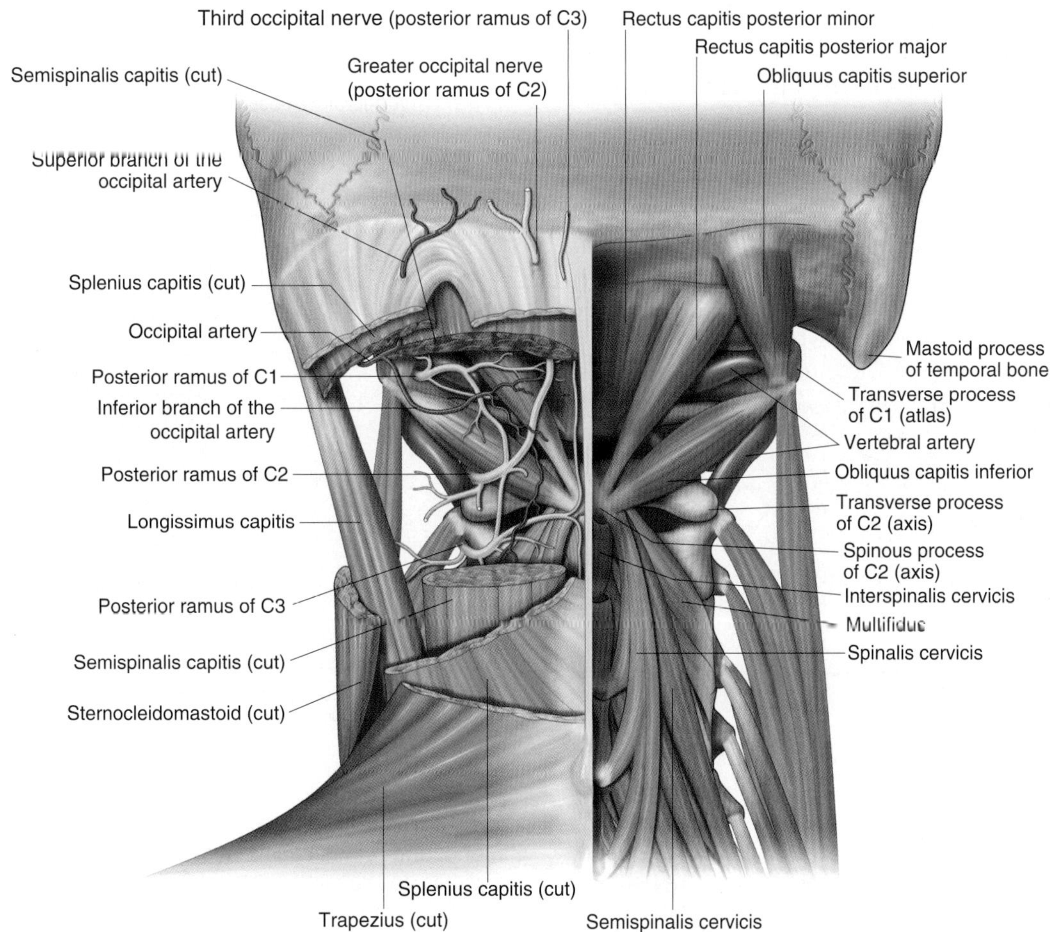

Plate 3.1 The suboccipital triangle and associated structures. (From Drake RL et al., *Gray's Atlas of Anatomy*, 3rd edition, Philadelphia, Elsevier, 2021, p. 43.)

- Expose the posterior arch of the atlas and identify a tough connective tissue layer joining the posterior arch of the atlas to the skull, the posterior atlanto-occipital membrane. Clean the loose connective tissue away from the arch and expose the vertebral artery, which lies in the sulcus of the posterior arch of the atlas. Between the sulcus of the posterior arch and the vertebral artery, identify the suboccipital nerve, which innervates the suboccipital muscles and overlying semispinalis capitis muscle (Fig. 3.17).
- Using a scalpel, cut the rectus capitis posterior major and inferior capitis oblique muscles from the spinous process of the axis and reflect them laterally (Fig. 3.18).
- Note the exit of the greater occipital nerve emerging from deeper tough connective tissue (Fig. 3.19).
- Remove this connective tissue surrounding the greater occipital nerve and expose its exit from the dura (Fig. 3.20).
- Retract the rectus capitis posterior minor superiorly and expose the spinal ganglion of the 2nd cervical (C2) spinal nerve (Fig. 3.21).

LAMINECTOMY

- In preparation for the laminectomy, reflect or cut away the muscles of the back from the spines and transverse processes of the vertebrae as completely as possible using a scalpel, scissors, and chisel (Fig. 3.22).
- Clean away as much as possible all of the intrinsic muscles of the back from the laminae of the lower

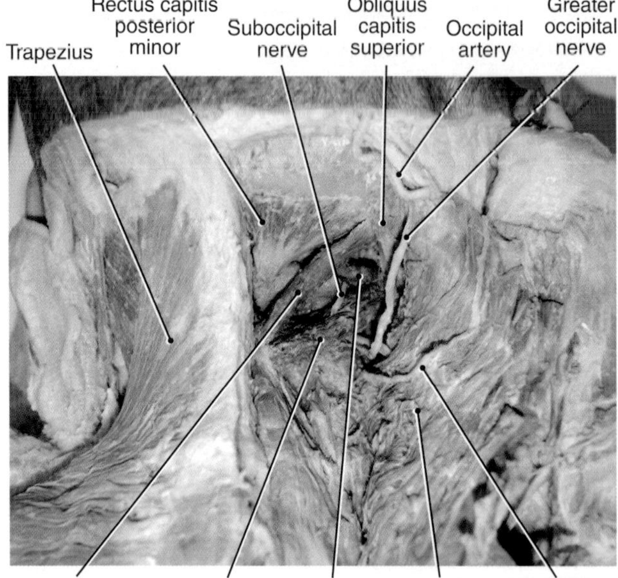

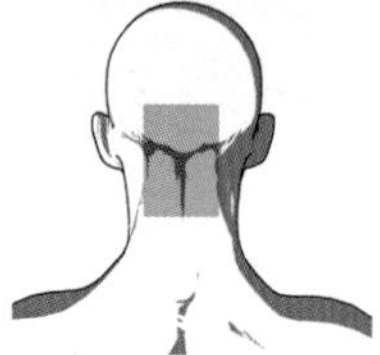

Fig. 3.17 Suboccipital triangle borders (rectus capitis posterior major, superior and inferior capitis oblique muscles) and contents (vertebral artery, suboccipital nerve).

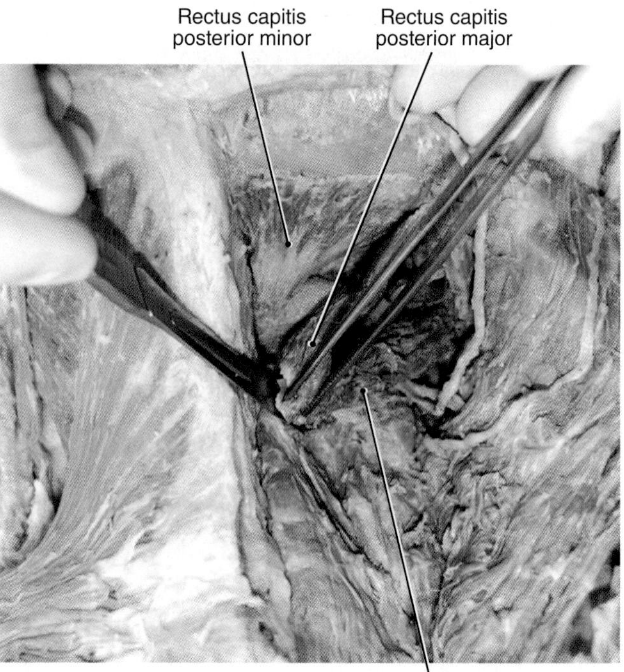

Fig. 3.18 Dissection of suboccipital triangle, reflecting rectus capitis posterior major and obliquus capitis inferior muscles laterally.

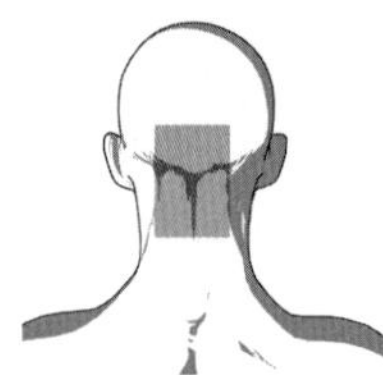

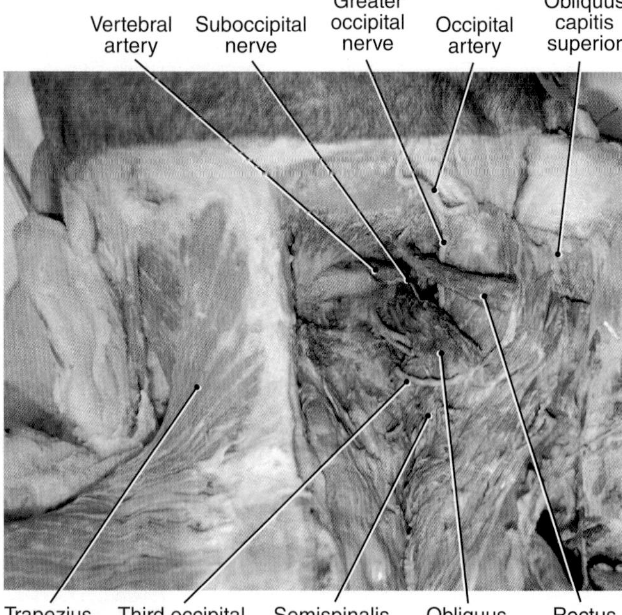

Fig. 3.19 Dissection of the suboccipital triangle illustrating the obliquus capitis inferior and rectus capitis posterior major muscles and revealing the suboccipital nerve and vertebral artery.

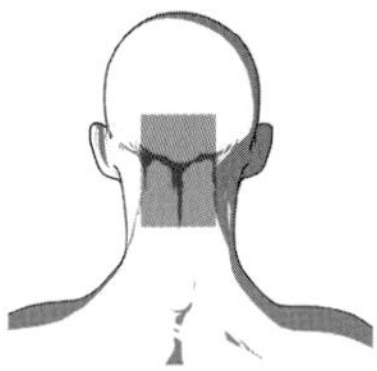

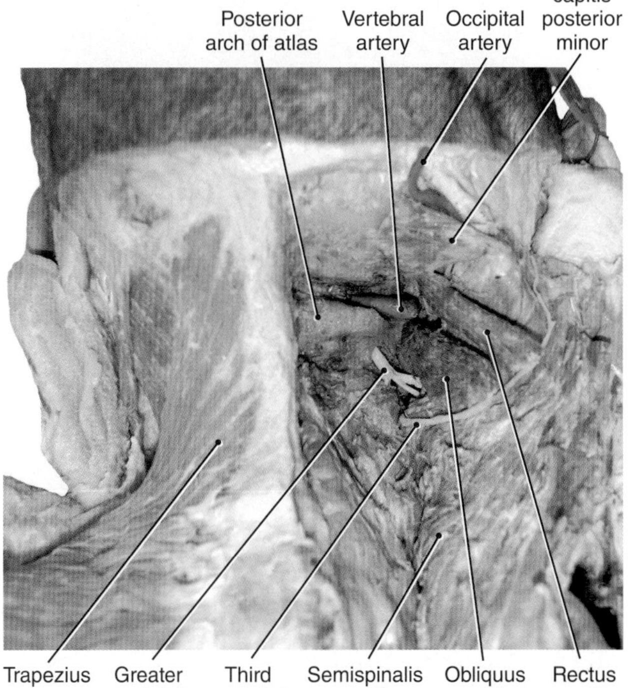

Fig. 3.20 Dissection of the suboccipital triangle, with reflected rectus capitis posterior minor exposing the posterior arch of atlas.

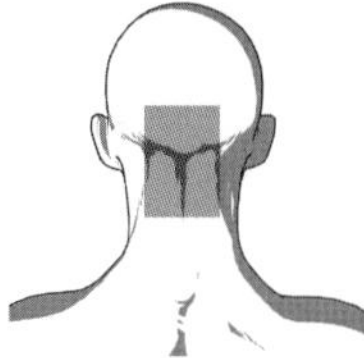

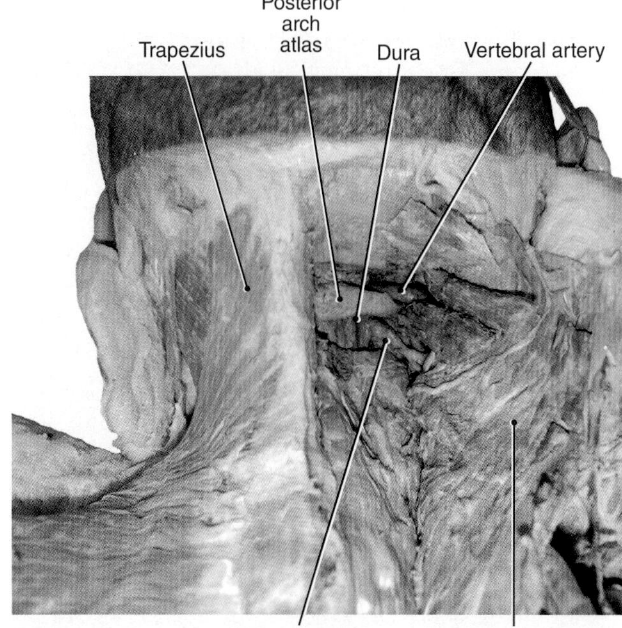

Fig. 3.21 Dissection of the suboccipital triangle exposing dura of spinal cord, spinal ganglion, vertebral artery, and posterior arch of the atlas.

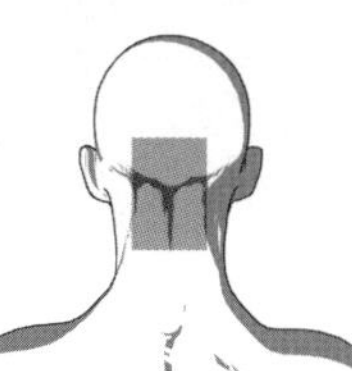

cervical, thoracic, and upper lumbar regions (Fig. 3.23).

- **With a bone saw or chisel and mallet, cut through the laminae longitudinally from the lower cervical to the lower lumbar regions (Figs. 3.24–3.26).**
- **Angle the saw or chisel laterally.**

DISSECTION **TIP**

If using a chisel and mallet, perform the surface fracturing technique. Short tapping blows of the mallet are used until the lamina is felt to fracture. Do not allow the chisel to be driven too deeply, or injury to the spinal cord or its rootlets will occur.

- **Direct the blade of the saw or chisel anteromedially to avoid cutting the spinal nerves (see Fig. 3.25 and Plate 3.2).**
- **Complete the dissection bilaterally (see Fig. 3.26).**
- **Using toothed forceps, gently lift the spinous process–lamina unit away from spinal canal, revealing dura, spinal ganglia, and spinal cord (Fig. 3.27).**
- **Remove the spinous process–lamina unit from the lumbar region, exposing dura (Fig. 3.28).**

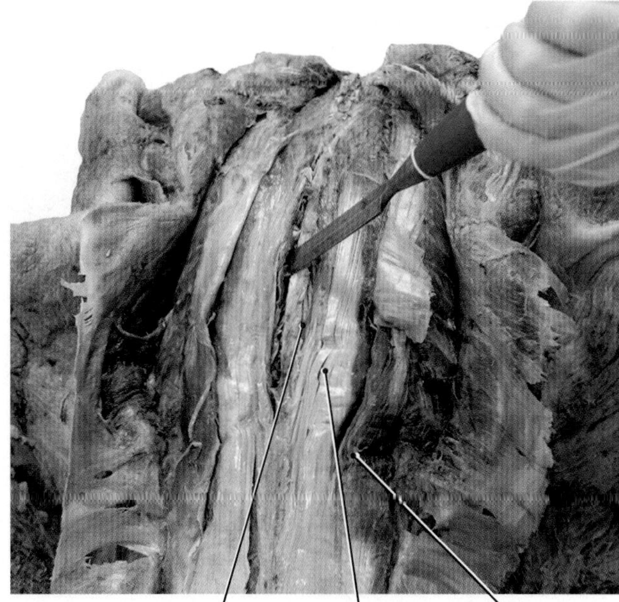

Fig. 3.22 Superficial and intermediate muscles of the back region reflected, revealing superficial layer of deep or native back muscles (erector spinae: spinalis, longissimus, iliocostalis).

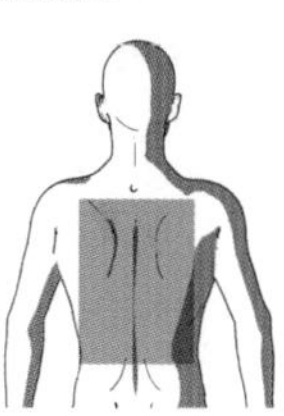

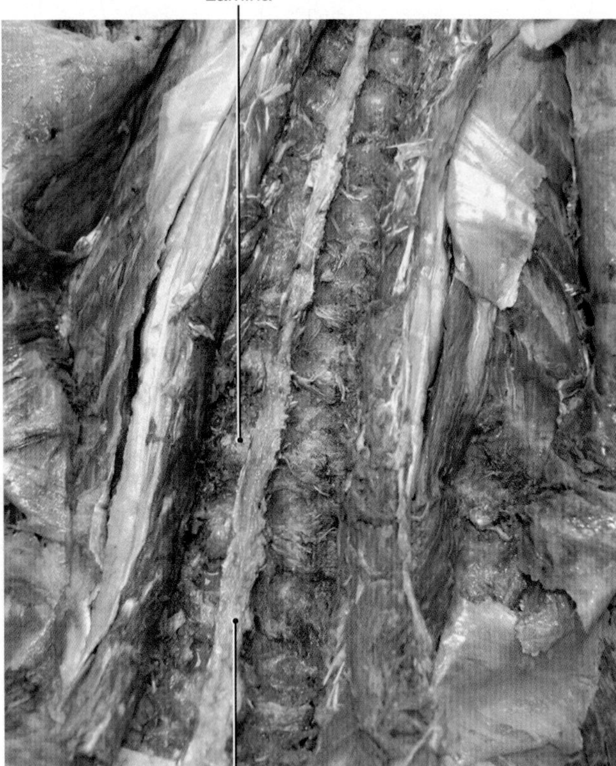

Fig. 3.23 After removal of all muscles from the paraspinous region, the spinous processes and laminae are seen.

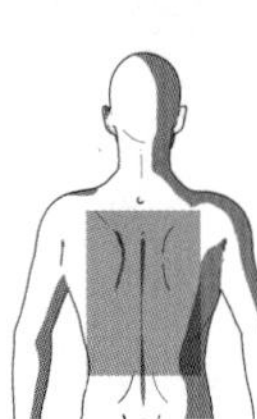

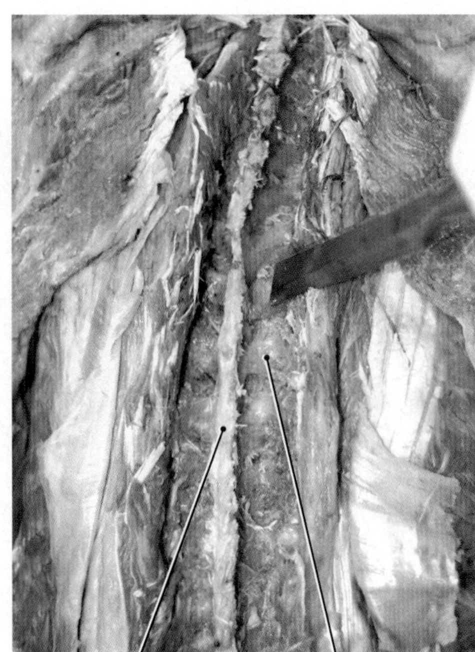

Fig. 3.24 The chisel is placed flat onto each lamina and angled away from the midline.

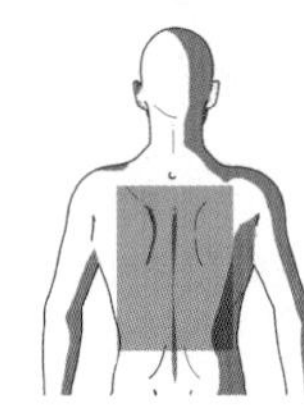

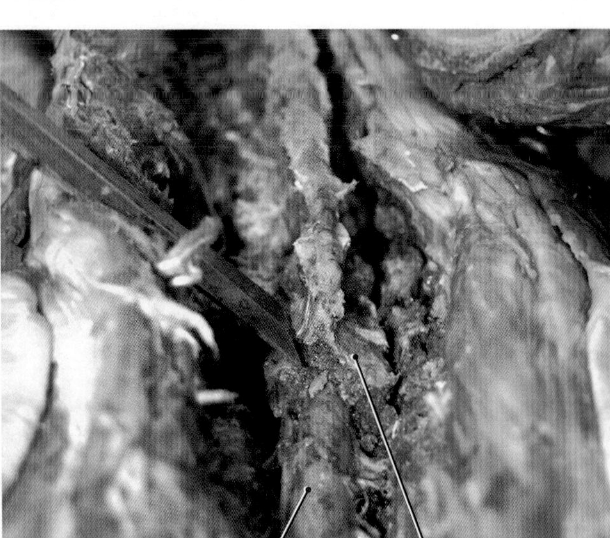

Fig. 3.25 Direct the blade of the saw or chisel anteromedially to avoid cutting the spinal nerves.

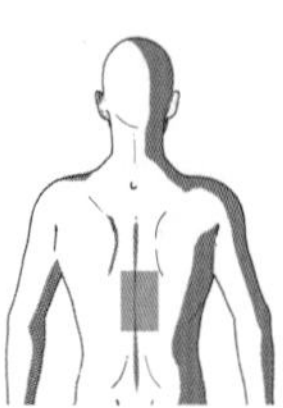

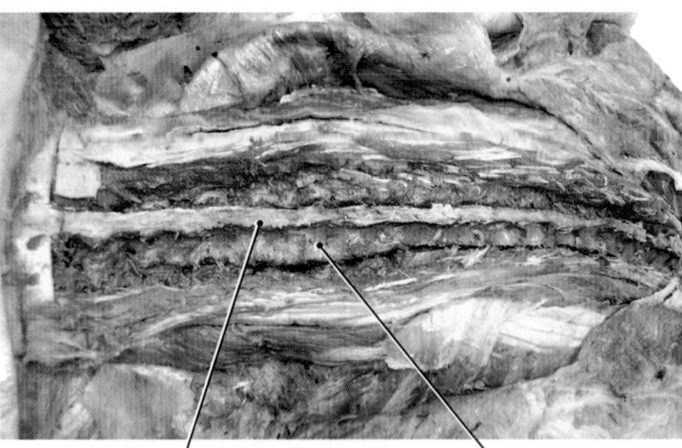

Fig. 3.26 Bilateral dissection through laminae of vertebrae using chisel and mallet technique to reveal dura and spinal cord (Stryker-type electric saw also can be used).

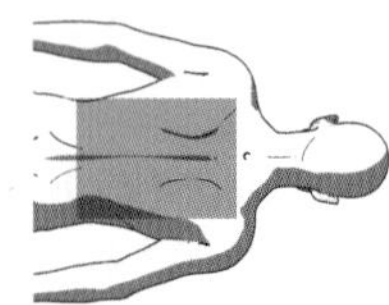

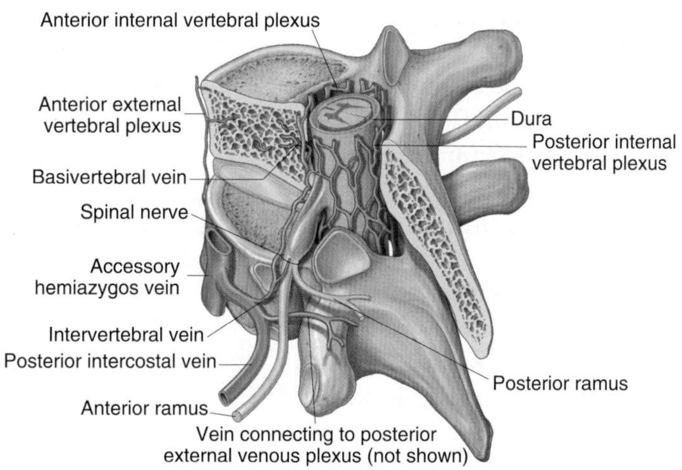

Plate 3.2 A lateral view of the hemisected vertebra exposing the spinal cord. (From Drake RL et al., *Gray's Atlas of Anatomy*, 3rd edition, Philadelphia, Elsevier, 2021, p. 47).

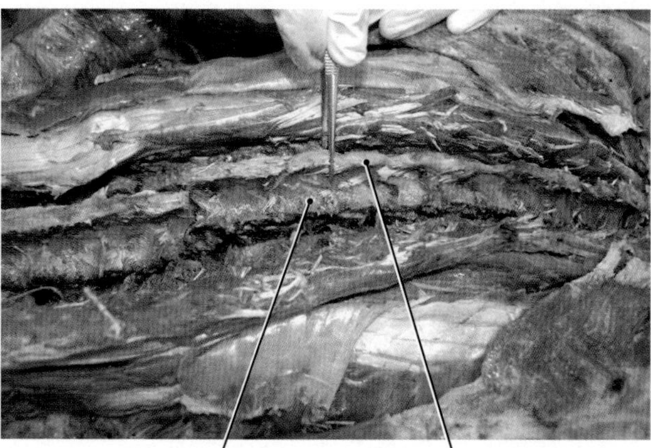

Fig. 3.27 Using toothed forceps, gently lift the spinous process–lamina unit away from spinal canal, revealing dura, spinal ganglia, and spinal cord.

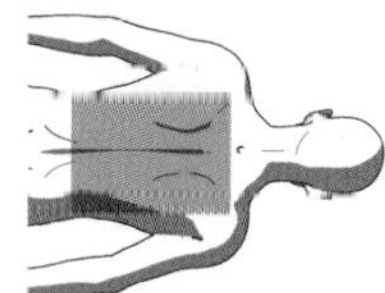

DISSECTION TIP

To facilitate the process, several laminae can be removed together as a block (see Figs. 3.26–3.28). After excision of the vertebral laminae and spinous processes, the vertebral canal may not be exposed widely enough for clear visualization of its contents. If this is the case, remove additional bone as necessary with bone rongeurs or with a mallet and chisel. Exercise particular care in the regions of the intervertebral foramina to avoid cutting or tearing away the spinal nerve rootlets. Sharply pointed edges of bone may be present in the dissection field after the laminectomy is completed. Identify any sharp spicules and remove them to avoid injuries to your hands.

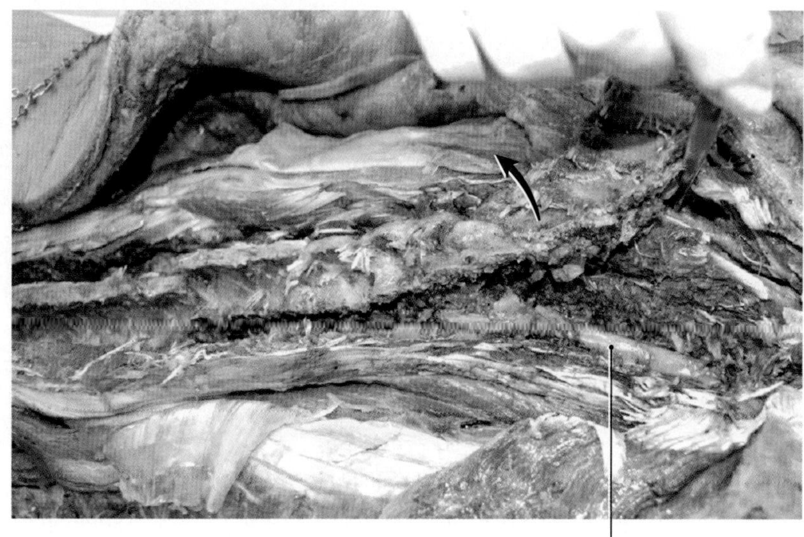

Fig. 3.28 Removal of the spinous process–lamina unit from the thoracolumbar region, exposing dura.

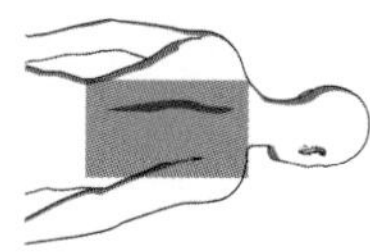

- Remove the spinous processes and the laminae en bloc from the spinal canal (Fig. 3.29).
- Note the contents of the spinal canal: the epidural fat and the vertebral venous plexus (of Batson) (Fig. 3.30).
- Remove the fat and the venous plexus from the epidural space to expose the dura. Lift a part of the dura in the midline and make a small, slit-like incision with scissors or a scalpel (Fig. 3.31).
- Continue the midline incision throughout the entire length of the dura (Fig. 3.32).
- If possible, avoid incising the underlying arachnoid layer by lifting and maintaining tension on the dura. Reflect the dura laterally to expose the contents of the dural sac. If the incision in the dura is made successfully, the arachnoid will appear as a thin, almost transparent layer (see Fig. 3.32).

DISSECTION TIP

Sometimes, arachnoid calcifications (plaques) may be present (Fig. 3.33). These are usually incidental findings and have been attributed to trauma, myelography, subarachnoid hemorrhage (see Fig. 3.32), and spinal anesthesia.

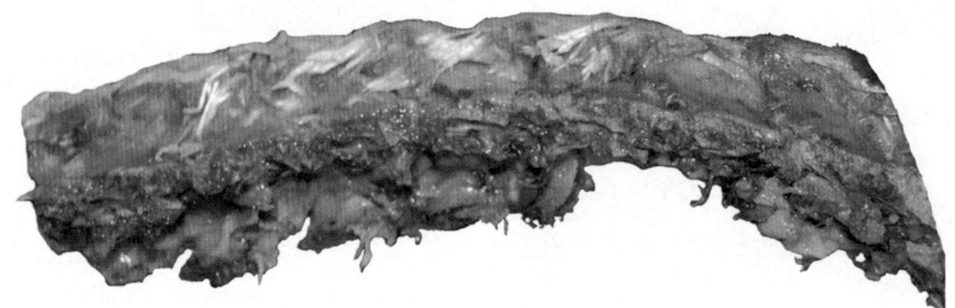

Fig. 3.29 Section of the spinous process–lamina unit removed from the vertebral column.

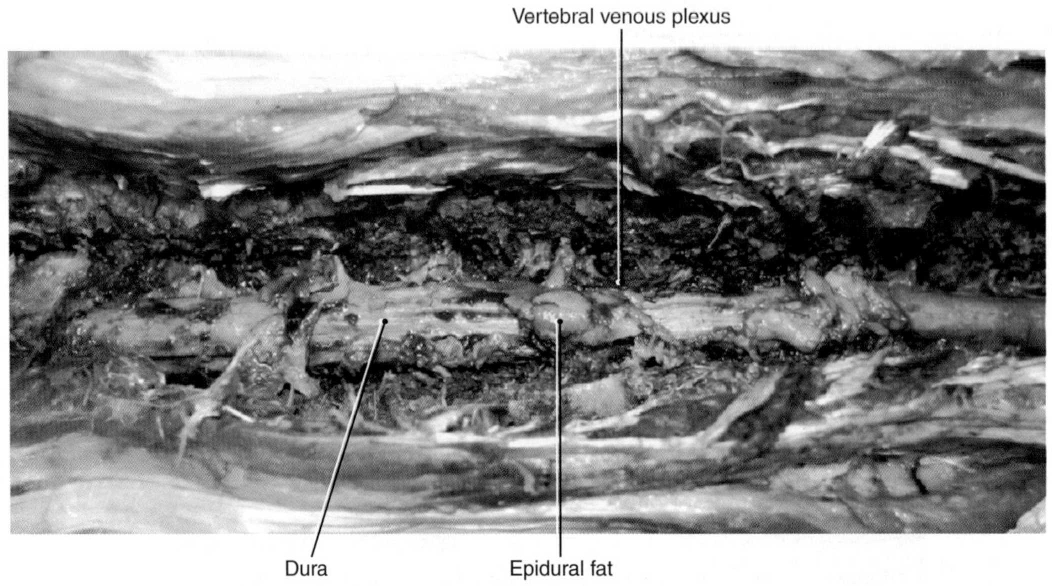

Fig. 3.30 Spinous process–lamina unit removed to expose epidural fat, dura, and vertebral venous plexus.

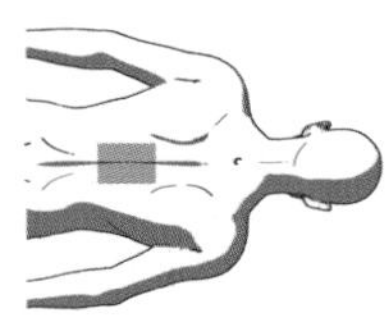

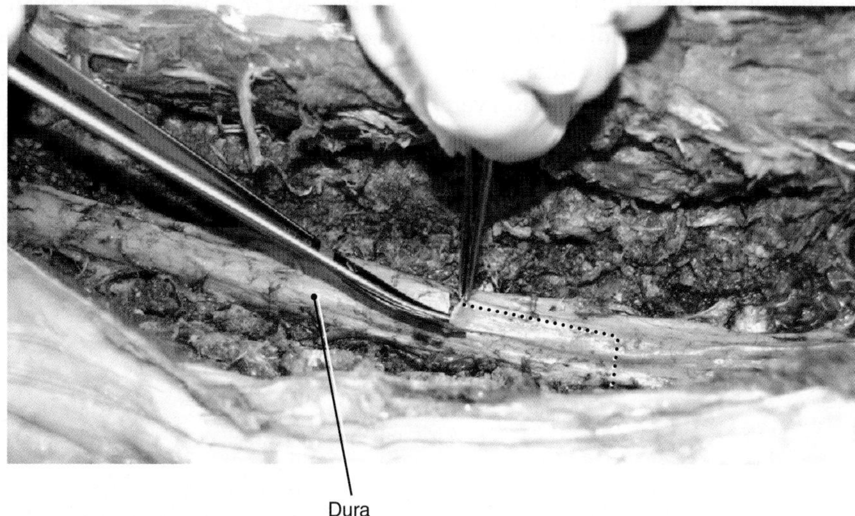

Fig. 3.31 Spinous process–lamina unit removed from the lumbar region, revealing dura covering spinal cord and cauda equina. Elevate the dura while making the transverse cut.

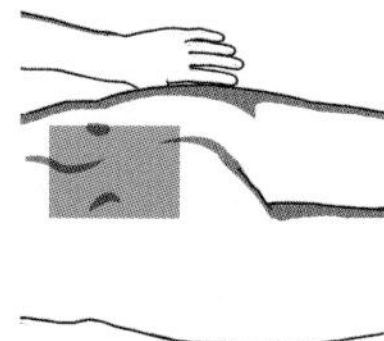

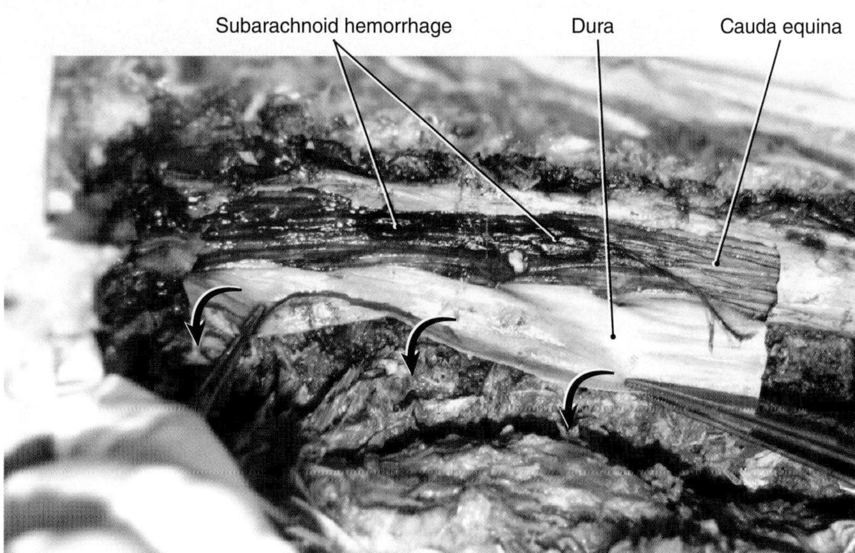

Fig. 3.32 Transverse and vertical incisions reflecting dura, revealing cauda equina and subarachnoid hemorrhage.

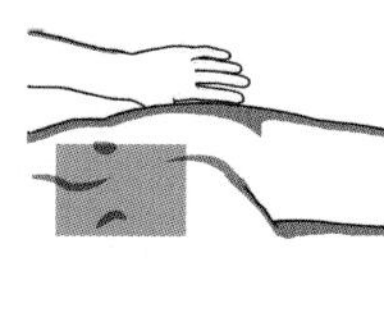

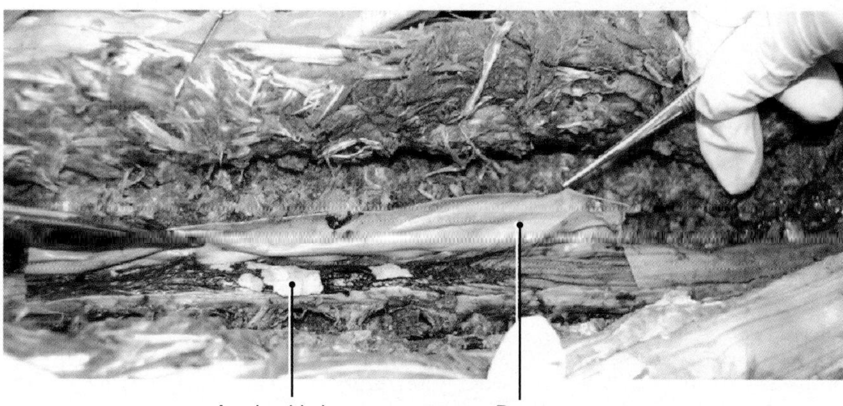

Fig. 3.33 Transverse and vertical incisions reflecting dura, revealing arachnoid plaque overlying the cauda equina.

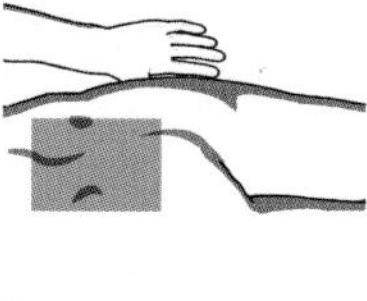

- Identify the spinal cord and its covering of pia. Observe the beginning of the filum terminale at its origin from the conus medullaris, the terminal part of the spinal cord. Note the cluster of nerve roots on either side of the conus medullaris, the *cauda equina* (Fig. 3.34; see also Figs. 3.31, 3.32, and 3.38).
- Transect and remove the spinal cord with its dural covering (Fig. 3.35).
- Look for the tooth-like denticulate ligaments on each side of the spinal cord, lifting the cord carefully with forceps for inspection. These projections occur from the occipital bone to the last thoracic spinal nerve. The denticulate ligaments pierce the arachnoid to attach to the dura (Figs. 3.36 and 3.37).
- Identify the posterior longitudinal ligament on the vertebral bodies after the removal of the spinal cord and dura (Fig. 3.38).

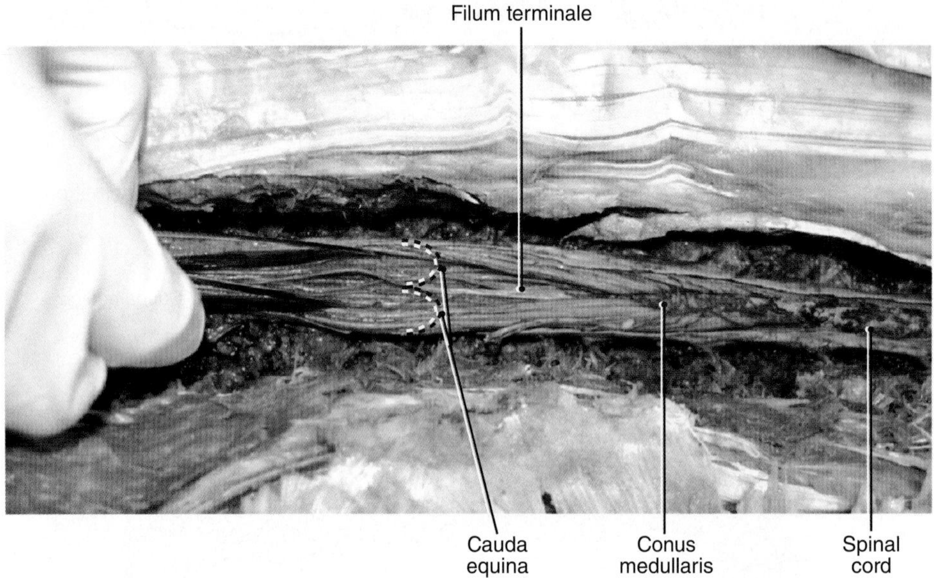

Fig. 3.34 Dura reflected to reveal the spinal cord, conus medullaris, filum terminale, and cauda equina.

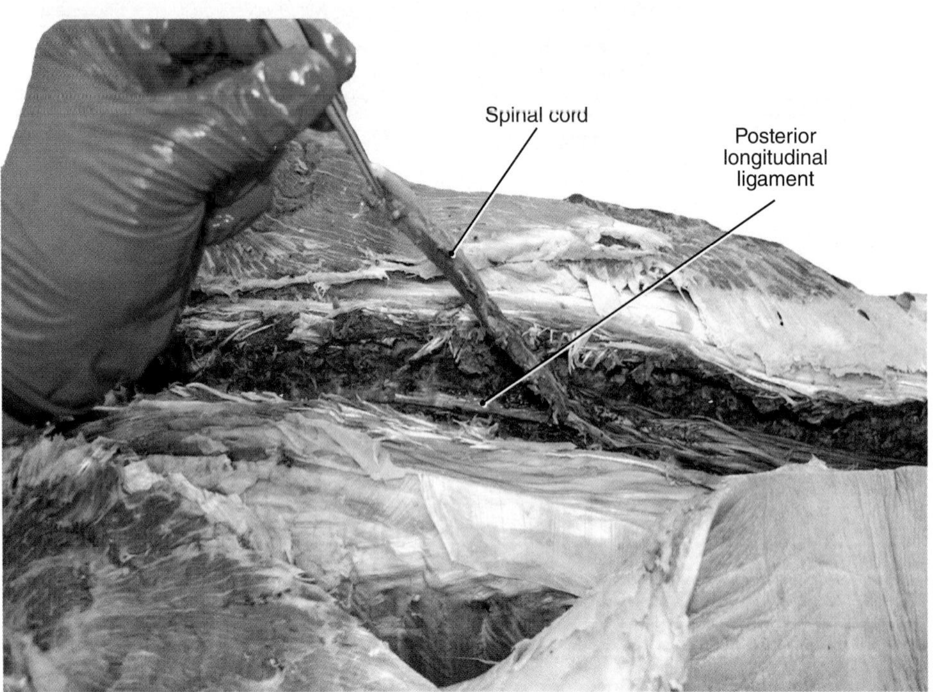

Fig. 3.35 Reflecting the spinal cord from cephalad to caudal to reveal the posterior longitudinal ligament.

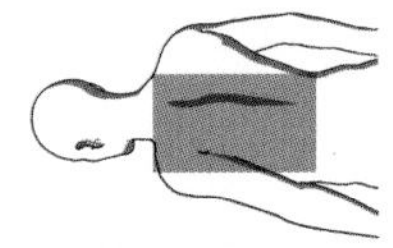

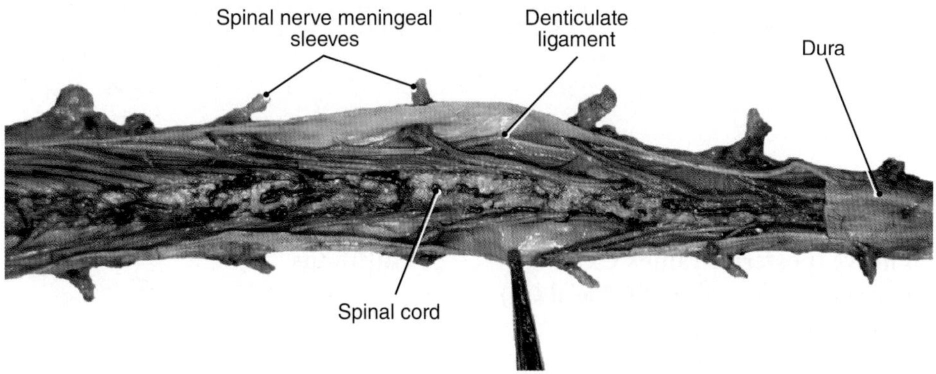

Fig. 3.36 Transverse and vertical incisions reflecting dura, revealing spinal cord, denticulate ligament, and spinal nerve dural sleeves.

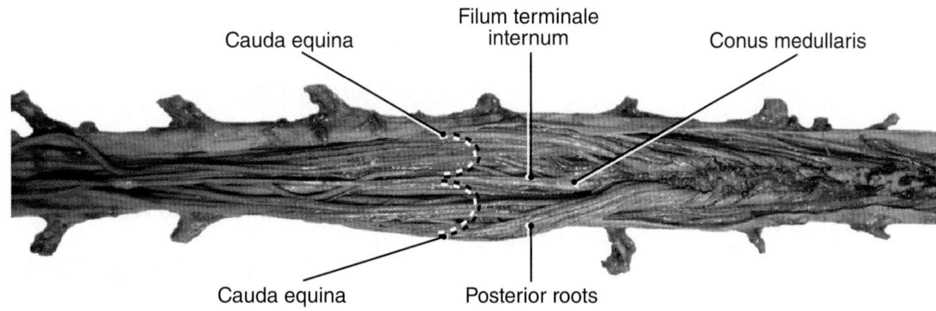

Fig. 3.37 Transverse and vertical incisions reflecting dura, revealing the conus medullaris, posterior roots, and filum terminale.

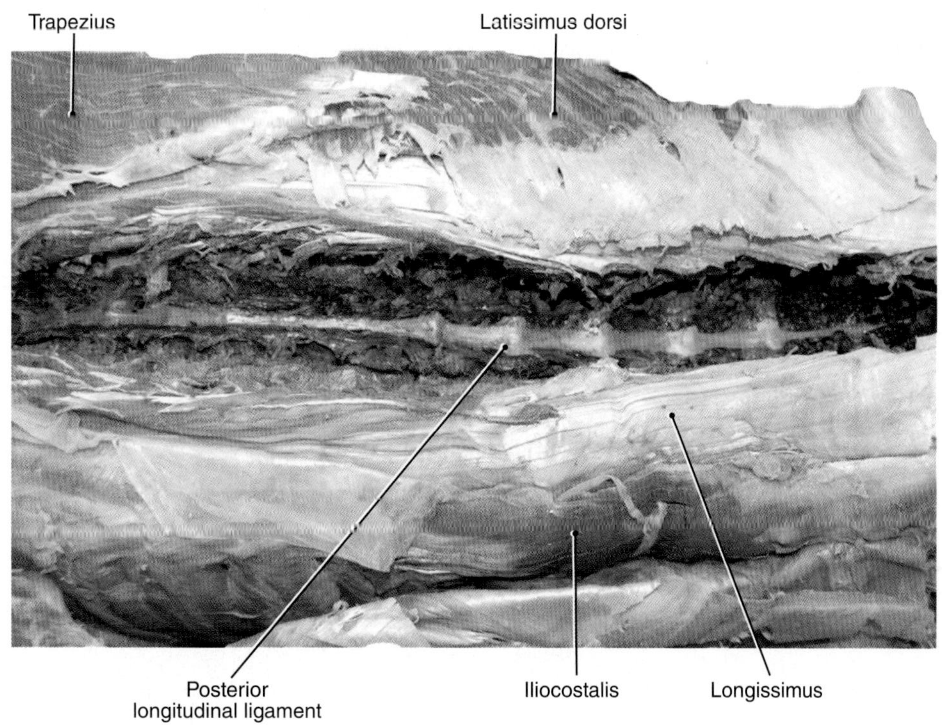

Fig. 3.38 Spinal cord and dura removed, revealing the posterior longitudinal ligament.

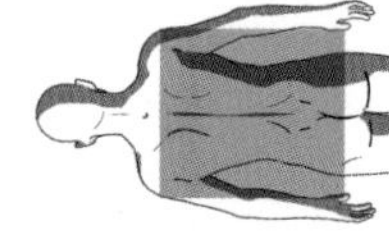

LABORATORY IDENTIFICATION CHECKLIST

NERVES

- ☐ Greater occipital nerve (posterior ramus C2)
- ☐ Lesser occipital nerve (anterior rami of C2 and C3)
- ☐ Third occipital nerve (posterior ramus C3)
- ☐ Suboccipital nerve (posterior ramus C1)
- ☐ Spinal ganglion
- ☐ Spinal nerve

ARTERIES

- ☐ Occipital artery
- ☐ Vertebral artery

VEIN

- ☐ Vertebral venous plexus (of Batson)

MUSCLES

- ☐ Trapezius
- ☐ Splenius capitis
- ☐ Semispinalis capitis
- ☐ Sternocleidomastoid
- ☐ Rectus capitis posterior major
- ☐ Rectus capitis posterior minor
- ☐ Obliquus capitis superior
- ☐ Obliquus capitis inferior
- ☐ Semispinalis capitis
- ☐ Spinalis
- ☐ Longissimus
- ☐ Iliocostalis
- ☐ Multifidus

BONES

- ☐ Atlas
  - ☐ Posterior arch
- ☐ Spinous processes
- ☐ Lamina(e)
- ☐ Transverse processes
- ☐ Body
- ☐ Vertebral foramen(foramina)

LIGAMENTS

- ☐ Nuchal ligament (ligamentum nuchae)
- ☐ Ligamentum flavum
- ☐ Posterior longitudinal ligament

SPINAL CORD AND MENINGES

- ☐ Dura
- ☐ Arachnoid
- ☐ Pia
- ☐ Denticulate ligaments
- ☐ Filum terminale (internum)
- ☐ Conus medullaris
- ☐ Cauda equina
- ☐ Spinal nerve meningeal sleeve

CLINICAL APPLICATIONS

LUMBAR PUNCTURE

Clinical Application

A lumbar puncture uses a spinal needle to access the subarachnoid space between the 2nd and 4th lumbar vertebrae (L2 and L4) to withdraw cerebrospinal fluid for analysis (Fig. II.1).

Anatomical Landmarks

- **Below the level of L2 vertebra, feel the spinous processes and the space between the processes (Fig. II.2).**
- **The imaginary transverse plane that originates at the iliac crest and crosses the L4/L5 junction is known as the supracristal plane. Puncture is safe just superior or inferior to this plane, which avoids the spinal cord.**
- **Superficial to deep:**
  Skin
  Subcutaneous tissue
  Supraspinous ligament
  Interspinous ligament
  Ligamentum flavum (provides increased resistance to needle)
  Dura
  Subarachnoid space–cerebrospinal fluid

EXTRADURAL ANESTHESIA (CAUDAL OR SACRAL BLOCK)

Clinical Application

Introduce anesthetic solutions into the epidural space, which will anesthetize the spinal nerves exiting the dura.

Anatomical Landmarks (Figs. II.4 and II.5)

- **Natal cleft**
- **Sacral horn**
- **Superficial to deep:**
  Skin
  Subcutaneous tissue
  Posterior sacrococcygeal ligament (increased resistance)
  Sacral canal
- **Sacralization is the variant fusion of the 5th lumbar vertebra (L5) to the 1st sacral vertebra (S1) (Fig. II.3).**

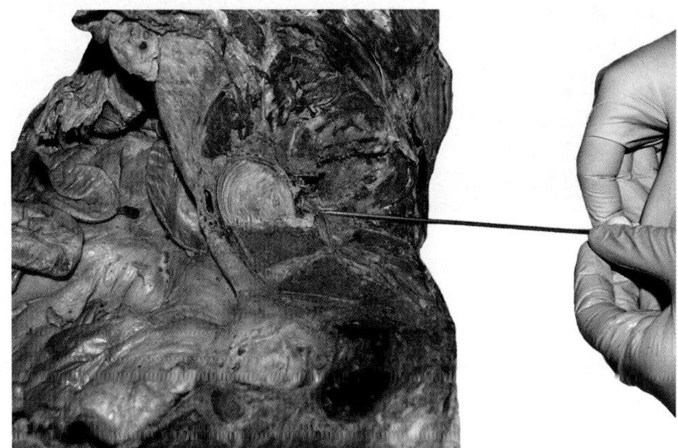

Fig. II.2

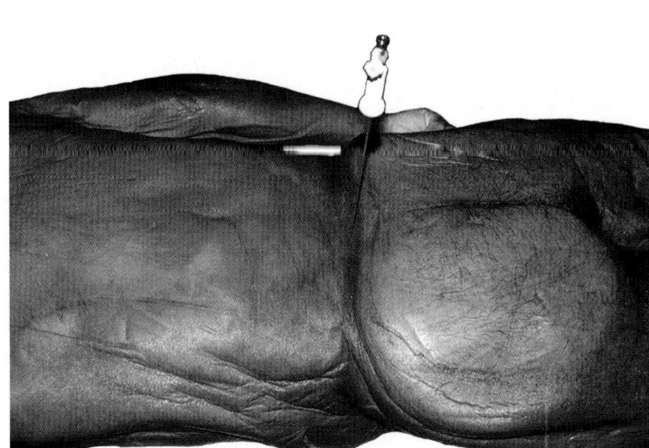

Fig. II.1

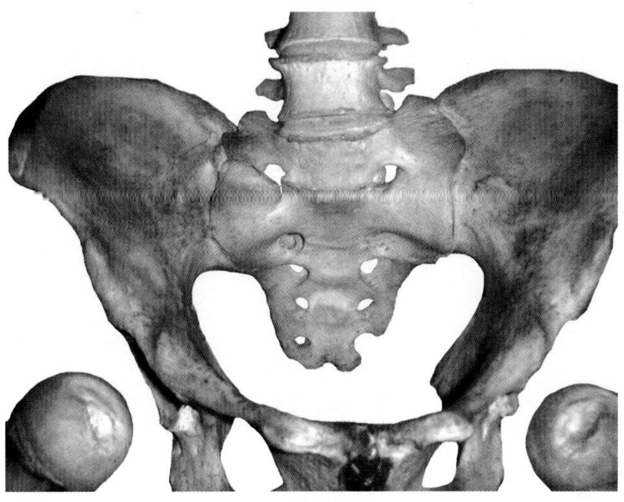

Fig. II.3

TRIANGLE OF AUSCULTATION

Clinical Application

The triangle of auscultation defines an area that allows better auscultation with a stethoscope (because of less overlying muscle mass), to maximize listening to the lungs, 6th intercostal space, and the gastroesophageal junction on the left and thus assessing the potential pathology.

Anatomical Landmarks

- **Medial border of scapula**
- **Lateral border of trapezius**
- **Superior border of latissimus dorsi**

Note: Area of triangle increases when arms are crossed and trunk is flexed.

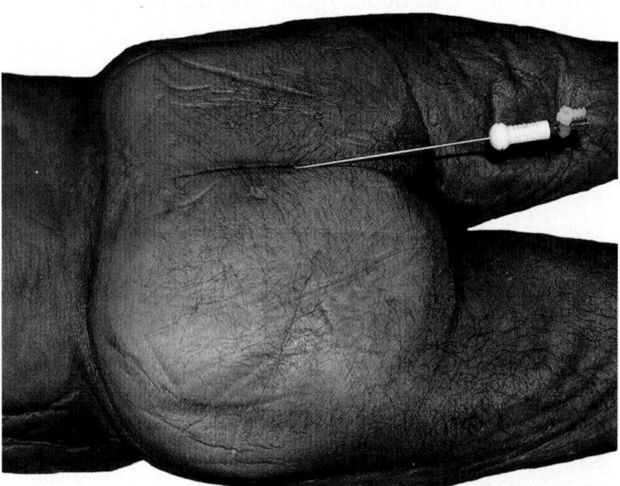

Fig. II.4

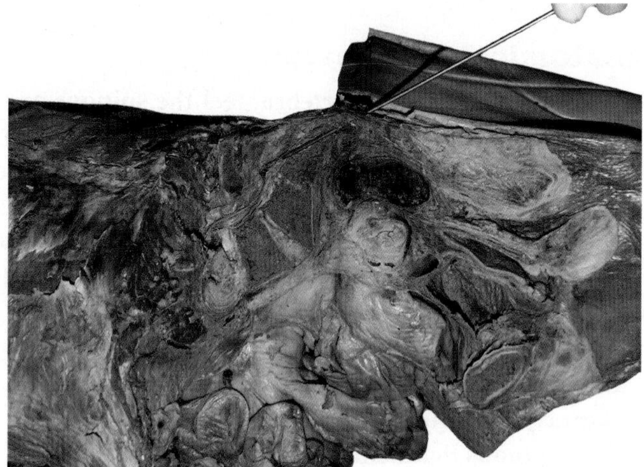

Fig. II.5

SECTION III

THORAX

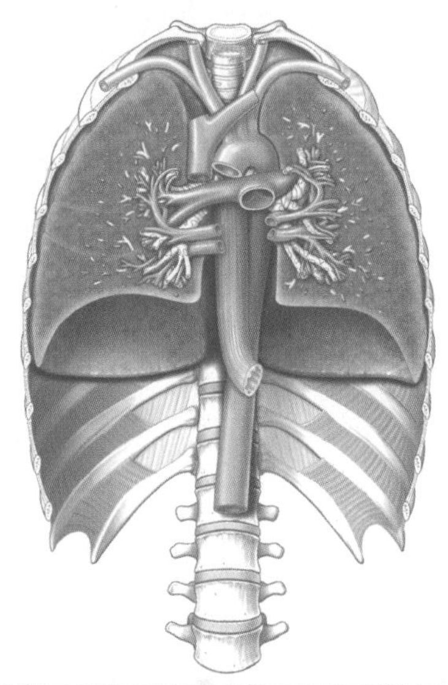

CHAPTER 4 PECTORAL REGION AND FEMALE BREAST

SKIN AND SUPERFICIAL FASCIA

- **Make an incision from the jugular notch of the sternum over the clavicle to the shoulder (Fig. 4.1a).**
- **Make a midline incision from the jugular notch of the sternum to the xiphoid process (Fig. 4.1b).**
- **Extend the incision across the border of the costal margin toward the midaxillary line (Fig. 4.1c).**
- **Continue the incision from the shoulder distally to the proximal one-third of the arm. An encircling incision around the midportion of the arm permits removal of the skin from the proximal arm (Fig. 4.1d).**
- **Start the dissection at the junction of the jugular notch of sternum and the clavicle. Reflect the skin of the anterior thoracic wall, medial to lateral using combined blunt and sharp dissection (Fig. 4.2).**

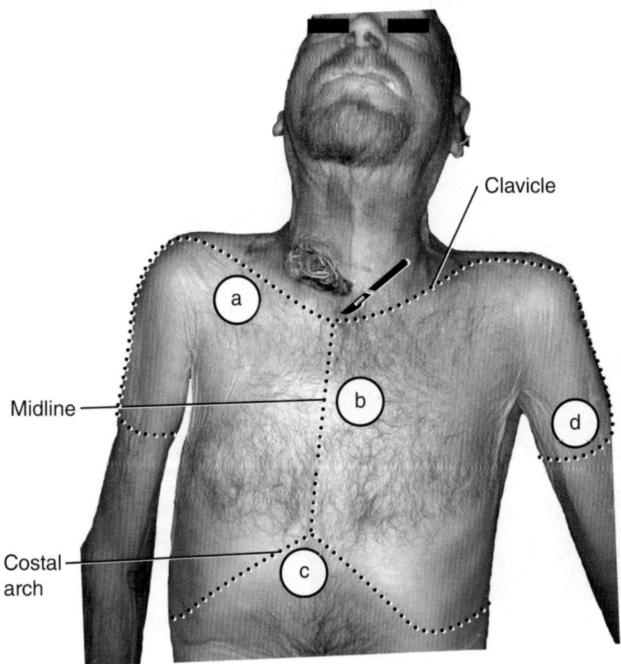

Fig. 4.1 Skin tracing of anterior thoracic wall for superficial dissection incisions. *a,* Clavicle; *b,* midline; *c,* xiphoid process; *d,* proximal arm.

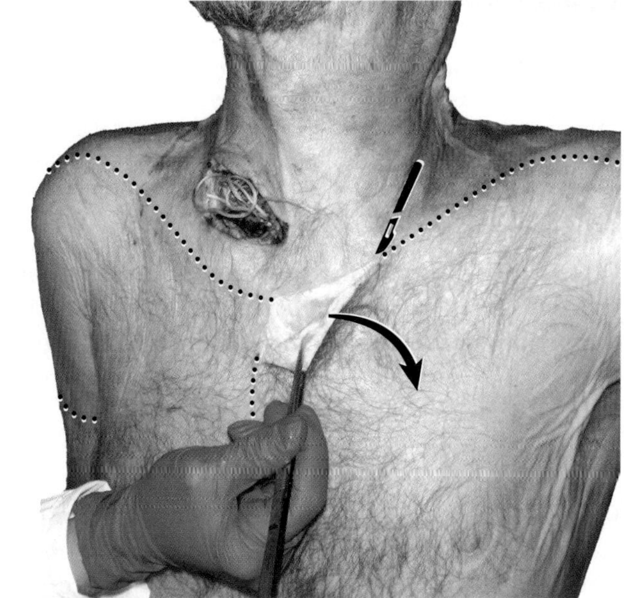

Fig. 4.2 Skin reflection of anterior thoracic wall.

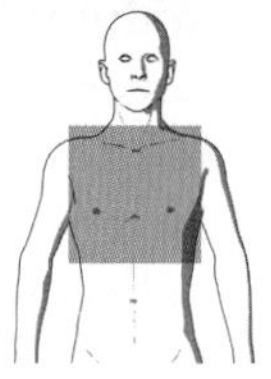

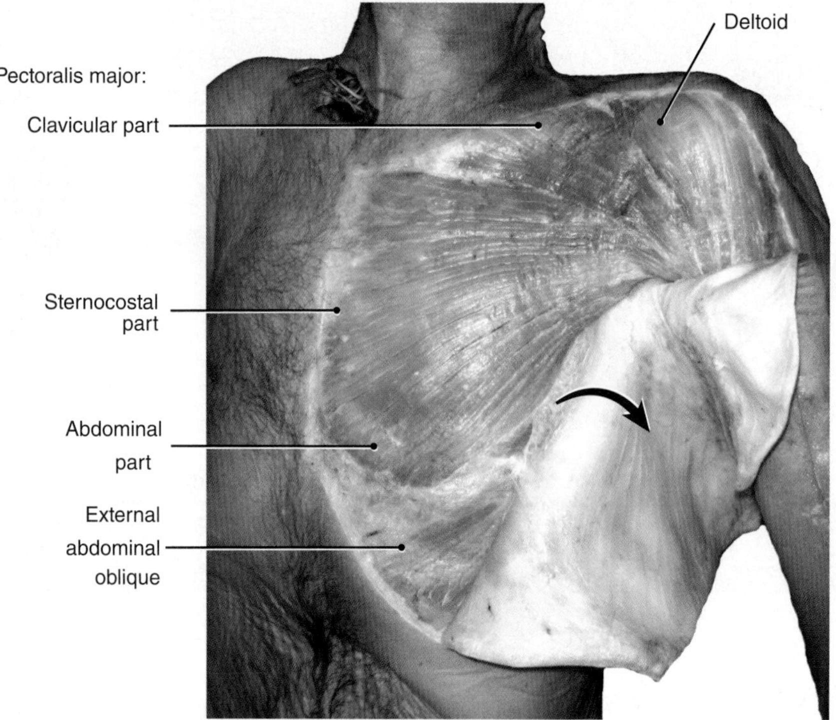

Fig. 4.3 Skin reflection of anterior thoracic wall, exposing the deltopectoral triangle, serratus anterior, and external abdominal oblique muscles.

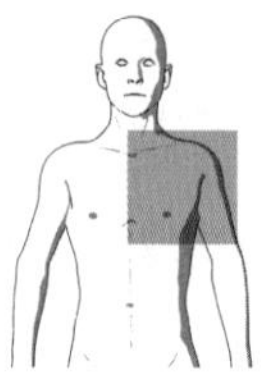

DISSECTION TIP

As the superficial fascia and skin are retracted, you will encounter anterior cutaneous branches of primary rami and vessels emerging near the sternum. The vessels are the perforating branches of the internal thoracic artery and the perforating tributaries to the internal thoracic vein. Cut through these cutaneous nerves and vessels.

- **Reflect the skin and remove the superficial fascia from the thorax, shoulders, axillae, and proximal portions of the arms medially to the axilla (Figs. 4.3 and 4.4). Continue to use combined blunt and sharp dissection.**

FEMALES

- **In addition to the aforementioned incisions described in the reflection of the skin, make an oblique incision through the skin of the breast from the midpoint of the clavicle toward the anterior axillary line, encircling the areola (Fig. 4.5).**
- **Lift the skin at the edge of the incision with your forceps and reflect laterally to the axilla.**
- **Reflect the adipose tissue from the pectoralis major with a scalpel (Figs. 4.6 and 4.7).**

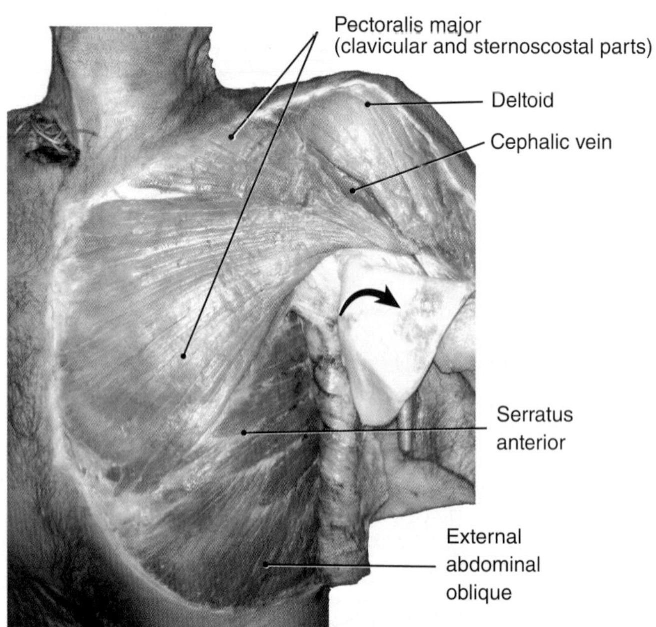

Fig. 4.4 Skin reflection of anterior thoracic wall, medial to lateral.

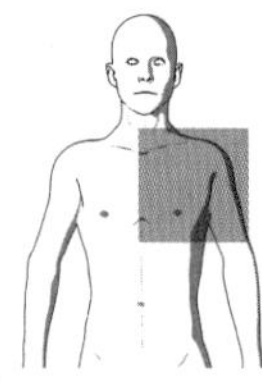

ANATOMY **NOTE**

Note the retinacula cutis, which begins at the dermis and extends deeply into the breast, forming fibrous septae and irregular bands of dense connective tissue.

- **Cut through the middle of the areola, making a sagittal incision through the nipple-areolar complex, and identify the glandular tissue, ducts, connective tissue, and fat of the breast (Fig. 4.8). Partially remove the breast (Fig. 4.9). Try to identify one or more lactiferous ducts (Fig. 4.10).**

ANATOMY **NOTE**

The lactiferous ducts may possess an expanded part (the lactiferous sinus or ampulla) deep to the nipple. The ducts become very narrow as they pass through the nipple, each terminating separately on its surface. In most aged cadavers, little will remain of the duct system or glandular tissue, being replaced with fibrous tissue infiltrated with adipose tissue.

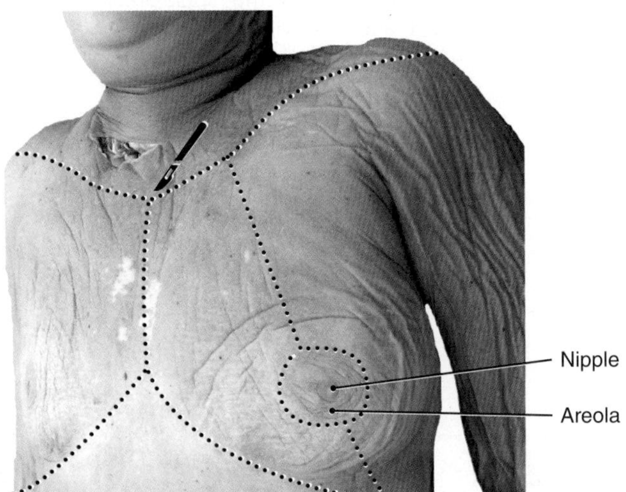

Fig. 4.5 Skin of female breast with nipple-areolar complex.

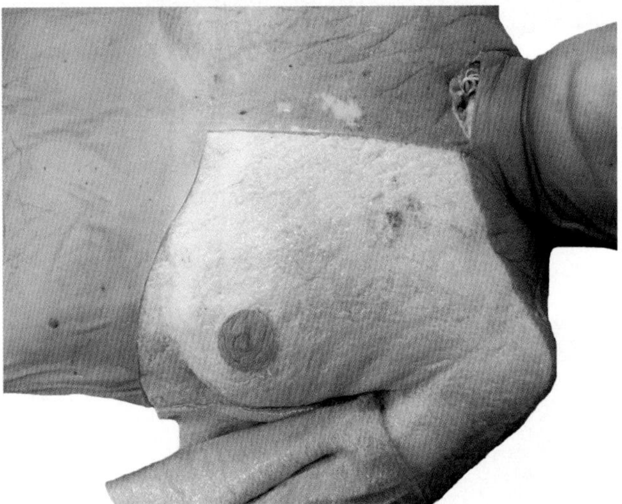

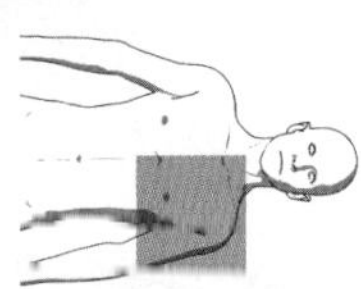

Fig. 4.6 Skin reflection from the anterior thoracic wall (same technique as Fig. 4.2), revealing superficial fascia and nipple-areolar complex.

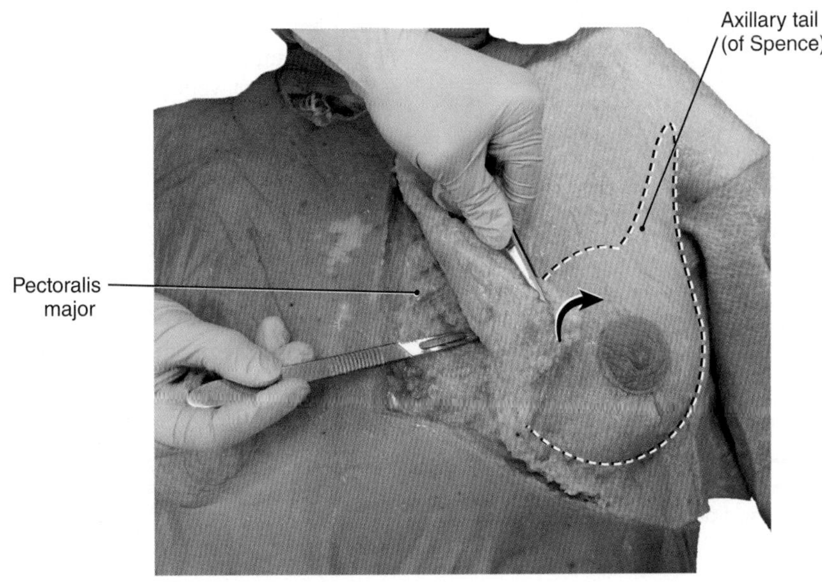

Fig. 4.7 Reflecting the left breast, deep to superficial fascia.

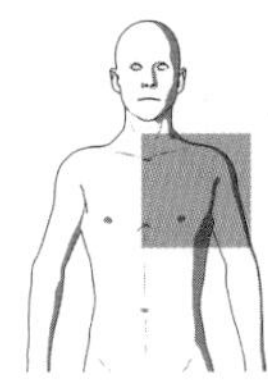

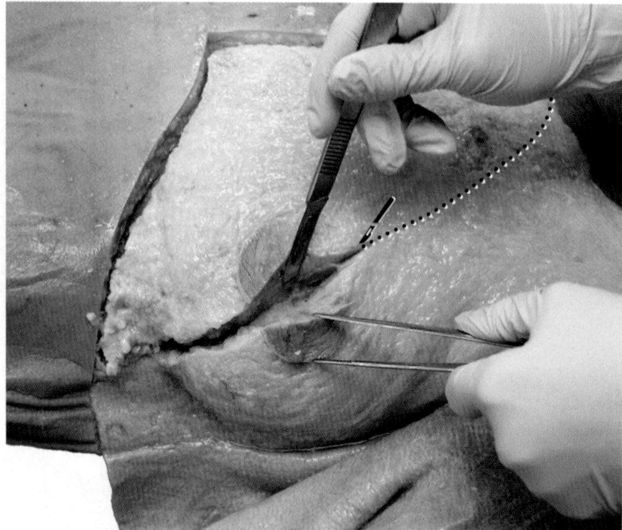

Fig. 4.8 Sagittal incision through the nipple-areolar complex, revealing glandular tissue, ducts, connective tissue, and fat of breast.

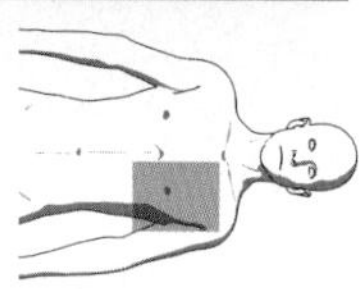

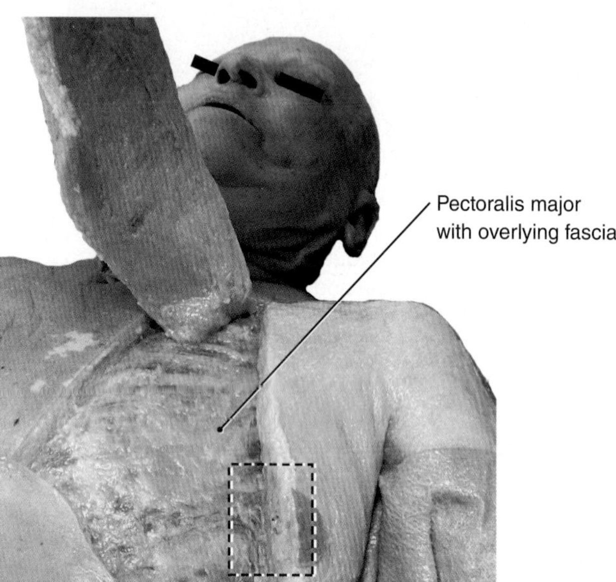

Fig. 4.9 Partial removal of left breast, revealing pectoralis major and fascia lying deep to breast.

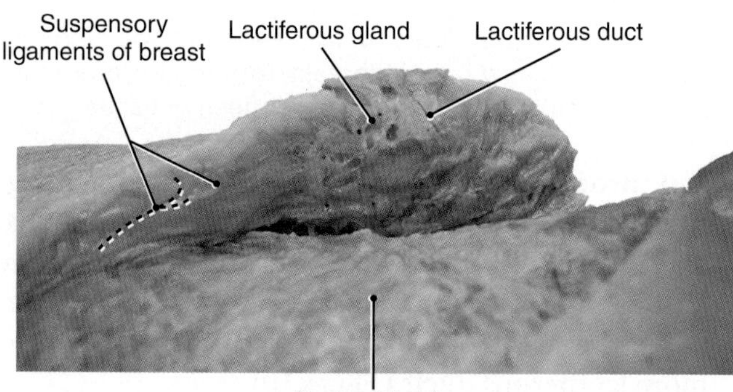

Fig. 4.10 Sagittal incision through the nipple-areolar complex, revealing gland, duct, and suspensory ligaments of breast (see *dashed square* in Fig. 4.9).

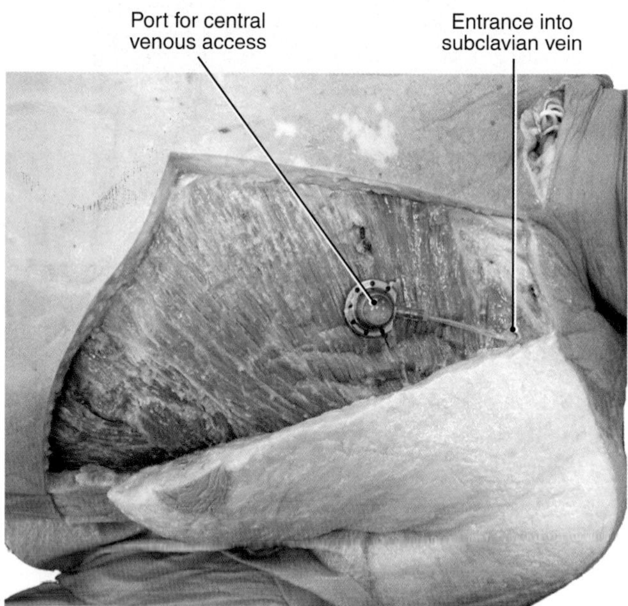

Fig. 4.11 Left pectoralis major with overlying central venous port.

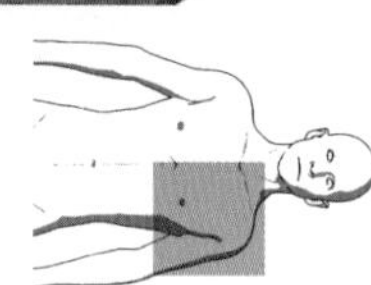

DISSECTION TIP

Sometimes it is possible to identify an injection reservoir under the subcutaneous tissue (Fig. 4.11). These allow direct access to a large vein without having to "stick" the vein each time and are used for long-term injections such as for chemotherapy.

SUPERFICIAL DISSECTION

- **Identify the pectoralis major muscle, which is invested in a thin tough fascia, the pectoral fascia (part of the deep fascia system) (Fig. 4.12).**
- **After cleaning the fascia from the pectoralis major, notice the separation of the pectoralis major from the deltoid muscle by the deltopectoral triangle (see Fig. 4.12).**

ANATOMY NOTE

The clavicle, the clavicular head of the pectoralis major muscle, and the deltoid muscle form this triangle. Within the deltopectoral triangle, the cephalic vein is found.

- **Dividing the fascia that lies superficial to it will expose the cephalic vein. The cephalic vein is an important landmark for identifying the first part of the axillary artery (see Fig. 4.12).**

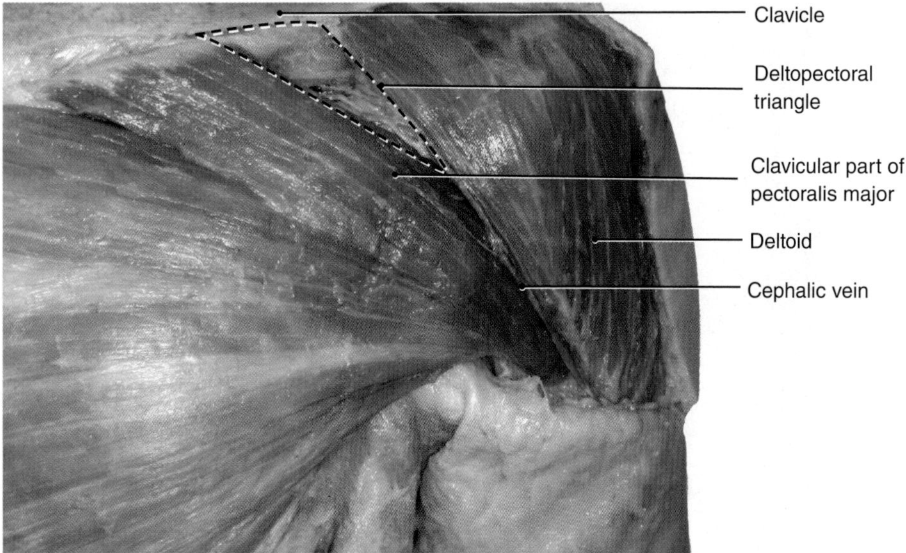

Fig. 4.12 Skin reflected from left anterolateral thoracic wall, revealing deltopectoral muscles, deltopectoral triangle, and cephalic vein.

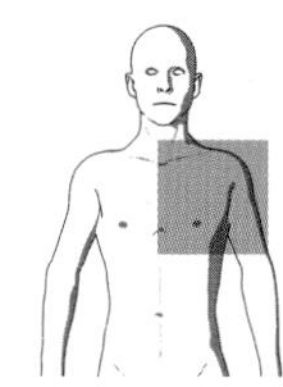

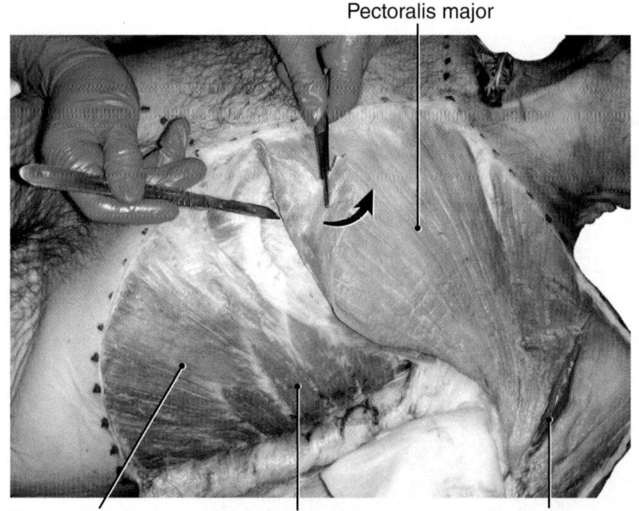

Fig. 4.13 Left pectoralis major muscle reflected from anterior thoracic wall.

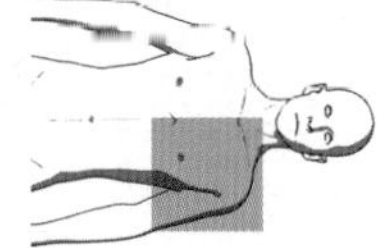

- **Detach the clavicular and sternocostal parts and abdominal part of the pectoralis major with a scalpel and reflect the muscle laterally to its insertion onto the humerus (Fig. 4.13).**

- **Transect the clavicular portion of the pectoralis major muscle to the midclavicular line to avoid cutting important vessels and nerves, including the medial and lateral pectoral nerves (Fig. 4.14).**

DISSECTION **TIP**

When the pectoralis major is reflected, pay special attention so as not to transect the medial pectoral nerve as it passes through (or lies lateral or inferior to) the pectoralis minor muscle to enter the pectoralis major.

DEEP DISSECTION

- **After the pectoralis major has been reflected, identify the upper border of pectoralis minor and dissect the clavipectoral fascia to expose the subclavian and axillary vein (Fig. 4.15).**

ANATOMY **NOTE**

The clavipectoral fascia attaches proximally to the clavicle and invests the subclavius muscle. It then passes as a sheet toward the pectoralis minor, invests it, and then blends distally with axillary fascia forming the so-called suspensory ligament of the axilla.

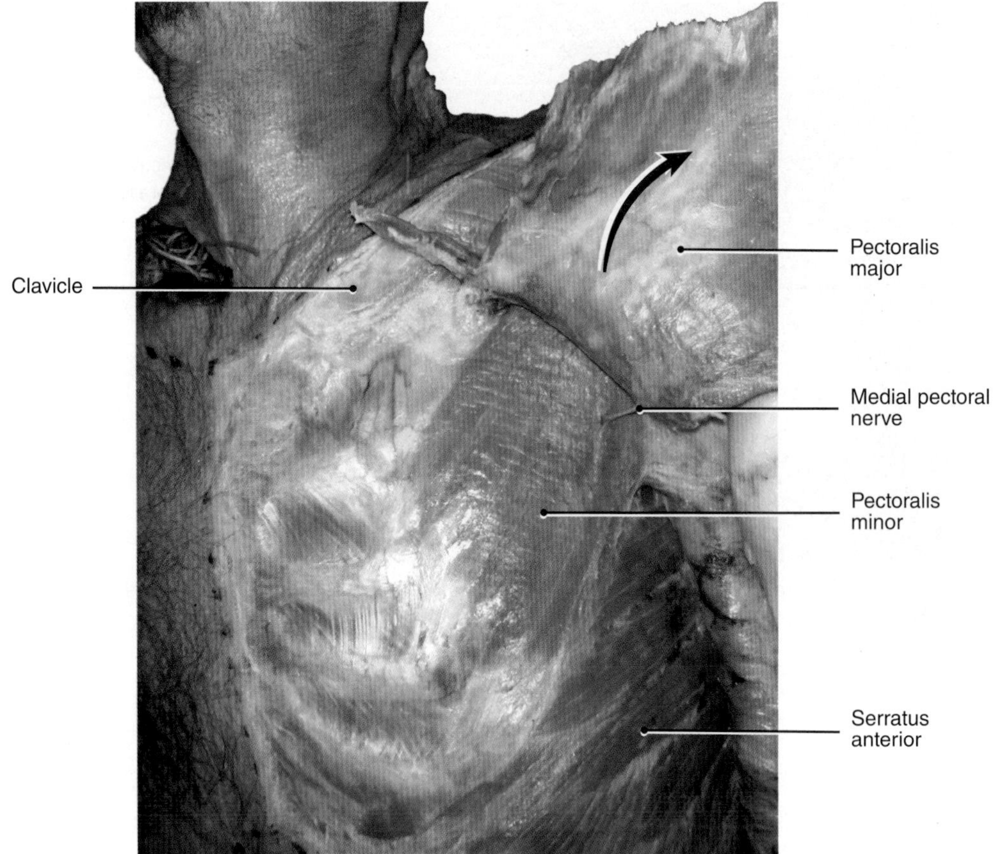

Fig. 4.14 Reflection of pectoralis major muscle highlighting pectoralis minor attachment to ribs 3 through 5.

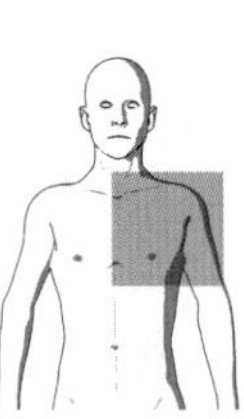

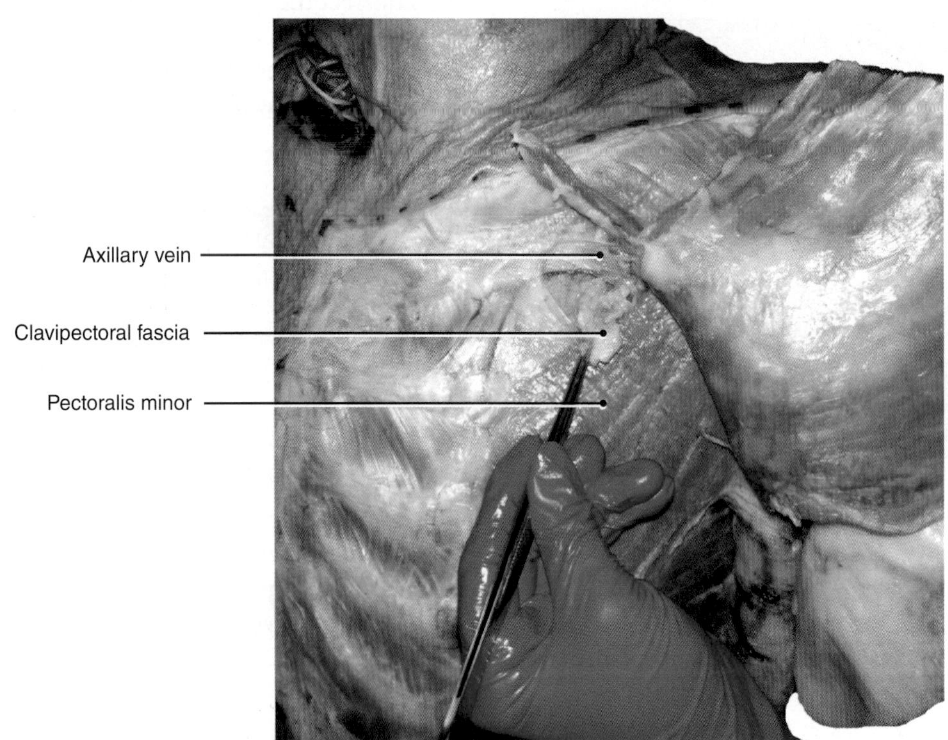

Fig. 4.15 Reflection of pectoralis major muscle and its fascia, revealing the clavipectoral fascia.

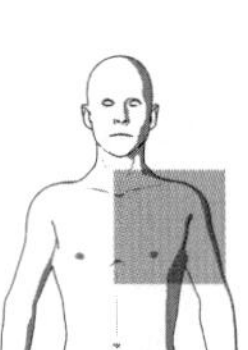

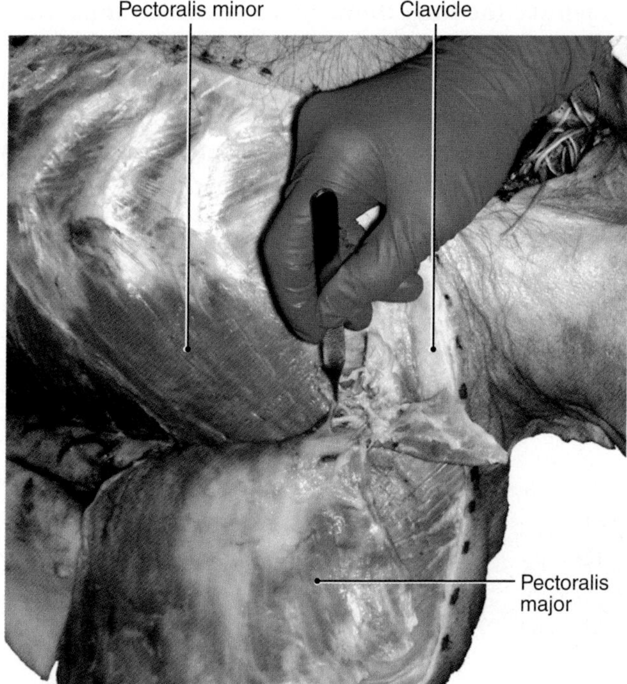

Fig. 4.16 Removal of clavipectoral fascia and identification of axillary vein.

- **Next, observe the subclavian vein, the lateral pectoral nerves, and the pectoral branches of the thoracoacromial artery as they emerge to reach the pectoralis major muscle (Figs. 4.16 and 4.17).**
- **Trace the pectoral arteries to their origin from the thoracoacromial artery and preserve these as the dissection proceeds.**
- **Insert the scissors under the inferior border of the pectoralis minor and cut the connective tissue underneath (Fig. 4.18). Reflect the pectoralis minor anteriorly.**
- **With a scalpel, reflect the pectoralis minor from ribs 3 through 5 (Fig. 4.19).**

DISSECTION **TIP**

Often, in older cadavers, large lymph nodes located deep to the pectoralis minor (retropectoral nodes) may be evident.

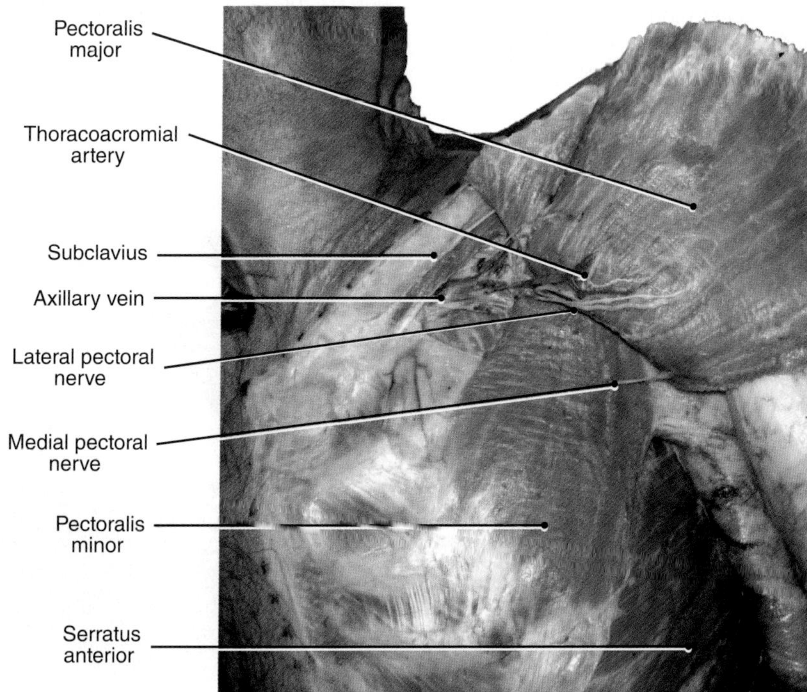

Fig. 4.17 Reflection of pectoralis major and its fascia, revealing medial and lateral pectoral nerves.

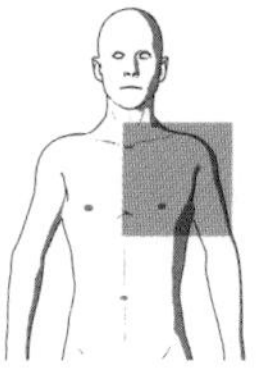

- As the superficial fascia is reflected from the anterolateral aspect of the thoracic wall, look for the thoracoepigastric vein. The thoracoepigastric vein is a tributary to the axillary vein by direct or indirect connections. During the reflection of the fascia near the midaxillary line, lateral cutaneous branches of anterior rami may be exposed where they enter the superficial fascia (Fig. 4.20). Try to preserve as many of these as possible.

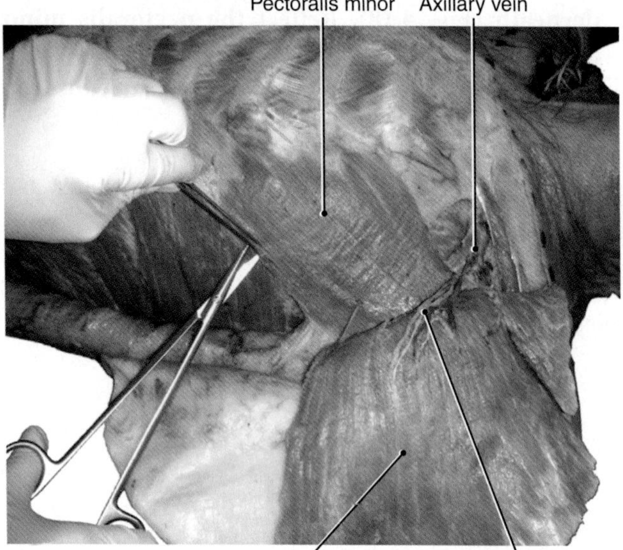

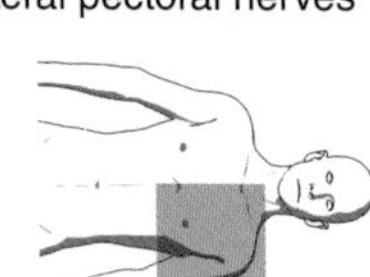

Fig. 4.18 Reflection of pectoralis major and its fascia, revealing pectoralis minor muscle. Scissors are positioned along the lateral inferior border of pectoralis minor.

- Identify the long thoracic nerve, which innervates the serratus anterior muscle (see Fig. 4.20). Trace the nerve a few centimeters inferior to the junction of the T2 anterior ramus (intercostobrachial nerve) and the thoracoepigastric vein at the midaxillary line over the serratus anterior muscle.

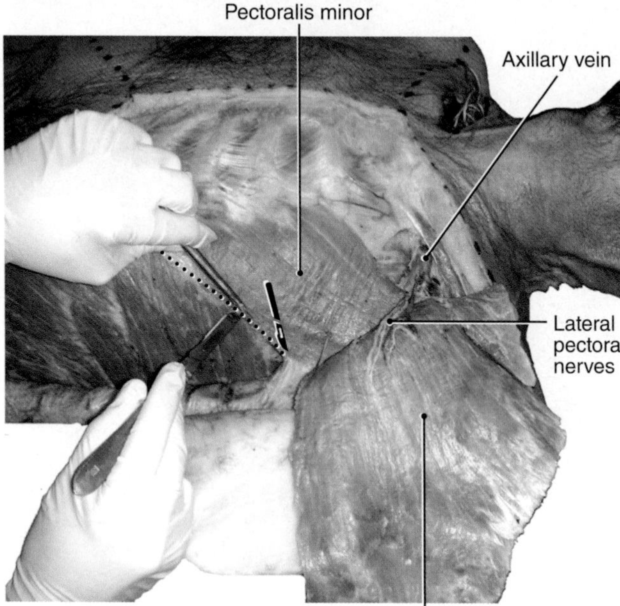

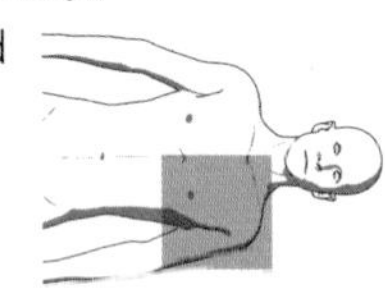

Fig. 4.19 Reflection of pectoralis major and its fascia, revealing pectoralis minor muscle. Place scalpel tip under lateral inferior border of pectoralis minor.

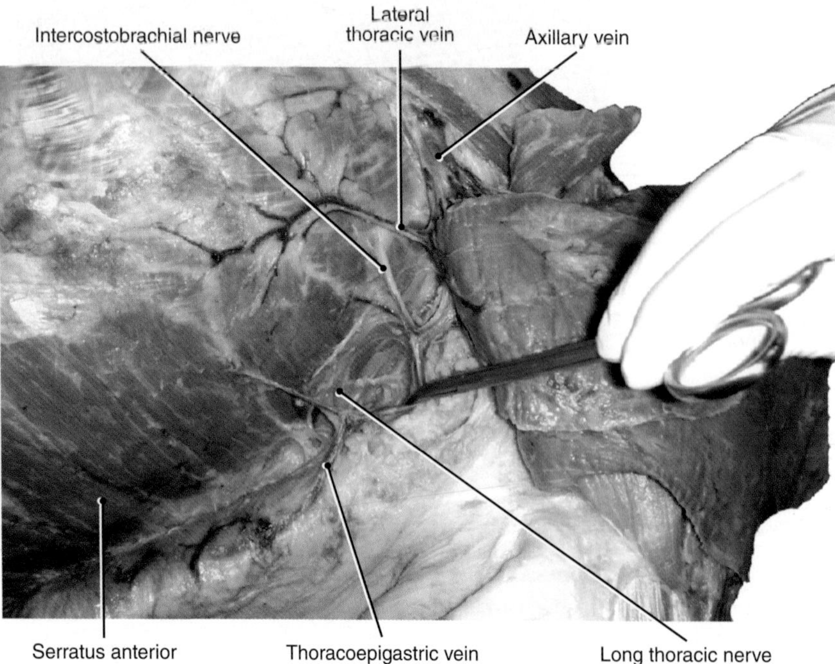

Fig. 4.20 Reflection of pectoralis major and minor muscles and deep fascia, revealing veins and intercostobrachial and long thoracic nerves.

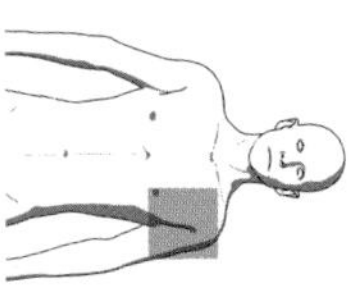

- Remove part of the axillary sheath and the axillary fascia deep to the pectoralis major. This tube-like fascia covers the axillary artery, axillary vein, and brachial plexus and is derived from the prevertebral fascia. With your scissors separate the fascia and remove most of it (Figs. 4.21 and 4.22). Once the fascia is removed, replace the pectoralis minor over the axillary artery.
- Clean the intercostobrachial nerve (T2), which emerges from the 2nd intercostal space. This nerve supplies the skin of the axilla and the proximal medial aspect of the arm. In some specimens, the 3rd intercostal nerve may communicate with the intercostobrachial nerve. Clean this nerve toward the skin of the axilla (Fig. 4.23).

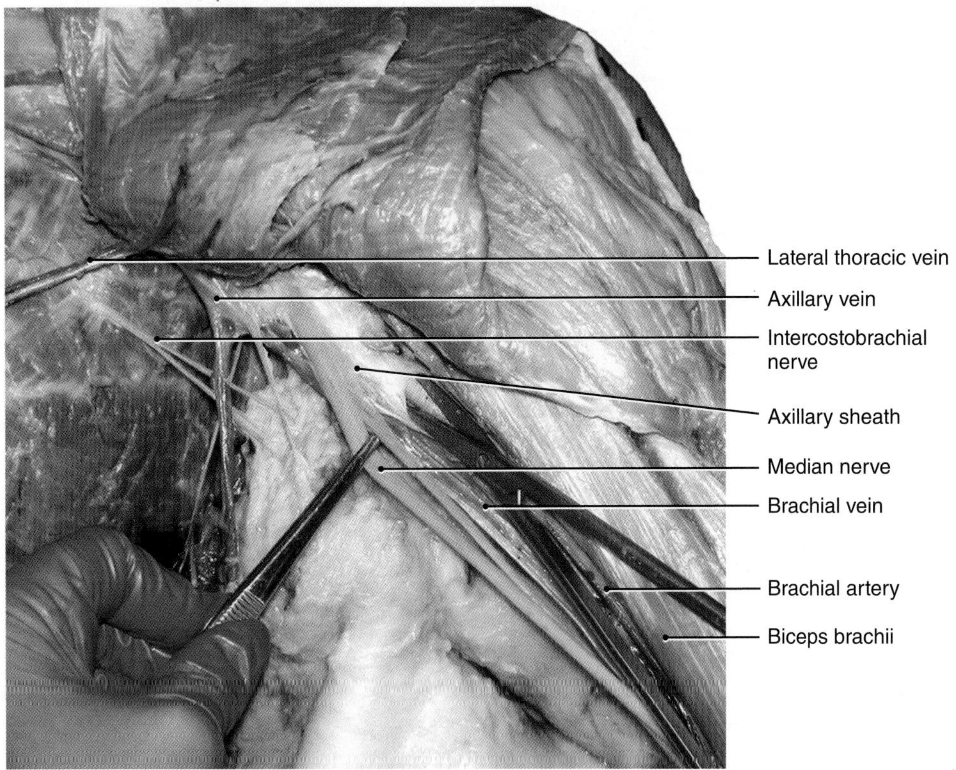

Fig. 4.21 Reflection of pectoralis major and minor muscles and deep fascia, revealing axillary sheath, axillary and brachial veins, and the median nerve.

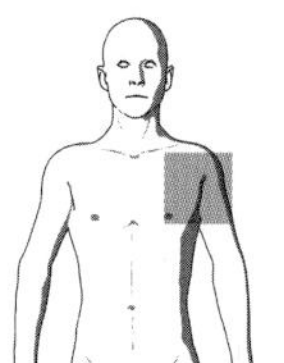

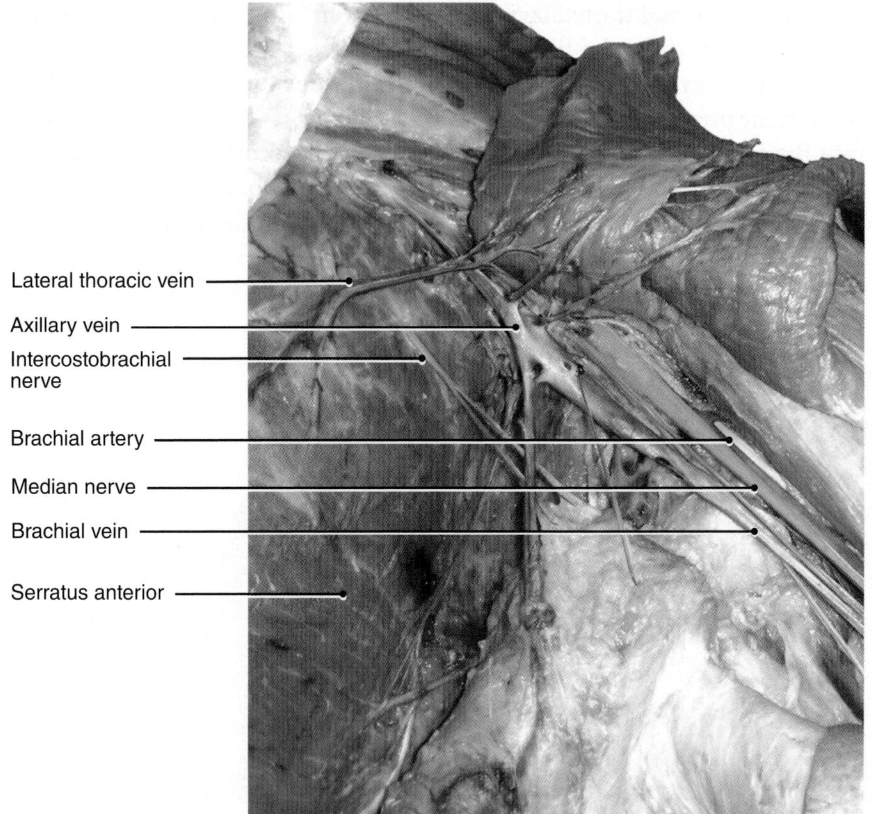

Fig. 4.22 Reflection of pectoralis major and minor muscles and deep fascia, revealing neurovascular structures of the axillary region.

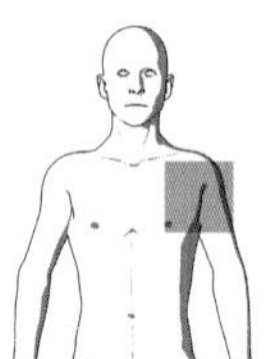

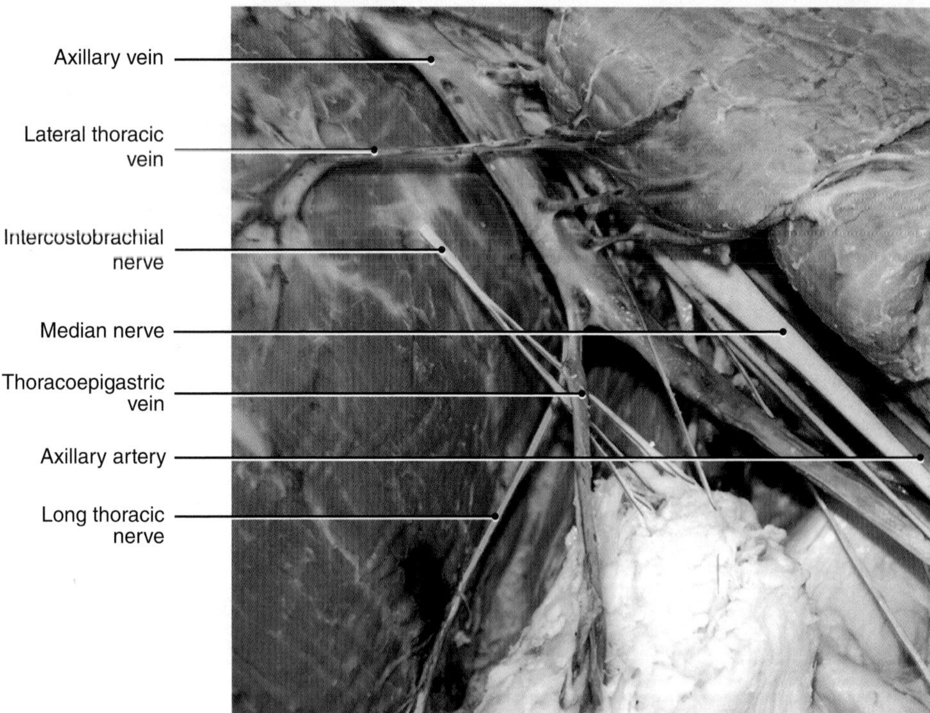

Fig. 4.23 Reflection of pectoralis major muscle and fascia, revealing pectoralis minor and relationship to axillary and long thoracic arteries.

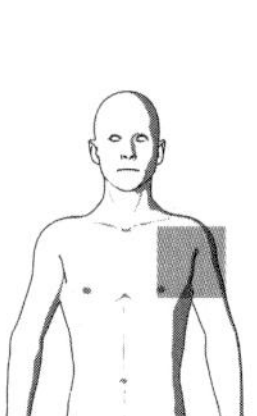

- The pectoralis minor muscle divides the axillary artery into three parts (Fig. 4.24).
- At the lateral border of the pectoralis minor on the surface of the serratus anterior, expose the lateral thoracic artery (see Fig. 4.24).
- Its origin is typically from the 2nd portion of the axillary artery; however, this may vary. Look carefully for a small artery penetrating the musculature of the 1st or 2nd intercostal space. This is the superior thoracic artery that arises from the first part of the axillary artery (Fig. 4.25, Plates 4.1 and 4.2).

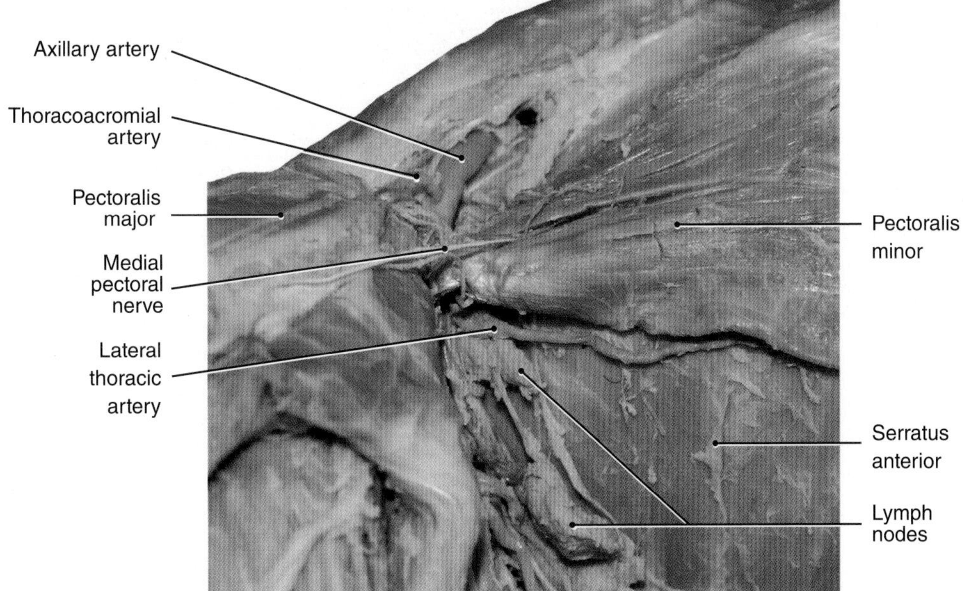

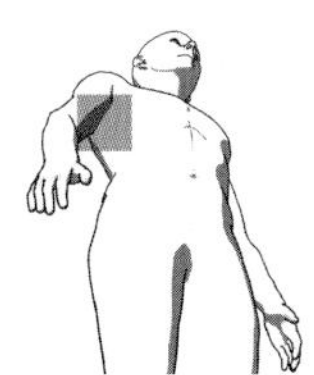

Fig. 4.24 Reflection of pectoralis major muscle exposing lateral thoracic artery, seen traveling along the lateral border of the pectoralis minor muscle.

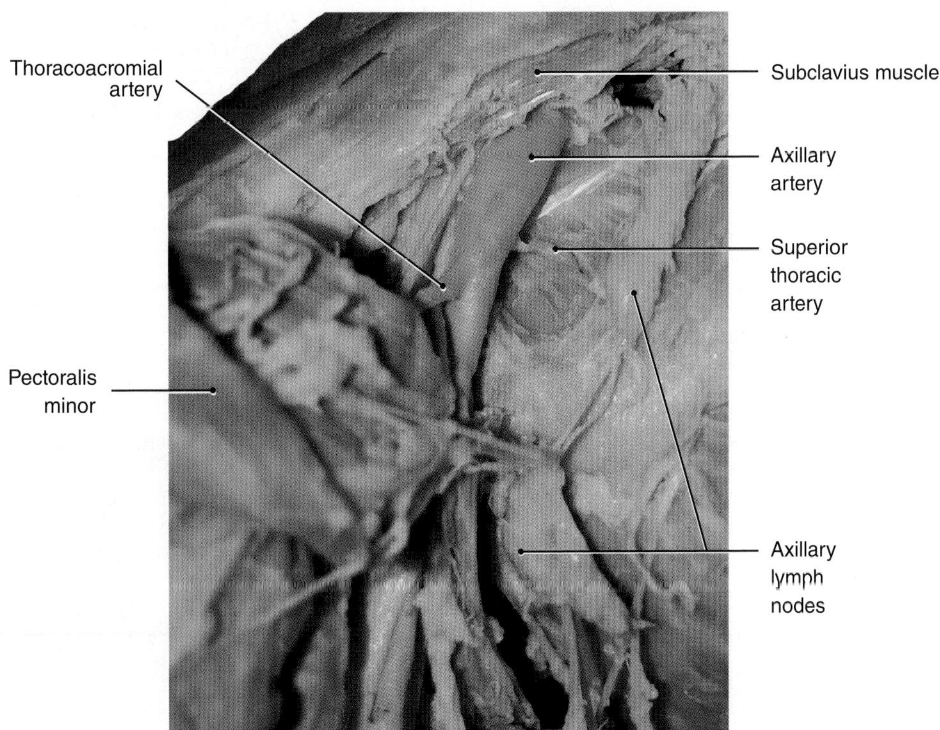

Fig. 4.25 Dissection of axillary region, revealing reflected pectoralis minor muscle, axillary and superior thoracic arteries, and axillary lymph nodes.

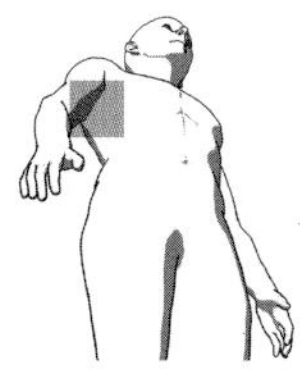

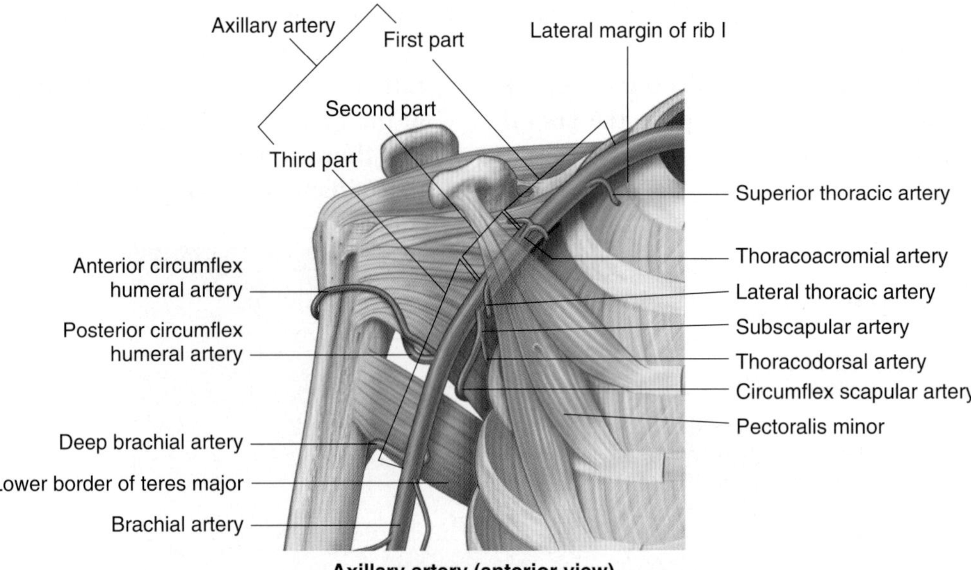

Plate 4.1 Divisions of axillary artery. (From Drake RL et al., *Gray's Atlas of Anatomy*, 3rd edition, Philadelphia, Elsevier, 2021, p. 403).

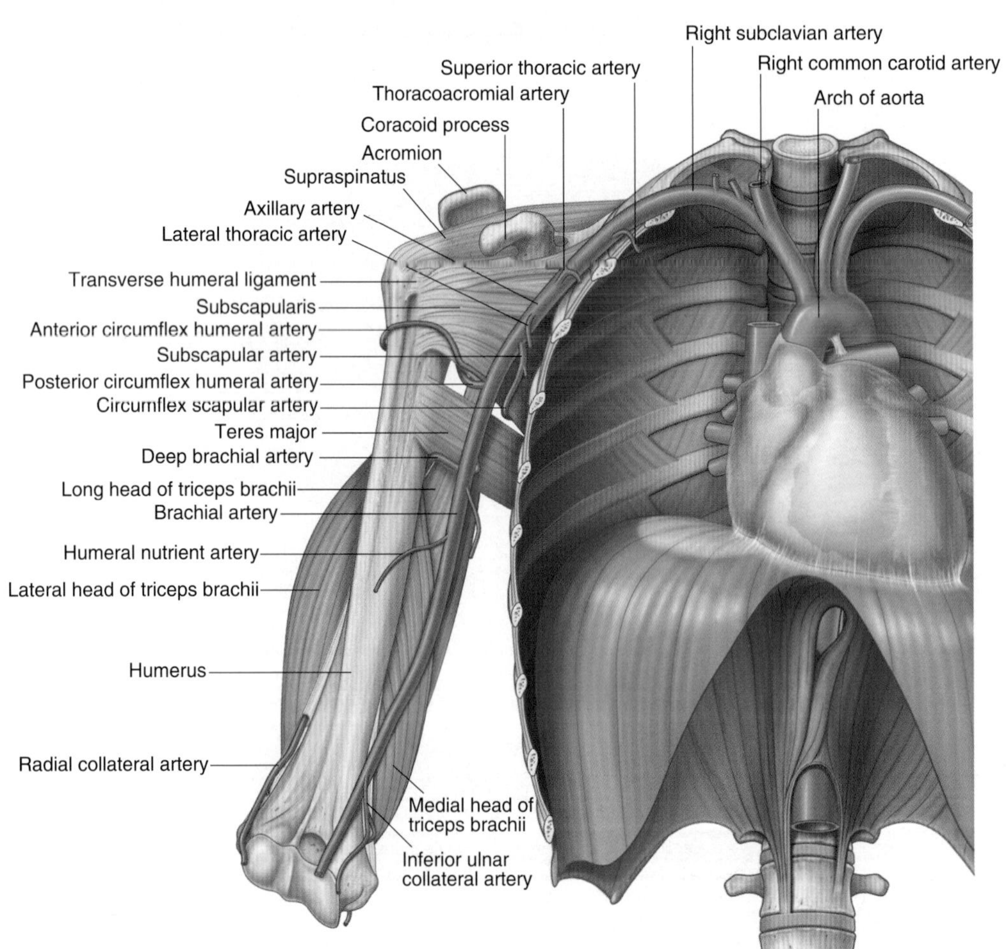

Plate 4.2 Branches of axillary artery. (From Drake RL et al., *Gray's Atlas of Anatomy*, 3rd edition, Philadelphia, Elsevier, 2021, p. 401).

- Place a probe or your scissors between the external intercostal membrane and the internal intercostal muscle (Fig. 4.26).

ANATOMY **NOTE**

The external intercostal membrane travels between the lateral border of the sternum and the midclavicular line.

- Cut this membrane and expose the internal intercostal muscle (Figs. 4.26 and 4.27).

ANATOMY **NOTE**

This muscle layer runs in a direction opposite to the external intercostals, like "hands in your back pockets." The external intercostal muscles are oriented in a direction medially and downward, like "hands in your front pockets" (Fig. 4.28). Near the sternum, the external intercostal muscles are continued medially as the external intercostal membrane.

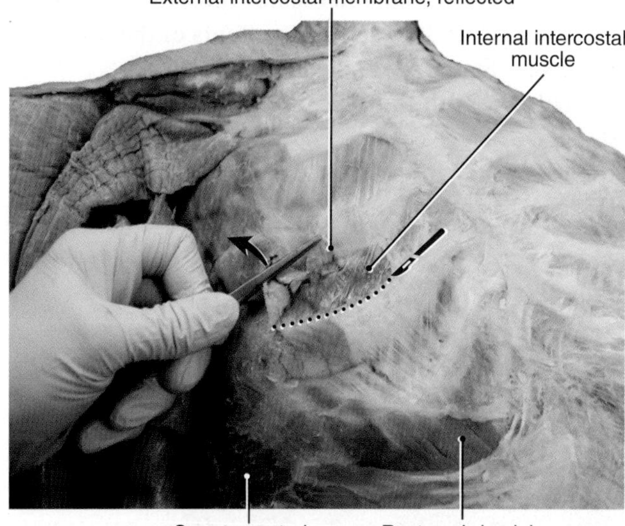

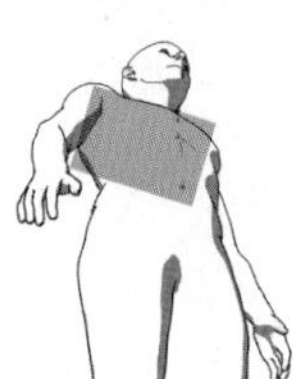

Fig. 4.27 The external intercostal membrane is cut and reflected laterally to reveal internal intercostal muscle.

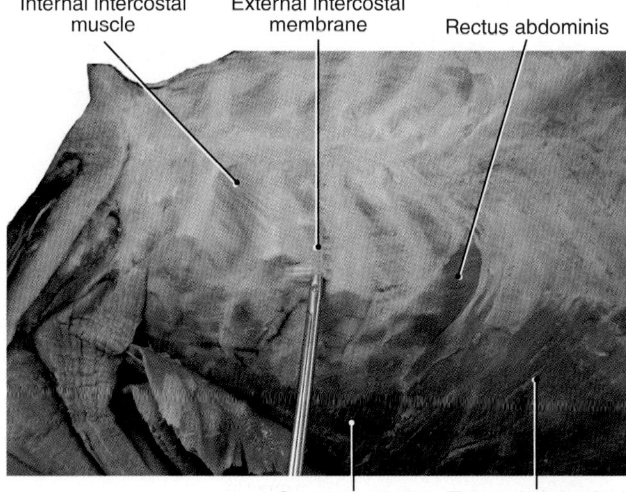

Fig. 4.26 Anterior thoracic wall musculature, revealing external intercostal membrane (over the scissors), internal intercostal, external abdominal oblique, rectus abdominis, and serratus anterior muscles.

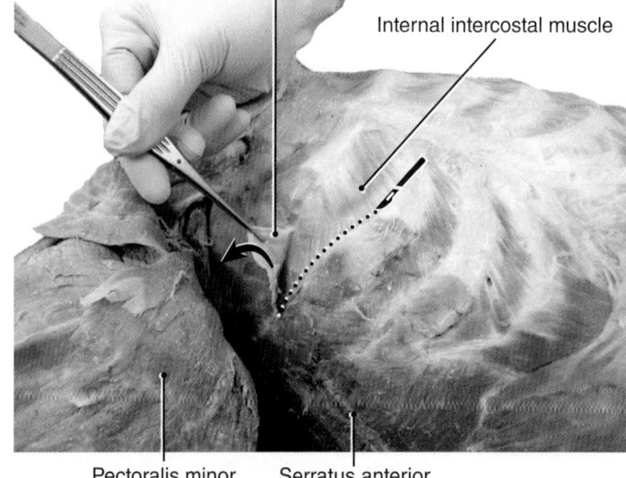

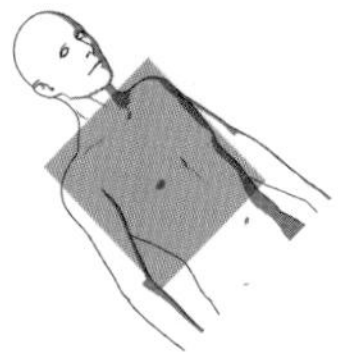

Fig. 4.28 Anterolateral thoracic wall with reflected pectoralis muscle and fascia, revealing external intercostal, internal intercostal, and serratus anterior muscles.

- **Reflect the internal intercostal muscle adjacent to the sternum and expose the contents of the intercostal space (Figs. 4.29 and 4.30).**
- **Identify the endothoracic fascia and carefully reflect it (Fig. 4.31).**
- **Identify the internal thoracic artery and vein (Figs. 4.32 and 4.33).**

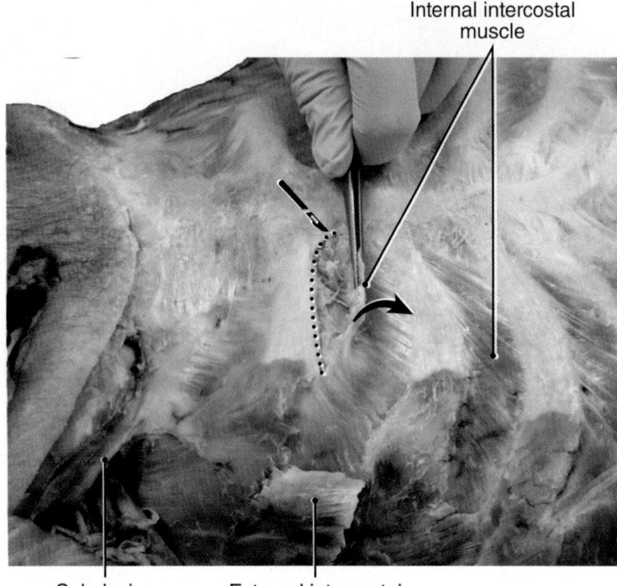

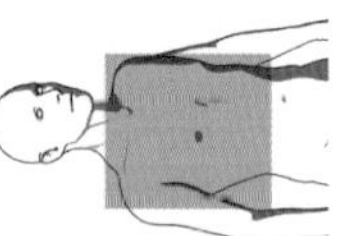

Fig. 4.29 Anterolateral thoracic wall revealing subclavius, external intercostal, and internal intercostal muscles. The internal intercostal muscle is cut superiorly and reflected inferiorly to expose the endothoracic fascia.

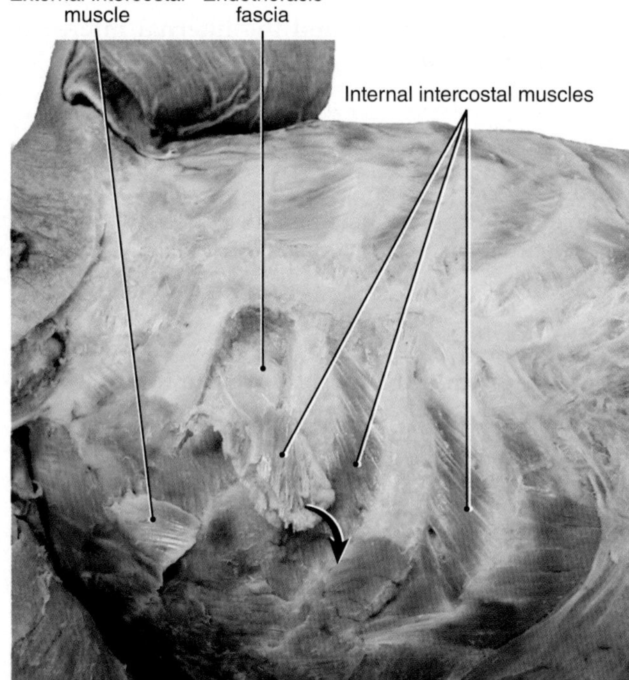

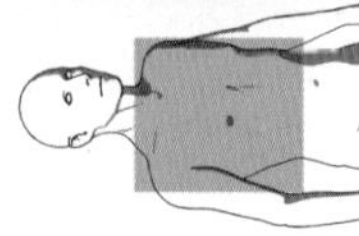

Fig. 4.30 Anterolateral thoracic wall with reflected internal intercostal, revealing endothoracic fascia and external and internal intercostal muscles.

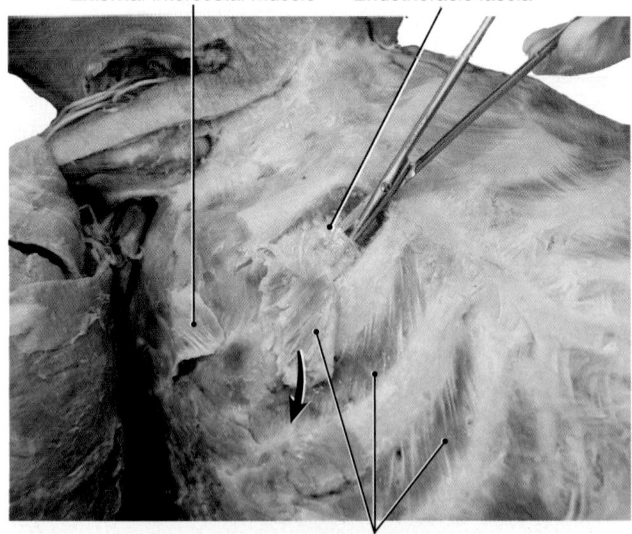

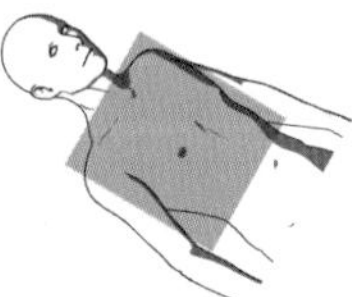

Fig. 4.31 Anterolateral thoracic wall with reflected internal intercostal, revealing endothoracic fascia with external and internal intercostal muscles.

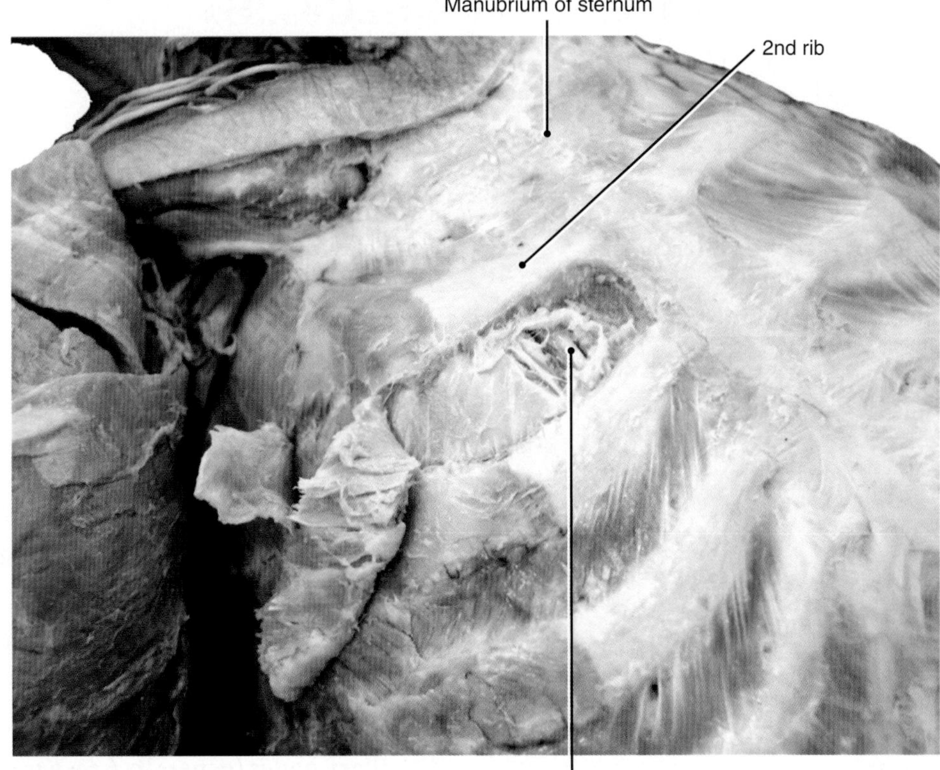

Fig. 4.32 Anterior thoracic wall with reflected internal intercostal muscle and endothoracic fascia, revealing internal thoracic artery and vein.

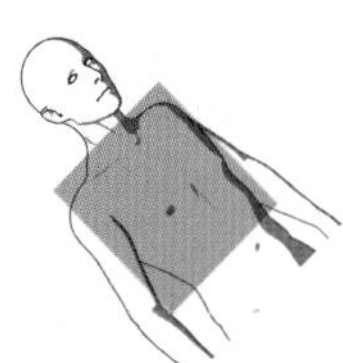

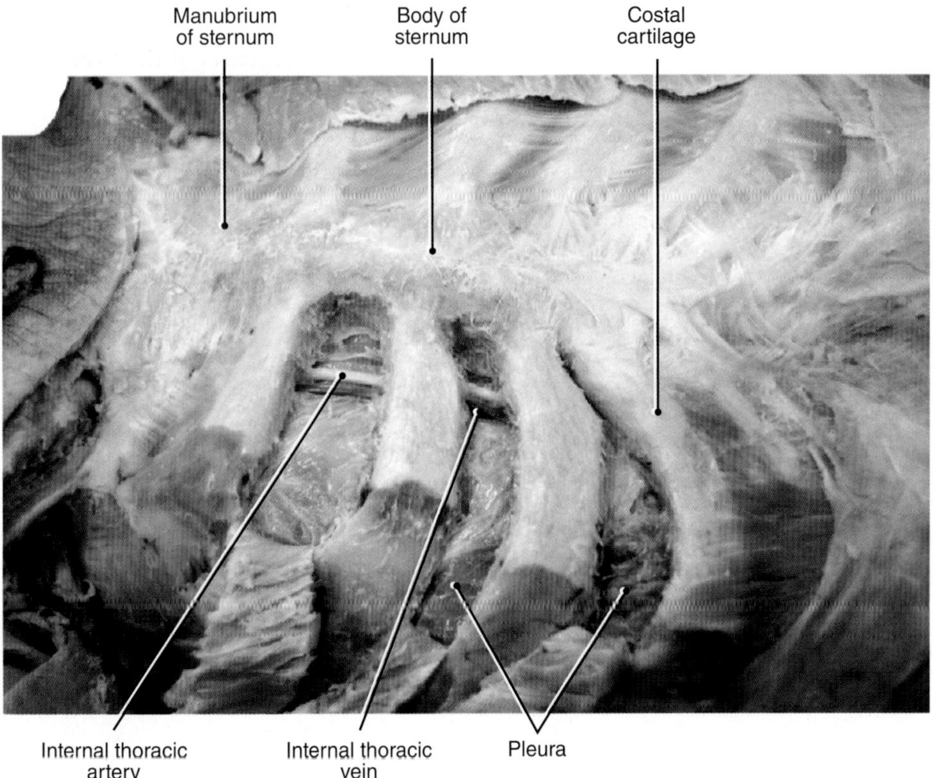

Fig. 4.33 Anterior thoracic wall with reflected internal intercostal muscle and endothoracic fascia, revealing internal thoracic artery and vein.

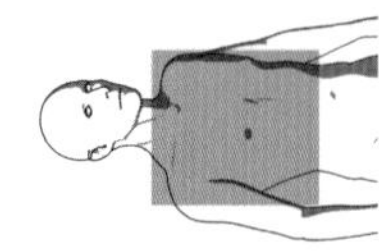

LABORATORY IDENTIFICATION CHECKLIST

Some of the nerves and arteries listed here will have been dissected during the laboratory for the superficial back (and upper limb) but also are seen when dissecting the breast.

NERVES

- ☐ Anterior cutaneous branches of intercostal
- ☐ Intercostobrachial (T2)
- ☐ Lateral cutaneous branches of intercostal (T3–T7)
- ☐ Lateral pectoral
- ☐ Medial pectoral
- ☐ Axillary
- ☐ Long thoracic
- ☐ Thoracodorsal
- ☐ Subscapular

ARTERIES

- ☐ Thoracoacromial
  - ☐ Pectoral branches
  - ☐ Deltoid branches
  - ☐ Clavicular branches
  - ☐ Acromial branches
- ☐ Internal thoracic
- ☐ Lateral thoracic
- ☐ Anterior intercostal
- ☐ Posterior intercostal

VEINS

- ☐ Axillary
- ☐ Internal thoracic
- ☐ Intercostal

MUSCLES

- ☐ Pectoralis major
  - ☐ Clavicular part
  - ☐ Sternocostal part
  - ☐ Abdominal part (not always present)
- ☐ Pectoralis minor
- ☐ Subclavius
- ☐ Serratus anterior
- ☐ External/internal intercostals

BONES

- ☐ Sternum
  - ☐ Manubrium
  - ☐ Body
  - ☐ Xiphoid process
  - ☐ Manubriosternal joint (angle of Louis, T4–T5)
- ☐ Clavicle
- ☐ 1st rib
- ☐ Ribs 2–12

LYMPHATICS

- ☐ Axillary nodes (generally 6 recognized nodal groups with a total of 35–40 nodes)
- ☐ Internal thoracic node drainage (~5 per side)
- ☐ Thoracic duct

LIGAMENTS

- ☐ Suspensory ligaments of the breast (of Cooper)

BREAST

- ☐ Areolar-nipple complex
- ☐ Superficial fascia (from anterior thoracic wall)
- ☐ Lobes (15–20)
- ☐ Tail of breast (Spence)
- ☐ Deep fascia

OPENING THE THORACIC CAVITY

Technique 1

- **With a scalpel, transect the intercostal muscles, serratus anterior muscle, and a portion of the external abdominal oblique muscle (Figs. 5.1 and 5.2).**
- **Make sure that you start your dissection above the emergence of the intercostobrachial nerve (T2) and then descend toward the midaxillary line.**
- **With a saw or bone cutter, carefully cut the intercostal musculature from the first intercostal space lateral to the manubrium, then extend these incisions downward, just anterior to the emergence of the anterior cutaneous branches of the intercostal nerves, cutting the ribs and intercostal musculature down to the level of the 10th rib (Fig. 5.3).**
- **Divide the manubrium transversely above the sternal angle using a bone saw, cutters, or scalpel (Fig. 5.4).**
- **After making the saw cuts, use a scalpel and bone cutters or mallet and chisel to free the anterior thoracic wall (Fig. 5.5).**

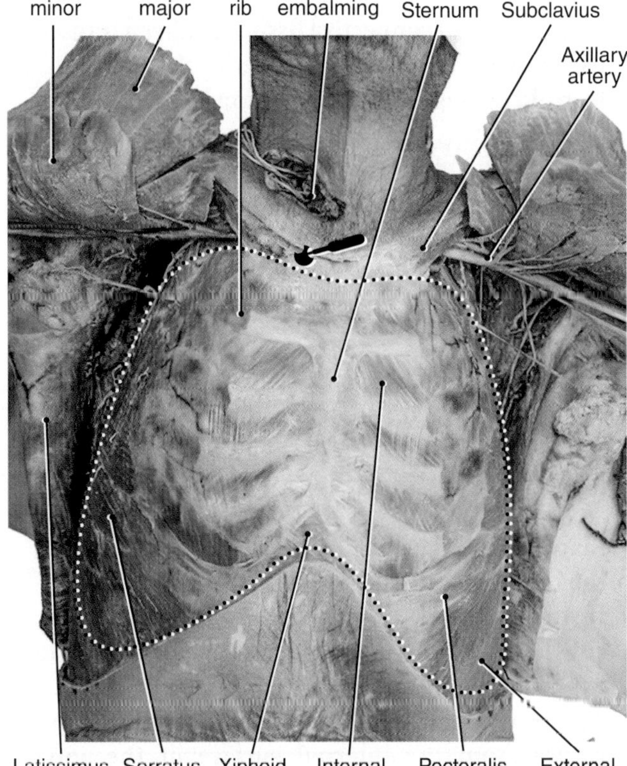

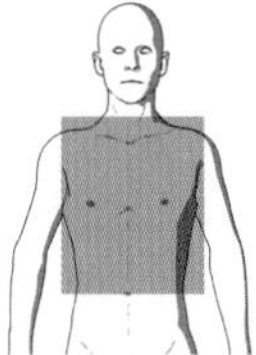

Fig. 5.1 Anterior thoracic wall with skin, fascia, and pectoralis major and minor reflected, revealing tracing of the anterior wall of the thorax for deep dissection of the thorax.

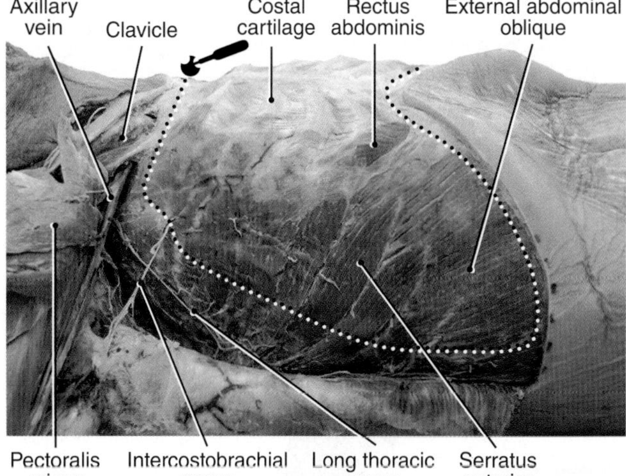

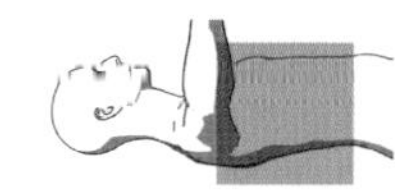

Fig. 5.2 Anterolateral view of thorax with tracing for incision to reveal internal structures.

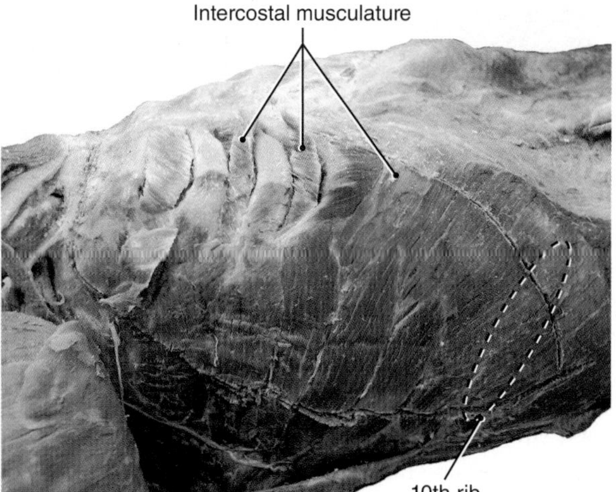

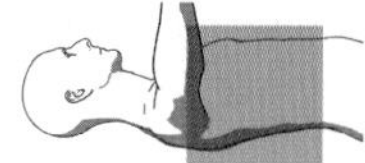

Fig. 5.3 Anterolateral view of thorax with incision to allow for thoracotomy.

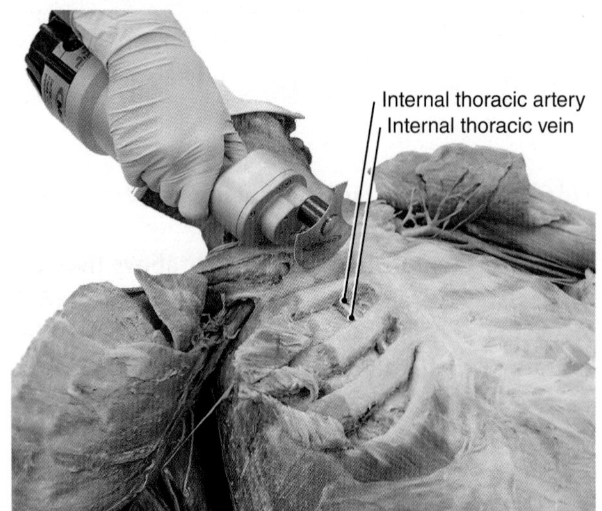

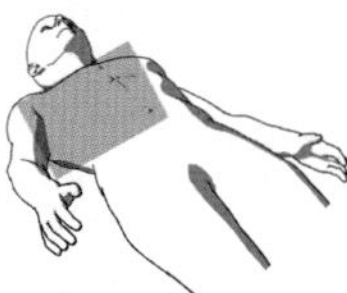

Fig. 5.4 Skin, fascia, and pectoral muscles reflected from anterior thoracic wall to reveal intercostal dissection of intercostal muscles, as well as internal thoracic artery and vein. Bone saw, cutters, or scalpel is used to make the bone cuts.

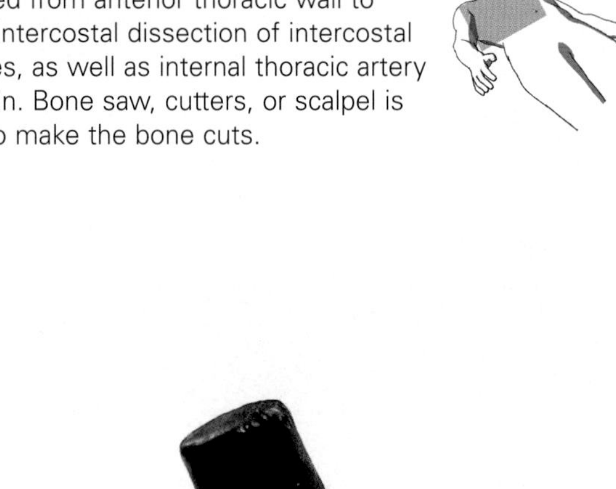

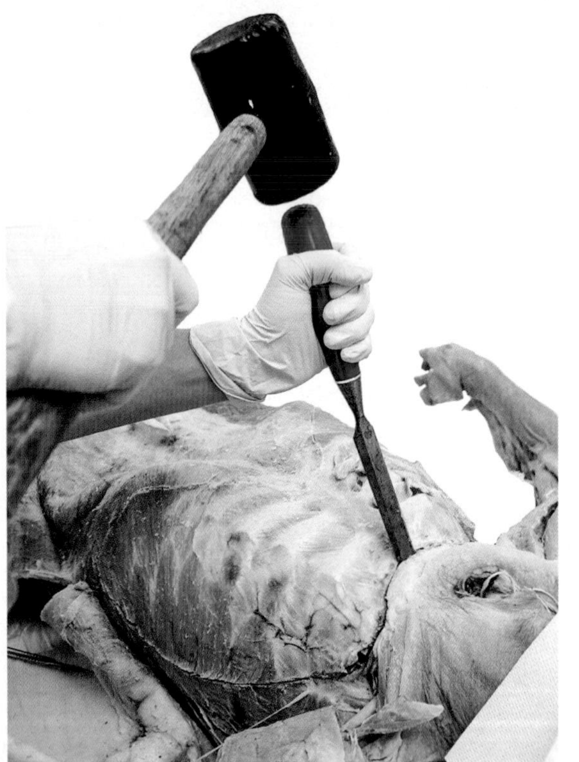

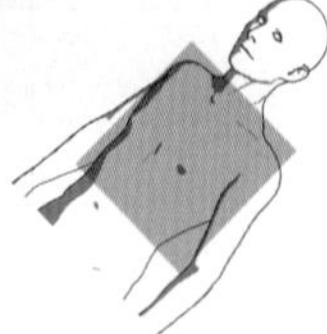

Fig. 5.5 Anterolateral view of chest with incision to reveal internal thoracic structures. Use mallet and chisel to release bone and connective tissue to allow removal of the anterior thoracic wall.

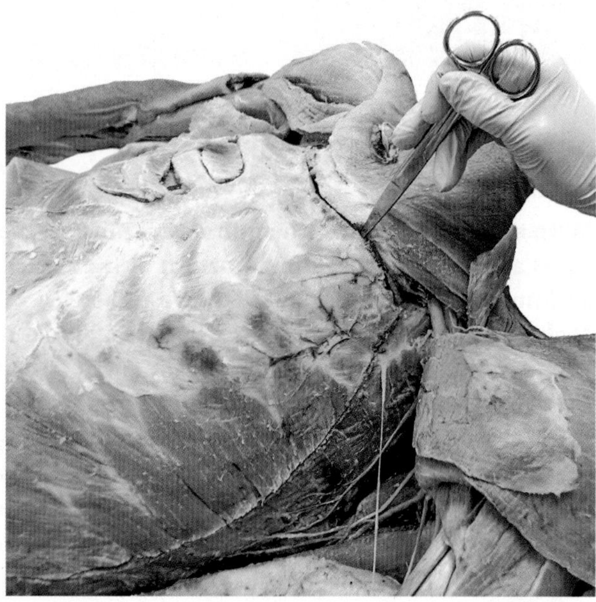

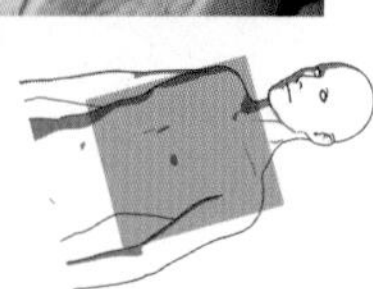

Fig. 5.6 Anterolateral view of thoracic wall with cuts to reveal deep thoracic structures. Once bone and connective tissue have been transected, use blunt scissors to lift anterior thoracic wall.

- **Once bone and connective tissue have been transected, use blunt scissors to lift the anterior thoracic wall. Try to avoid damage to the underlying lungs (Fig. 5.6).**

DISSECTION **TIP**

Often, in the first and second intercostal spaces, you will be able to place your fingertips underneath the internal surface of the anterior thoracic wall and lift it up (Fig. 5.7).

If some parts are still connected to the wall, use a scalpel and bone cutters to free the anterior thoracic wall (Fig. 5.8).

Be careful when you place your fingertips under the exposed ribs; sharp bone spicules are often present and may cause injury. Use a bone cutter or rongeur to remove these.

- **Place your fingertips underneath the openings of the thoracic wall and pull up (Fig. 5.9).**
- **If the internal thoracic vessels are still intact, cut them and then pull the thoracic wall inferiorly, exposing the thoracic contents.**
- **As you reflect the wall inferiorly, incise the parietal pleura from the internal surface of the anterior thoracic wall with a scalpel, leaving it intact over the lungs (Fig. 5.10).**
- **Cut the sternopericardial ligaments that connect the pericardial sac to the posterior surface of the sternum.**
- **Continue the reflection of the anterior thoracic wall downward until the thoracic viscera can be clearly seen (Fig. 5.11).**

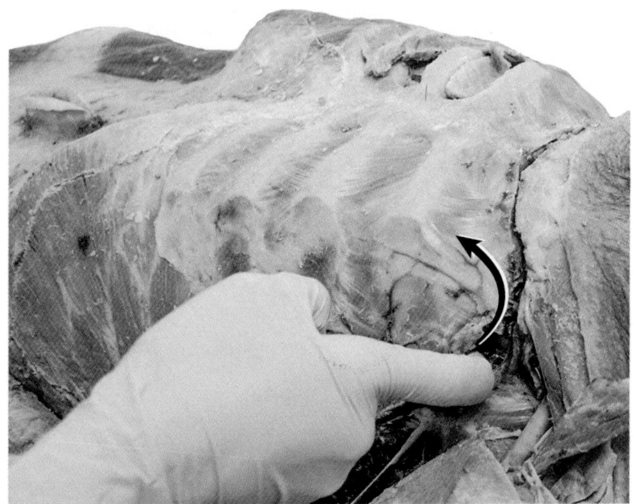

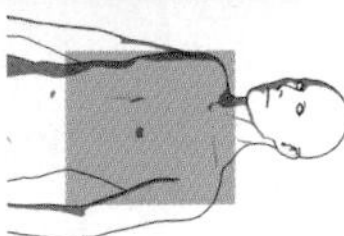

Fig. 5.7 Anterolateral thoracic wall can be removed manually.

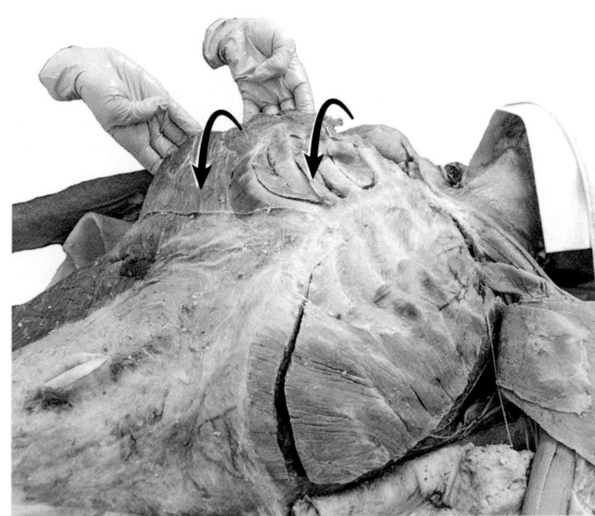

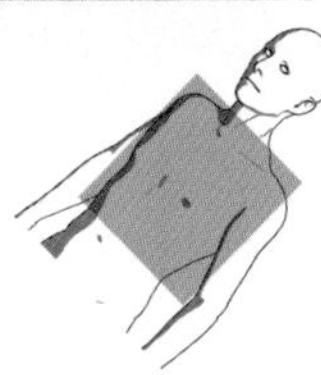

Fig. 5.9 Anterolateral thoracic wall reflected manually. Release connective tissue deep to anterior thoracic wall bilaterally.

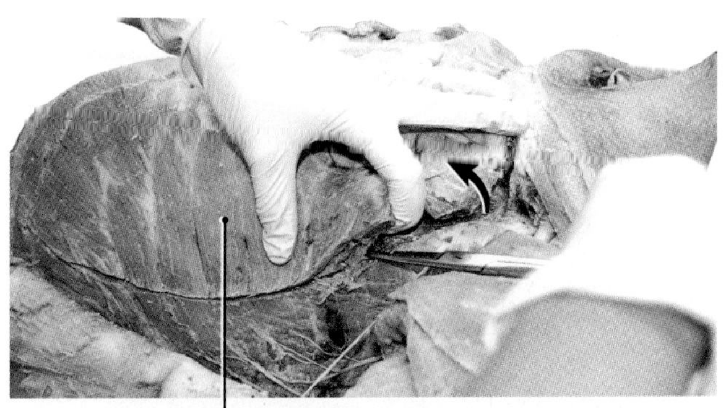

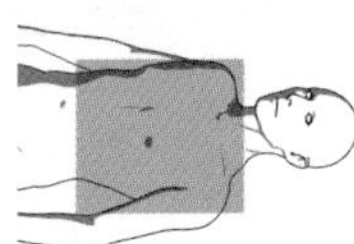

Fig. 5.8 Anterolateral view of thorax with cuts to reveal deeper structures. Use blunt dissection with scissors to remove the anterior thoracic wall.

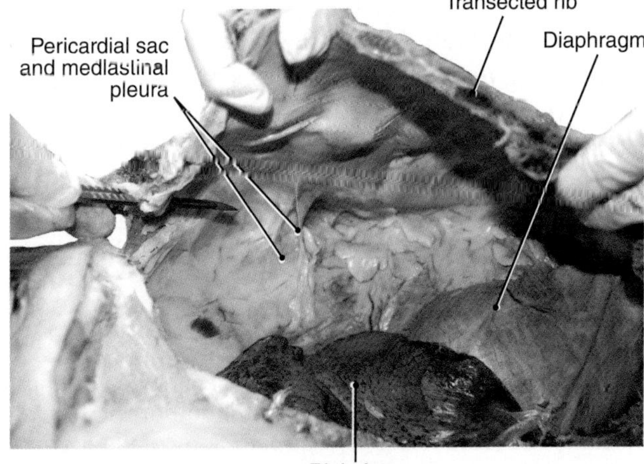

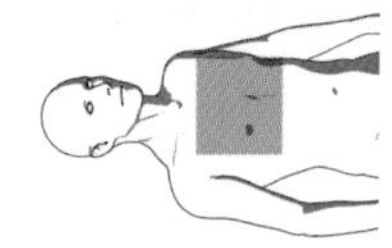

Fig. 5.10 Partial reflection of anterior thoracic wall, revealing internal structures.

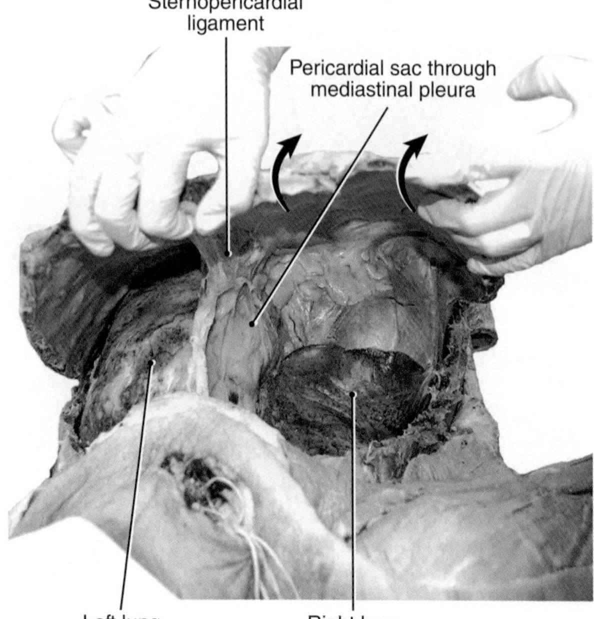

Fig. 5.11 Bilateral reflection of anterior thoracic wall, revealing internal structures.

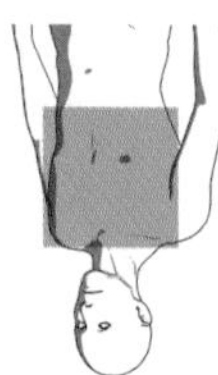

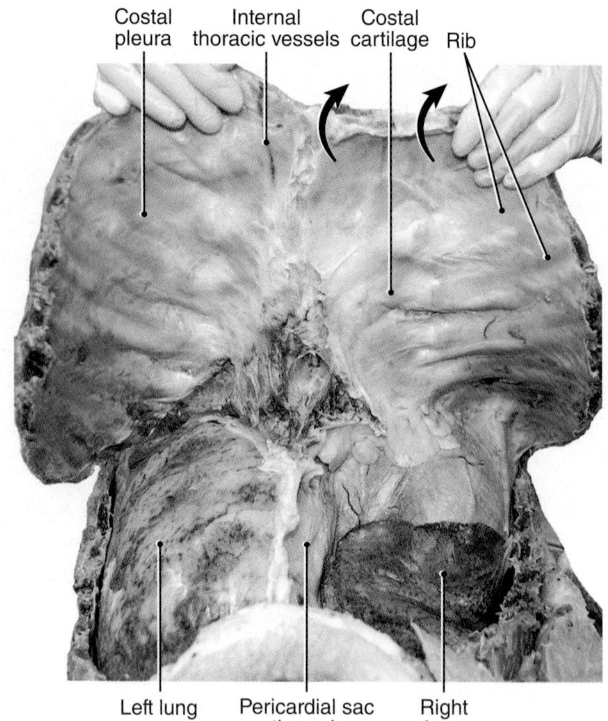

Fig. 5.12 Bilateral reflection of anterior thoracic wall, revealing internal structures.

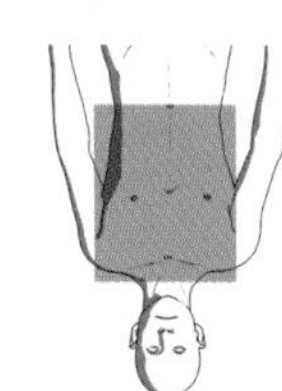

- **Keep the anterior thoracic wall turned downward as the dissection proceeds (Fig. 5.12).**
- **Forcing the wall down usually results in sufficient stretching or tearing of tissues so that the anterior wall remains reflected inferiorly. If this is not the case, you can remove the anterior thoracic wall (Fig. 5.13). Using blunt dissection with your hand or blunt-ended scissors from superior to inferior helps guide the anterior connective tissue as desired.**

DISSECTION TIP

The pleura is attached to the thoracic wall by a continuous layer of connective tissue, the endothoracic fascia. In some cadavers with previous pathology of the thorax, such as infections, the pleura may be thickened and adherent to the thoracic walls, making efforts to preserve it difficult.

- **Observe the internal surface of the anterior thoracic wall and identify the internal thoracic arteries and veins and their branches (Fig. 5.14).**
- **Reflect the parietal pleura to expose the intercostal muscles.**
- **Reflecting the parietal pleura in the 1st and 2nd intercostal spaces exposes the internal thoracic artery. Identify it.**
- **To expose the internal thoracic artery and vein further, reflect the transversus thoracis muscles.**

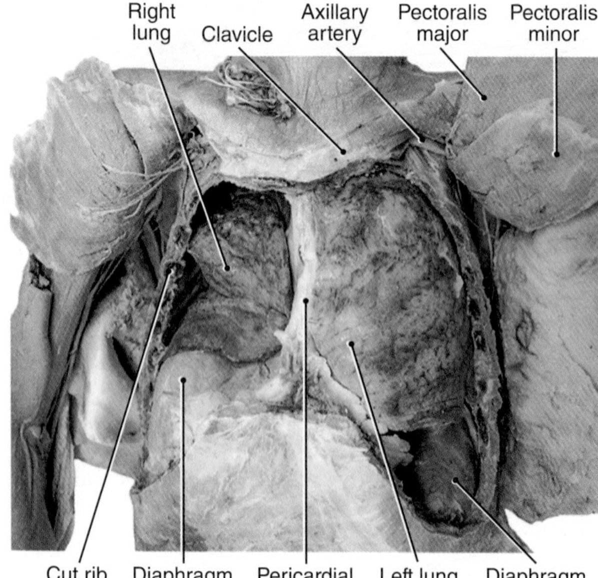

Fig. 5.13 Anterior thoracic wall removed, revealing internal thoracic structures. Note that the right lung is collapsed. This is probably due to a pneumothorax that occurred during life.

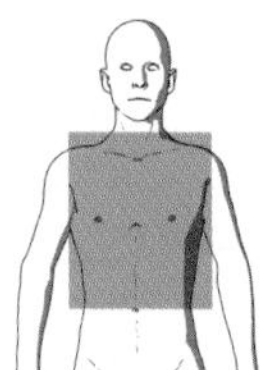

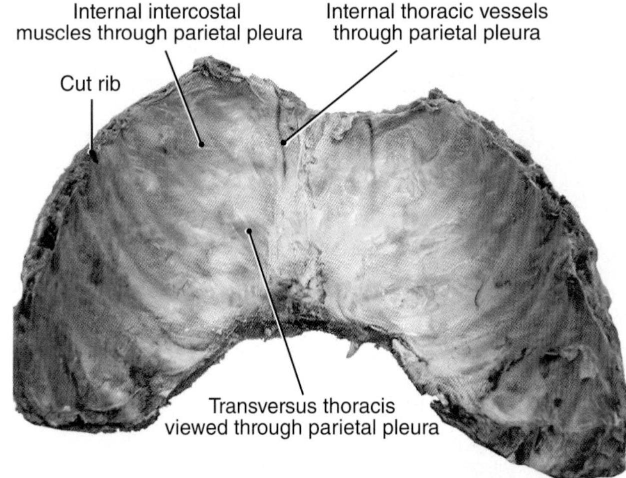

Fig. 5.14 Undersurface of the removed anterior thoracic wall, revealing structures intimate with it.

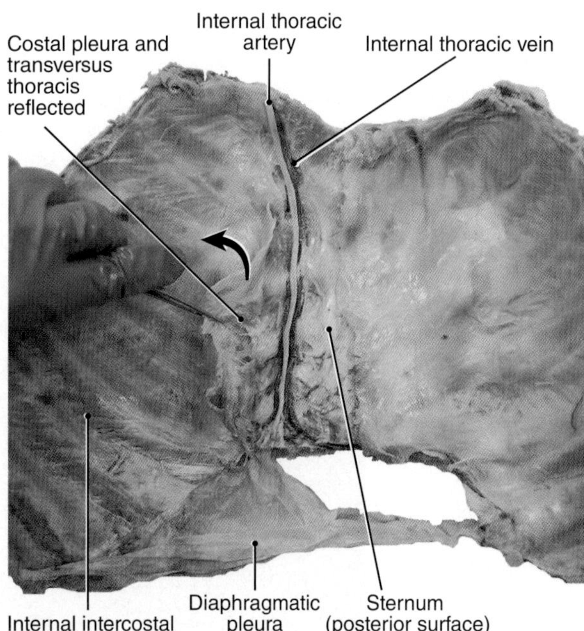

Fig. 5.15 Undersurface of removed anterior thoracic wall, highlighting internal thoracic artery.

- **Identify the branches of the internal thoracic artery, such as the perforating and anterior intercostal branches (Fig. 5.15).**

ANATOMY **NOTE**

Typically, the terminal branches of the internal thoracic artery—the superior epigastric and musculophrenic branches—are located near the xiphoid process.

Technique 2

- **With a scalpel, transect the intercostal muscles, serratus anterior muscle, and a portion of the external abdominal oblique muscle as shown in Figs. 4.26 to 4.32. At the costodiaphragmatic recess, identify the peritoneum below the diaphragm and slowly cut it across (Figs. 5.16 and 5.17). Once the peritoneum has been cut, continue the lateral incisions from the midaxillary line toward the anterior iliac spine (Fig. 5.18). Lift and reflect the anterior thoracic wall and the anterior abdominal wall en bloc (Fig. 5.19).**

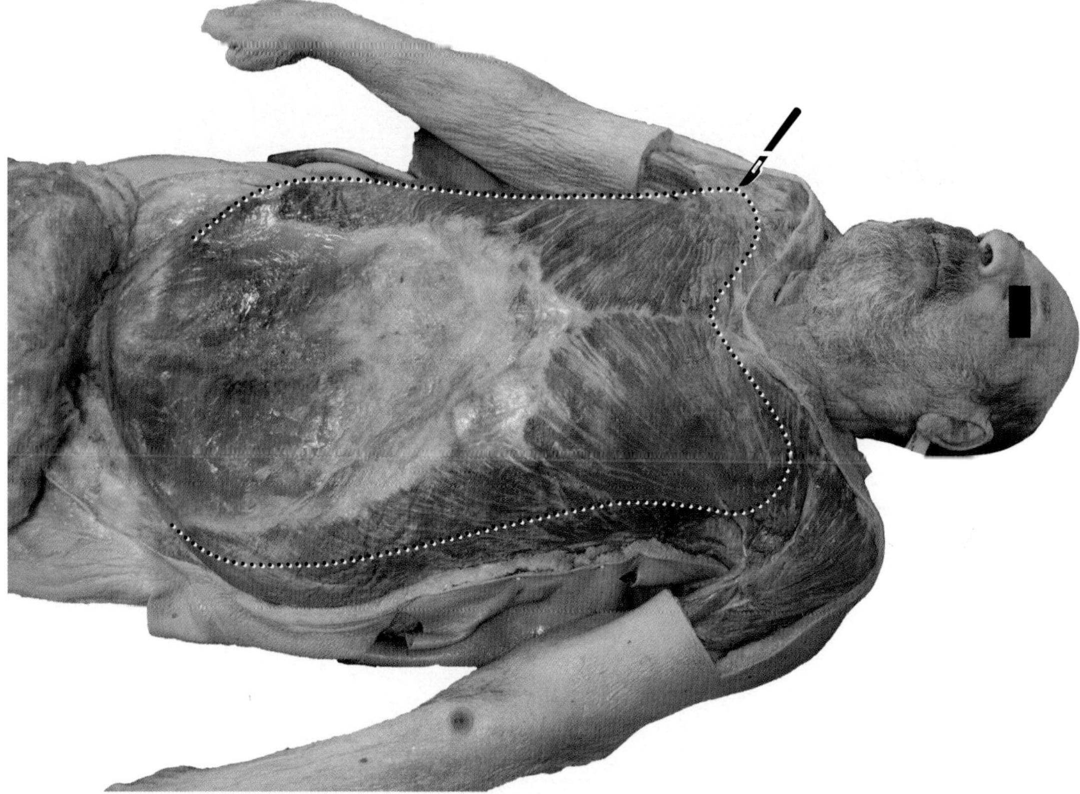

Fig. 5.16 Outline of cuts used to reflect anterior thoracic and abdominal walls.

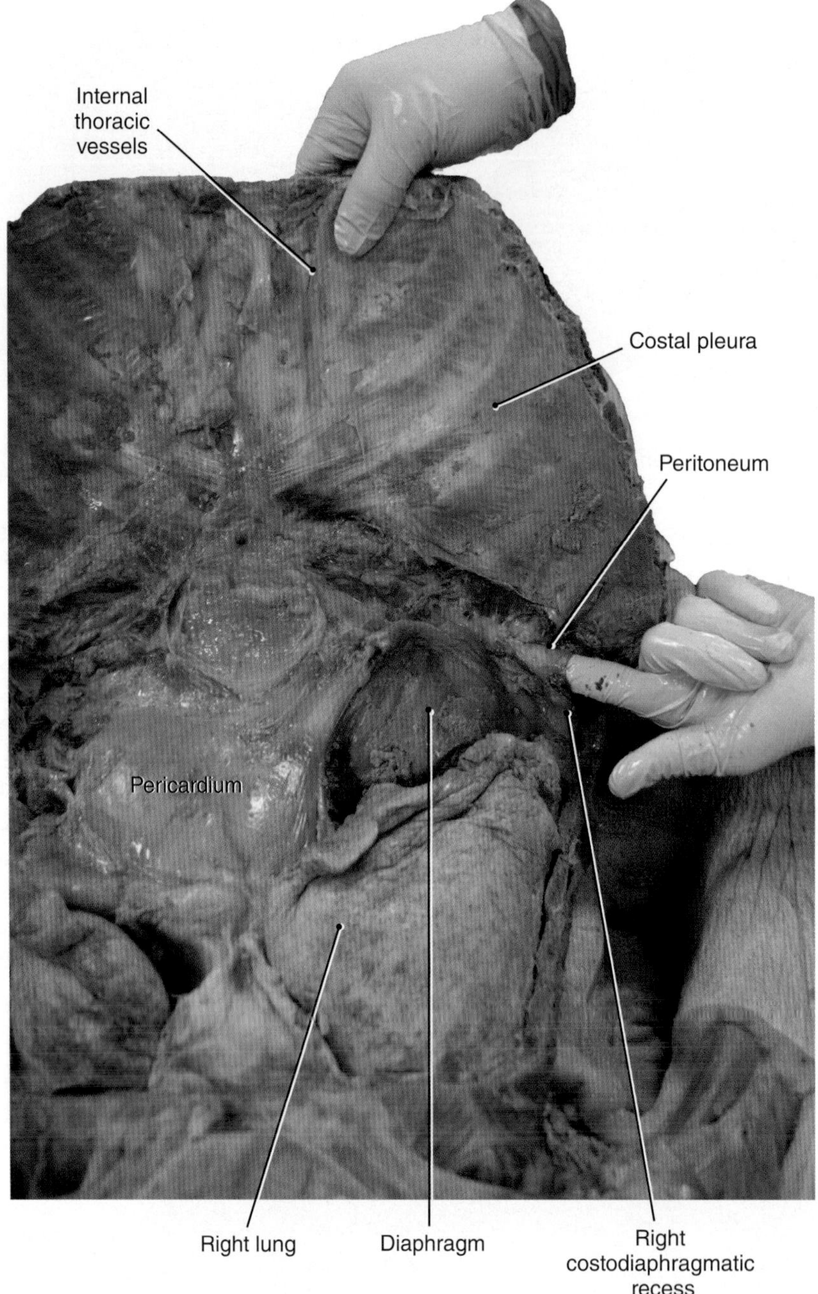

Fig. 5.17 Elevation of the anterior thoracic wall noting the identification of the adjacent parietal peritoneum.

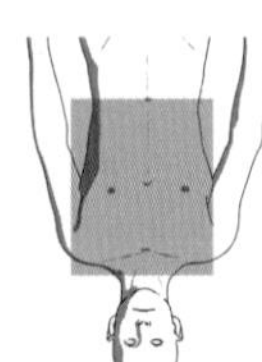

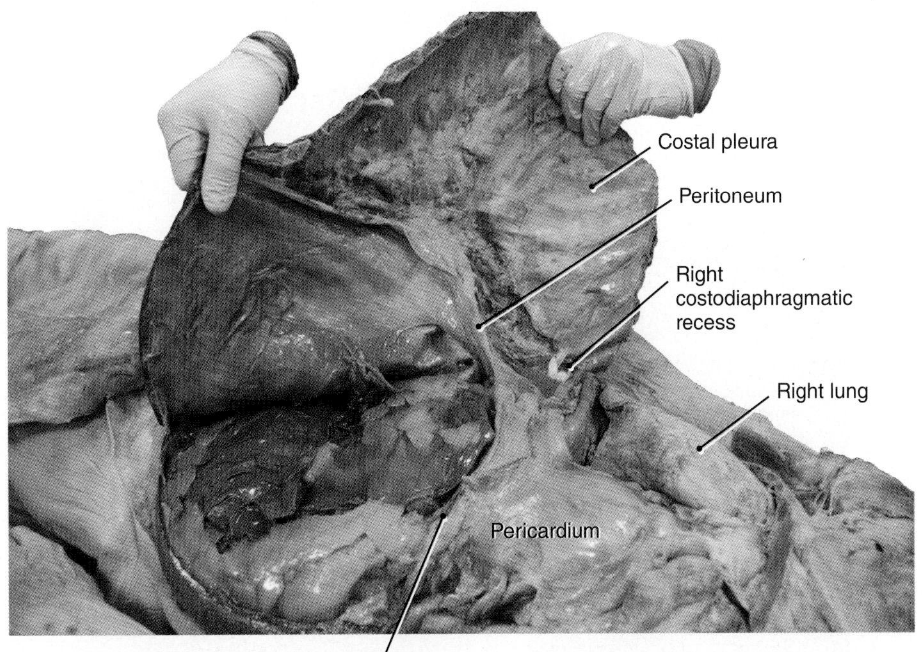

Fig. 5.18 Elevation of the anterior thoracic and abdominal walls.

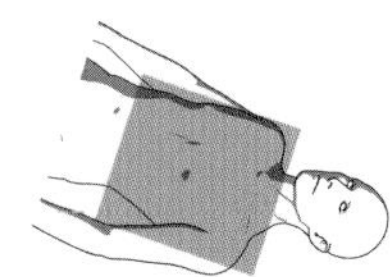

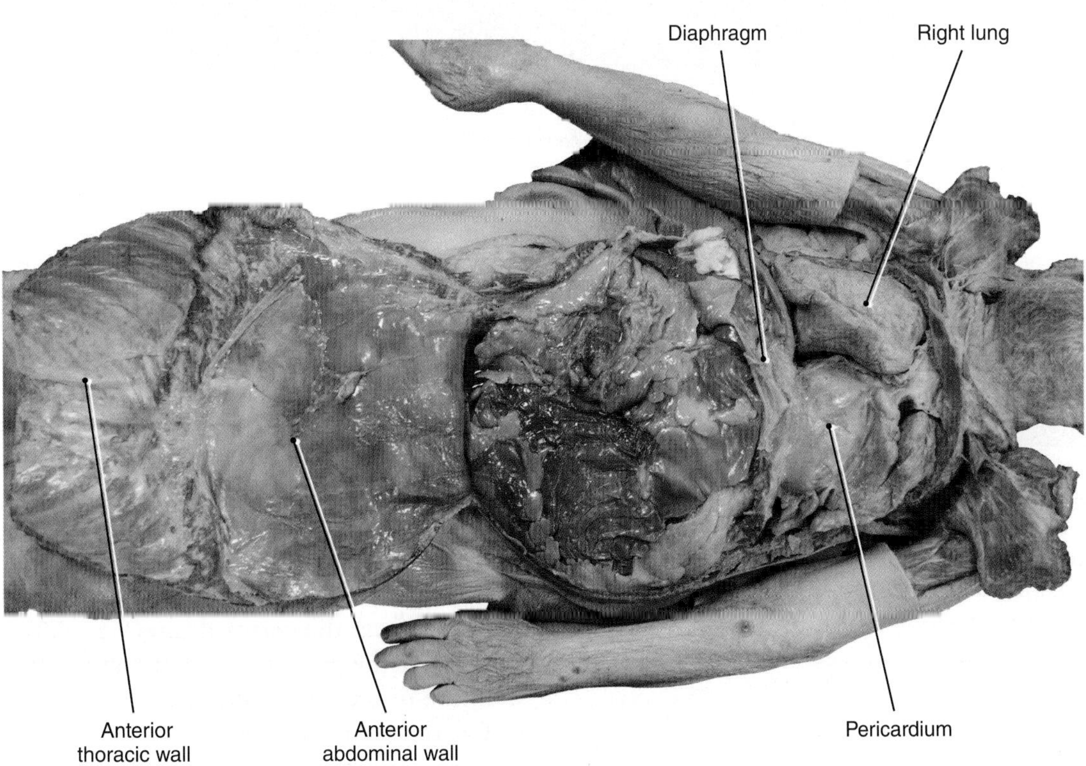

Fig. 5.19 Complete reflection of the anterior thoracic and abdominal walls.

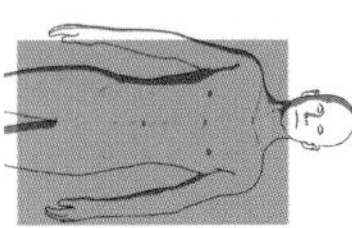

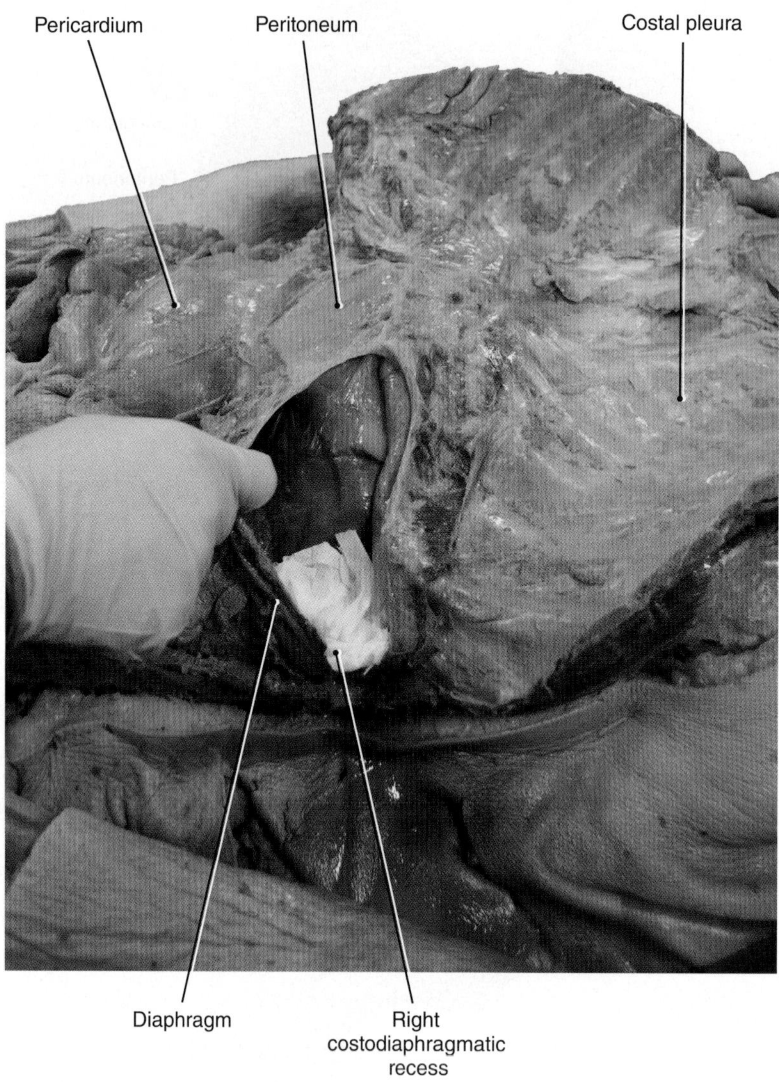

Fig. 5.20 Paper towel placed into the right costodiaphragmatic recess.

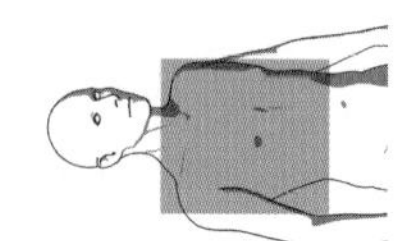

DISSECTION TIP

Place your finger at the costodiaphragmatic recess just underneath the peritoneum and slowly start separating the tissues next to it. In some specimens there may be attachments between the transverse colon and the peritoneum. Separate these carefully. Place paper towels in the costodiaphragmatic recess to absorb the fluid collections (Fig. 5.20).

- **Identify the costodiaphragmatic and costomediastinal recesses.**
- **After inspecting the subdivisions of the parietal pleura, push the lung away from the heart with your fingertips.**
- **Identify the mediastinal pleura separating the lung from the pericardial sac.**
- **Insert the scissors and separate the mediastinal pleura from the pericardium (Figs. 5.21 and 5.22).**
- **Identify the phrenic nerve traveling anterior to the hilum of the lung and preserve it (Fig. 5.23).**
- **Use the separation technique to expose the pulmonary arteries and veins (Fig. 5.24).**
- **Use the same technique for the contralateral lung (Figs. 5.25 and 5.26).**

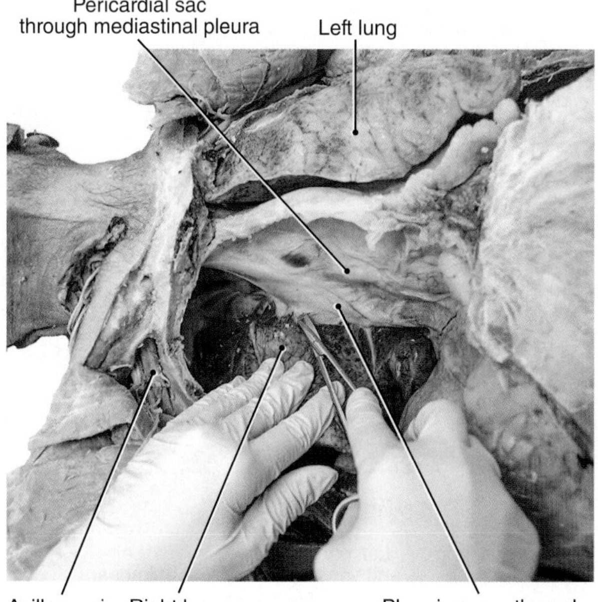

Fig. 5.21 Anterior thoracic structures with right lung reflected to expose mediastinum to dissect for lung removal.

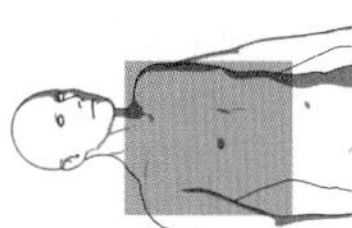

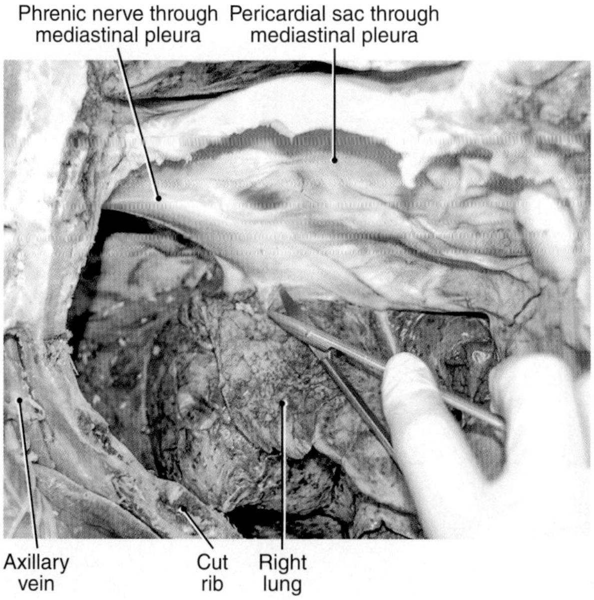

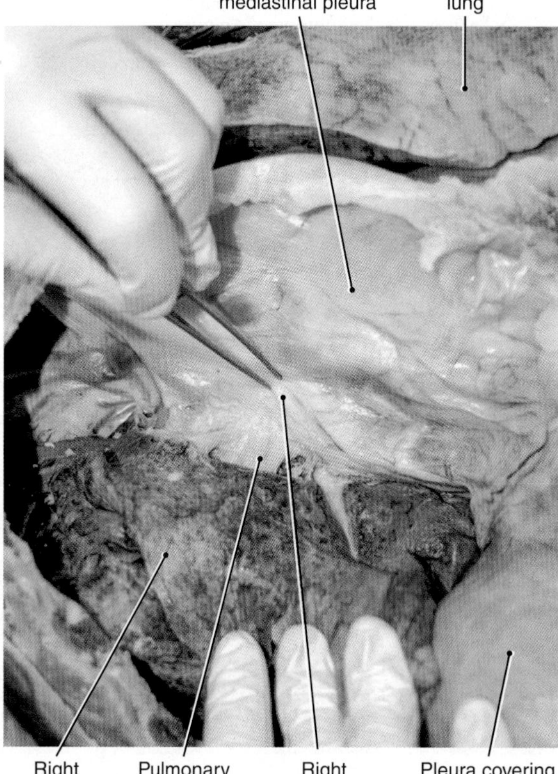

Fig. 5.23 Anterior structures of the thorax with right lung reflected to reveal mediastinum, highlighting phrenic nerve through the mediastinal pleura.

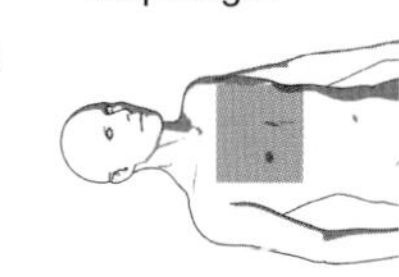

Fig. 5.22 Thoracic structures with right lung reflected to expose mediastinum.

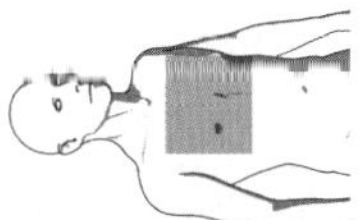

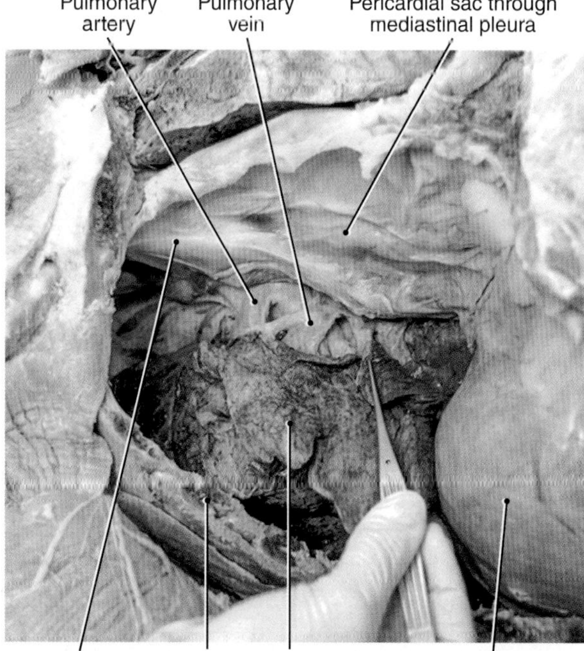

Fig. 5.24 In the right pleural cavity, the pulmonary artery and vein are seen.

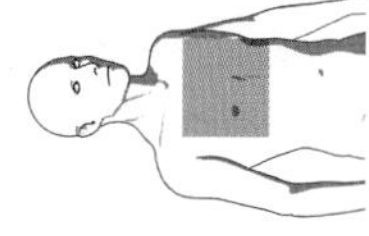

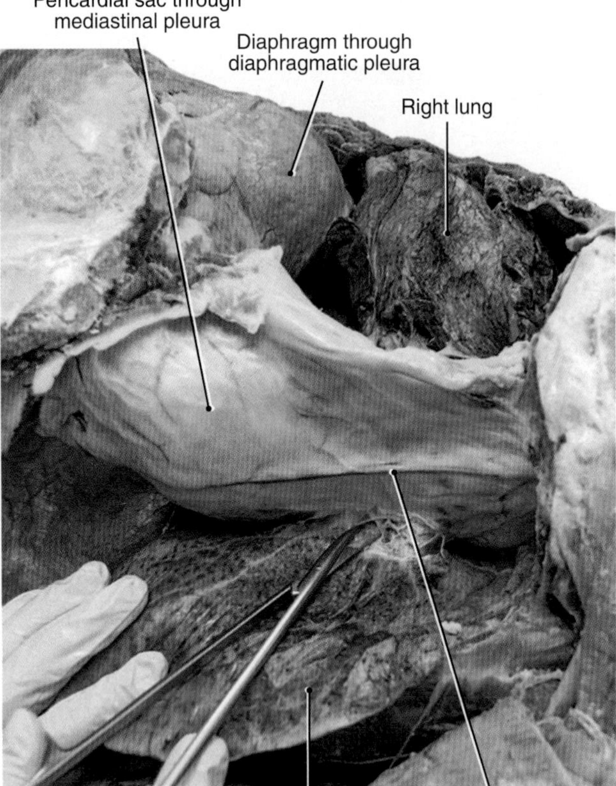

Fig. 5.25 Anterior thoracic structures with left lung reflected for hilar dissection.

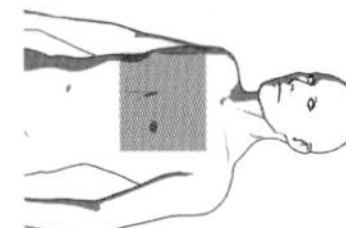

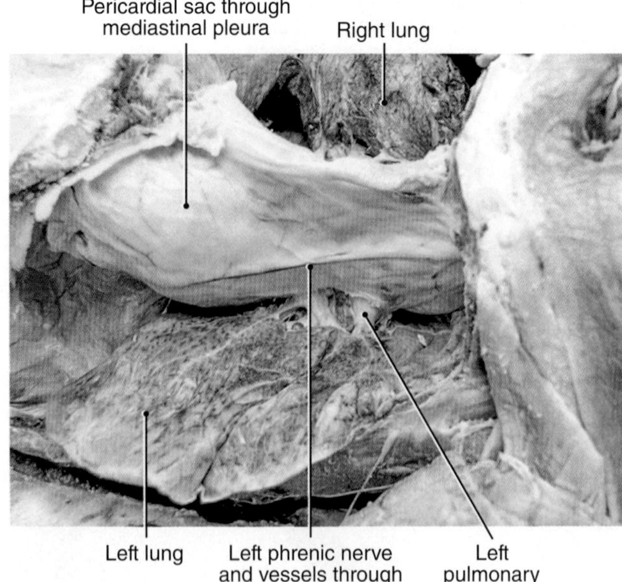

Fig. 5.26 Anterior thoracic structures with left lung reflected for hilar dissection, revealing pulmonary vessels.

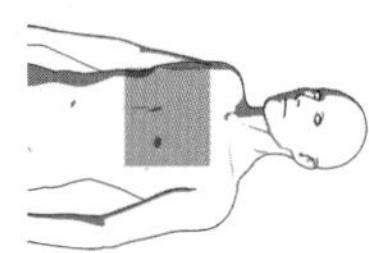

DISSECTION **TIP**

The costodiaphragmatic recess is usually the location where excess embalming fluids accumulate during dissection. Drain the fluid using a syringe and place paper towels into the recess (Figs. 5.27 and 5.28). Also, once the lungs are removed, holes can be made in the posterior intercostal spaces so that fluid exits onto the dissection table. This method may necessitate placing a wedge or block under the thorax to lift the body slightly off the dissecting table.

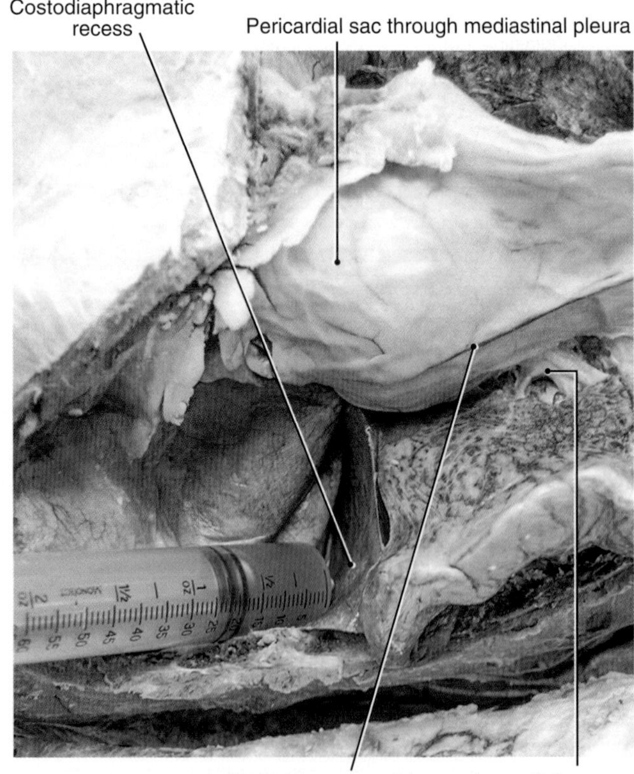

Fig. 5.27 Anterolateral view of deep thoracic dissection. Syringe is placed into the costodiaphragmatic recess, and excess fluid is aspirated.

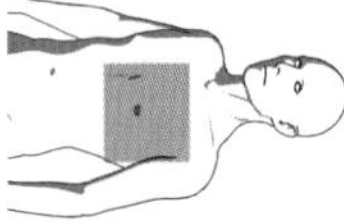

- **After exposing the pulmonary veins, pulmonary arteries, and primary bronchi at the hila of the left and right lungs, transect them with scissors or a scalpel (Figs. 5.29–5.31 and Plate 5.1).**
- **Remove the lungs from the thoracic cavity and observe the posterior mediastinum covered with parietal pleura (Figs. 5.32–5.35).**

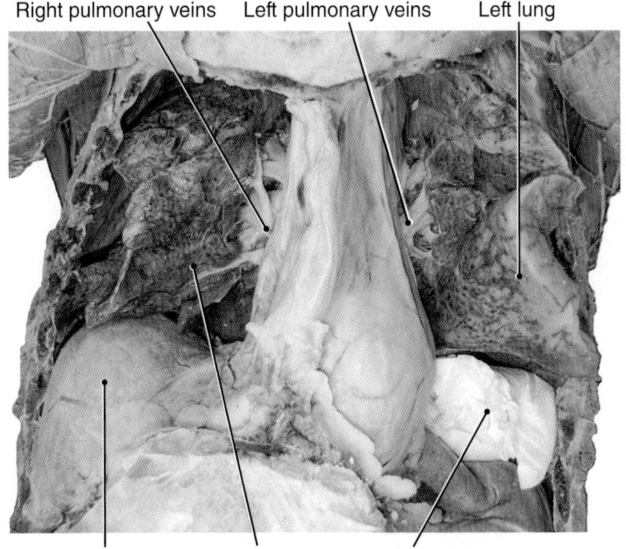

Fig. 5.28 Anterior thoracic wall removed, revealing deep structures. Right and left pulmonary veins are exposed.

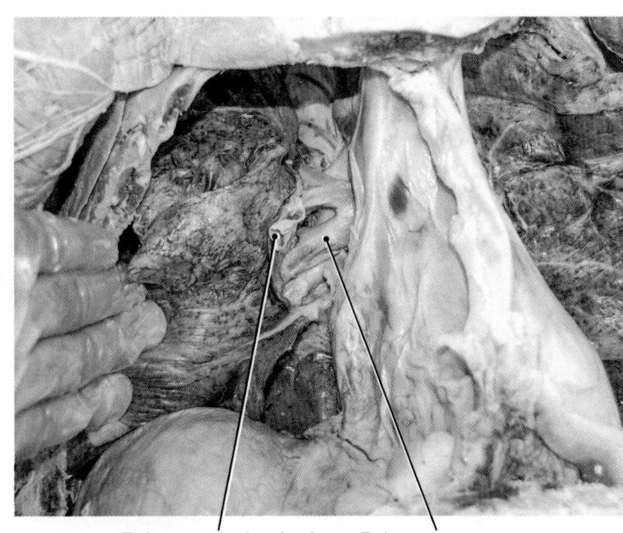

Fig. 5.30 Right lung retraction revealing pulmonary artery after pulmonary veins have been cut.

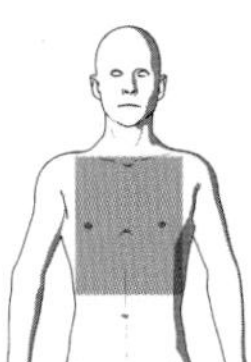

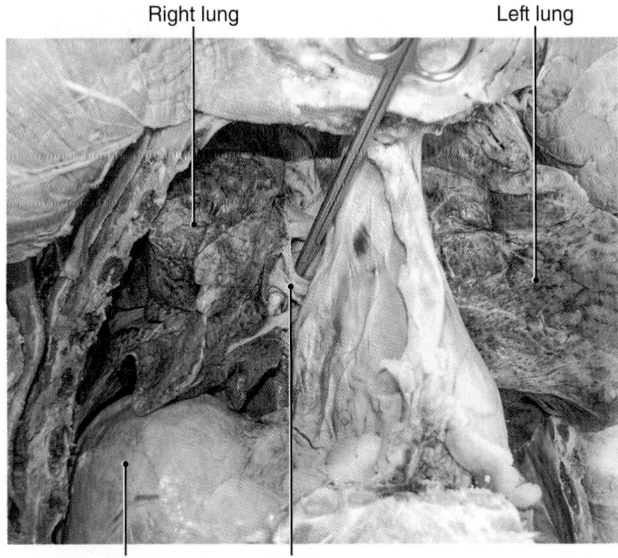

Fig. 5.29 Right pulmonary vein exposed and lifted upward for transection.

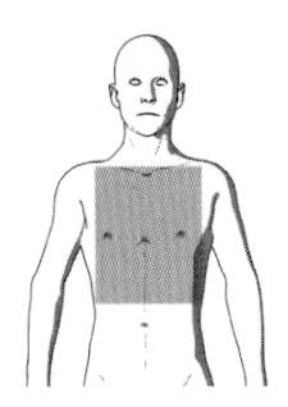

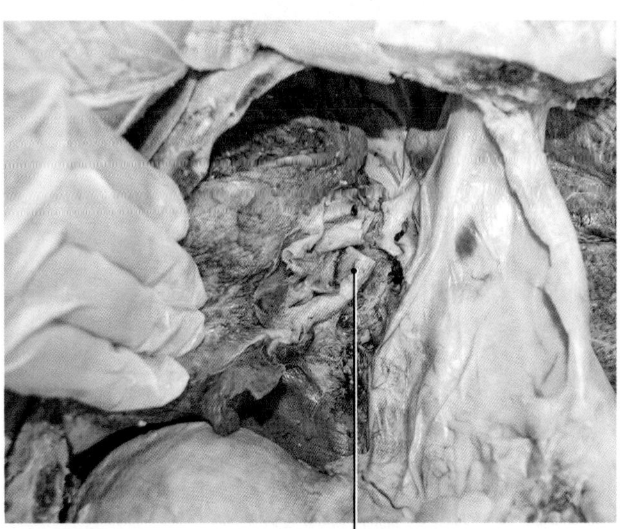

Fig. 5.31 Right lung pulmonary vasculature and airway (primary bronchus) transected.

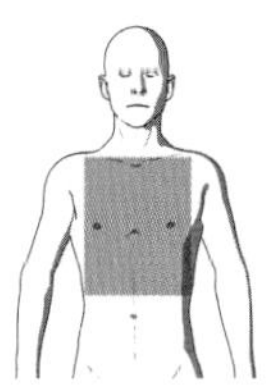

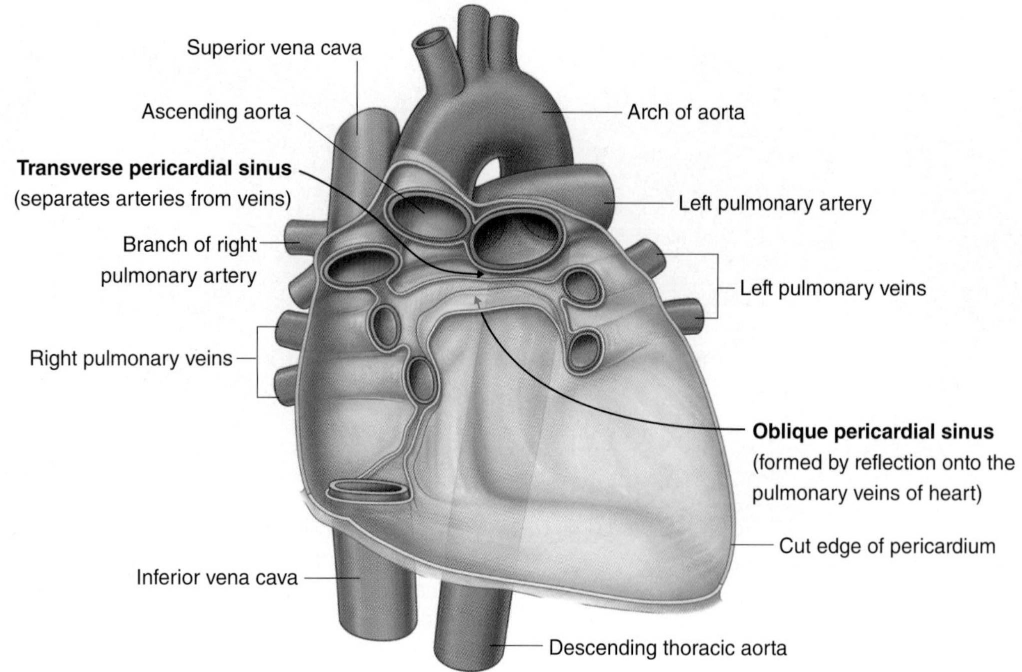

Plate 5.1 Pericardial sac with heart removed. (From Drake et al., *Gray's Anatomy for Students*, 5th edition, Philadelphia, Elsevier, 2024, Figure 3.63, p. 189.)

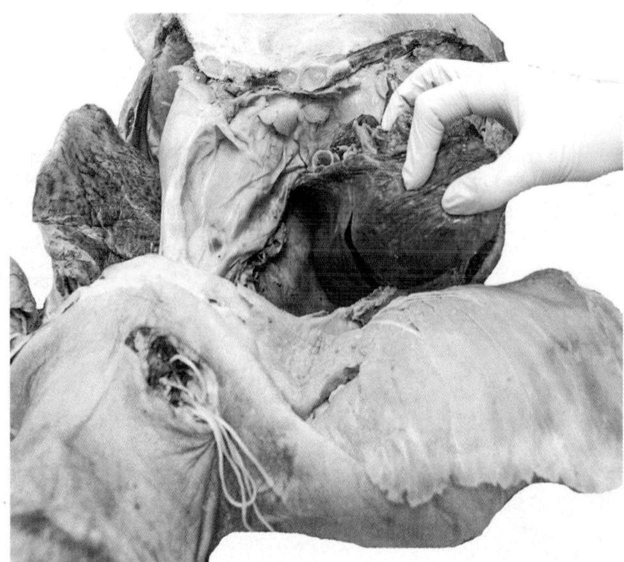

Fig. 5.32 Removal of right lung from superior to inferior with lateral retraction.

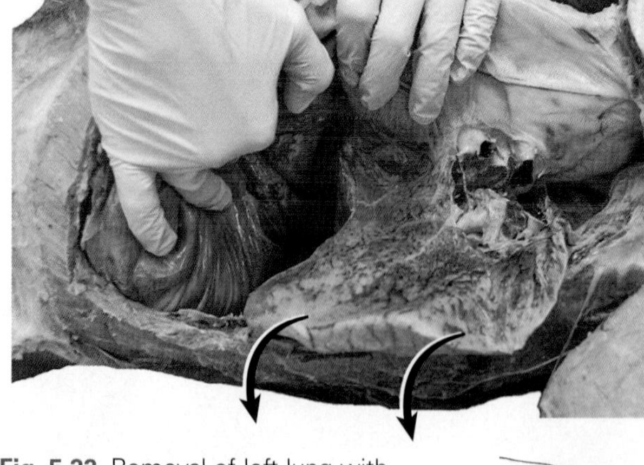

Fig. 5.33 Removal of left lung with pulmonary vasculature and bronchi transected, using medial retraction.

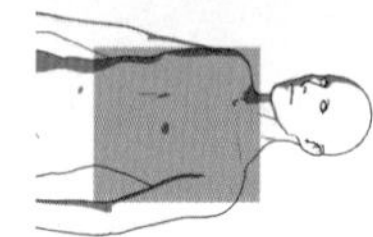

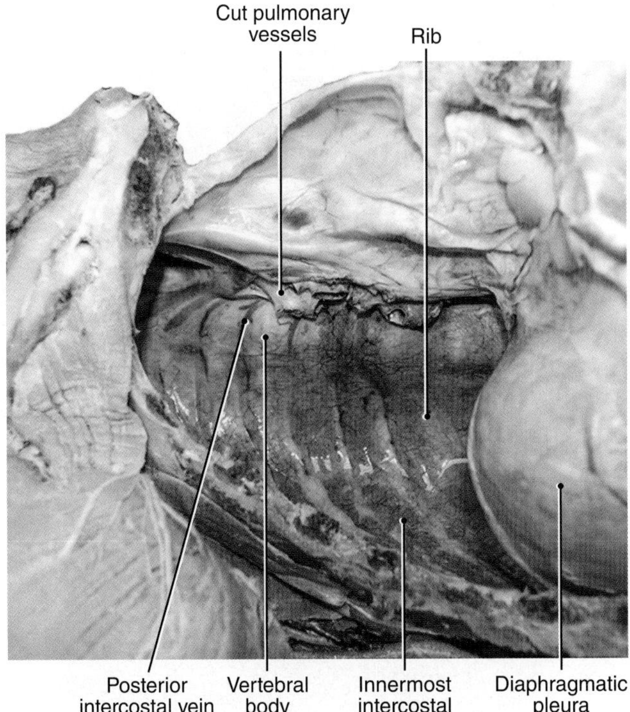

Fig. 5.34 Right hemithorax with lung removed, revealing vertebral column and posterior thoracic wall.

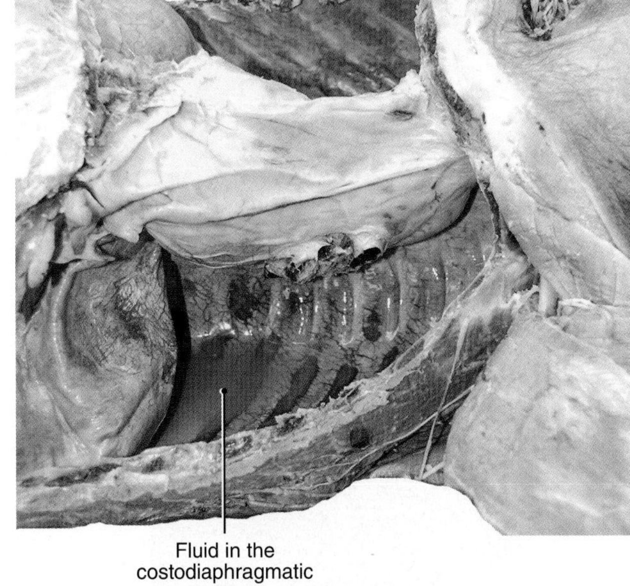

Fig. 5.35 Bilateral lung removal with intact pericardial sac and contents.

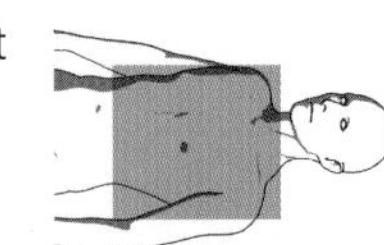

DISSECTION TIP

Often the lungs have adhesions far inferior and posterior to the hilum of the lung. To remove the lung completely, push the diaphragm inferiorly and explore with your fingertips the area posterior and inferior to the hilum so that such adhesions can be dissected free (see Fig. 5.35).

- **Place the lungs onto a tray and examine the internal surface of each lung separately. For the right lung, identify the oblique and horizontal fissures and their corresponding upper, middle, and lower lobes (Fig. 5.36).**
- **Inspect the hilum of the lung and identify the pulmonary arteries, pulmonary veins, and primary bronchi (Fig. 5.37).**

DISSECTION TIP

Note that the horizontal fissure often appears to be incomplete in the right lungs. To identify the pulmonary arteries and pulmonary veins at the hilum of the lung, note that the pulmonary veins are located along the anterior aspect of the hilum, where the pulmonary arteries usually are located superior and anterior to the bronchi (see Fig. 5.37).

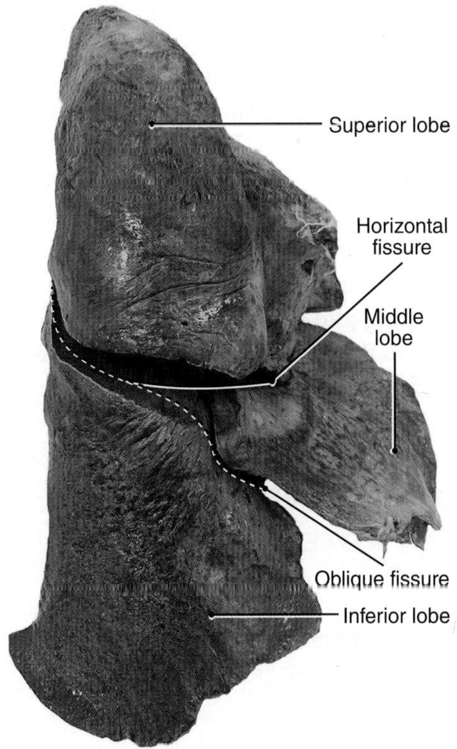

Fig. 5.36 Right lung with anterolateral surfaces.

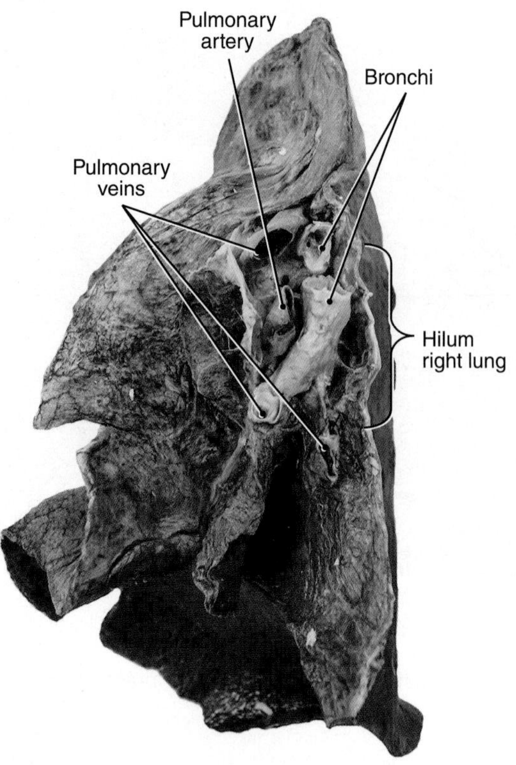

Fig. 5.37 Right lung (medial view) highlighting structures of the hilum.

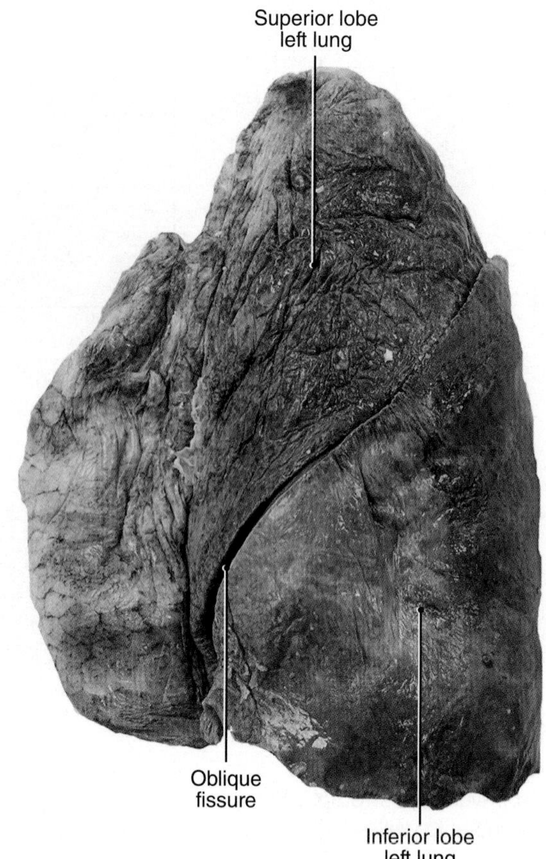

Fig. 5.38 Left lung.

- **Similar to the right lung, identify the oblique fissure in the left lung and the corresponding upper and lower lobes (Fig. 5.38).**
- **Inspect the hilum of the lung and identify the pulmonary arteries, pulmonary veins, and primary bronchi (Fig. 5.39).**
- **Identify the cardiac notch on the superior lobe of the left lung and lingula.**
- **Inferior to the hilum, trace the two layers of visceral pleura fusing together to form the pulmonary ligament (Fig. 5.40).**

OPTIONAL LUNG DISSECTION

ANATOMY **NOTE**

The lung contents can be dissected to expose a single segmental bronchus, segmental artery, and segmental vein. The portion of lung supplied by the segmental bronchus, artery, and vein is defined as a *bronchopulmonary segment.*

- **With your forceps, lift the bronchus, and using blunt dissection, separate it from the lung parenchyma.**
- **Remove most of the internal lung parenchyma with your forceps and scissors, leaving its borders and lateral walls intact (Fig. 5.41).**
- **In the right lung, you will be able to dissect the superior, middle, and inferior lobar bronchi.**

ANATOMY **NOTE**

Each lobar bronchus branches off into several segmental bronchi, and each of these supplies one bronchopulmonary segment. The right lung contains 10 to 12 bronchopulmonary segments, and the left lung contains 10.

ANATOMY **NOTE**

When you reach a bronchopulmonary segment, note the relationships among the artery, vein, and bronchus. The segmental arteries are located posterior to the segmental bronchi, and the segmental veins are between two adjacent bronchopulmonary segments.

ANATOMY **NOTE**

As it passes superior to the right pulmonary artery, the right superior lobar bronchus is termed the *eparterial bronchus.*

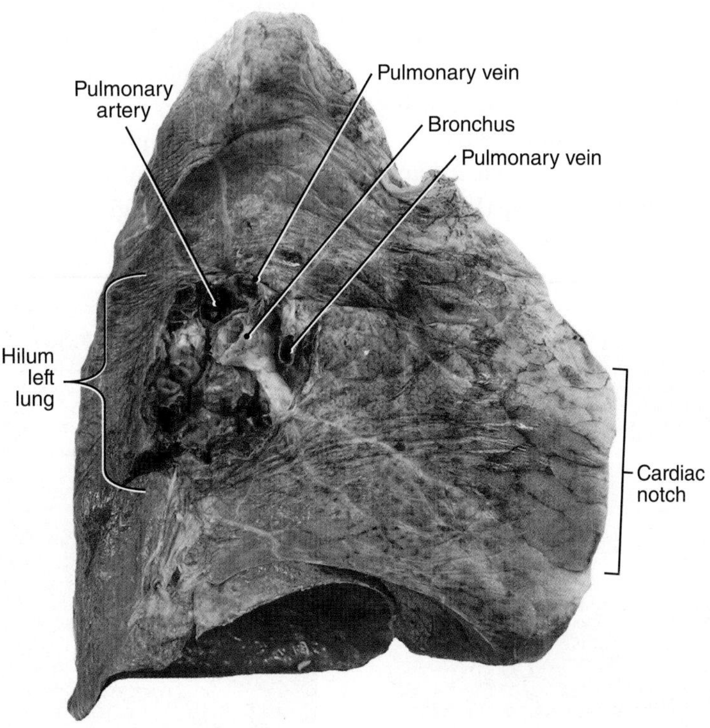

Fig. 5.39 Removal of left lung with medial view highlighting structures at the hilum.

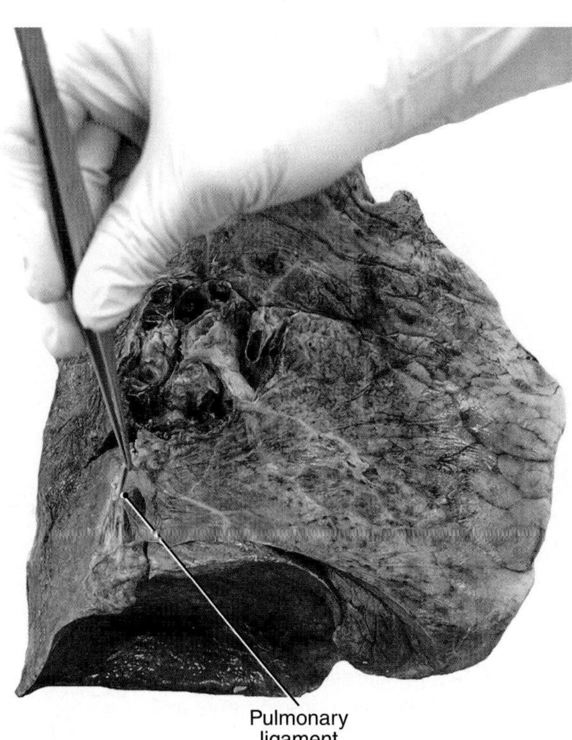

Fig. 5.40 Removal of left lung with medial view highlighting the pulmonary ligament.

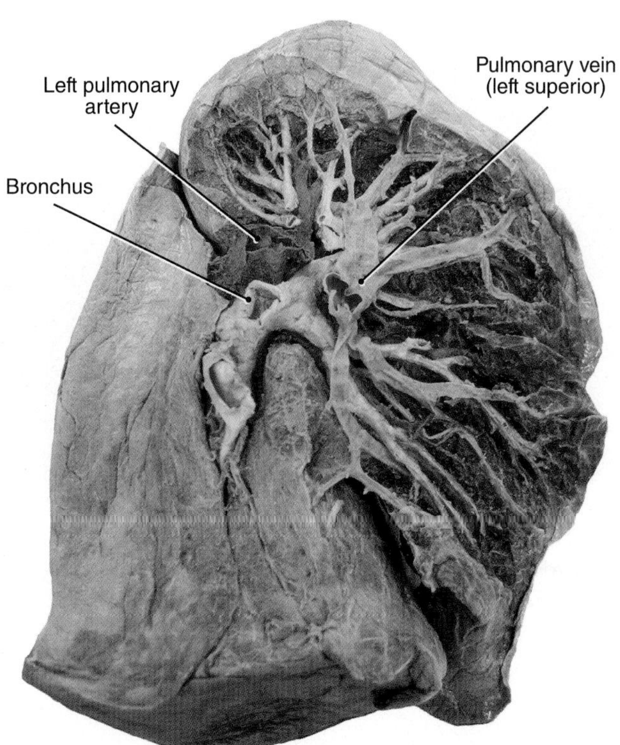

Fig. 5.41 Removal of left lung with medial view illustrating bronchopulmonary segments.

REMOVAL OF THE HEART

- **Before removing the heart from the pericardial cavity, the phrenic nerves must be identified and preserved. Observe the pericardiacophrenic vein at the lateral border of the pericardial sac bilaterally.**
- **Dissect the pericardium next to the pericardiacophrenic vein and identify the phrenic nerve (Figs. 5.42 and 5.43).**

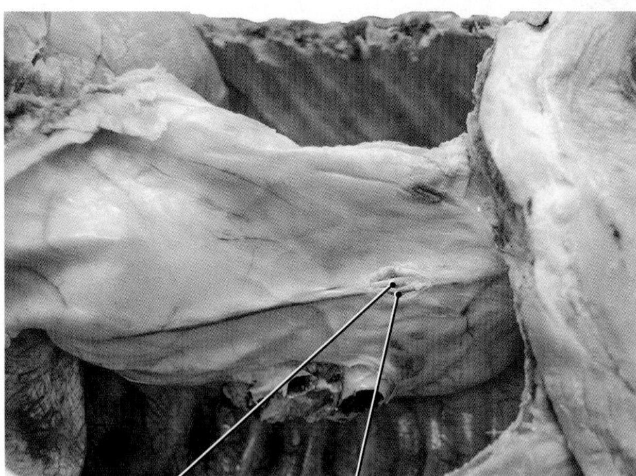

Fig. 5.42 Bilateral lung removal with intact pericardial sac and contents.

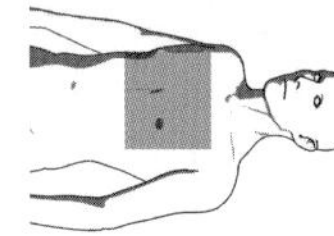

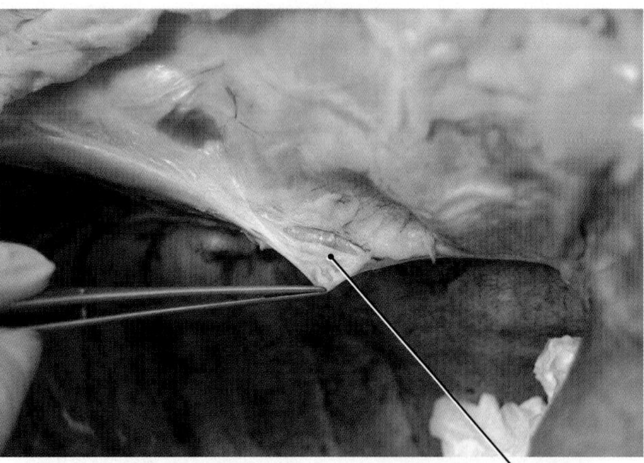

Fig. 5.43 Left side of the thorax with intact pericardial sac, revealing left phrenic nerve.

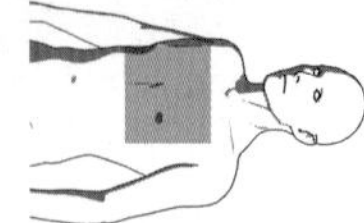

ANATOMY NOTE

The phrenic nerve is accompanied by the pericardiacophrenic artery, a branch of the internal thoracic artery.

- **Dissect the phrenic nerve along its entire length, from the top of the thoracic cavity to its penetration of the diaphragm (Figs. 5.44 and 5.45).**

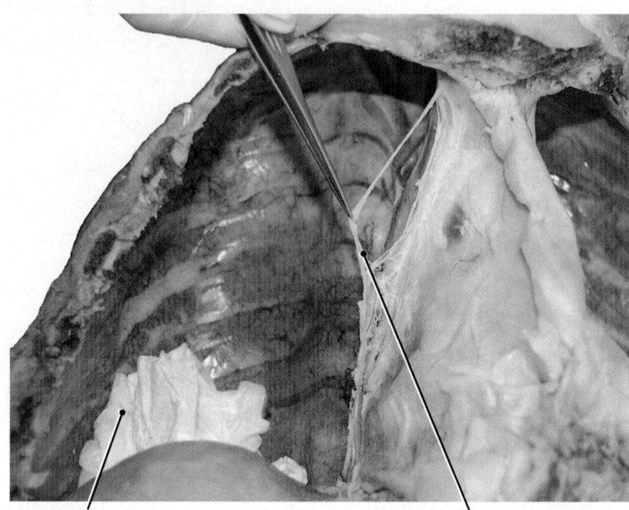

Fig. 5.44 Bilateral lung removal with intact pericardial sac and contents, exposing the right phrenic nerve.

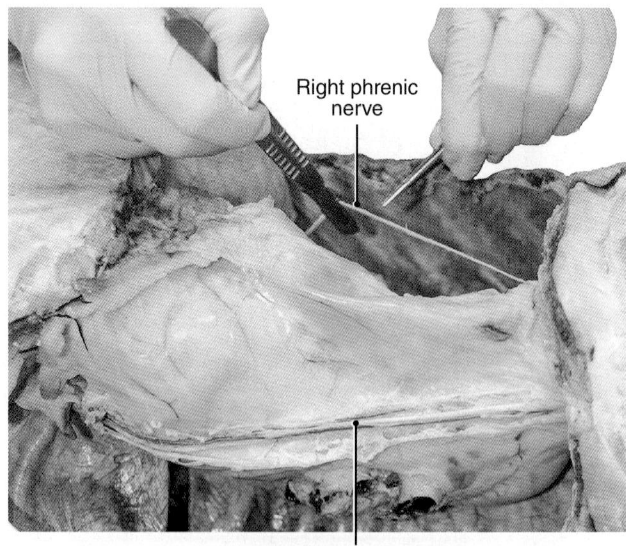

Fig. 5.45 Intact pericardial sac and contents with dissected phrenic nerve and pericardiacophrenic vessels.

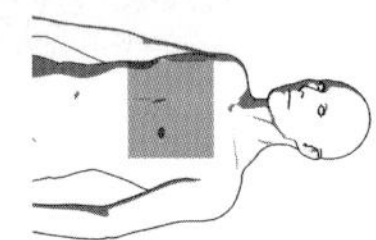

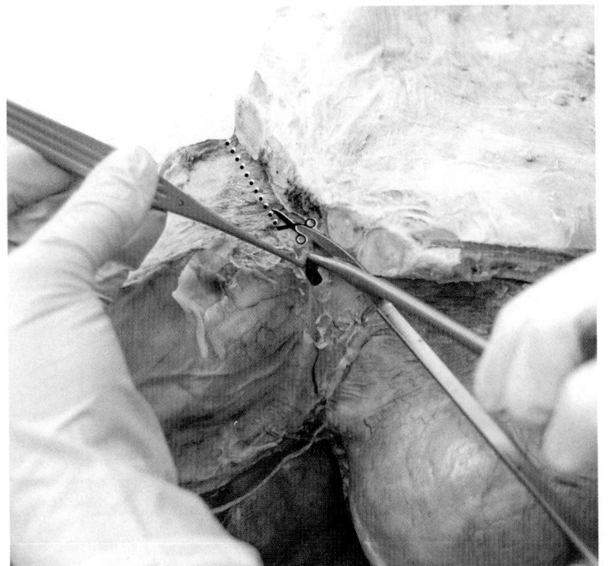

Fig. 5.46 Anterior view of pericardial sac with tracing for transverse incision *(dotted line)* of pericardial sac.

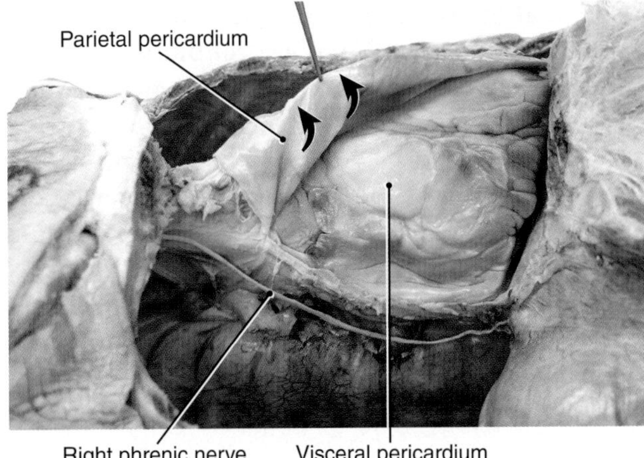

Fig. 5.48 Reflected pericardial sac revealing visceral pericardium of heart.

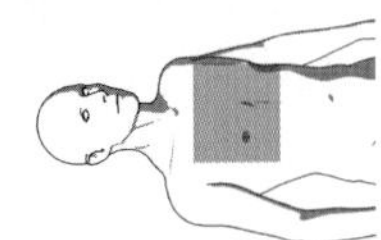

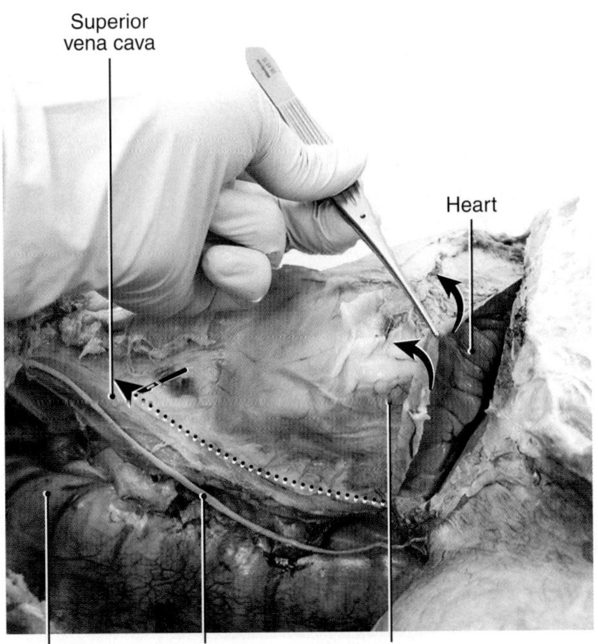

Fig. 5.47 Anterolateral view of pericardial sac with base reflected *(black arrows)* and tracing for lateral vertical incision *(dotted line)*.

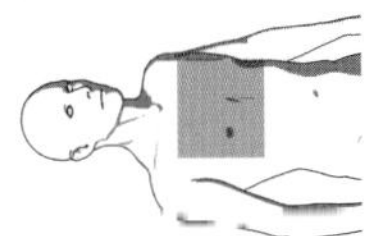

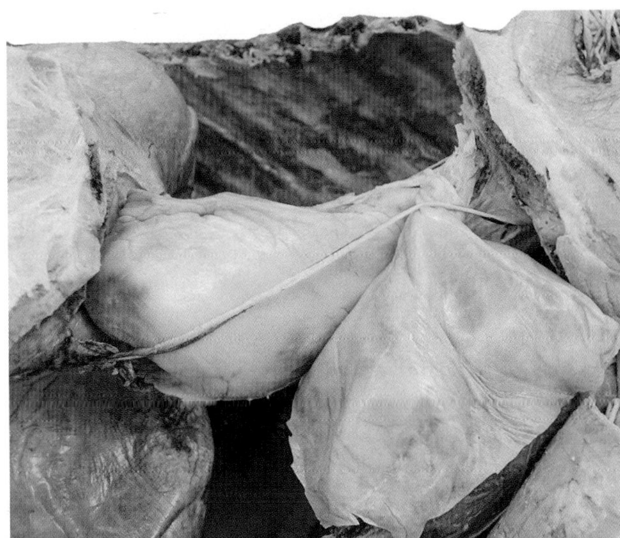

Fig. 5.49 Anterolateral reflection of pericardial sac while maintaining an intact left phrenic nerve.

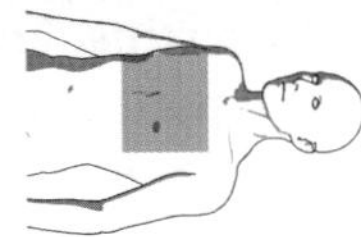

- **With toothed forceps, lift the right inferolateral edge of the pericardium near the diaphragm and make a small incision (Fig. 5.46).**
- **Note the attachment of the pericardium to the central tendon of the diaphragm.**
- **Make a transverse incision in the pericardium parallel to the diaphragmatic surface (Fig. 5.47).**

DISSECTION TIP

When the pericardial sac is first opened, a small amount of serous fluid is often seen.

- **Make a second, connecting vertical incision through the pericardium along the side of the right atrium (Fig. 5.48) and along the side of the left ventricle (Fig. 5.49).**

○ Note that the parietal pericardium and the visceral pericardium (epicardium) are continuous with the great vessels as they pierce the fibrous pericardium.

EXTERNAL INSPECTION

○ For orientation of the heart within the pericardial cavity, observe the position of the right atrium, right auricle, right ventricle and its outflow tract, and pulmonary trunk. Note the left atrium, left ventricle and apex of the heart, and anterior and posterior interventricular grooves.

ANATOMY **NOTE**

The right ventricle forms the sternocostal surface and part of the diaphragmatic surface of the heart. The left or pulmonary surface is composed mainly of the left ventricle. The right ventricle forms the sternocostal surface and part of the diaphragmatic surface of the heart. Note that the right ventricle is the most anterior part of the heart and is almost in contact with the sternum.

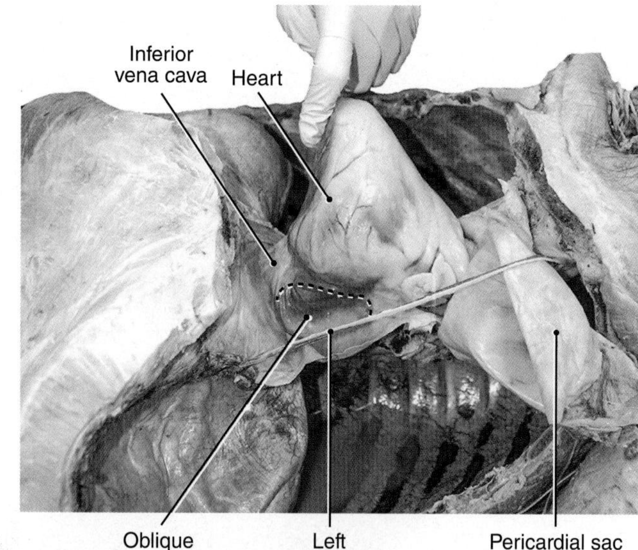

Fig. 5.50 Reflected pericardial sac with apex of heart reflected anteriorly to reveal the oblique sinus *(dotted line)*.

SINUSES

ANATOMY **NOTE**

Note the position of the inferior vena cava, which is located inferior and to the right between the heart and the diaphragm.

ANATOMY **NOTE**

The reflections of the pericardium lead to the formation of two so-called sinuses within the pericardial cavity, the transverse and oblique pericardial sinuses.

○ To identify the oblique pericardial sinus, lift the apex of the heart laterally and to the right with your fingertips, and expose the blindly ending space in the pericardial cavity behind the heart great vessels (Fig. 5.50).

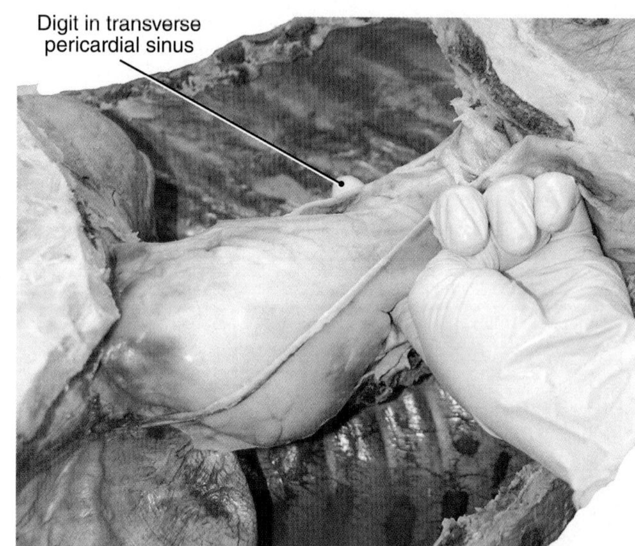

Fig. 5.51 Reflected pericardial sac with placement of digit through transverse sinus.

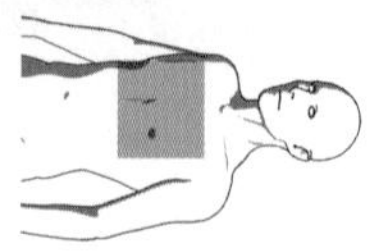

ANATOMY **NOTE**

The venous hilum contains the four pulmonary veins and the superior and inferior vena cava. The sleeve-like investment of visceral pericardium around these vessels and the roof of the left atrium reflects to show the parietal pericardial sac, forming the inverted, U-shaped oblique sinus.

○ If you place your fingers in front of the atria and directly behind the aorta and pulmonary artery, you will occupy the space known as the *transverse pericardial sinus* (Fig. 5.51).

TECHNIQUE

○ To remove the heart, first lift its apex upward and expose the inferior vena cava, then transect it (Figs. 5.52 and 5.53).

○ With scissors, separate the adhesions between the heart (posteriorly) and pericardium and lift the heart upward to expose the left atrium (Figs. 5.54 and 5.55).

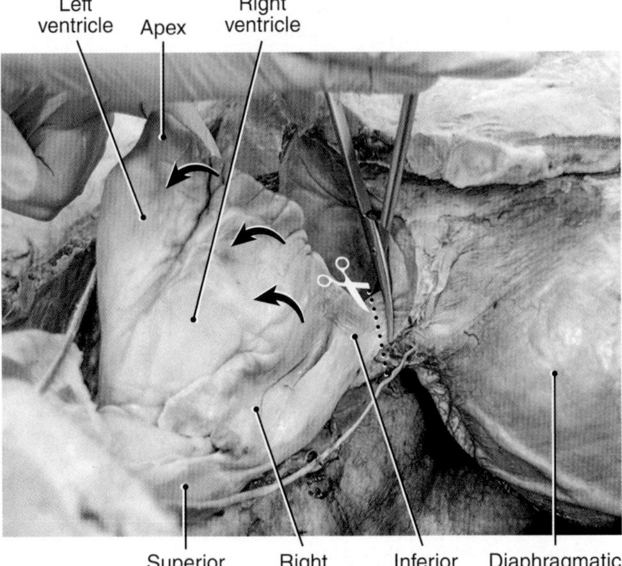

Fig. 5.52 Apex of heart reflected anteriorly to allow transection of the inferior vena cava.

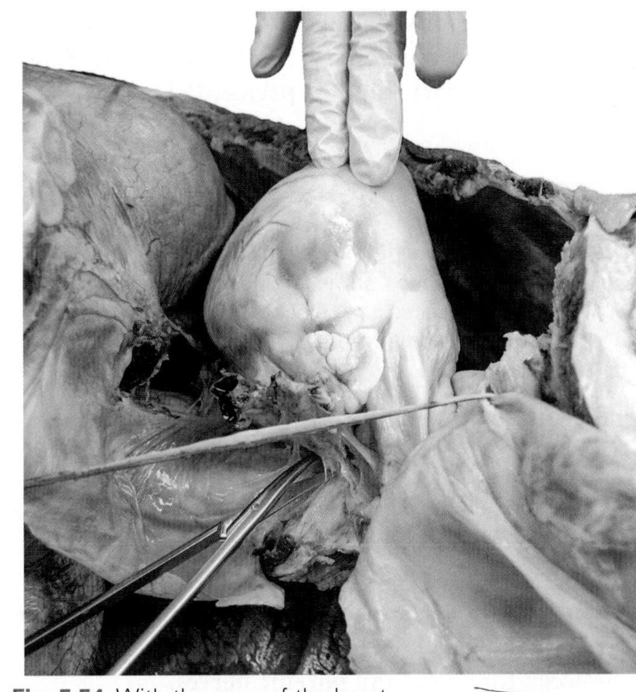

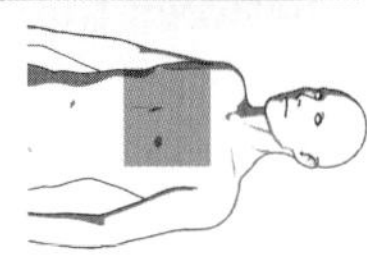

Fig. 5.54 With the apex of the heart elevated, scissors are used to separate the pericardium from the posterior surface of the heart.

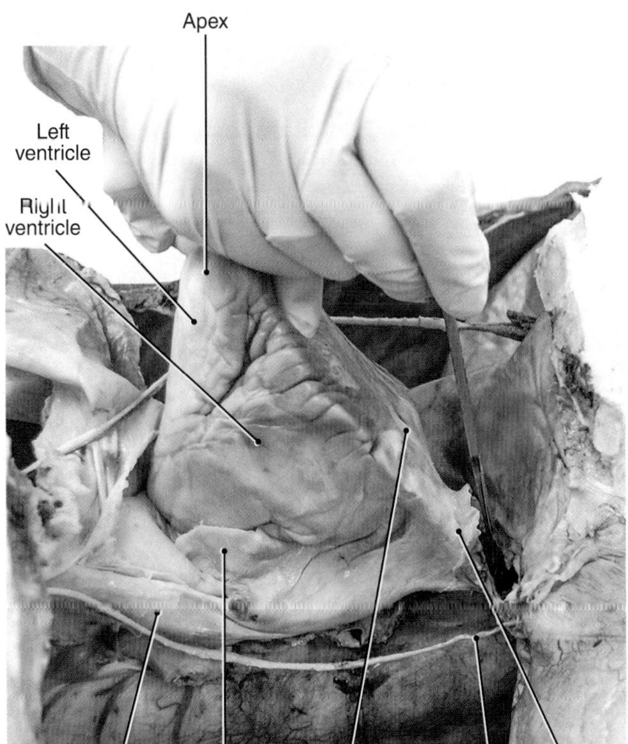

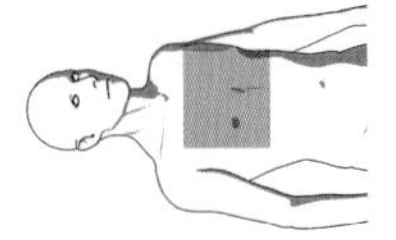

Fig. 5.53 Apex of heart reflected anteriorly to allow transection of the inferior vena cava.

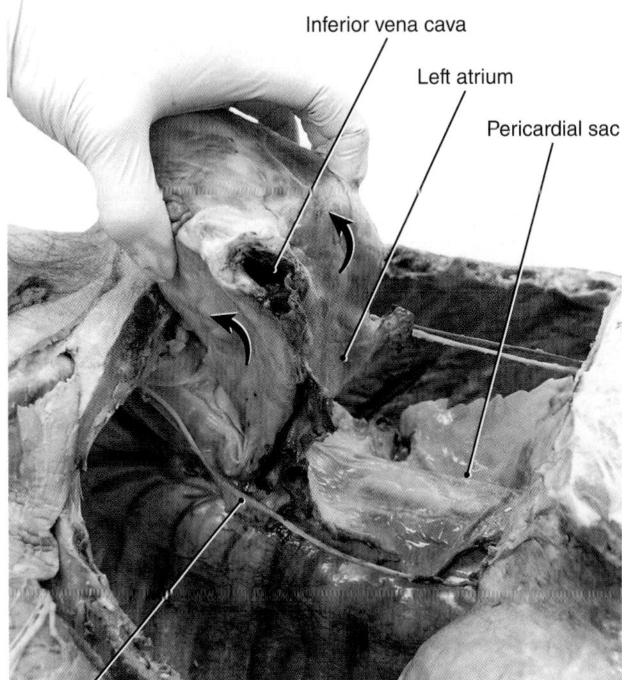

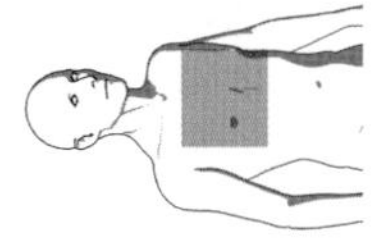

Fig. 5.55 Apex of heart reflected anterosuperiorly, revealing cut inferior vena cava, left atrium, and posterior pericardial structures.

- **Cut the superior vena cava. Next, cut the ascending aorta and the pulmonary trunk (Figs. 5.56–5.58). Remove the heart from the pericardial cavity.**

DISSECTION **TIP**

In some hearts, the pulmonary veins are adherent to the pericardium. Place some tension on the heart and lift it upward. If necessary, place the scissors between the pulmonary veins and the pericardium and separate the two.

- **Observe the left side of the thoracic cavity, specifically the lateral side of the aortic arch and the pulmonary trunk (Figs. 5.59 and 5.60).**
- **Identify and trace the left vagus nerve over the arch of the aorta (Fig. 5.61). Note the relationship between the vagus and phrenic nerves.**

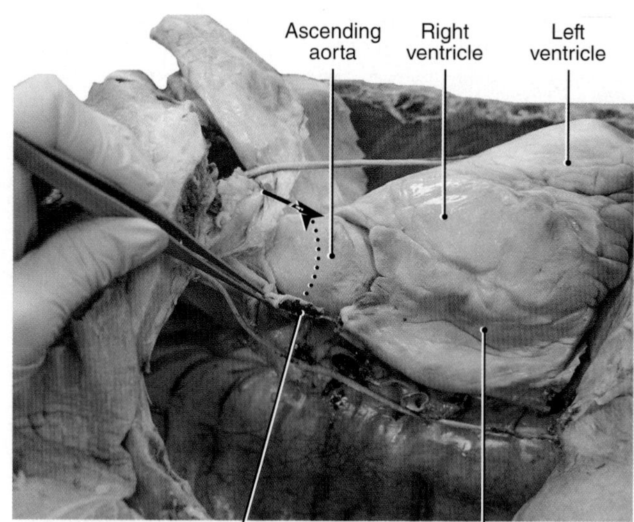

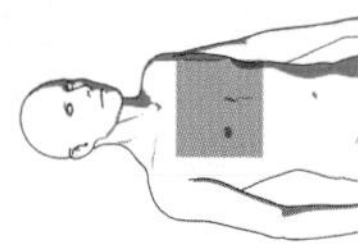

Fig. 5.56 With the pericardial sac displaced laterally and the superior vena cava cut, the ascending aorta is identified. The *dotted line* notes the region of the aorta to be transected.

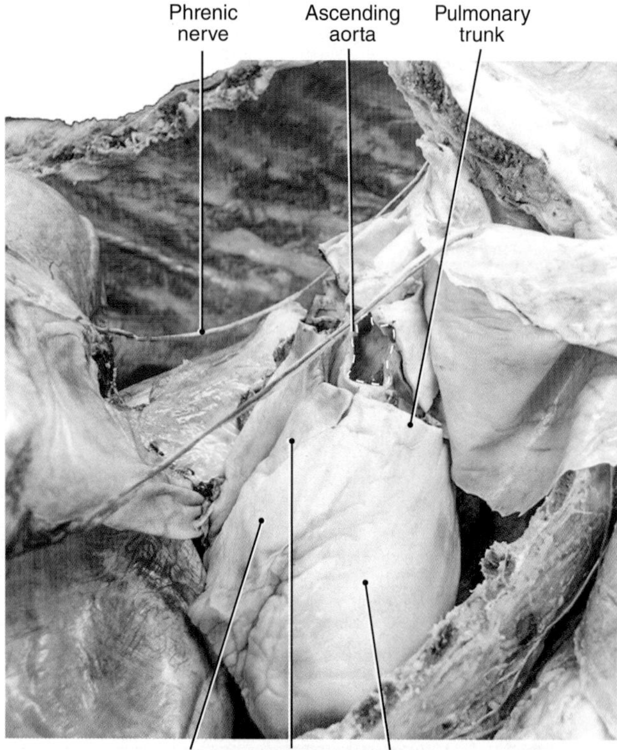

Fig. 5.57 External view of heart with transected great vessels.

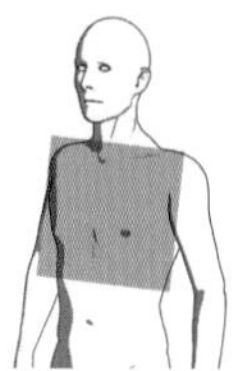

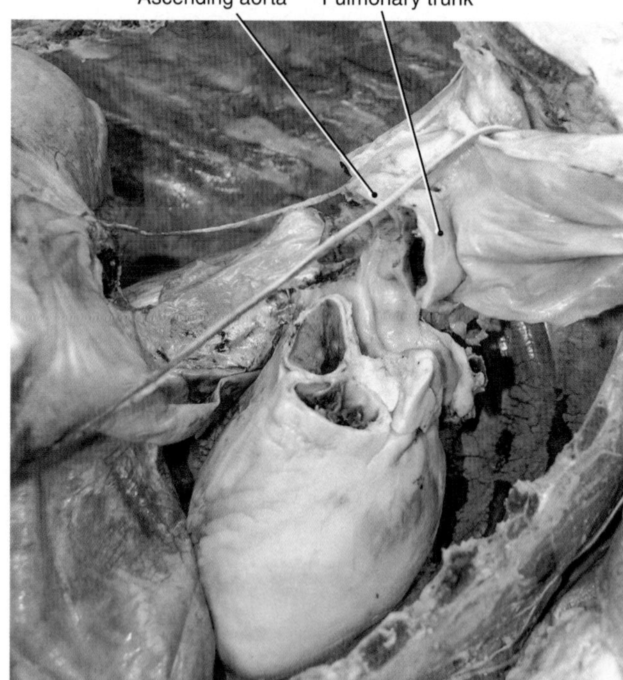

Fig. 5.58 External view of heart with transected great vessels.

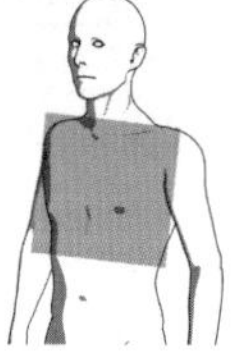

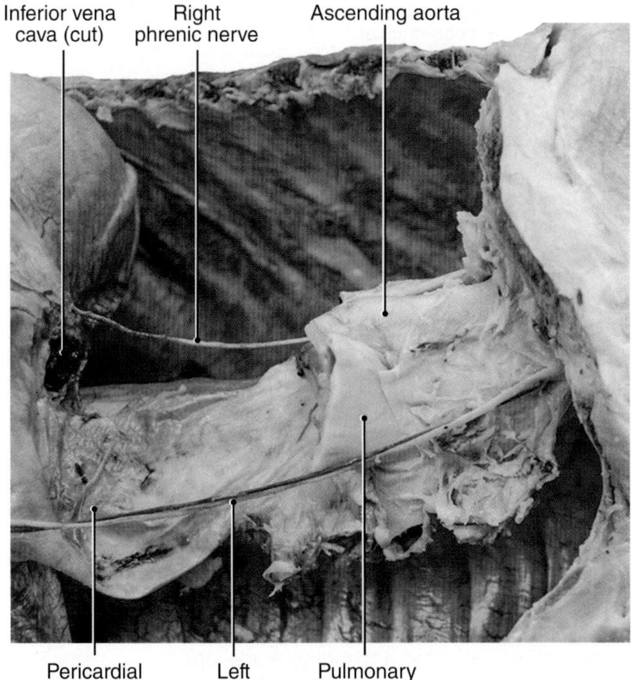

Fig. 5.59 Bilateral lung removal, with the anterior part of the pericardial sac and heart removed.

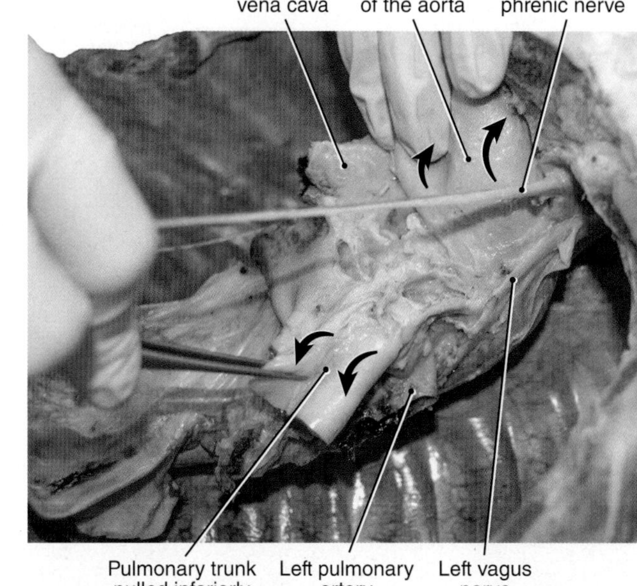

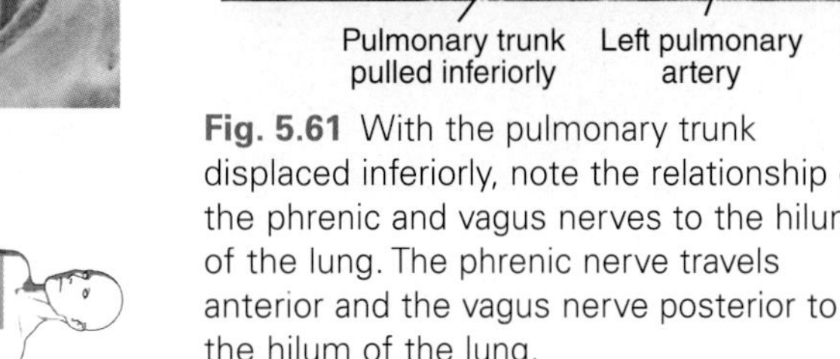

Fig. 5.61 With the pulmonary trunk displaced inferiorly, note the relationship of the phrenic and vagus nerves to the hilum of the lung. The phrenic nerve travels anterior and the vagus nerve posterior to the hilum of the lung.

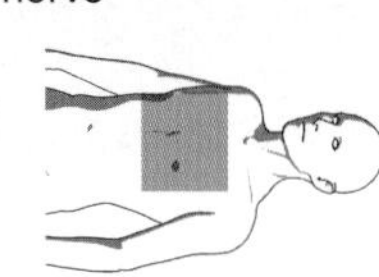

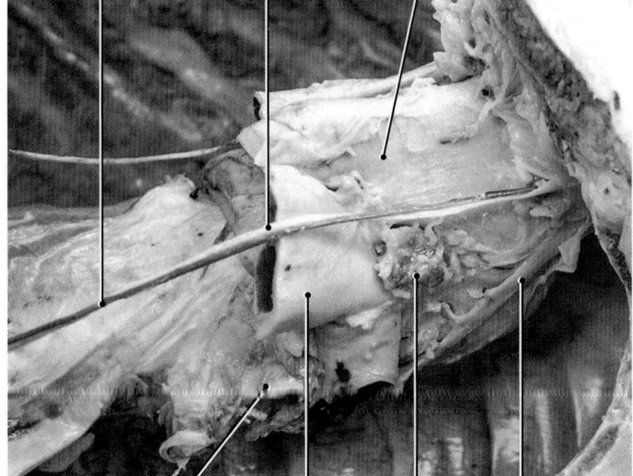

Fig. 5.60 A closer view of Fig. 5.59 shows the left vagus nerve and a regional lymph node.

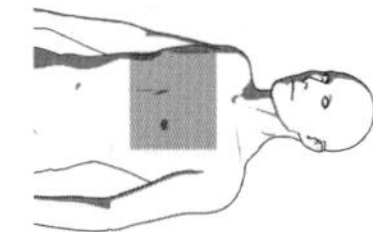

ANATOMY **NOTE**

Identify the ligamentum arteriosum, the connection between the left pulmonary artery and the arch of the aorta. Identify the trachea and its bifurcation into the left and right bronchi. The vagus nerves give rise to the recurrent laryngeal nerves. On the left side, as the nerve crosses the aorta, it gives rise to the recurrent laryngeal nerve (Figs. 5.62 and 5.63).

- **Clean the left vagus nerve, and where the left vagus crosses the aortic arch, locate the left recurrent laryngeal nerve.**

ANATOMY **NOTE**

The left recurrent laryngeal nerve passes under the ligamentum arteriosum and courses upward between the trachea/esophagus and the ascending aorta in the tracheoesophageal groove. The right recurrent laryngeal nerve arises from the right vagus nerve at the level of the right subclavian artery and turns back superiorly behind this vessel to pass upward and medially toward the larynx to enter the tracheoesophageal groove.

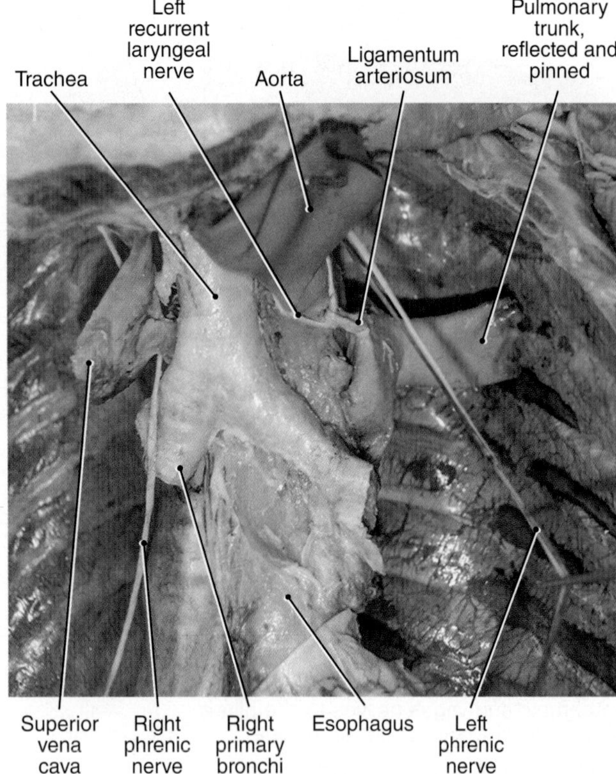

Fig. 5.62 Anterior view of mediastinal structures, including the aorta, trachea, and esophagus.

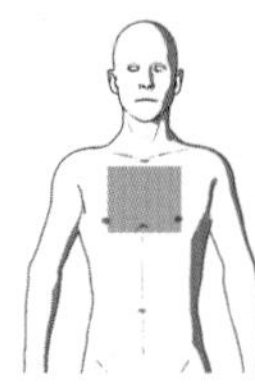

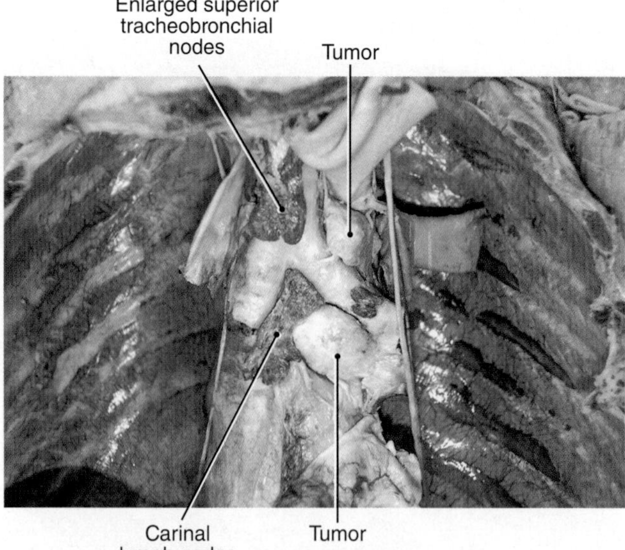

Fig. 5.64 Anterior view of mediastinal structures, revealing lymph nodes, right and left bronchus, reflected ascending aorta, and tumor intimate with left bronchus.

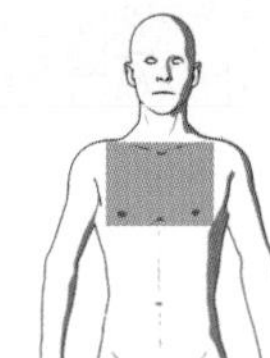

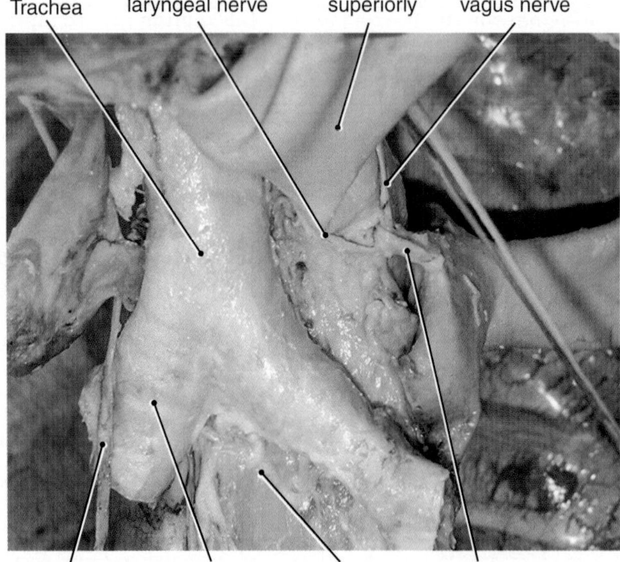

Fig. 5.63 Deep mediastinal structures include right and left bronchus and vagus, phrenic, and recurrent laryngeal nerves.

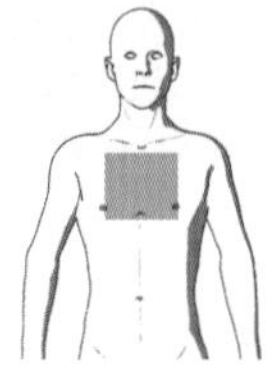

- **Along the right side of the trachea (or esophagus), identify and clean the right vagus nerve. This nerve can be found by probing between the azygos vein and the lateral aspect of the trachea, at which point the right vagus nerve begins to pass posterior to the root of the right lung.**
- **Expose the tracheal bifurcation and identify the carinal (inferior tracheobronchial) nodes. A nerve plexus anterior to the carina can be seen by cutting into the trachea at its bifurcation. The nerves represent the deep cardiac plexus formed by sympathetic and vagal fibers.**

DISSECTION TIP

Dissect the tracheobronchial lymph nodes; these nodes often are enlarged from malignant disease (Fig. 5.64).

- **Remove the pericardium over the esophagus. With forceps, lift the esophagus and remove the pleura from over the esophagus and the vertebral column (Figs. 5.65 and 5.66).**

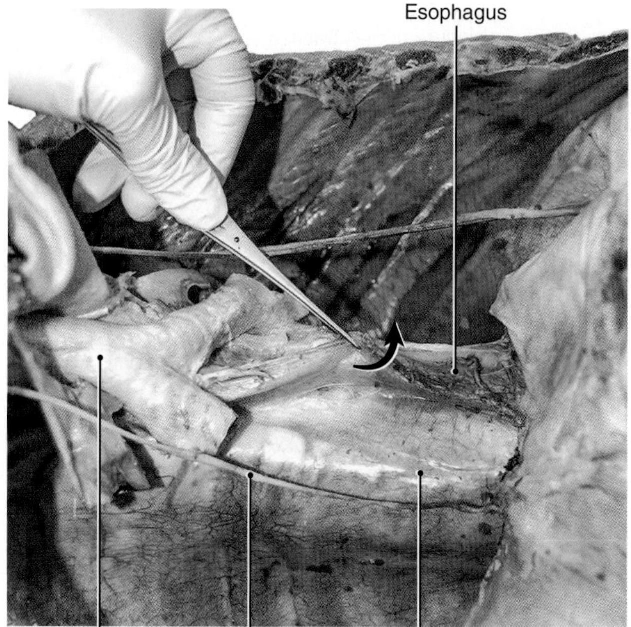

Fig. 5.65 Anterolateral view of the posterior mediastinum. Note that the esophagus is being retracted laterally.

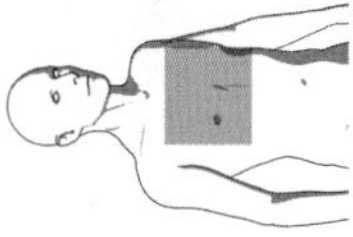

- **After removal of the pleura, dissect the fatty layer present over the vertebral bodies. Dissect between the esophagus and the vertebral bodies to identify the thoracic duct (Fig. 5.67), which often looks similar to adipose tissue.**
- **Clean and preserve the thoracic duct (Fig. 5.68).**
- **With forceps, lift the pleura, and with the aid of scissors, separate the pleura from the underlying tissues over the ribs (Figs. 5.69 and 5.70).**

DISSECTION **TIP**

To reflect the pleura, use the tip of the scissors or a probe and scrape the tissue between the pleura and the ribs. Do not cut any tissue with the forceps; use it as a probe (see Figs. 5.69 and 5.70).

- **Remove the majority of pleura from the thoracic cavity (Fig. 5.71). Trace the intercostal vein, artery, and nerve traveling in one of the posterior intercostal spaces.**

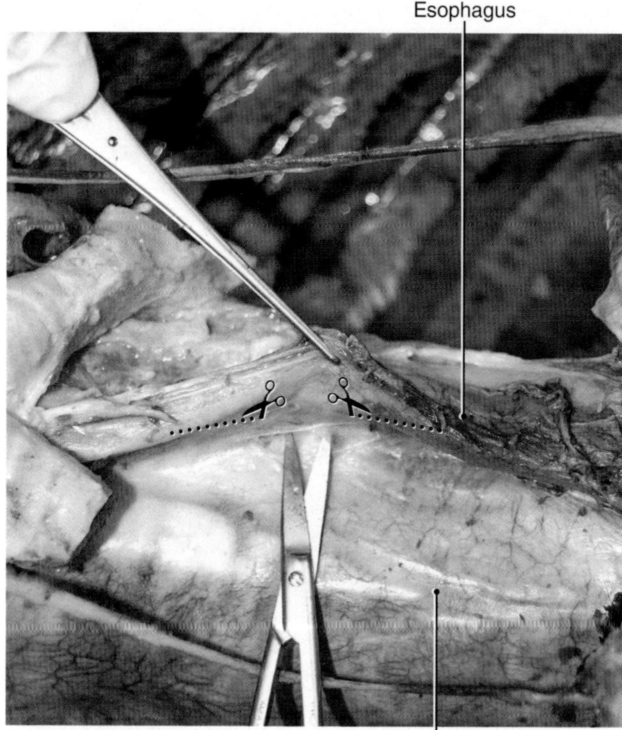

Fig. 5.66 Anterolateral view of deep posterior mediastinal structures with tension on mediastinal pleura.

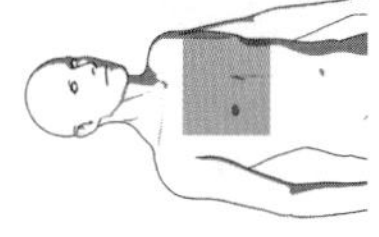

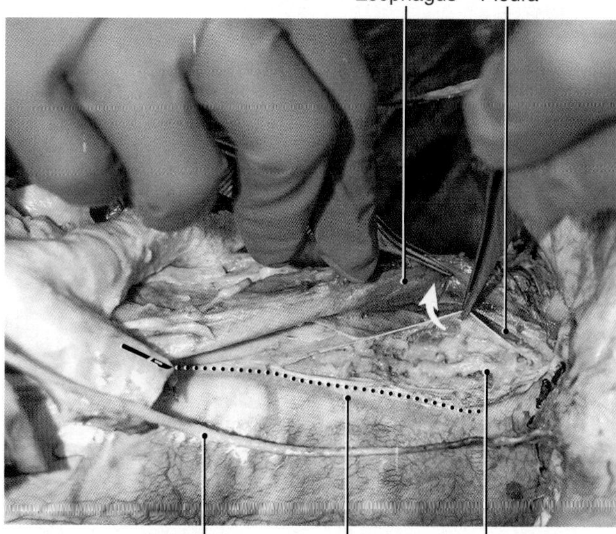

Fig. 5.67 Anterolateral view of deep posterior mediastinal structures, highlighting the thoracic duct, esophagus, and azygos vein.

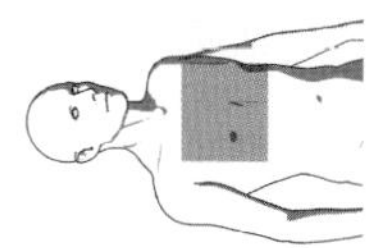

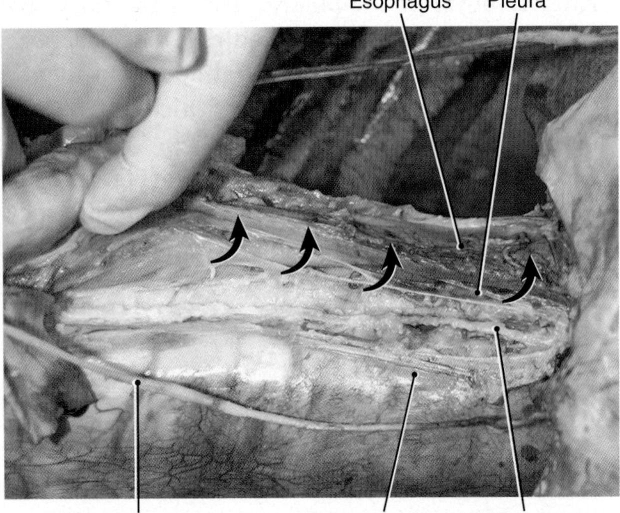

Fig. 5.68 Anterolateral view of deep posterior mediastinal structures, demonstrating the thoracic duct, esophagus, and azygos vein.

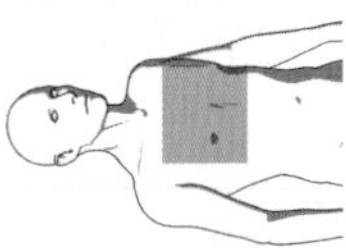

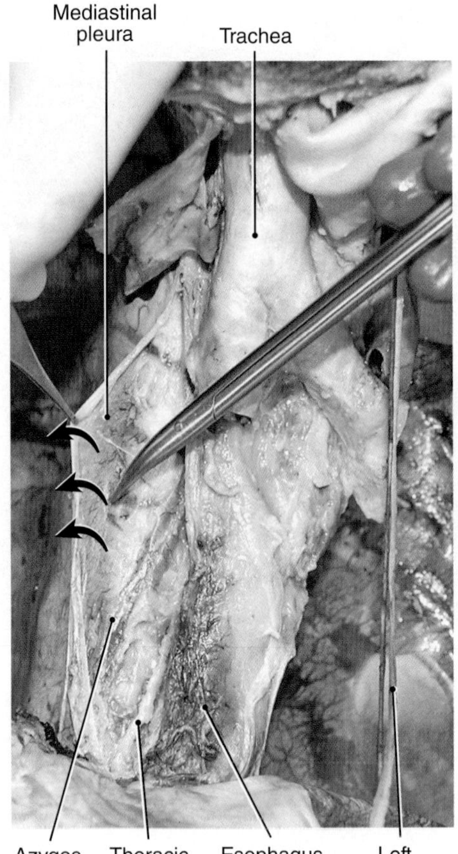

Fig. 5.69 Anterior view of deep mediastinal structures, revealing azygos vein, thoracic duct, and esophagus.

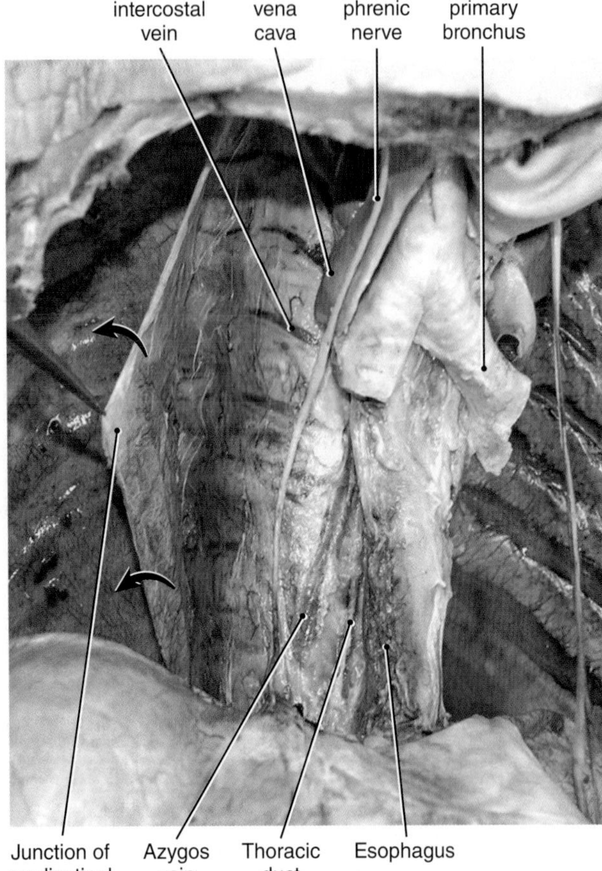

Fig. 5.70 Anterior view of posterior thoracic wall structures, revealing posterior intercostal vein, azygos vein, superior vena cava, and interface between mediastinal and costal pleurae.

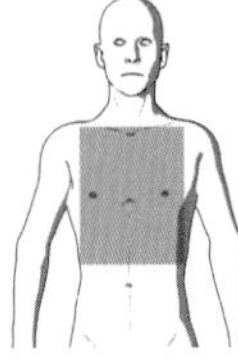

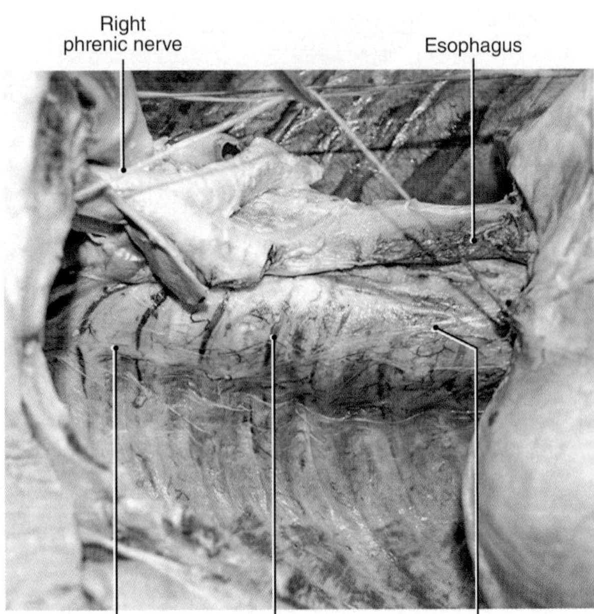

Fig. 5.71 Right lateral view of posterior thoracic wall, revealing sympathetic trunk, greater thoracic splanchnic nerves, and posterior intercostal vein.

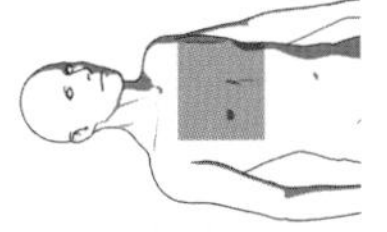

DISSECTION **TIP**

Use the handle of your scissors to remove fat over the intercostal space (Fig. 5.72).

- **Trace and identify the sympathetic trunk that runs along the junction between the vertebral bodies and ribs and appears as a white line. Near the mid-portion of the thoracic vertebral column, identify a bundle of nerve fibers originating from the sympathetic chain and running obliquely toward the midline (Fig. 5.73). This is the *greater thoracic splanchnic nerve*, arising from the sympathetic trunk.**
- **Clean the sympathetic trunk and identify the greater (T5–T9), lesser (T10–T11), and least (T12) thoracic splanchnic nerves (Fig. 5.74, Plate 5.2).**

DISSECTION **TIP**

The origin of the greater, lesser, and least thoracic splanchnic nerves is subject to variation. Also, the lesser and least thoracic splanchnic nerves are often difficult to see in the thorax before removal of the liver on the right and because of an immobile descending thoracic aorta on the left.

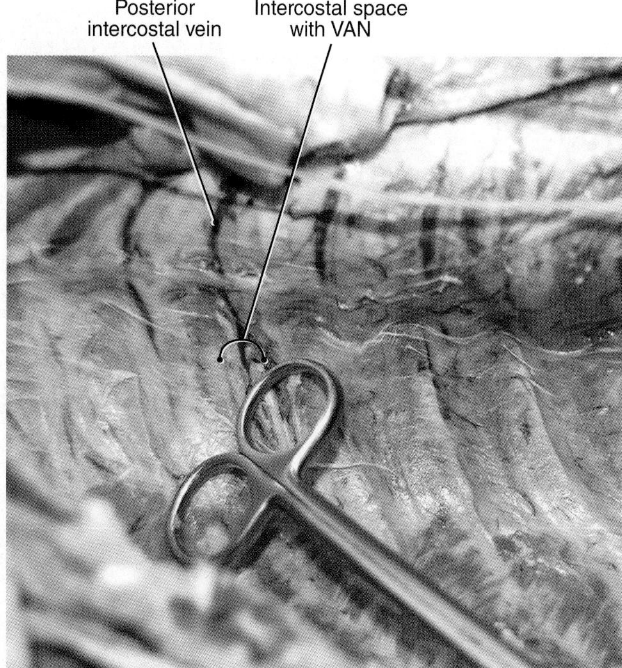

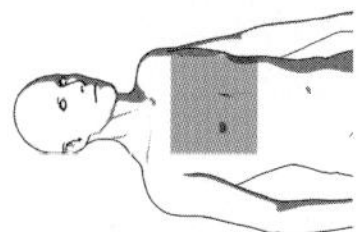

Fig. 5.72 Right lateral view of posterior thoracic wall, revealing neurovascular structures of the intercostal space at T4. *VAN,* Vein, artery, nerve.

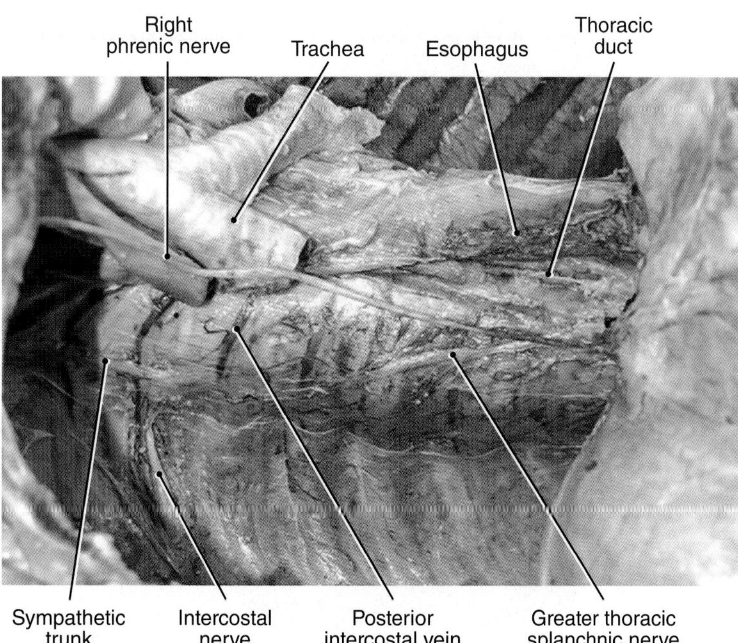

Fig. 5.73 Right lateral view of posterior thoracic wall, demonstrating the sympathetic trunk, greater thoracic splanchnic nerve, and intercostal nerve.

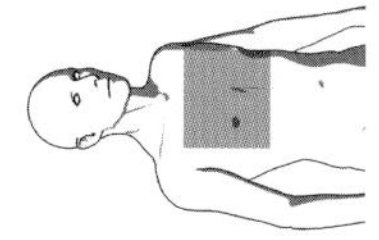

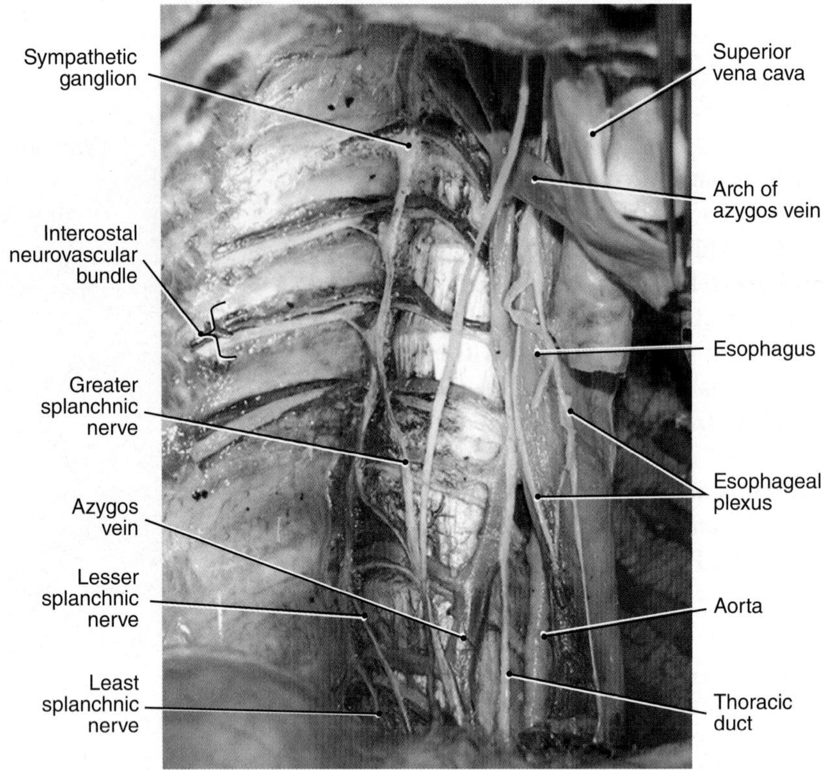

Fig. 5.74 Right lateral view of posterior thoracic wall, highlighting sympathetic trunk, sympathetic ganglion, and greater and lesser thoracic splanchnic nerves.

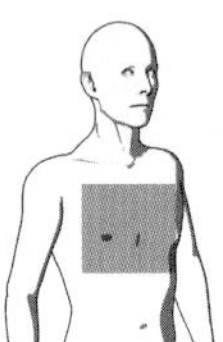

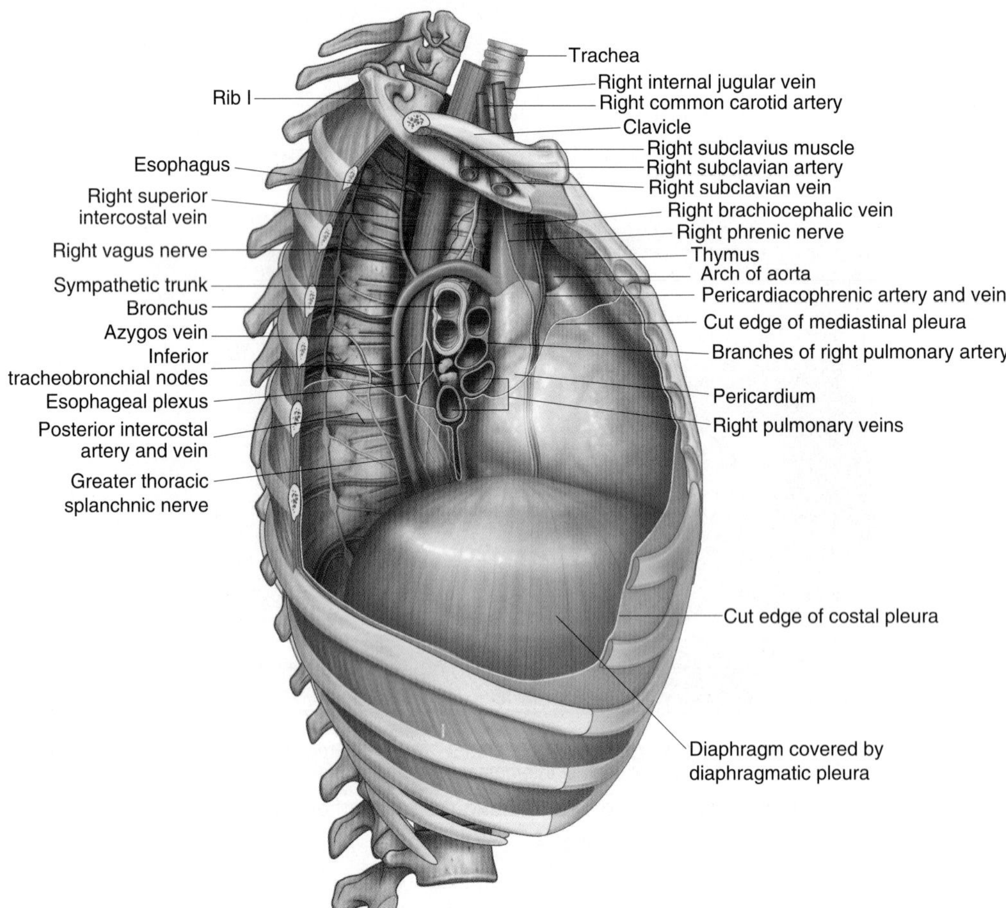

Plate 5.2 Right side of hemithorax and mediastinum. (From Drake et al., *Gray's Anatomy for Students*, 5th edition, Philadelphia, Elsevier, 2024, Figure 3.72, p. 157.)

- After cleaning out the sympathetic trunk and thoracic splanchnic nerves, dissect and clean the communicating rami connecting the sympathetic trunk with the intercostal nerves. Identify the white and gray rami communicantes (Fig. 5.75).
- Trace the left and right vagus nerves as they descend behind the right and left primary bronchi to form the esophageal plexus on the anterior surface of the esophagus (Fig. 5.76).
- Trace the superior vena cava and the veins draining into it. To the right of the superior vena cava, find the azygos vein draining into it (see Fig. 5.76). Identify the right posterior intercostal veins anterior and superior to the vertebral bodies.
- On the left side of the thorax, identify the hemiazygos vein with the lowest three or four left posterior intercostal venous tributaries. Lift the esophagus at the midline and note the accessory hemiazygos vein crossing the midline to join the azygos vein (Fig. 5.77).

DISSECTION TIP

The arch of the aorta and the descending thoracic aorta can be displaced or atherosclerotic, making the dissection of the left posterior thorax difficult. Often the greater, lesser, and least thoracic splanchnic nerves, as well as the hemiazygos and accessory hemiazygos veins, are hidden behind the aorta.

- Lift the midportion of the thoracic aorta and note the origin of the posterior intercostal arteries. Identify the esophageal and bronchial arteries arising from the anterior aspect of the aorta (Figs. 5.78 and 5.79).

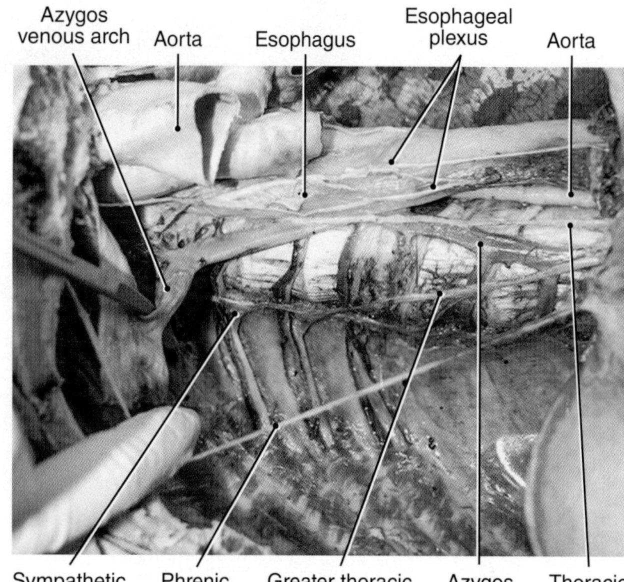

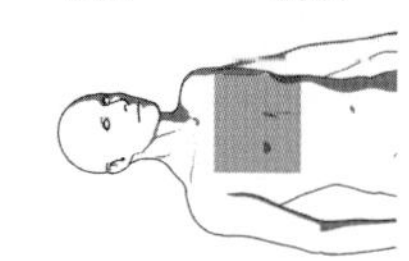

Fig. 5.76 Right lateral view of posterior thoracic wall, revealing azygos vein, sympathetic trunk, ganglia, and greater thoracic splanchnic nerve.

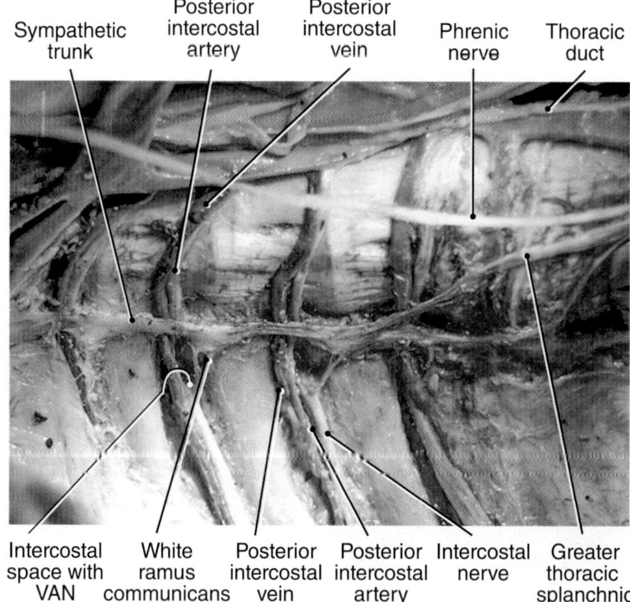

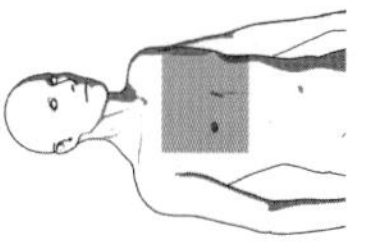

Fig. 5.75 Right lateral view of posterior thoracic wall with sympathetic trunk, white ramus communicans, and intercostal nerve. *VAN,* Vein, artery, nerve.

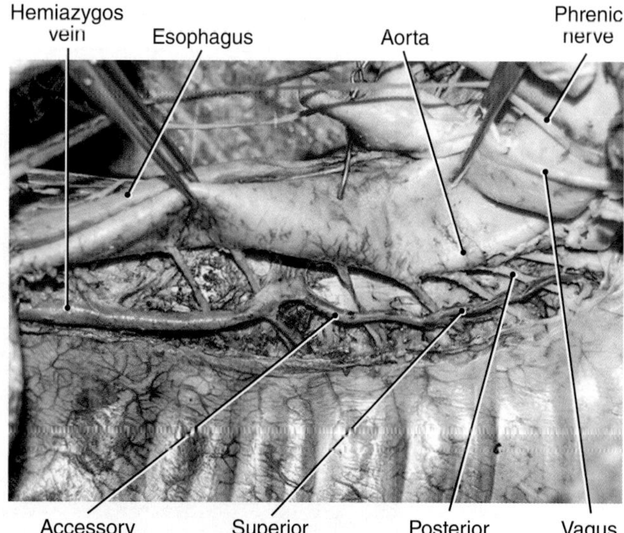

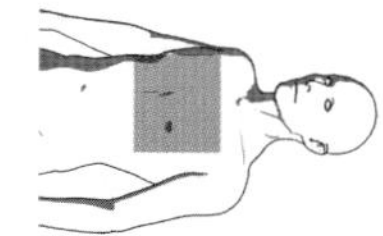

Fig. 5.77 Left lateral view of posterior thoracic wall, revealing accessory hemiazygos and accessory hemiazygos veins.

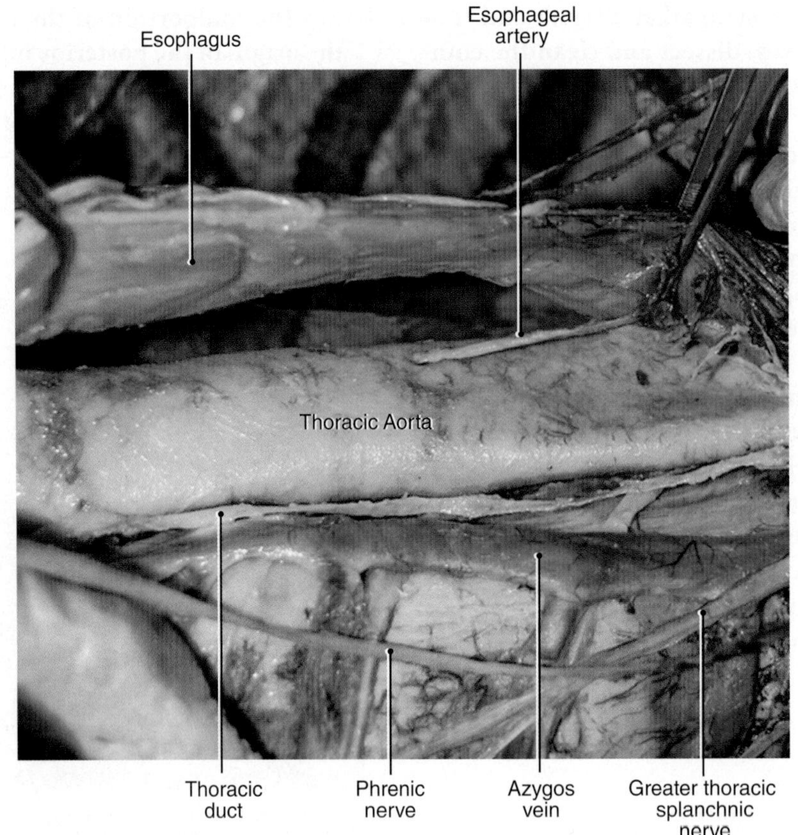

Fig. 5.78 Right lateral view of posterior thoracic wall, demonstrating the esophagus, esophageal artery, aorta, thoracic duct, and azygos vein.

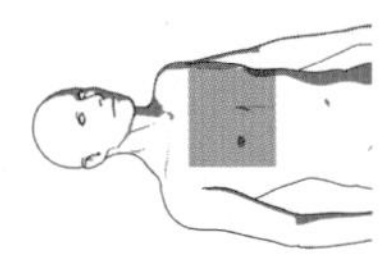

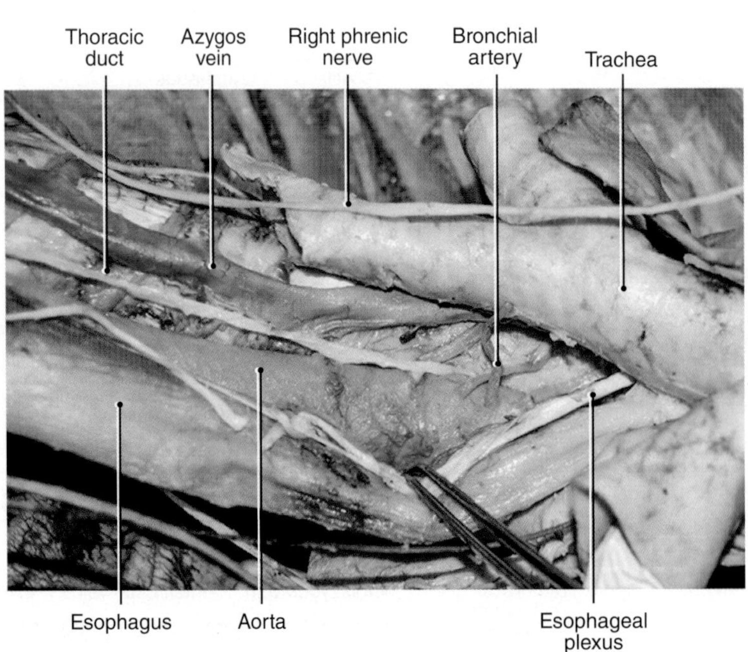

Fig. 5.79 Left lateral view of posterior mediastinum with the esophagus and esophageal plexus reflected, demonstrating the aorta, thoracic duct, and azygos vein.

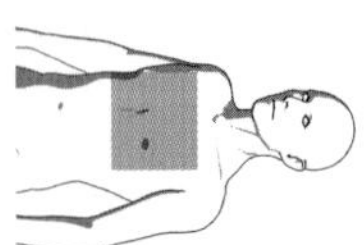

LABORATORY IDENTIFICATION CHECKLIST

NERVES

- ☐ Anterior intercostal
- ☐ Intercostobrachial (T2)
- ☐ Lateral intercostal T3–T7
- ☐ Intercostal
- ☐ Sympathetic trunk
- ☐ Sympathetic ganglia
- ☐ Greater thoracic splanchnic
- ☐ Lesser thoracic splanchnic
- ☐ Least thoracic splanchnic
- ☐ Gray and white rami communicantes
- ☐ Stellate ganglion
- ☐ Phrenic
- ☐ Vagus
- ☐ Right recurrent laryngeal
- ☐ Left recurrent laryngeal
- ☐ Esophageal plexus
- ☐ Cardiac plexus

ARTERIES

- ☐ Aorta
- ☐ Subclavian
- ☐ Internal thoracic
- ☐ Superior epigastric
- ☐ Musculophrenic
- ☐ Pericardiacophrenic
- ☐ Pulmonary
- ☐ Bronchial
- ☐ Esophageal
- ☐ Anterior intercostal
- ☐ Posterior intercostal

VEINS

- ☐ Superior vena cava
- ☐ Inferior vena cava
- ☐ Subclavian
- ☐ Internal thoracic
- ☐ Superior epigastric
- ☐ Brachiocephalic
- ☐ Anterior intercostal
- ☐ Posterior intercostal
- ☐ Azygos
- ☐ Accessory hemiazygos
- ☐ Hemiazygos

MUSCLES

- ☐ External intercostal
- ☐ Internal intercostal
- ☐ Innermost intercostal
- ☐ Transversus thoracis
- ☐ Subcostals
- ☐ Diaphragm

LYMPHATICS

- ☐ Thoracic duct

LIGAMENT

- ☐ Ligamentum arteriosum

ORGAN TISSUES

- ☐ Lung
  - ☐ Hilum
  - ☐ Lingula
  - ☐ Oblique fissure
- ☐ Parietal pleura
- ☐ Visceral pleura
- ☐ Pulmonary ligament
- ☐ Lobes of right and left lungs
- ☐ Primary bronchi
- ☐ Secondary bronchi
- ☐ Tertiary bronchi
- ☐ Apex of heart
- ☐ Base of heart
- ☐ Esophagus
- ☐ Thymus

BONES

- ☐ Sternum
- ☐ Ribs
- ☐ Bodies of thoracic vertebrae with intervertebral discs

BEFORE YOU BEGIN

Inspection

Inspect the heart externally and identify the following:

- Right atrium
- Right auricle
- Superior vena cava (SVC)
- Inferior vena cava (IVC)
- Subpulmonary infundibulum or conus
- Pulmonary artery
- Ascending aorta
- Left atrium
- Pulmonary veins
- Anterior interventricular sulcus
- Inferior interventricular sulcus
- Coronary sulcus
- Sulcus terminalis
- Left auricle (Figs. 6.1–6.4)

Identify the *sulcus terminalis*, a shallow sulcus on the surface of the right atrium, which extends between the right side of the orifice of the SVC and that of the IVC.

DISSECTION **TIP**

The dissection typically begins with the exposure and identification of the coronary arteries. Note the apex of the heart and the *acute* (right and inferior) (see Fig. 6.1) and *obtuse* (left) (see Fig. 6.4) margins of the heart.

CORONARY ARTERIES

- **To remove the epicardium (visceral pericardium) and the fat covering the right coronary artery, identify the right auricle and retract it laterally.**
- **Palpate the space between the right auricle and the atrioventricular (AV, coronary) sulcus and expose the proximal part of the right coronary artery (Fig. 6.5).**

DISSECTION **TIP**

Most of the coronary arteries in adults can be felt with palpation because of their increased hardening from atherosclerotic calcified plaques.

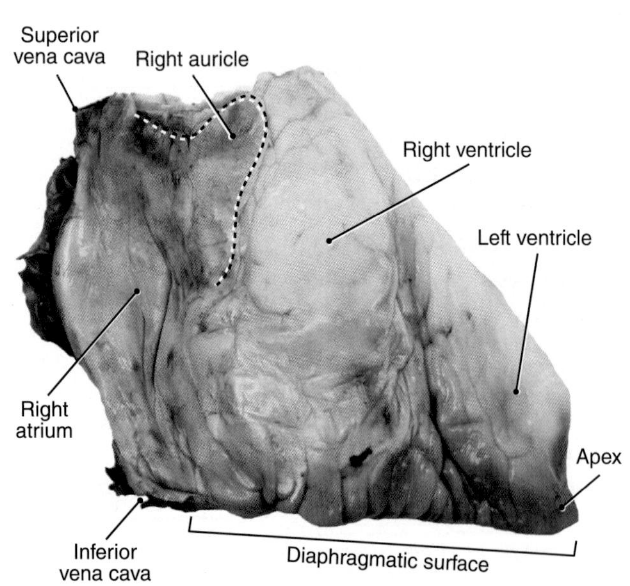

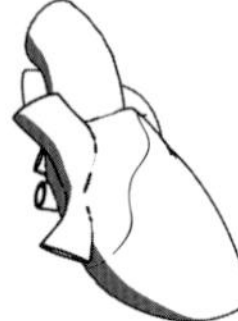

Fig. 6.1 Anterior view of external surfaces of the heart; *dotted outline*, right auricle.

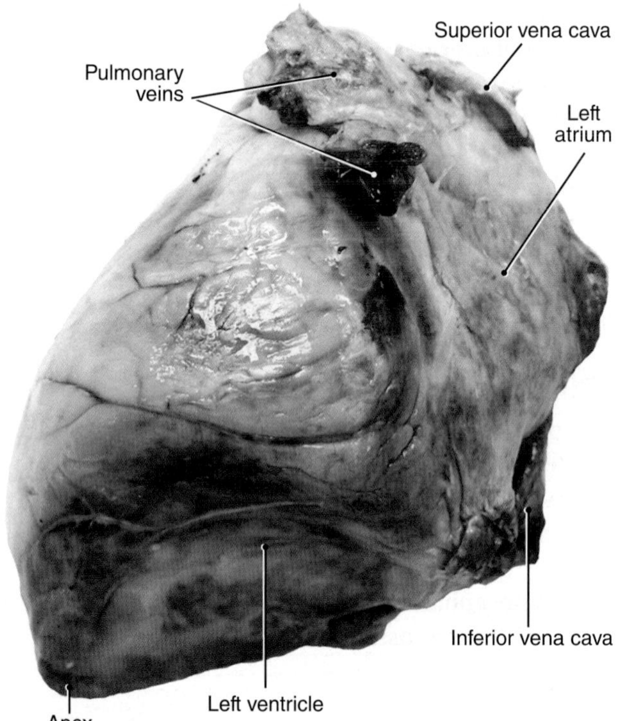

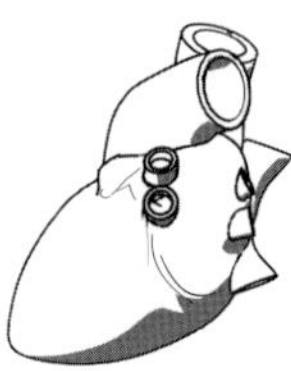

Fig. 6.2 Topographic view of left atrium and ventricle.

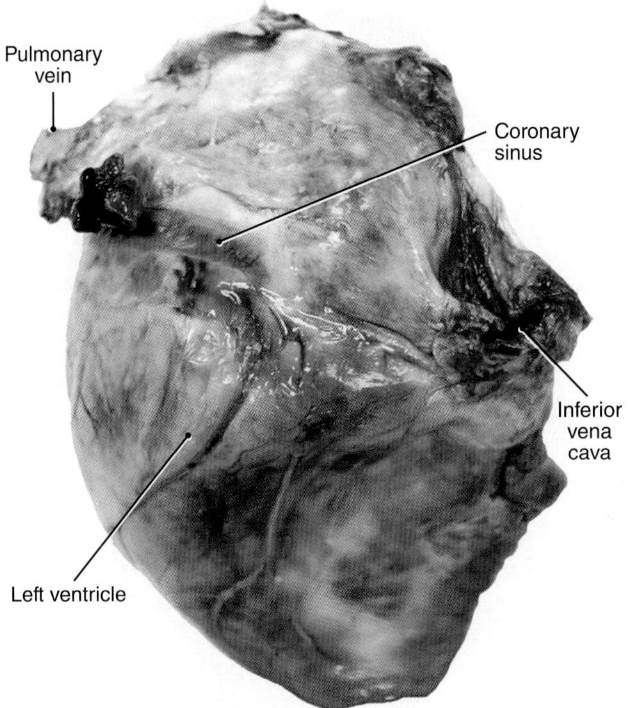

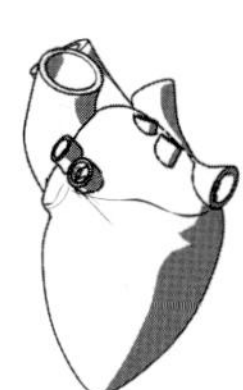

Fig. 6.3 Topographic view of the posterior heart.

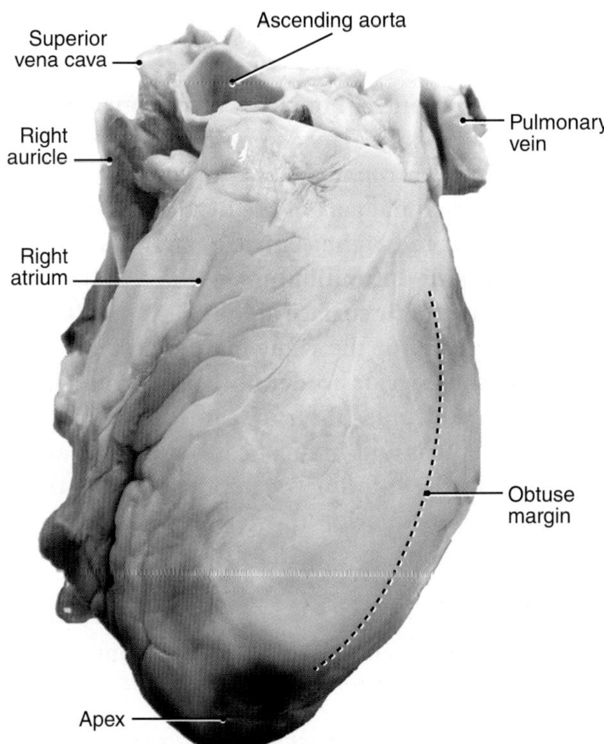

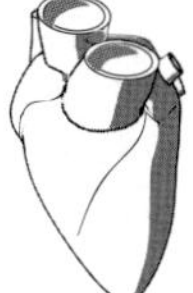

Fig. 6.4 Base, margin, and apex of the heart; *dotted line,* obtuse margin (left border).

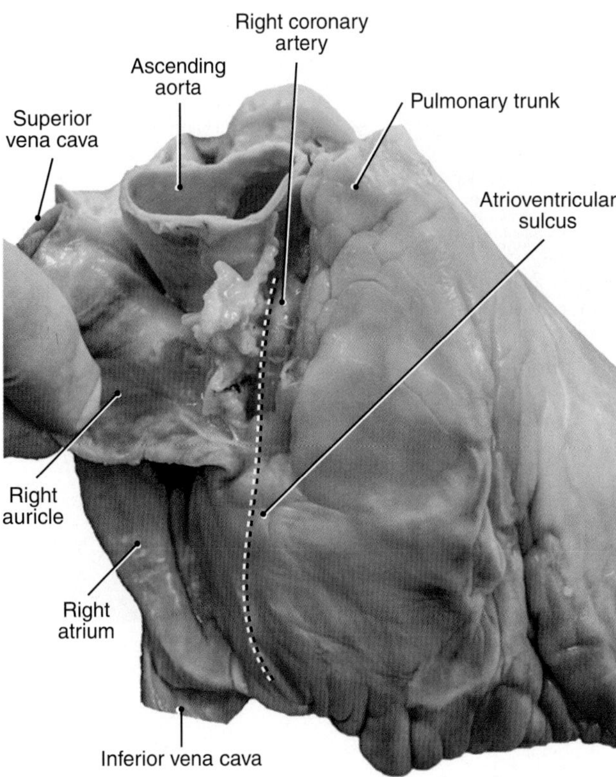

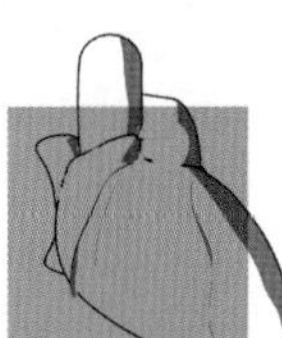

Fig. 6.5 Topographic view of anterolateral heart; *dotted line,* tracing of right coronary artery.

ANATOMY **NOTE**

The terms *atrium* and *auricle* are not synonymous. The auricles are appendages of the atria.

- **Expose the superficial portion of the *right coronary artery* (RCA) by cleaning away the epicardium and fat covering the vessel (Fig. 6.6).**
- **Trace the RCA toward the right side of the diaphragmatic surface of the heart, taking care to protect its branches.**
- **As the artery passes near the edge of the right auricle, it usually gives off the artery of the sinuatrial node (Fig. 6.7).**

ANATOMY **NOTE**

The sinuatrial (SA) nodal artery arises from the proximal portion of the RCA in 65% of cases, traveling upward to the right atrium at the junction of the SVC and the right auricle, where it enters the SA. In the remaining cases, the SA nodal artery arises from the proximal portion of the left coronary artery.

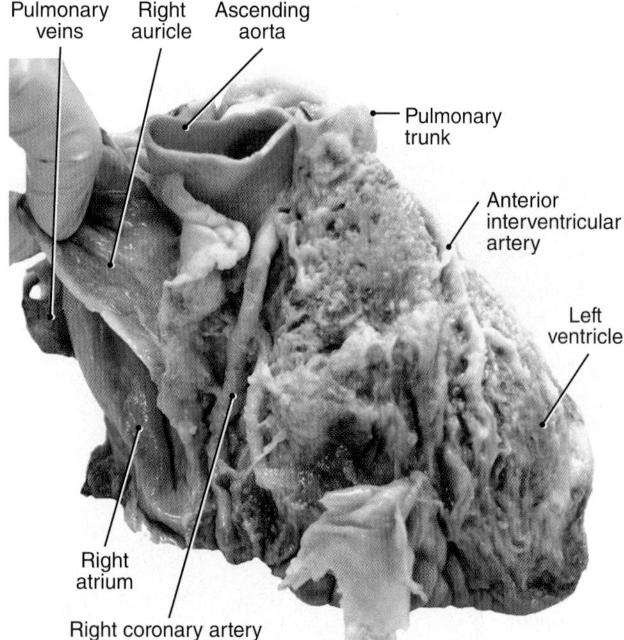

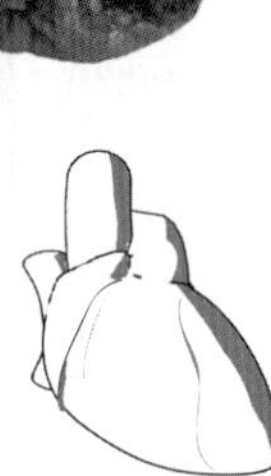

Fig. 6.6 Dissection of right coronary artery from its origin.

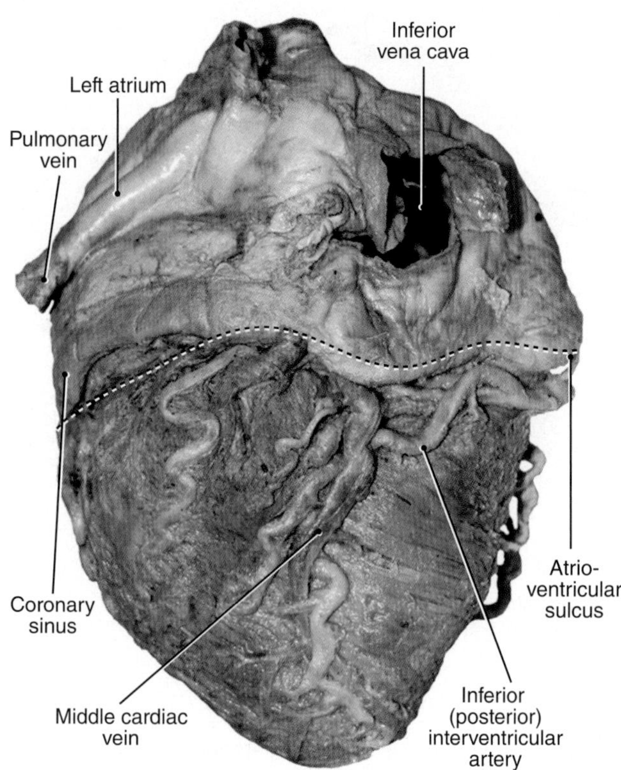

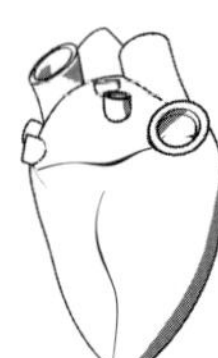

Fig. 6.8 Inferior view of heart with the inferior interventricular artery and middle cardiac vein exposed.

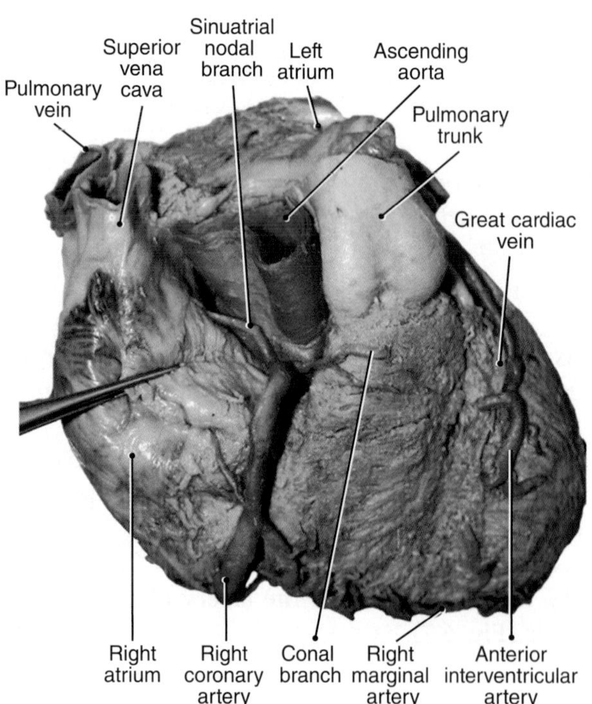

Fig. 6.7 Dissection of right coronary artery from its origin.

- **The second branch of the RCA is the conal branch of the right coronary artery sometimes also referred to as the conus, or *conal artery*. The conal artery arises from the proximal part of the RCA and passes to the left, around the right ventricle, at the level of the subpulmonary infundibulum (see Fig. 6.7). Close to the diaphragmatic surface of the heart, the RCA typically gives rise to the right marginal artery, which supplies the inferior border of the right ventricle.**
- **The RCA continues inferiorly in the AV (atrioventricular) sulcus and in most cases descends and terminates in the inferior (posterior) interventricular sulcus as the inferior (posterior) interventricular (descending) artery (Fig. 6.8).**

ANATOMY **NOTE**

This artery supplies the inferior third of the interventricular septum and a portion of the inferior wall of the left ventricle.

The nomenclature of posterior interventricular artery has been replaced with the anatomically correct attitudinal terminology of inferior interventricular artery, since the left ventricle lies inferiorly on top of the diaphragm and the true posterior structures of the heart are the left atrium and the corresponding pulmonary veins.

- **Before it becomes the inferior interventricular artery, the RCA will give off the artery of the atrioventricular (AV) node at the crux of heart.**

ANATOMY **NOTE**

In 80% of specimens, the AV nodal artery arises from the RCA near the inferior interventricular sulcus as it crosses the "crux" of the heart (Fig. 6.9). The crux of the heart is the center point of the anatomic base where the atria and ventricles are most closely approximated posteriorly and inferiorly.

DISSECTION **TIP**

To identify the artery to the AV node, carefully lift the left atrium at the inferior AV sulcus and clean away the fat (see Fig. 6.9B).

- **To remove the epicardium (visceral pericardium) and the fat covering the left coronary artery, identify the left auricle and retract it laterally (Figs. 6.10 and 6.11).**
- **Palpate the space between the left auricle and the AV (coronary) sulcus and expose the proximal part of the left coronary artery (Figs. 6.12 and 6.13).**
- **The left coronary artery is typically very small in length (a few centimeters) and divides into the anterior interventricular artery (left anterior descending [LAD] as many clinicians will refer to) and circumflex artery.**
- **Palpate the anterior interventricular sulcus and feel for the anterior interventricular artery. Use the separation technique to expose the anterior interventricular artery. This vessel gives off relatively large diagonal branches to the anterior surface of the left ventricle (Fig. 6.14).**

ANATOMY **NOTE**

An often-encountered variation is the presence of myocardial bridges covering the anterior interventricular artery, which penetrates the myocardium for a few centimeters and emerges distally as an epicardial artery (see Fig. 6.14).

- **Deeply penetrating septal branches arise from the deep surface of the anterior interventricular artery**

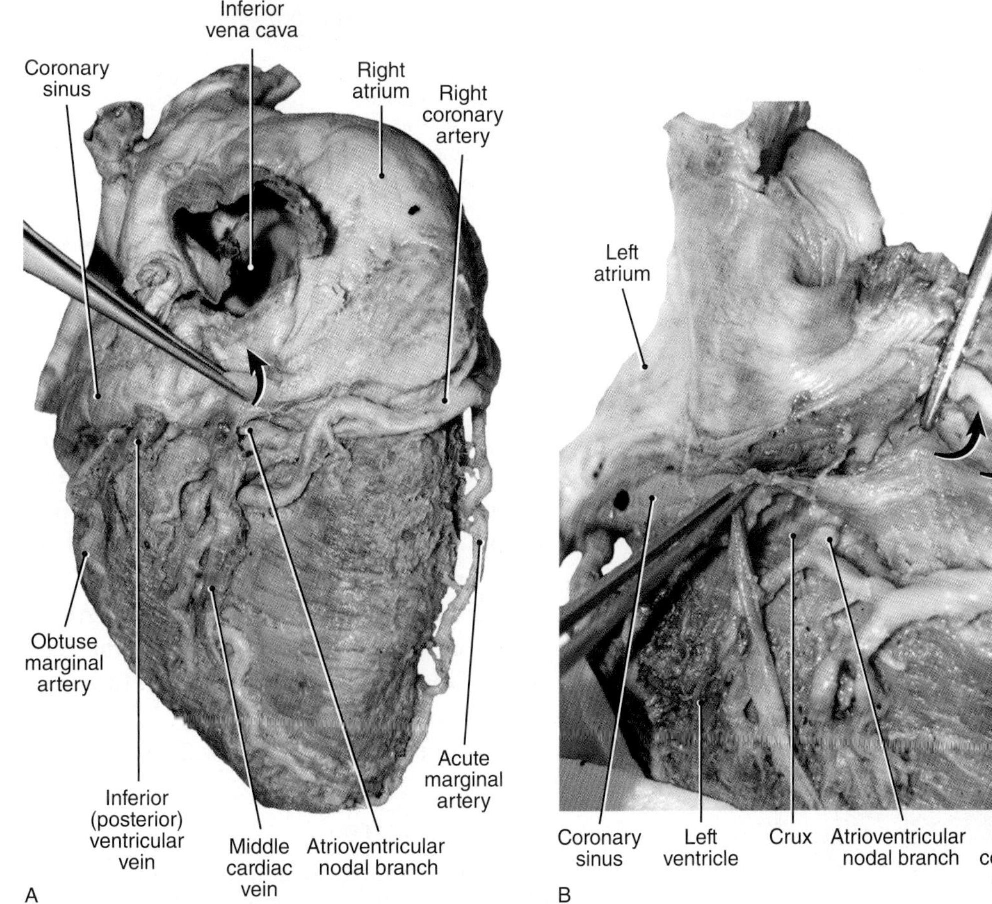

Fig. 6.9 A, Inferior view of heart with inferior interventricular artery and artery to the atrioventricular *(AV)* node exposed. B, Left atrium pulled back to reveal the AV nodal artery within the crux of the heart.

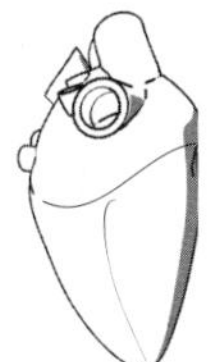
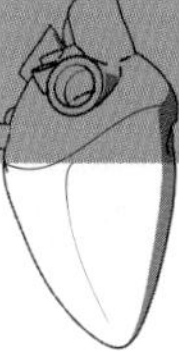

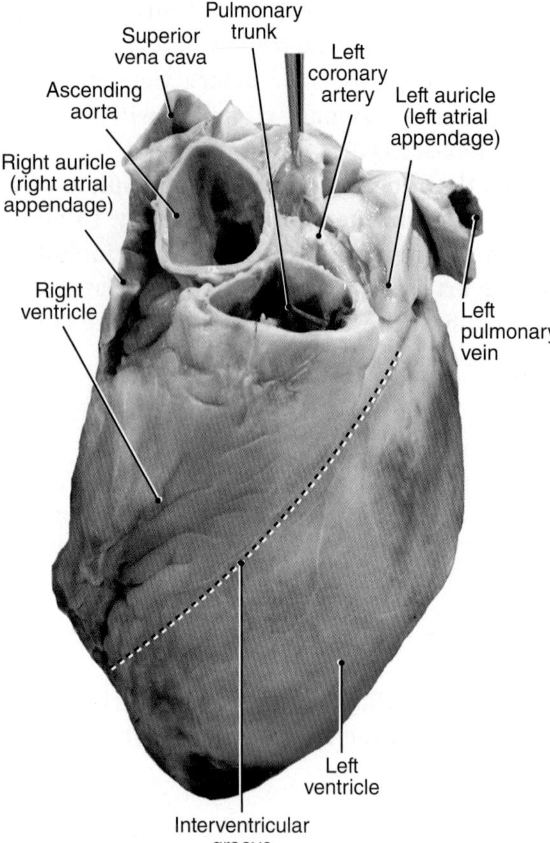

Fig. 6.10 Vertical tilt of heart showing the right and left ventricles, as well as the apex of the heart.

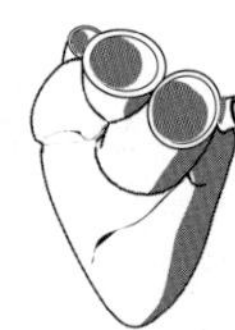

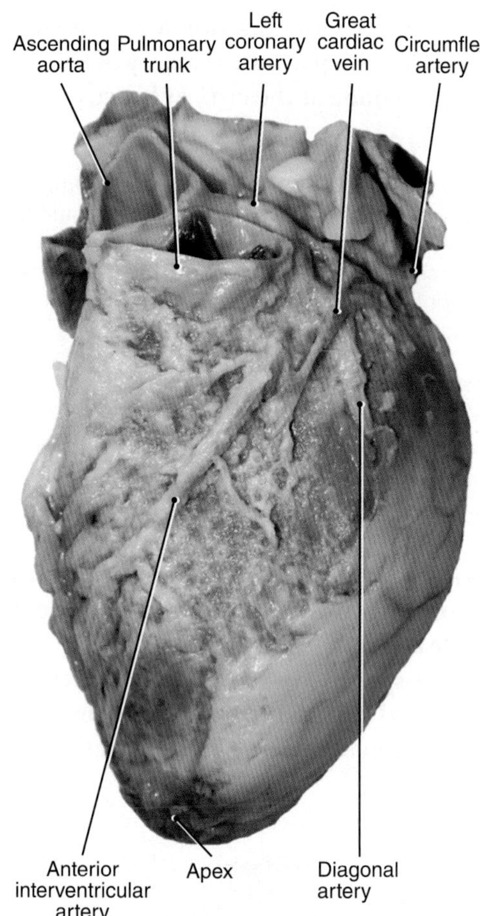

Fig. 6.12 Epicardial fat is removed from the surface of the left ventricle and the anterior interventricular artery is exposed.

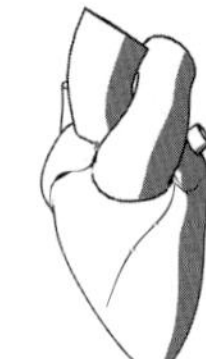

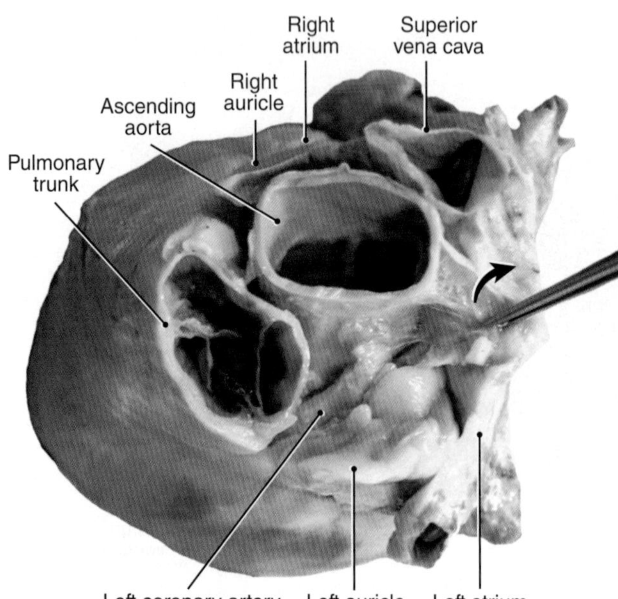

Fig. 6.11 Superior view of the great vessels. To the left of the great vessels, fat is reflected and the origin of the left coronary artery is exposed.

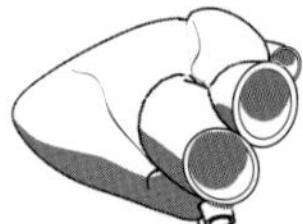

and enter the muscular interventricular septum (Figs. 6.15 and 6.16). Specifically, at the level of the subpulmonary infundibulum, the septal perforators supply the proximal parts of the left and right bundle branches.

- **The circumflex artery runs in the left AV sulcus toward the left border and around the base of the heart. This vessel typically gives off the left marginal artery crossing the left border of the heart, supplying the left ventricular free wall (Fig. 6.17).**

ANATOMY **NOTE**

Numerous variations exist in the pattern of distribution of the right and left coronary arteries. Among the most common variations of the origin of the coronary arteries is the source of the inferior interventricular coronary artery. In the majority of cases, the RCA provides the source for this artery. In about 15% of cases, however, the circumflex artery gives off this branch.

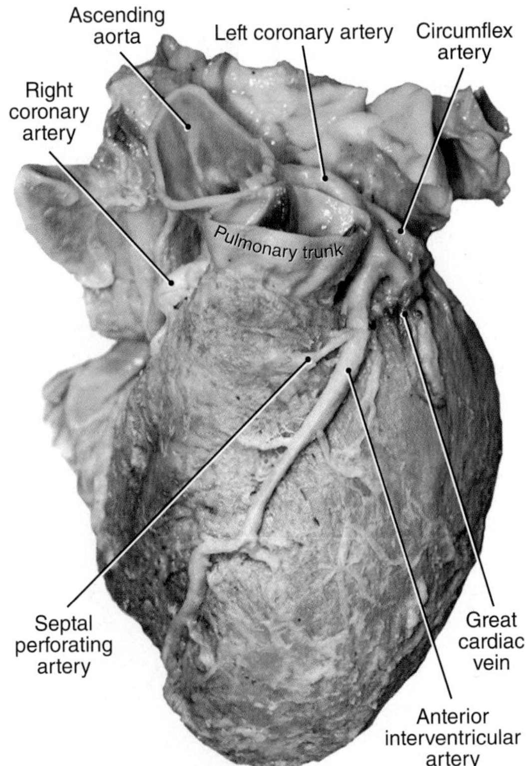

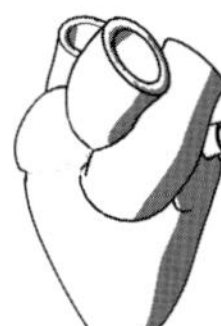

Fig. 6.13 Epicardial fat removed from left ventricle with the anterior interventricular artery exposed.

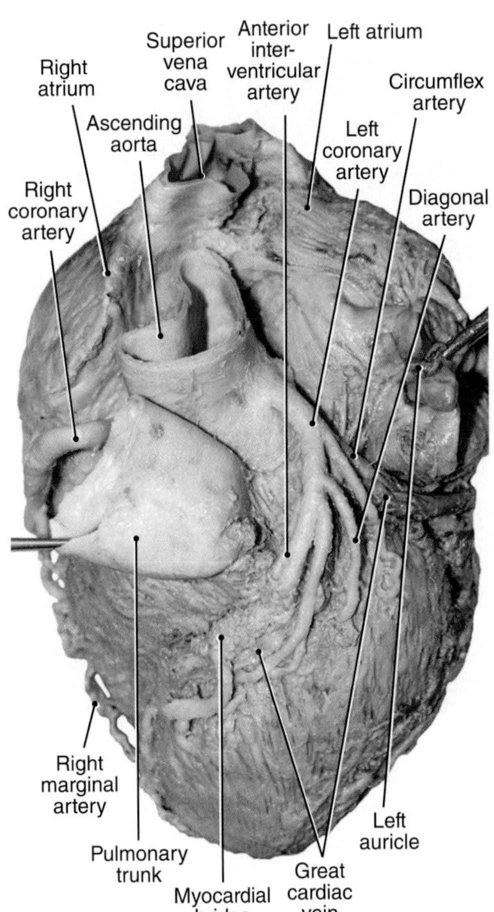

Fig. 6.14 Removing epicardial fat from the left ventricle and exposing the anterior interventricular artery to reveal diagonal branches and a myocardial bridge.

DISSECTION **TIP**

At many times during this dissection, it is possible to identify hearts that have undergone coronary artery bypass graft (CABG) procedures (Figs. 6.18 and 6.19).

- **Try to expose the graft vessel and identify to which vessel it is connected.**
- **On the posterior and inferior surface of the heart at the AV sulcus between the IVC and the left atrium, identify the *coronary sinus*, a small confluence of veins approximately 2 cm long.**

ANATOMY **NOTE**

The coronary sinus receives the great cardiac vein, the middle cardiac vein, the small cardiac vein, and the oblique vein of the left atrium.

- **Identify the great cardiac vein, which lies in the anterior interventricular sulcus, accompanying the anterior interventricular artery.**
- **The middle cardiac vein lies in the inferior interventricular sulcus and accompanies the inferior interventricular artery.**

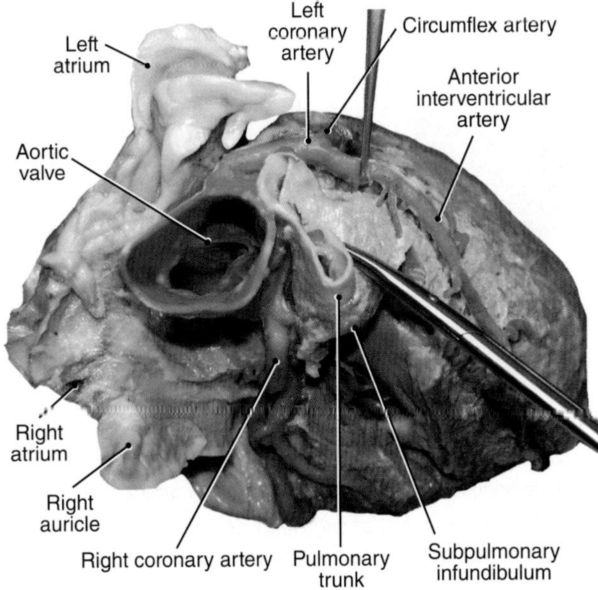

Fig. 6.15 Anterior interventricular artery is retracted, and septal perforating branches are exposed.

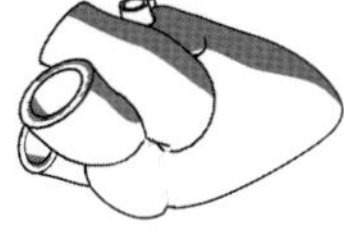

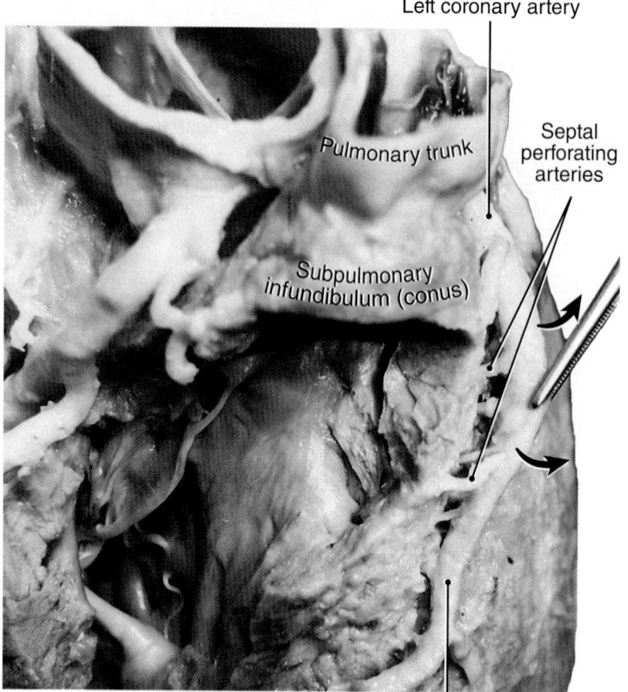

Fig. 6.16 Left coronary artery with septal and anterior interventricular branches.

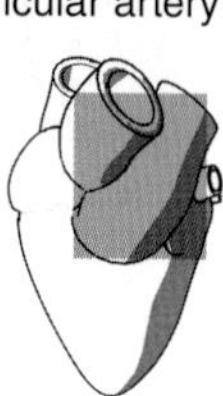

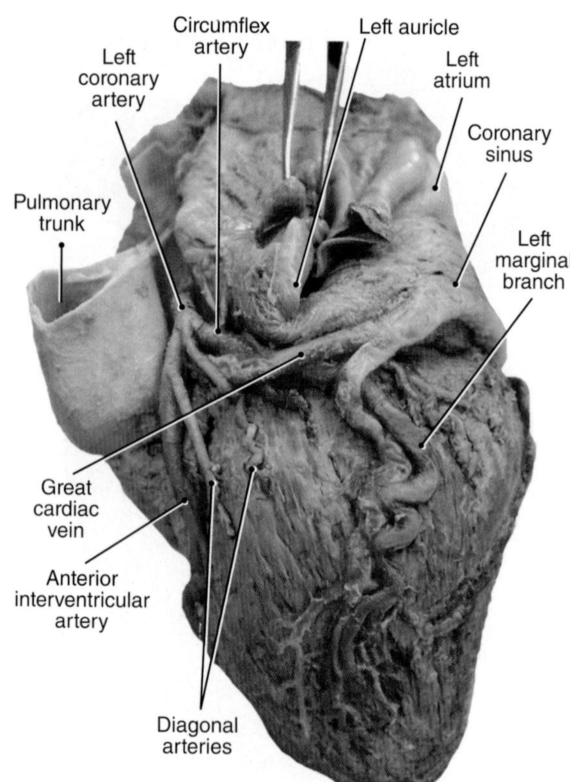

Fig. 6.17 Lateral view with vertical tilt revealing left coronary artery, circumflex, and marginal branches.

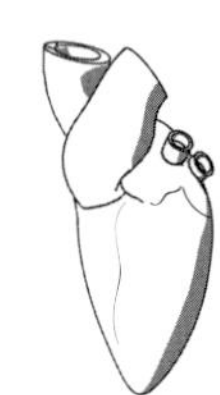

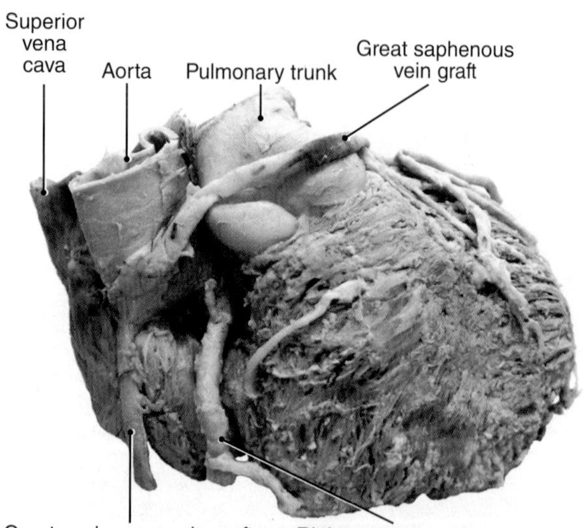

Fig. 6.18 Anterior view of the heart demonstrating a great saphenous vein graft used for coronary artery bypass graft (CABG).

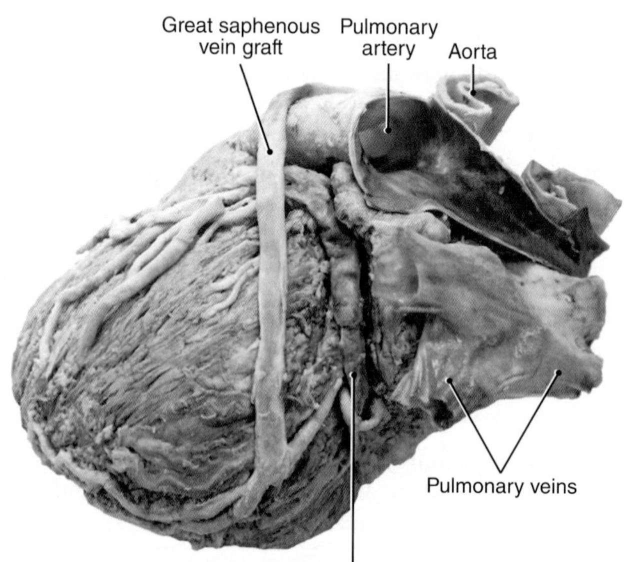

Fig. 6.19 Inferolateral view revealing the great saphenous vein graft.

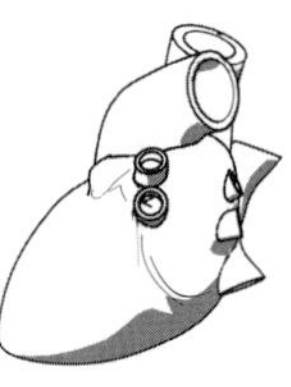

- The small cardiac vein lies in the AV sulcus next to the opening of the coronary sinus. This vein usually joins the right marginal vein or separately opens into the right atrium.

DISSECTION **TIP**

The cardiac veins have very thin walls and are often damaged during dissection.

DISSECTION OF HEART

Right Atrium

Technique 1

- Incise the right atrium laterally, making a vertical incision from the inferior vena cava to the superior vena cava (Fig. 6.20), and avoid cutting the valve of the IVC (eustachian valve).
- With forceps, reflect the flap made by the lateral incision in the right atrium, and observe the muscular ridge within the chamber, the *crista terminalis* (Fig. 6.21 and Plate 6.1).
- Note the pectinate muscles arising from the crista terminalis and fanning out through the wall of the right auricle.
- Observe the smooth roof of the right atrium between the orifices of the two venae cavae, the *sinus venarum.*
- Within the right atrium, note the valve of the IVC (eustachian valve), medial to the opening of the IVC. Note the valve (thebesian valve) and ostium of the coronary sinus.
- Note also the venae cordis minimae (thebesian veins), which are small openings in the internal surface of the right atrium.
- The interatrial septum forms the medial wall of the right atrium.
- Within the septum is a depressed region, the *fossa ovalis of the right atrium,* bordered by a thicker rim of muscle, the limbus fossae ovalis (Fig. 6.22).

Technique 2

- Incise the right atrium in a semicircular fashion starting 1 to 2 cm above the IVC as shown in Fig. 6.20, to avoid cutting the valve of the IVC (eustachian valve).
- With forceps, reflect the flap made by this incision in the right atrium and observe all the structures of therein as described earlier (Fig. 6.22).

ANATOMY **NOTE**

The fossa ovalis of the right atrium represents the only true atrial septum separating the right from the left atria. Any other musculature between the right and left atria separates the two structures by a thick layer of extracardiac fat.

The fossa ovalis of the right atrium also marks the line of fusion between the original embryonic septum secundum with the septum primum, closing the ostium secundum. In 20% of cases, the area of fusion in the interatrial septum is incomplete, and an oblique fissure of communication between the two atria is retained. This is known as a "probe-patent foramen ovale" (Fig. 6.23).

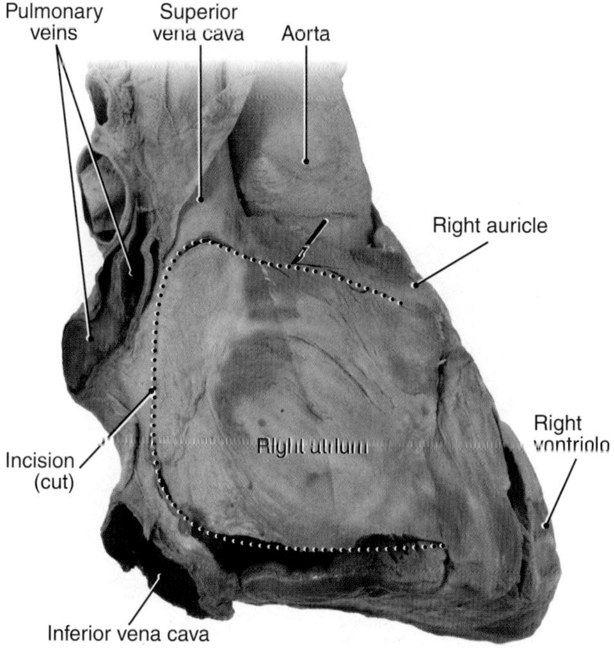

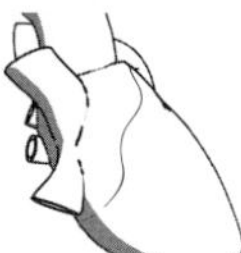

Fig. 6.20 Anterior view of the right atrium with incision landmark between the inferior and superior venae cavae.

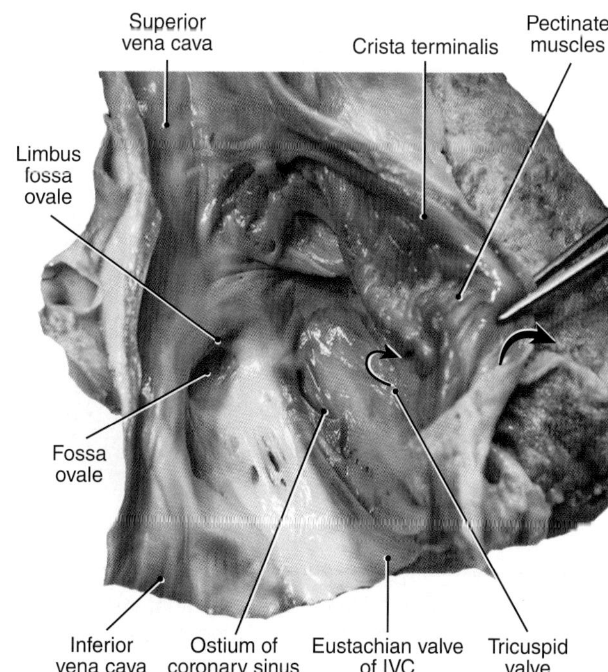

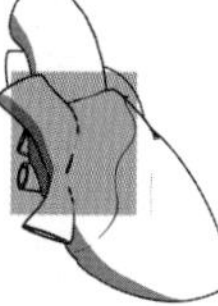

Fig. 6.21 Superior and inferior venae cavae opened with a vertical incision, revealing internal structures of the right atrium. *IVC,* Inferior vena cava.

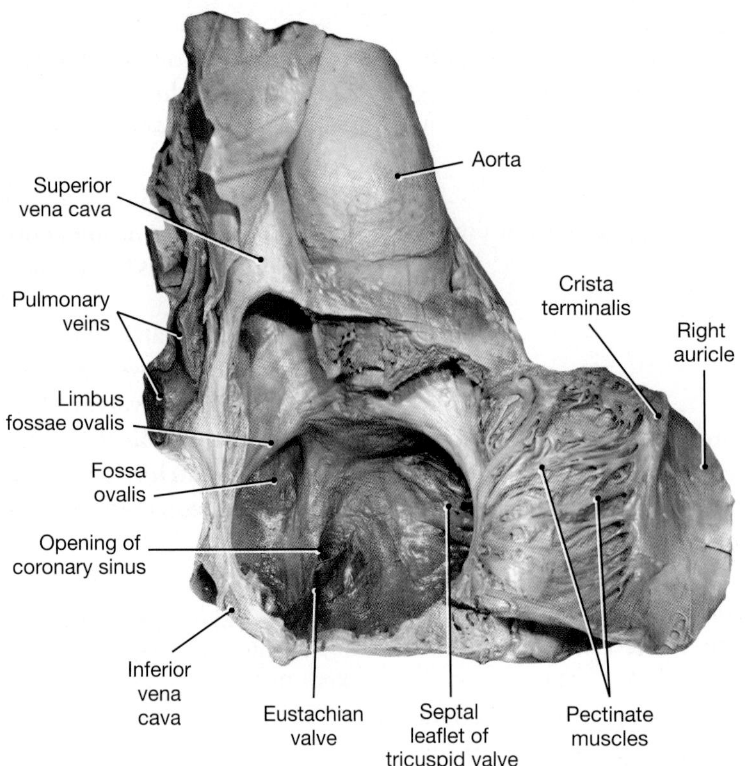

Fig. 6.22 Internal aspect of the heart and superior vena cava.

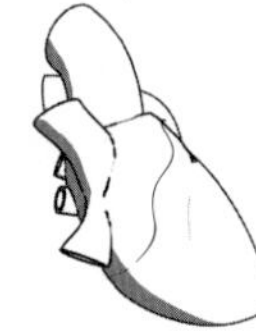

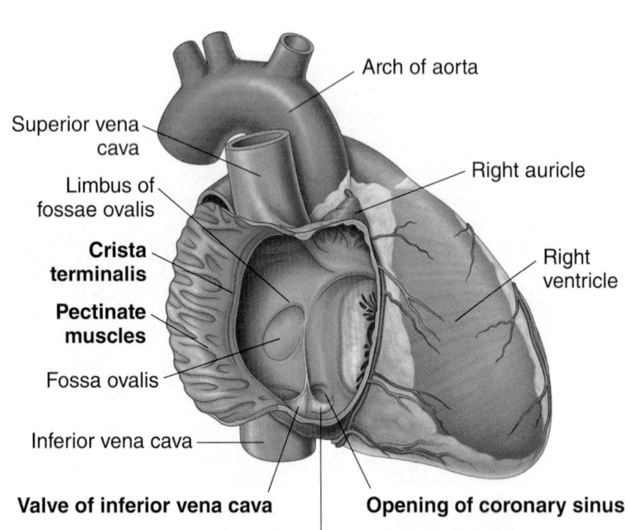

Plate 6.1 A view of the structures of the right atrium. (From Drake RL et al. *Gray's Anatomy for Students*, 5th edition, Philadelphia, Elsevier, 2024, Figure 3.72, p. 197.)

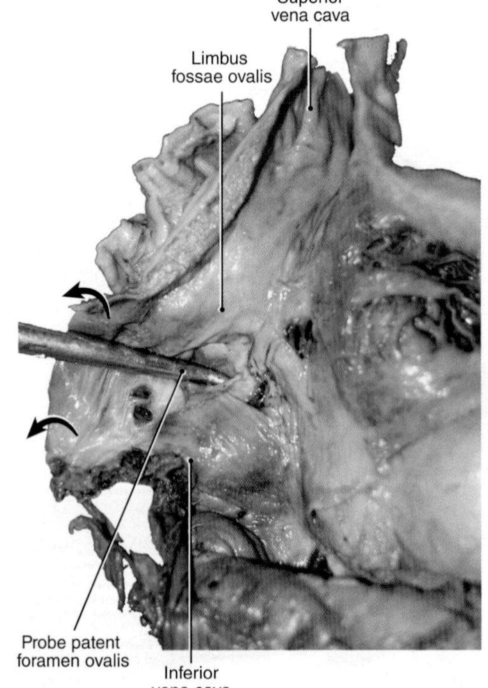

Fig. 6.23 Right atrium reflected to reveal patent foramen ovale.

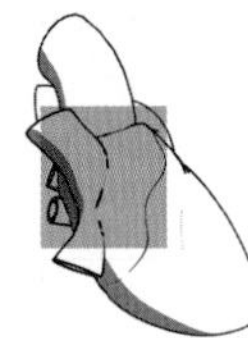

- **Turn the right atrium upward and note the *tricuspid valve* and its three leaflets: septal, anterior, and inferior.**
- **The separation of the three leaflets may not be well delineated.**
- **Identify the membranous septum between the septal and anterior leaflets of the tricuspid valve.**
- **Place index finger deeply within the aorta (below the level of its valve) while palpating the base of the interatrial septum with the thumb of the same hand. The small area where the thumb and the finger are separated by the thinnest amount of tissue marks the site of the membranous septum (Figs. 6.24 and 6.25).**

Left Atrium

- **Incise the left atrium laterally, making a horizontal incision from the right to the left pulmonary veins (Fig. 6.26).**
- **With forceps, reflect the flap made by the lateral incision in the left atrium and observe within the chamber a smooth surface and limited number of pectinate muscles in the left auricle (Fig. 6.27 and Plate 6.2).**

Right Ventricle

The following two techniques are used to expose the contents of the right ventricle:

Technique 1

- **Open the right ventricle by making an incision through the right atrium to expose fully the tricuspid valve toward the right ventricle (ventricular inlet) (Fig. 6.28).**
- **Make a second incision from the pulmonary valve to the apex of the right ventricle (ventricular outlet). The major problem with this technique is that the septomarginal trabecula and RCA are often cut (Fig. 6.29).**

Technique 2

- **Make a small, circular incision a few centimeters below the subpulmonary infundibulum. This area typically is occupied by the right ventricular free wall (Fig. 6.30).**
- **Carefully, start cutting larger pieces of the right ventricular free wall, keeping in mind not to cut the septomarginal trabecula (Fig. 6.31 and Plate 6.3).**
- **Identify the septomarginal trabecula (also referred to as moderator band), cut around the papillary muscle toward the tricuspid valve, and expose as much of the right ventricle as possible (Fig. 6.32).**

Membranous part of interventricular septum
Pectinate muscles
Superior vena cava
Fossa ovalis
Inferior vena cava
Septal leaflet
Anterior leaflet

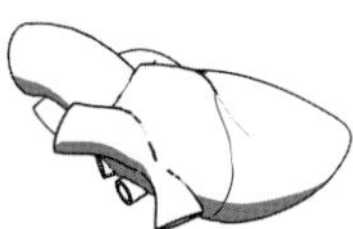

Fig. 6.24 Anterior atrial wall is lifted upward, and with a light behind it (transillumination), the membranous septum is seen.

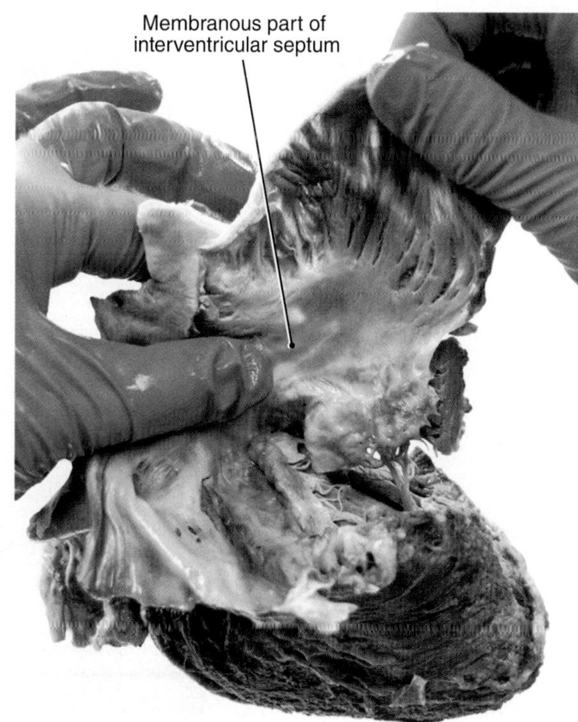

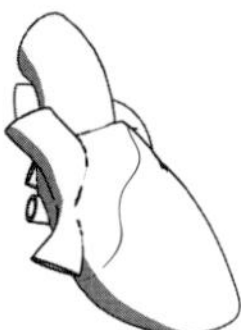

Fig. 6.25 Right atrium reflected with dissector's left thumb palpating the membranous septum.

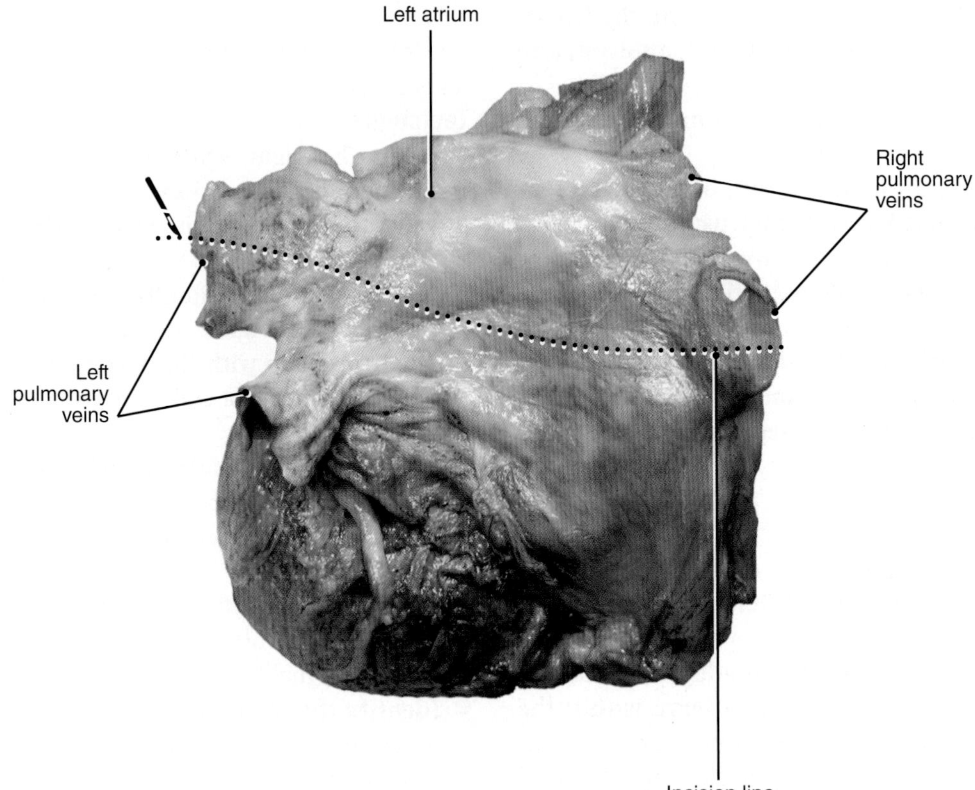

Fig. 6.26 Base of heart with outline used for making incision to see contents of the left atrium.

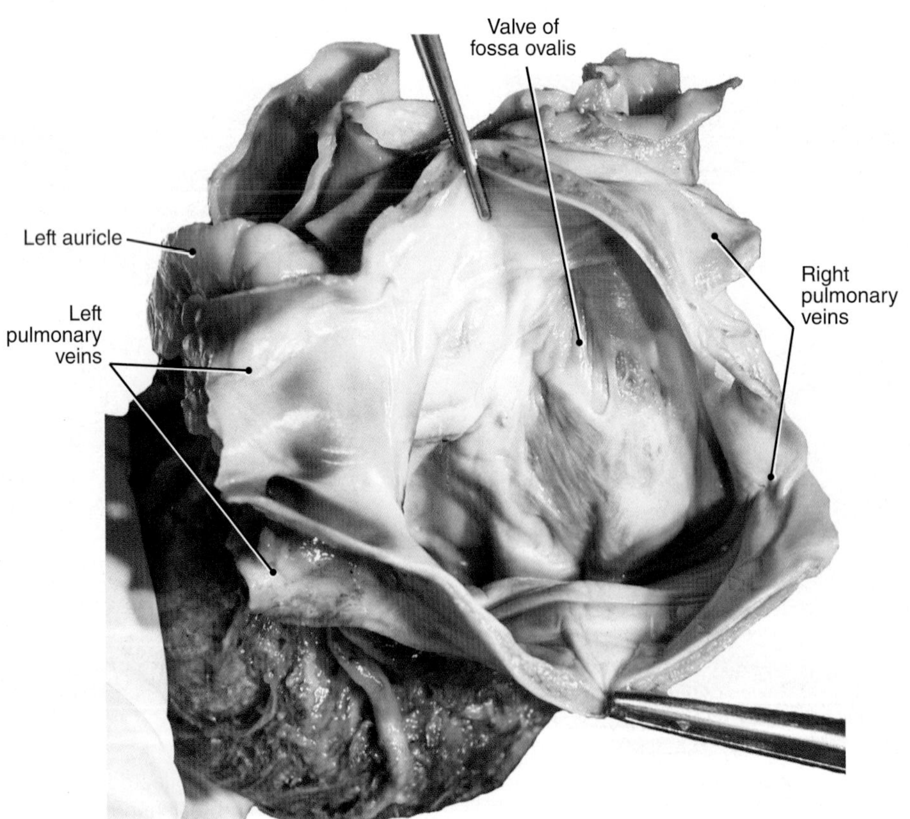

Fig. 6.27 Left atrium incised superiorly, revealing internal structures.

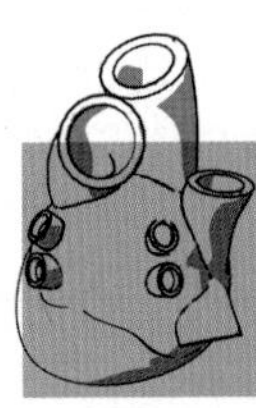

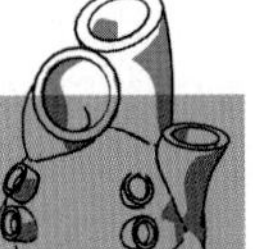

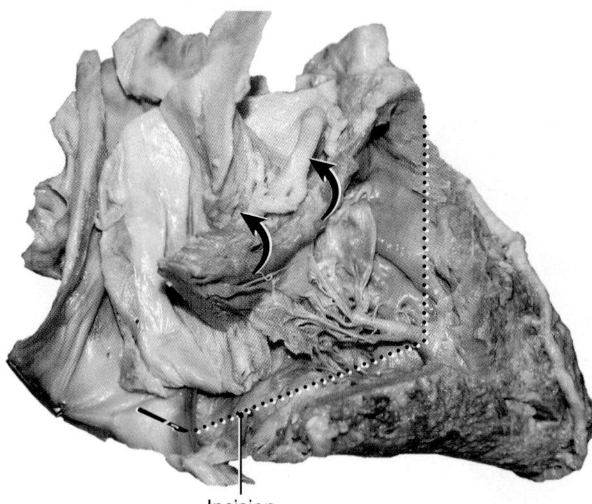

Fig. 6.28 Deep dissection of right ventricle using V-shaped incisions revealing internal structures.

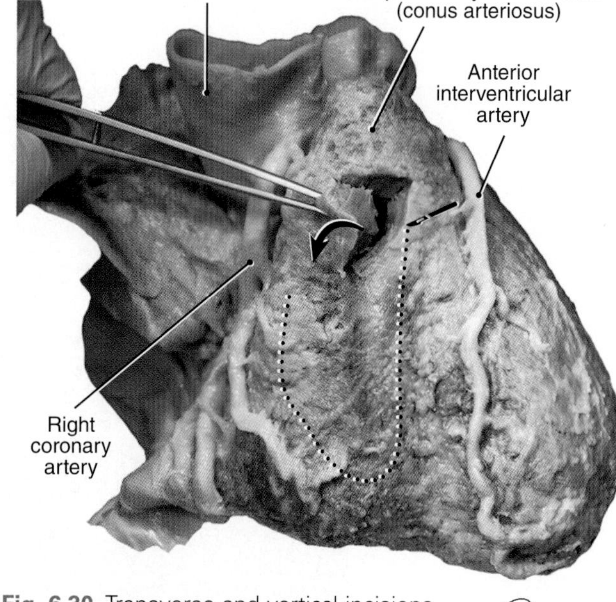

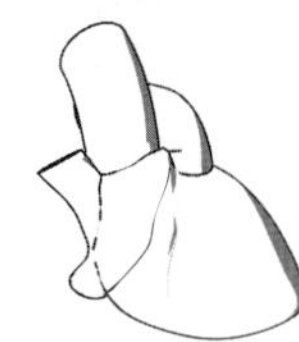

Fig. 6.30 Transverse and vertical incisions into the right ventricle, creating a window into the conus arteriosus; *dotted line* shows continuation of incision.

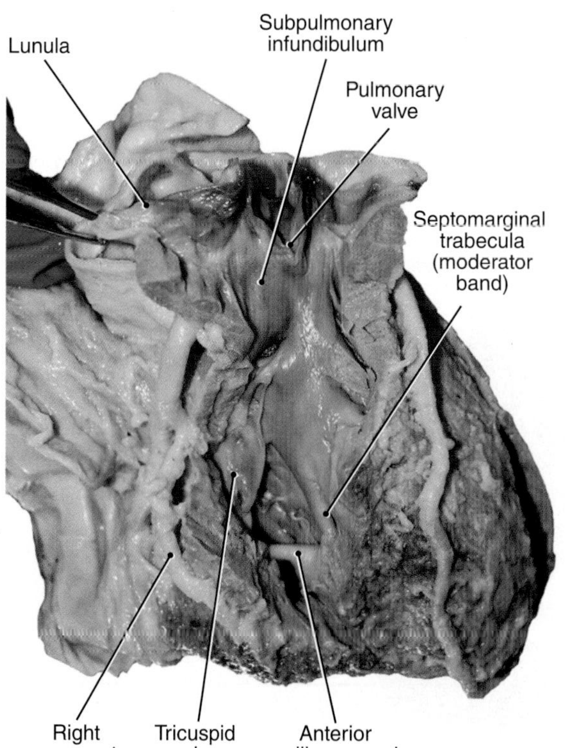

Fig. 6.29 Right ventricle reflected away from apex and in line with the pulmonary valve; anterior interventricular artery.

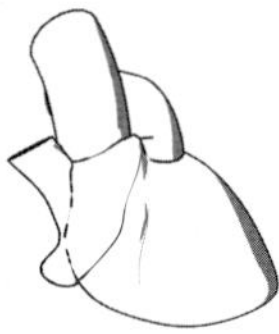

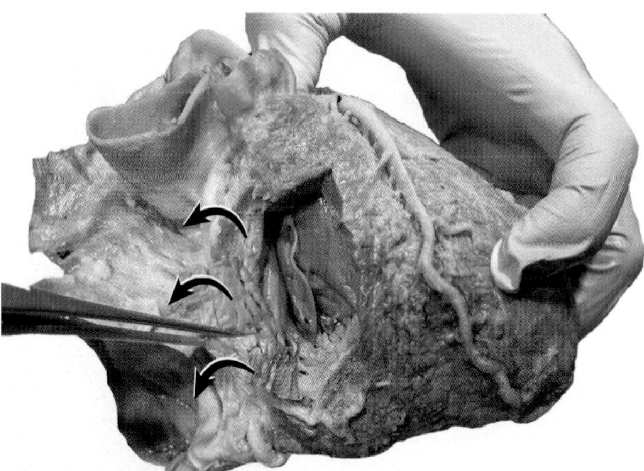

Fig. 6.31 Reflected anterior wall of the right ventricle revealing internal structures.

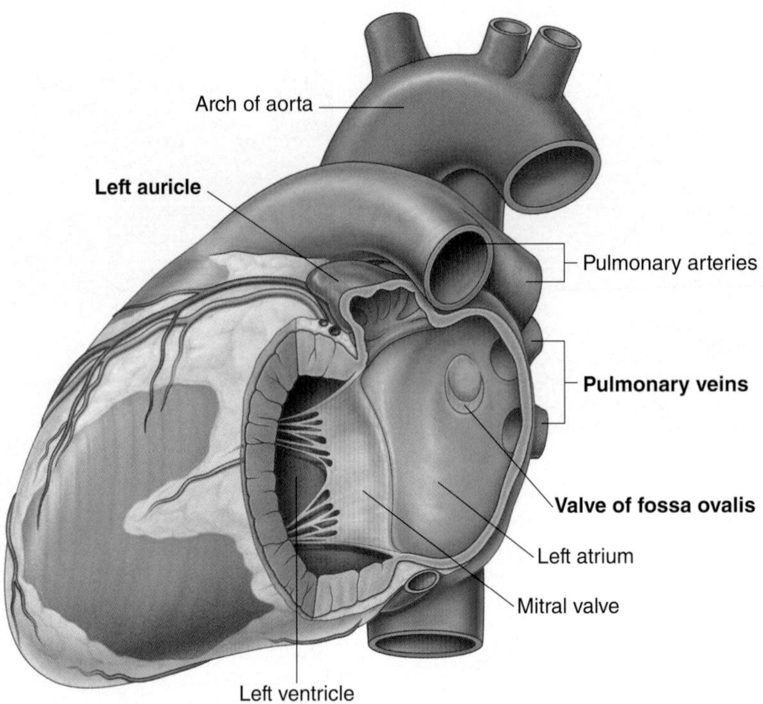

Plate 6.2 A view of the structures of the left atrium. (From Drake RL et al. *Gray's Anatomy for Students*, 5th edition, Philadelphia, Elsevier, 2024, Figure 3.75A, p. 201.)

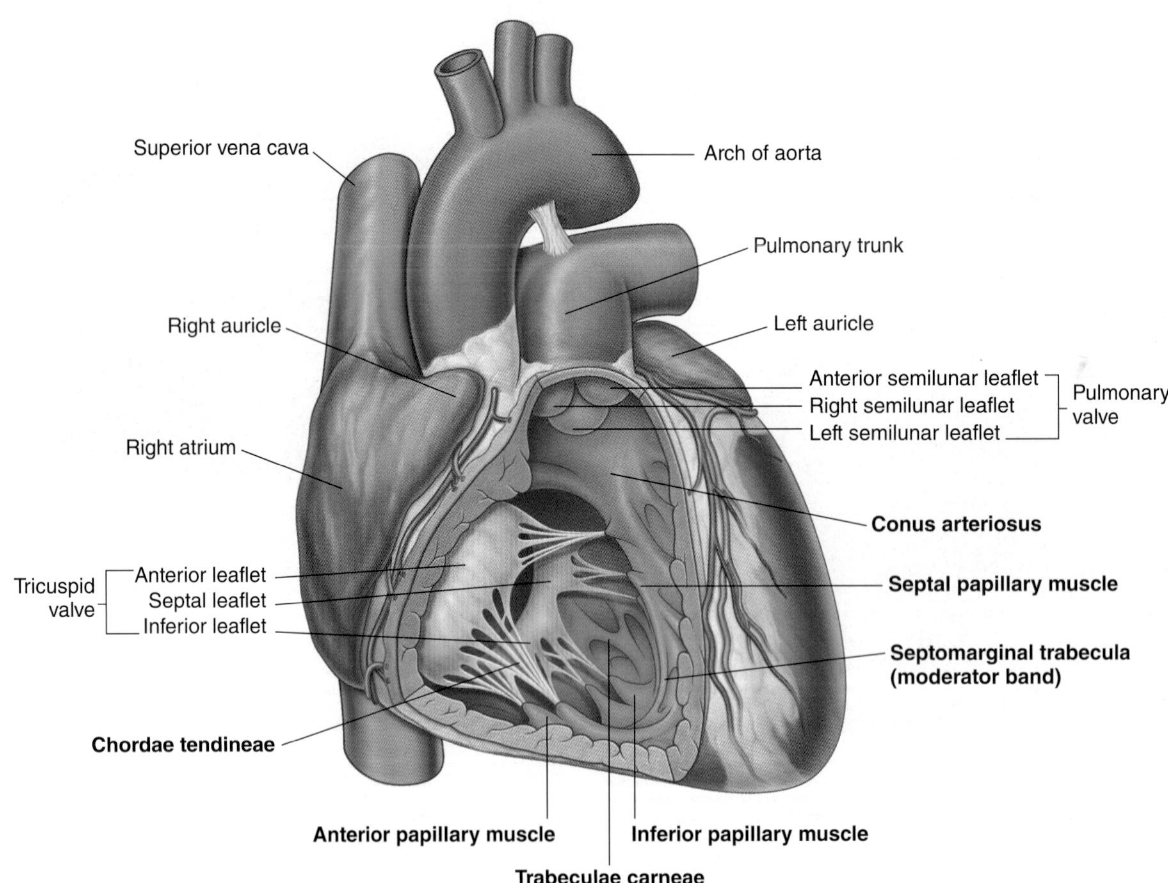

Plate 6.3 A view of the structures of the right ventricle. (From Drake RL et al. *Gray's Anatomy for Students*, 5th edition, Philadelphia, Elsevier, 2024, Figure 3.73, p. 199.)

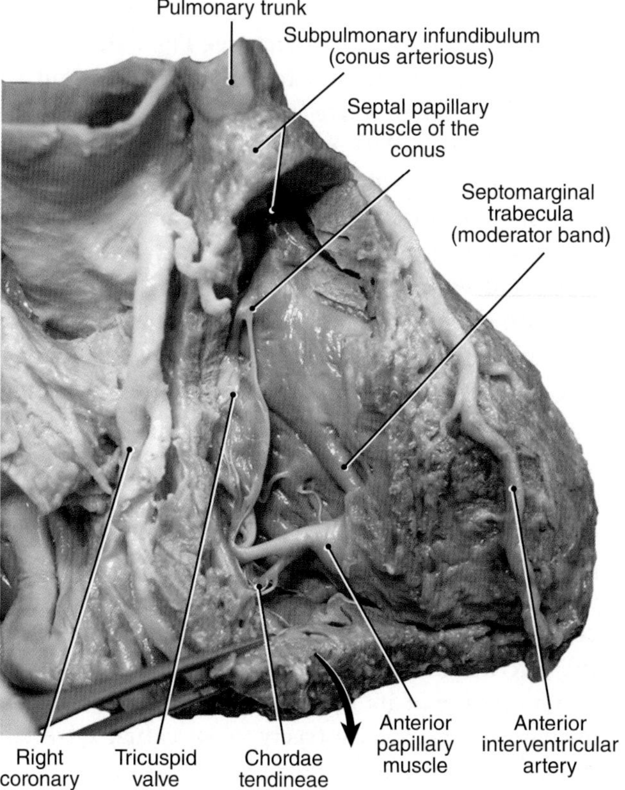

Fig. 6.32 Reflected anterior wall of right ventricle revealing internal structures.

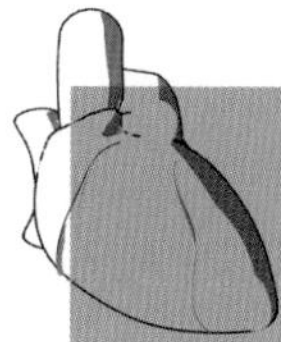

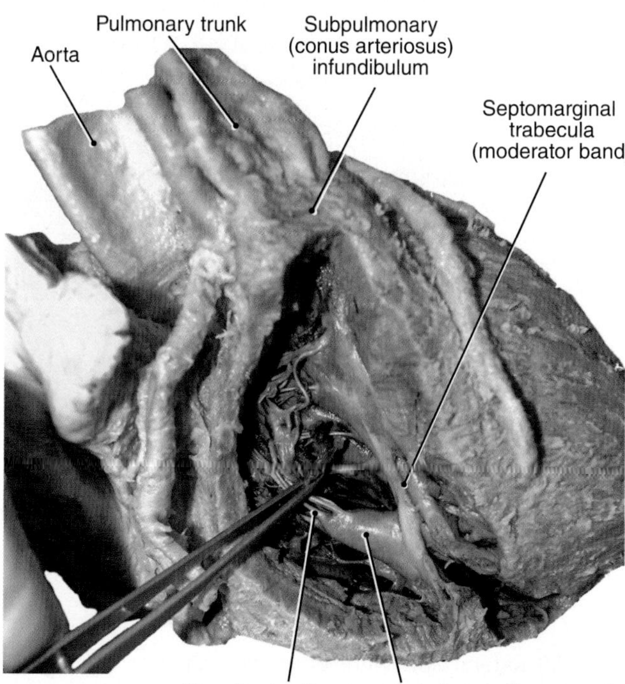

Fig. 6.33 Reflected anterior wall of the right ventricle revealing internal structures.

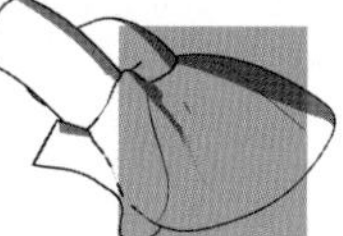

DISSECTION TIP

The majority of hearts have a significant amount of coagulated blood around the cordae tendineae and the papillary muscles (Fig. 6.33). With forceps, carefully clean out the coagulated blood (Fig. 6.34). Water also may be run through the heart to aid in this cleaning process.

- **Identify the anterior, inferior, and septal leaflets of the tricuspid valve. Observe that the leaflets are anchored to papillary muscles within the ventricle by slender chordae tendineae (see Fig. 6.34).**
- **Identify the large anterior papillary muscle.**
- **Posterior and inferior to this muscle is the inferior papillary muscle.**
- **The septal papillary muscle may consist of several small, septal papillary muscles arising from the interventricular septum, with short chordae tendineae passing to the septal leaflet of the valve. The highest and largest is called the septal papillary muscle of the conus, or of Luschka or Lancisi (see Fig. 6.34).**
- **Note the thick, irregular-shaped bundles of muscle within the right ventricle, the *trabeculae carneae*. The *septomarginal trabecula* (or septomarginal trabeculation or moderator band) passes from the**

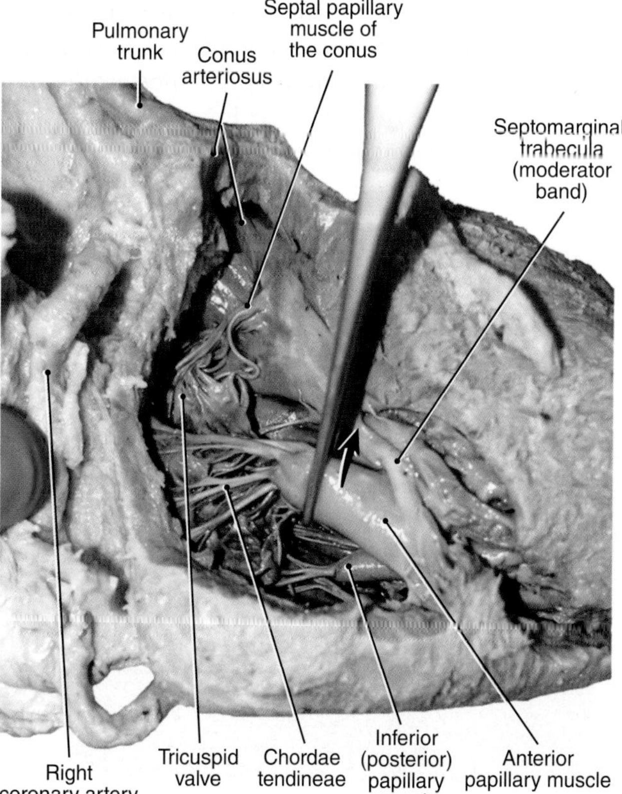

Fig. 6.34 Reflected anterior wall of the right ventricle revealing internal structures.

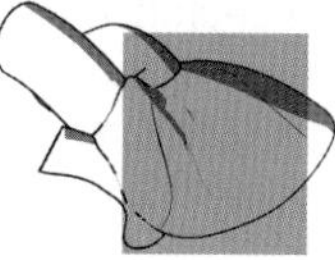

muscular interventricular septum to the base of the anterior papillary muscle.

- If Technique 2 was used to open the right ventricle, now cut through the pulmonary trunk.
- Refer to Fig. 6.29. Note that the three semilunar-shaped leaflets join together at the commissures.
- Note the *lunula* (free margin) and nodule of each leaflet. Observe the horizontal muscle tissue in which the pulmonary valve sits; this is the subpulmonary muscular infundibulum.
- The area between the septal papillary muscle of the conus and subpulmonary infundibulum is demarcated by the crista supraventricularis.

Left Ventricle

- Identify the right coronary leaflet, the noncoronary leaflet (also known as nonadjacent), and the left coronary leaflet of the aortic valve (Fig. 6.35).
- Make a parallel incision from the anterior interventricular artery to the bifurcation of the left coronary artery into anterior interventricular and circumflex arteries (Figs. 6.36 and 6.37).
- With your fingers or a retractor, open the left ventricle and observe the muscular ridges, the trabeculae carneae (Fig. 6.38).
- Identify the mitral valve (left AV valve) with its two leaflets, an anterior (aortic) and a posterior leaflet (mural) attaching by chordae tendineae to two papillary muscles, the inferoseptal (posteromedial) papillary muscle (closer to the intraventricular septum, *septophilic*) and the superolateral (anterolateral) papillary muscle (farther away from the intraventricular septum, *septophobic*) (see Fig. 6.38).
- Make a vertical incision toward the aorta and cut through the aortic valve (Fig. 6.39).
- Identify the leaflets of the aortic valve and the lunula (free margin) and nodule of each leaflet. Identify the ostia of the coronary arteries and the depressions in the wall of the aorta, the "aortic sinuses of Valsalva."
- Beneath the junction of the noncoronary leaflet and the right coronary leaflet of the aortic valve, identify the membranous portion of the interventricular septum (Fig. 6.40).
- Observe the leaflets of the mitral valve and the aortic-mitral valve continuity (Fig. 6.40).
- Notice the layer of lighter-colored tissue, which appears to travel inferiorly down the interventricular septum, between the coronary leaflet and the noncoronary leaflet of the aortic valve. This tissue forms the left bundle branch of the cardiac conduction system. Some of its fibers may be seen crossing the left ventricular cavity freely as so-called false tendons (see Figs. 6.40 and 6.41 and Plate 6.4).

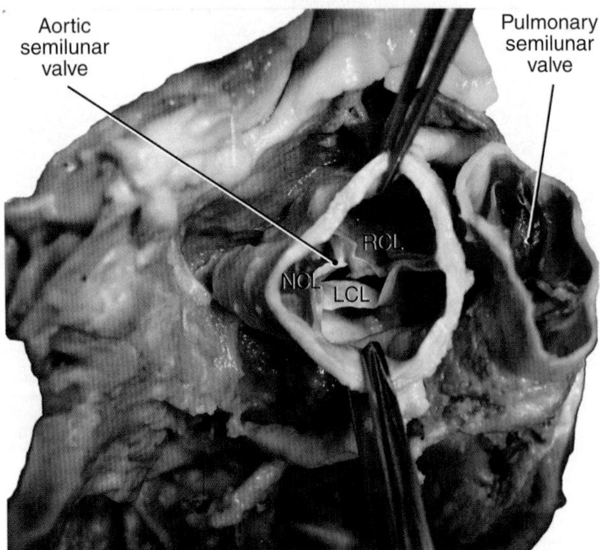

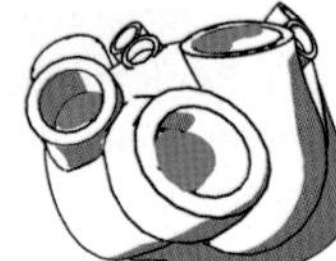

Fig. 6.35 Aorta and pulmonary vessels transected superior to base of heart revealing their valves, respectively. *LCL*, Left coronary leaflet; *NCL*, noncoronary leaflet; *RCL*, right coronary leaflet.

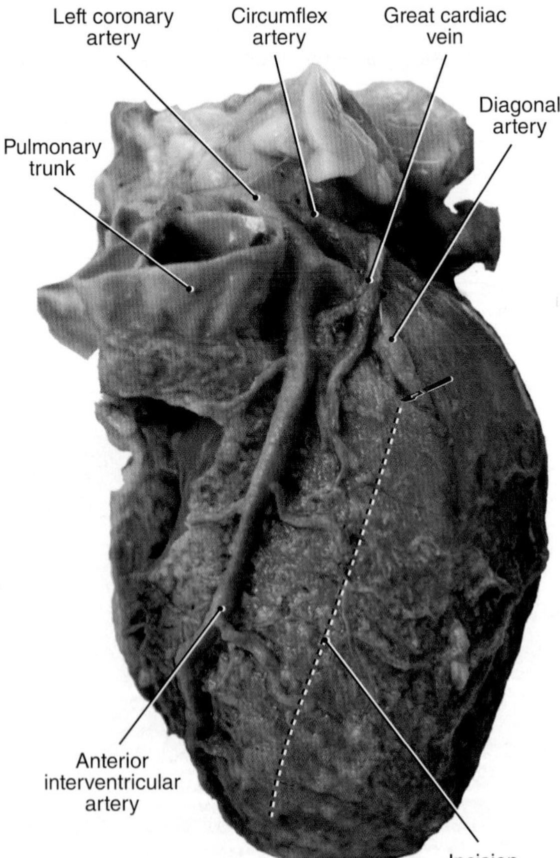

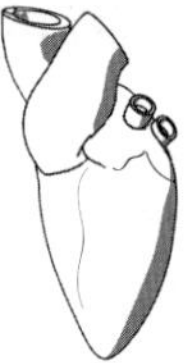

Fig. 6.36 Lateral view with vertical tilt revealing the left coronary artery and dominant branches, with tracing *(dotted line)* for incision into the left ventricle.

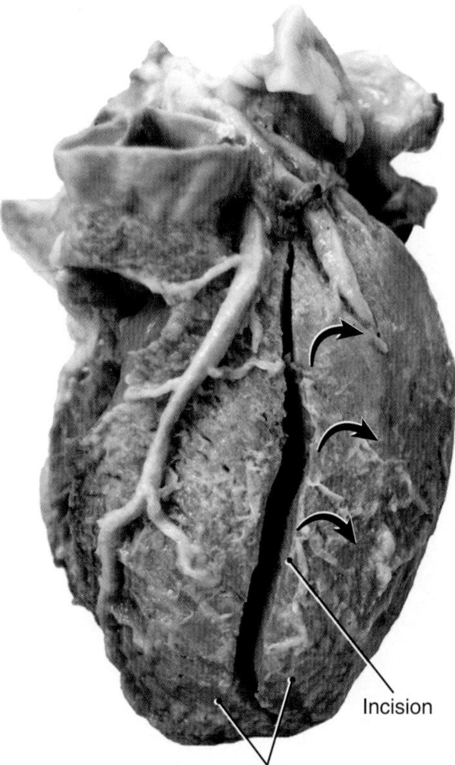

Fig. 6.37 Lateral view with vertical tilt revealing the left coronary artery and dominant branches, with incision into the left ventricle.

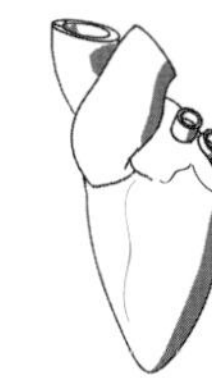

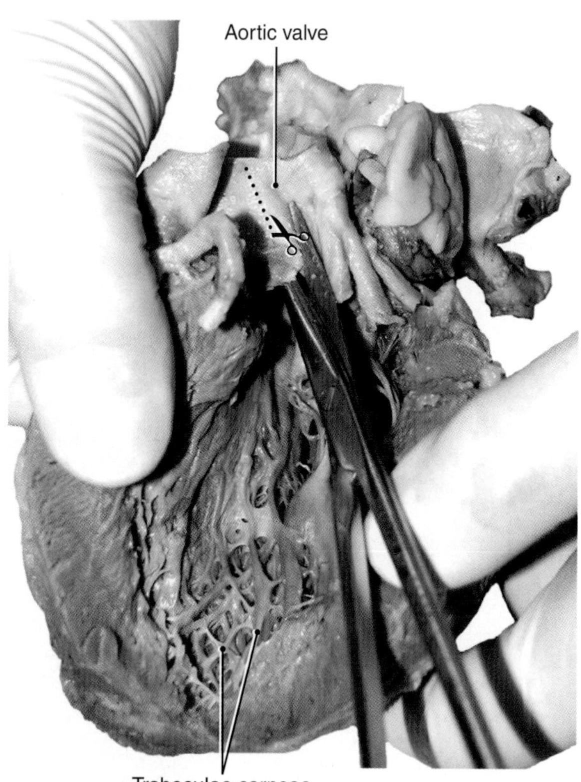

Fig. 6.39 Opened left ventricle demonstrating internal structures and the scissors incising aortic valve.

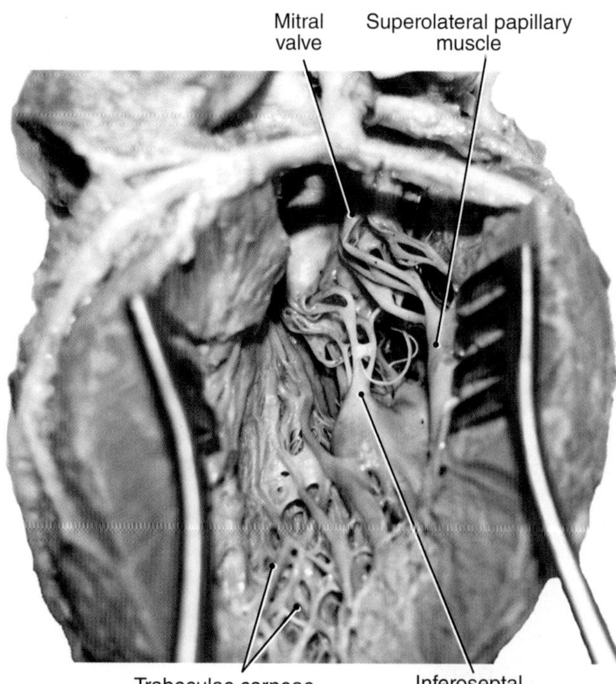

Fig. 6.38 Lateral view with vertical tilt revealing internal structures of the left ventricle.

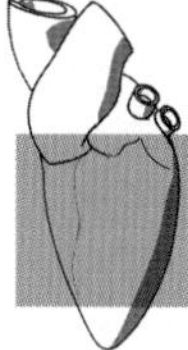

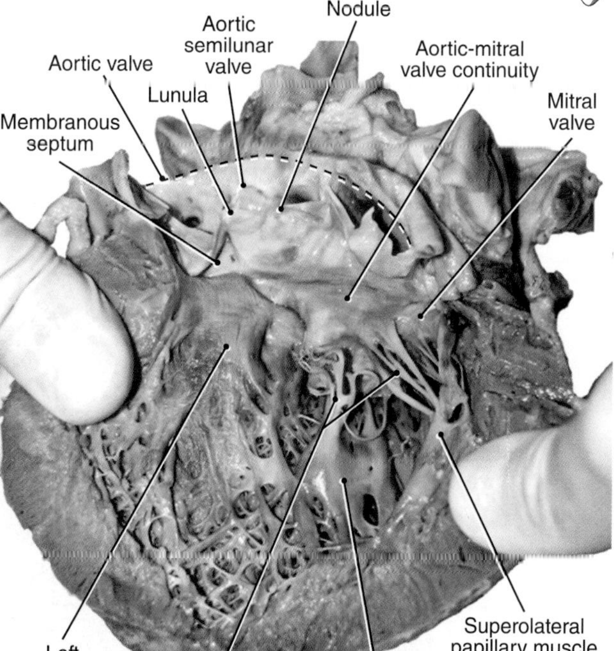

Fig. 6.40 Left ventricle reflected revealing internal structures and highlighting the aortic and mitral valves.

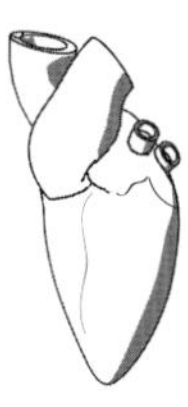

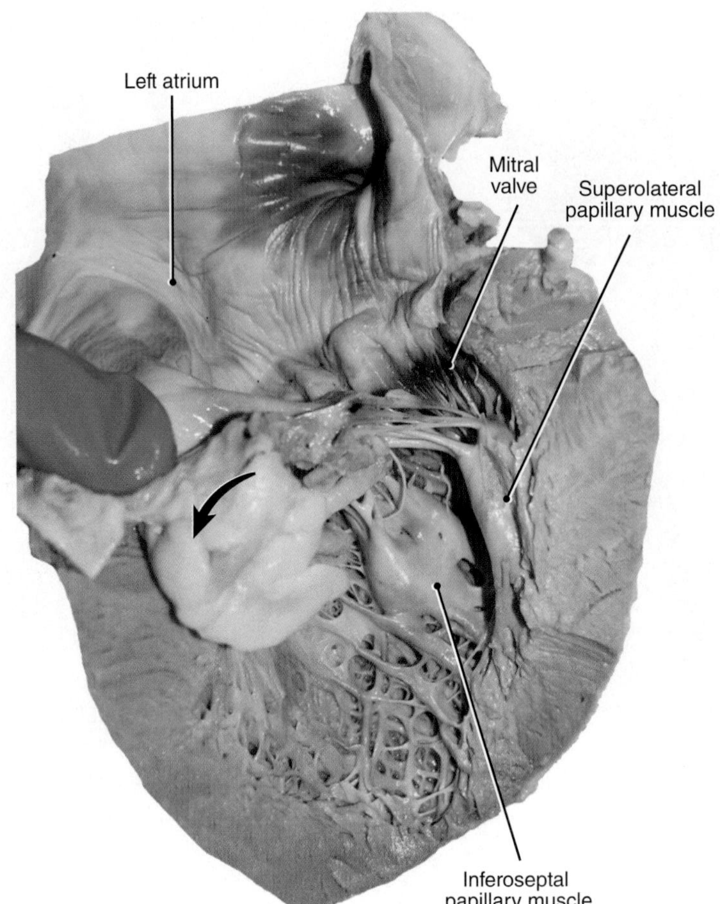

Fig. 6.41 Left ventricle opened and reflected revealing left atrioventricular valve and papillary muscles.

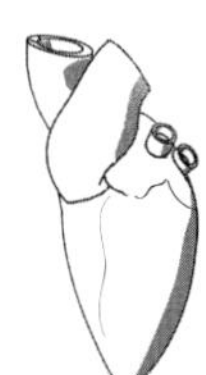

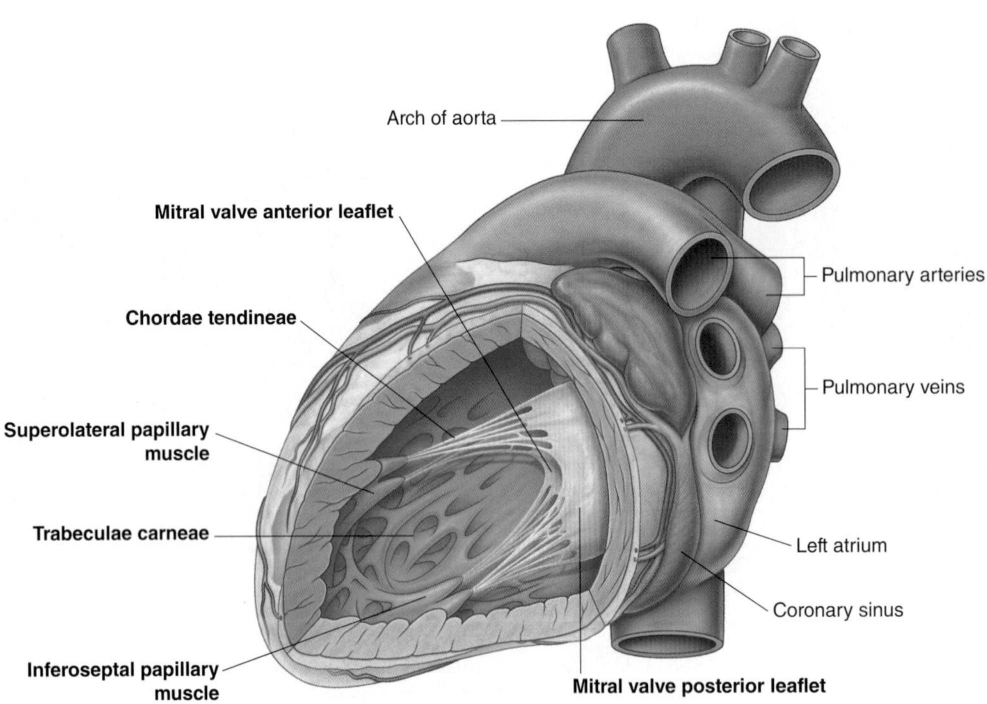

Plate 6.4 A view of the structures of the left ventricle. (From Drake RL et al. *Gray's Anatomy for Students*, 5th edition, Philadelphia, Elsevier, 2024, Figure 3.76, p. 202.)

LABORATORY IDENTIFICATION CHECKLIST

ARTERIES

- ☐ Aorta
- ☐ Common carotid
- ☐ Brachiocephalic trunk
- ☐ Pulmonary
- ☐ Left coronary
- ☐ Anterior interventricular
- ☐ Circumflex
- ☐ Interventricular septal branches
- ☐ Right coronary
- ☐ Marginal
- ☐ Sinuatrial (SA) nodal
- ☐ Atrioventricular (AV) nodal
- ☐ Inferior interventricular

VEINS

- ☐ Superior vena cava
- ☐ Inferior vena cava and eustachian valve
- ☐ Right and left pulmonary veins
- ☐ Coronary sinus and thebesian valve
- ☐ Great cardiac
- ☐ Middle cardiac
- ☐ Small cardiac

HEART

- ☐ Right atrium
  - ☐ Right auricle
  - ☐ Superior vena cava
  - ☐ Inferior vena cava
  - ☐ Fossa ovalis
  - ☐ Opening of coronary sinus
  - ☐ Crista terminalis
  - ☐ Pectinate muscle
  - ☐ Sinus venosus region
- ☐ Right ventricle
  - ☐ Right atrioventricular (AV) valve or tricuspid valve
  - ☐ Chordae tendineae
  - ☐ Anterior papillary muscle
  - ☐ Inferior papillary muscle
  - ☐ Septal papillary muscle
  - ☐ Septomarginal trabecula (septomarginal trabeculation or moderator band)
  - ☐ Interventricular septum
  - ☐ Trabeculae carneae
- ☐ Subpulmonary infundibulum (conus arteriosus)
  - ☐ Pulmonary valve
- ☐ Left atrium
- ☐ Left auricle
- ☐ Right and left pulmonary veins
- ☐ Left atrioventricular (AV) valve, or bicuspid/mitral valve
  - ☐ Anterior leaflet (aortic)
  - ☐ Inferior leaflet (mural)
- ☐ Left ventricle
- ☐ Aortic valve
  - ☐ Right coronary leaflet
  - ☐ Noncoronary leaflet
  - ☐ Left coronary leaflet
  - ☐ Superolateral papillary muscle
  - ☐ Inferoseptal papillary muscle
  - ☐ Chordae tendineae
  - ☐ Trabeculae carneae
  - ☐ Anterior interventricular sulcus
  - ☐ Inferior interventricular sulcus
  - ☐ Coronary sulcus
  - ☐ Sulcus terminalis

CLINICAL APPLICATIONS

THORACENTESIS

Clinical Application

Introduce a needle or trocar into the pleural cavity, creating a conduit to allow air (pneumothorax) to escape or to help remove fluid.

Anatomical Landmarks

- *Needle:* **2nd intercostal space at midclavicular line**
  - **Skin**
  - **Subcutaneous tissues**
  - **External intercostal fascia/muscle**
  - **Internal intercostal fascia/muscle**
  - **Parietal pleura**
- *Tube:* **5th intercostal space at the midaxillary line**
  - **Skin**
  - **Subcutaneous tissues**
  - **Inferior angle of the scapula**
  - **Lateral border of pectoralis major**
  - **Lateral border of breast**
  - **Intercostal muscles**
  - **Parietal pleura**

Note: Needle placement for pneumothorax is 2nd intercostal space at the midclavicular line; tube placement is at the midaxillary line (Fig. III.1).

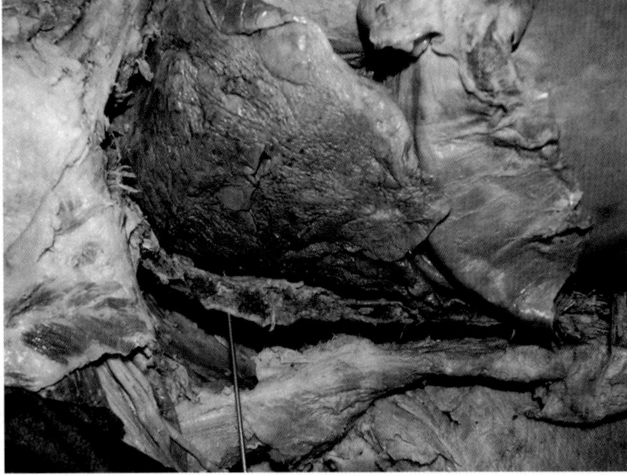

Fig. III.1

CENTRAL VENOUS LINE (CATHETERIZATION OF SUBCLAVIAN VEIN OR INTERNAL JUGULAR VEIN)

Clinical Application

Introduce a line (catheter) into the internal jugular vein above and behind the clavicle and medial to the sternocleidomastoid muscle for long-term infusion of fluids or medicines (Fig. III.2).

Anatomical Landmarks

- **Skin**
- **Subcutaneous tissues**
- **Sternocleidomastoid muscle**
- **Clavicle**
- **Costoclavicular ligament**
- **Subclavian vein**
- **Anterior scalene, phenic nerve, lymphatic ducts**
- **Pleura**

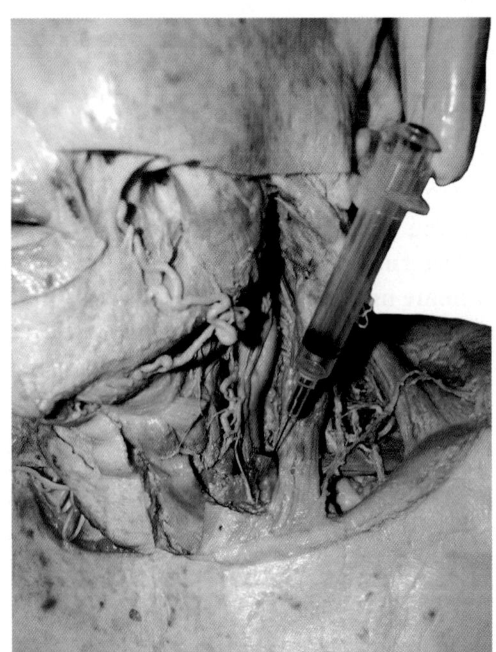

Fig. III.2

PERICARDIOCENTESIS

Clinical Application

Withdraw fluid from the pericardial space (Fig. III.3). *Note:* The liver, stomach, and internal thoracic artery may be in danger of injury (Fig. III.4).

Anatomical Landmarks

Subxiphoid Approach

- **Xiphoid process of sternum**
- **Skin**
- **Subcutaneous tissue**
- **Rectus abdominis**
- **Pericardium**
- **Pericardial space**

Parasternal Approach

- **Left 5th intercostal space**
- **Left sternal border**
- **Skin**
- **Subcutaneous tissue**
- **External intercostal muscle**
- **Internal intercostal muscle**
- **Innermost intercostal muscle**
- **Pleura**
- **Pericardial space**

OTHER LANDMARKS AND OBSERVATIONS

- Fig. III.5 shows an example of enlarged malignant lymph nodes in the axilla.
- The sternalis muscle is one of the most common variations found in the musculature of the anterior thoracic wall (Fig. III.6).
- Fig. III.7 shows a cadaver with a pacemaker.
- See Figs. III.8 to III.11 for examples of lungs with malignant lesions.
- The *myocardial bridge* is a muscular bridge that covers the anterior interventricular artery for a short distance within the myocardium. It is a common finding during dissection (Fig. III.12).
- Figs. III.13 and III.14 show the effects of myocardial infarction of the heart.

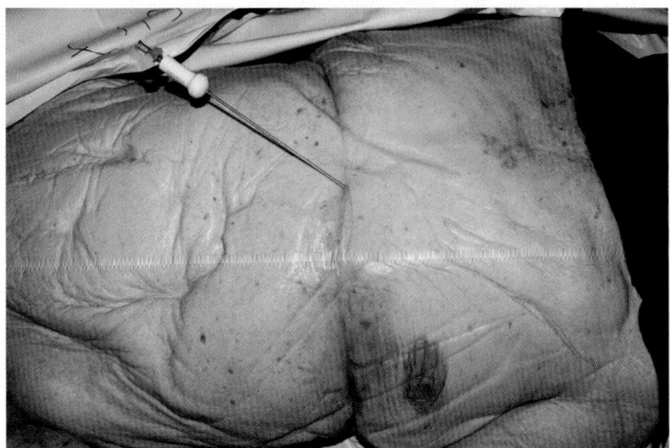

Fig. III.3

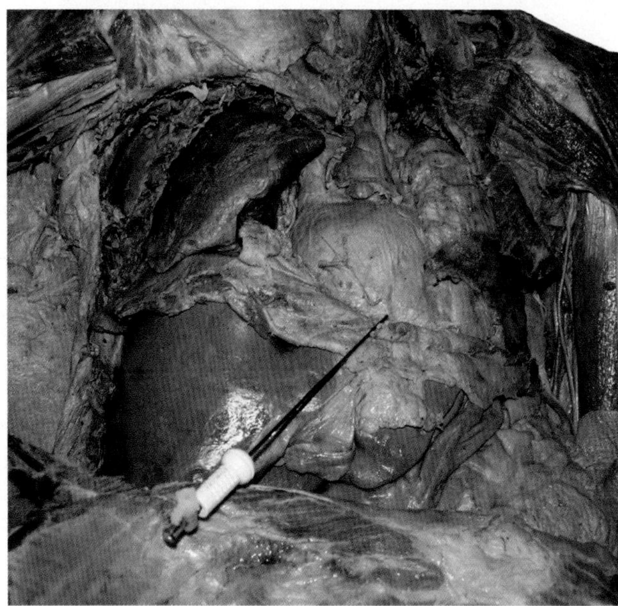

Fig. III.4

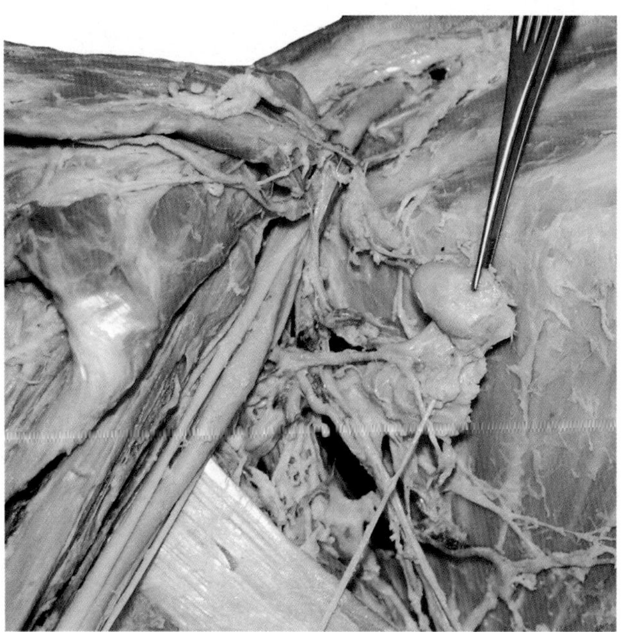

Fig. III.5

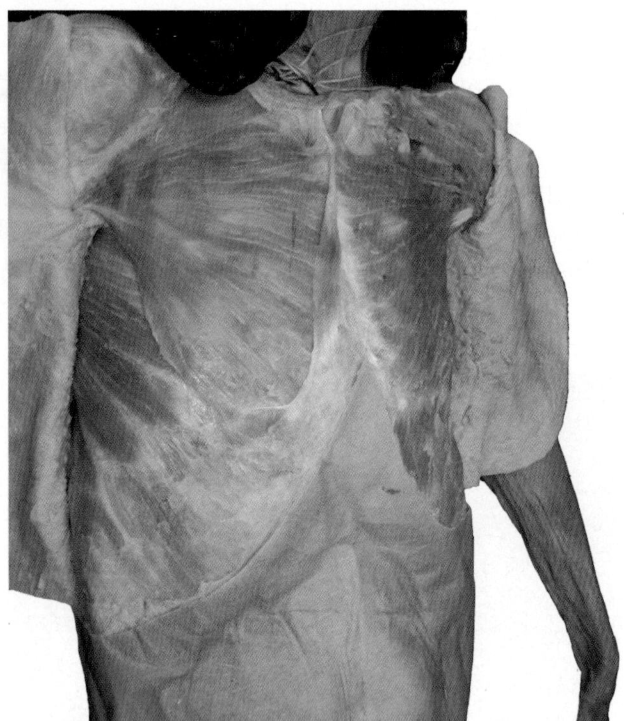

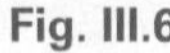

Fig. III.6

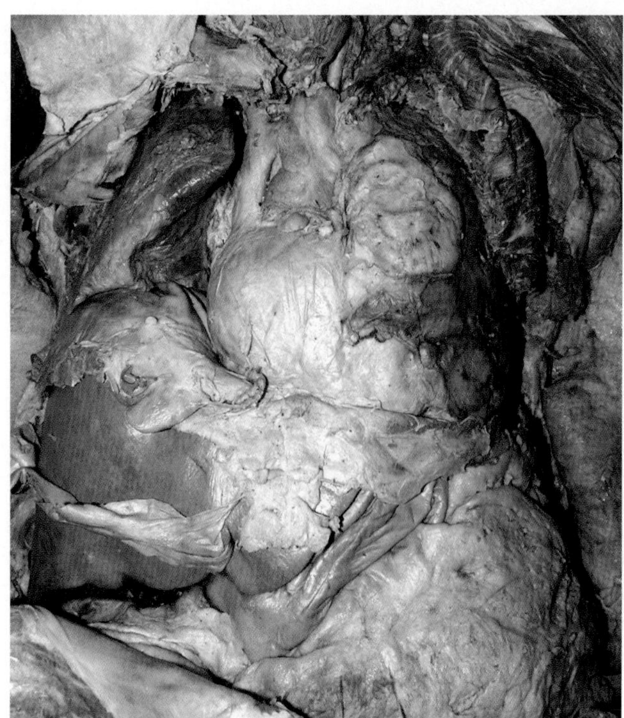

Fig. III.8

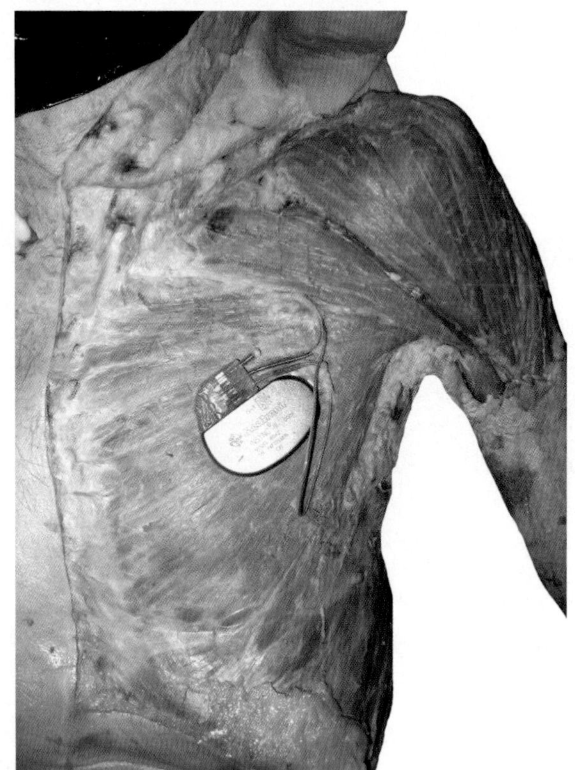

Fig. III.7

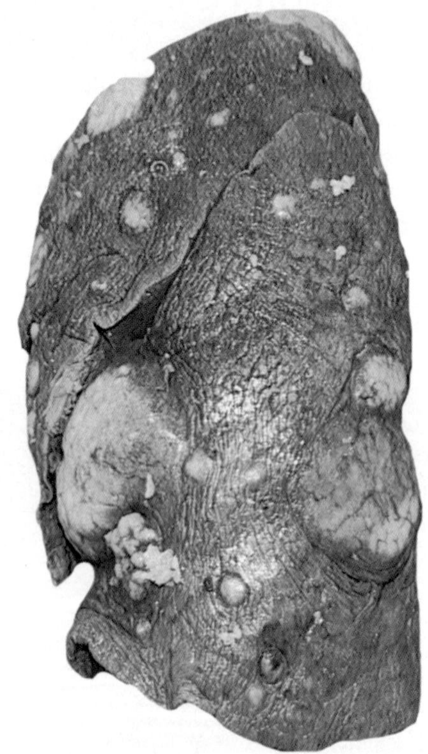

Fig. III.9

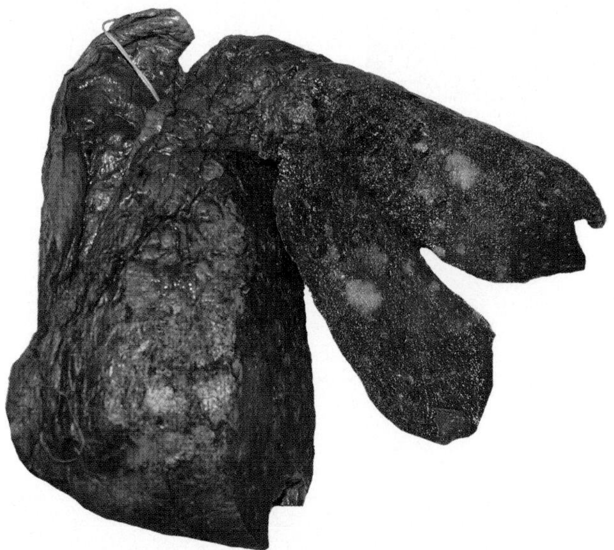

Fig. III.10

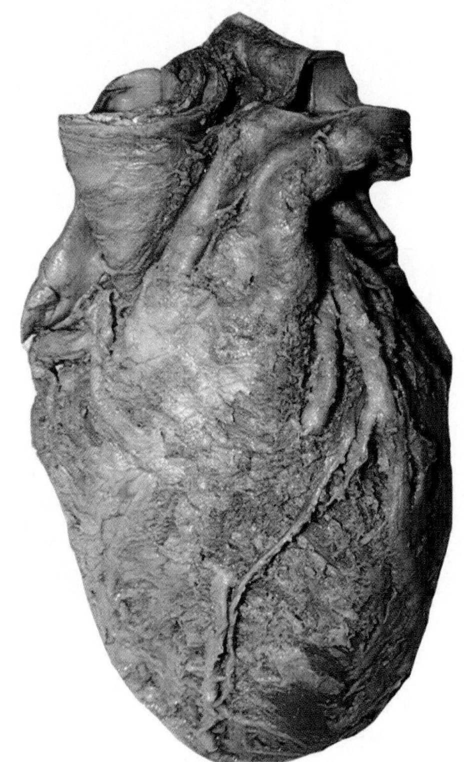

Fig. III.12

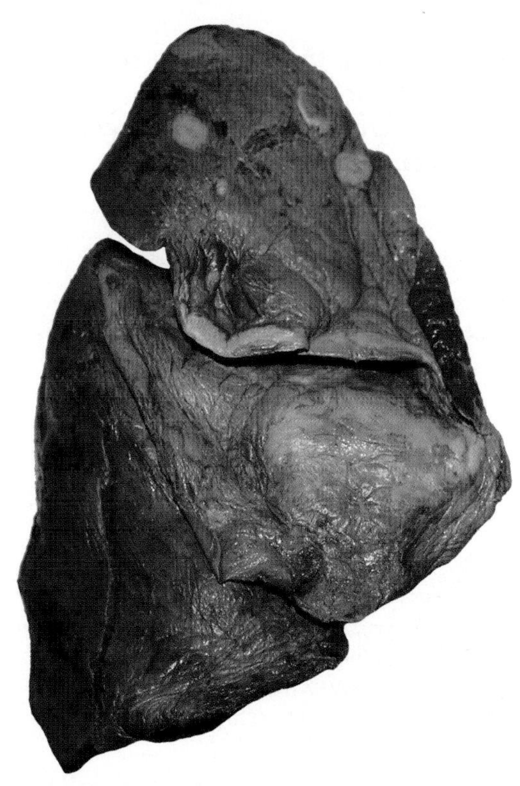

Fig. III.11

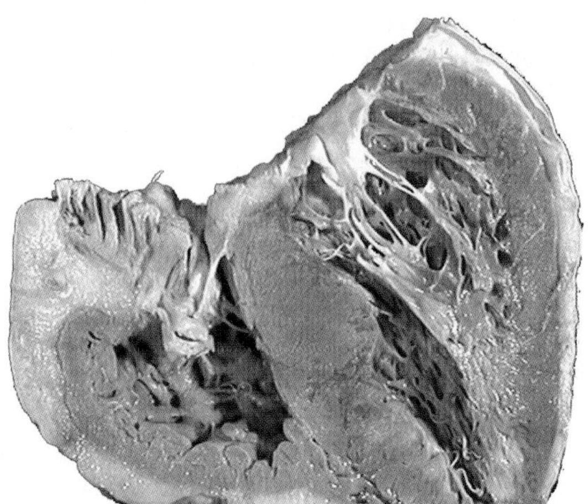

Fig. III.13

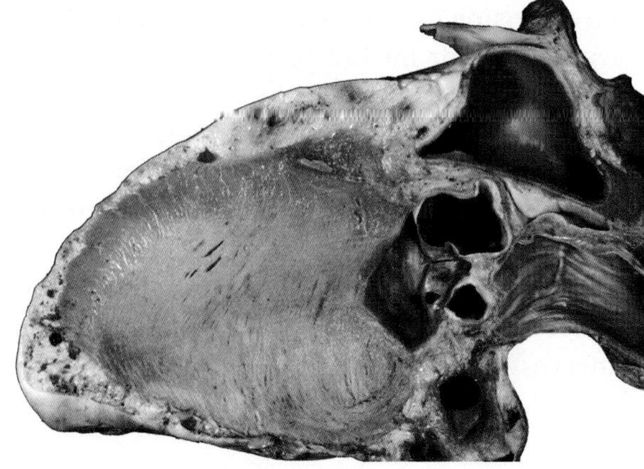

Fig. III.14

SECTION IV

UPPER LIMB

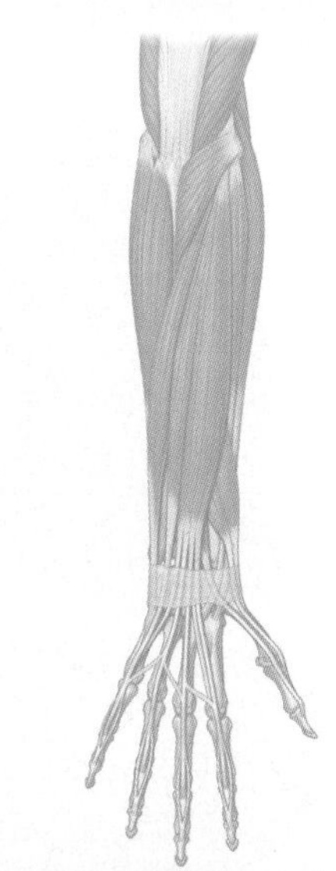

CHAPTER 7 AXILLA AND ARM

BEFORE YOU BEGIN

Axillary Borders

The pectoral region should have been dissected before the study of the axilla is begun. Refer to Chapter 4 for the regional anatomy of the pectoral region and breast. Review the following borders of the axilla:

- **Anterior wall:** Pectoralis major and minor muscles and clavipectoral fascia
- **Posterior wall:** Latissimus dorsi, teres major, and subscapularis muscles
- **Lateral wall:** Humerus, short head of biceps brachii muscle, and coracobrachialis muscle
- **Medial wall:** Upper five ribs, their intercostal muscles, and adjacent serratus anterior muscle
- **Base:** Axillary fascia
- **Apex** *(cervicoaxillary canal):* Superior border of scapula, 1st rib, and clavicle

DISSECTION STEPS

- **Make a skin incision from the shoulder distally to a point 2 to 3 inches (5–7.5 cm) above the elbow.**
- **An encircling incision around the midportion of the arm allows for medial retraction of the skin from the proximal arm.**
- **Reflect the skin from the thorax, shoulders, axillae, and proximal portions of the arms medially to the axillary space (as shown previously in Fig. 4.4).**
- **See Chapter 8 for the incisions used in the forearm.**
- **Reflect the pectoralis muscles, better exposing the intercostobrachial and long thoracic nerves.**
- **Identify the long thoracic nerve running over the serratus anterior muscle.**
- **Note the intercostobrachial nerve emerging from the 2nd intercostal space.**

ANATOMY NOTE

The intercostobrachial nerve emerging from the 2nd intercostal space is usually the lateral cutaneous branch of the 2nd thoracic (T2) nerve crossing over the long thoracic nerve, that supplies the skin of the proximal, medial aspect of the arm and axilla (Fig. 7.1).

- **Preserve these two nerves.**

DISSECTION TIP

Adipose tissue and lymphatics occupy most of the space in the axilla. Do not attempt to remove them at this stage. Push them away from the structures you identify and remove them at a later stage.

- **Identify the fascia that invests the axillary artery, axillary vein, and brachial plexus. This is the *axillary sheath.***
- **Excise the axillary sheath between the axillary artery and the brachial plexus by gently pulling away the nerves (Fig. 7.2).**
- **Remove the axillary sheath and clean the adipose tissue away from the brachial plexus (Fig. 7.3).**
- **Identify and clean the axillary artery and vein (Fig. 7.4).**

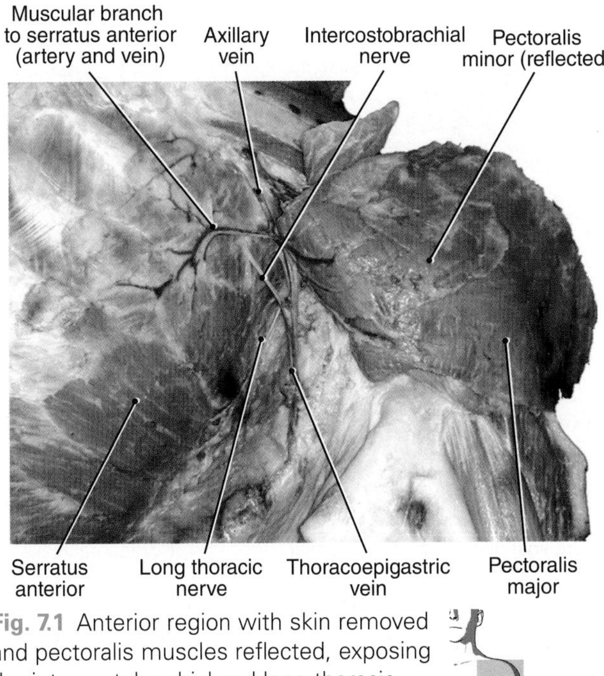

Fig. 7.1 Anterior region with skin removed and pectoralis muscles reflected, exposing the intercostobrachial and long thoracic nerves.

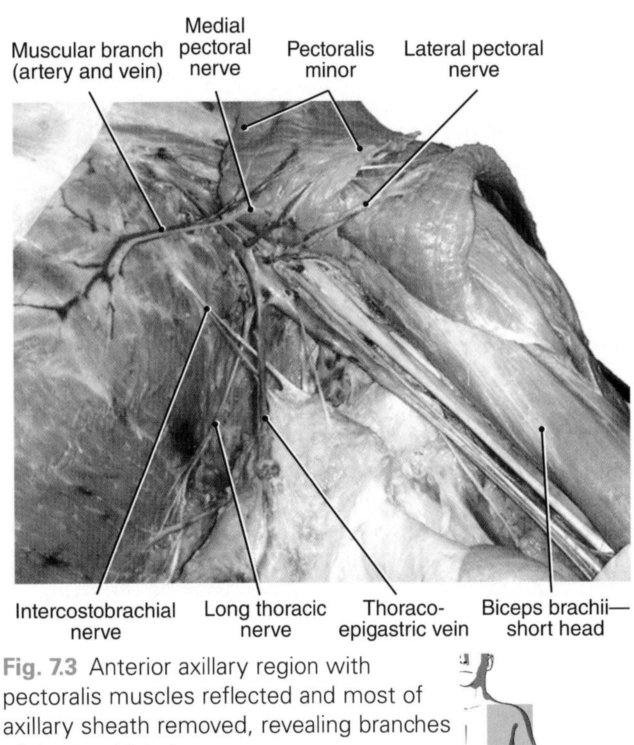

Fig. 7.3 Anterior axillary region with pectoralis muscles reflected and most of axillary sheath removed, revealing branches of the brachial plexus.

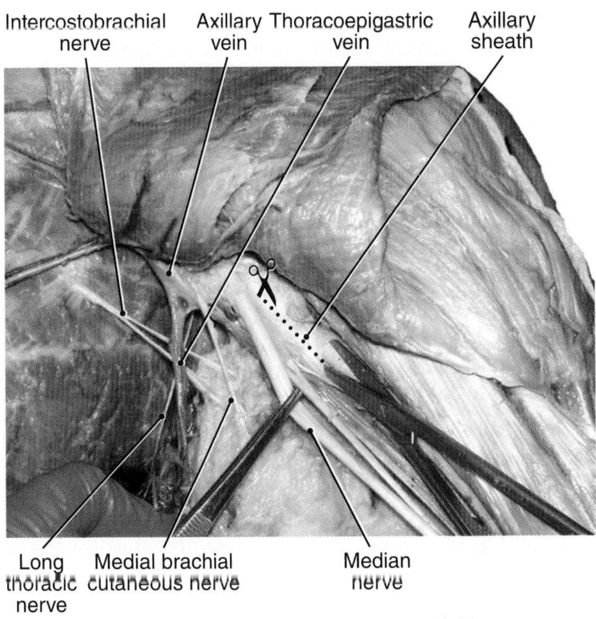

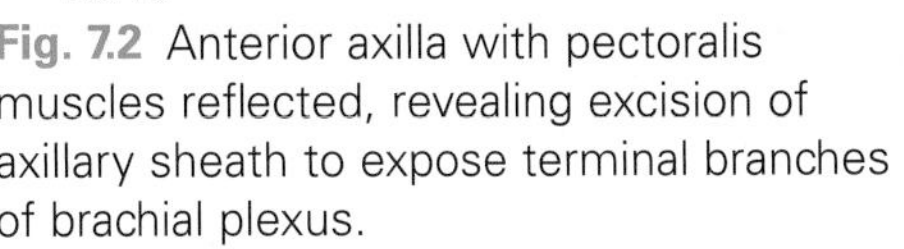

Fig. 7.2 Anterior axilla with pectoralis muscles reflected, revealing excision of axillary sheath to expose terminal branches of brachial plexus.

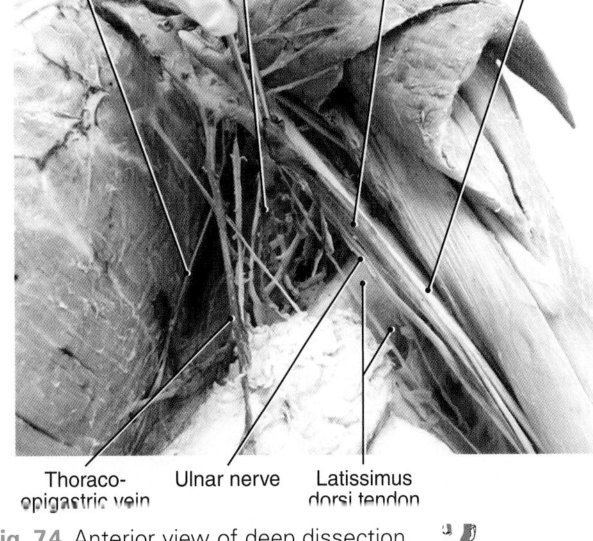

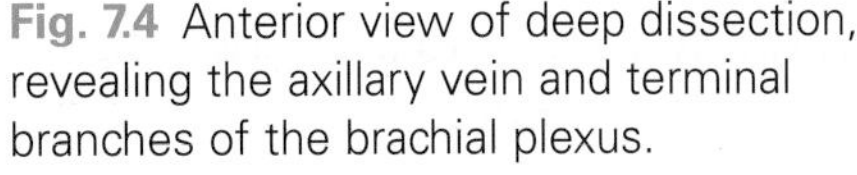

Fig. 7.4 Anterior view of deep dissection, revealing the axillary vein and terminal branches of the brachial plexus.

ANATOMY **NOTE**

The axillary vein is formed at the base of the axilla by the confluence of the venae comitantes of the brachial vein with the basilic vein. (Large arteries, such as the axillary or femoral, are accompanied by a single vein. Medium and smaller arteries, such as the brachial, have two or more accompanying veins, which are found on either side of the artery and are called the *venae comitantes.*)

DISSECTION **TIP**

Do not attempt to identify any lymph nodes associated with the axillary vein and its tributaries. Nodes are evident and easily dissected only in cadavers with pathologies (e.g., cancer). Similarly, do not attempt to identify the central axillary nodes within the fat of the central portion of the axilla. Smaller tributaries to the axillary vein that obscure the dissecting field can be removed.

- **Clean the adipose tissue between the pectoralis minor muscle and brachial plexus (see Fig. 7.4).**

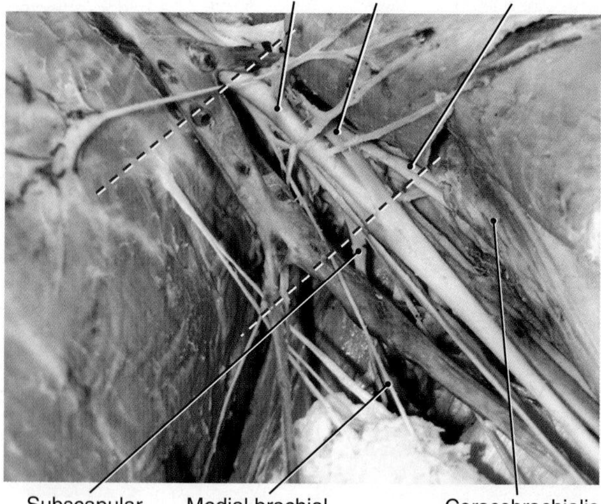

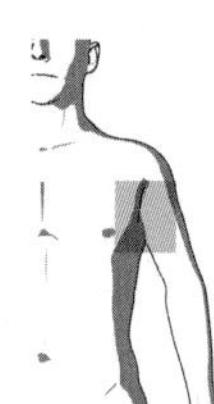

Fig. 7.5 Anterior view of the axilla revealing the second part of the axillary artery, thoracoacromial artery, and lateral cord. *Red dashed lines* represent the borders on the pectoralis minor muscle over the axillary artery, dividing into three portions.

ANATOMY **NOTE**

The axillary artery extends from the lateral border of the 1st rib to the inferior border of the teres major muscle. Just before it crosses the 1st rib, the artery is named the *subclavian artery.* Distal to the teres major, the name of the vessel changes to the *brachial artery.*

DISSECTION **TIP**

Typically, the arteries are named based on the structures they supply, not according to their origin.

- **Identify the axillary artery and its three divisions, demarcated with its relationship to the pectoralis minor muscle (Fig. 7.5).**
- **Identify the superior thoracic artery arising from the first part of the axillary artery. To identify this vessel, look for an artery penetrating the musculature of the 1st or 2nd intercostal space.**
- **From the second part of the axillary artery (deep to pectoralis minor muscle), identify the thoracoacromial artery and the lateral thoracic artery (see Fig. 7.5).**
- **Look for the pectoral branches of the thoracoacromial artery supplying the pectoralis major and minor muscles. The remaining branches of the thoracoacromial artery (deltoid, acromial, and clavicular) may be challenging to dissect out since there are several arterial variations.**

DISSECTION **TIP**

The following anatomical landmarks may be helpful when identifying the branches of the axillary artery.

- **Superior thoracic artery:** 1st or 2nd intercostal spaces.
- **Lateral thoracic artery:** Lateral border of pectoralis minor muscle. Often the lateral thoracic artery arises as a branch of the thoracoacromial artery.
- **Thoracoacromial artery:** Second part of the axillary artery.
- **Pectoral branches:** Look for these on the internal surface of the pectoralis major and minor muscles and trace them backward to the axillary artery and thoracoacromial artery. The pectoral branches often originate directly from the second part of the axillary artery.
- Separate the axillary artery from the branches of the brachial plexus and remove fat from the latissimus dorsi muscle (Fig. 7.6).
- Continue removing the axillary sheath from the brachial artery and vein and expose the median nerve distally to the midportion of the arm (Fig. 7.7).

DISSECTION **TIP**

Exposing the branches of the brachial plexus to the midportion of the humerus allows greater mobility and facilitates the identification of structures deep in the axilla.

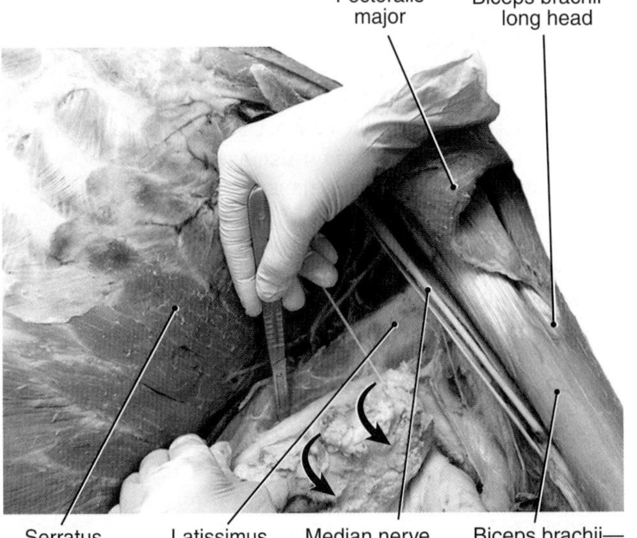

Fig. 7.6 Anterior view illustrating removal of the fat from the latissimus dorsi muscle.

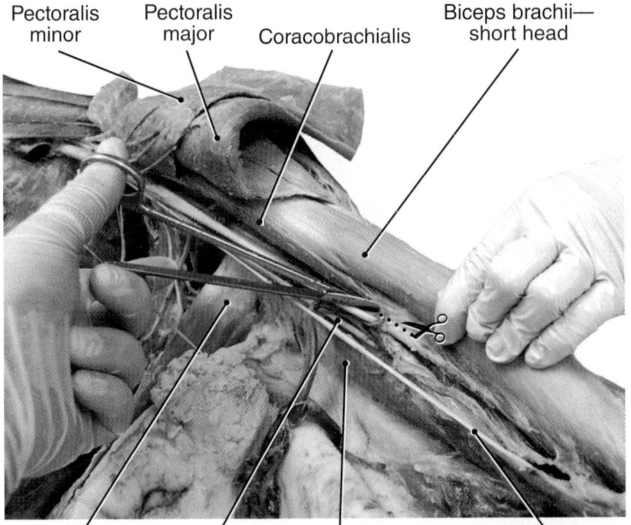

Fig. 7.7 Removing the axillary sheath and soft tissues.

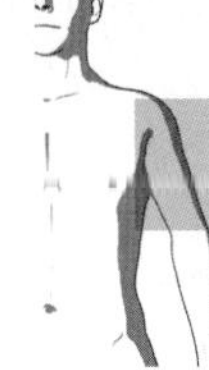

- **Cut the axillary vein at the point where the first part of the axillary artery originates and reflect the vein and its tributaries toward the forearm.**
- **Do not completely remove the vein from the cadaver.**
- **Distal to the pectoralis minor muscle, from the third portion of the axillary artery, identify the anterior**

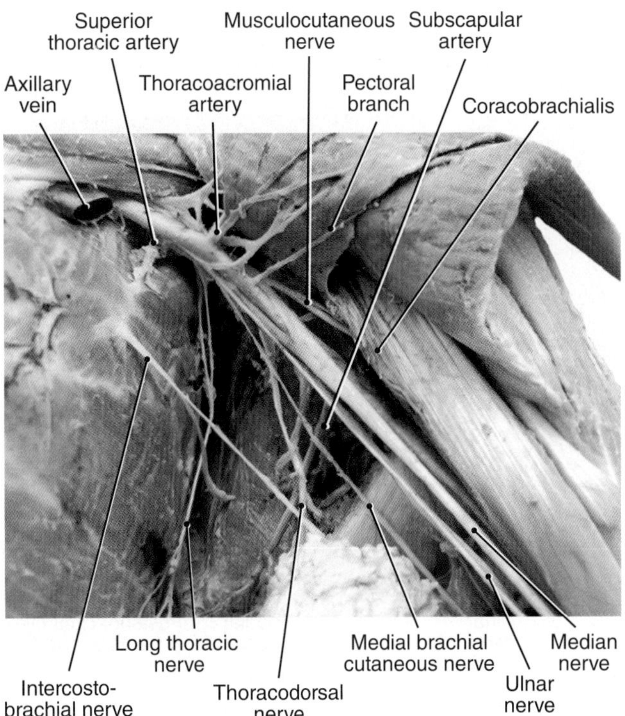

Fig. 7.8 Anterior view of the axilla with reflected pectoralis muscles, removed axillary vein, illustrating the axillary artery and associated nerves.

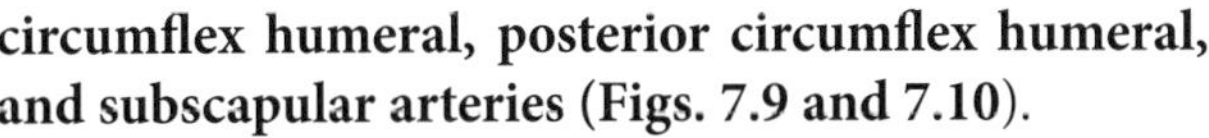

circumflex humeral, posterior circumflex humeral, and subscapular arteries (Figs. 7.9 and 7.10).

ANATOMY **NOTE**

The subscapular artery runs vertically toward the latissimus dorsi and branches into the thoracodorsal artery, supplying the latissimus dorsi muscle, and the circumflex scapular artery, traveling posteriorly to the muscles of the posterior scapula (Figs. 7.8 and 7.9).

- **Identify the subscapular artery and thoracodorsal arteries.**
- **Identify and clean the branches of the medial cord: the medial pectoral nerve, ulnar nerve, medial root of the median nerve, medial brachial cutaneous nerve, and medial antebrachial cutaneous nerve.**
- **Alongside the medial antebrachial cutaneous nerve, identify the basilic vein (formed at the medial aspect of the dorsal venous arch of the hand; see Chapters 8 and 9 for hand structures).**
- **Trace and expose the median nerve to the elbow (see Fig. 7.9).**

Fig. 7.9 Axillary artery and ulnar and median nerves are pulled medially to expose the radial nerve and anterior and posterior circumflex humeral arteries.

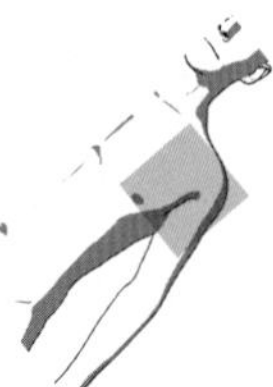

DISSECTION **TIP**

ANATOMICAL LANDMARKS

- **Subscapular artery:** Arises from the third part of the axillary artery (pull the medial cord upward to expose it) and runs vertically down between the latissimus dorsi and subscapularis muscles.
- **Thoracodorsal artery:** Arises from the subscapular artery and continues to run downward to supply the latissimus dorsi muscle. This artery is found on the surface of the latissimus dorsi and is accompanied by the thoracodorsal nerve (also known as middle subscapular nerve) (trace the artery backward to its origin).

ANATOMY **NOTE**

The brachial plexus is divided into rami, trunks, divisions, cords, and terminal branches. The rami, trunks, and divisions are identified later in the root of the neck dissection. In this dissection, you will be able to identify the cords and terminal branches of the brachial plexus. The cords are named in respect to their positions in relationship to the axillary artery. As a result, the *lateral cord* is situated lateral to the axillary artery, the *medial cord* medial to the axillary artery, and the *posterior cord* posterior (deep) to the axillary artery. The lateral cord gives off two branches: the lateral pectoral nerve supplies the pectoralis major muscle and the musculocutaneous nerve supplies the biceps brachii, coracobrachialis, and brachialis muscles (see Fig. 7.8) (Plate 7.1).

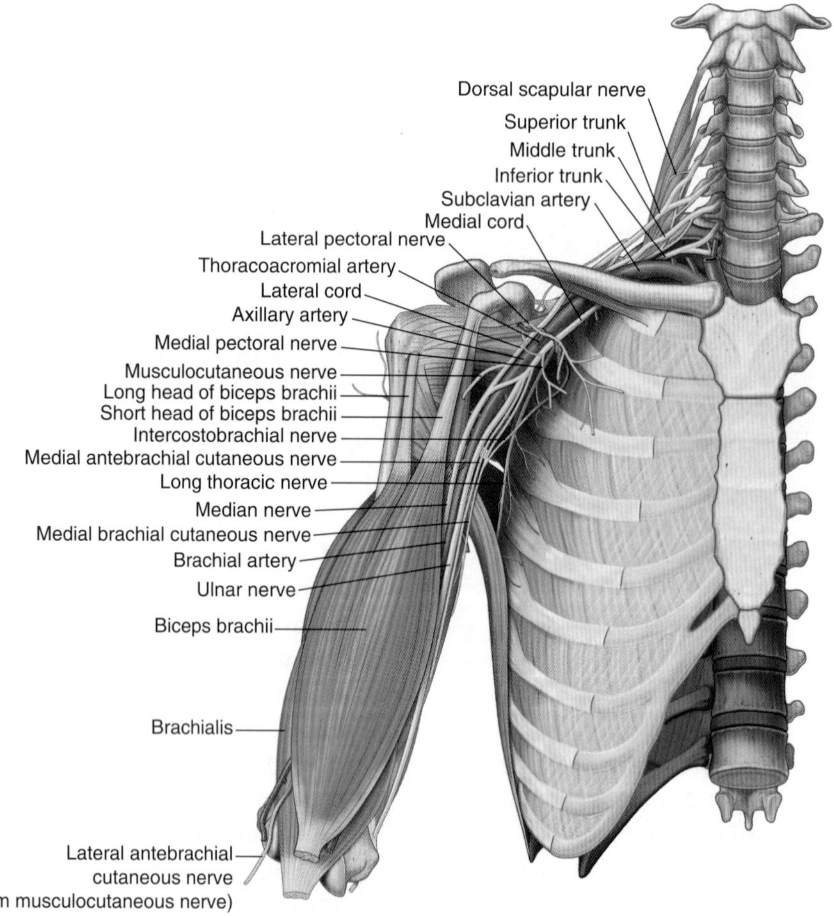

Plate 7.1 Lateral and medial cords of the brachial plexus. (From Drake RL et al., *Gray's Atlas of Anatomy*, 3rd edition, Philadelphia, Elsevier, 2021, p. 406.)

DISSECTION TIP

A landmark for identifying the musculocutaneous nerve is that the nerve often pierces the proximal portion of the coracobrachialis muscle.

DISSECTION TIP

ANATOMICAL LANDMARKS

- **Ulnar nerve:** Look for the nerve traveling along the medial aspect of the arm, not providing any branches to the arm, and crossing posterior to the medial epicondyle.
- **Median nerve:** Look for the nerve traveling along the medial aspect of the arm without giving off any branches to the arm. It is found easily as it travels underneath the bicipital aponeurosis.
- **Medial brachial cutaneous nerve:** Runs parallel for a short distance in the arm with the medial antebrachial cutaneous nerve and is distributed to the skin of the medial surface of the arm. This nerve is often cut when the skin of the arm is reflected.
- **Medial antebrachial cutaneous nerve:** Runs parallel and superficial to the ulnar nerve and is distributed to the skin of the forearm. The basilic vein runs alongside this nerve.

DISSECTION TIP

The medial brachial cutaneous nerve (medial cutaneous nerve to the arm) is often severed during the removal of the skin over the arm. The medial antebrachial cutaneous nerve (medial cutaneous nerve to the forearm) runs parallel to the ulnar nerve. The landmark for identifying the ulnar nerve is to trace it as it crosses posterior to the medial epicondyle of the humerus. In contrast, the medial antebrachial cutaneous nerve runs more superficially and terminates in the skin of the forearm (see Fig. 7.14).

ANATOMY NOTE

The posterior cord gives rise to the following branches: superior, inferior subscapular nerves; thoracodorsal nerve; axillary nerve; and radial nerve.

DISSECTION TIP

To identify the posterior cord, pull the medial cord and the axillary artery, laterally, away from the coracobrachialis muscle (Figs. 7.9, 7.10). Look posteriorly and deep to it for the posterior cord.

- Deep to the axillary artery, identify the posterior cord.
- Identify and trace the radial nerve as it penetrates the triceps brachii.
- At the level of the surgical neck of the humerus, dissect and expose the anterior and posterior circumflex humeral arteries (see Fig. 7.10).

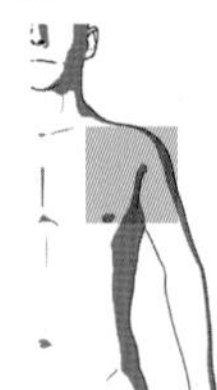

Fig. 7.10 Anterior axillary view with reflected pectoralis muscles, traction from the axillary artery, revealing the lateral cord, posterior cord, and musculocutaneous nerve. *Red dashed line* shows the level of the surgical neck of the humerus.

DISSECTION TIP

ANATOMICAL LANDMARKS

Radial nerve: Look at the medial surface of the arm for the nerve innervating the triceps brachii muscle (see Fig. 7.15). Trace the nerve backward to the axilla and posterior cord.

DISSECTION TIP

ANATOMICAL LANDMARKS

Posterior circumflex humeral artery: Pull the axillary artery away from the coracobrachialis at the level of the surgical neck of the humerus and identify the artery. It runs alongside the axillary nerve.

DISSECTION TIP

The posterior circumflex humeral artery is typically much larger than the anterior circumflex humeral artery. In some specimens, the posterior circumflex humeral artery may arise from the subscapular artery.

- Identify the axillary nerve running alongside the posterior circumflex humeral artery passing posterior to the surgical neck of the humerus to reach the quadrangular space.
- Trace the nerve backward to the posterior cord.
- Pull the medial cord upward and observe the subscapular artery and the posterior cord of the brachial plexus (Fig. 7.11).

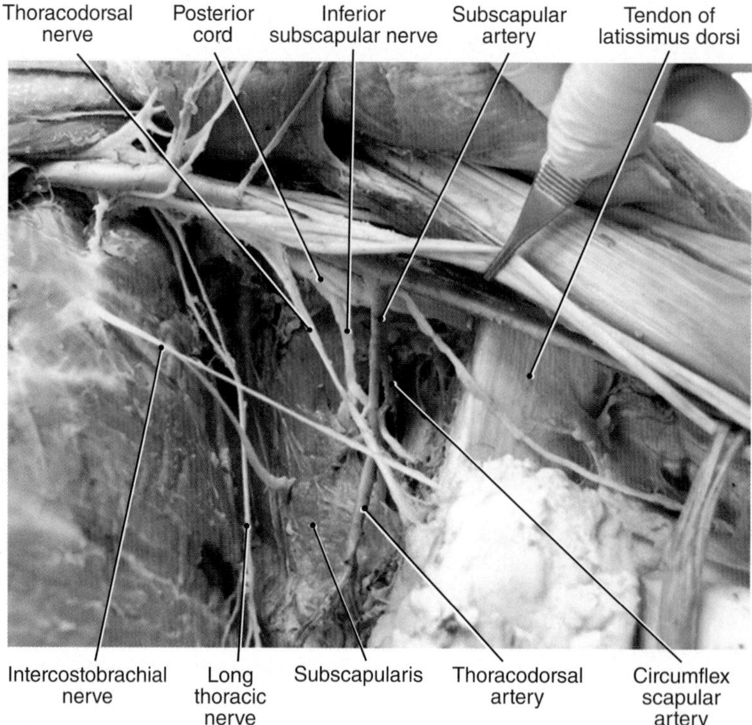

Fig. 7.11 Anterior view revealing posterior structures of the axilla.

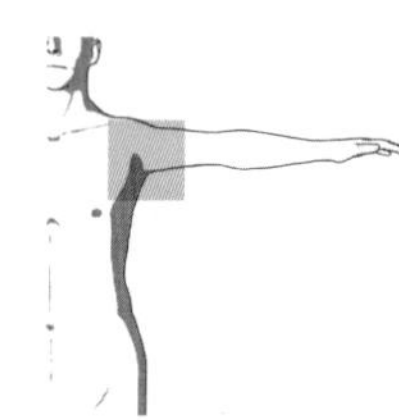

- **Identify the thoracodorsal nerve that supplies the latissimus dorsi muscle and runs alongside the thoracodorsal artery, which also supplies the latissimus dorsi (see Figs. 7.11 and 7.12).**
- **Distal to the origin of the thoracodorsal nerve, identify the inferior subscapular nerve running at the lateral border of subscapularis with the circumflex scapular artery.**
- **Identify the circumflex scapular artery.**
- **Clean out the subscapularis muscle and at its deeper portion, identify the superior subscapular nerve supplying the subscapularis muscle (Figs. 7.12 and 7.13).**

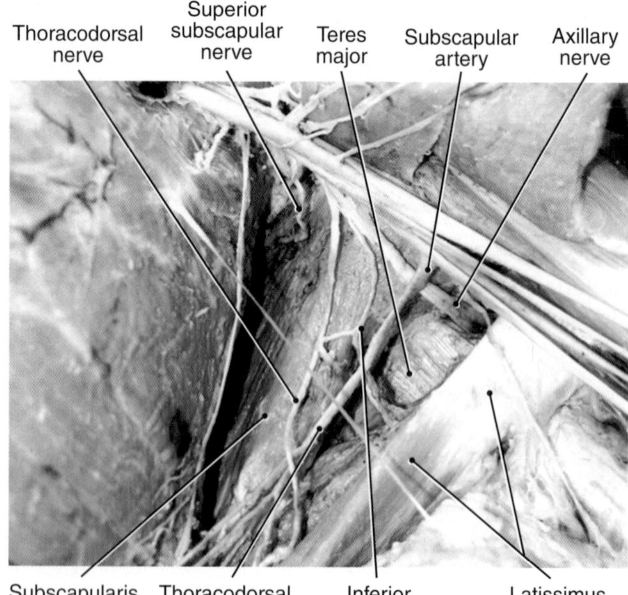

Fig. 7.12 Deep anterior axillary view showing the superior and inferior subscapular nerves and thoracodorsal nerve.

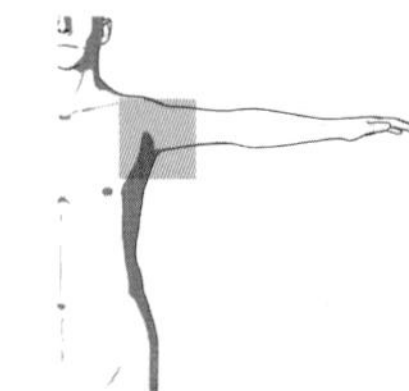

DISSECTION **TIP**

ANATOMICAL LANDMARKS

Thoracodorsal nerve: Found on the surface of the latissimus dorsi muscle running alongside the thoracodorsal artery.

ANATOMY **NOTE**

The inferior subscapular nerve supplies part of the subscapularis and the entire teres major muscle.

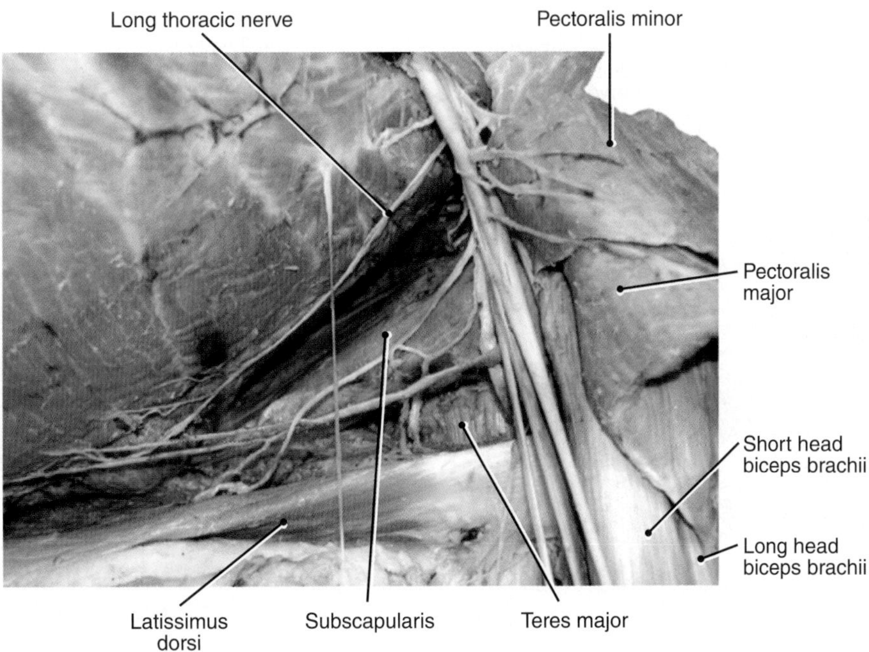

Fig. 7.13 Deep anterior view revealing the posterior nerves.

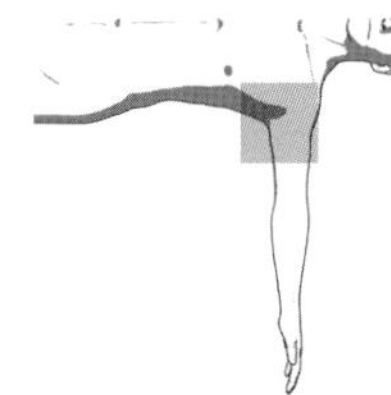

DISSECTION TIP

ANATOMICAL LANDMARKS

- **Circumflex scapular artery:** Arises from the subscapular artery and turns around to enter the gap between the lateral border of the subscapularis and latissimus dorsi muscles alongside the inferior subscapular nerve (trace the nerve proximally to its origin from the posterior cord).
- **Inferior subscapular nerve:** It runs with the circumflex scapular artery in the gap between the lateral border of the subscapularis and latissimus dorsi muscles.

DISSECTION TIP

ANATOMICAL LANDMARKS

Superior subscapular nerve: Look deep in the axilla for the nerve that penetrates the subscapularis muscle. It is located deep and medial to the subscapularis muscle.

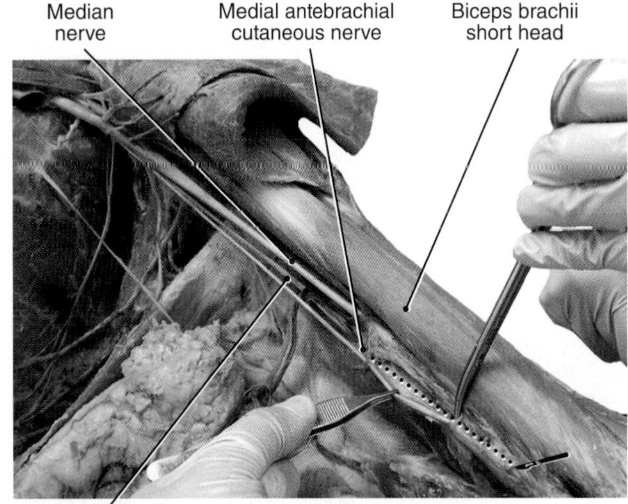

Fig. 7.14 Complete exposure of the median, ulnar, and medial antebrachial cutaneous nerves in the arm.

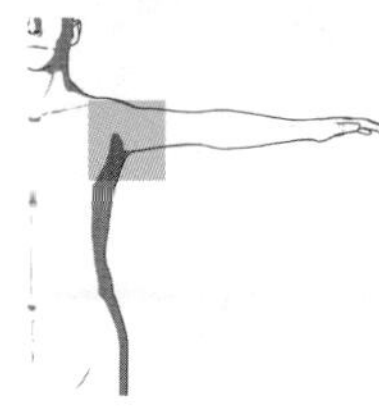

- **Continue the dissection by exposing the terminal branches of the brachial plexus in the arm (Figs. 7.14 and 7.15).**
- **The *axillary* artery changes its name to *brachial* artery as it crosses the inferior border of the teres major.**
- **Identify the first branch of the brachial artery, the *deep* brachial artery running deep to the triceps brachii muscle with the radial nerve.**
- **Continue the dissection, reflecting the skin over the medial portion of the triceps brachii muscle, and expose all the branches of the radial nerve (Fig. 7.16).**
- **Reflect the skin medially over the biceps brachii muscle (Figs. 7.16 and 7.17).**
- **Identify the long and short heads of the biceps brachii.**

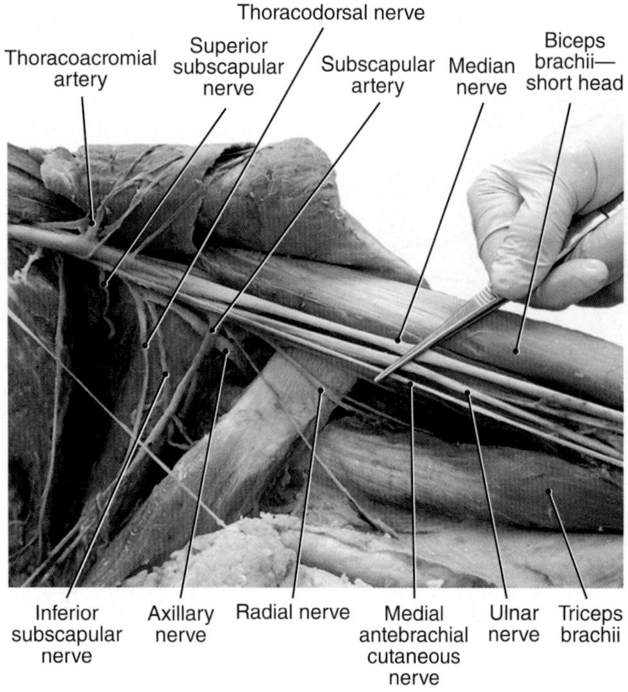

Fig. 7.15 Axillary and proximal arm view with skin reflected, revealing muscles and nerves.

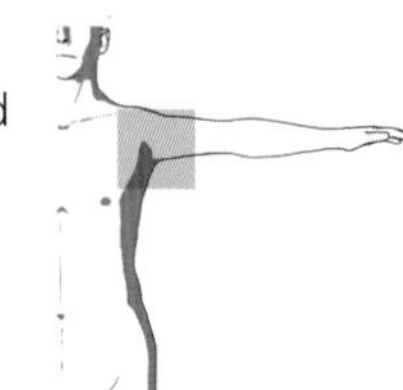

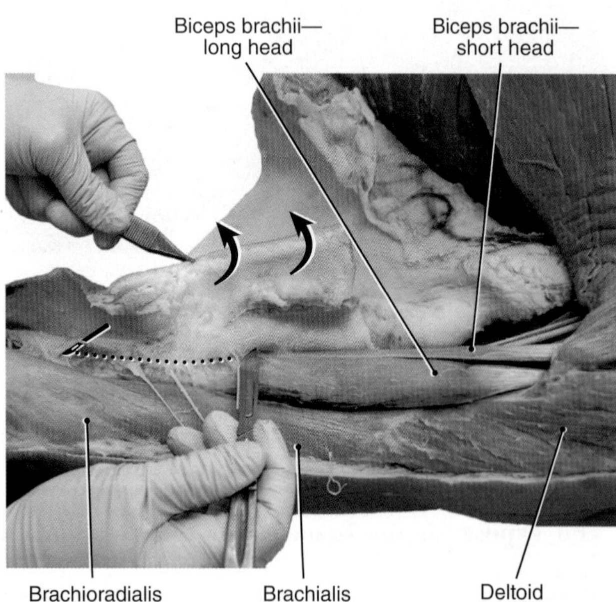

Fig. 7.16 Anterior arm with skin reflected, revealing biceps brachii, brachialis, and deltoid muscles.

Biceps brachii—long head

Pectoralis major

Brachioradialis

Brachialis

Deltoid

Fig. 7.17 Anterior arm with the skin reflected, revealing the biceps brachii, brachialis, and deltoid muscles.

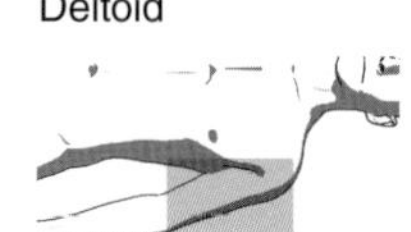

DISSECTION **TIP**

If time permits, expose the short head of the biceps brachii from its origin at the coracoid process of the scapula. The tendon of the long head of the biceps brachii lies lateral to the short head. You may expose the tendon of the long head of the biceps brachii muscle from the supraglenoid tubercle, just above the glenoid fossa of the scapula.

- **Just inferior to the biceps brachii, identify the brachialis muscle (see Fig. 7.17).**
- **Identify the coracobrachialis muscle, noting the musculocutaneous nerve passing through the muscle.**

ANATOMY **NOTE**

The brachialis muscle is innervated primarily by the musculocutaneous nerve; however, the radial nerve also may contribute to its innervation.

- **Reflect the skin over the lateral aspect of the arm inferiorly (Fig. 7.18).**
- **Identify the posterior antebrachial cutaneous nerve (branch of radial nerve) emerging between the brachialis and triceps brachii muscles (Fig. 7.19).**
- **Trace the origin of the posterior antebrachial cutaneous nerve by separating the brachialis from the triceps brachii (Fig. 7.20).**
- **Lift the distal portion of the deltoid muscle off the humerus.**
- **Reflect the fascia covering the triceps brachii and expose its lateral head (Fig. 7.21).**

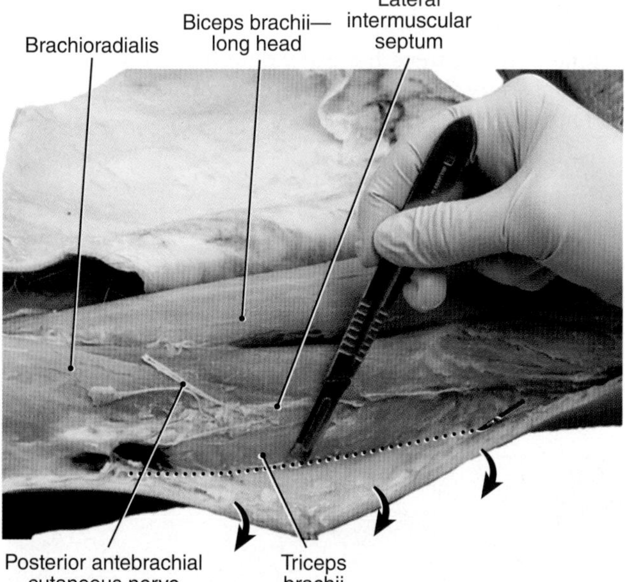

Fig. 7.18 Dissection and reflection of skin over the lateral head of triceps brachii, with exposure of the posterior antebrachial cutaneous nerve.

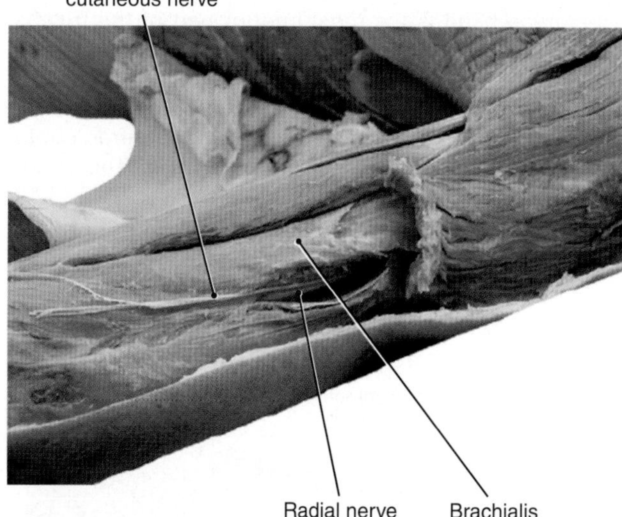

Fig. 7.20 Reflection of deltoid muscle and exposure of the origin of the posterior antebrachial cutaneous nerve.

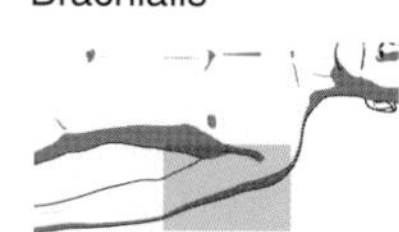

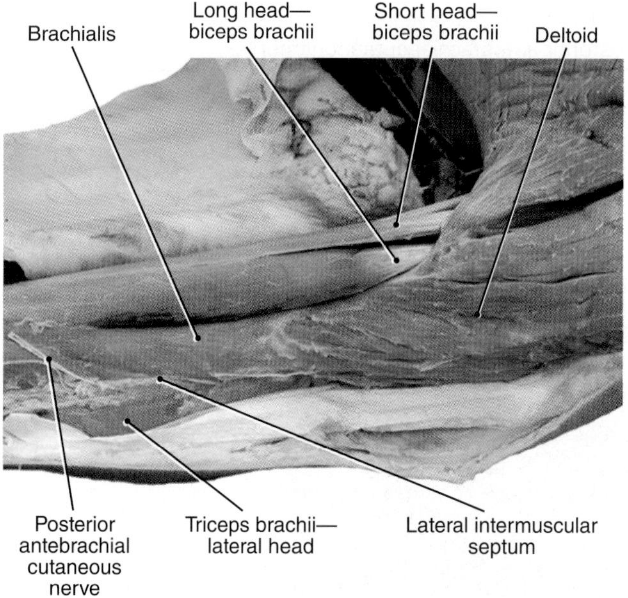

Fig. 7.19 Anterior arm with skin reflected, revealing superficial musculature.

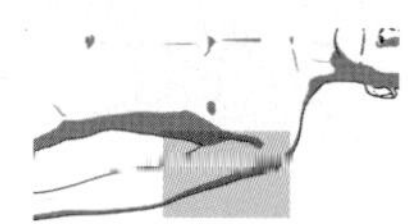

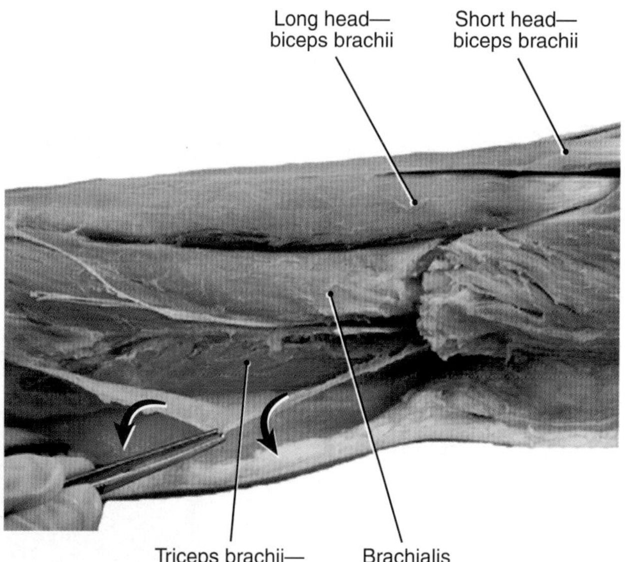

Fig. 7.21 Reflection of deltoid and lateral head of triceps brachii, with exposure of posterior brachial cutaneous nerve.

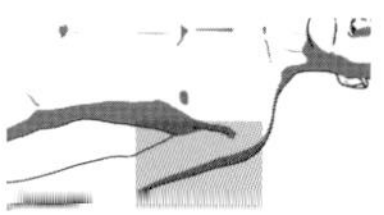

- **Trace the radial nerve to the radial groove of the humerus between the medial and long heads of the triceps brachii muscle (Fig. 7.22).**
- **Trace the musculocutaneous nerve as it penetrates the coracobrachialis muscle; then lift the biceps brachii up and observe the course of the musculocutaneous nerve (Fig. 7.23).**
- **Clean all soft tissues between the biceps brachii and brachialis muscles and dissect the musculocutaneous nerve to the lateral aspect of the arm as it emerges to become the lateral antebrachial cutaneous nerve (Fig. 7.24 and Plate 7.2).**
- **Identify the three heads of the triceps brachii muscle.**

ANATOMY NOTE

The *lateral* head is the most inferior part of the triceps brachii muscle and is recognizable on the lateral surface of this muscle. The *medial* head arises from the posterior and medial surfaces of the humerus distal to the radial groove. The *long* head arises from the infraglenoid tubercle of the scapula and is located medial and proximal to the radial groove.

DISSECTION TIP

If time permits, trace the ascending branch of the deep brachial artery and look for its anastomosis with the posterior circumflex humeral artery.

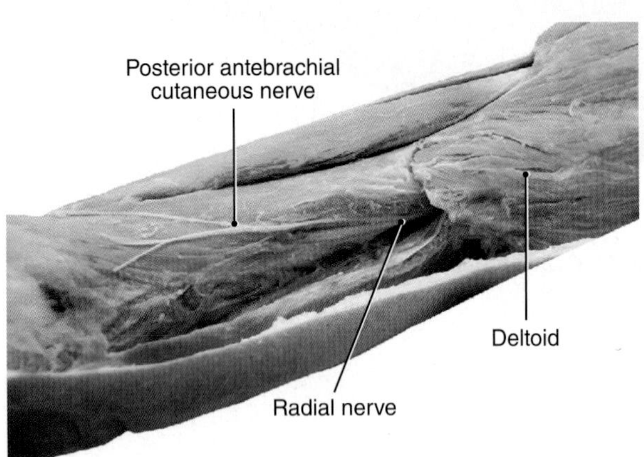

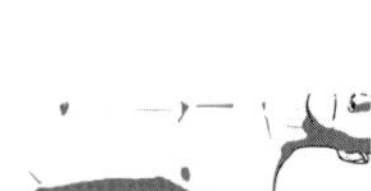

Fig. 7.22 Reflection of deltoid and lateral head of triceps, with exposure of posterior antebrachial cutaneous nerve and radial nerve.

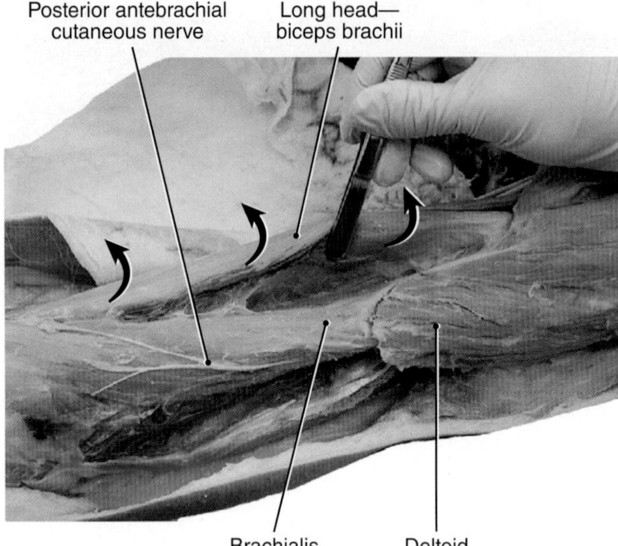

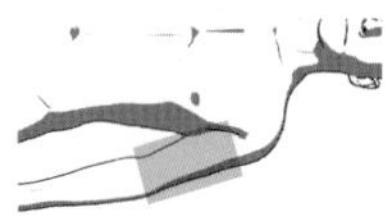

Fig. 7.23 Anterior arm, with retraction of the biceps brachii revealing brachialis and posterior antebrachial cutaneous nerve.

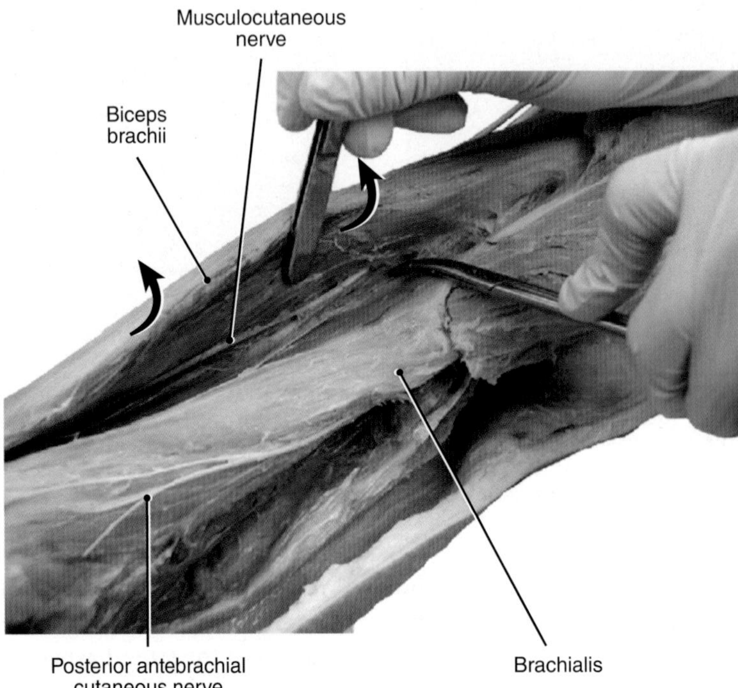

Fig. 7.24 Anterior view of the arm with elevation of the biceps brachii, demonstrating the underlying musculocutaneous nerve.

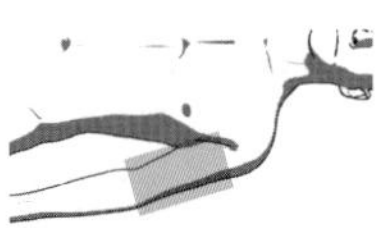

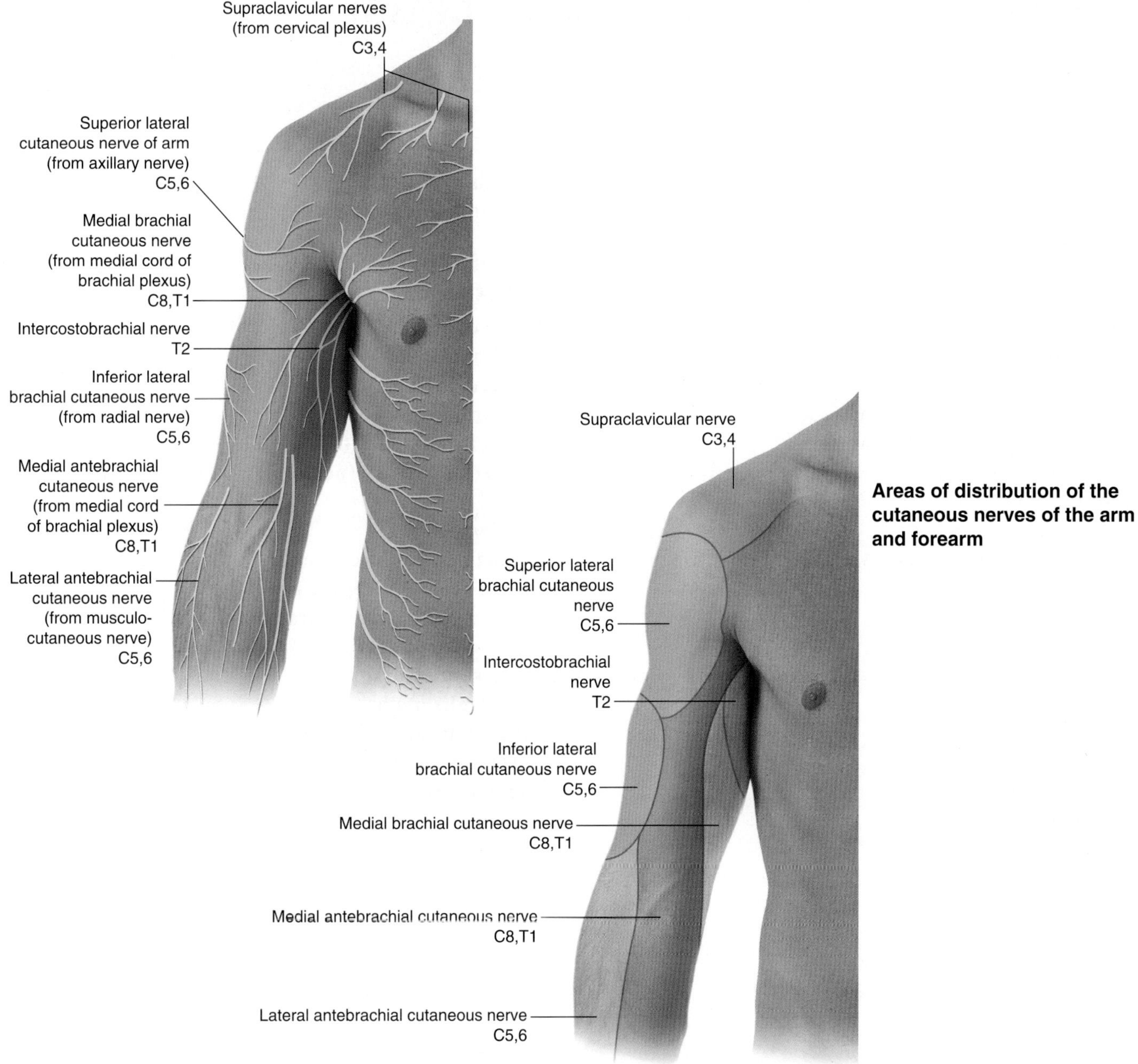

Plate 7.2 Cutaneous innervation of the anterior arm. (From Drake RL et al., *Gray's Atlas of Anatomy*, 3rd edition, Philadelphia, Elsevier, 2021, p. 420.)

LABORATORY IDENTIFICATION CHECKLIST

NERVES

Lateral Cord

- ☐ Median
- ☐ Musculocutaneous
- ☐ Lateral pectoral

Medial Cord

- ☐ Median
- ☐ Medial pectoral
- ☐ Medial brachial cutaneous
- ☐ Medial antebrachial cutaneous
- ☐ Ulnar nerve

Posterior Cord

- ☐ Axillary
- ☐ Superior subscapular
- ☐ Inferior subscapular
- ☐ Thoracodorsal
- ☐ Radial

ARTERIES

- ☐ Axillary
- ☐ Superior thoracic
- ☐ Thoracoacromial
- ☐ Pectoral
- ☐ Lateral thoracic
- ☐ Subscapular
- ☐ Thoracodorsal
- ☐ Circumflex scapular
- ☐ Anterior circumflex humeral
- ☐ Posterior circumflex humeral

VEINS

- ☐ Axillary
- ☐ Thoracoepigastric
- ☐ Cephalic
- ☐ Brachial
- ☐ Venae comitantes

LYMPH NODES (IF EVIDENT IN YOUR CADAVER)

- ☐ Infraclavicular
- ☐ Apical axillary
- ☐ Lateral axillary
- ☐ Central axillary
- ☐ Posterior axillary (subscapular)
- ☐ Anterior axillary (pectoral)

MUSCLES

- ☐ Short head of biceps brachii
- ☐ Long head of biceps brachii
- ☐ Long head of triceps brachii
- ☐ Lateral head of triceps brachii
- ☐ Latissimus dorsi
- ☐ Pectoralis major
- ☐ Pectoralis minor
- ☐ Serratus anterior
- ☐ Subclavius
- ☐ Deltoid
- ☐ Subscapularis
- ☐ Teres major
- ☐ Teres minor

FASCIA

- ☐ Clavipectoral fascia

BONES

- ☐ Clavicle
- ☐ Humerus
- ☐ Scapula

BEFORE YOU BEGIN

Palpate the following bony landmarks on the cadaver or on yourself:

- Lateral and medial epicondyles of the humerus
- Styloid process of the radius
- Head, styloid process, olecranon, and body of the ulna
- Carpal bones

GETTING STARTED

- **Continue the incision from the lateral side of the shoulder with a vertical incision across the length of the forearm toward the wrist.**
- **Make an encircling incision around the wrist (Fig. 8.1).**
- **Reflect the skin medially from the anterior compartment of the forearm and expose the antebrachial fascia and the extensor retinaculum (Fig. 8.2).**
- **Identify the posterior posterior antebrachial nerve (see Fig. 8.2).**
- **Identify the lateral antebrachial cutaneous nerve and medial antebrachial cutaneous nerve (Fig. 8.3).**

DISSECTION TIP

Preserve as many of the cutaneous nerve branches as possible. Typically, the posterior antebrachial cutaneous nerve emerges between the triceps brachii and brachialis muscles; the lateral cutaneous nerve to the forearm emerges lateral to the bicipital aponeurosis between the biceps brachii and brachioradialis muscles; and the medial antebrachial cutaneous nerve can be traced proximally to the medial cord of the brachial plexus.

CUBITAL FOSSA

- **Reflect the skin over the bicipital aponeurosis and expose the cubital fossa. The biceps brachii tendon enters the cubital fossa as an aponeurotic expansion.**

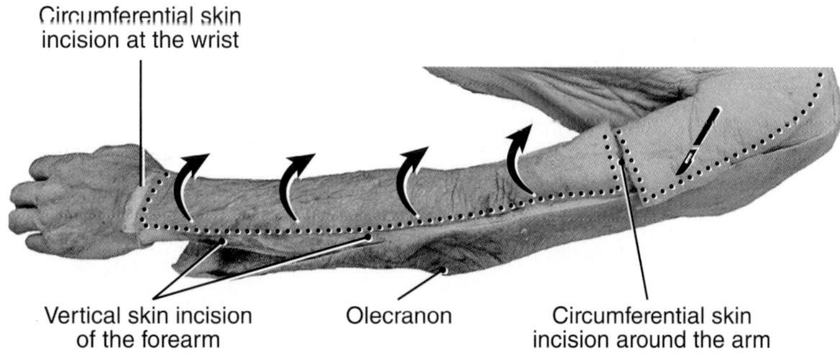

Fig. 8.1 Skin incisions for arm and forearm dissections.

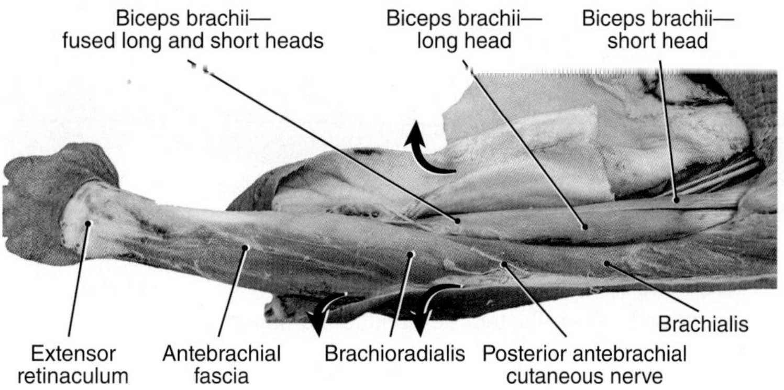

Fig. 8.2 Lateral arm and posterior forearm with skin reflected, demonstrating superficial structures.

- Remove the deep fascia and the fat over the cubital fossa, preserving the bicipital aponeurosis.
- Observe how the lateral and medial antebrachial cutaneous nerves relate to the bicipital aponeurosis (Fig. 8.4).
- Lateral to the tendon of the biceps brachii, separate the brachioradialis muscle from the brachialis muscle and identify the radial nerve as it enters the forearm.
- Reflect the bicipital aponeurosis laterally, and identify the brachial artery, just deep to the veins of the cubital fossa.
- Retract the brachial artery laterally, and on its medial side, identify the median nerve.

LATERAL ARM AND EXTENSOR COMPARTMENT OF THE FOREARM

- Continue the dissection by reflecting the skin over the extensor compartment of the forearm and identify the distribution of the medial and lateral antebrachial cutaneous nerves (Fig. 8.5).
- Identify the superficial branch of the radial nerve just proximal to the lateral side of the wrist (Fig. 8.6).
- With a pair of scissors, make a small incision into the antebrachial fascia (deep fascia) near the lateral epicondyle of the humerus (Fig. 8.7).
- Reflect the antebrachial fascia and expose the underlying musculature of the extensor compartment of the forearm (Figs. 8.8–8.10).
- Remove all remnants of deep fascia covering the extensor surface.

Fig. 8.3 Lateral arm with skin reflected, demonstrating superficial structures.

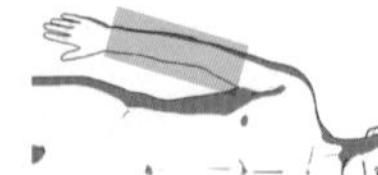

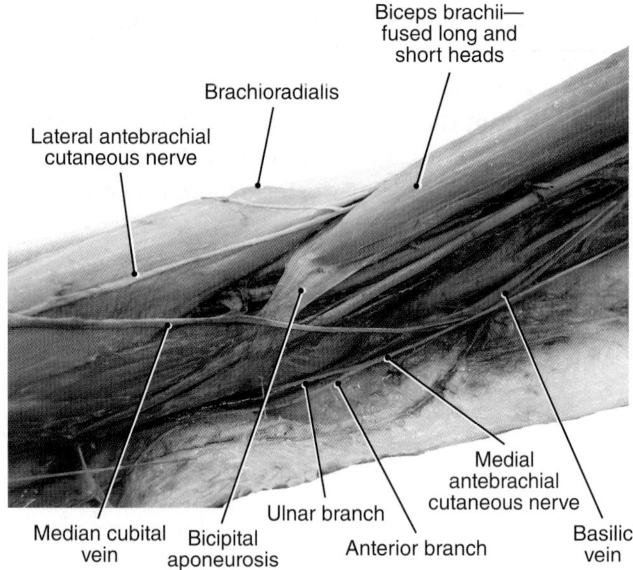

Fig. 8.4 View of the cubital fossa with skin reflected, showing superficial structures.

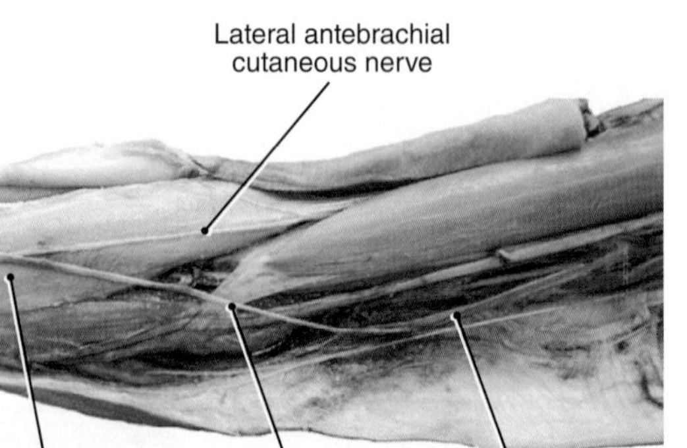

Fig. 8.5 Anterior arm and forearm with skin reflected, demonstrating superficial structures.

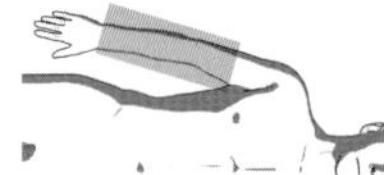

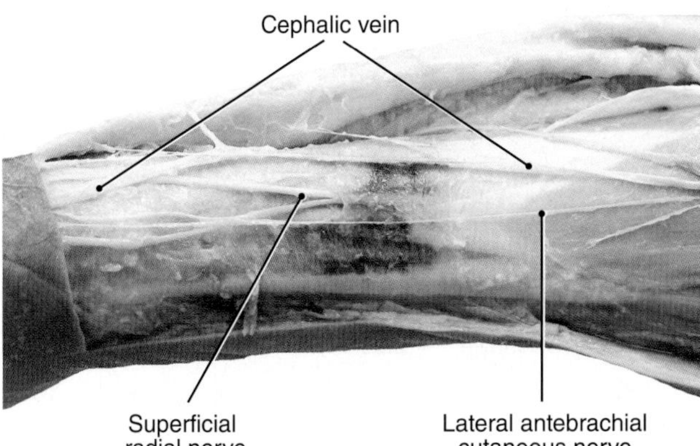

Fig. 8.6 View of the cubital fossa with skin reflected, showing superficial structures.

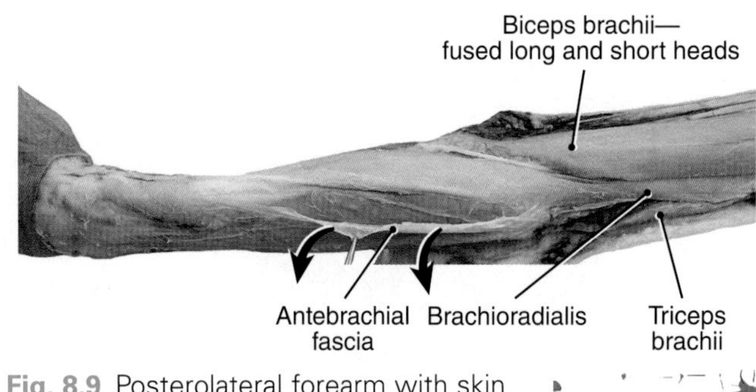

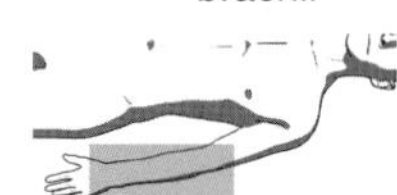

Fig. 8.9 Posterolateral forearm with skin removed demonstrating fascia and superficial structures.

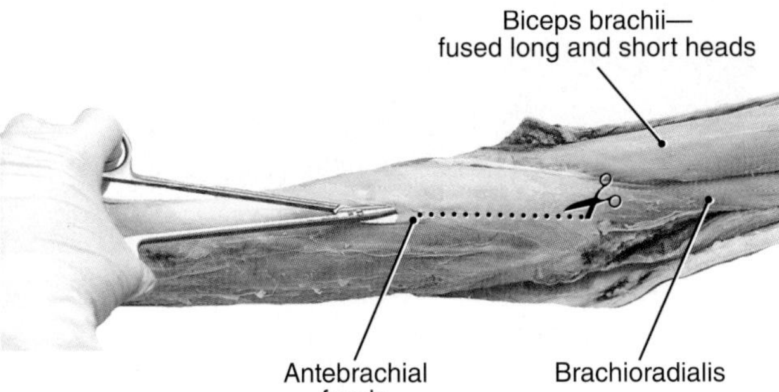

Fig. 8.7 Anterior forearm and cubital fossa with skin removed, demonstrating fascia.

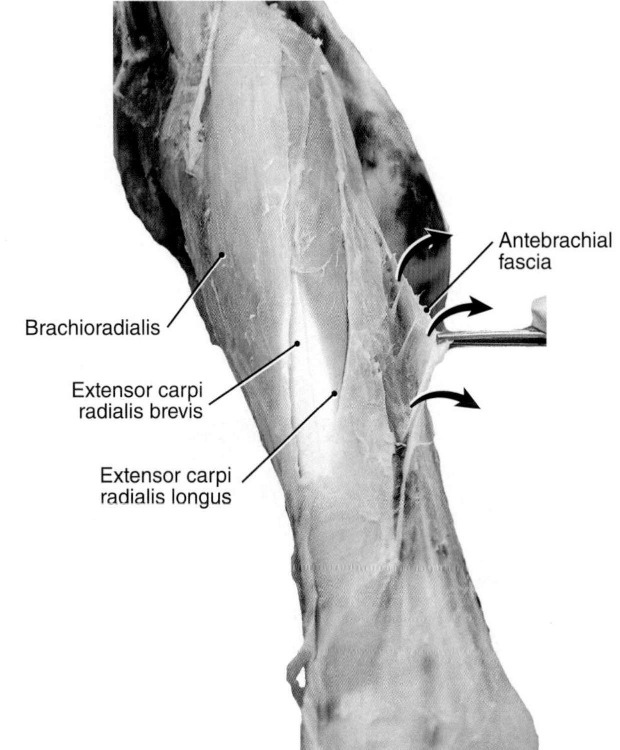

Fig. 8.10 Posterior forearm view with skin reflected showing fascia and superficial structures.

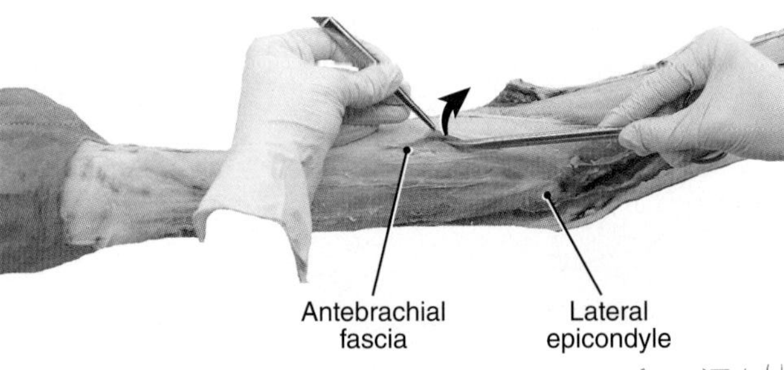

Fig. 8.8 Posterior forearm with skin removed, showing fascia.

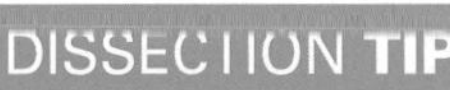

DISSECTION **TIP**

Take special care when the deep fascia is removed. In the majority of cases, the deep fascia adheres tightly to the muscles of the extensor compartment (Fig. 8.11). To identify the tendinous insertions of the muscles of the extensor compartment, the skin over the dorsum of the hand also is removed.

- **Make a vertical incision at the midpoint of the wrist to the midline of the 3rd digit (Fig. 8.12).**
- **With a pair of forceps, lift the skin over the dorsum of the hand and detach it from the underlying dermis (Fig. 8.13).**
- **Reflect the skin laterally without cutting any of the nerves and tributaries of the dorsal venous arch (Figs. 8.14 and 8.15).**
- **With a fine pair of scissors, expose the dorsal venous arch (Fig. 8.16).**
- **As the subcutaneous tissue is removed, pay special attention to identifying the cutaneous nerves running alongside the dorsal venous arch (Fig. 8.17).**

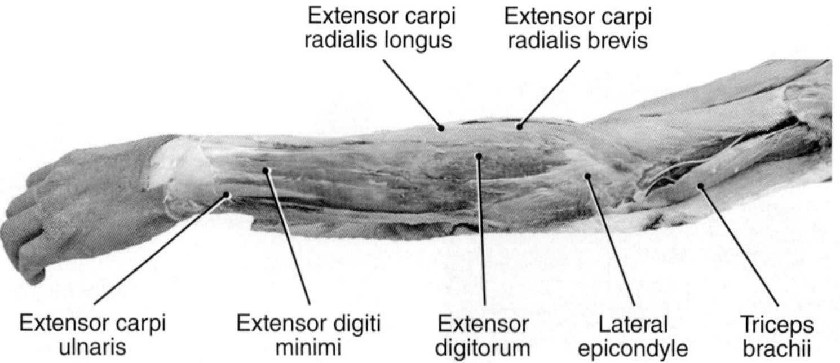

Fig. 8.11 Posterior arm and forearm with skin removed demonstrating fascia.

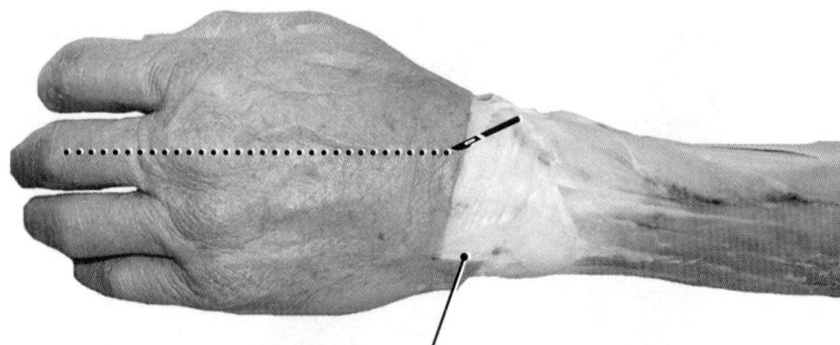

Fig. 8.12 Posterior wrist with skin removed showing extensor retinaculum.

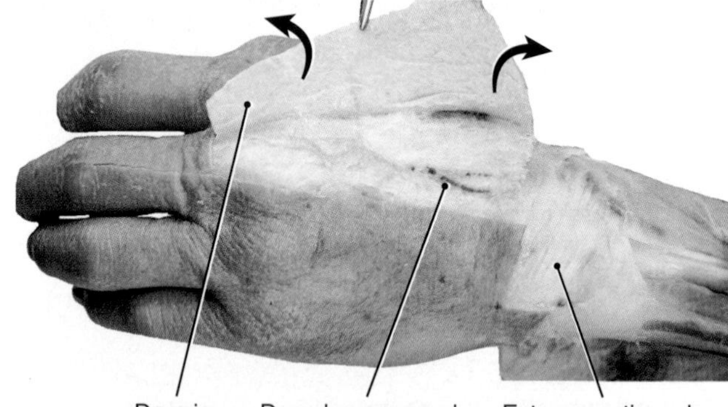

Fig. 8.14 Dorsal hand after skin reflection.

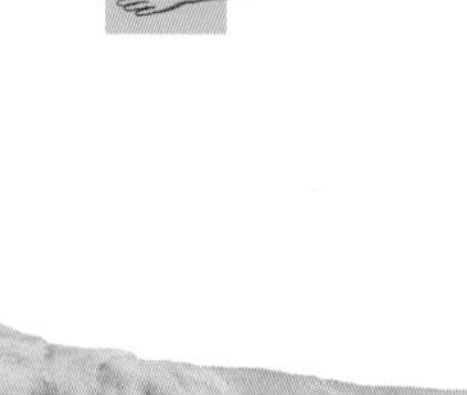

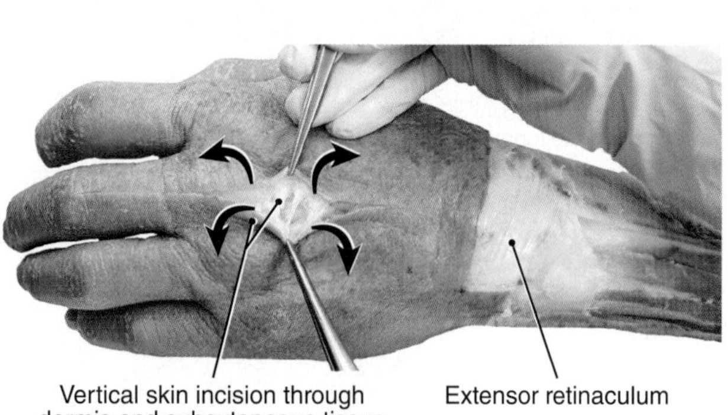

Fig. 8.13 Posterior wrist with skin removed demonstrating extensor retinaculum.

Dorsal venous arch
Dermis and subcutaneous tissue
Extensor retinaculum

Fig. 8.15 Dorsal hand and wrist with skin reflected demonstrating superficial structures.

DISSECTION **TIP**

Exposing the dorsal venous arch and the cutaneous nerves on the dorsum of the hand can take some time (see Fig. 8.17). If time does not permit, skip this step and remove the subcutaneous tissue, dorsal venous arch, and cutaneous branches en bloc.

- **Continue the reflection of the skin over the 3rd digit (Fig. 8.18).**
- **Identify the *extensor retinaculum*, a thick fibrous band of the antebrachial fascia that holds the tendons of the extensor compartment in place (Fig. 8.19).**
- **Place a probe or scissors underneath the extensor retinaculum (Fig. 8.20) and release it from the underlying tendons.**
- **Make a vertical incision and retract the retinaculum laterally to expose the tendons of the extensor compartment (Fig. 8.21).**
- **Identify the extensor digitorum muscle (see Fig. 8.21).**
- **Lift its tendons and clean away its tendinous sheath (Fig. 8.22).**

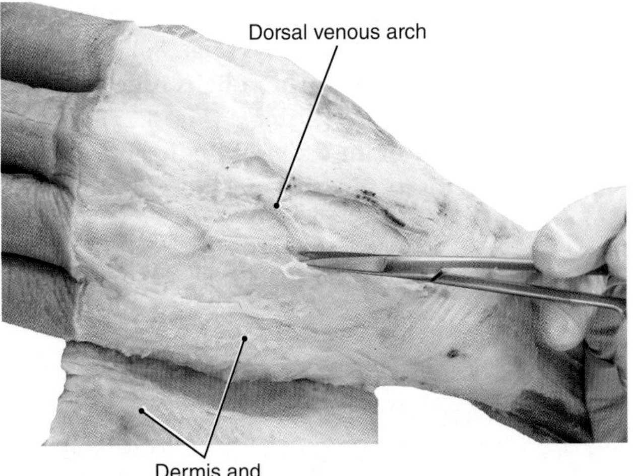

Fig. 8.16 Dorsal hand and wrist with skin reflected showing dorsal venous arch.

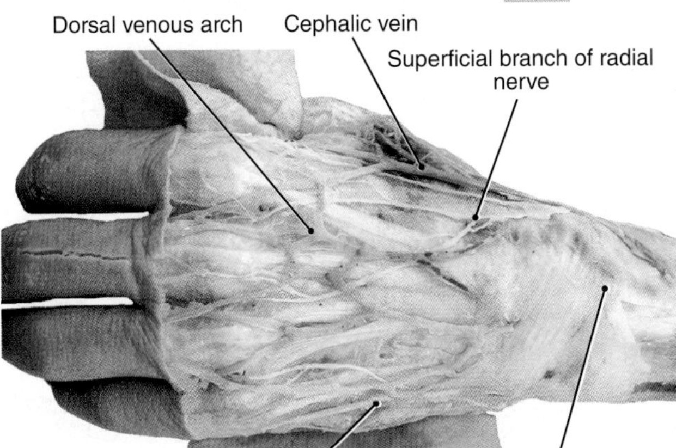

Fig. 8.17 Dorsal hand and wrist with skin reflected highlighting superficial nerves and veins.

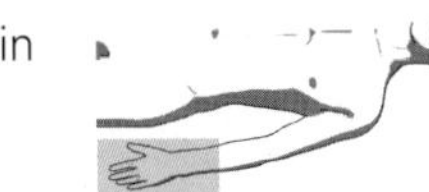

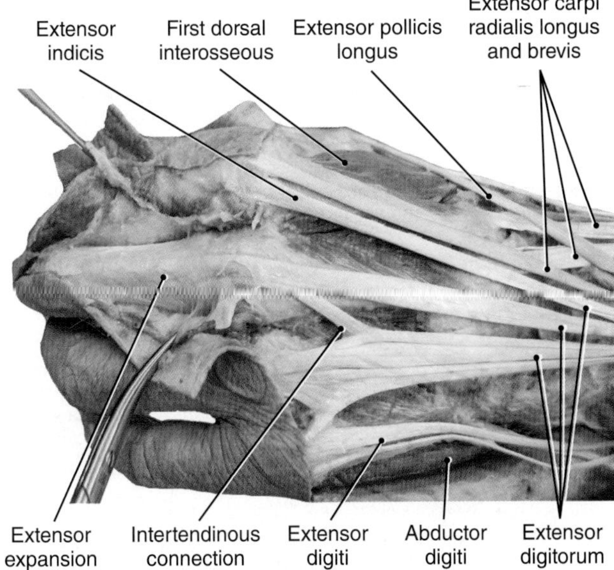

Fig. 8.18 Dorsal hand and wrist with skin reflected exposing extensor tendons.

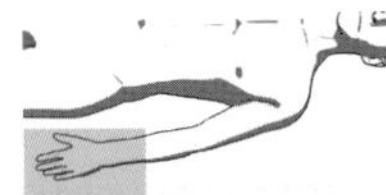

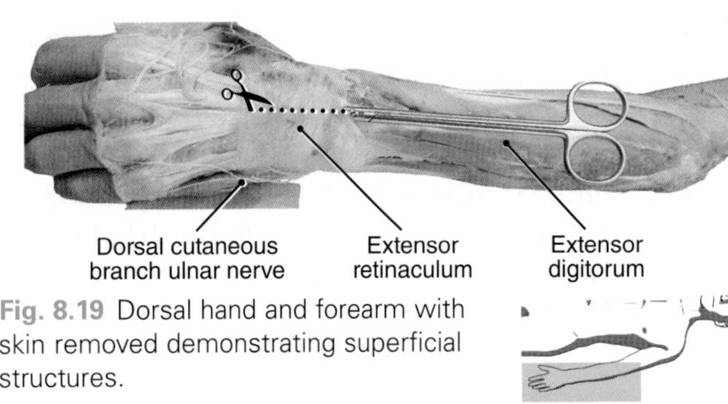

Fig. 8.19 Dorsal hand and forearm with skin removed demonstrating superficial structures.

Extensor retinaculum
Extensor digitorum
Dorsal cutaneous branch ulnar nerve
Extensor digiti minimi
Extensor carpi ulnaris

Fig. 8.20 Dorsal hand and forearm with skin removed showing superficial structures.

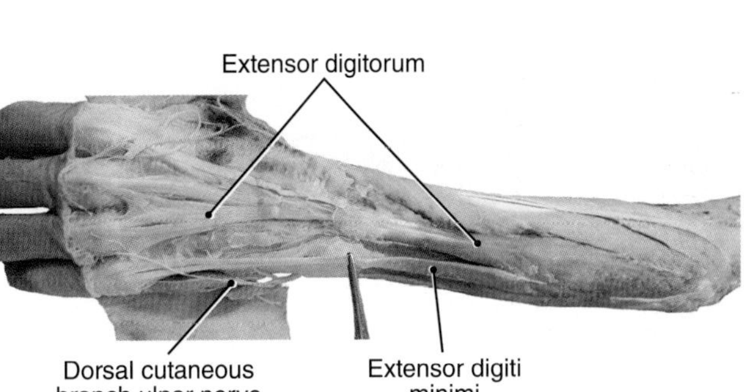

Fig. 8.21 Dorsal hand and forearm with skin removed, highlighting superficial structures.

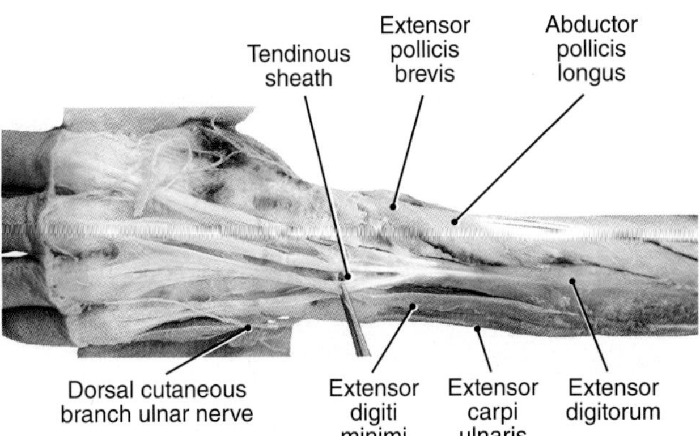

Fig. 8.22 Dorsal hand and forearm with skin reflected, demonstrating musculotendinous structures.

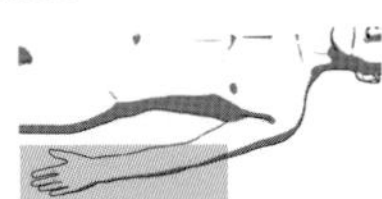

- On the radial side of the extensor digitorum muscle, identify the tendons of the abductor pollicis longus, extensor pollicis brevis, and extensor pollicis longus muscles (see Fig. 8.22).
- On its ulnar side, identify the extensor digiti minimi muscle, which is seen traveling to the 5th digit. In the majority of specimens, this muscle belly is fused with the extensor digitorum muscle (Fig. 8.23).

DISSECTION TIP

In the majority of specimens, the muscle bellies of the abductor pollicis longus and extensor pollicis brevis muscles are fused. Use your scissors to separate them (see Fig. 8.23).

- Lift the extensor digitorum muscle and identify the extensor indicis muscle deep to it (Fig. 8.24). The extensor indicis typically runs along the ulnar side of the tendon from the extensor digitorum to the 2nd digit.
- At the distal third of the forearm, lift the extensor pollicis longus and extensor pollicis brevis muscles, and underneath them, identify the extensor carpi radialis longus and brevis muscles (Figs. 8.25 and 8.26).
- Medial to the extensor carpi radialis brevis muscle, palpate dorsal tubercle (Lister's) (Fig. 8.27).
- On the ulnar side of the extensor digitorum, identify the extensor digiti minimi and the extensor carpi ulnaris muscles (Fig. 8.28).

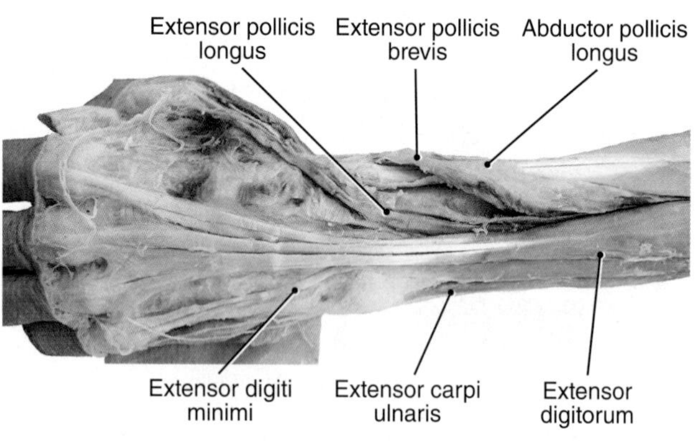

Fig. 8.23 Dorsal hand and forearm with skin reflected, highlighting musculotendinous structures.

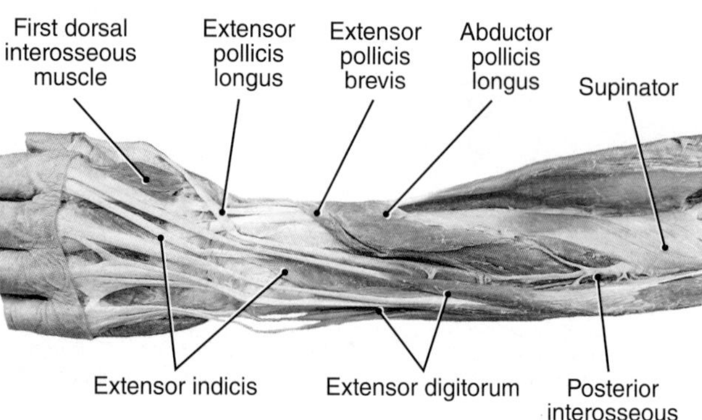

Fig. 8.24 Posterior forearm and hand with brachioradialis muscle reflected, demonstrating muscles and tendons.

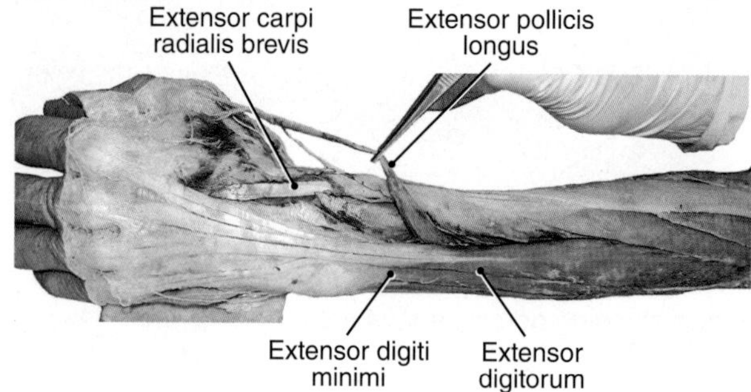

Fig. 8.25 Dorsal hand and forearm with skin reflected.

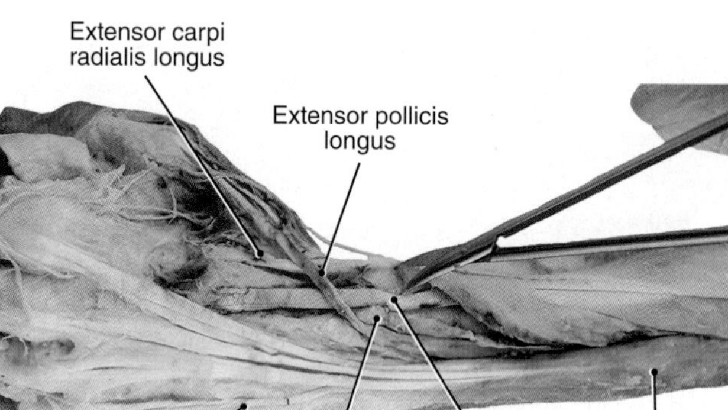

Fig. 8.26 Dorsal hand and forearm with skin reflected.

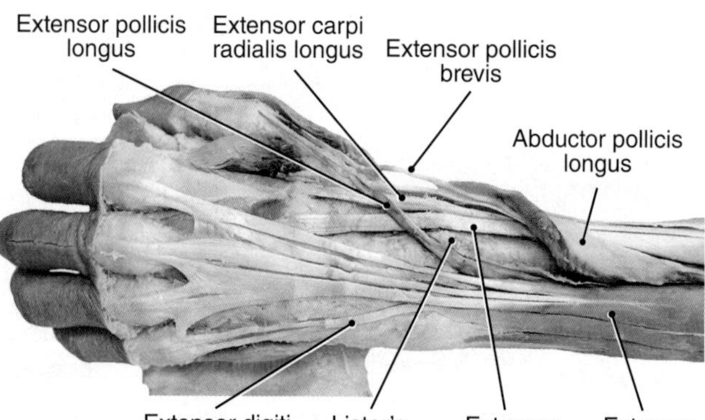

Fig. 8.27 Dorsal hand and forearm with skin reflected.

- Follow the extensor carpi ulnaris to the wrist. Cut the extensor retinaculum (Fig. 8.29) and release the tendons underneath it (Fig. 8.30).
- Retract the extensor carpi ulnaris muscle and separate it from the adjacent extensor digiti minimi muscle (Figs. 8.31 and 8.32).
- On the radial aspect of the proximal part of the forearm, identify and separate the brachioradialis, extensor carpi radialis longus, extensor carpi radialis brevis, and extensor digitorum muscles (Fig. 8.33).
- Lift the brachioradialis from the underlying extensor carpi radialis longus muscle. Use a probe or scissors to complete the separation of these two muscles (Figs. 8.34 and 8.35).
- Reflect or lift the brachioradialis muscle anteriorly and identify the radial nerve (Fig. 8.36). Lift the brachioradialis muscle to allow maximum exposure of the radial nerve.
- Clean the radial nerve and identify its division into superficial and deep branches. The superficial branch runs beneath the brachioradialis to reach the dorsum of the hand. The deep branch of the radial nerve runs through the supinator muscle.
- With a pair of scissors, cut between the fibers of the extensor carpi radialis brevis and extensor digitorum muscles and expose the supinator muscle lying underneath (Fig. 8.37).

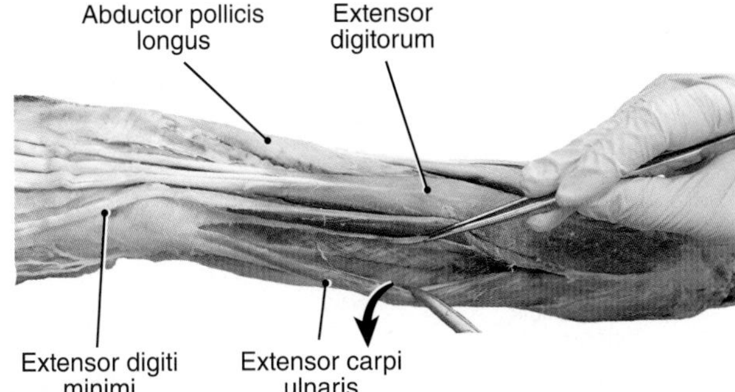

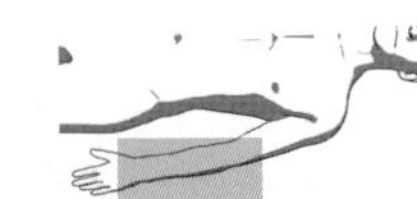

Fig. 8.28 Posterior forearm.

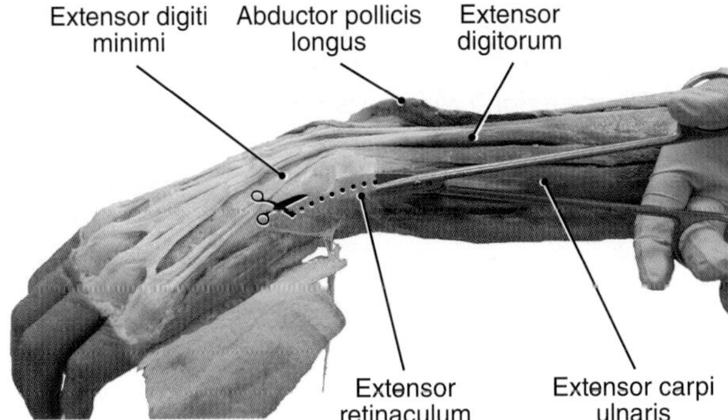

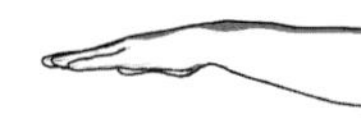

Fig. 8.29 Posteromedial wrist demonstrating superficial structures.

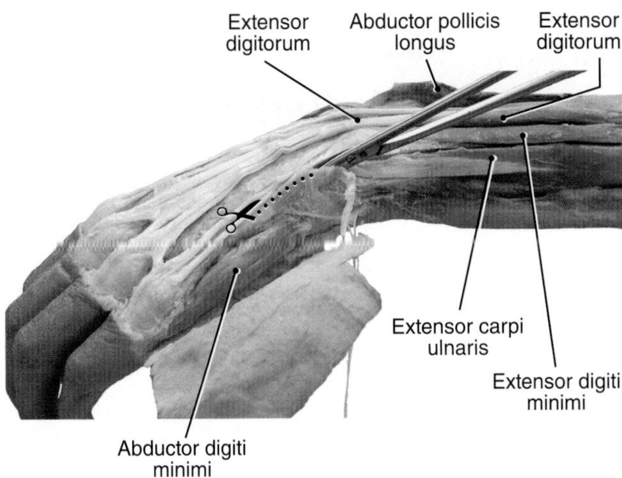

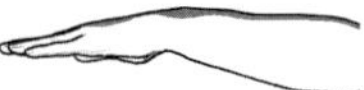

Fig. 8.30 Posteromedial wrist demonstrating superficial structures.

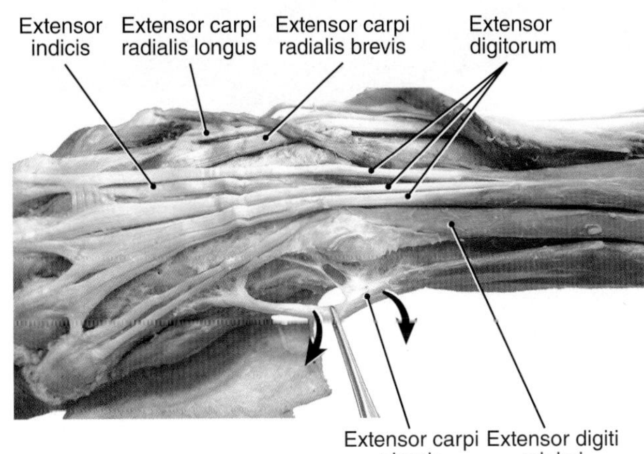

Fig. 8.31 Posteromedial view of wrist showing muscle and tendons.

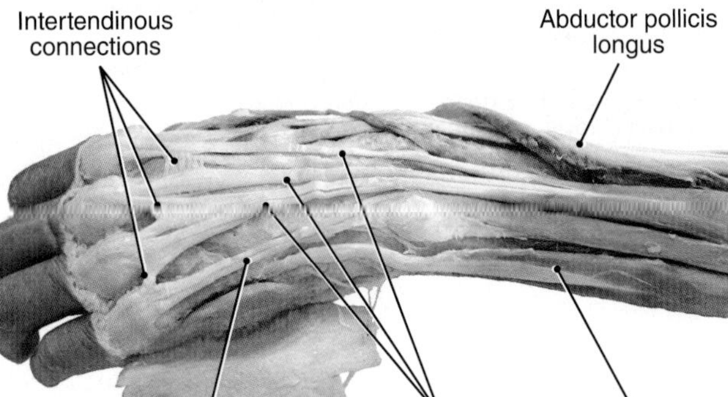

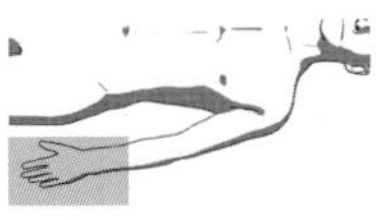

Fig. 8.32 Posteromedial view of wrist exposing muscle and tendons.

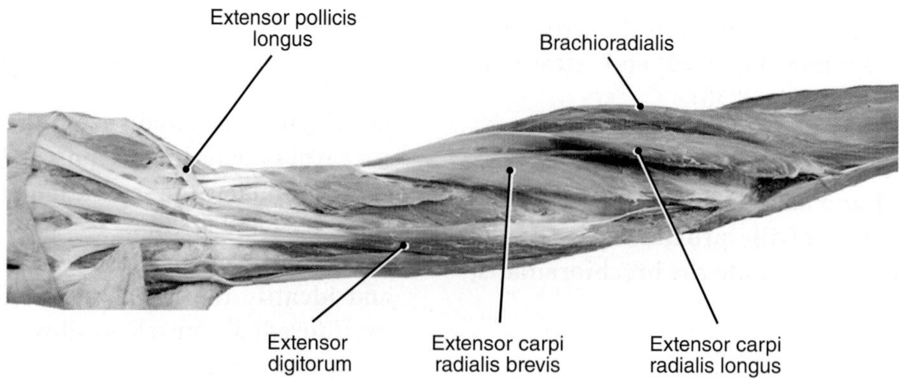

Fig. 8.33 Posterior view of forearm highlighting musculature.

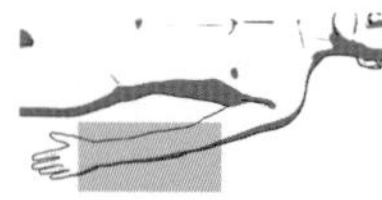

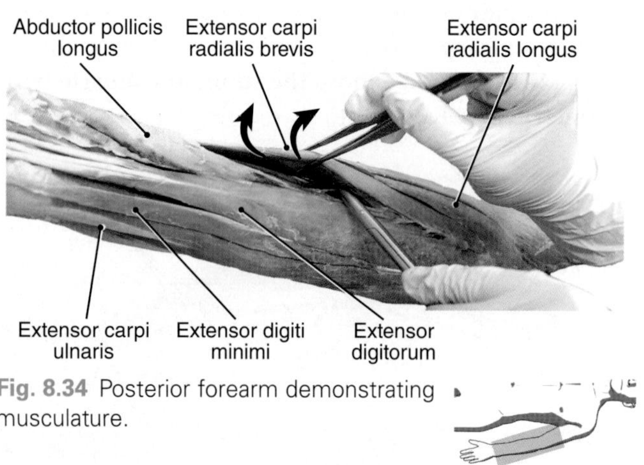

Fig. 8.34 Posterior forearm demonstrating musculature.

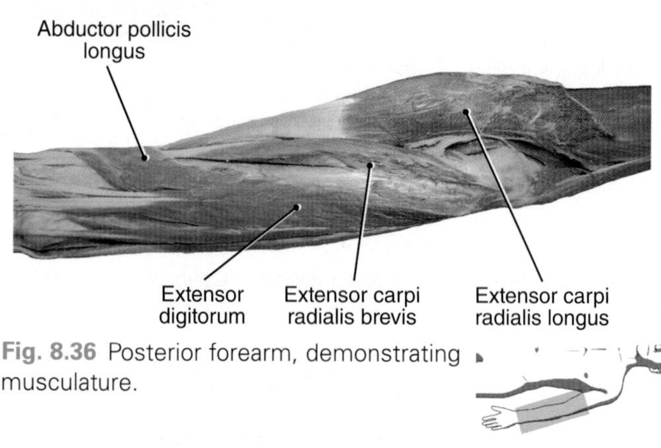

Fig. 8.36 Posterior forearm, demonstrating musculature.

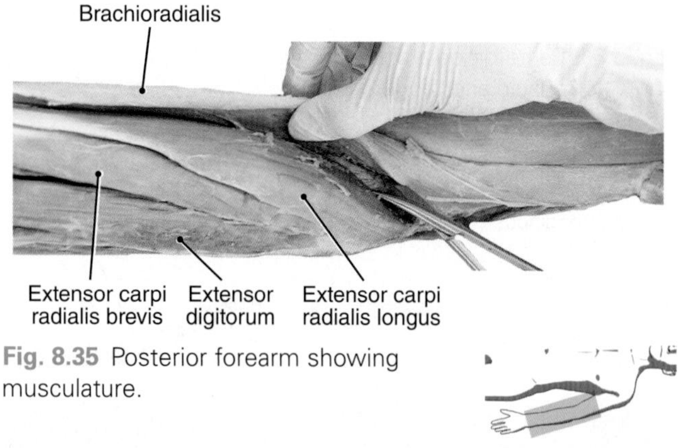

Fig. 8.35 Posterior forearm showing musculature.

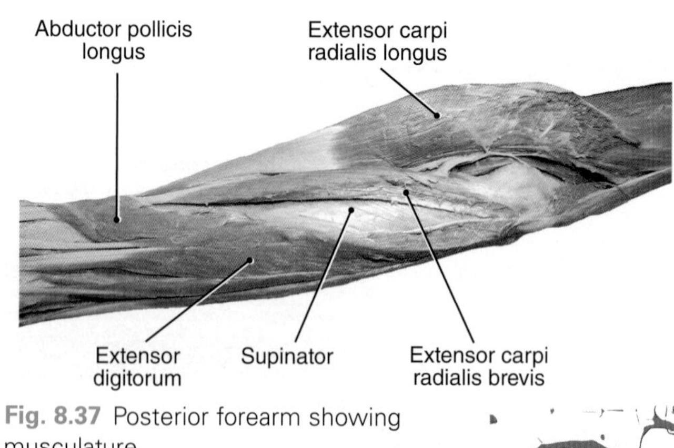

Fig. 8.37 Posterior forearm showing musculature.

- Reflect the extensor digitorum away from the supinator muscle to expose the supinator's borders (Fig. 8.38).
- At the inferior border of the supinator, trace and expose the deep radial nerve (Fig. 8.39, Plate 8.1). With a scalpel, make an incision in the supinator where the deep branch of the radial nerve first enters it (Fig. 8.40).
- Reflect the supinator and expose the deep radial nerve (Fig. 8.41, Plate 8.2).
- Make an incision on the posterior border of the ulna and detach the extensor carpi ulnaris muscle. Look for the emergence of the posterior interosseous artery running parallel to the deep branch of the radial nerve between the radius and the ulna.

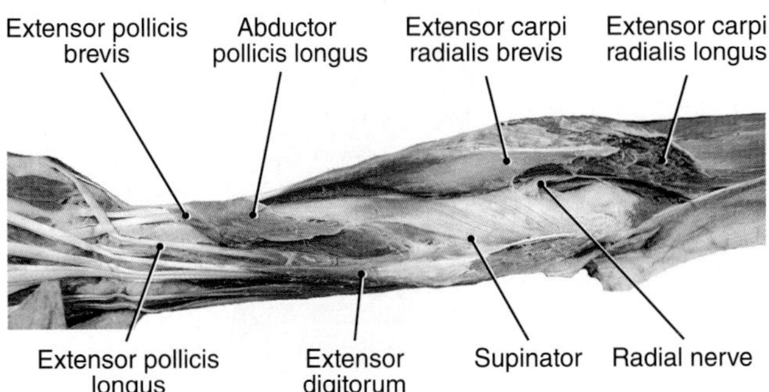

Fig. 8.38 Posterior forearm with brachioradialis muscle cut demonstrating radial nerve and supinator muscle.

DISSECTION TIP

The recurrent interosseous artery can be found between the anconeus and supinator muscles. Remove the anconeus, which travels from the lateral epicondyle to the lateral aspect of the olecranon. Just beneath it, on the anterior surface of the supinator, identify the recurrent interosseous artery. This artery is usually small and often is cut during routine dissection.

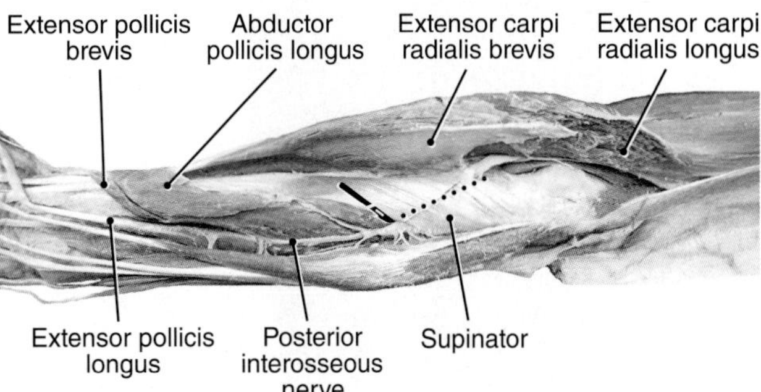

Fig. 8.40 Posterior forearm with brachioradialis cut demonstrating supinator muscle.

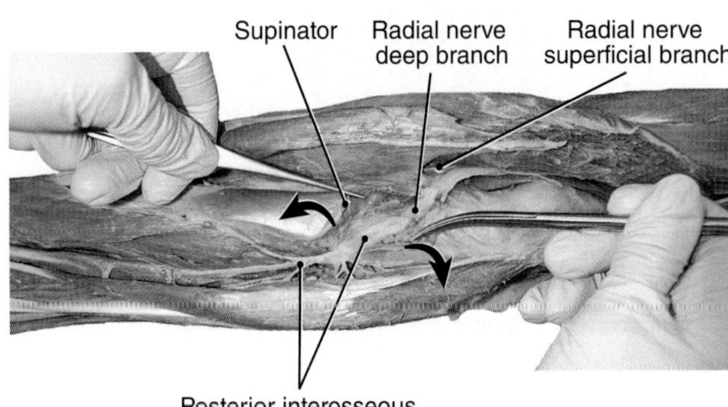

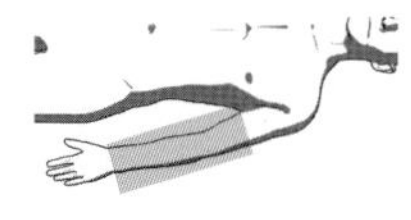

Fig. 8.41 Posterior forearm with brachioradialis cut demonstrating radial nerve branches, supinator muscle, and posterior interosseous nerve.

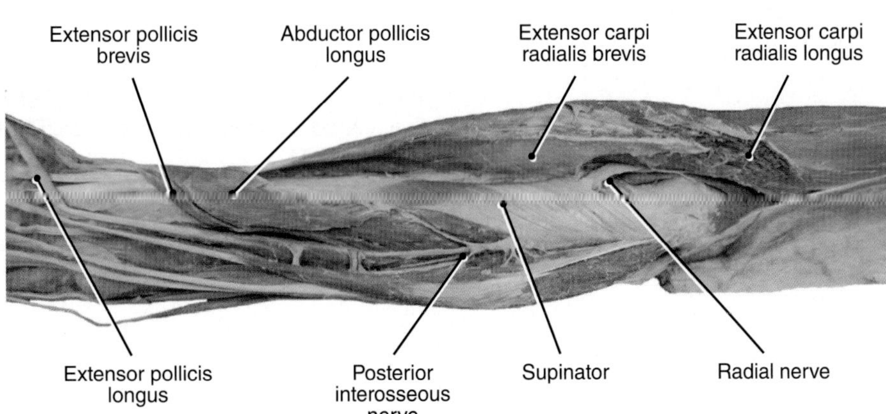

Fig. 8.39 Posterior forearm with brachioradialis muscle cut showing radial nerve and supinator muscle.

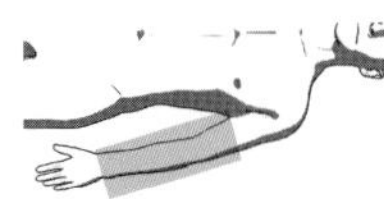

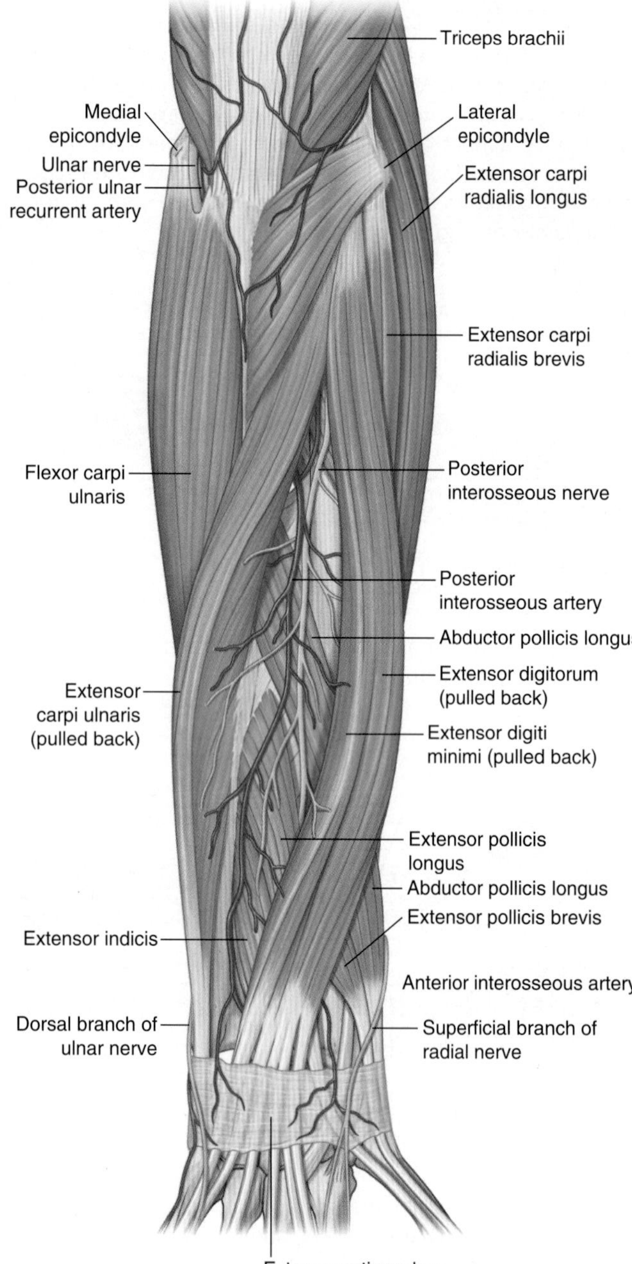

Plate 8.1 Arteries and nerves of the extensor compartment of the forearm. (From Drake RL et al. *Gray's Atlas of Anatomy*, 3rd edition, Philadelphia, Elsevier, 2021, p. 439).

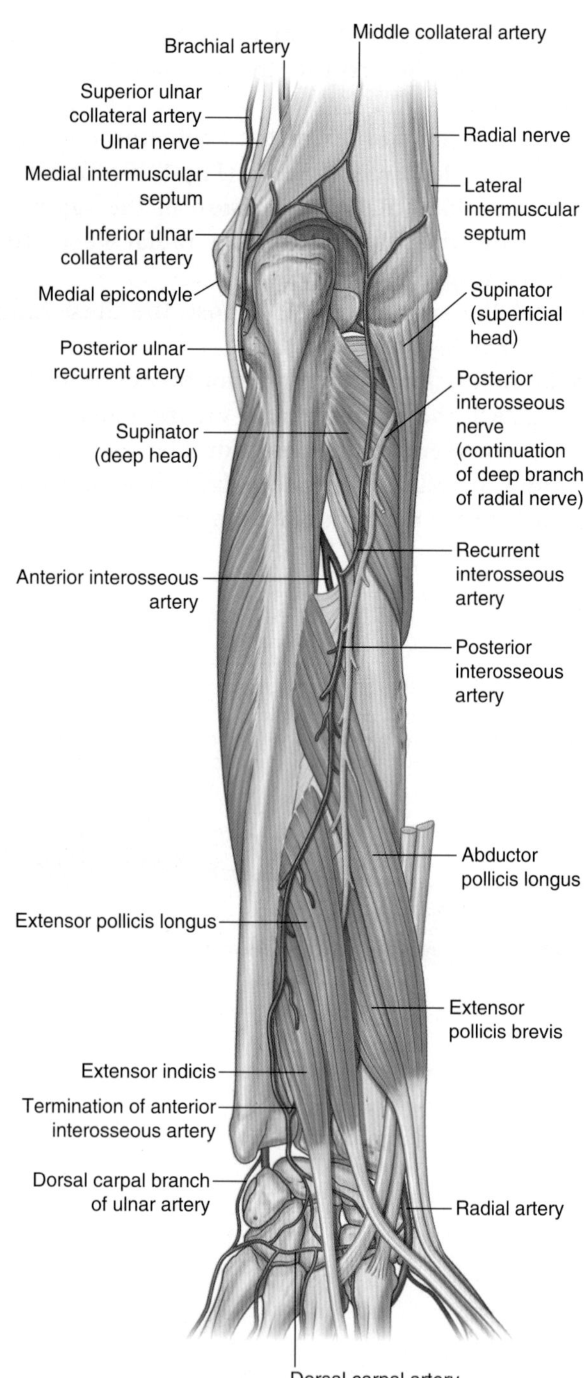

Plate 8.2 Arteries and nerves of the extensor compartment of the forearm (deeper dissection). (From Drake RL et al. *Gray's Atlas of Anatomy*, 3rd edition, Philadelphia, Elsevier, 2021, p. 439.)

FLEXOR COMPARTMENT

- **After completion of the dissection of the extensor compartment, rotate the upper limb and visualize the flexor compartment (Fig. 8.42).**
- **Make a vertical incision across the length of the forearm toward the wrist. Make an encircling incision around the cubital fossa and the wrist (see Fig. 8.42).**
- **Reflect the skin medially and laterally from the flexor compartment and expose the antebrachial fascia and the flexor retinaculum (Fig. 8.43). Continue the vertical midline incision toward the 3rd digit. Chapter 9 details the dissection of the hand.**
- **Identify the veins in the flexor compartment and in the cubital fossa. Trace the tributaries of the basilic vein.**
- **Identify the median cubital vein connecting the basilic and cephalic veins (Fig. 8.44).**
- **Once you identify the cephalic vein, trace it proximally to the arm. Lateral to the cephalic vein, identify the lateral antebrachial cutaneous nerve.**
- **This nerve is the cutaneous branch of the musculocutaneous nerve and supplies the lateral aspect of the forearm (see Fig. 8.44).**

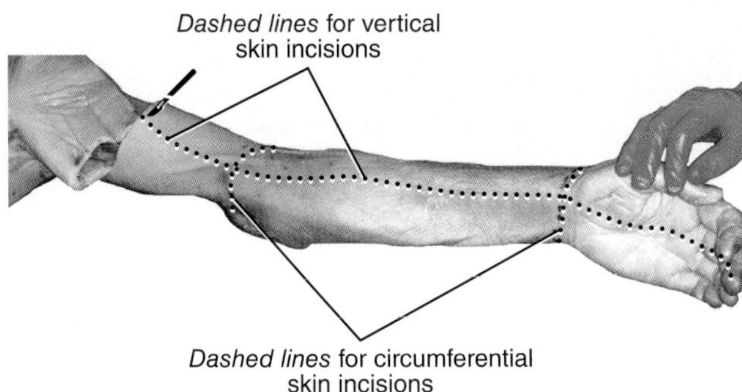

Fig. 8.42 Anterior view of the arm, forearm, and hand, with *dashed lines* for incisions.

- **Notice the thick, flat connective tissue aponeurosis of the biceps brachii muscle, the *bicipital aponeurosis.***
- **An easy way to identify the muscles of the forearm is to expose them from the wrist toward the cubital fossa.**
- **At the wrist, the tendons of each muscle are fairly evident and require minimal dissection.**
- **The following three muscles occupy the superficial layer of the muscles of the flexor compartment.**
  - On the radial side of the forearm, identify the flexor carpi radialis muscle (**Fig. 8.45**). The flexor carpi radialis attaches to the 2nd metacarpal bone, and some of its fibers may radiate to the adjacent 3rd metacarpal.
  - Medial to the flexor carpi radialis, note the palmaris longus muscle inserting into the palmar aponeurosis.
  - On the ulnar side of the forearm, identify the flexor carpi ulnaris muscle.

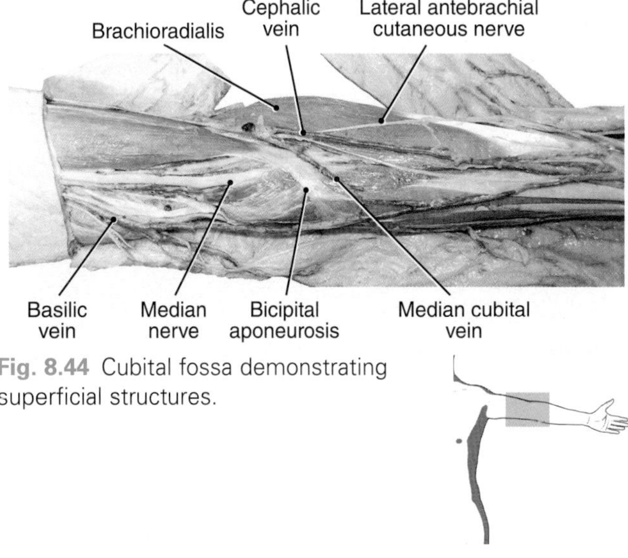

Fig. 8.44 Cubital fossa demonstrating superficial structures.

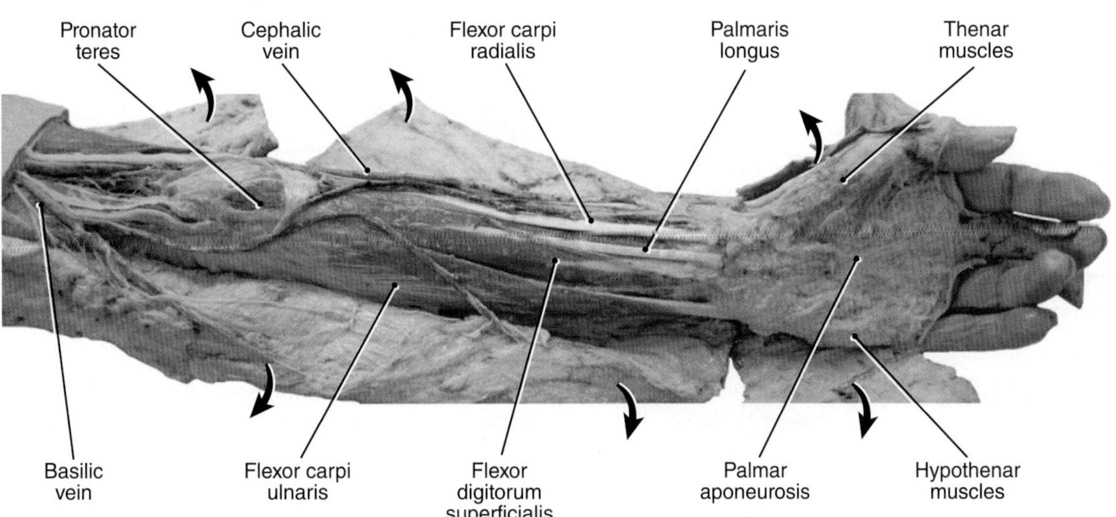

Fig. 8.43 Anterior view of the forearm and hand with skin reflected, demonstrating superficial structures.

DISSECTION **TIP**

The palmaris longus muscle is absent in roughly 10% of the population.

- **Dissect the deep fascia and the connective tissue over the tendons and the muscles of the flexor compartment (Figs. 8.46 and 8.47).**
- **Expose the tendon insertions of the flexor carpi ulnaris and flexor carpi radialis muscles (Fig. 8.48).**
- **Deep to the palmaris longus muscle, note the flexor digitorum superficialis muscle.**

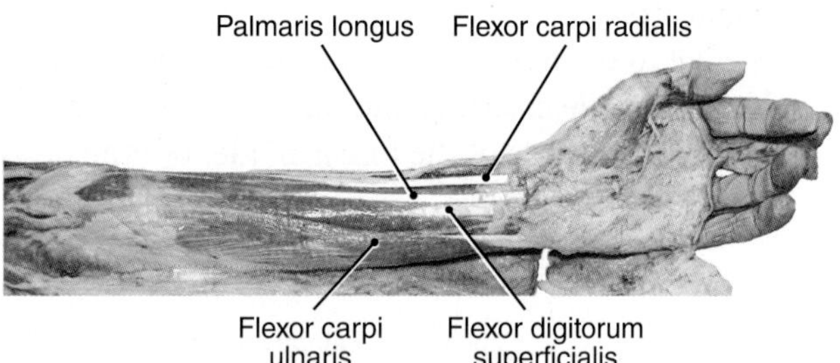

Fig. 8.45 Anterior view of the forearm showing muscles and tendons.

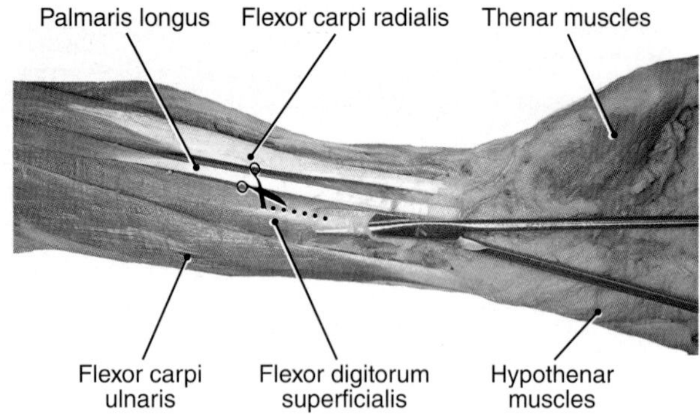

Fig. 8.46 Anterior view of the forearm demonstrating muscles and tendons.

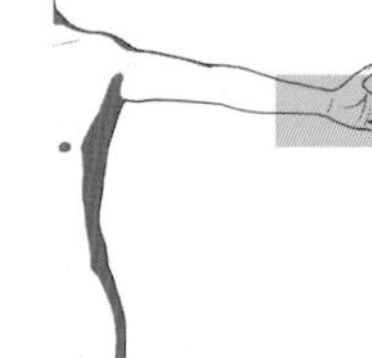

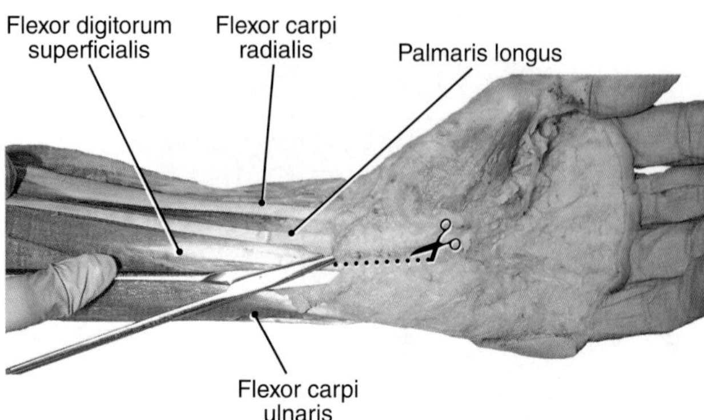

Fig. 8.47 Anterior view of the forearm, highlighting muscles and tendons.

- **Retract the flexor carpi ulnaris, and in the space between it and the flexor digitorum superficialis, identify a thick bundle of connective tissue encircling the ulnar artery and nerve (Fig. 8.49).**
- **With the aid of scissors, separate the connective tissue over the ulnar artery and nerve (Fig. 8.50).**
- **Further retract the flexor digitorum superficialis muscle and clean and expose the ulnar artery and nerve along the entire length of the forearm (Figs. 8.51 and 8.52).**
- **Underneath the flexor digitorum superficialis, identify the flexor digitorum profundus muscle.**
- **Clean the loose connective tissue over the flexor digitorum profundus (Fig. 8.53).**
- **Identify the radial artery between the brachioradialis and flexor carpi radialis muscles (Fig. 8.54).**
- **Further retract the brachioradialis muscle and expose the radial artery in the forearm (Figs. 8.55 and 8.56).**
- **Parallel to the radial artery, identify and expose the superficial branch of the radial nerve (Fig. 8.57).**

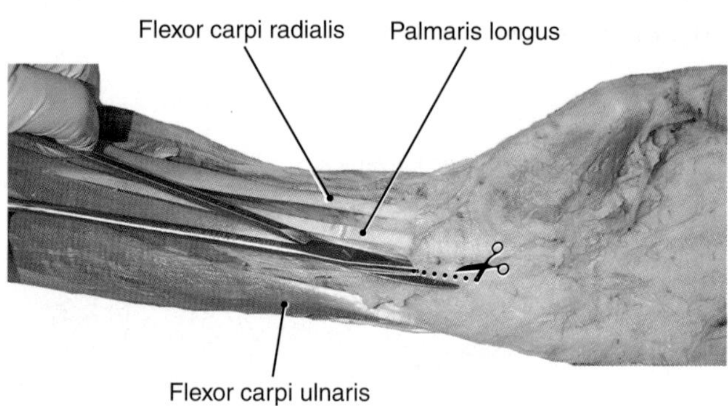

Fig. 8.48 Anterior view of the forearm showing muscles and tendons.

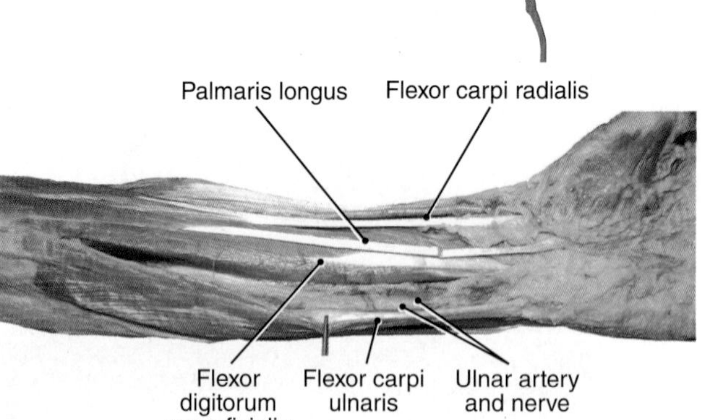

Fig. 8.49 Anterior view of the forearm demonstrating muscle-tendon units, with traction of flexor carpi ulnaris.

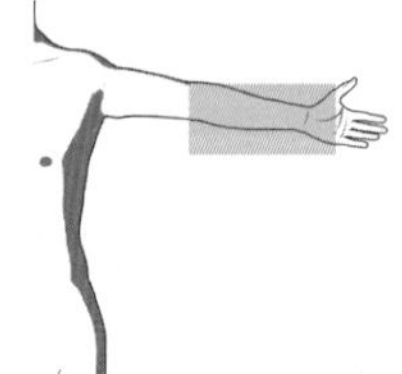

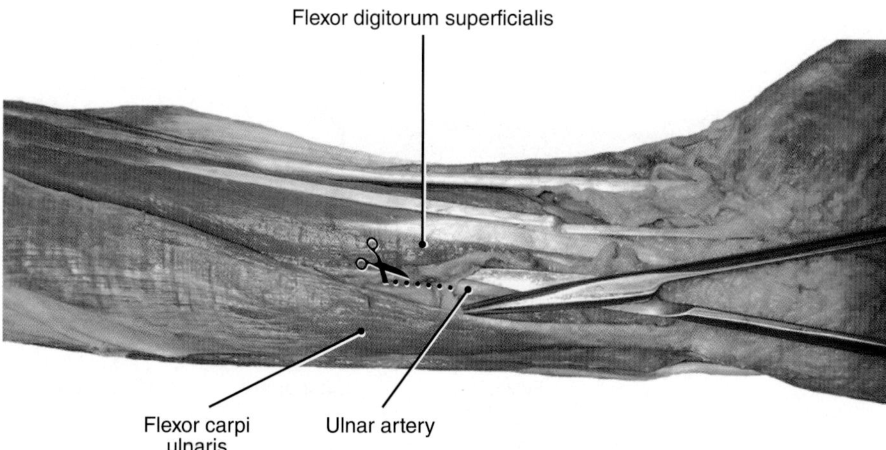

Fig. 8.50 Anterior view of the forearm and wrist demonstrating muscles and tendons.

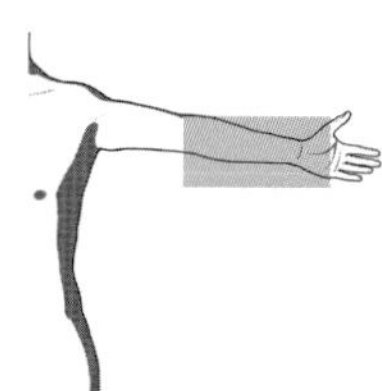

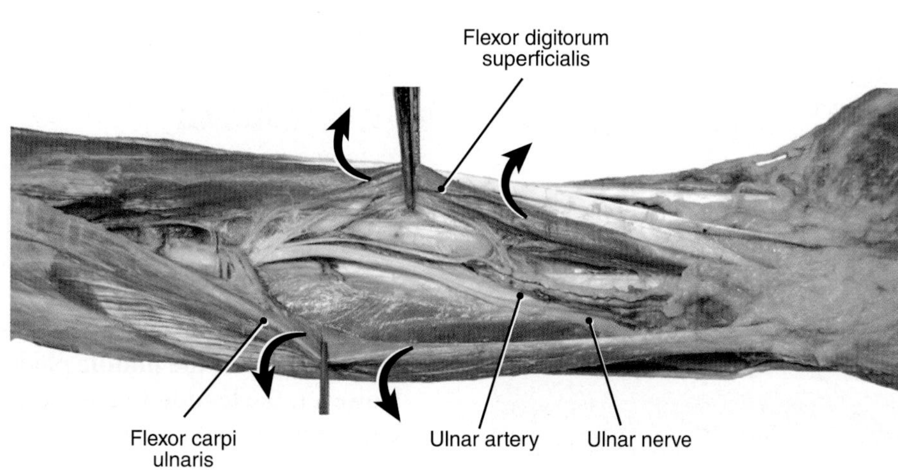

Fig. 8.51 Anterior forearm with traction on the flexor digitorum superficialis muscle showing intermediate layer.

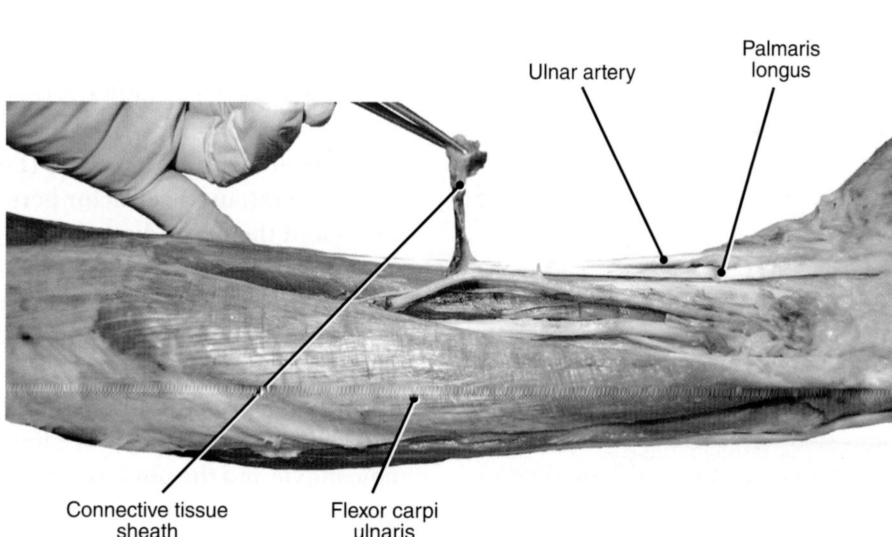

Fig. 8.52 Anterior forearm noting the flexor carpi ulnaris and palmaris longus muscles.

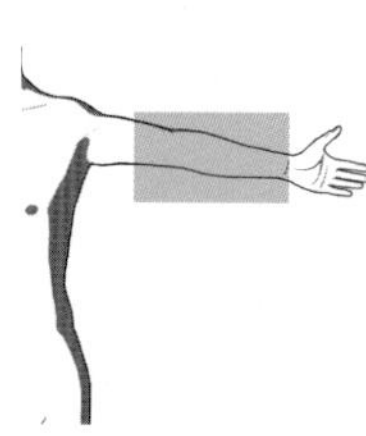

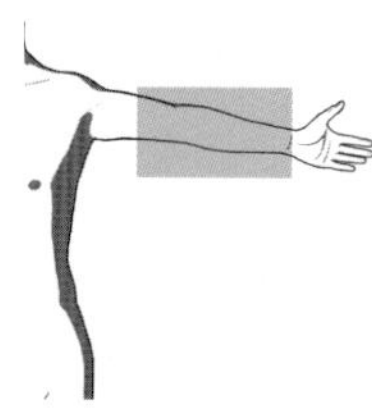

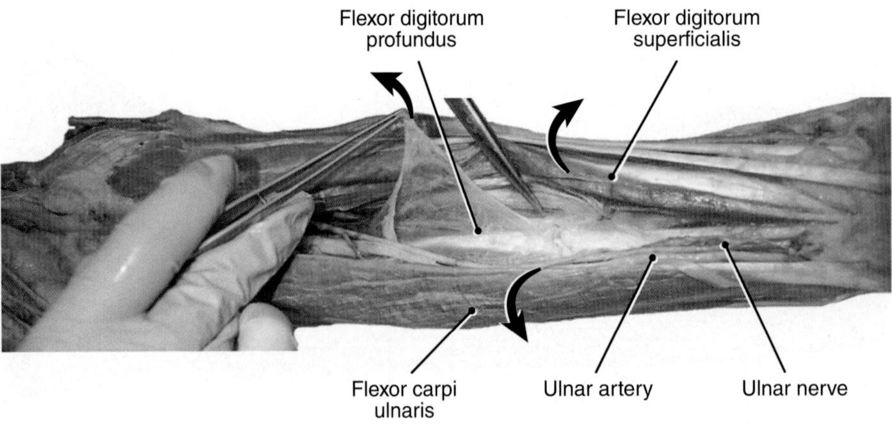

Fig. 8.53 Anterior view of the forearm with traction on flexor digitorum superficialis muscle, exposing the flexor digitorum profundus.

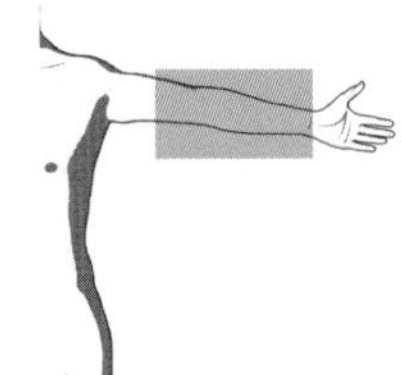

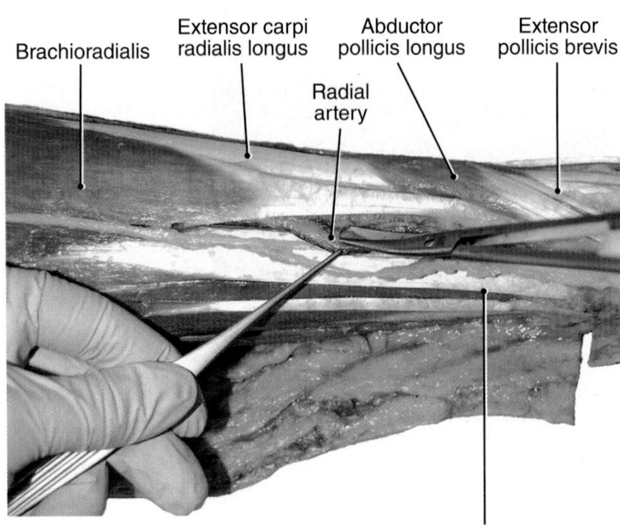

Fig. 8.54 Anterior view of distal forearm demonstrating radial neurovascular bundle.

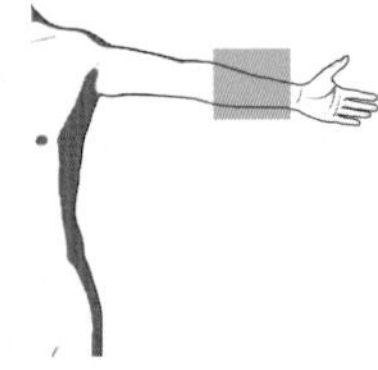

DISSECTION TIP

Note the following landmarks in the course of the radial artery:

- Passes superficial to the pronator teres muscle.
- Travels deep to the brachioradialis muscle.

At the wrist, the radial artery is found between the tendons of the flexor carpi radialis and the brachioradialis muscles. This point is used to feel the radial pulse or to perform arterial catheterization.

- **The flexor digitorum profundus muscle inserts onto the bases of the distal phalanx of each of the medial four digits.**

DISSECTION TIP

A common variation of the flexor digitorum profundus is that its tendon to the 2nd digit may form an independent muscle. The flexor pollicis longus muscle inserts onto the distal phalanx of the 1st digit.

- **The flexor digitorum superficialis muscle inserts onto the base of the middle phalanx of digits 2 to 5. However, the tendon to the 5th digit may be absent.**
- **Expose the radial artery (Fig. 8.58).**

CUBITAL FOSSA AND FLEXOR COMPARTMENT OF THE FOREARM

- **Cut the bicipital aponeurosis (Fig. 8.59) to trace the radial artery to its branch point from the brachial artery.**
- **Coursing with the ulnar artery, identify the median nerve and the vena comitans (Fig. 8.60).**
- **Lift the brachial and radial arteries and expose the ulnar artery with its branches (Fig. 8.61).**
- **At this point, use a retractor between the brachioradialis and the flexor digitorum superficialis muscles to expose deeper structures (Fig. 8.62).**
- **Follow the course of the ulnar and radial arteries and identify the recurrent ulnar and recurrent radial arteries.**
- **Identify the pronator teres and its two heads; the humeral (superficial) head is attached to the medial epicondyle and the ulnar (deep) head to the coronoid process of the ulna.**
- **Trace the course of the medial nerve as it travels from the cubital fossa and then enters the forearm between the two heads of the pronator teres (see Fig. 8.62).**
- **Note the ulnar artery entering the forearm deep to the ulnar (deep) head of the pronator teres muscle (see Fig. 8.62).**

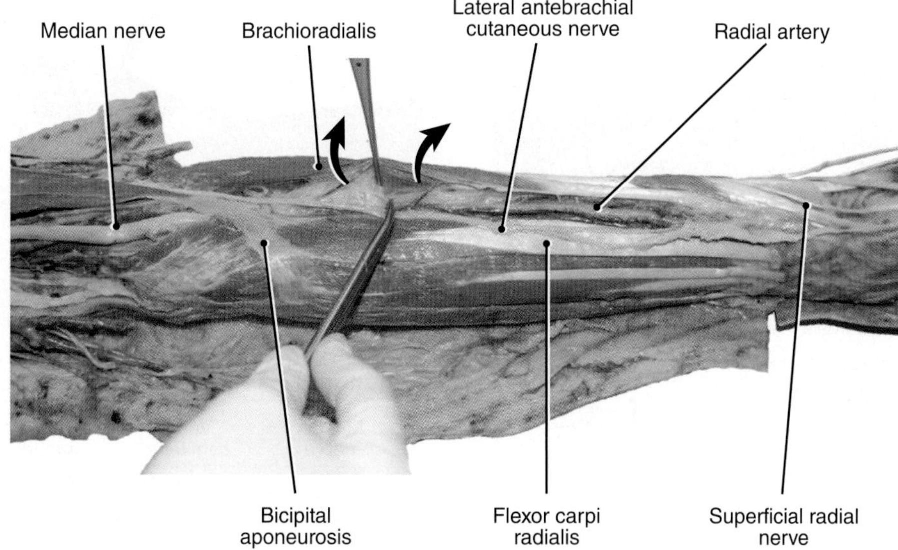

Fig. 8.55 Anteromedial view of forearm with skin reflected demonstrating the radial artery and vein.

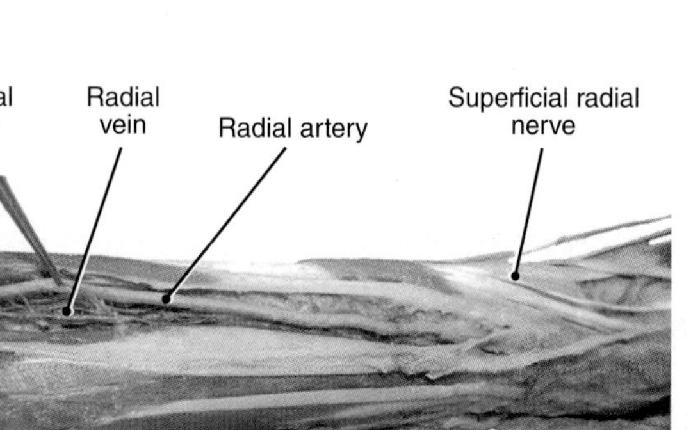

Fig. 8.56 Anterior forearm view with skin reflected demonstrating the radial artery and vein.

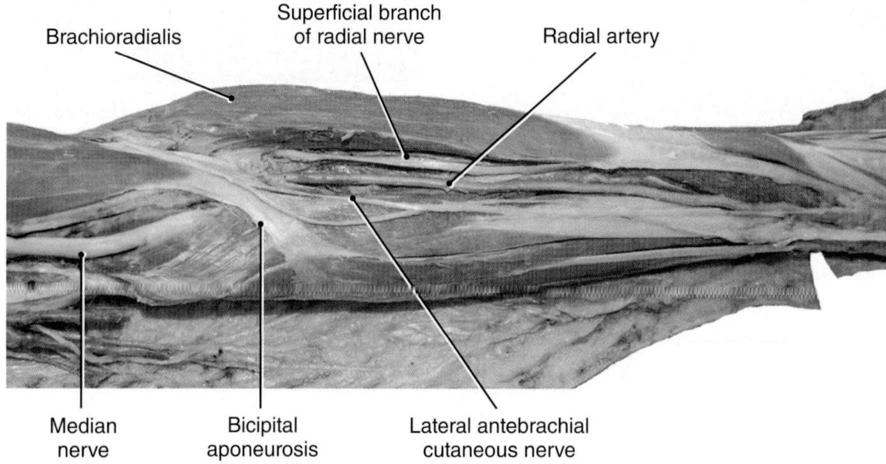

Fig. 8.57 Anterior forearm view showing the radial artery, vein, and nerve.

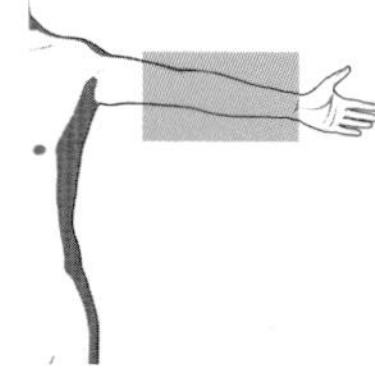

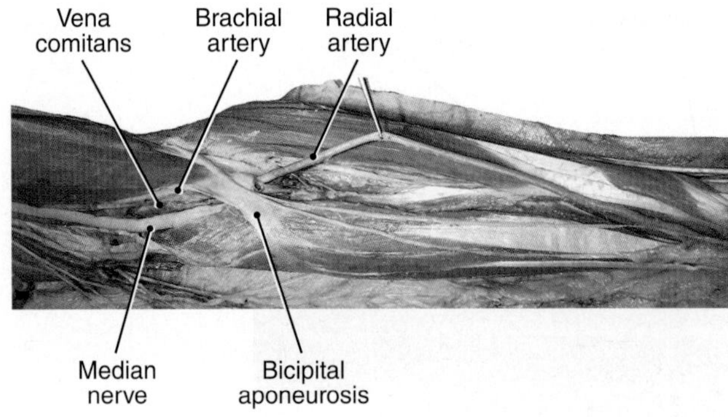

Fig. 8.58 Anterior forearm with radial artery and traction demonstrating musculature.

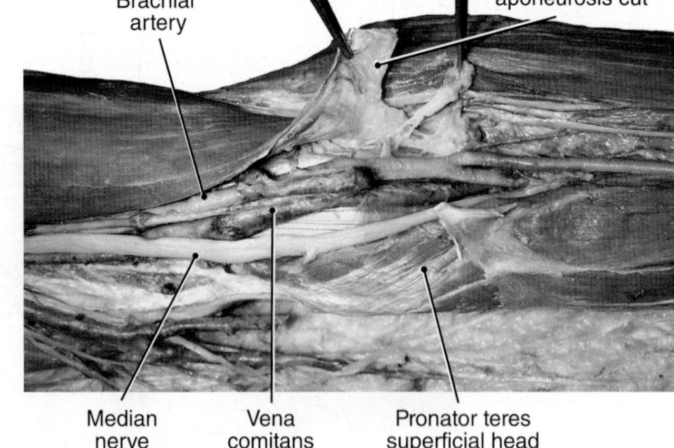

Fig. 8.60 Cubital fossa with bicipital aponeurosis reflected highlighting brachial artery and median nerve.

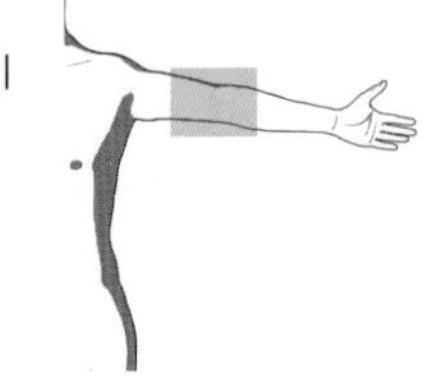

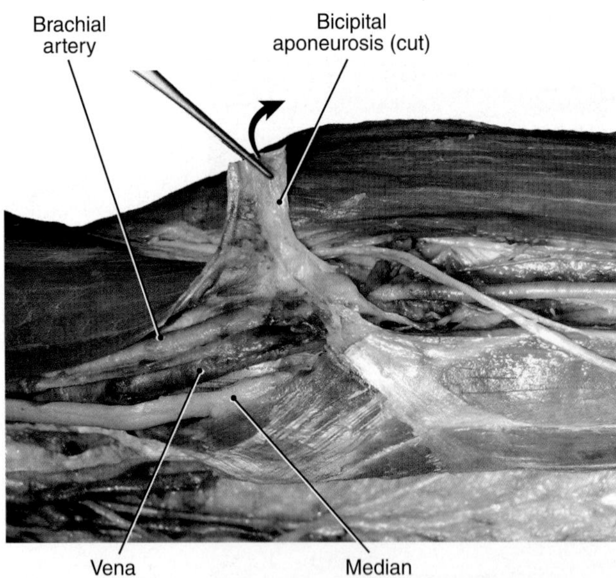

Fig. 8.59 Cubital fossa with bicipital aponeurosis reflected demonstrating brachial artery and median nerve.

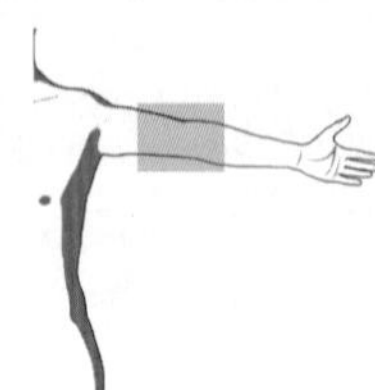

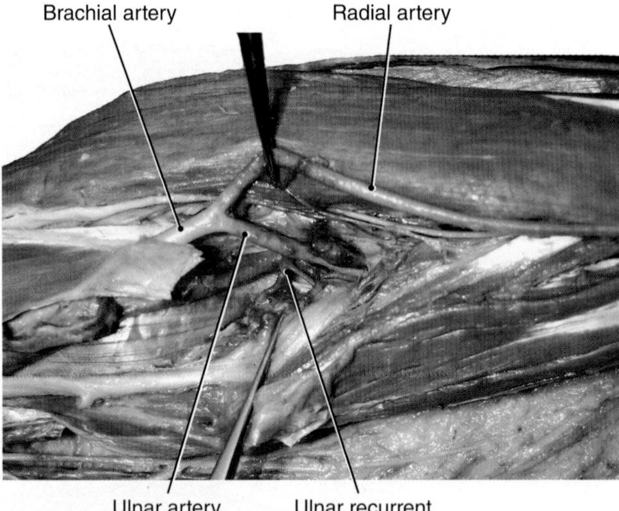

Fig. 8.61 Cubital fossa with bicipital aponeurosis cut demonstrating the bifurcation of the brachial artery.

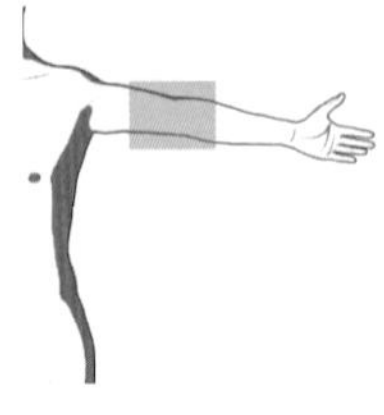

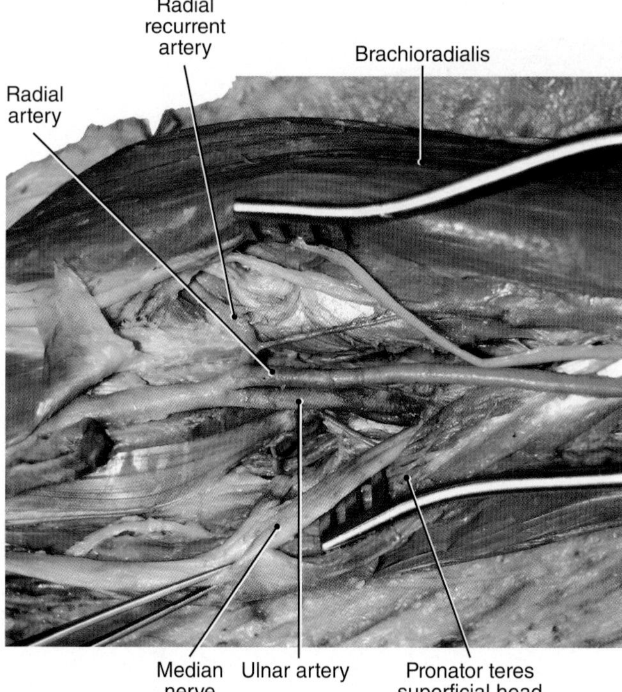

Fig. 8.62 Cubital fossa view with bicipital aponeurosis reflected exposing neurovascular structures.

- **Lift up the median nerve and identify its muscular branches (Fig. 8.63).**

DISSECTION TIP

To continue the dissection, the vena comitans must be removed (Fig. 8.64). Cut the veins in the cubital fossa and as distal as possible in the forearm. Use paper towels to absorb any fluid that issues from the cut veins.

- **Expose the borders of the pronator teres and retract the radial artery (Fig. 8.65).**
- **Carefully split the humeral head of the pronator teres (Fig. 8.66) from the underlying ulnar (deep) head and flexor digitorum superficialis muscle (Figs. 8.67 and 8.68).**
- **Lift the median nerve and expose its course in the deep flexor compartment of the forearm (Fig. 8.69).**
- **Dissect distally the ulnar artery and identify the common interosseous artery (Fig. 8.70).**
- **The common interosseous artery arises from the ulnar artery and then divides into the anterior and posterior interosseous branches (Fig. 8.71).**

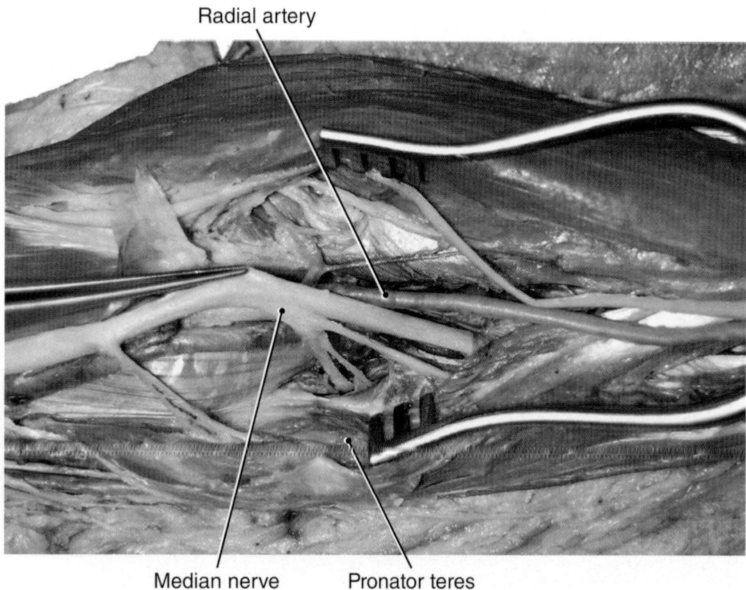

Fig. 8.63 Cubital fossa view with bicipital aponeurosis reflected demonstrating neurovascular structures.

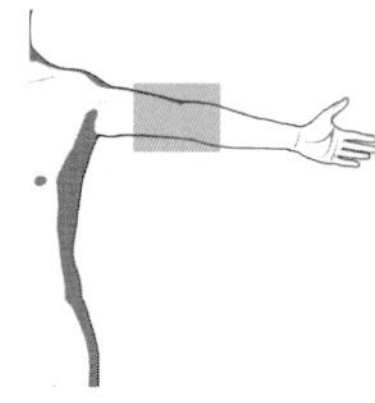

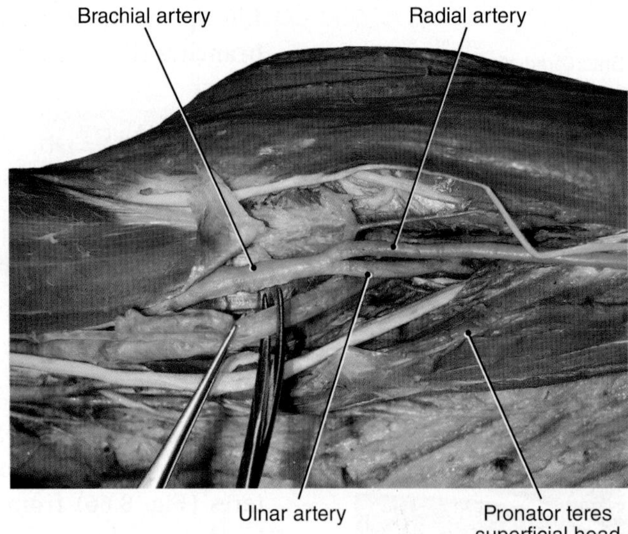

Fig. 8.64 Anterior view of the cubital fossa with the bicipital aponeurosis reflected, highlighting neurovascular structures.

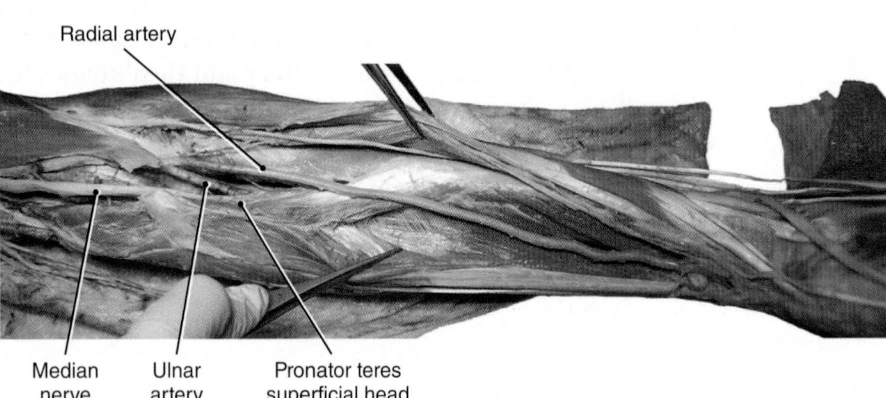

Fig. 8.65 View of the anterolateral forearm with skin reflected, demonstrating the radial artery and musculature.

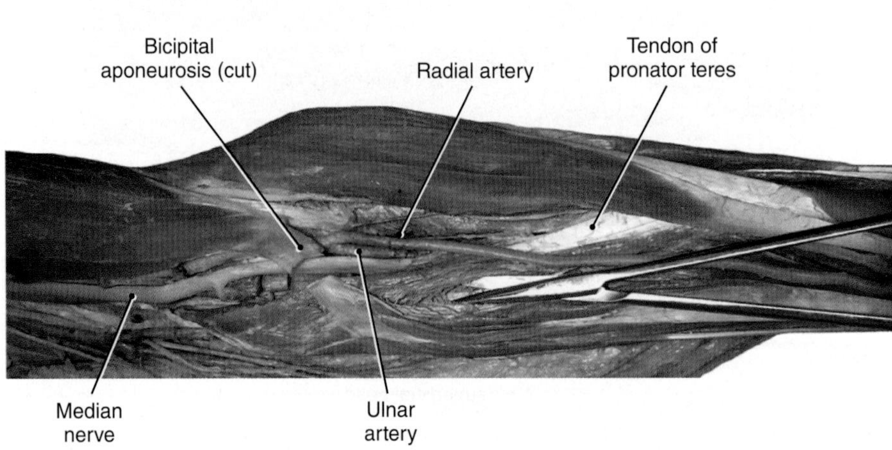

Fig. 8.66 Anterior cubital fossa with bicipital aponeurosis cut, exposing the median nerve, radial artery, and pronator teres muscle.

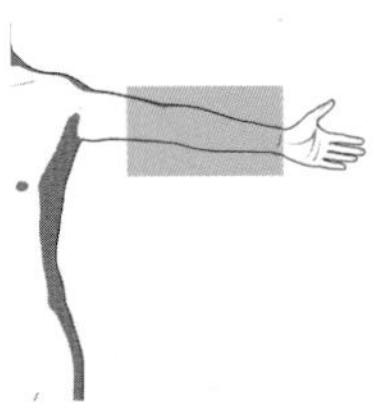

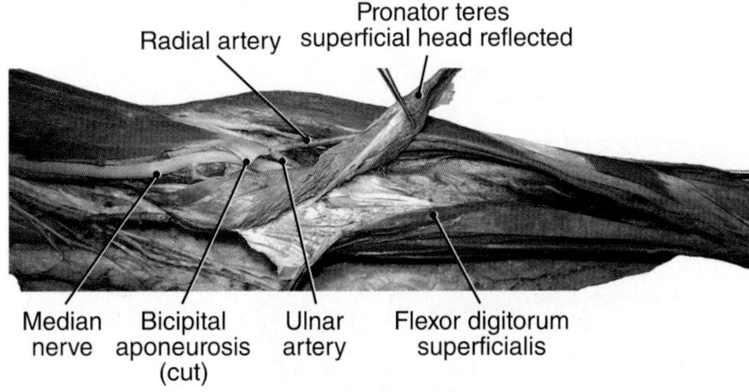

Fig. 8.67 Anterior view of lateral cubital fossa and forearm with reflected pronator teres.

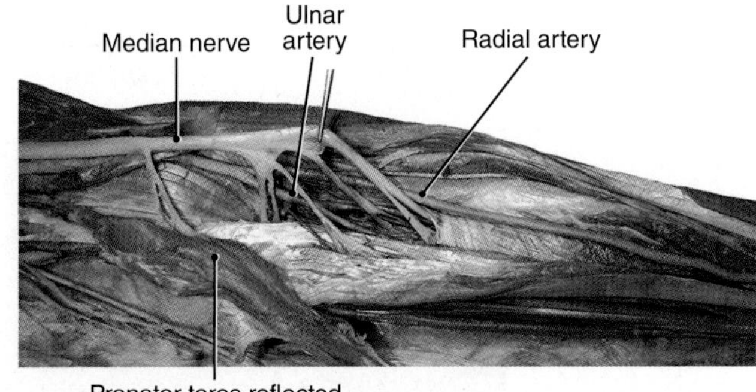

Fig. 8.69 Cubital fossa view with the superficial (humeral) head of pronator teres muscle reflected, and median nerve traction demonstrating the deep (ulnar) head of pronator teres.

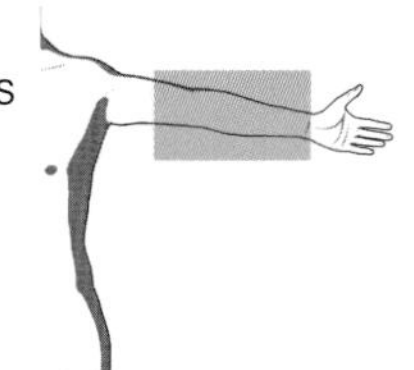

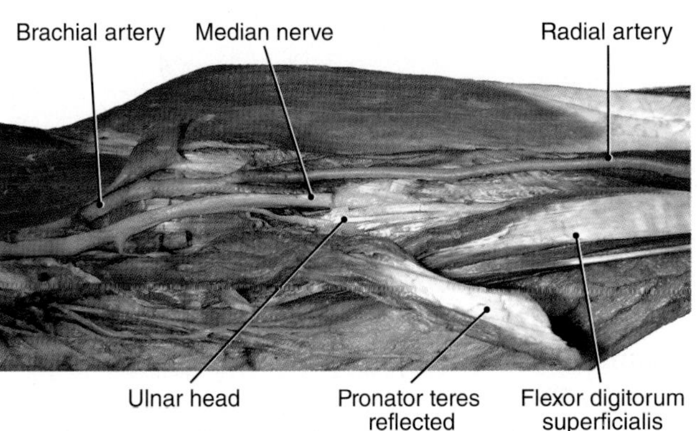

Fig. 8.68 Cubital fossa with pronator teres muscle reflected, demonstrating deeper structures.

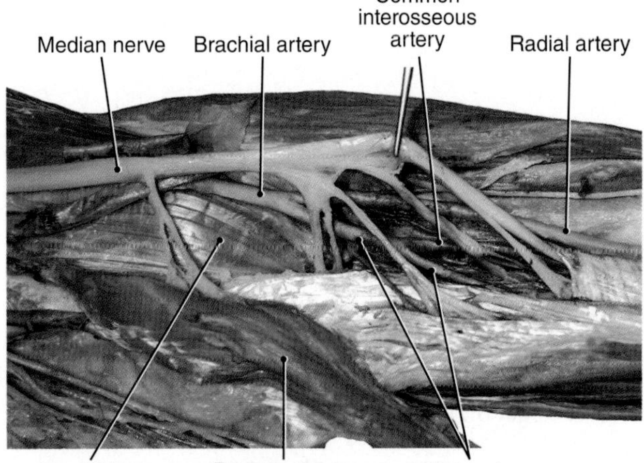

Fig. 8.70 Cubital fossa view with the superficial pronator teres head reflected, and median nerve traction demonstrating the deep pronator teres head, and radial and ulnar arteries.

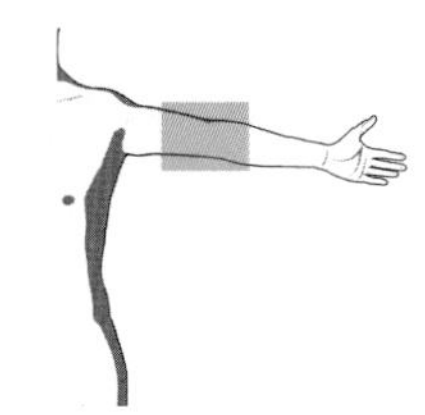

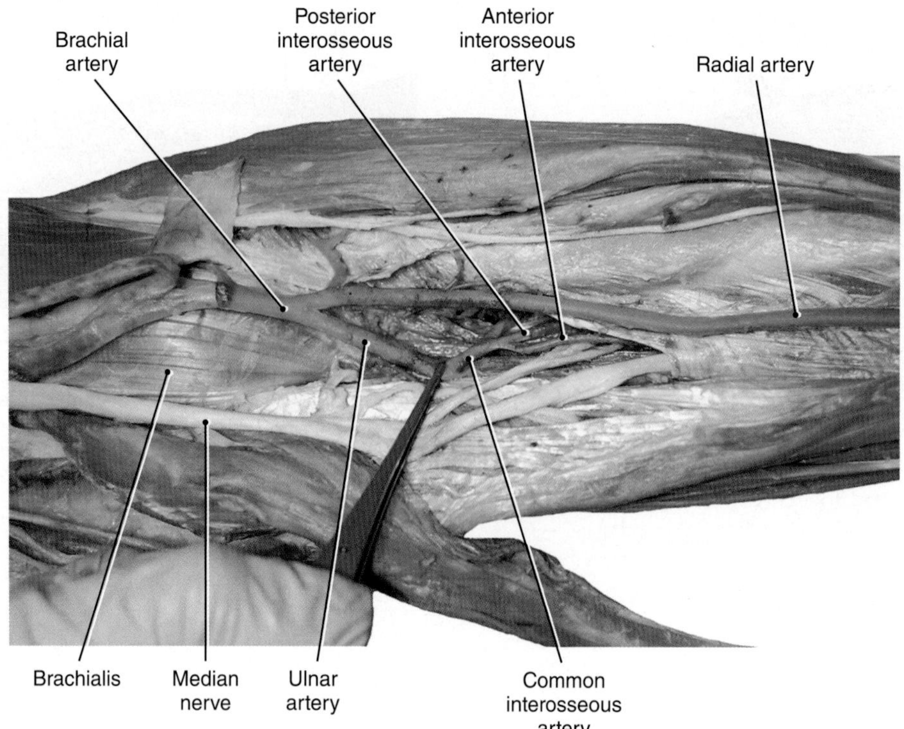

Fig. 8.71 Cubital fossa with the superficial head of pronator teres reflected, and median nerve traction demonstrating the deep head of pronator teres and radial and ulnar arteries.

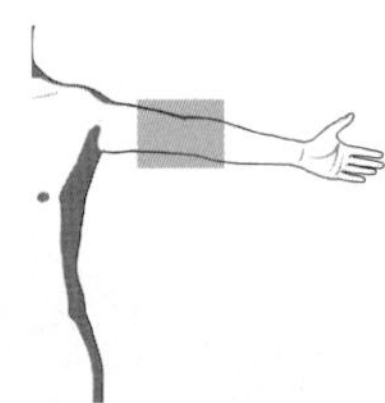

- **The posterior interosseous artery passes through the interosseous membrane to reach the extensor compartment of the forearm.**
- **As the median nerve is lifted, identify the anterior interosseous nerve, which arises from the median nerve just proximal to the pronator teres muscle (see Figs. 8.70 and 8.71, Plate 8.3).**

DEEP FLEXOR COMPARTMENT

- **Cut the tendons of the flexor digitorum superficialis, or widely retract them, and identify the flexor digitorum profundus and flexor pollicis longus muscles (Fig. 8.72).**
- **Finally, identify the pronator quadratus, which connects the distal portions of the ulna and radius (Fig. 8.73).**
- **In the space between the flexor pollicis longus and flexor digitorum profundus muscles, trace the course of the anterior interosseous artery and anterior interosseous nerve, a branch of the median nerve (see Figs. 8.72 and 8.73).**

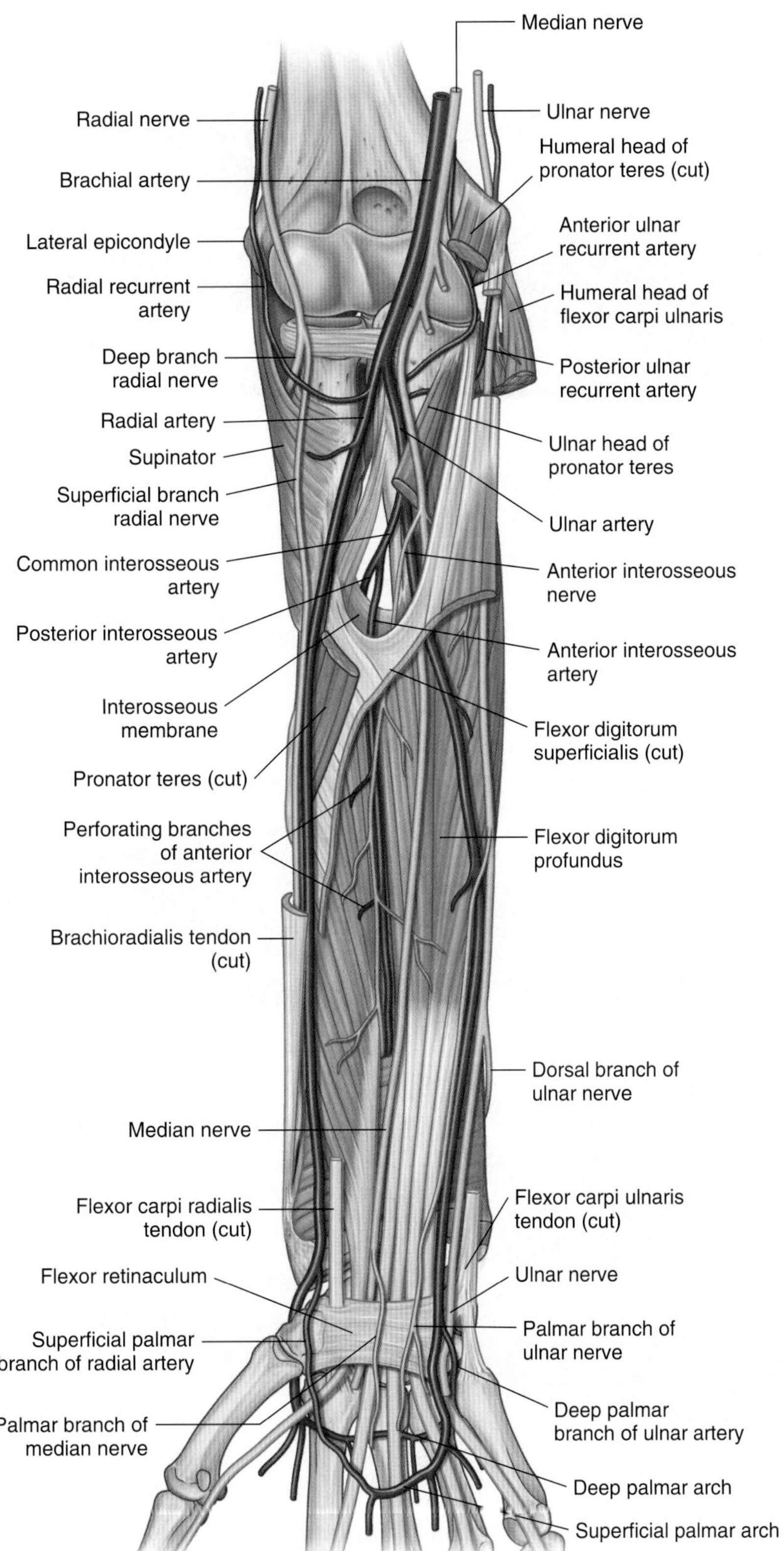

Plate 8.3 Arteries and nerves of the flexor compartment of the forearm. (From Drake RL et al. *Gray's Atlas of Anatomy*, 3rd edition, Philadelphia, Elsevier, 2021, p. 436).

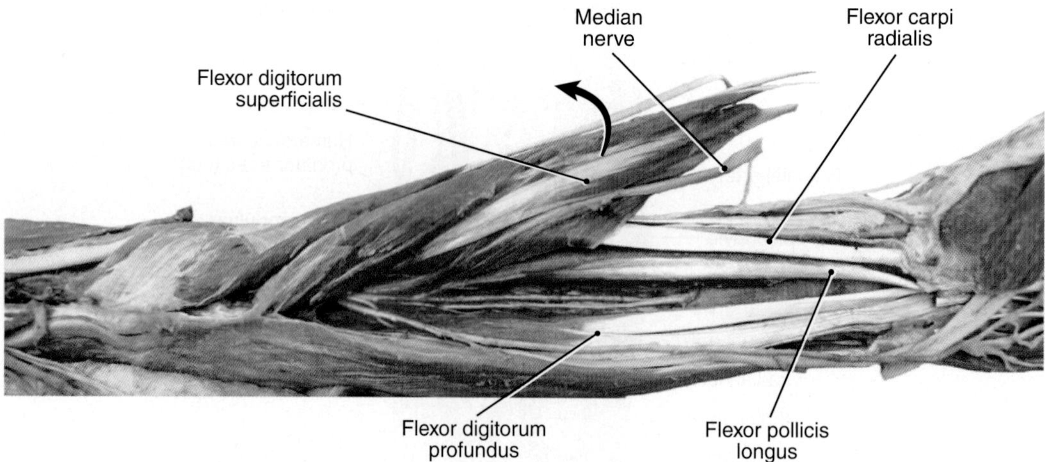

Fig. 8.72 Anterior forearm with superficial and intermediate muscle layers cut and reflected, exposing deeper structures.

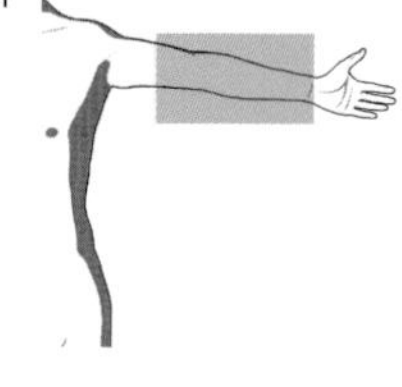

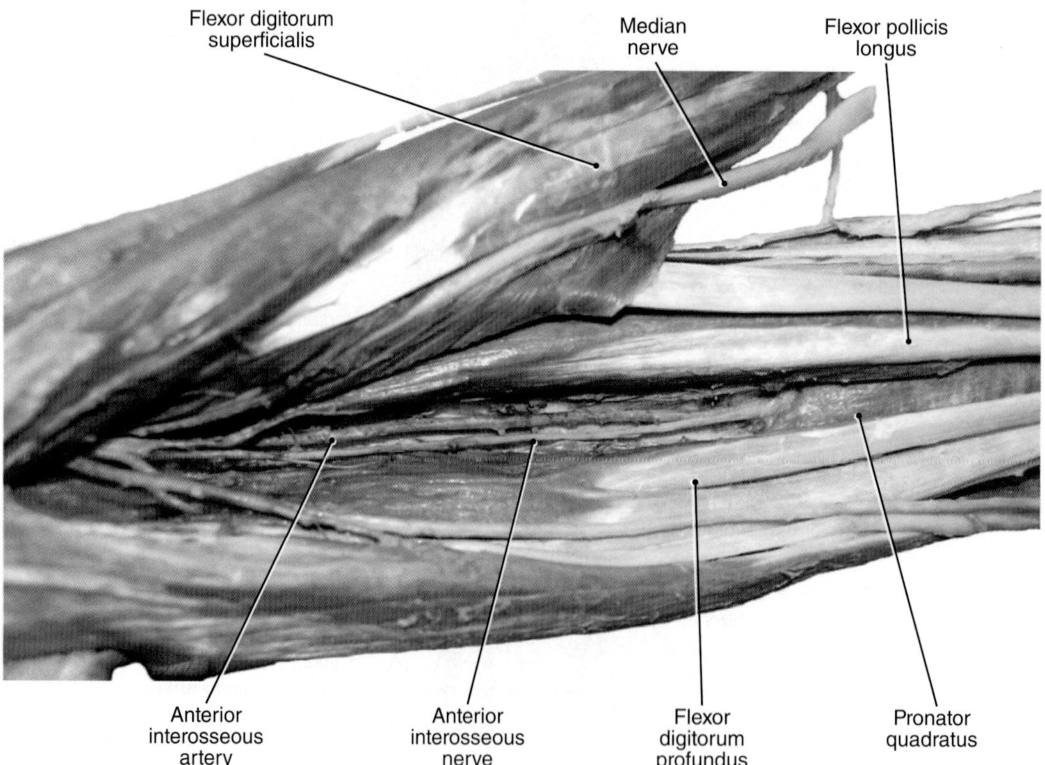

Fig. 8.73 Anterior view of forearm with superficial and intermediate muscle layers cut and reflected, demonstrating deeper structures.

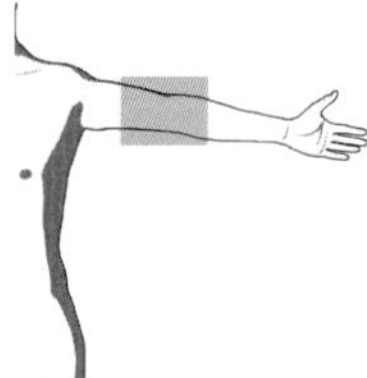

LABORATORY IDENTIFICATION CHECKLIST

NERVES

- ☐ Musculocutaneous
- ☐ Lateral antebrachial cutaneous
- ☐ Median
- ☐ Anterior interosseous
- ☐ Medial brachial cutaneous
- ☐ Medial antebrachial cutaneous
- ☐ Ulnar
- ☐ Radial
- ☐ Posterior interosseous

ARTERIES

- ☐ Brachial
- ☐ Radial
- ☐ Radial recurrent
- ☐ Interosseous recurrent
- ☐ Ulnar
- ☐ Common interosseous
- ☐ Anterior interosseous
- ☐ Posterior interosseous
- ☐ Ulnar anterior recurrent
- ☐ Ulnar posterior recurrent

VEINS

Superficial

- ☐ Cephalic
- ☐ Basilic
- ☐ Cubital

Deep

- ☐ Brachial
- ☐ Radial
- ☐ Ulnar

MUSCLES

Anterior Compartment of Arm

- ☐ Coracobrachialis
- ☐ Biceps brachii
  - ☐ Long head
  - ☐ Short head
- ☐ Brachialis

Posterior Compartment of Arm

- ☐ Triceps brachii
  - ☐ Long head
  - ☐ Lateral head
  - ☐ Medial head
- ☐ Anconeus

Anterior Compartment of Forearm

Superficial Layer

- ☐ Pronator teres
  - ☐ Superficial (humeral) head
  - ☐ Deep (superficial) head
- ☐ Flexor carpi radialis
- ☐ Palmaris longus
- ☐ Flexor carpi ulnaris

Intermediate Layer

- ☐ Flexor digitorum superficialis

Deep Layer

- ☐ Flexor digitorum profundus
- ☐ Flexor pollicis longus
- ☐ Pronator quadratus

Posterior Compartment of Forearm

Superficial Layer

- ☐ Brachioradialis
- ☐ Extensor carpi radialis longus
- ☐ Extensor carpi radialis brevis
- ☐ Extensor digitorum
- ☐ Extensor digiti minimi
- ☐ Extensor carpi ulnaris

Deep Layer

- ☐ Supinator
- ☐ Abductor pollicis longus
- ☐ Extensor pollicis longus
- ☐ Extensor pollicis brevis
- ☐ Extensor indicis

LIGAMENTS

- ☐ Ulnar collateral
- ☐ Radial collateral
- ☐ Annular

CONNECTIVE TISSUES

- ☐ Bicipital aponeurosis
- ☐ Antebrachial fascia
- ☐ Flexor retinaculum
- ☐ Extensor retinaculum

BONES

- ☐ Scapula
- ☐ Humerus
- ☐ Radius
- ☐ Ulna
- ☐ Carpals
- ☐ Metacarpals
- ☐ Phalanges

BEFORE YOU BEGIN

Palpation

Flex and extend your digits, noting the movements of the tendons beneath the skin. On the dorsal side of your hand, identify the tendons of the extensor digitorum muscle. At the flexor aspect of the palm, note the distal skin crease (crease between wrist and forearm), marking the proximal edge of the flexor retinaculum (Fig. 9.1).

- At the ulnar side of the distal skin crease, palpate the pisiform bone. At the radial side of the distal skin crease, palpate the scaphoid bone. Immediately beneath the radial and ulnar sides of the distal skin crease, palpate the **radial** and **ulnar styloid processes**, respectively.
- By flexing the closed fist against resistance, you should be able to identify several tendons at the anterior wrist, from medial to lateral: the flexor carpi ulnaris, flexor digitorum superficialis, palmaris longus, and flexor carpi radialis. However, the most prominent tendons are those of the palmaris longus, lying at the midline, and the flexor carpi radialis, lying on the radial side. Lateral to the tendon of the flexor carpi radialis, you can palpate the radial artery. The pulsations of the ulnar artery are more difficult to detect but usually are felt about 3 cm proximal to the pisiform bone, lateral to the flexor carpi ulnaris muscle. Note the thenar and hypothenar eminences, which contain muscles of the 1st and 5th digits, respectively.

On the dorsum surface of the hand, extend the 1st digit, noting the tendons of the abductor pollicis longus (to base of 1st metacarpal bone), the extensor pollicis brevis (to base of 1st phalanx), and the extensor pollicis longus muscles (to base of distal phalanx of 1st digit) forming the "anatomical snuffbox" (Fig. 9.2). This anatomic area is important because the radial artery lies on the scaphoid bone and passes to reach the dorsum of the 1st digit.

If the dorsum of the hand has not been dissected already on your cadaver as it was in Chapter 8, then refer to Chapter 8, Figs. 8.12 to 8.16 before proceeding to the palmar dissection (Fig. 9.3).

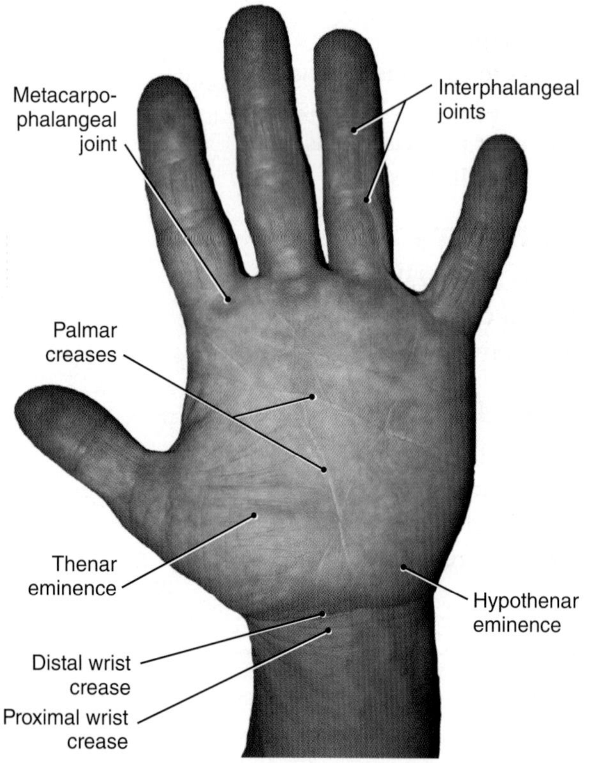

Fig. 9.1 Anterior view of palmar surface of hand. Note positioning of interphalangeal and metacarpal phalangeal joints, palmar and wrist creases, and thenar and hypothenar eminences.

PALMAR HAND

- **Make a similar midline incision on the palmar surface, starting from the distal palmar crease to the base of**

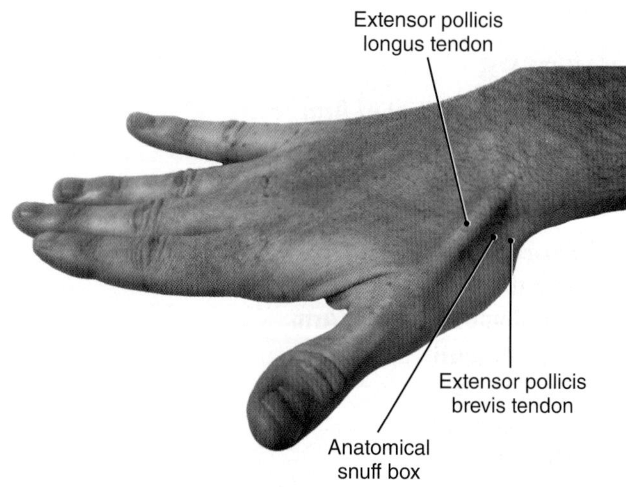

Fig. 9.2 Dorsolateral view of wrist, noting "anatomical snuffbox," which is bordered by the underlying extensor pollicis longus and brevis tendons.

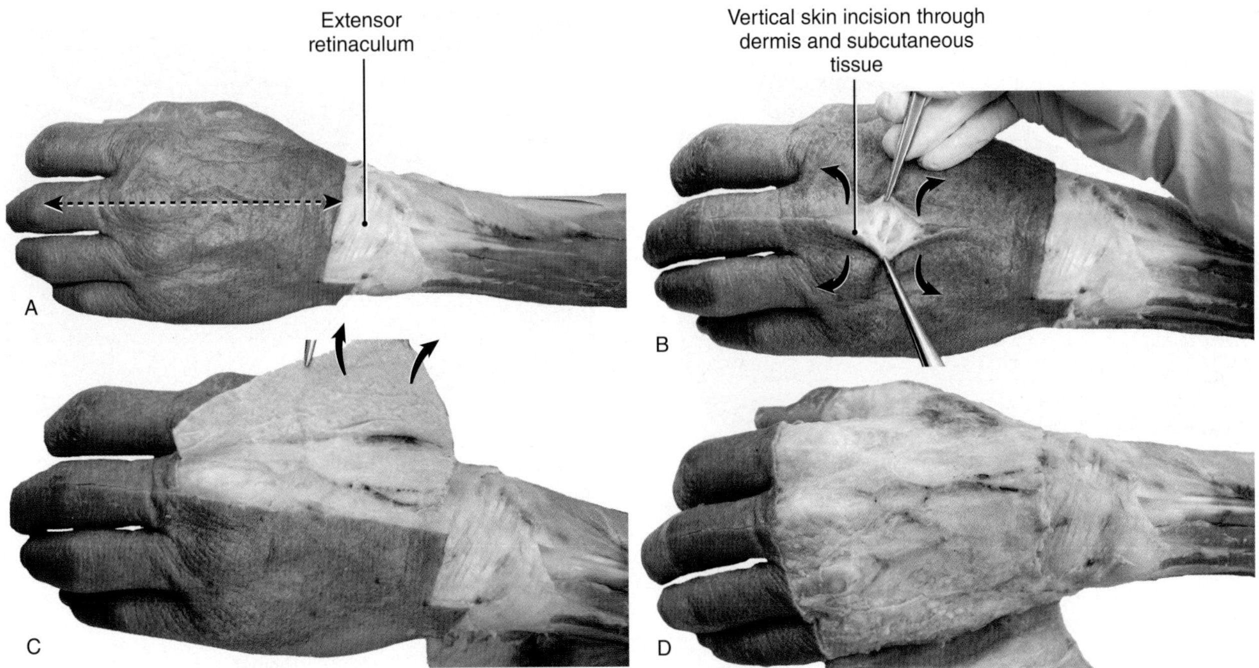

Fig. 9.3 Make a midline incision on the dorsal surface of the hand as indicated in Chapter 8 (Figs. 8.12–8.16).

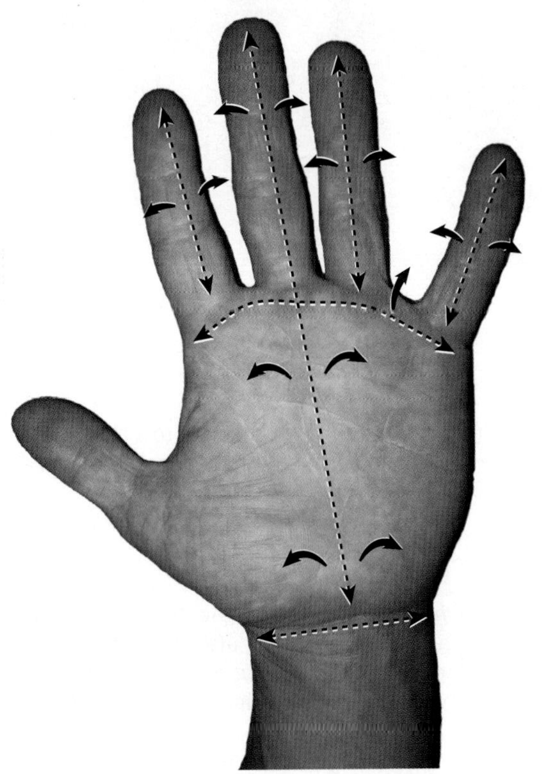

Fig. 9.4 Anterior view of the hand, with *dashed lines* showing skin incision sites.

the 3rd digit (Fig. 9.4). Make a second midline incision on the palmar surface of each digit. Join these with transverse incisions at the bases of the digits.

- **With additional incisions as necessary, reflect and remove the skin from the hand (Fig. 9.5).**

DISSECTION TIP

The skin on the dorsum of the hand is very thin, whereas the skin on the palmar surface is thick and tightly bound to the underlying palmar aponeurosis. Make a shallow incision on the dorsum of the hand, and with the aid of dissecting scissors, separate the skin from the underlying tissues. Make a deeper incision on the palmar surface of the hand, using the palmaris longus muscle as a guide to remove the skin with sharp dissection.

- **After removal of the skin on the palmar surface of the hand, trace the continuation of the palmaris longus muscle to the palmar aponeurosis (see Fig. 9.5).**
- **Note the thenar eminence with the flexor pollicis brevis and abductor pollicis muscles (Fig. 9.6).**
- **Lift the palmar aponeurosis (Fig. 9.7) and with the aid of dissecting scissors separate it from the underlying structures (Fig. 9.8).**

ANATOMY NOTE

The *palmar aponeurosis* is composed of longitudinal and transversely oriented fibers of dense connective tissue. The longitudinal fibers form digital bands that attach to the bases of the proximal phalanges and become continuous with the fibrous digital sheaths (ligamentous tubes enclosing the synovial sheaths).

- **With scissors, cut the attachments of the longitudinal bands from the bases of the proximal phalanges. Reflect the palmaris longus muscle and the palmar aponeurosis toward the forearm (Fig. 9.9).**

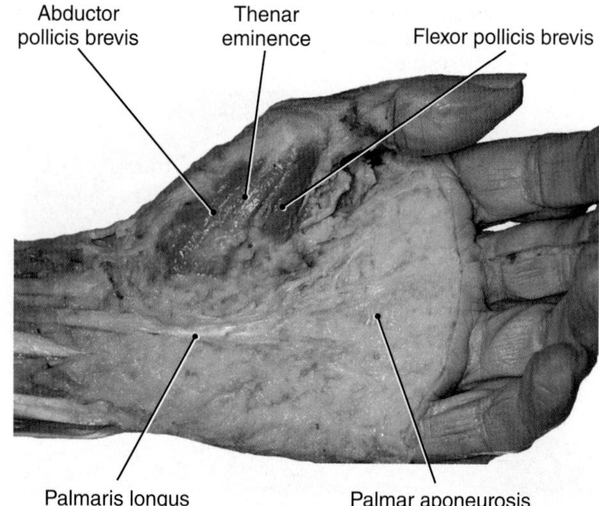

Fig. 9.5 Palmar hand with skin reflected, noting superficial structures, including muscles of the thenar eminence and the palmar aponeurosis. Note the palmaris longus muscle inserting into the palmar aponeurosis.

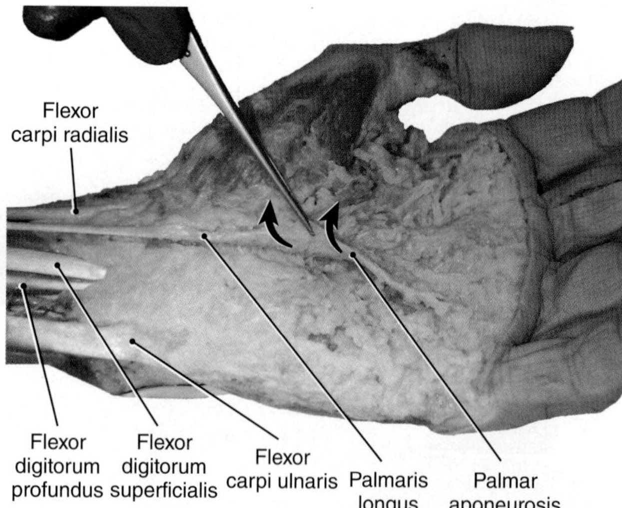

Fig. 9.7 Palmar hand with skin reflected and traction on the palmar aponeurosis. The aponeurosis is reflected to reveal deeper structures.

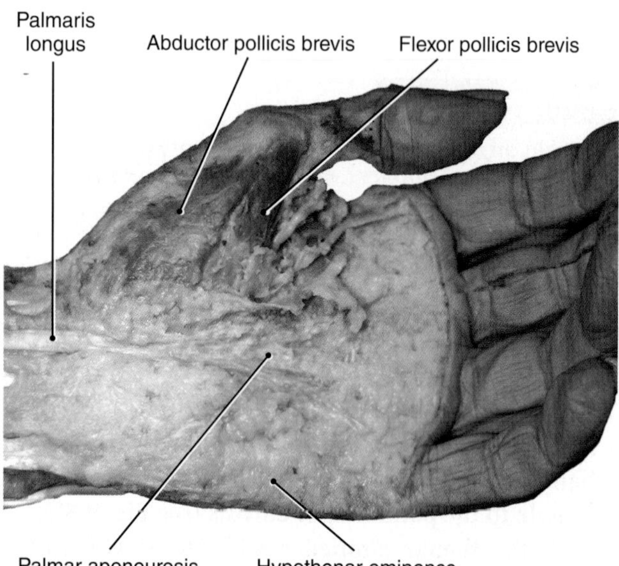

Fig. 9.6 Palmar hand with skin reflected, illustrating subcutaneous fat covering muscles that make up the hypothenar eminence.

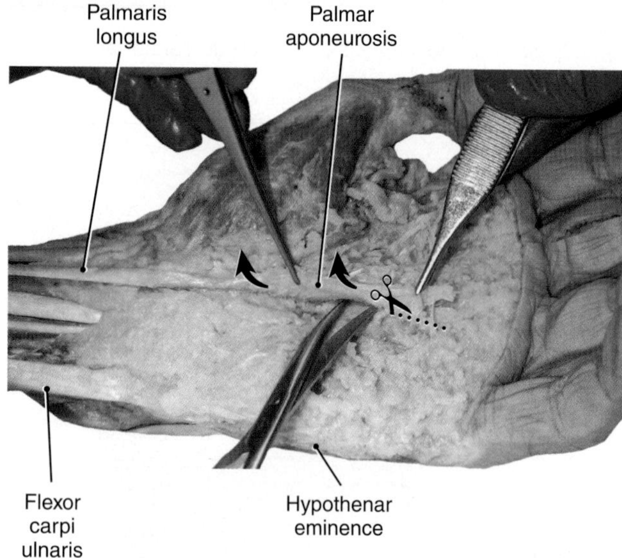

Fig. 9.8 Palmar hand with skin reflected, revealing the palmar aponeurosis. Constant tension on the aponeurosis will allow scissors to be inserted deep to it.

DISSECTION **TIP**

The removal of the palmar aponeurosis takes time. Pay special attention to using the scalpel as little as possible so as not to injure the palmar digital nerves and the superficial palmar arch. These structures travel deep to the palmar aponeurosis.

- **After removal of the palmar aponeurosis, start exposing the superficial palmar arch (Figs. 9.10 and 9.11, Plate 9.1).**

ANATOMY **NOTE**

The *superficial palmar arch* is the termination of the superficial branch of the ulnar artery, which gives rise to three common palmar digital arteries. These arteries anastomose with the palmar metacarpal branches from the deep palmar arterial arch. The common palmar digital arteries then divide into a pair of proper digital arteries, supplying the adjacent sides of the 2nd to 4th digits.

DISSECTION **TIP**

The superficial palmar arch is related to the superficial venous arch, as well as with common palmar digital branches of the median nerve. With scissors, separate the nerves from the superficial palmar arch (see Figs. 9.10–9.12). Also, remove the veins from this area.

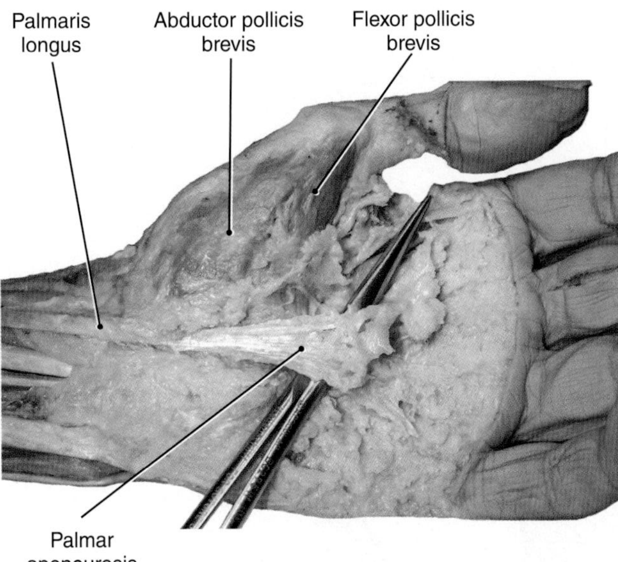

Fig. 9.9 Palmar hand with skin reflected, revealing the palmar aponeurosis. Once the aponeurosis is cut distally, it can be reflected to demonstrate deeper structures.

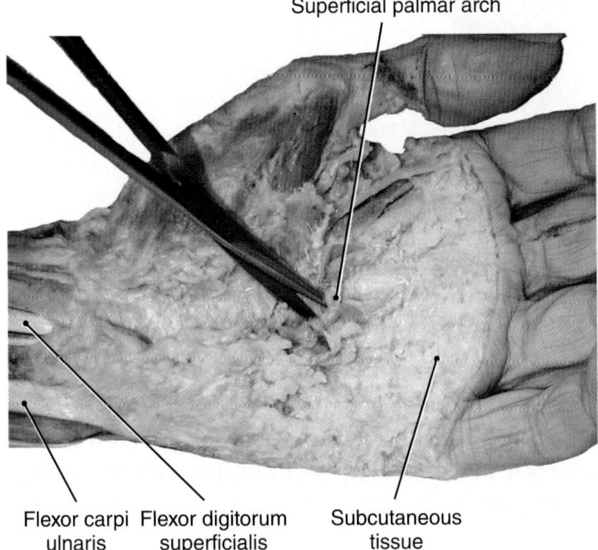

Fig. 9.10 Palmar hand with skin and the palmar aponeurosis reflected, revealing deeper structures such as the superficial palmar arch.

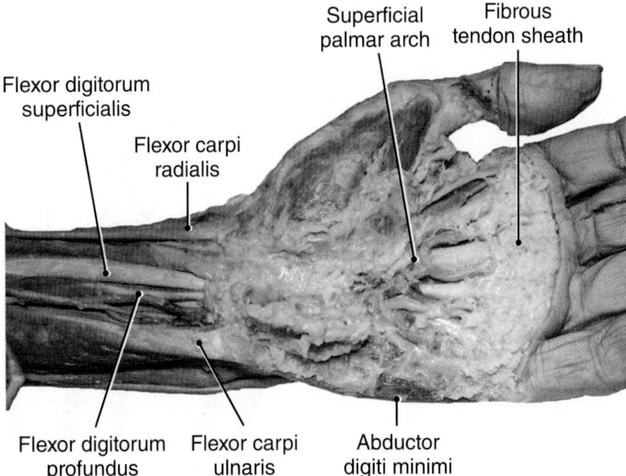

Fig. 9.11 Palmar hand with skin and the palmar aponeurosis reflected, showing tendon sheaths and neurovascular structures such as the superficial palmar arch.

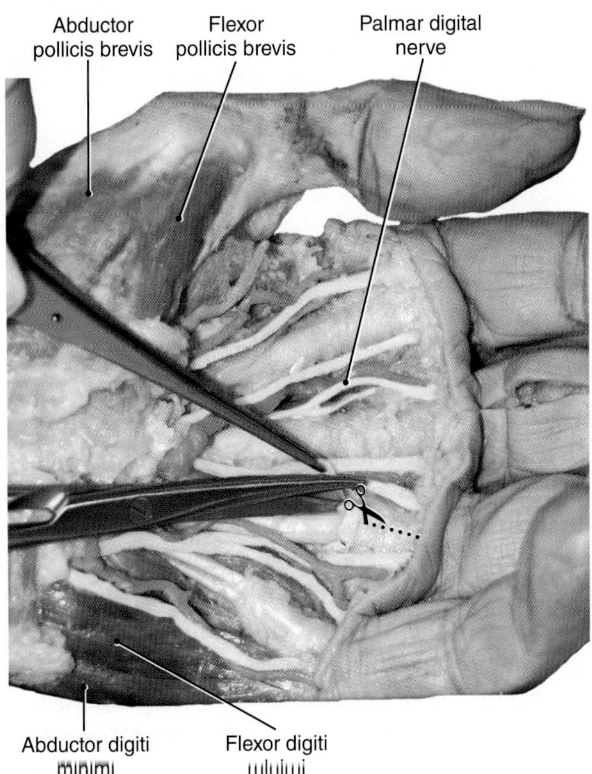

Fig. 9.12 Palmar hand with skin and the palmar aponeurosis reflected, revealing tendon sheaths and adjacent neurovascular structures.

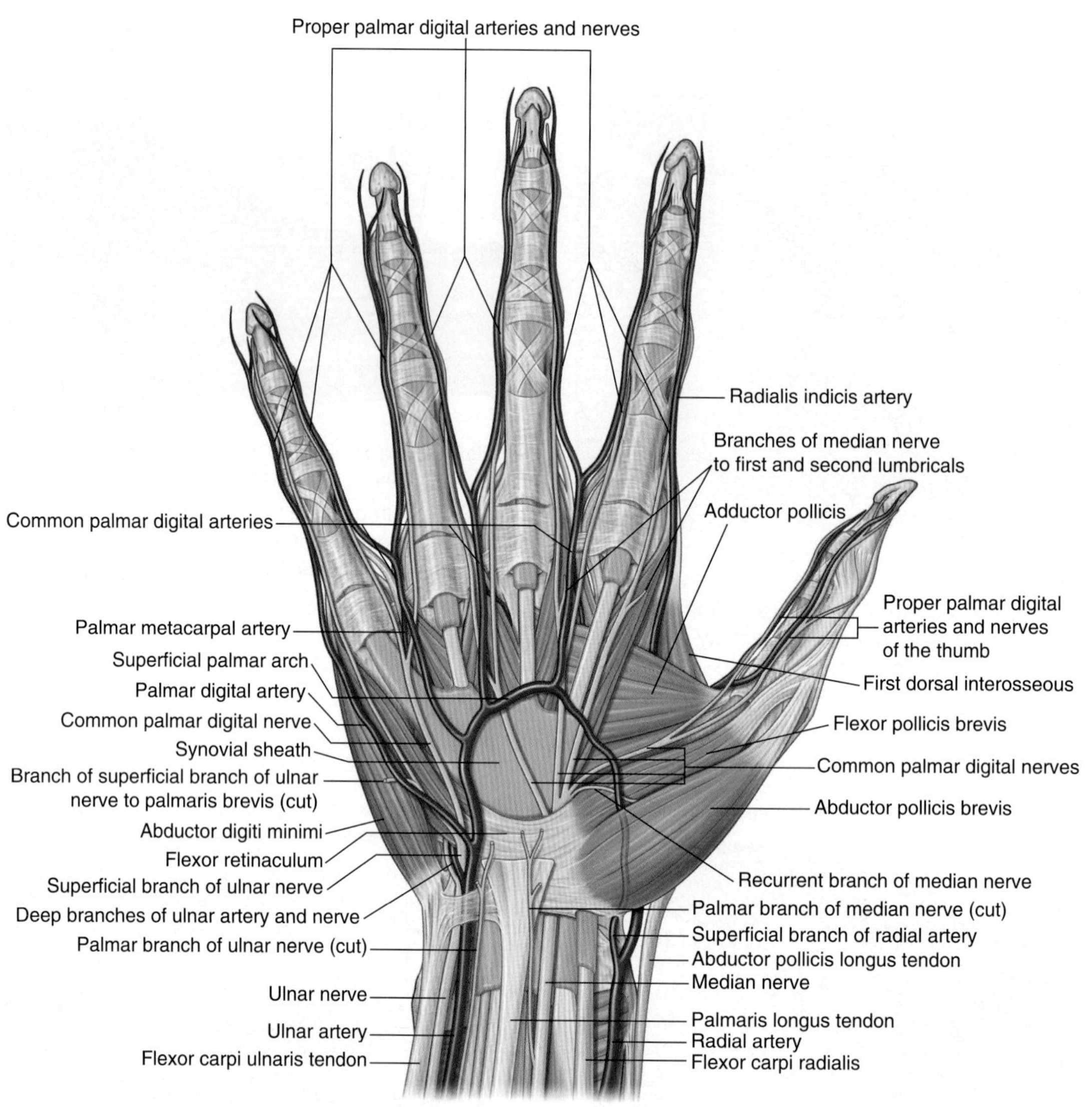

Plate 9.1 Superficial muscles, arteries, and nerves of the palmar hand. (From Drake RL et al. *Gray's Atlas of Anatomy*, 3rd edition, Philadelphia, Elsevier, 2021, p. 450.)

- **Immediately after its passage through the carpal tunnel, the median nerve gives rise to several smaller branches: the recurrent branch of the median nerve and the common palmar digital branches. At this point in the dissection, identify the common palmar digital branches of the median nerve running alongside the common palmar digital arteries (Fig. 9.13, Plate 9.2).**
- **Continue the dissection toward the phalanges and expose the separation of the common palmar digital branches of the median nerve into proper palmar digital nerves of the digits.**
- **Similarly, expose the site at which the common palmar digital arteries give rise to the palmar digital arteries (Fig. 9.14).**
- **Clean away the fascia investing the abductor and flexor digiti minimi muscles over the hypothenar region.**
- **Continue the removal of fat and remnants of the palmar aponeurosis at the medial aspect of the palm, the *hypothenar eminence* (see Fig. 9.8). Identify the flexor digiti minimi and the abductor digiti minimi muscles (see Fig. 9.12). Expose the palmar digital branches to the 5th digit and medial half of the 4th digit (see Fig. 9.14).**

DISSECTION **TIP**

The most superficially placed muscle in the hypothenar eminence is the *palmaris brevis.* This muscle is extremely thin and often blended with adipose tissue, arising from the palmar aponeurosis to insert into the skin. It is rather difficult to expose the palmaris brevis because it is detached during removal of the palmar aponeurosis and skin.

DISSECTION **TIP**

In about 65% of hands, a communication between the ulnar and median nerves exists distal to the flexor retinaculum.

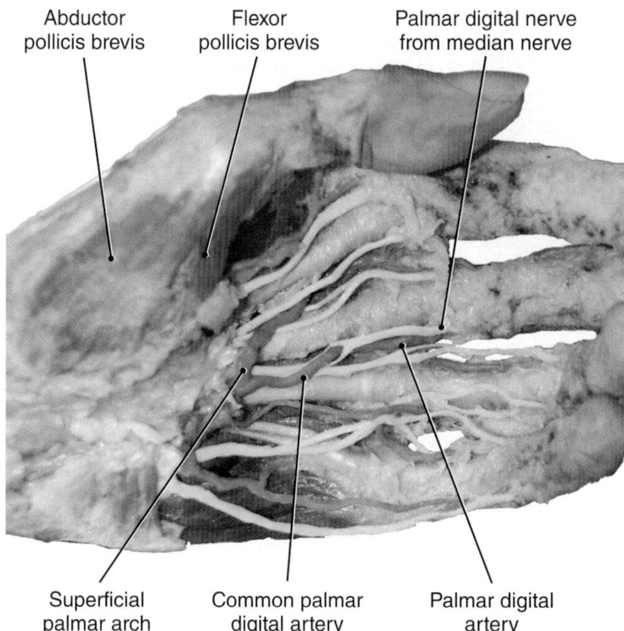

Fig. 9.13 Palmar hand with skin and the palmar aponeurosis reflected, highlighting tendon sheaths and neurovascular structures such as palmar digital nerves and arteries.

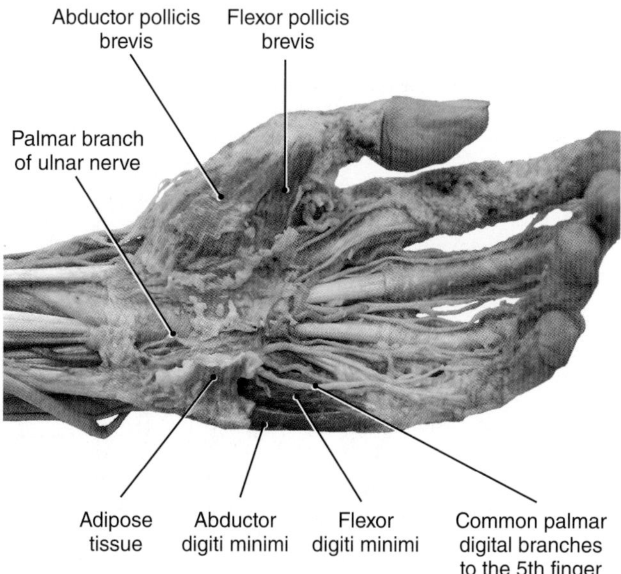

Fig. 9.15 Palmar hand with the skin and aponeurosis reflected, revealing the thenar and hypothenar muscles.

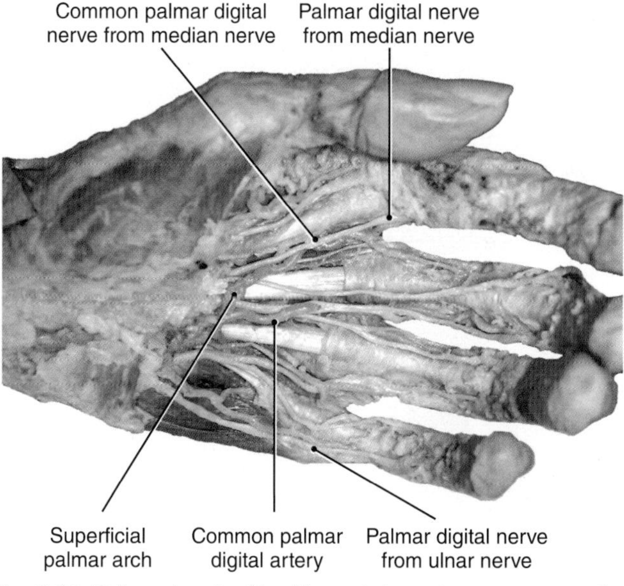

Fig. 9.14 Palmar hand with skin and the palmar aponeurosis reflected, revealing tendon sheaths and neurovascular structures. Note common palmar arteries arising from superficial palmar arch.

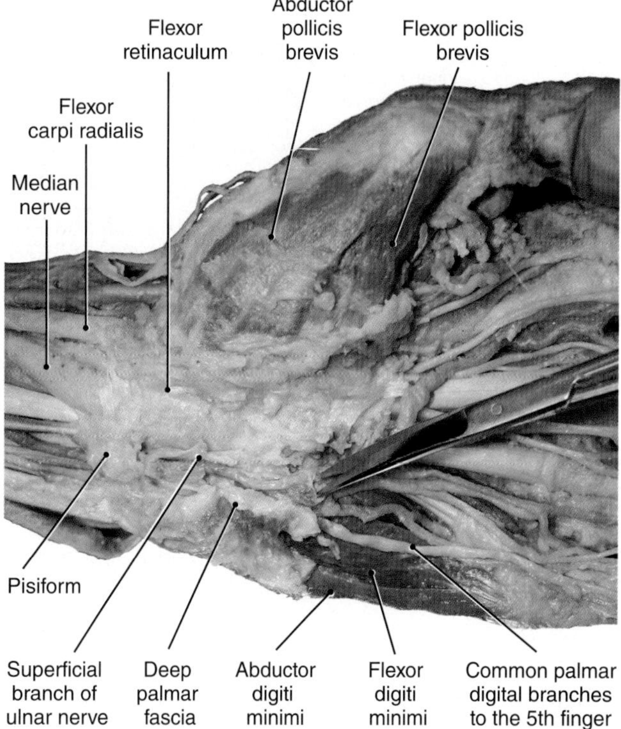

Fig. 9.16 Palmar hand with skin and the palmar aponeurosis reflected, revealing thenar and hypothenar muscles. Note median nerve traveling deep to flexor retinaculum within the carpal tunnel.

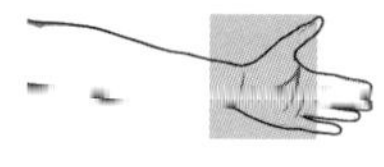

- **Trace the palmar digital branches to the 5th digit and medial half of the 4th digit toward their origin from the superficial branch of the ulnar nerve (Fig. 9.15).**
- **Remove the deep fascia at the ulnar side of the wrist, and using scissors (Fig. 9.16) expose the superficial branch of the ulnar nerve (Fig. 9.17). The ulnar artery and nerve travel lateral to the pisiform bone to enter the deep palm.**

ANATOMY **NOTE**

Guyon's canal (or tunnel) is formed by the pisiform bone, and an extension of the deep fascia of the forearm (palmar carpal ligament).

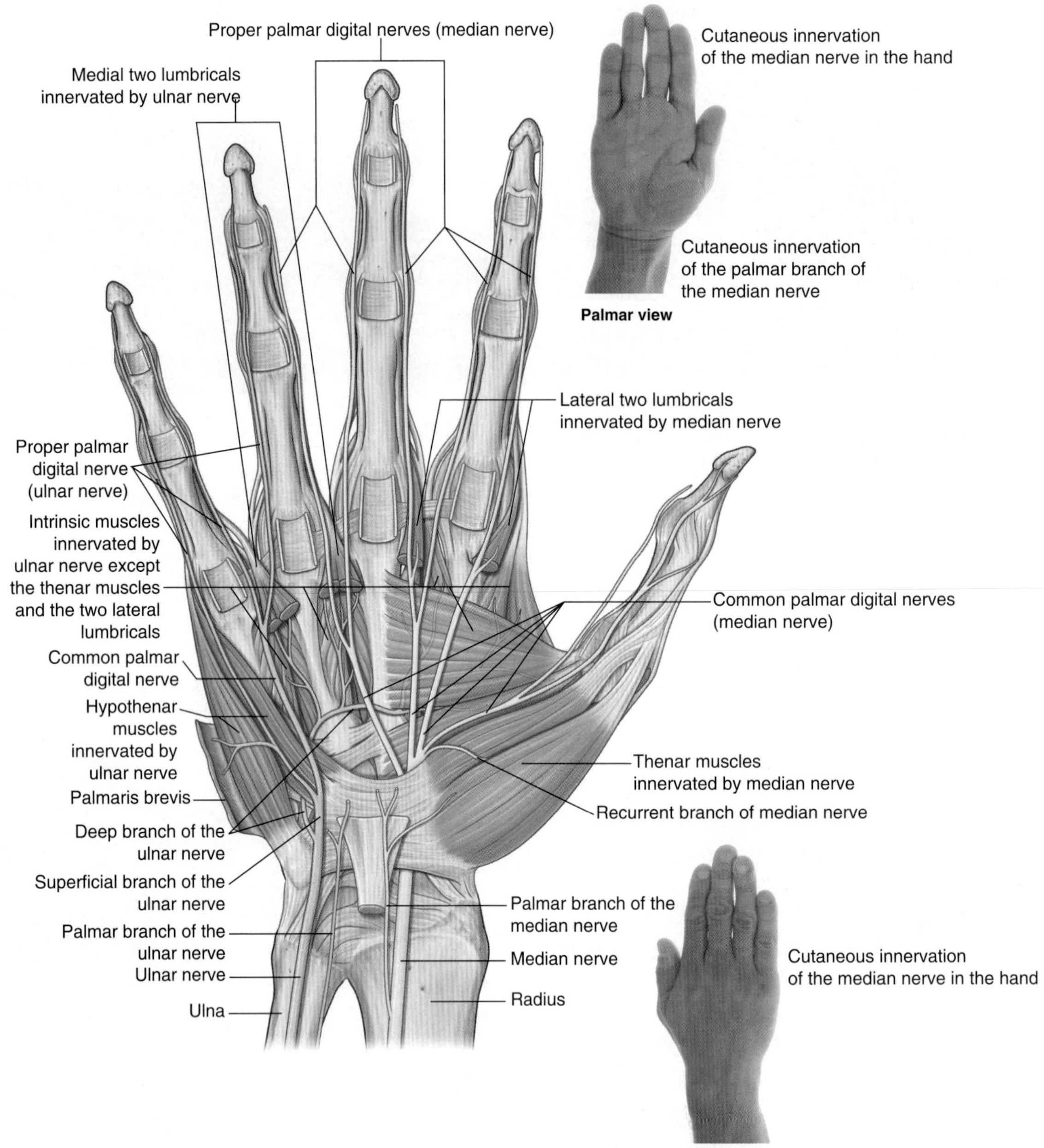

Plate 9.2 Innervation of the hand by the median and ulnar nerves. (From Drake RL et al. *Gray's Atlas of Anatomy*, 3rd edition, Philadelphia, Elsevier, 2021, p. 453.)

- **Expose the superficial ulnar artery and nerve toward the pisiform bone (Fig. 9.18).**
- **Clean the adipose tissue and remnants of the palmar aponeurosis surrounding the superficial palmar arch distally to the carpal tunnel and flexor retinaculum (see Fig. 9.18).**

ANATOMY **NOTE**

The primary contributor to the superficial palmar arch is the ulnar artery.

- **Expose the ulnar artery and clean the surface of the flexor retinaculum (Fig. 9.19).**

DISSECTION **TIP**

The tendons of the flexor digitorum superficialis and flexor digitorum profundus muscles are enclosed by a synovial sheath, the *ulnar bursa*. The tendon of the flexor pollicis longus is also enclosed by a synovial sheath, the *radial bursa*.

- **To free up the superficial palmar arch and nerve structures from the underlying long flexor tendons, use scissors to incise the fibrous tendinous sheaths longitudinally. Identify the tendons of the flexor digitorum superficialis and profundus muscles (Fig. 9.20).**

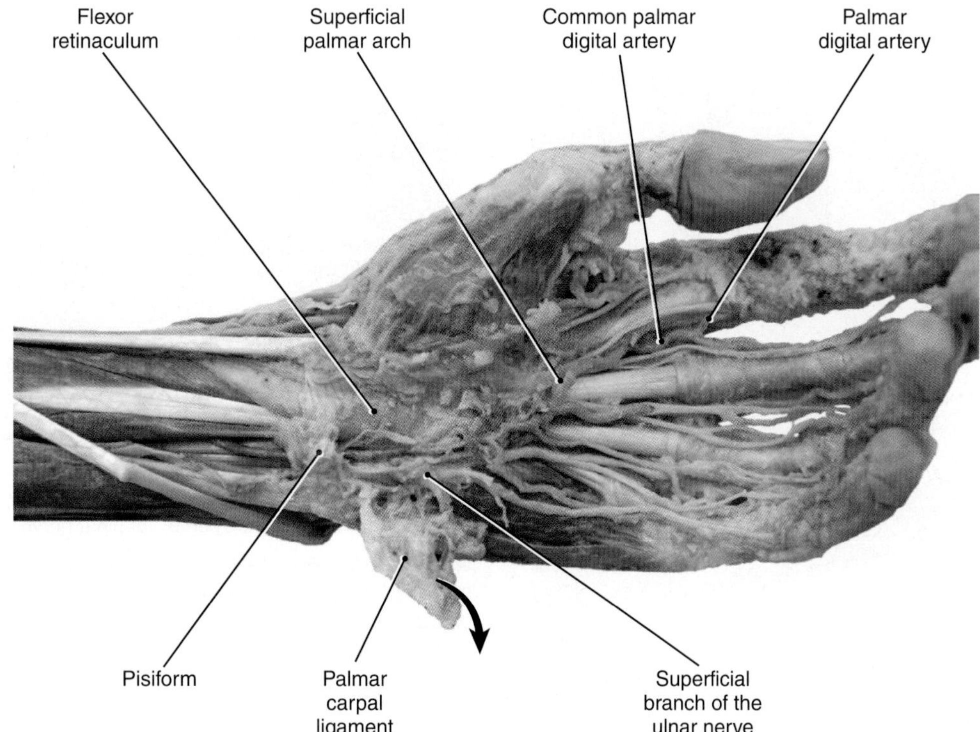

Fig. 9.17 Palmar hand with skin and the palmar aponeurosis reflected, revealing thenar and hypothenar muscles. Note the palmar carpal ligament that has been reflected to better illustrate the deeper flexor retinaculum.

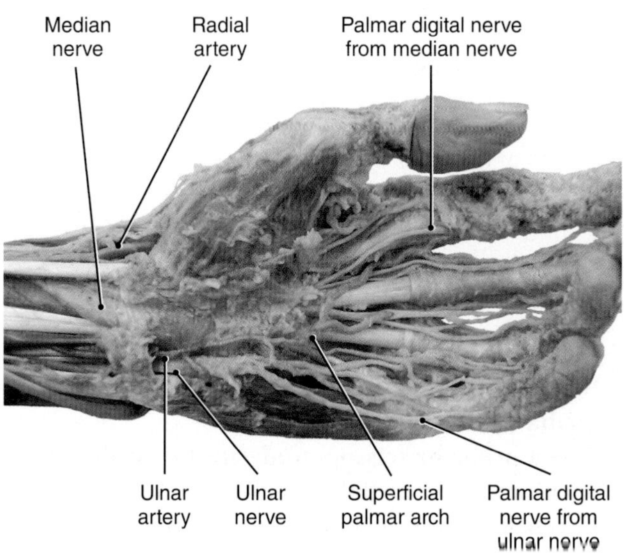

Fig. 9.18 Palmar hand with skin and the palmar aponeurosis removed, revealing superficial palmar arch.

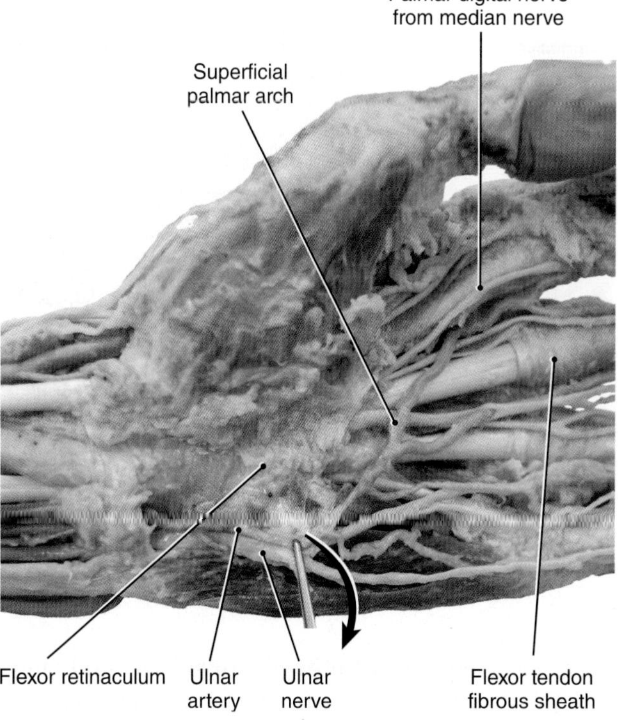

Fig. 9.19 Palmar hand with skin and the palmar aponeurosis removed, revealing superficial palmar arterial arch and branches to the digits.

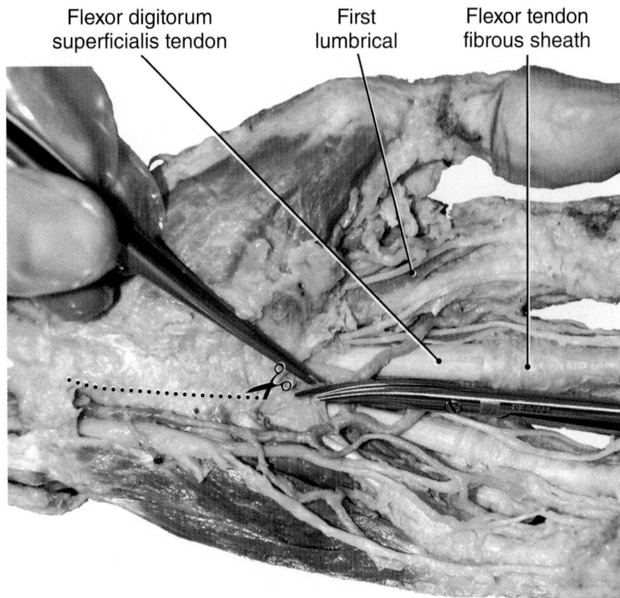

Fig. 9.20 Palmar hand with skin and the palmar aponeurosis removed. Use scissors to open the fibrous tendon sheaths to identify tendons of flexor digitorum superficialis and profundus muscles.

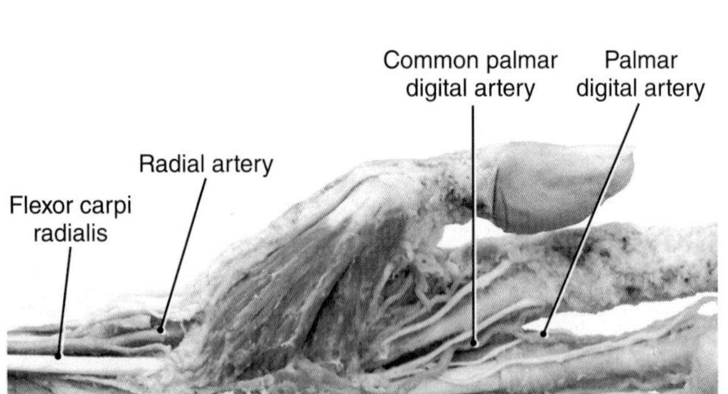

Fig. 9.21 Palmar hand with skin and the aponeurosis removed, revealing digital arteries and nerves and superficial branches of ulnar nerve and artery (superficial palmar arch).

- **Immediately distal to the pisiform bone and lateral to the flexor retinaculum, expose the division of the ulnar artery and nerve into deep and superficial branches (Fig. 9.21).**
- **The deep branches dive deeply between the abductor and flexor digiti minimi muscles of the 5th digit.**

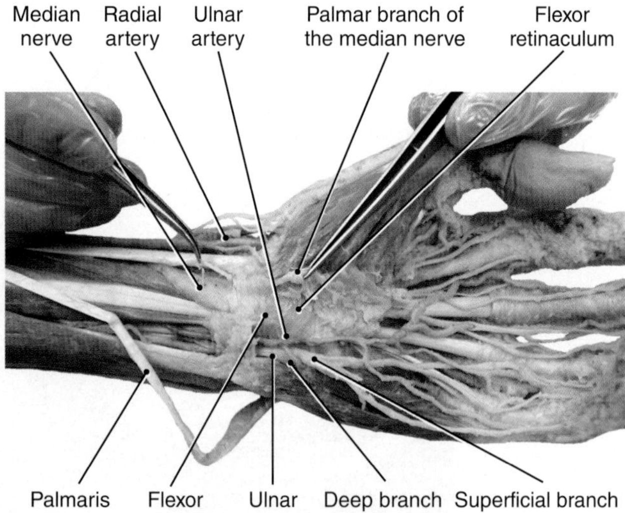

Fig. 9.22 Palmar hand with skin and the aponeurosis removed, revealing palmar branch of median nerve, which passes superficial to the flexor retinaculum to supply the skin over the thenar eminence.

DISSECTION **TIP**

The palmar branch of the median nerve is often cut during routine dissection. The median nerve is seen at the distal forearm between the tendons of the palmaris longus and flexor carpi radialis and supplies the skin over the central portion of the palm.

ANATOMY **NOTE**

The *flexor retinaculum* is a dense connective tissue band that helps create a tunnel *(carpal tunnel)* for the tendons of the flexor digitorum superficialis, flexor digitorum profundus, flexor pollicis longus, and the median nerve to reach the palm.

- **Carefully expose the flexor retinaculum and identify its borders. Look for the palmar branch of the median nerve (Fig. 9.22).**
- **Pass a probe or scissors underneath the flexor retinaculum in the carpal tunnel (Fig. 9.23).**
- **Leave the probe within the carpal tunnel and with scissors divide the flexor retinaculum on top of the probe (Fig. 9.24). This retinaculum is transected by inserting the scissors into the carpal tunnel upwardly, cutting in a proximal-to-distal manner.**
- **Remove the probe and retract the flexor retinaculum to expose the median nerve and tendons of the flexor digitorum superficialis (Figs. 9.25 and 9.26).**
- **Remove the connective tissue sheath over the median nerve and the underlying flexor digitorum superficialis muscle (Fig. 9.27).**

- **Continue exposing the median nerve within the carpal tunnel. Identify the recurrent branch of the median nerve (Fig. 9.28). Finish the exposure of the common palmar digital branches of the median nerve.**

DISSECTION TIP

The recurrent branch of the median nerve usually travels deep to the thenar muscles, and tracing its course anteriorly may be difficult. In such cases, gently retract the median nerve (within exposed carpal tunnel) laterally and identify the recurrent branch of the median nerve. You also may dissect between the flexor pollicis brevis and the underlying adductor pollicis muscle to trace the recurrent branch of the median nerve.

DISSECTION TIP

In some cases, branches of the superficial palmar arch travel close to the common palmar digital branches or penetrate them. Use special care when you dissect these structures (Fig. 9.29).

- **With forceps, retract the abductor digiti minimi muscle laterally and expose the flexor digiti minimi brevis and the opponens digiti minimi muscles (Fig. 9.30).**
- **You may cut and reflect the abductor digiti minimi near its origin to expose the underlying opponens digiti minimi muscle.**

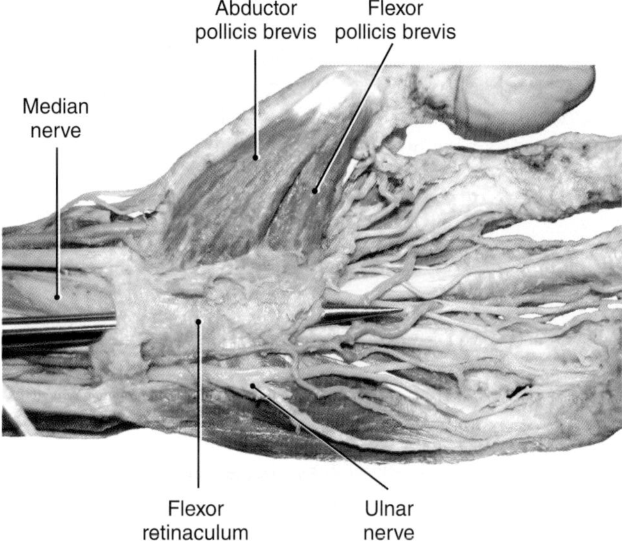

Fig. 9.23 Palmar hand with removed skin and the palmar aponeurosis showing the flexor retinaculum. Note that the ulnar nerve and artery travel superficial to the flexor retinaculum but deep to the palmar carpal ligament.

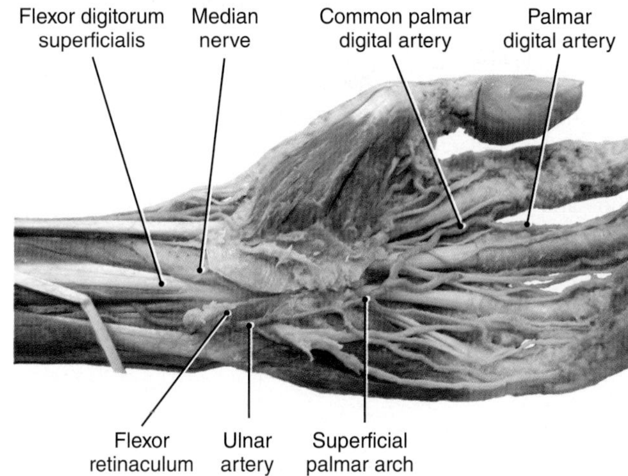

Fig. 9.25 Palmar hand with transection of the flexor retinaculum. Deeper dissection will reveal the nine tendons and one nerve that course through the carpal tunnel.

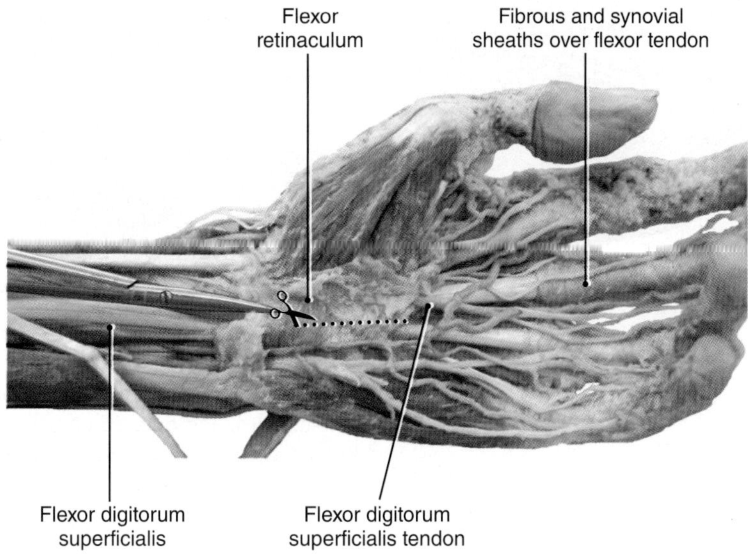

Fig. 9.24 Palmar hand with removed skin and palmar aponeurosis revealing the flexor retinaculum.

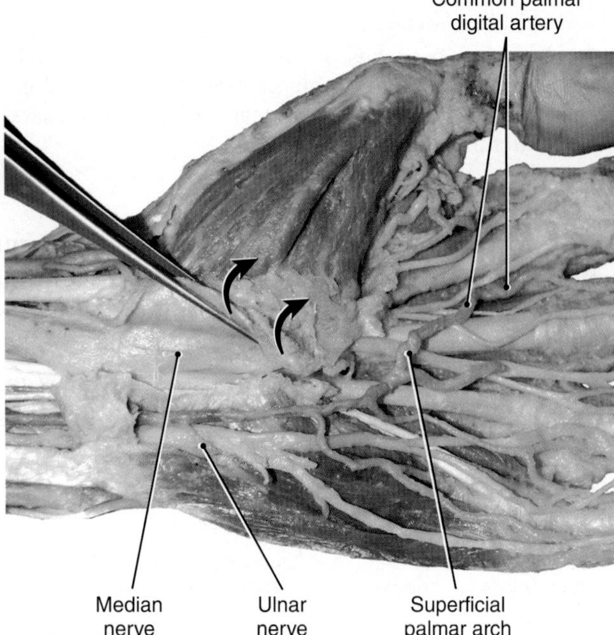

Fig. 9.26 Palmar hand with the flexor retinaculum reflected. The median nerve can be traced from the distal forearm to the hand through the exposed carpal tunnel. Distal to the flexor retinaculum, note the branching pattern of the median nerve.

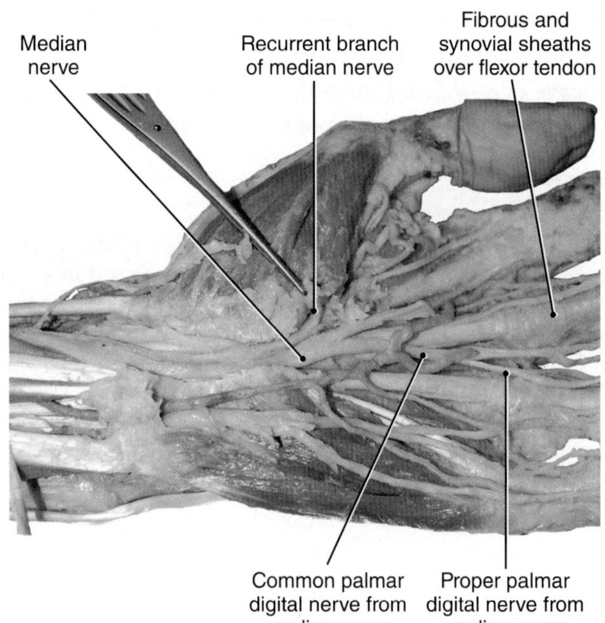

Fig. 9.28 Palmar hand with cut flexor retinaculum revealing the carpal tunnel. The median nerve can be traced through the tunnel and its recurrent branch is identified near the distal end of the flexor retinaculum.

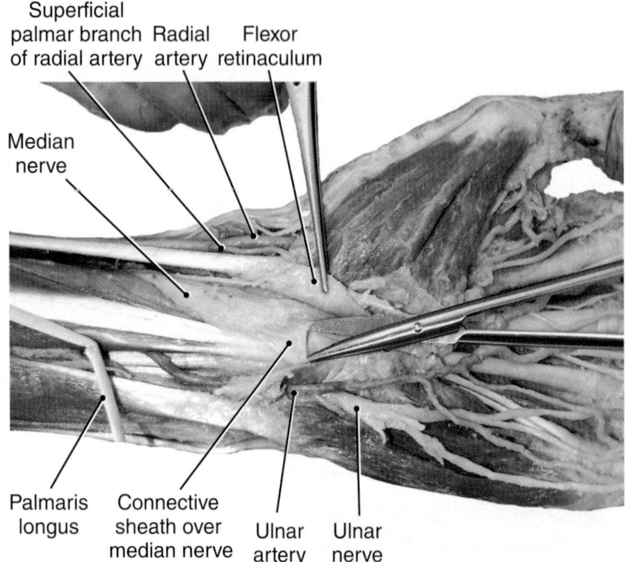

Fig. 9.27 Palmar hand after transection of the flexor retinaculum, revealing the carpal tunnel.

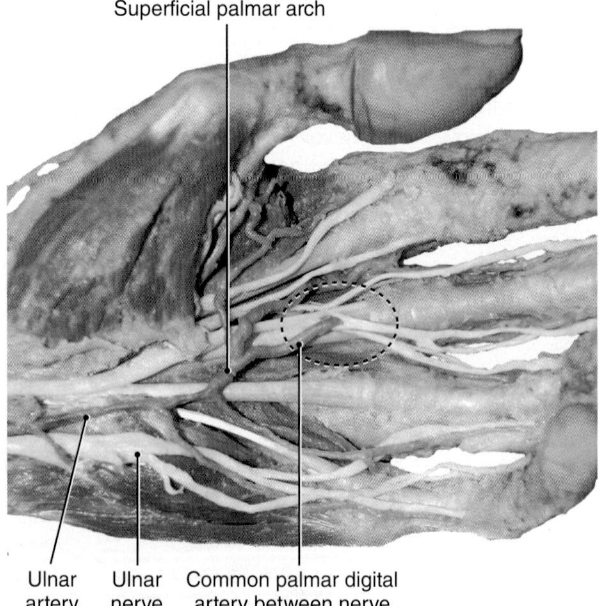

Fig. 9.29 Palmar hand with removed aponeurosis, cut flexor retinaculum, and opened carpal tunnel. Note the relationship between common palmar digital arteries and nerves *(circled)*.

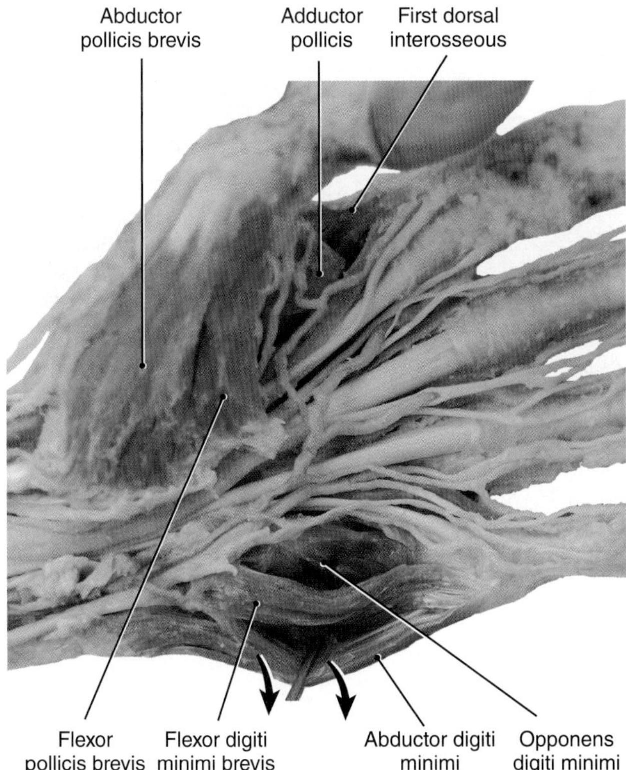

Fig. 9.30 Palmar hand with removed skin and aponeurosis and cut flexor retinaculum revealing the carpal tunnel. With separation, muscular components of the hypothenar eminence are seen.

DISSECTION TIP

In the majority of the specimens, the flexor digiti minimi muscle is difficult to separate from the abductor digiti minimi muscle. Follow the deep branch of the ulnar nerve to the hypothenar muscles. This nerve runs between the flexor digiti minimi and abductor digiti minimi muscles, facilitating their identification. The deepest of the hypothenar muscles is the opponens digiti minimi muscle.

- **Trace the superficial palmar arch laterally in the space between the 1st and 2nd digits.**

DISSECTION TIP

There is usually an anastomosis between the superficial palmar arch and a branch of the radial artery, the *radialis indicis*, and a branch to the 1st digit, the *princeps pollicis* (Fig. 9.31).

- **Identify the *abductor pollicis brevis muscle,* lying at the lateral side of the base of the proximal phalanx of the 1st digit (see Fig. 9.31).**
- **Medial and next to the abductor pollicis brevis muscle, identify the flexor pollicis brevis muscle, which is passing along the radial side of the tendon of the flexor pollicis longus muscle. Retract the abductor pollicis brevis muscle laterally from the flexor pollicis brevis muscle and identify the opponens pollicis muscle (Fig. 9.32). Flexor pollicis brevis has two heads. Its deep head can be mistaken for the opponens pollicis brevis. Reflect both heads.**

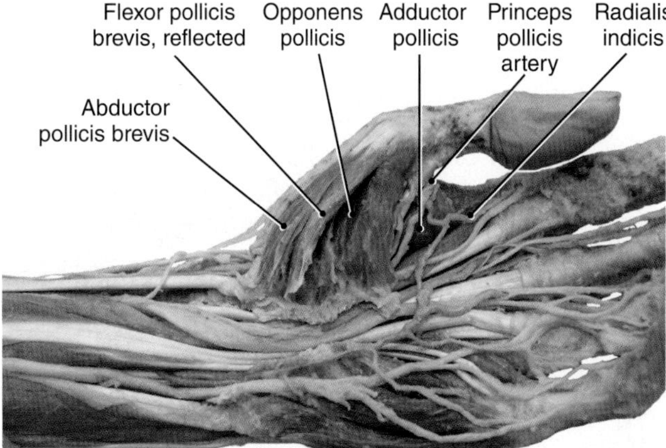

Fig. 9.31 Palmar hand with removed skin and aponeurosis and cut flexor retinaculum revealing the carpal tunnel. With separation, muscles of the thenar eminence are seen.

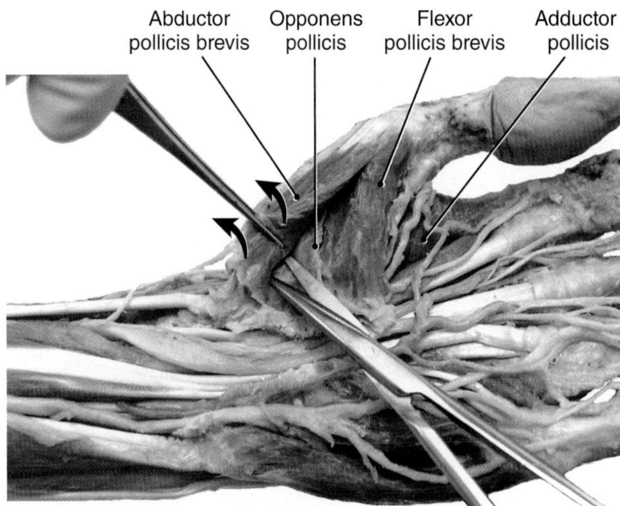

Fig. 9.32 Palmar hand with skin and aponeurosis removed and flexor reticulum cut revealing the thenar muscles. Scissors are used to transect the origin of the abductor pollicis brevis muscle.

- **Finally, identify the adductor pollicis muscle, which can be seen between the bases of the 2nd and 1st digits.**

DISSECTION TIP

You may also transect the abductor pollicis brevis and identify the opponens pollicis muscle just underneath it (Fig. 9.33). Another way to distinguish the opponens pollicis brevis muscle from the abductor pollicis brevis and the flexor pollicis muscles is its insertion point. The opponens pollicis brevis muscle inserts on the 1st metacarpal.

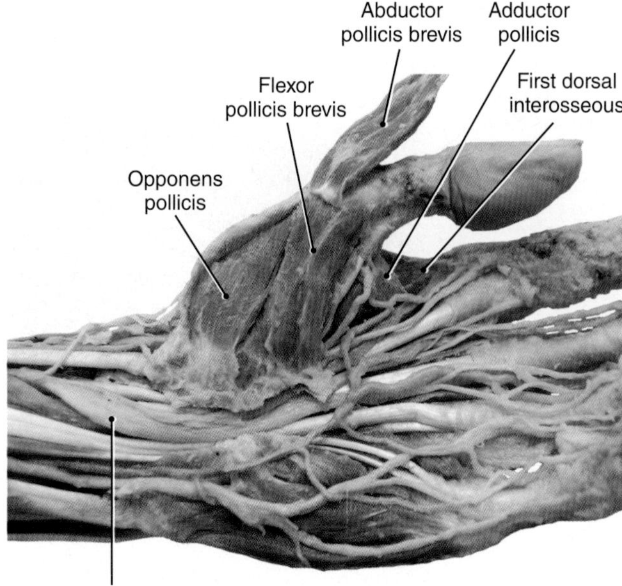

Fig. 9.33 Palmar hand with skin and aponeurosis removed and flexor reticulum cut revealing the thenar structures. With the abductor pollicis brevis reflected, the deeper-lying opponens pollicis is visualized.

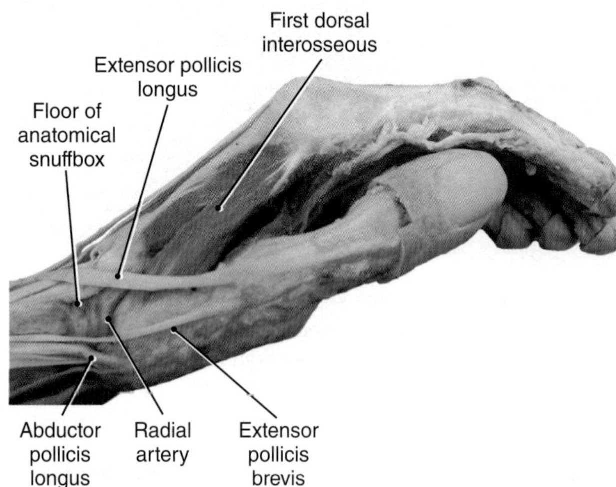

Fig. 9.34 Region of "anatomical snuffbox," with borders and contents, including radial artery. Note the 1st dorsal interosseous muscle between the 1st and 2nd digits.

- On the dorsum of the hand, clean and expose the tendinous insertions of the abductor pollicis longus, the extensor pollicis brevis, and the extensor pollicis longus (Fig. 9.34).

ANATOMY **NOTE**

The tendons of these three muscles (abductor pollicis longus, the extensor pollicis brevis, and the extensor pollicis longus) form the boundaries of the anatomical snuffbox, through which the radial artery passes to reach the dorsum of the 1st digit.

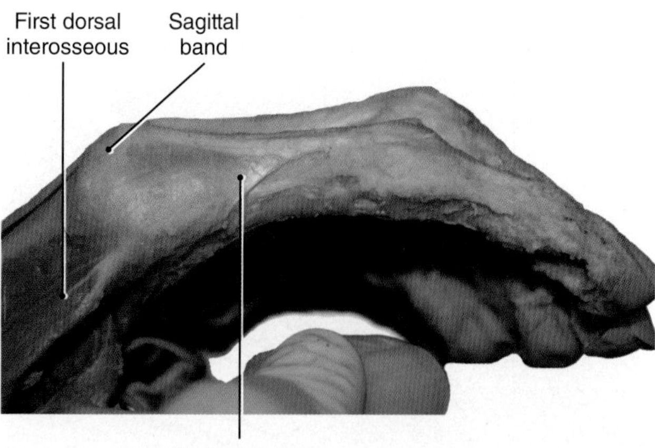

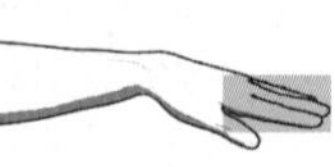

Fig. 9.35 Dorsal view of the 1st and 2nd digits with skin removed, revealing superficial structures. Note components of the extensor expansion, including the sagittal and lateral bands.

DORSAL HAND

- **Identify the radial artery and trace it as it passes between the two heads of the 1st dorsal interosseous muscle (see Fig. 9.34).**
- **Observe the radial side of the 2nd digit. At the level of the proximal interphalangeal joint, note the extensor expansion splitting into three parts (Fig. 9.35).**
- **At the palmar side of the digits, observe the fibrous synovial sheaths surrounding the tendons of the long flexor muscles (Fig. 9.36).**

DISSECTION **TIP**

These fibrous sheaths are thin at the interphalangeal joints (cruciate fibers) and thick over the phalanges (annular fibers/ligament).

RETURN TO PALMAR HAND AND ANTERIOR FOREARM

- **With a scalpel, cut at the midline the fibrous synovial sheath and expose the tendon of the flexor digitorum superficialis and flexor digitorum profundus (Figs. 9.37 and 9.38).**
- **Extend the distal interphalangeal joint. Observe the tendon of the flexor digitorum superficialis dividing before inserting at the base of the middle phalanx. In addition, the tendon of the flexor digitorum profundus passes through the divided tendon of the flexor digitorum superficialis to insert onto the distal phalanges (Figs. 9.39 and 9.40). Note the vinculum longum,**

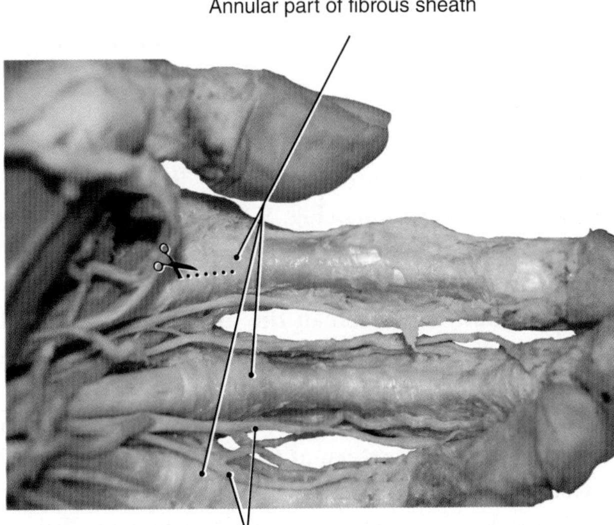

Fig. 9.36 View illustrating the fibrous digital sheaths and related structures (e.g., palmar digital nerves).

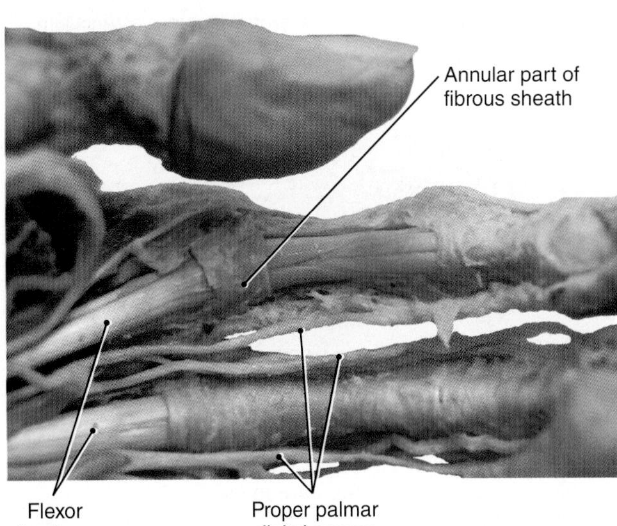

Fig. 9.38 Palmar view of the 1st to 3rd digits. Note the annular part of the fibrous digital sheath and the deeper-lying flexor tendons.

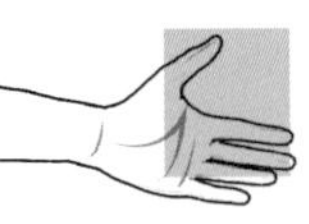

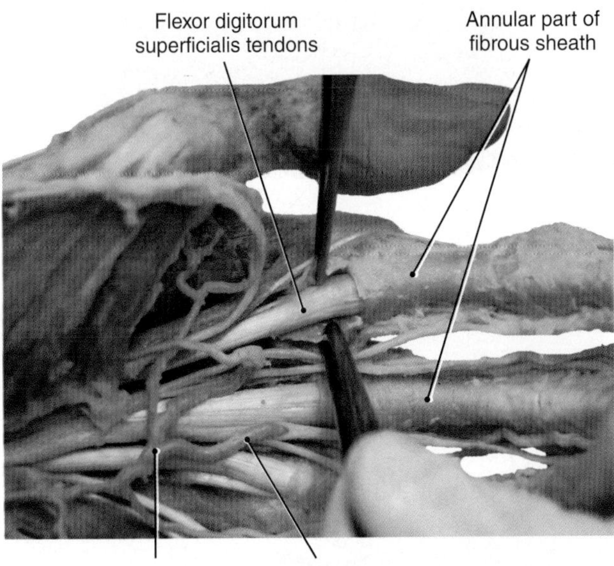

Fig. 9.37 Palmar view of the hand after partial opening of flexor digital sheaths of the 2nd and 3rd digits. Note the annular components of the fibrous sheaths and the internally located flexor tendons.

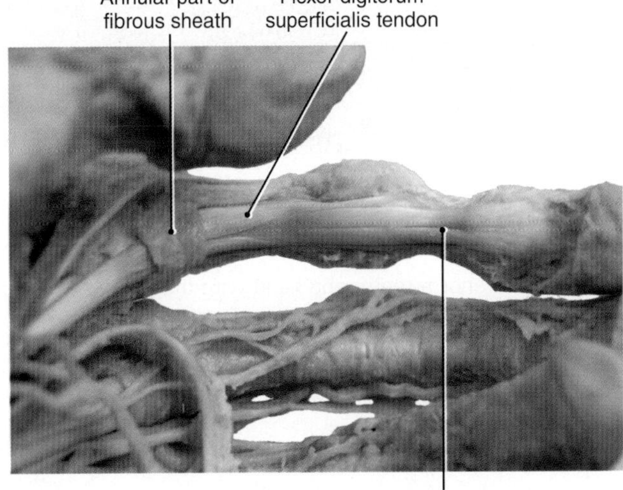

Fig. 9.39 View of the 1st to 4th digits with portions of fibrous digital sheaths removed. Note the deeper-lying flexor tendons of flexor digitorum superficialis and profundus muscles.

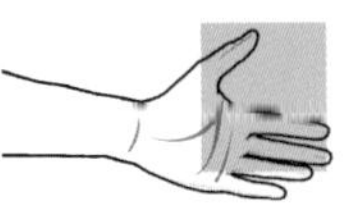

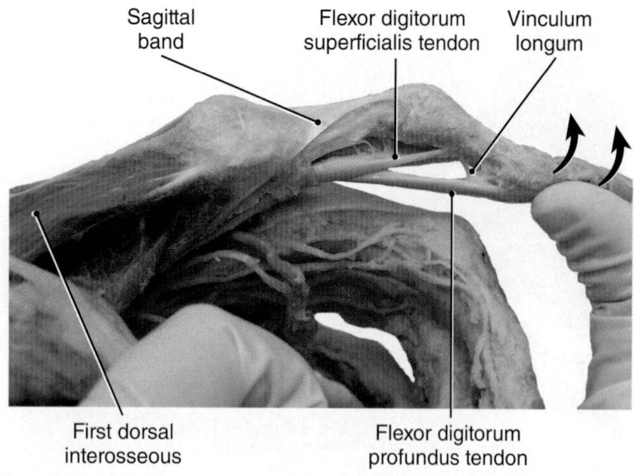

Fig. 9.40 Lateral view of the interspace between 1st and 2nd digits. Note the flexor digitorum profundus tendon passing through the split tendon of flexor digitorum superficialis muscle.

a thin ligament that adds support for the attachments of the flexor digitorum superficialis and flexor digitorum profundus.

- Once all muscles, nerves, and arteries of the hand have been identified (Fig. 9.41), pass a probe or a pair of scissors underneath the flexor digitorum superficialis tendons (Fig. 9.42) and transect them at the level of the carpal tunnel (Fig. 9.43).
- Lift the flexor digitorum superficialis and expose the median nerve. Clean the median nerve and its surrounding muscles from any loose connective tissue (Figs. 9.44 and 9.45).
- Transect the median, ulnar, and radial nerves, as well as the ulnar artery, at the same level (Fig. 9.46).
- Retract the neurovascular bundles distally to expose the tendons of the flexor digitorum superficialis. Lift the tendons of the flexor digitorum superficialis and expose all four lumbrical muscles (Fig. 9.47).

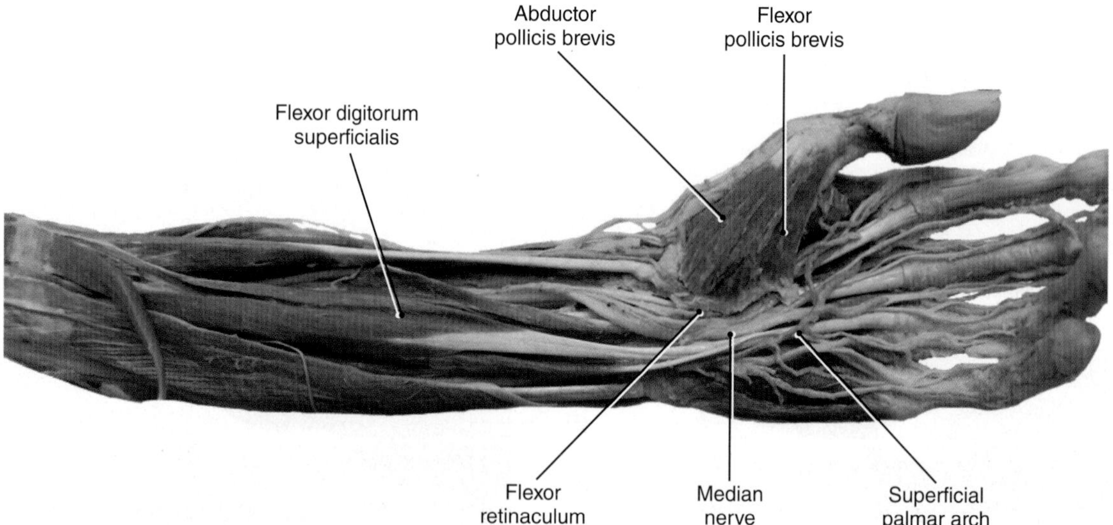

Fig. 9.41 Anterior forearm and hand with the palmar aponeurosis removed, revealing the superficial and intermediate musculature.

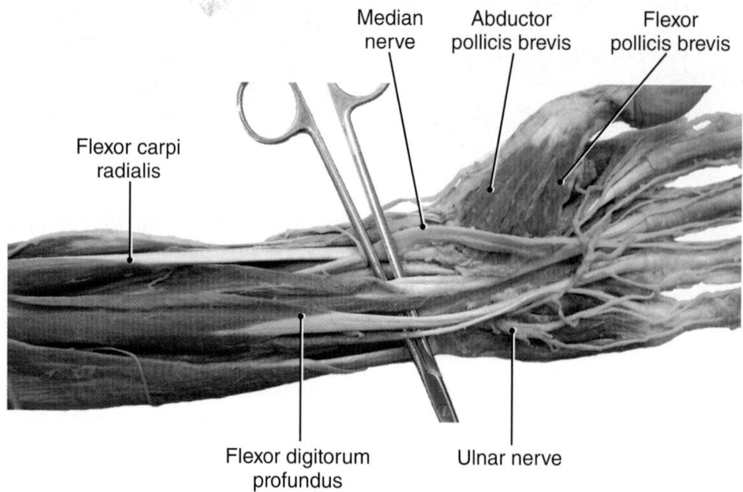

Fig. 9.42 Anterior view of the forearm and hand with the palmar aponeurosis removed, revealing the superficial and intermediate musculature. The median nerve is pulled from between the flexor digitorum superficialis and profundus muscles; these muscles are pulled forward and scissors placed deep to them.

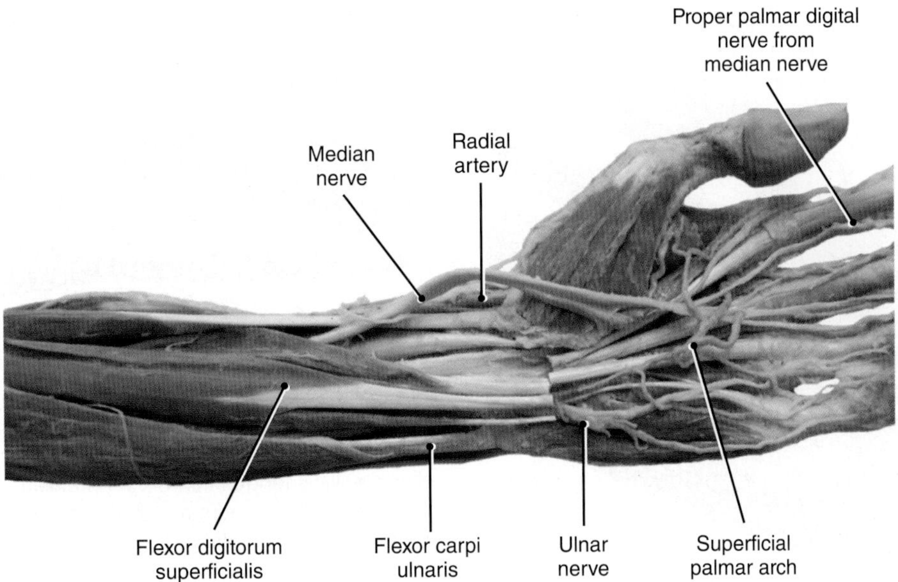

Fig. 9.43 Anterior forearm and hand with the skin and palmar aponeurosis removed; superficial and intermediate muscles are cut at the wrist. The median nerve is retracted.

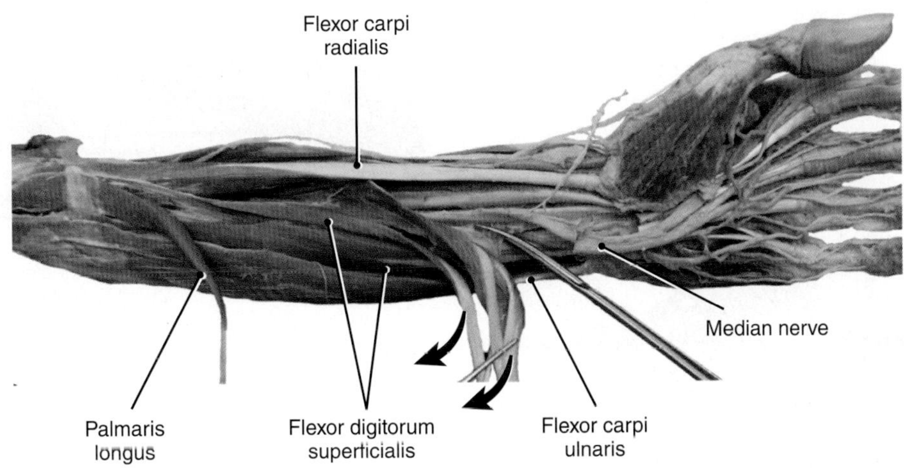

Fig. 9.44 Anterior forearm and hand with the skin and palmar aponeurosis removed and the superficial muscles reflected, revealing neurovascular structures.

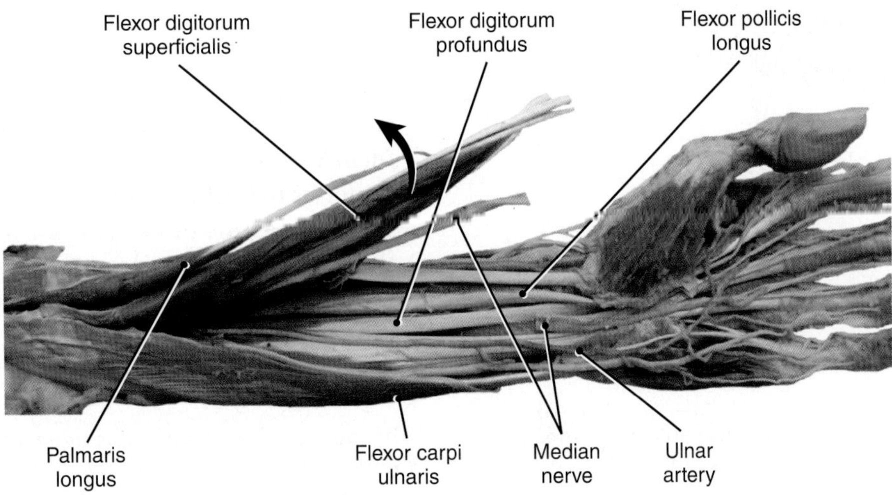

Fig. 9.45 Palmar hand with the skin and the palmar aponeurosis removed and the flexor retinaculum cut, revealing tendons and muscles. The median nerve has been transected in the distal forearm.

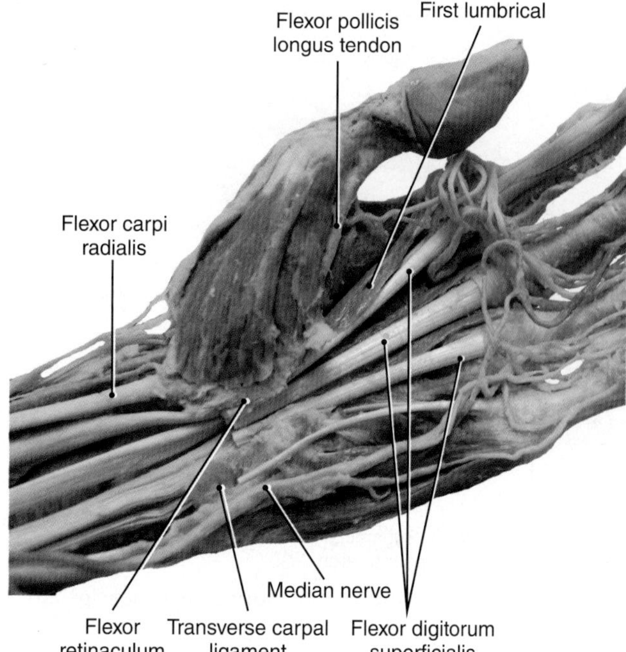

Fig. 9.46 Palmar hand with the skin and the palmar aponeurosis removed and flexor retinaculum cut, revealing tendons and muscles. The flexor pollicis longus tendon is exposed, and the superficial neurovascular structures are reflected distally.

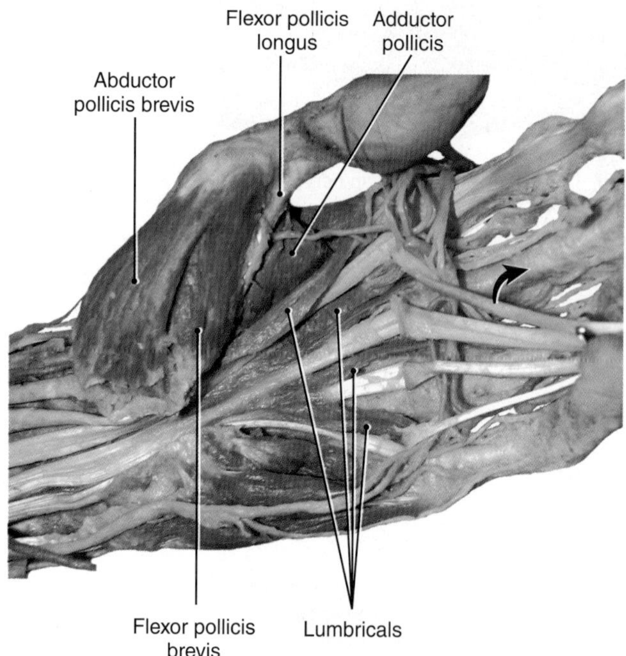

Fig. 9.47 Palmar hand with the skin and the palmar aponeurosis removed, revealing deeper muscles (e.g., adductor pollicis and lumbricals).

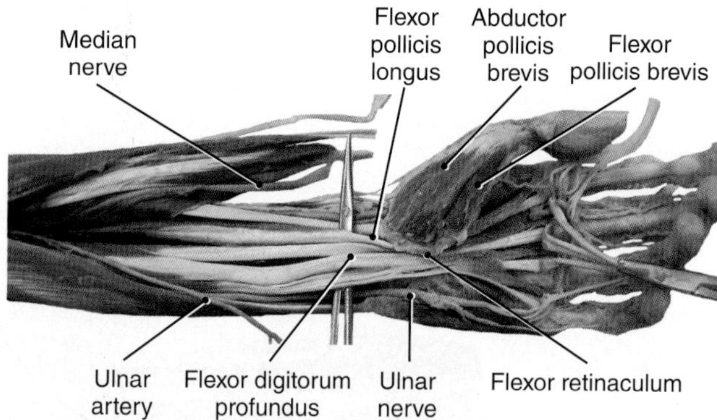

Fig. 9.48 Anterior forearm and hand with the skin and the palmar aponeurosis removed; superficial and intermediate muscles reflected, revealing deep muscles. The tendon of the flexor pollicis longus can be seen entering and exiting the carpal tunnel. Scissors are placed deep to nine tendons that travel through the carpal tunnel.

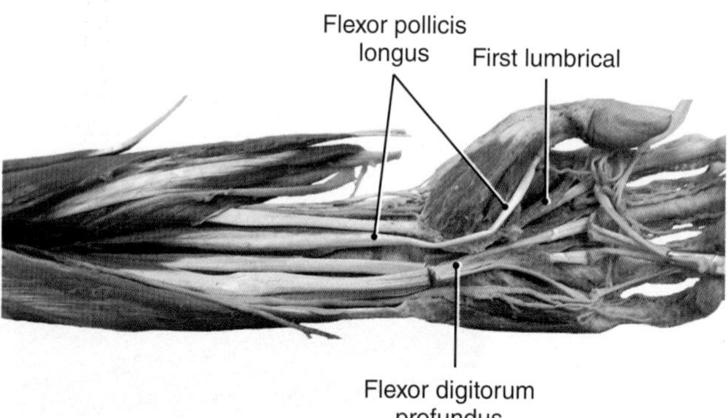

Fig. 9.49 Palmar view of the hand and wrist with the skin and the palmar aponeurosis removed and flexor retinaculum cut, revealing tendons within the carpal tunnel.

- **Clamp the tendons of the flexor digitorum superficialis with a hemostat and retract the tendons distally.**
- **Pass a probe or scissors underneath the flexor digitorum profundus (Fig. 9.48) and transect it at the level of the carpal tunnel (Fig. 9.49).**
- **Lift this part of the flexor digitorum profundus from the palm and separate it from the underlying structures with scissors (Fig. 9.50).**
- **Identify the adductor pollicis muscle, and at the center of the palm, observe the loose connective tissue covering the underlying structures (Fig. 9.51).**
- **With sharp scissors, clean the connective tissue and expose the deep palmar arch and the deep branch of the ulnar nerve (Fig. 9.52).**

ANATOMY NOTE

The lumbricals arise from the tendons of the flexor digitorum profundus muscle and travel to the radial side of the medial four digits to insert into the extensor expansion of each digit.

ANATOMY NOTE

The radial artery enters the deep portion of the hand between the two heads of the first dorsal interosseous muscle and anastomoses with the deep branch of the ulnar artery.

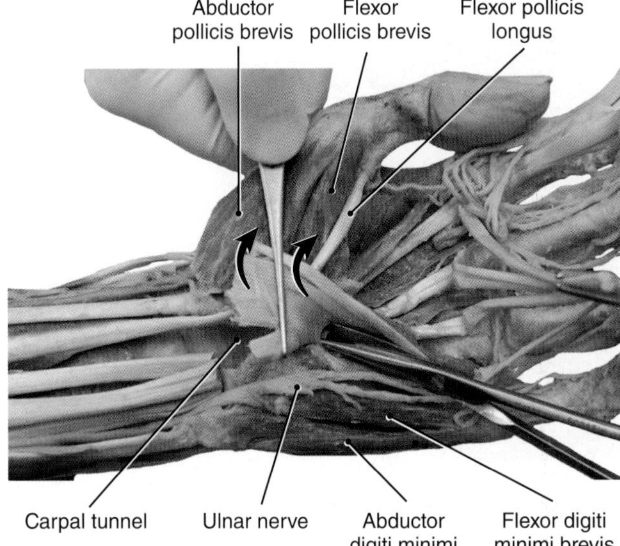

Fig. 9.50 Palmar hand with the skin and the palmar aponeurosis removed; superficial and deep tendons cut and reflected, revealing carpal tunnel and its contents. The tendons of the flexor digitorum superficialis and profundus are cut and reflected.

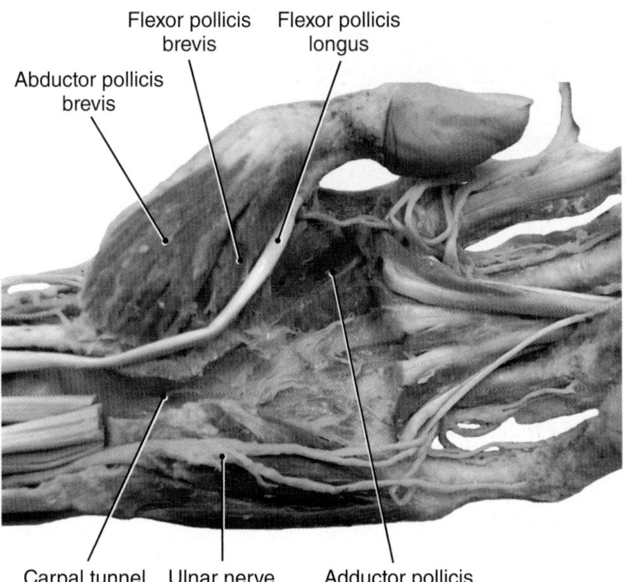

Fig. 9.51 Palmar hand with the skin and the palmar aponeurosis removed; tendons reflected from carpal tunnel revealing the thenar and palmar muscles.

- **Continue exposing the deep palmar arch and the ulnar nerve and identify the interossei muscles. Identify four dorsal and three palmar interossei muscles (Fig. 9.53).**
- **Reflect the flexor digitorum profundus and superficialis and note the pronator quadratus muscle. This muscle requires no dissection (Fig. 9.54).**
- **At the end of the dissection, place all structures back in their original anatomical position (Fig. 9.55). By following this dissection technique, you will be able to examine the specimen with all the structures in their original position.**

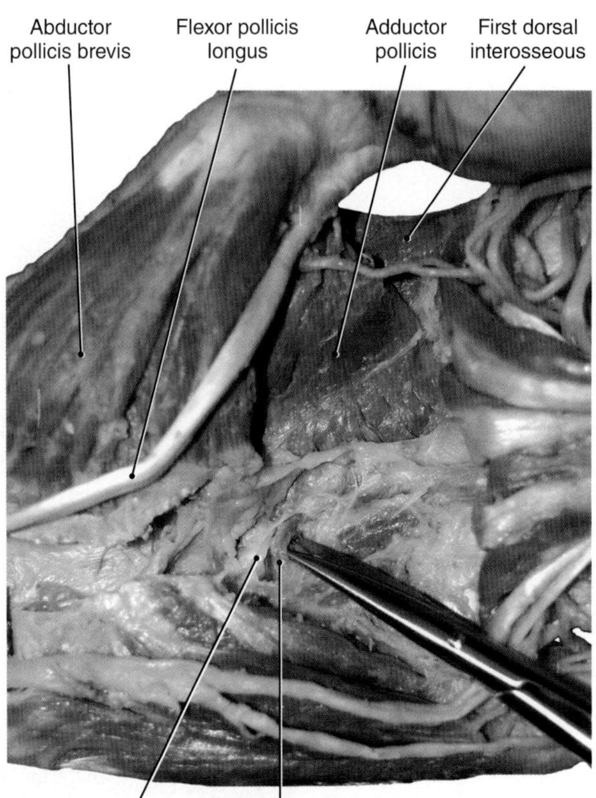

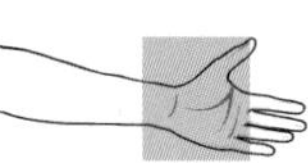

Fig. 9.52 Palmar hand with the skin and the palmar aponeurosis removed; tendons cut and reflected to reveal the deep palmar arch, contributed primarily by the radial artery.

DISSECTION TIP

The dorsal and palmar interossei muscles insert partially on the base of the proximal phalanx of each of the medial four digits and into their extensor expansions:

- 1st dorsal interosseous muscle inserts on the radial side of the 2nd digit.
- 2nd and 3rd dorsal interossei insert on either side of the 3rd digit.
- 4th dorsal interosseous muscle inserts on the ulnar side of the 4th digit.
- 1st palmar interosseous muscle inserts on the ulnar side of the 2nd digit.
- 2nd palmar interosseous muscle inserts on the radial side of the 4th digit.
- 3rd palmar interosseous muscle inserts on the radial side of the 5th digit.

DISSECTION TIP

The palmar fascial spaces are **potential spaces**, which are clinically important as routes of infection spread. These are not dissected in routine dissection.

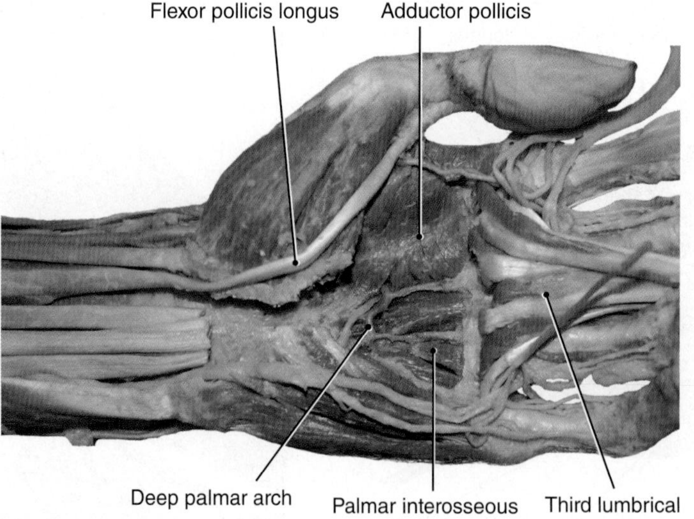

Fig. 9.53 Anterior forearm and hand with the skin and the palmar aponeurosis removed; superficial muscles reflected, revealing the deep structures, including the deep palmar arch and interosseous muscles.

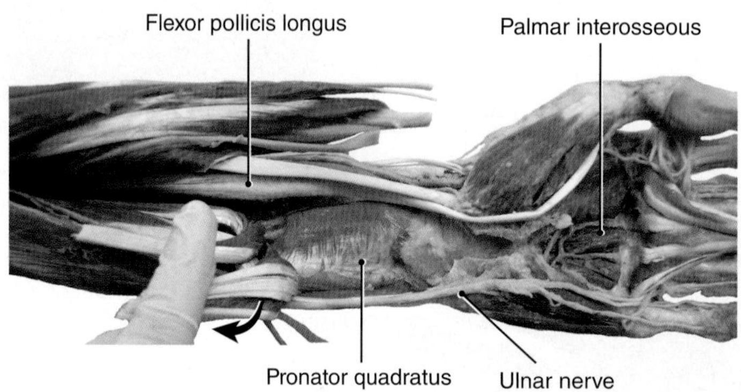

Fig. 9.54 Palmar hand and wrist with the skin and the palmar aponeurosis removed and tendons cut, revealing the deeper structures such as the pronator quadratus muscle.

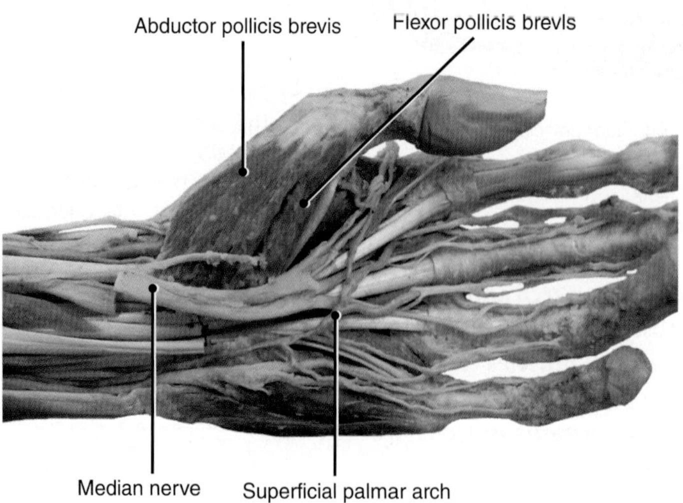

Fig. 9.55 Palmar hand and wrist with the skin and the palmar aponeurosis removed. The median nerve is transected in distal anterior forearm. Note the palmar branch of the median nerve crossing superficial to the flexor retinaculum.

LABORATORY IDENTIFICATION CHECKLIST

NERVES

- ☐ Median
  - ☐ Palmar branch
  - ☐ Recurrent branch
- ☐ Common palmar digital
  - ☐ Palmar digital
- ☐ Ulnar
  - ☐ Superficial branch
  - ☐ Deep branch
- ☐ Common palmar digital
  - ☐ Palmar digital
  - ☐ Dorsal branch
  - ☐ Dorsal digital
- ☐ Radial
  - ☐ Superficial branch
  - ☐ Dorsal digital branches

ARTERIES

- ☐ Ulnar
  - ☐ Superficial palmar arch
    - ☐ Common palmar digital
    - ☐ Palmar digital
- ☐ Radial
  - ☐ Deep arch
- ☐ Princeps pollicis
- ☐ Radialis indicis
- ☐ Palmar metacarpal
  - ☐ Palmar digital
  - ☐ Dorsal arterial arch
- ☐ Dorsal metacarpal
  - ☐ Dorsal digital

VEINS

- ☐ Dorsal digital
- ☐ Dorsal metacarpal
- ☐ Dorsal venous arch
  - ☐ Cephalic
  - ☐ Basilic
- ☐ Palmar digital

MUSCLES

Thenar Muscles

- ☐ Abductor pollicis brevis
- ☐ Flexor pollicis brevis
- ☐ Opponens pollicis brevis

Hypothenar Muscles

- ☐ Abductor digiti minimi
- ☐ Flexor digiti minimi
- ☐ Opponens digiti minimi
- ☐ Palmaris brevis

Palmar Muscles

- ☐ Adductor pollicis
- ☐ Palmar interossei
- ☐ Dorsal interossei
- ☐ Lumbricals

LIGAMENTS

- ☐ Ulnar collateral
- ☐ Radial collateral
- ☐ Palmar carpal

CONNECTIVE TISSUE

- ☐ Digital fibrous sheath with annular and cruciate regions
- ☐ Palmar aponeurosis
- ☐ Flexor retinaculum
- ☐ Extensor retinaculum
- ☐ Vinculum longum

BONES

Carpal Bones

- ☐ Scaphoid
- ☐ Lunate
- ☐ Triquetrum
- ☐ Hamate
- ☐ Capitate
- ☐ Trapezium
- ☐ Trapezoid
- ☐ Pisiform
- ☐ Metacarpals
- ☐ Phalanges
  - ☐ Proximal
  - ☐ Middle
  - ☐ Distal

CLINICAL APPLICATIONS

SUBACROMIAL BURSITIS INJECTION

Clinical Application

Provides relief for frequently inflamed bursa lying beneath the acromion near the supraspinatus tendon.

Anatomical Landmarks (Fig. IV.1)

- **Anterior acromion**
- **Lateral acromion**
- **Posterior acromion**
- **Scapular spine**
- **Humeral head**

ACROMIOCLAVICULAR JOINT INSPECTION

Clinical Application

Relieve pain from acromioclavicular joint irritation.

Anatomical Landmarks

- **Anterior acromion**
- **Lateral acromion**
- **Acromioclavicular joint**

Fig. IV.1

GLENOHUMERAL JOINT INJECTION

Clinical Application

Relieve the pain from the glenohumeral joint irritation.

Anatomical Landmarks (Figs. IV.2 and IV.3) **(Posterior Approach)**

- **Skin**
- **Subcutaneous tissues**
- **Infraspinatus**
- **Joint capsule**
- **Glenoid fossa**
- **Humeral head**

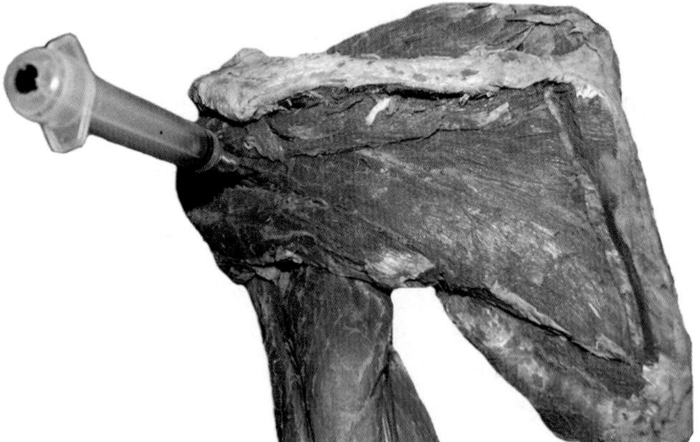

Fig. IV.2

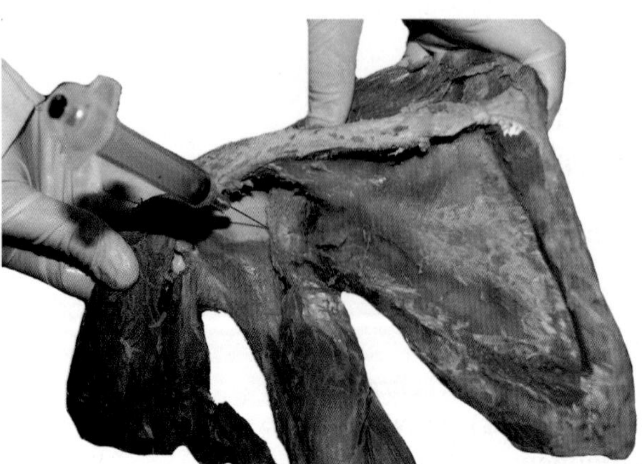

Fig. IV.3

STERNOCLAVICULAR JOINT INJECTION

Clinical Application

Relieve pain from sternoclavicular joint irritation.

Anatomical Landmarks

- **Skin**
- **Subcutaneous tissue**
- **Anterior sternoclavicular ligament**
- **Articular disc**
- **Medial clavicle**
- **Manubrium**
- **Brachiocephalic vein**
- **Subclavian artery**

BICIPITAL TENOSYNOVITIS INJECTION

Clinical Application

Acute trauma or chronic overuse of the biceps brachii tendon (usually long head); relieves pain and may prevent further shoulder pathology.

Anatomical Landmarks (Fig. IV.4)

- **Supinated upper limb**
- **Inferior border of pectoralis major**
- **Biceps brachii long head**
- **Humerus**

ULNAR NERVE BLOCK FOR CUBITAL TUNNEL SYNDROME

Clinical Application

For relief of pain caused by irritation of the ulnar nerve.

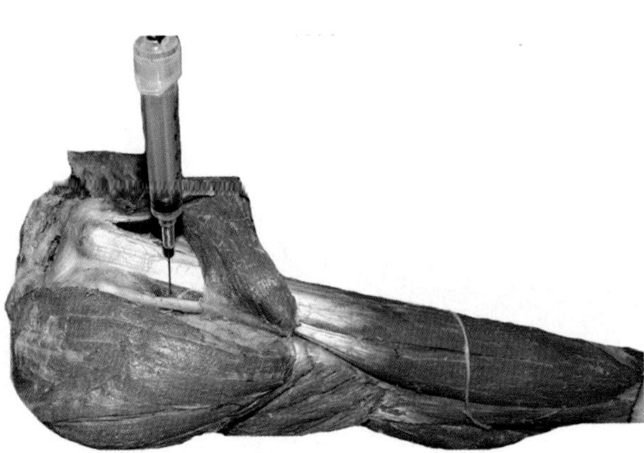

Fig. IV.4

Anatomical Landmarks

- **Laterally rotated upper limb**
- **Medial epicondyle**
- **Groove for ulnar nerve**
- **Olecranon**
- **Flexor carpi ulnaris**
- **Tendinous arch connecting the two heads of flexor carpi ulnaris**

Needle is advanced parallel to the ulnar nerve.

MEDIAN NERVE BLOCK (INJECTION AT WRIST)

Clinical Application

Median nerve block anesthetizes the lateral palmar 3½ digits.

Anatomical Landmarks (Figs. IV.5 and IV.6)

- **Skin**
- **Proximal palmar skin crease**
- **Subcutaneous tissue**
- **Flexor retinaculum**
- **Palmaris longus muscle (absent in approximately 20%)**

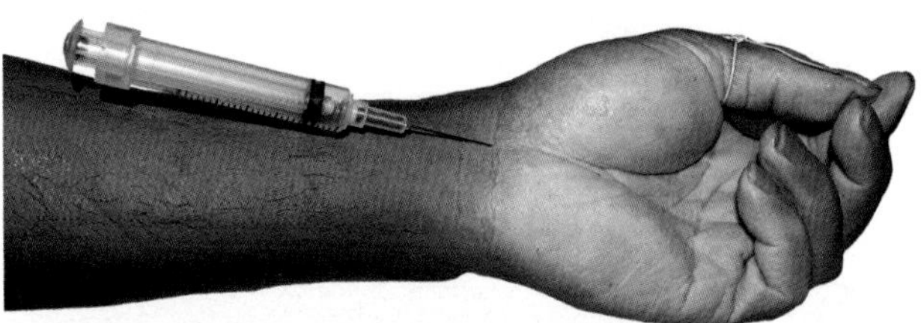

Fig. IV.5

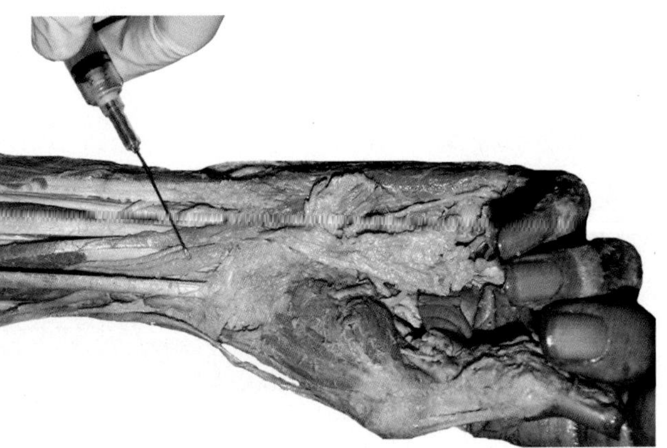

Fig. IV.6

- Flexor carpi radialis muscle
- Median nerve

DE QUERVAIN TENOSYNOVITIS INJECTION

Clinical Application

Relieve pain associated with stenosing tenosynovitis of the extensor pollicis brevis muscle.

Anatomical Landmarks (Figs. IV.7 and IV.8)

- Skin
- Subcutaneous tissue
- 1st dorsal compartment retinaculum
- Cephalic vein
- Radial artery branches
- 1st metacarpal base
- 1st metacarpophalangeal joint
- Extensor pollicis brevis

MEDIAL EPICONDYLITIS (GOLFER'S ELBOW) INJECTION

Clinical Application

Relief of pain caused by strain to the attachment of the wrist flexors at the medial epicondyle region.

Anatomical Landmarks

- Skin
- Subcutaneous tissue
- Common flexor tendon
- Medial epicondyle

LATERAL EPICONDYLITIS (TENNIS ELBOW) INJECTION

Clinical Application

Relief of pain caused by strain to the attachment of the forearm flexors at the lateral epicondyle region.

Anatomical Landmarks (Figs. IV.9 and IV.10)

- Skin
- Subcutaneous tissue
- Common extensor tendon
- Lateral epicondyle

DIGITAL NERVE BLOCK (HAND)

Clinical Application

Anesthetize the palmar or dorsal side of a single or multiple digits to perform invasive procedures.

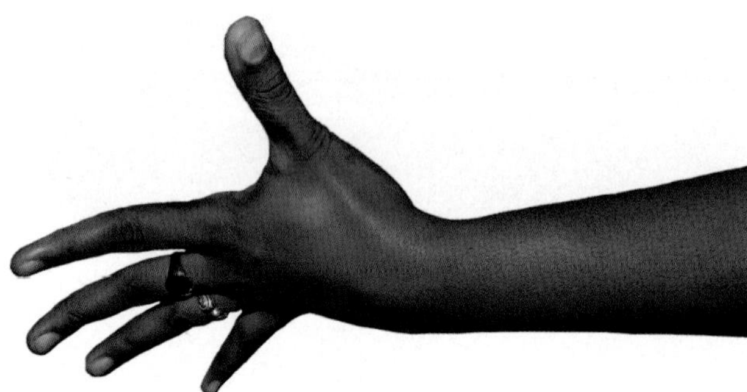

Fig. IV.7

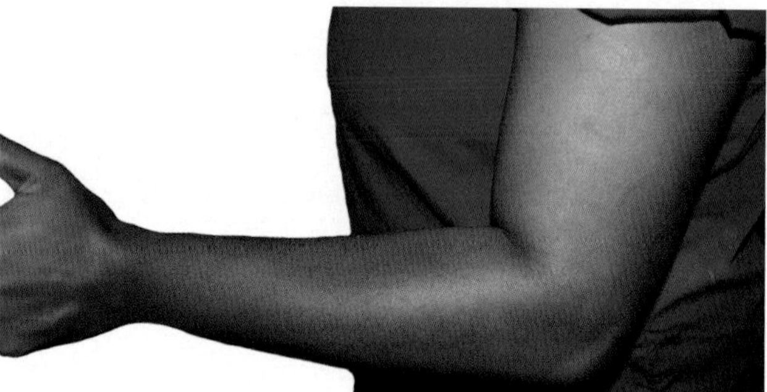

Fig. IV.9

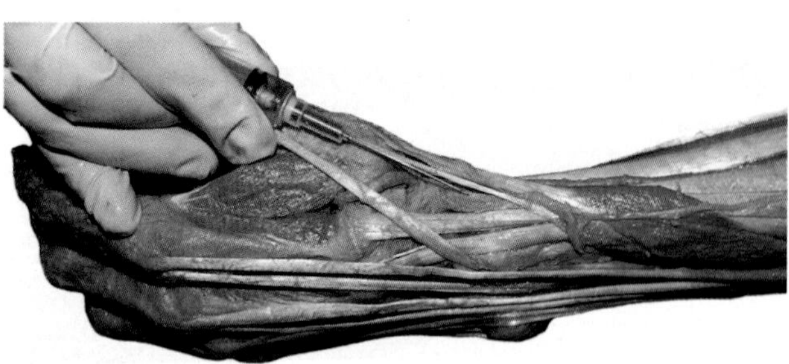

Fig. IV.8

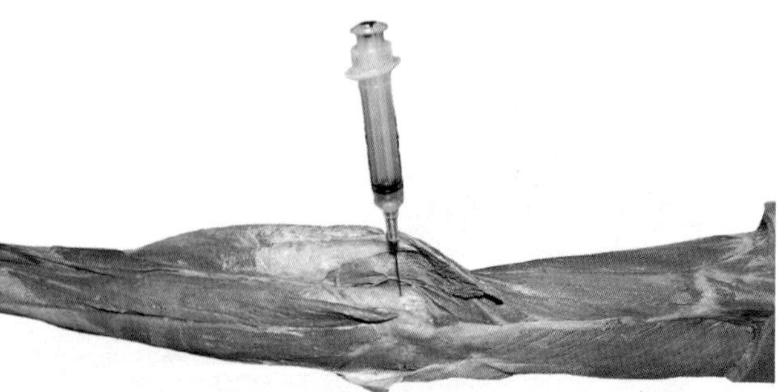

Fig. IV.10

Anatomical Landmarks (Figs. IV.11 and IV.12)

- **Skin**
- **Subcutaneous tissue**
- **Common digital nerves/arteries**
- **Palmar digital nerves/arteries**
- **Dorsal digital nerves/arteries**
- **Metacarpophalangeal joints**
- **Proximal interphalangeal joints**

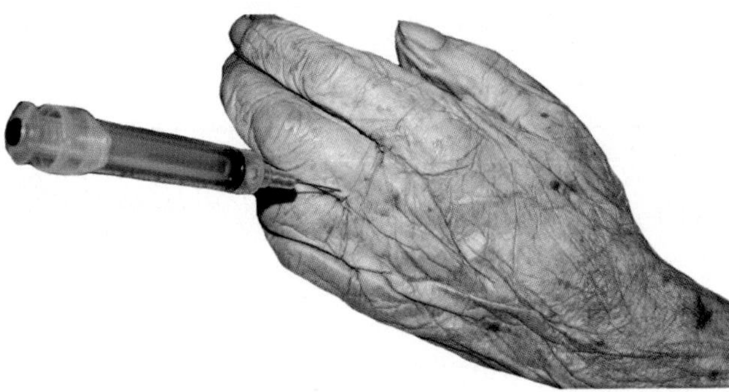

Fig. IV.11

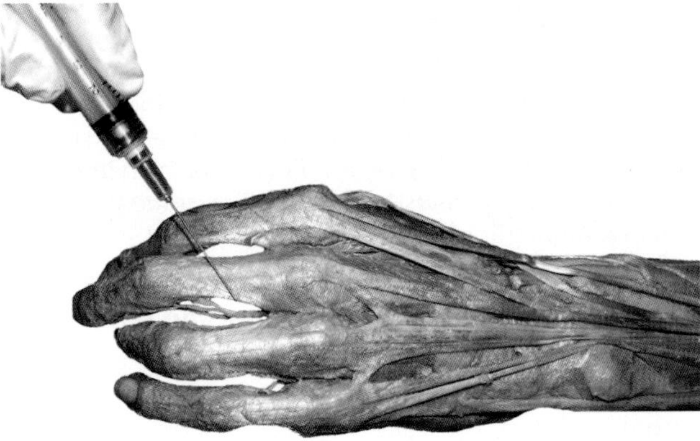

Fig. IV.12

VENIPUNCTURE OR PHLEBOTOMY

Clinical Application

To withdraw venous blood through needle penetration, or to insert intravenous (IV) cannula.

Anatomical Landmarks (Fig. IV.13)

- **Skin**
- **Subcutaneous tissue**

  Elbow: **Cubital vein**
  Forearm: **Cephalic vein**
  Basilic vein
  Hand dorsum: **Cephalic vein**
  Basilic vein
  Dorsal venous arch
  Metacarpal veins

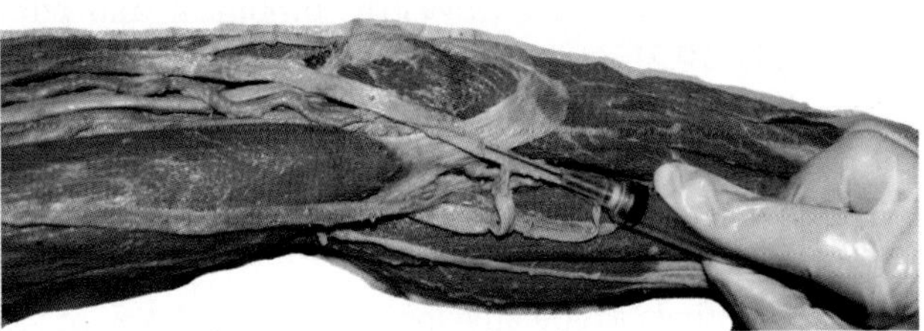

Fig. IV.13

SECTION V

ABDOMEN

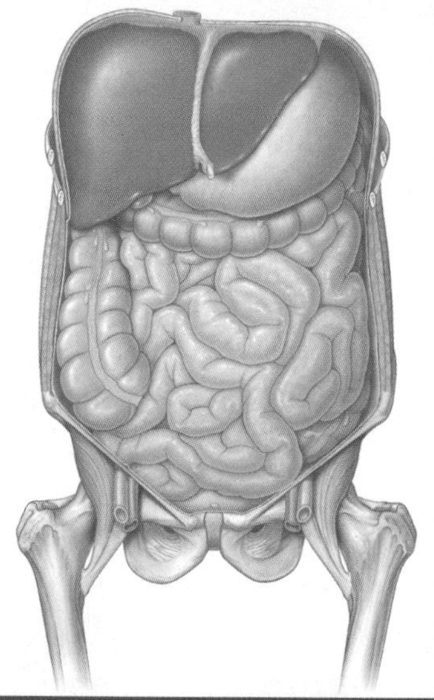

CHAPTER 10 ANTEROLATERAL ABDOMINAL WALL AND INGUINAL REGION

BEFORE YOU BEGIN

In general, the abdomen can be divided into right and left superior (upper) quadrants and right and left inferior (lower) quadrants. This division is based on drawing vertical and horizontal lines through the umbilicus (Fig. 10.1). More specifically, the anterior abdominal wall can be divided into regions: the right and left *hypochondriac* regions; the right and left *lateral* regions; the right and left *inguinal* regions; and the epigastric, umbilical, and pubic regions (Fig. 10.2).

Identify and palpate the following:

- Xiphoid process
- The lower costal margins, which form the subcostal plane
- The umbilicus (typically located at the level of 4th lumbar vertebra)
- Anterior superior iliac spines
- Pubic symphysis
- Pubic crests
- Iliac crests
- Tubercles of the iliac crests, which form the intertubercular plane when connected. This plane is located at the L5 level just inferior to the bifurcation of the abdominal aorta

SKIN AND SUPERFICIAL FASCIA

From the xiphoid process, make a midline vertical skin incision from the xiphoid process to the pubic symphysis. Do not cut through the umbilicus; make a circumferential incision around it. From the costal margins make a second incision following this margin from the midaxillary line to the xiphoid process. Finally, make an incision from the anterior superior iliac spine to the pubic symphysis (Fig. 10.3).

DISSECTION TIP

An alternate method is to make a vertical incision from the midaxillary line to 2 inches (5 cm) inferior to the anterior superior iliac spine. Make a transverse incision inferior to the inguinal ligament. Reflect the skin inferiorly to the level of the anterior superior iliac spine to expose the inguinal region.

- **Dissect the skin from the midline and reflect it laterally (Fig. 10.4).**
- **Expose the superficial fascia beneath the skin (Fig. 10.5).**

ANATOMY NOTE

The fatty layer of the superficial fascia is also known as *Camper's fascia*, whereas the membranous layer is known as *Scarpa's fascia*.

- **As the superficial fascia is reflected (Fig. 10.6), note a superficial fatty layer and a deeper membranous layer.**
- **Reflect the superficial fatty layer similar to the previously made skin incision.**
- **Make a shallow incision with the scalpel and place your index finger into the incision so that lateral traction can be applied and reflection performed.**
- **Continue with blunt dissection to identify the deep membranous fascia over the abdominal muscles.**
- **Once this is achieved, continue the dissection using a scalpel.**

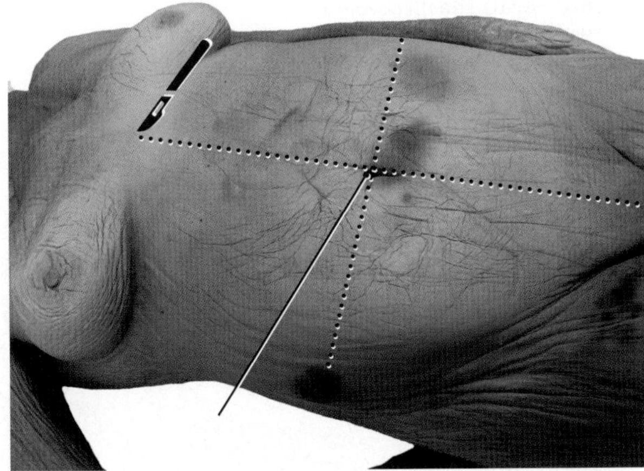

Fig. 10.1 Anterior view of abdomen showing simplified division into quadrants.

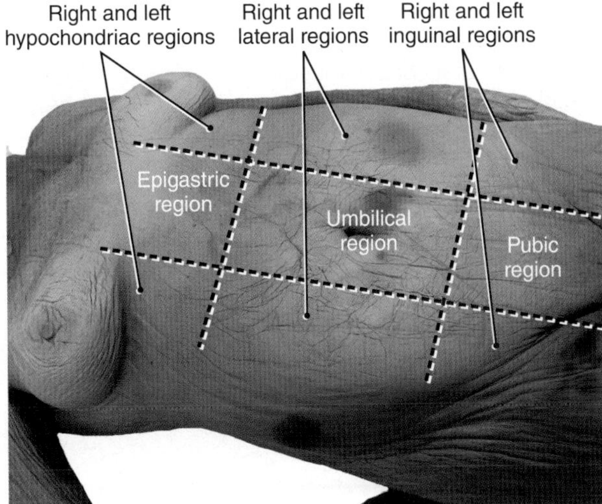

Fig. 10.2 Anterior view of abdomen showing division into regions.

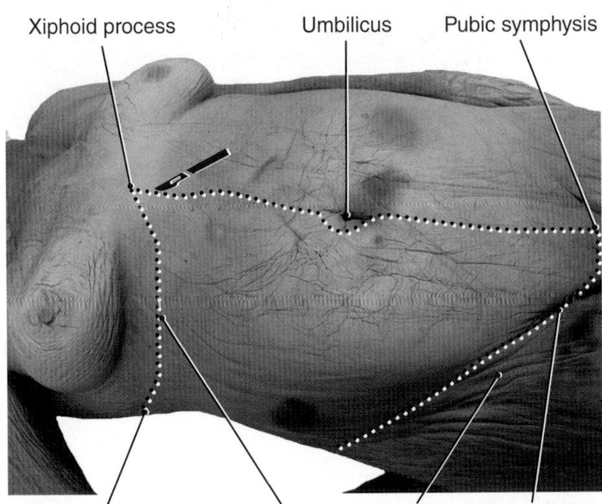

Fig. 10.3 Anterior view of the abdomen showing the skin incisions *(dashed lines)* used to begin the dissection. *ASIS*, Anterior superior iliac spine.

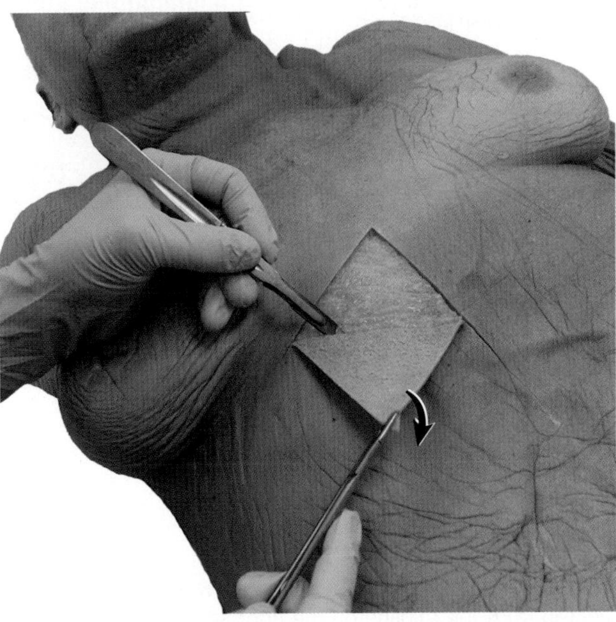

Fig. 10.4 Method used to reflect the skin from the underlying fascia. Note tension is placed on the corner of the skin flap as the scalpel liberates this layer from the underlying fascia.

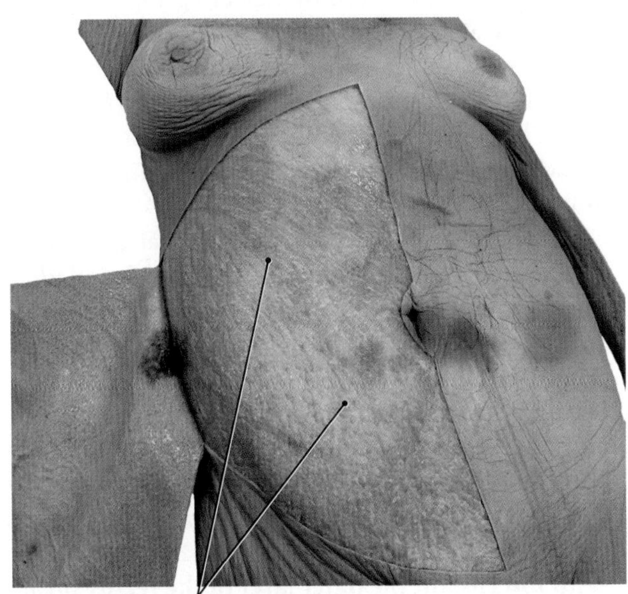

Fig. 10.5 Anterior view of the abdomen showing the skin reflection with the underlying subcutaneous tissues.

MUSCLES OF THE ANTEROLATERAL ABDOMINAL WALL

ANATOMY **NOTE**

The three flat muscles of the anterolateral abdominal wall—external abdominal oblique, internal abdominal oblique, and transversus abdominis—are covered by a superficial fascia and a deep fascia. The outermost fascia covering the external abdominal oblique muscle (deep) is called the *fascia of Gallaudet*.

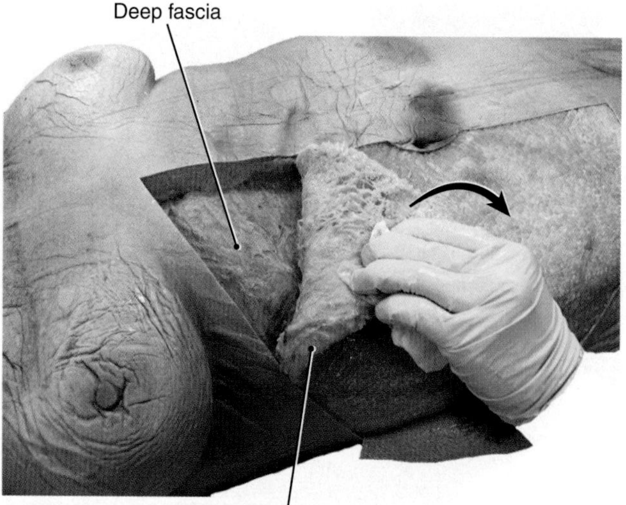

Fig. 10.6 Anterior view of the abdomen with skin and fascia reflected from the midline on the right side.

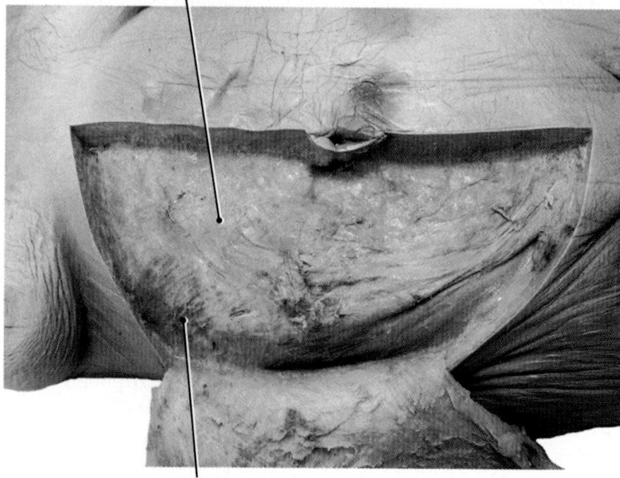

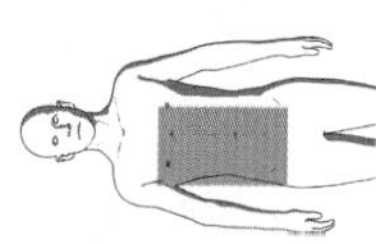

Fig. 10.7 With additional dissection, the external abdominal oblique muscle is identified with its contribution to the outer rectus sheath.

- Continue the dissection by reflecting the superficial fatty layer and exposing the muscles of the anterior abdomen (covered with deep fascia) and the outer layer of the rectus sheath (anterior lamina) (Fig. 10.7).
- At the level of the midaxillary line, remove the deep fascia and expose the external abdominal oblique muscle (Fig. 10.8).
- Clean the deep fascia over the external abdominal oblique and outer layer of the rectus sheath and identify the linea alba, linea semilunaris (at the lateral border of the rectus sheath), and inguinal ligament (Figs. 10.9 and 10.10).
- Once the external abdominal oblique muscle is exposed at the midabdomen on both sides, continue the reflection of the deep fascia over the pubic symphysis and inguinal ligament to further expose the external abdominal oblique muscle (Fig. 10.11).
- With forceps, lift the outer layer of the rectus sheath (anterior lamina) at the level of the xiphoid process.
- With scissors, make a small incision into the rectus sheath (anterior lamina) (Fig. 10.12).
- Lift the rectus sheath upward and identify the rectus abdominis muscle underneath it (Fig. 10.13).
- With your scalpel, detach the outer layer of the rectus sheath (anterior lamina) alongside its border with the external abdominal oblique muscle (Fig. 10.14).

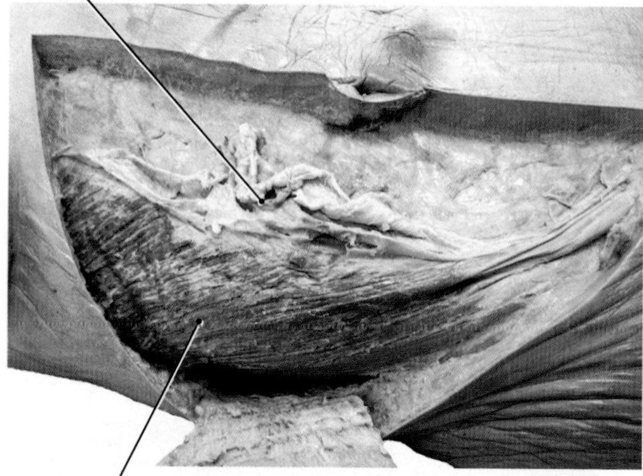

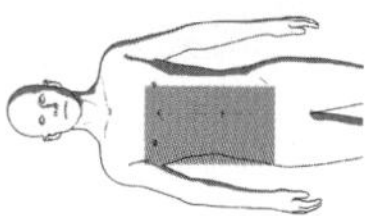

Fig. 10.8 Anterior view of the abdomen noting the exposed external abdominal oblique muscle and contributions medially into the outer rectus sheath.

DISSECTION TIP

An alternative method is to make a vertical incision at the midline and reflect the outer layer of the rectus sheath laterally from the linea alba.

DISSECTION TIP

The tendinous intersections attach firmly to the anterior lamina of the rectus sheath. Employ sharp dissection when necessary to remove the anterior lamina. Observe the linea alba becoming wider and thicker above the umbilicus.

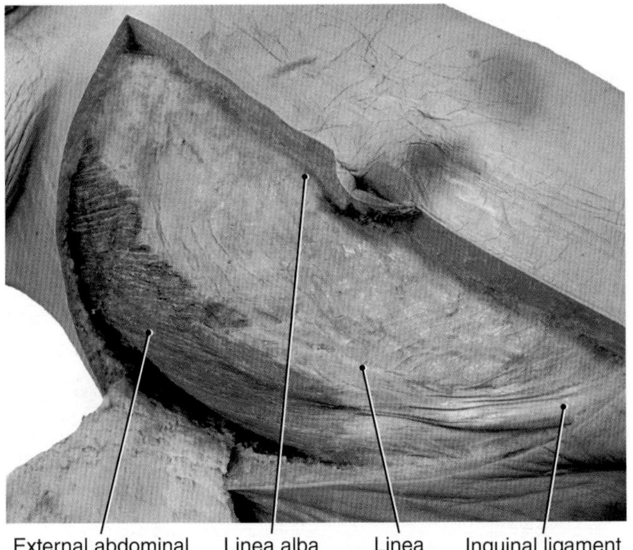

Fig. 10.9 Anterior view of the abdomen noting the exposed external abdominal oblique muscle and contributions medially into the outer rectus sheath.

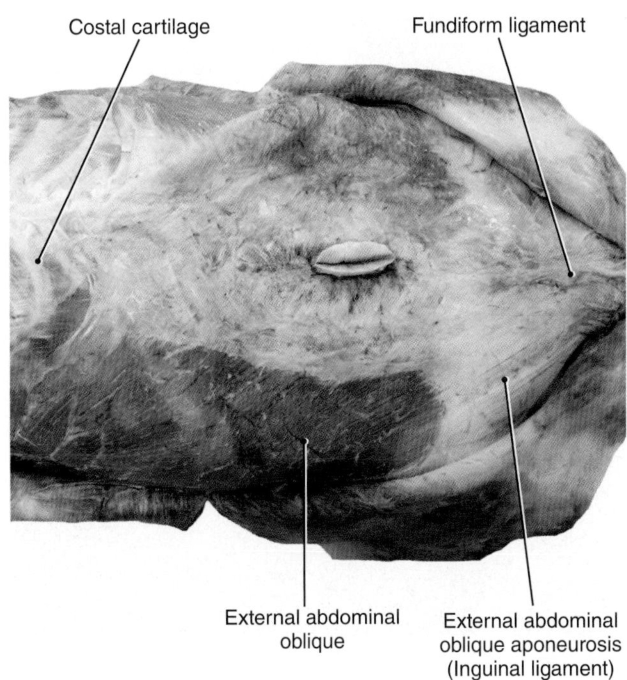

Fig. 10.11 Anterior view of the abdomen noting upper attachments of external abdominal oblique muscle along the costal margin and inferiorly with specialization of its aponeurosis, the inguinal ligament.

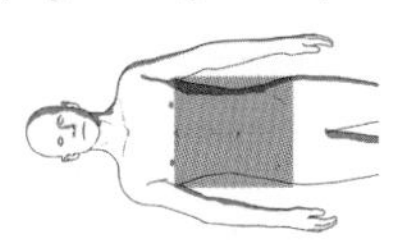

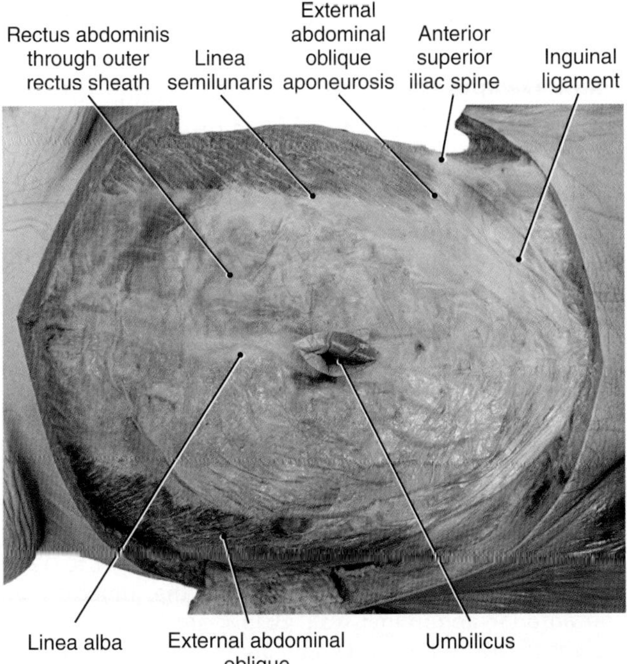

Fig. 10.10 Anterior view of the full abdominal exposure showing anatomical landmarks. Note the linea alba in the midline with the interposed umbilicus.

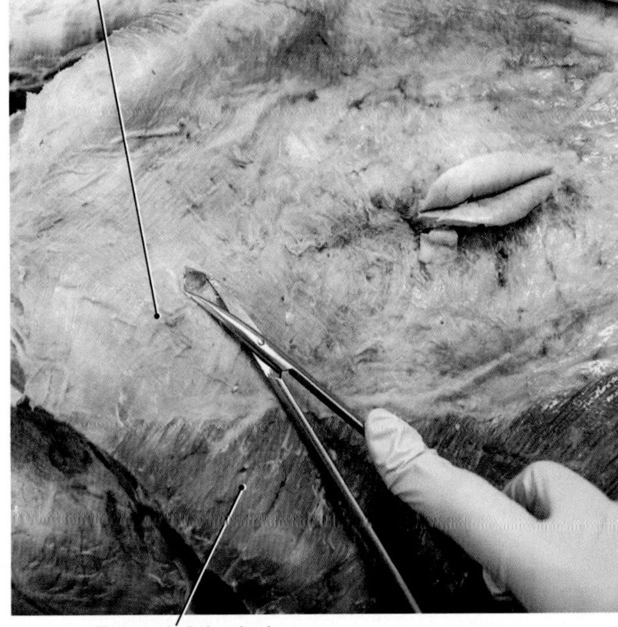

Fig. 10.12 Anterior view of the abdomen showing the outer rectus fascia.

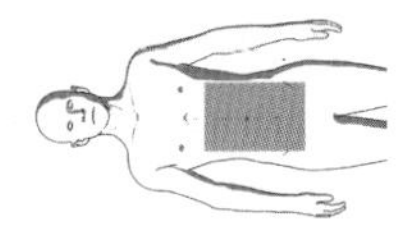

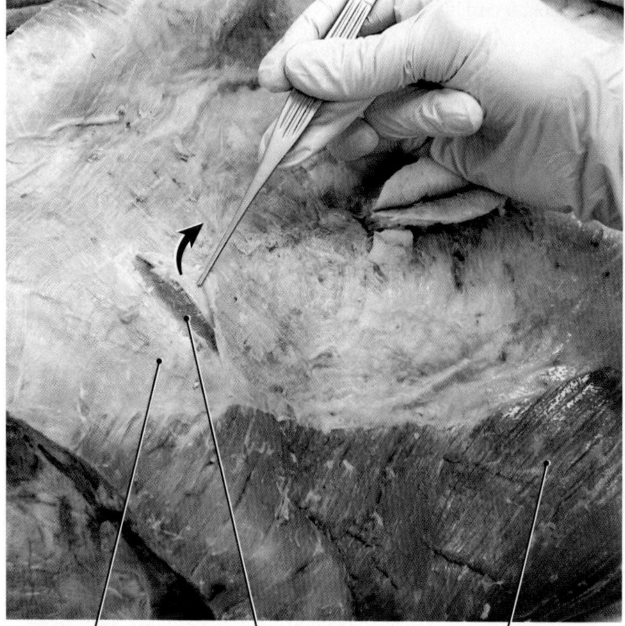

Fig. 10.13 Anterior view of the abdomen noting continued opening of the outer rectus sheath.

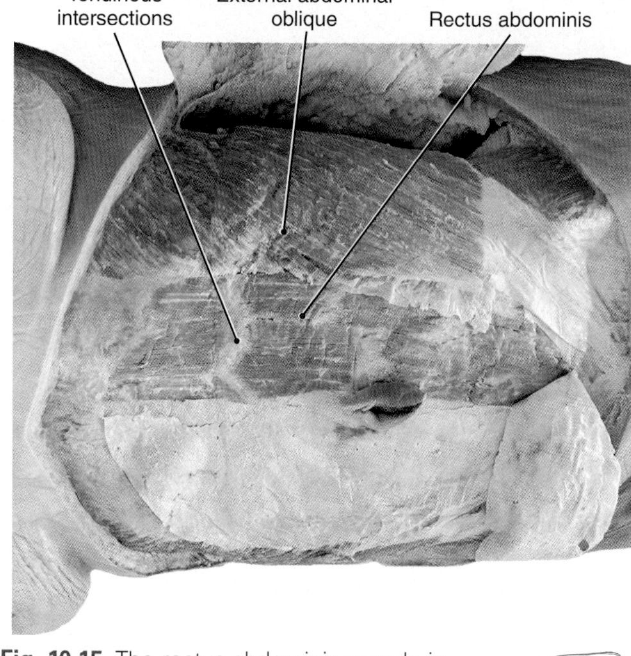

Fig. 10.15 The rectus abdominis muscle is exposed more or less along its entirety.

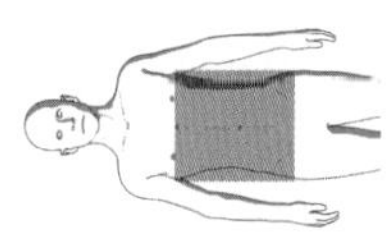

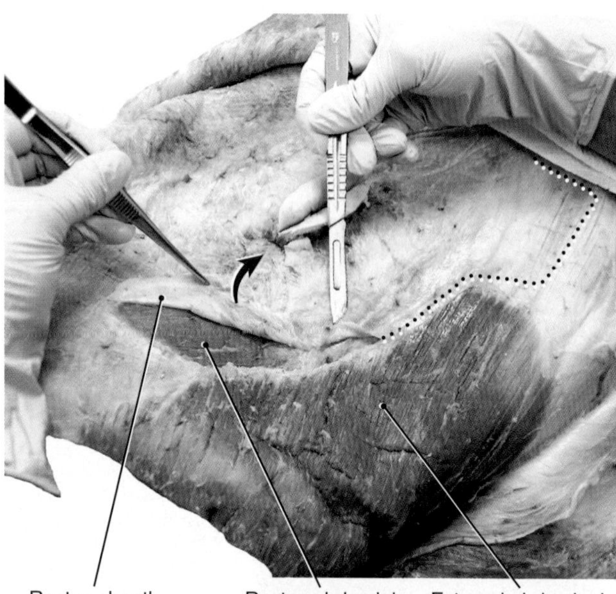

Fig. 10.14 Outer sheath is exposed along the lateral edge of the junction of the external abdominal oblique muscle with its aponeurosis.

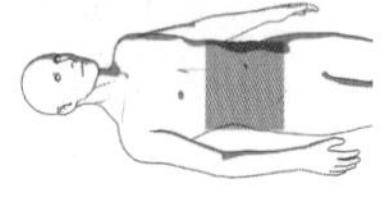

- **Reflect the outer layer of the rectus sheath (anterior lamina) from the xiphoid process to pubic symphysis and completely expose the rectus abdominis muscle. Leave a small part of the rectus sheath intact (Fig. 10.15).**
- **Identify the tendinous intersections, formed by the tendinous inscriptions of the rectus abdominis muscle and its segmentation, and the *linea alba,* the avascular fusion point of the aponeuroses of the muscles of the anterior abdominal wall at the midline extending from the xiphoid process to the pubic symphysis (Fig. 10.16).**
- **At the inferior portion of the rectus abdominis muscle and anterior to it, identify the pyramidalis muscle (see Fig. 10.16).**

DISSECTION TIP

The pyramidalis muscle is absent in about 20% of cases.

DISSECTION TIP

During the dissection of the anterolateral abdominal wall, note the anterior primary rami of the 7th to 12th thoracic nerves (T7–T12) supplying the muscles of the anterior abdominal wall. Below are five important nerves in this region and some anatomical landmarks:

1. T7, usually found just inferior to the xiphoid process.
2. T10, at the level of the umbilicus.
3. T12, at the level just above the pubis.
4. Ilioinguinal nerve, at the level of the anterior superior iliac spine, underneath the external abdominal oblique muscle.

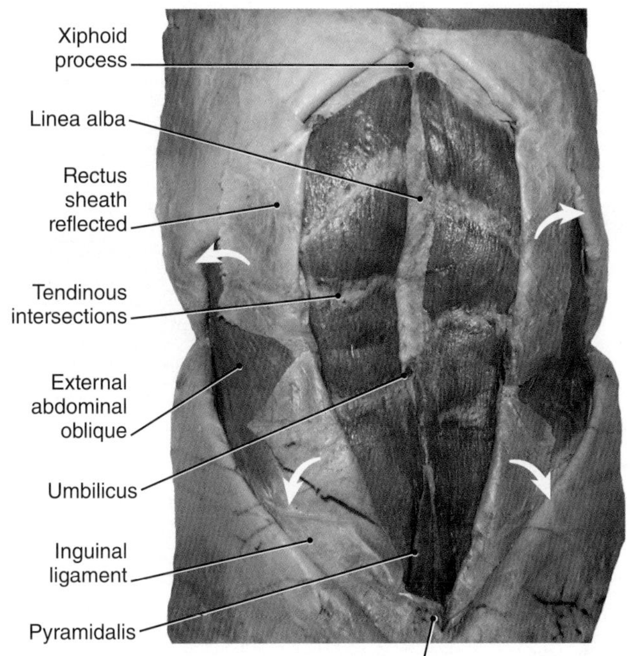

Fig. 10.16 Continued exposure of the outer rectus sheath.

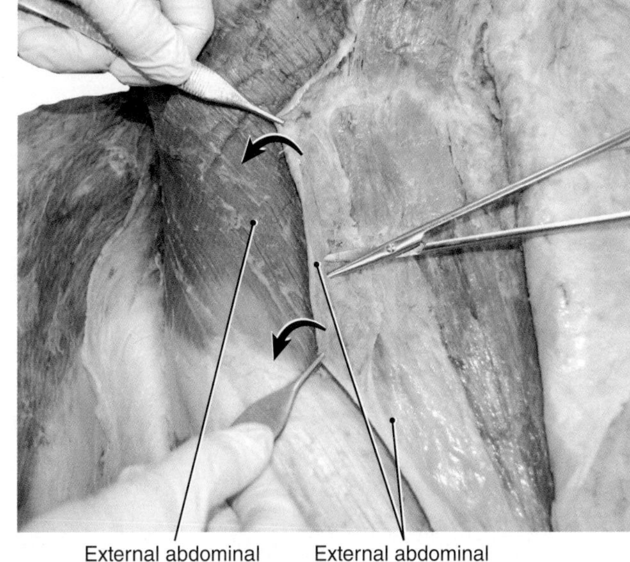

Fig. 10.17 Continued exposure of the outer rectus sheath.

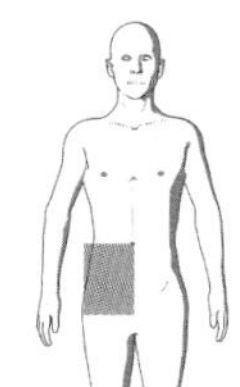

5. Iliohypogastric nerve, 3 to 4 cm above the ilioinguinal nerve at the level of the anterior superior iliac spine.

- **At the level of the linea semilunaris, make a small incision between the external abdominal oblique and rectus abdominis muscles (Fig. 10.17).**
- **Retract the external abdominal oblique muscle laterally and expose the fibers of the underlying internal abdominal oblique muscle (Fig. 10.18).**
- **Similarly, cut the internal abdominal oblique muscle at the level of the linea semilunaris and expose the underlying transversus abdominis muscle (Fig. 10.19).**
- **Note the difference in the muscle fiber orientation between the external abdominal oblique, internal abdominal oblique, and transversus abdominis muscles.**
- **Cut the transversus abdominis muscle and reflect it to expose the underlying transversalis fascia (Fig. 10.20).**
- **Between the internal abdominal oblique and transversus abdominis muscles, identify anterior primary rami from T7 to T12 (see Fig. 10.20).**
- **Note that the fascia that lies deep to the transversus abdominis (at its deepest surface) is the *transversalis fascia* (see Fig. 10.20).**

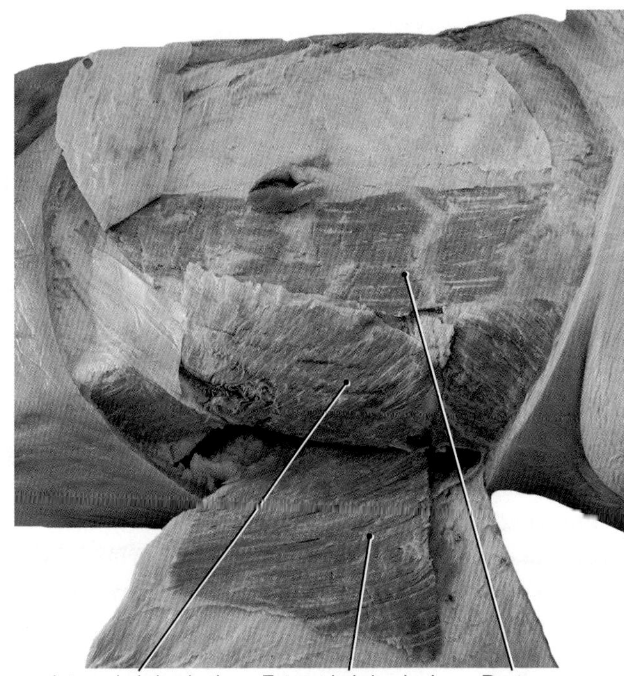

Fig. 10.18 After reflecting part of the external abdominal oblique muscle, the deeper layer composed of the internal abdominal oblique muscle is visualized.

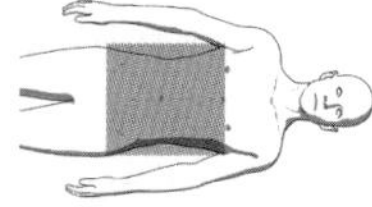

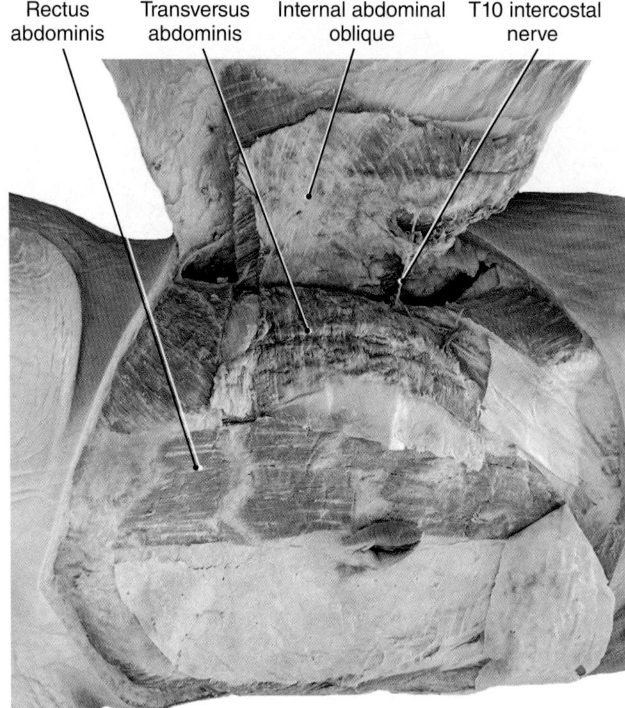

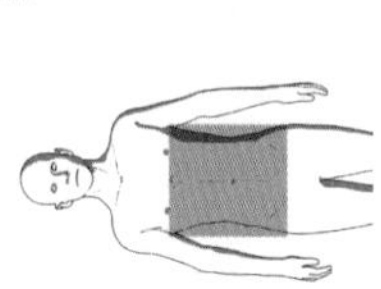

Fig. 10.19 After part of the internal abdominal oblique is reflected, the deeper transversus abdominis muscle is visible.

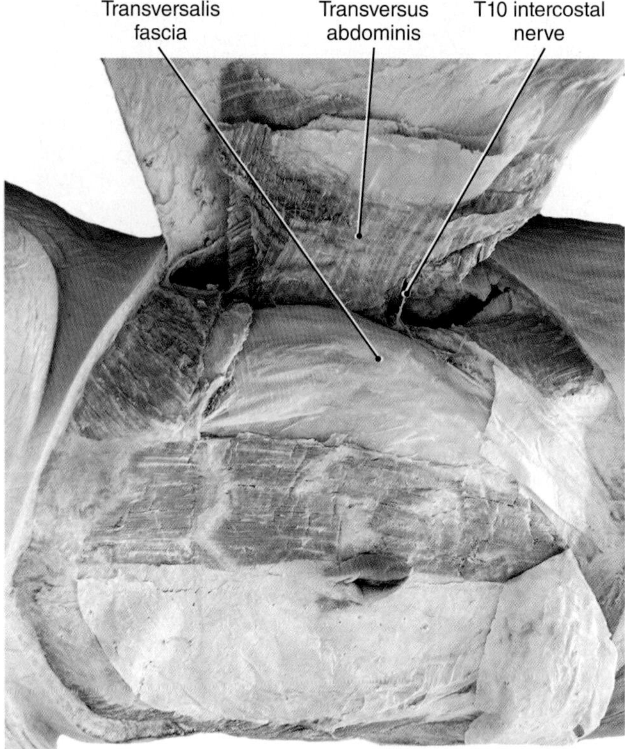

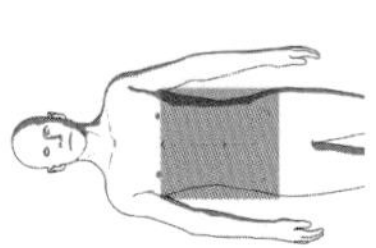

Fig. 10.20 After reflecting part of the transversus abdominis muscle, the deeper transversalis fascia is observed.

DISSECTION **TIP**

An alternate method is to make a vertical incision at the external abdominal oblique muscle on the midaxillary line, where the underlying internal abdominal oblique and transversus abdominis muscles are usually the thickest. Reflect the external abdominal oblique muscle and identify the internal abdominal oblique muscle. Continue the same process with the internal abdominal oblique and identify the transversus abdominis muscle (Figs. 10.21 and 10.22).

- **At the level of the xiphoid process, make a shallow transverse incision at the rectus abdominis muscle (Fig. 10.23).**
- **Lift the rectus abdominis from its posterior lamina of the rectus sheath and reflect it downward (see Fig. 10.23 and Plate 10.1).**
- **Identify the anterior rami of T7 to T12 penetrating the posterior lamina of the rectus sheath (Fig. 10.24).**
- **Reflect the rectus abdominis muscle superiorly from the posterior lamina of the rectus sheath and identify, on its deep surface, the superior and inferior epigastric arteries (Fig. 10.25).**

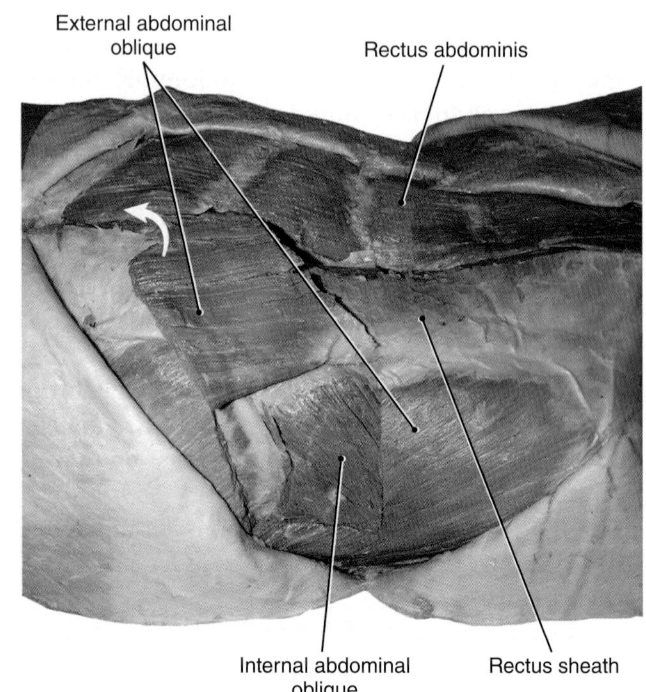

Fig. 10.21 Anterior view showing the external abdominal oblique and rectus abdominis muscles.

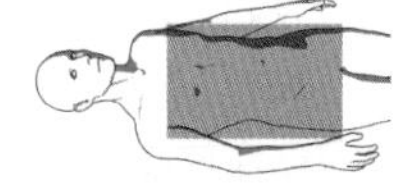

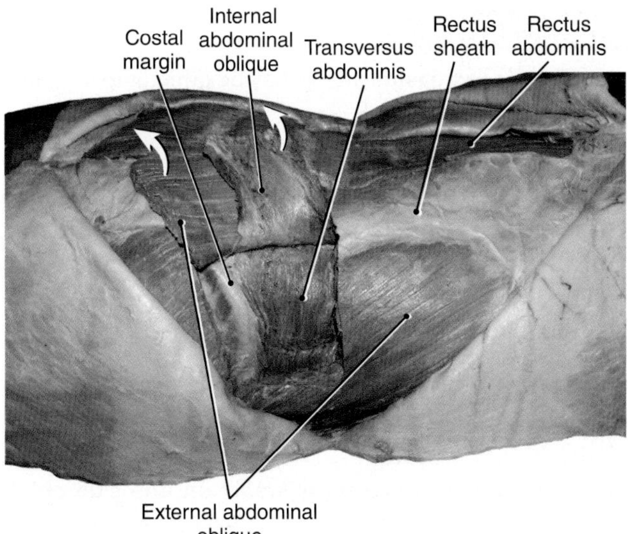

Fig. 10.22 Additional view after muscular flap cuts showing the outermost external abdominal oblique muscle and reflected, deeper-lying internal abdominal oblique muscle. Deep to the reflected internal abdominal oblique, the transversus abdominis muscle is seen.

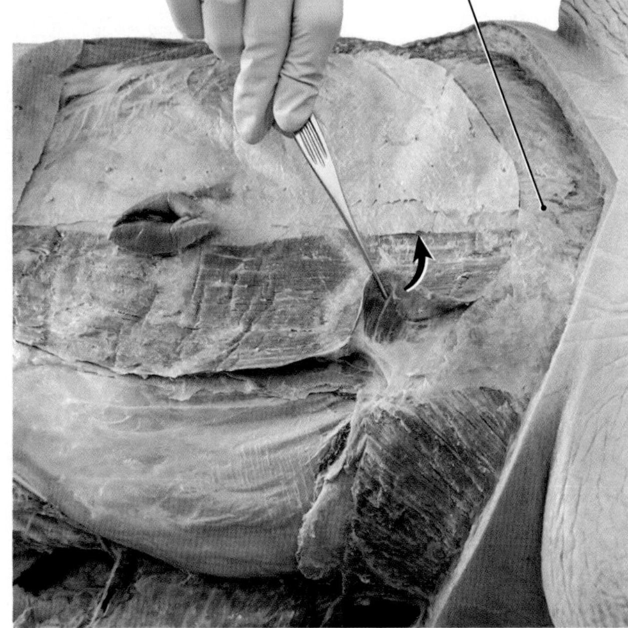

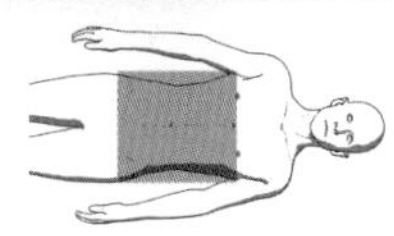

Fig. 10.23 The rectus abdominis muscle is reflected inferiorly.

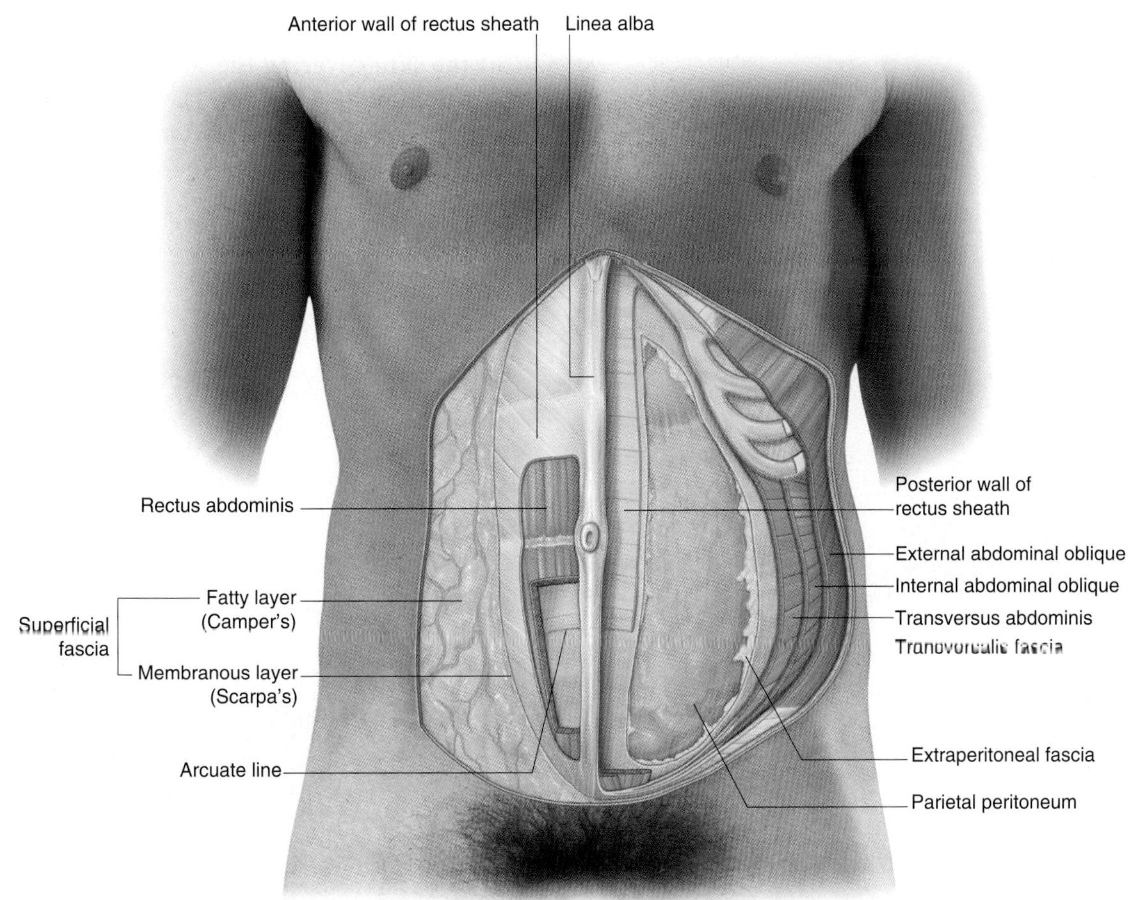

Plate 10.1 Layers of the anterior abdominal wall. (From Drake RL et al. *Gray's Atlas of Anatomy*, 3rd edition, Philadelphia, Elsevier, 2021, p. 136.)

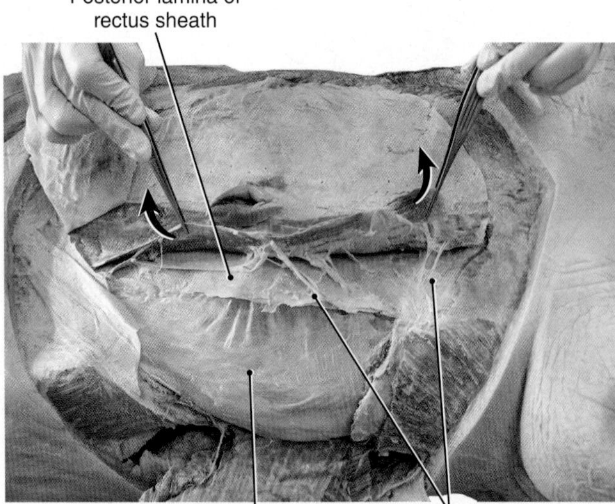

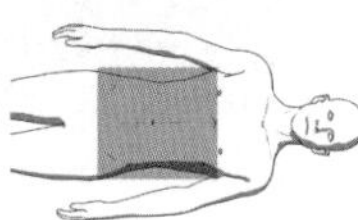

Fig. 10.24 With reflection of the rectus abdominis muscle, the segmental nerves of this region are appreciated.

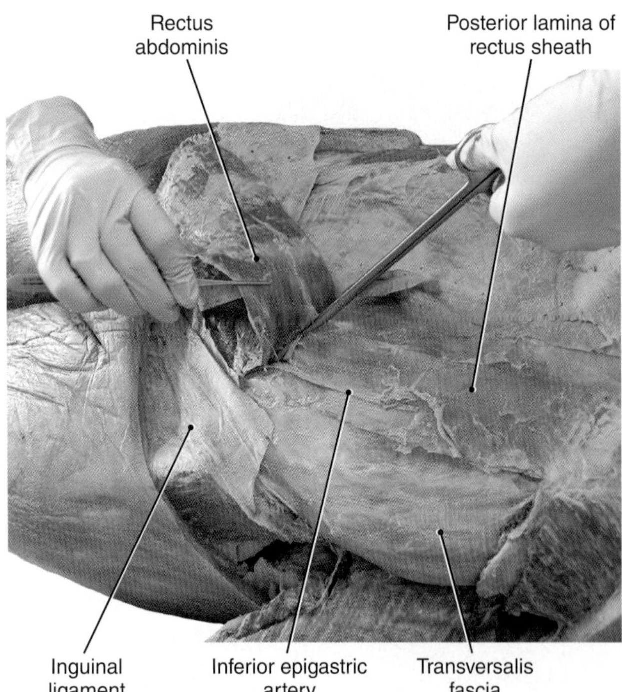

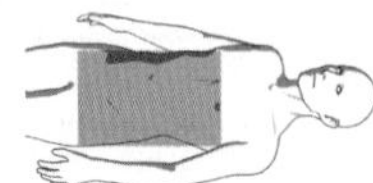

Fig. 10.25 With continued reflection of the rectus abdominis muscle, the inferior epigastric vessels are seen.

DISSECTION **TIP**

The superior epigastric artery may be difficult to identify.

- **Just inferior to the umbilicus, identify the arcuate line of the rectus sheath, where the posterior lamina of the sheath is formed only by transversalis fascia (Figs. 10.26–10.28).**

INGUINAL REGION

DISSECTION **TIP**

Complete this dissection preferably on one side only! It is important to leave one side intact so that you can compare sides.

- **Identify the inferior edge of the aponeurosis of the external abdominal oblique muscle, the *inguinal ligament* (Fig. 10.28, Plate 10.2).**
- **Reflect part of the skin over the superior portion of the thigh and identify the great saphenous vein (Fig. 10.29).**
- **Extend the skin flap medially and expose the inferior border of the inguinal ligament (Fig. 10.30).**
- **Cut the skin covering the spermatic cord inferiorly toward the testis (Fig. 10.31).**
- **Clean the adipose tissue and identify the superficial inguinal ring and the spermatic cord covered**

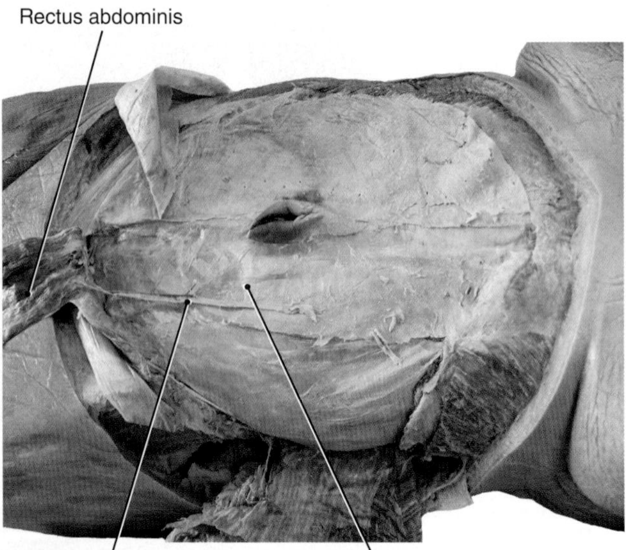

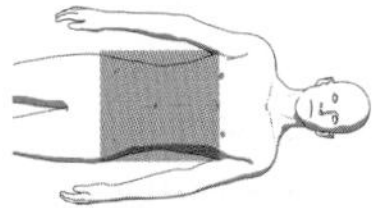

Fig. 10.26 Rectus abdominis muscle is reflected superiorly, and the inferior epigastric vessels are seen. Note the arcuate line.

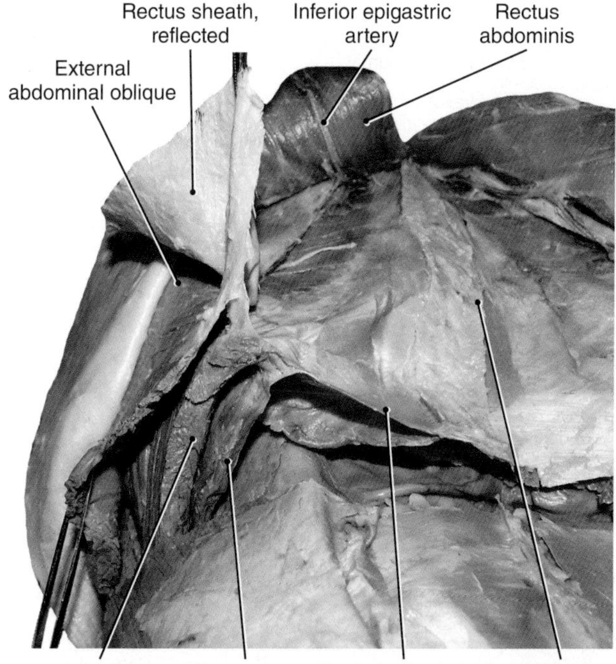

Fig. 10.27 Anterolateral view of the left abdominal wall muscles. Note that rectus abdominis muscles are reflected inferiorly and shown laterally are the external and internal oblique and transversus abdominis muscles.

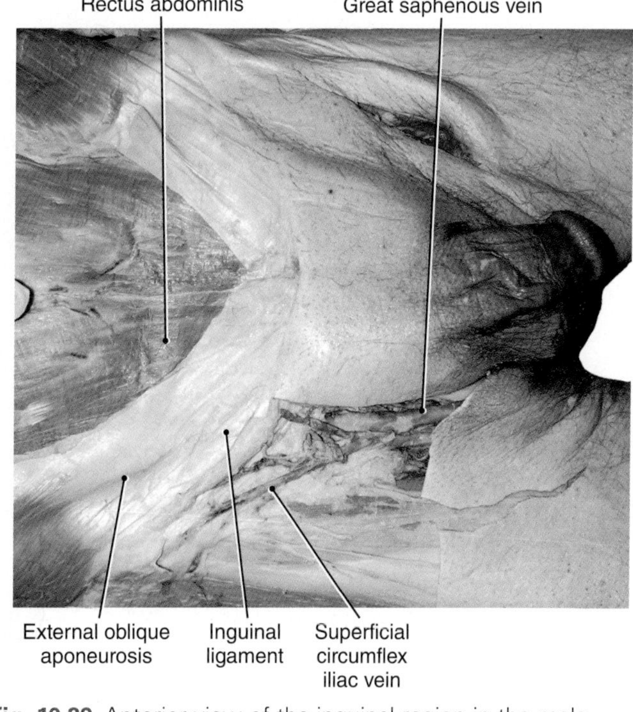

Fig. 10.29 Anterior view of the inguinal region in the male.

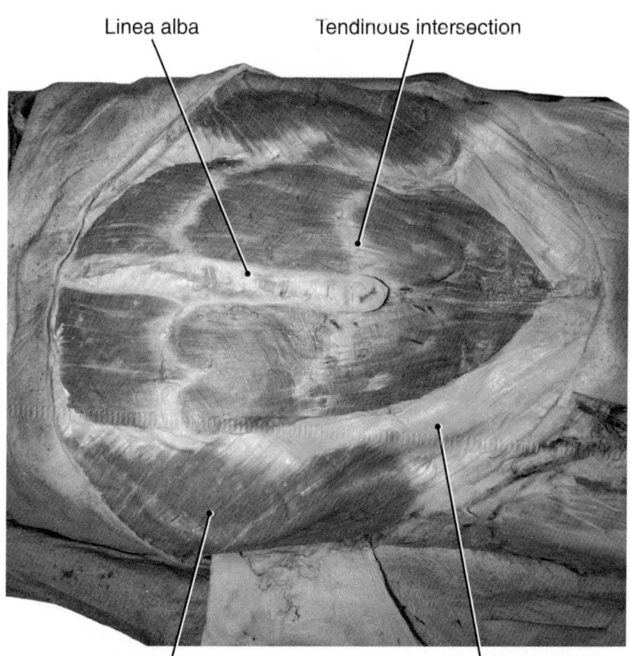

Fig. 10.28 Anterior view of the anterior abdominal wall. With muscles intact, note the linea alba and external abdominal oblique muscle and its aponeurosis.

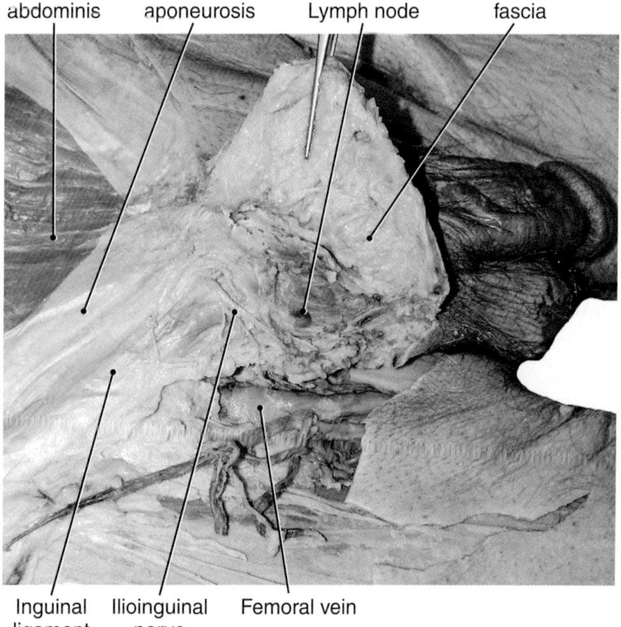

Fig. 10.30 Anterior view of the inguinal region in the male showing the ilioinguinal nerve.

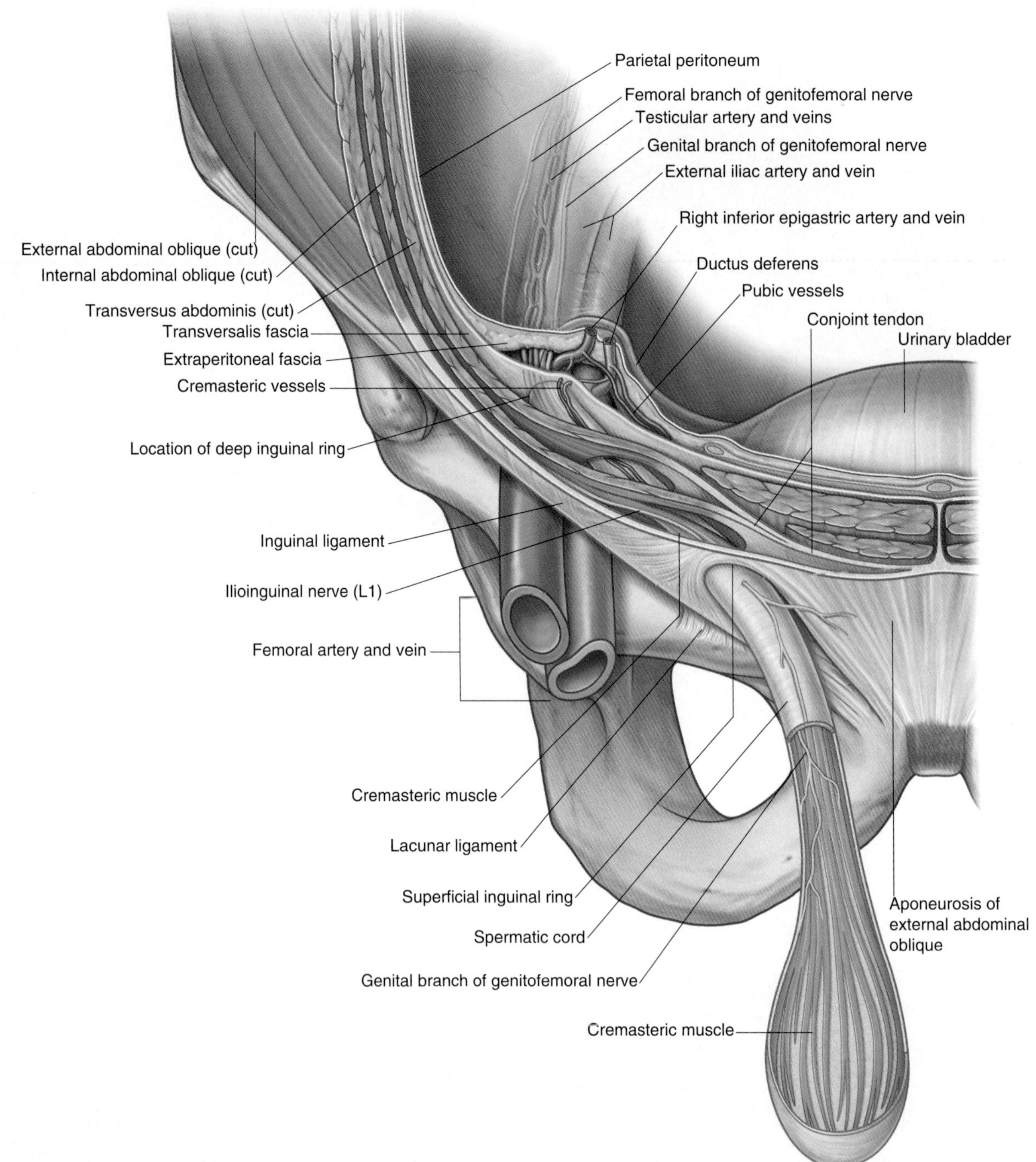

Plate 10.2 Inguinal canal and spermatic cord. (From Drake RL et al. *Gray's Atlas of Anatomy*, 3rd edition, Philadelphia, Elsevier, 2021, p. 148.)

by the external spermatic fascia (see Figs. 10.31 and 10.32).

- Identify the superomedial part of the inguinal ligament, the *superior crus*, and the inferolateral part, the *inferior crus* (Fig. 10.33).
- Just superior and anterior to the superior crus, identify the ilioinguinal nerve.
- Look for the genital branch of the genitofemoral nerve as it travels through the deep and the superficial inguinal rings within the spermatic cord.
- Retract the testis laterally (see Fig. 10.33).
- With scissors, cut the aponeurosis of the external abdominal oblique muscle between the two crura at the superficial inguinal ring (Fig. 10.34).
- Place the scissors underneath the external spermatic fascia and make a small incision (Fig. 10.35) to expose the contents of the spermatic cord (Fig. 10.36).

DISSECTION TIP

Place your index finger in the opening of the superficial inguinal ring to appreciate the oblique course of the *spermatic cord* through the body wall toward the deep ring.

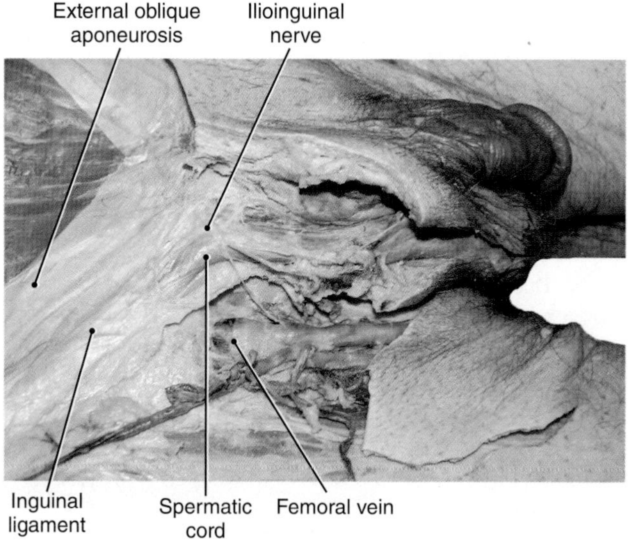

Fig. 10.31 Anterior view of the inguinal region in the male.

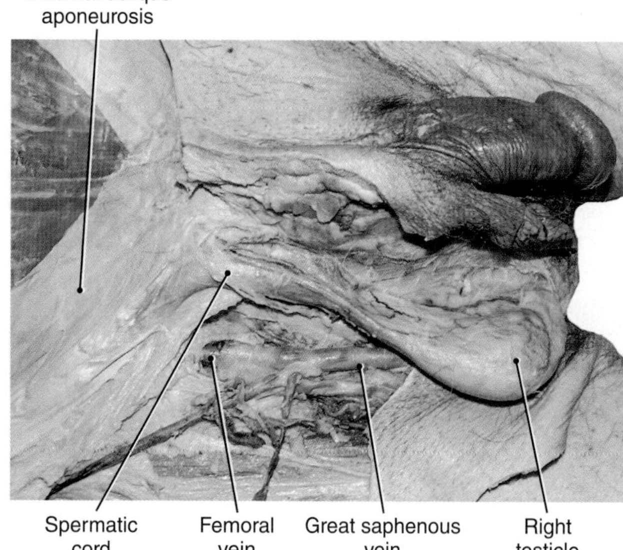

Fig. 10.33 Inguinal region, noting the superficial ring of inguinal canal and spermatic cord and right testicle.

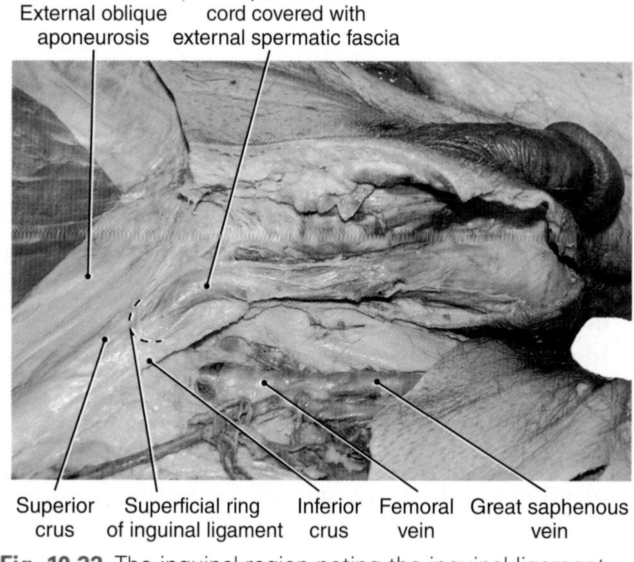

Fig. 10.32 The inguinal region noting the inguinal ligament.

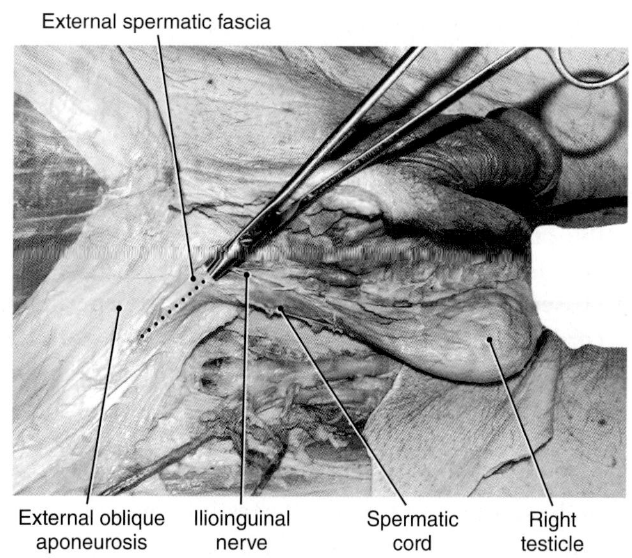

Fig. 10.34 Inguinal and proximal femoral regions.

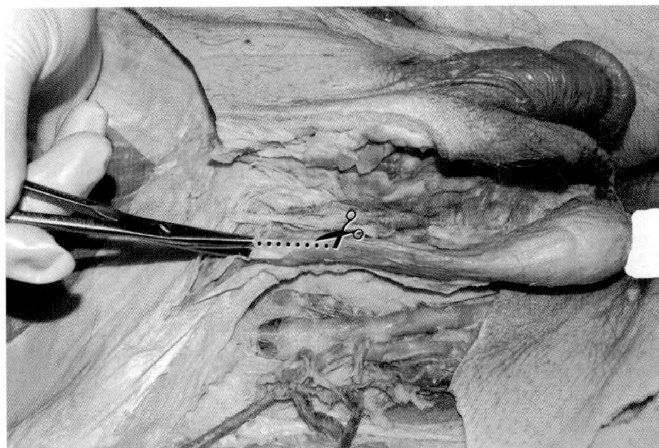

Fig. 10.35 Inguinal and proximal femoral regions.

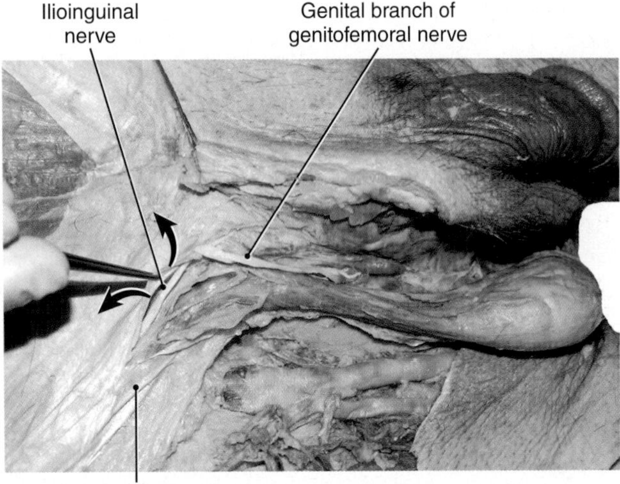

Fig. 10.36 Inguinal region. Note the genital branch of the genitofemoral nerve.

ANATOMY **NOTE**

In the female, the *round ligament* of the uterus replaces the spermatic cord in the inguinal canal. The fascia covering the spermatic cord, and specifically its superolateral aspect, is named the *cremasteric fascia.*

- **Incise the external spermatic fascia, formed by the external abdominal oblique muscle.**
- **Trace the pampiniform venous plexus, and incise the cremasteric fascia, derived from the internal abdominal oblique muscle.**
- **Dissect the deepest fascial layer of the spermatic cord, the *internal spermatic fascia,* formed from the transversalis fascia, and identify the ductus deferens (Fig. 10.37, Plate 10.3).**
- **Identify the cremasteric artery (Fig. 10.38).**
- **Continue the incision of the external spermatic fascia to the scrotum and expose the testis in the scrotal sac.**
- **Lift the spermatic cord and liberate the testis from the scrotum (Fig. 10.39).**

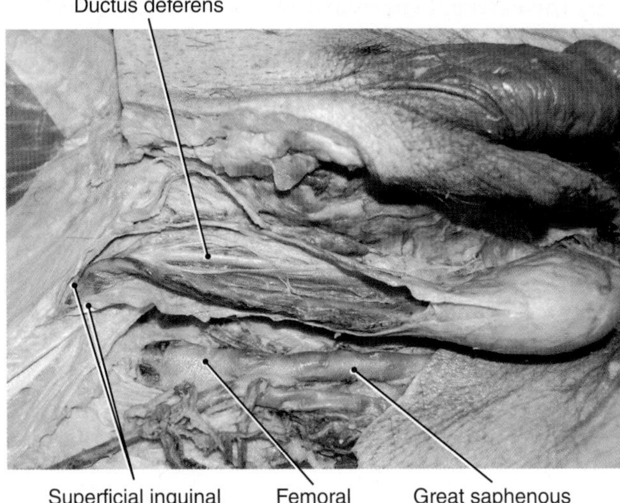

Fig. 10.37 With deeper dissection within the spermatic cord, note the ductus deferens.

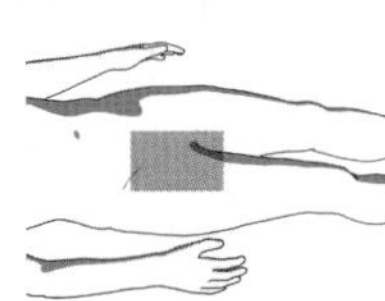

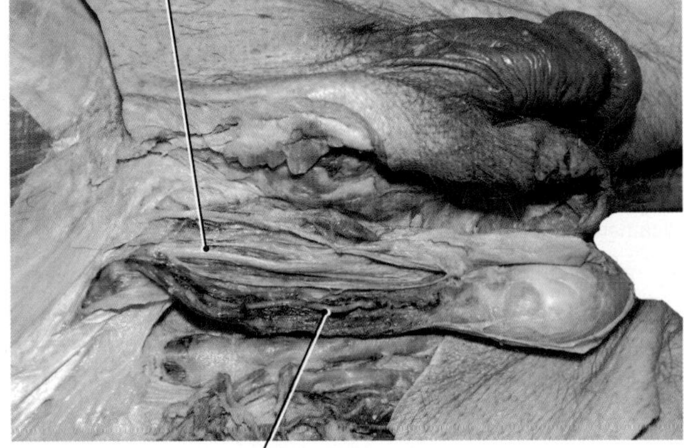

Fig. 10.38 Inguinal region in the male showing cremasteric artery.

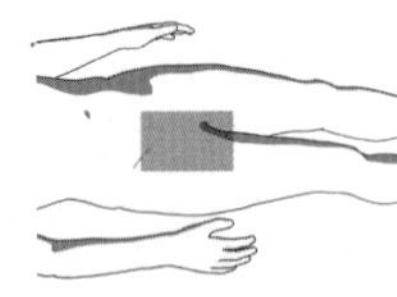

- **Note the outermost layer, called the parietal layer, and the inner, visceral layer of the tunica vaginalis, connecting the epididymis to the testis (with a distinct fold).**
- **Identify the epididymis, and note its head, body, and tail (see Fig. 10.39).**
- **Hold the testis and with a scalpel make a longitudinal incision to open its coverings (Fig. 10.40).**
- **Identify the dense capsule of the testis, the *tunica albuginea*, and the septae, which arise from the capsule, and divide the testis into several compartments.**

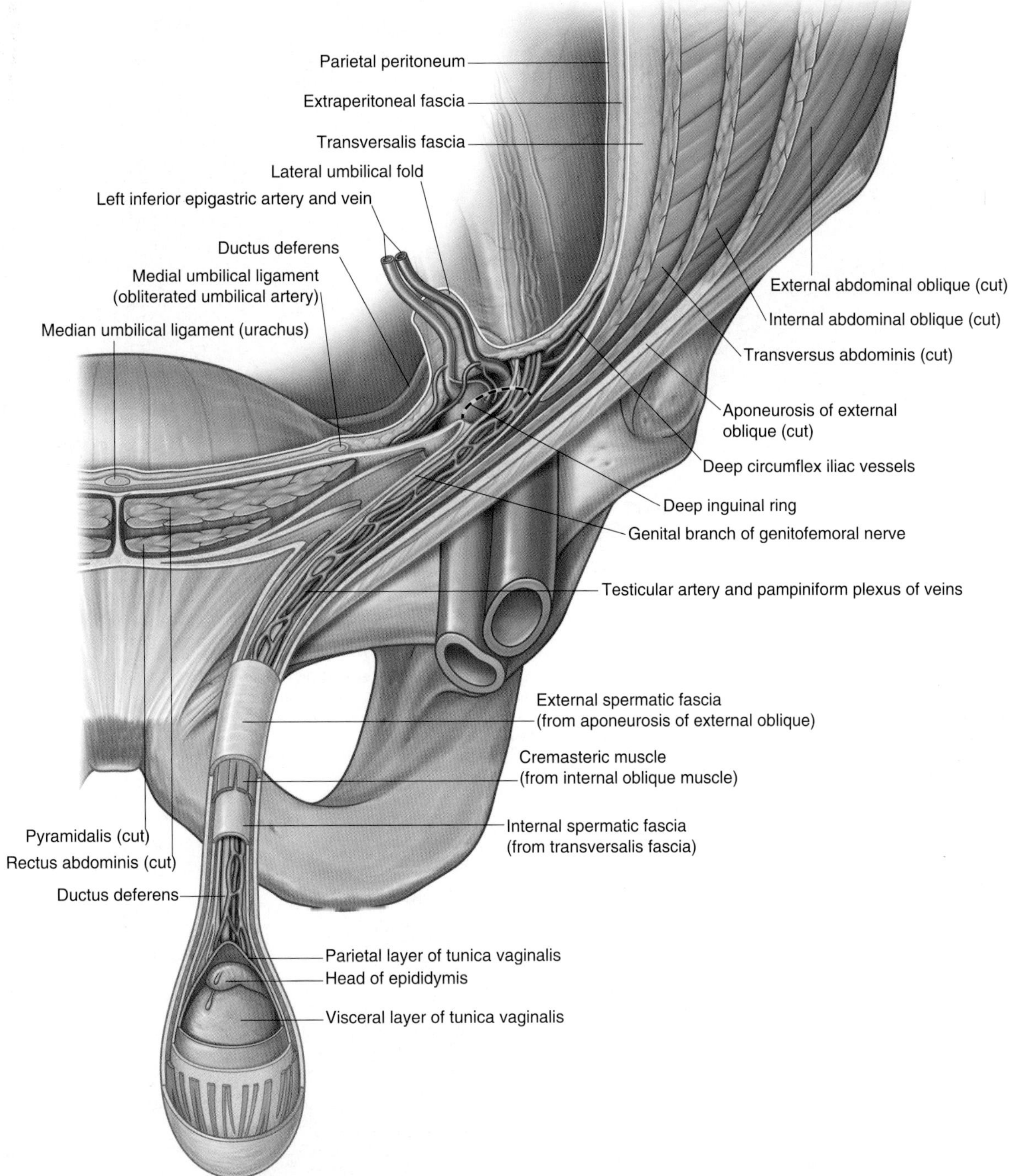

Plate 10.3 Inguinal canal and contents of spermatic cord. (From Drake RL et al. *Gray's Atlas of Anatomy*, 3rd edition, Philadelphia, Elsevier, 2021, p. 149.)

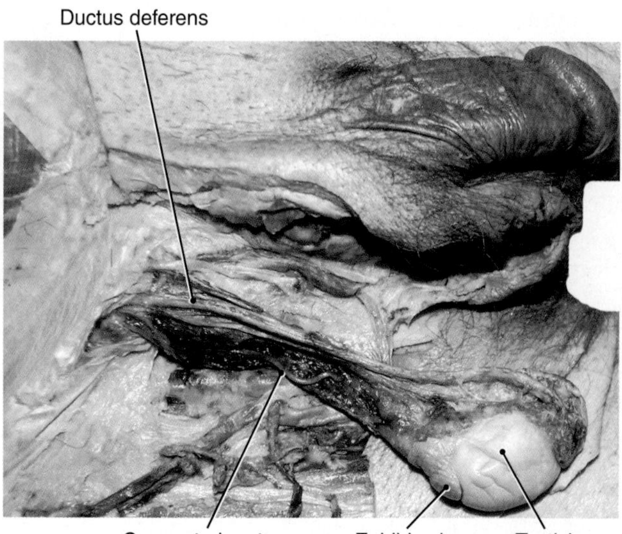

Fig. 10.39 Inguinal region showing epididymis and its relationship to ductus deferens.

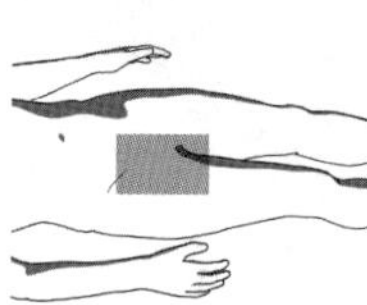

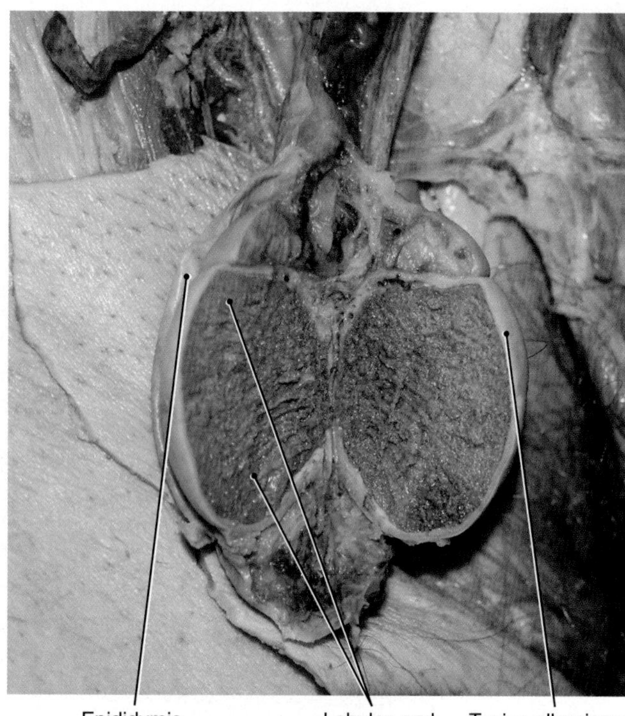

Fig. 10.40 Coronal section through the proximal testis noting its layers and components.

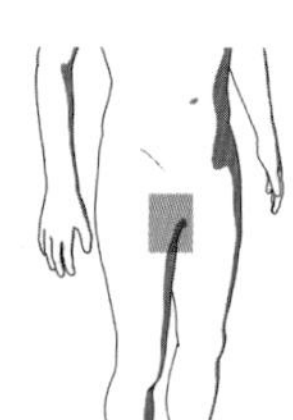

DISSECTION **TIP**

If you dissect a female cadaver and a uterus is present, identify the round ligament of the uterus.

ANATOMY **NOTE**

The round ligament (ligamentum teres) of the uterus is a fibrous cord traveling from the uterus through the inguinal canal to attach to the labia majora. Identify the round ligament at the superficial ring and follow it toward the labia majora.

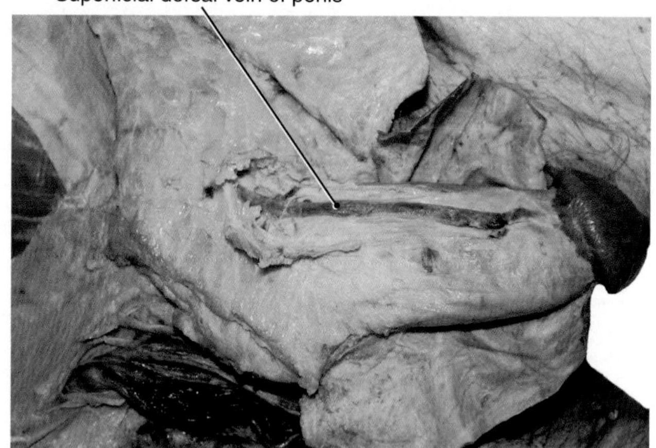

Fig. 10.41 Deeper dissection of the dorsal penis shows superficial dorsal vein of penis.

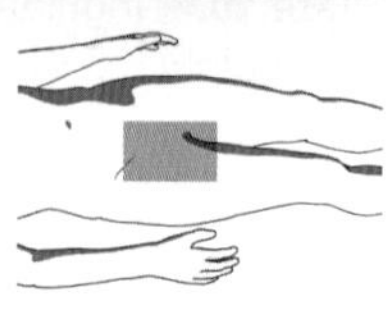

- **Cut the skin covering the penis.**
- **Continue to remove fat and skin over the pubic symphysis and the penis.**
- **Identify the superficial dorsal vein of the penis embedded in the superficial fascia of the penis (Fig. 10.41).**
- **Dissect out and reflect the superficial fascia of the penis laterally (Fig. 10.42).**
- **Notice the deep fascia, *Buck's fascia*, of the penis deep to the superficial fascia.**
- **On the dorsal surface of the penis, note the separation between the superficial and deep dorsal veins of the penis by Buck's fascia (Fig. 10.43).**
- **Separate Buck's fascia and identify the dorsal artery of the penis, which is located bilaterally on the dorsum of the penis medial to the dorsal nerves of the penis (Fig. 10.44).**
- **Continue the removal of the fat toward the pubic symphysis and expose the fundiform ligament of the penis arising from the superficial fascia (Fig. 10.45).**
- **Insert scissors or a probe into the superficial ring just underneath the tendon of the external abdominal oblique muscle, directed toward the anterior superior iliac spine (Fig. 10.46).**

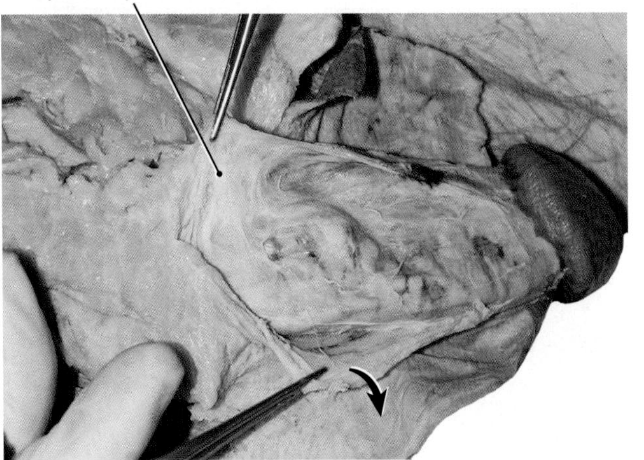

Fig. 10.42 Dorsal view of penis and its related fascia.

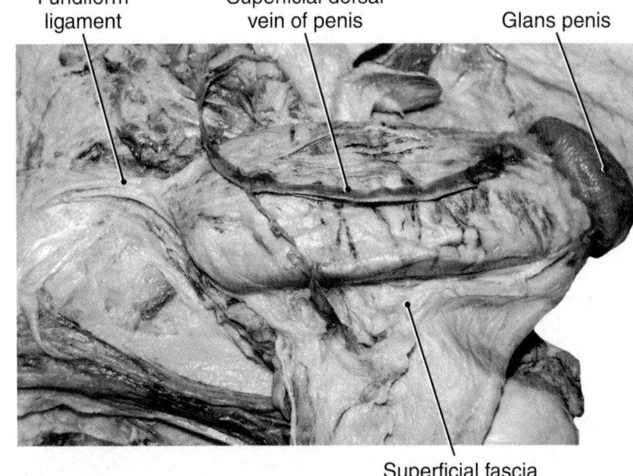

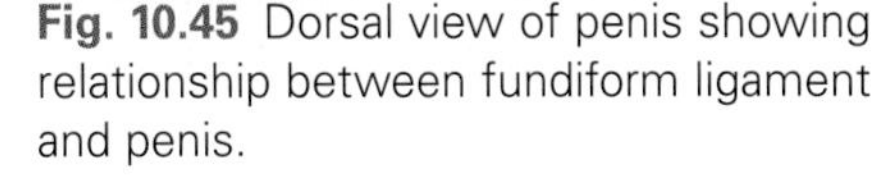

Fig. 10.45 Dorsal view of penis showing relationship between fundiform ligament and penis.

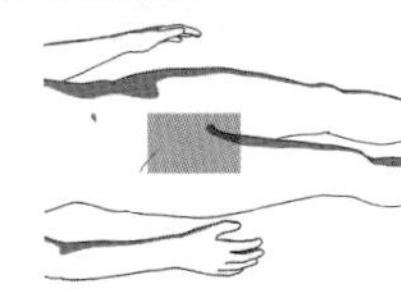

Dorsal nerve of penis
Superficial dorsal vein of penis
Buck's fascia
Ductus deferens
Deep dorsal vein of penis

Fig. 10.43 Dorsal view of penis showing relationship between the superficial and deep fasciae. Note the position of the superficial dorsal vein of penis.

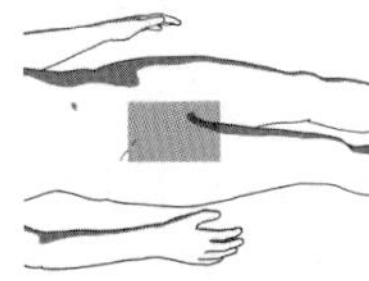

Anterior superior iliac spine
Inguinal ligament
Superficial inguinal ring

Fig. 10.46 The superficial inguinal ring is opened, revealing deeper structures of the inguinal canal.

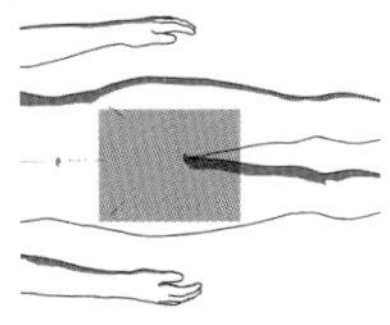

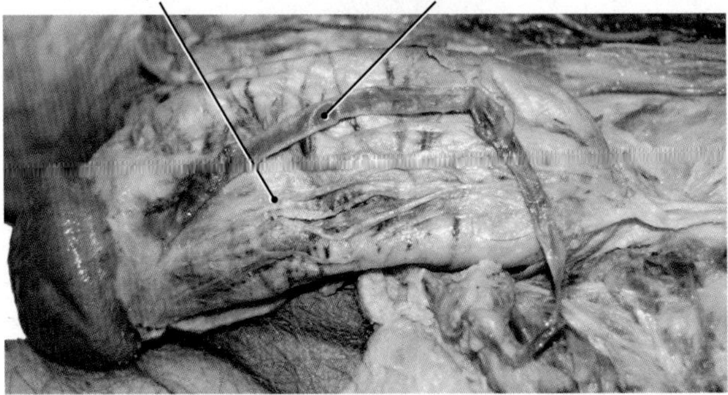

Fig. 10.44 Dorsal view of the penis with deeper dissection, showing the underlying dorsal nerve of penis and its branches.

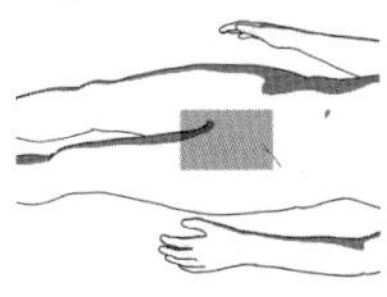

- **Incise the inguinal ligament over the probe or scissors that was previously inserted and reflect its borders laterally (Fig. 10.47).**
- **Pull the spermatic cord laterally and expose the lacunar ligament (Gimbernat's ligament), which represents the medial triangular expansion of the inguinal ligament to the pectineal line of the pubis (Figs. 10.48 and 10.49).**
- **Locate the pectineal ligament (Cooper's ligament), which is a strong fibrous band that extends laterally from the lacunar ligament along the pectineal line of the pubis (see Figs. 10.48 and 10.49).**

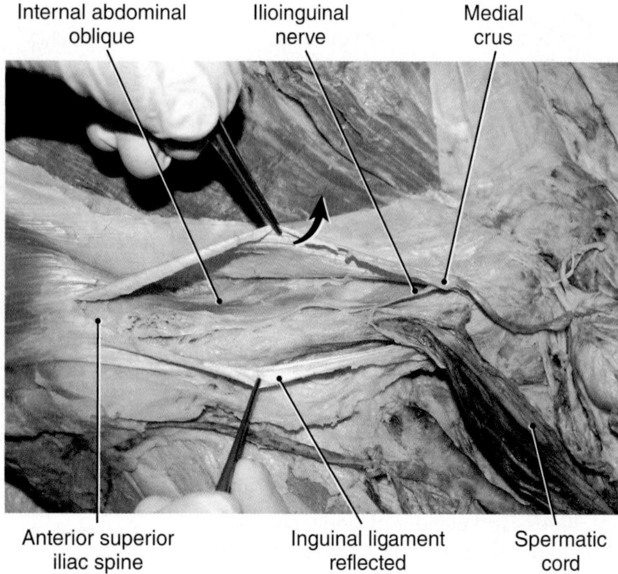

Fig. 10.47 Inguinal region on the right side, showing the exposed inguinal canal and its contents.

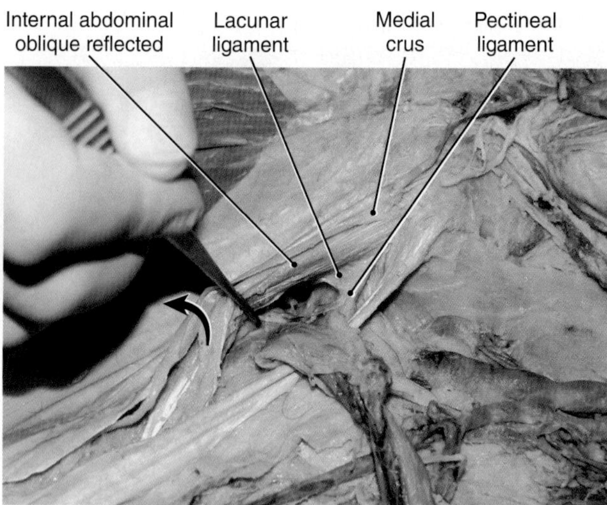

Fig. 10.49 Inguinal region on the right side, showing specializations of the inguinal ligament, the lacunar and pectineal ligaments.

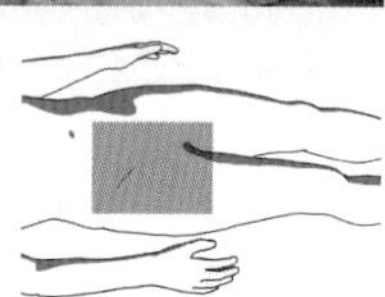

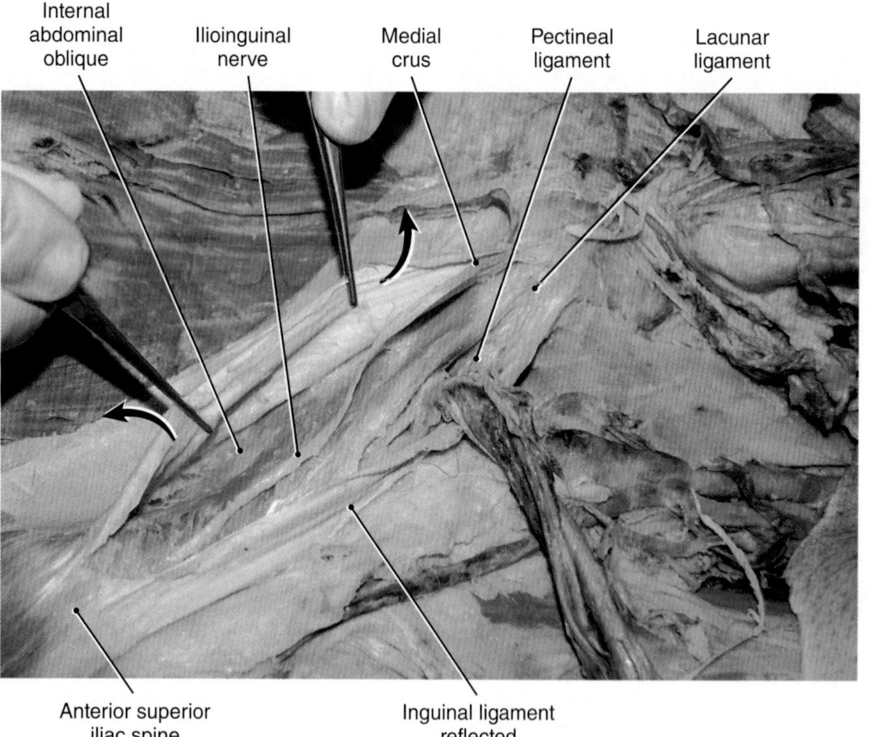

Fig. 10.48 Inguinal region on the right side. Note the specializations of the inguinal ligament—the lacunar and pectineal ligaments.

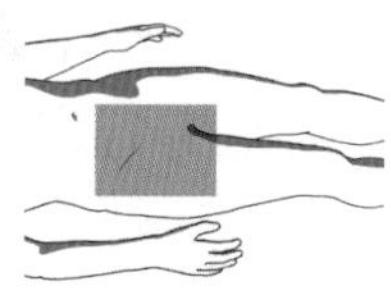

LABORATORY IDENTIFICATION CHECKLIST

NERVES

- ☐ Iliohypogastric
- ☐ Ilioinguinal
- ☐ Genitofemoral
  - ☐ Genital branch
  - ☐ Femoral branch
- ☐ Dorsal, of penis
- ☐ Femoral

ARTERY

- ☐ Cremasteric
- ☐ Inferior epigastric

VEINS

- ☐ Inferior epigastric
- ☐ Superficial external pudendal
- ☐ Superficial dorsal, of penis
- ☐ Femoral
- ☐ Great saphenous

MUSCLES

- ☐ External abdominal oblique
  - ☐ External abdominal oblique aponeurosis
- ☐ Internal abdominal oblique
- ☐ Cremasteric
- ☐ Transversus abdominis
- ☐ Rectus abdominis
  - ☐ Tendinous intersections
  - ☐ Linea alba

BONES

- ☐ Pubis
  - ☐ Pubic tubercle
  - ☐ Pubic crest
- ☐ Ischium
- ☐ Ilium
  - ☐ Anterior superior iliac spine

LIGAMENTS

- ☐ Inguinal
  - ☐ Superficial ring
  - ☐ Deep ring
- ☐ Lacunar
- ☐ Pectineal
- ☐ Fundiform

FASCIA

- ☐ Superficial
  - ☐ Fatty or Camper's layer
  - ☐ Membranous or Scarpa's layer
- ☐ External spermatic
- ☐ Cremasteric
- ☐ Superficial, of penis
- ☐ Deep, of penis

OTHER STRUCTURES

- ☐ Spermatic cord
- ☐ Testes
  - ☐ Lobules
  - ☐ Septae
- ☐ Epididymis
- ☐ Ductus deferens
- ☐ Tunica vaginalis
- ☐ Tunica albuginea

THREE DIFFERENT TECHNIQUES FOR OPENING THE PERITONEAL CAVITY

DISSECTION TIP

All cuts with the scalpel should be made carefully to avoid cutting too deeply into the peritoneal cavity and underlying viscera.

Technique 1

- **After removal of the skin over the anterolateral abdominal wall, palpate the most inferior costal cartilages and the xiphoid process (Fig. 11.1).**
- **With scissors or a scalpel, cut the attachments of the rectus abdominis and external abdominal oblique muscles over the right and left hypochondriac areas (Fig. 11.2).**
- **Continue the incision of the muscles from the xiphoid process toward the midaxillary line on both sides of the cadaver (Fig. 11.3). A variation of this technique is the continuation of the reflection of the anterior thoracic wall with the anterior abdominal wall as one block toward the pubic symphysis.**
- **Reflect the rectus abdominis and abdominal oblique muscles inferiorly (Fig. 11.4).**

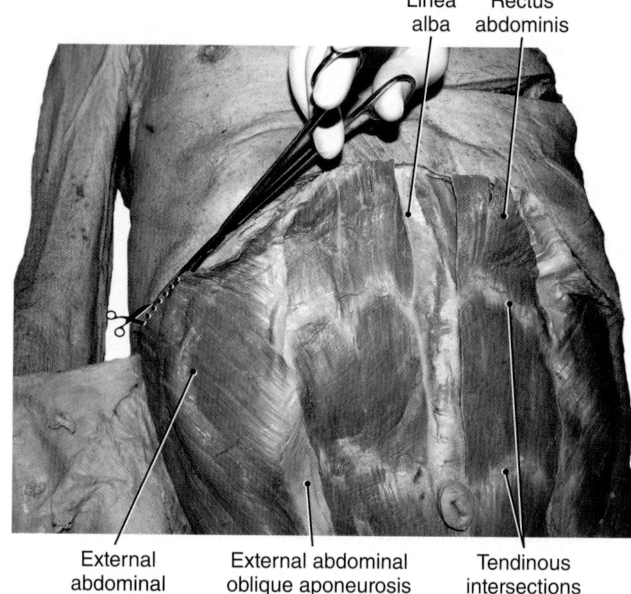

Fig. 11.2 Attachments of the rectus abdominis and external oblique muscles incised over the right and left hypochondriac areas.

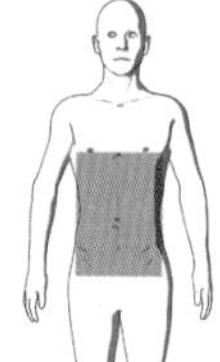

Fig. 11.1 Anterior abdomen with skin and subcutaneous tissue reflected revealing the rectus abdominis and external oblique muscles.

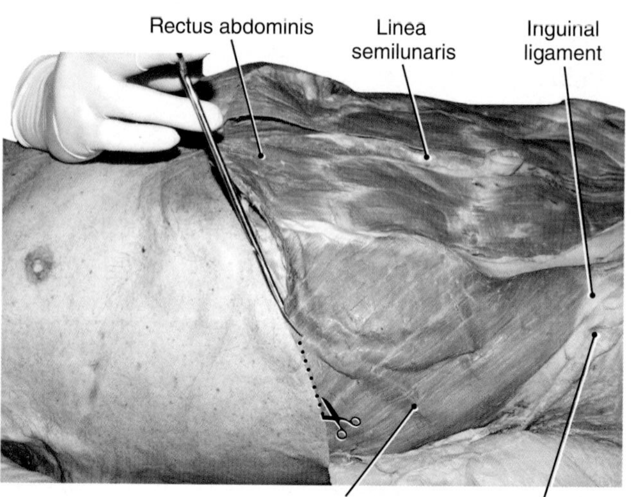

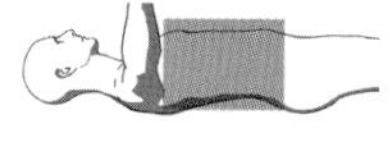

Fig. 11.3 Incision of the muscles from the xiphoid process to the midaxillary line on both sides.

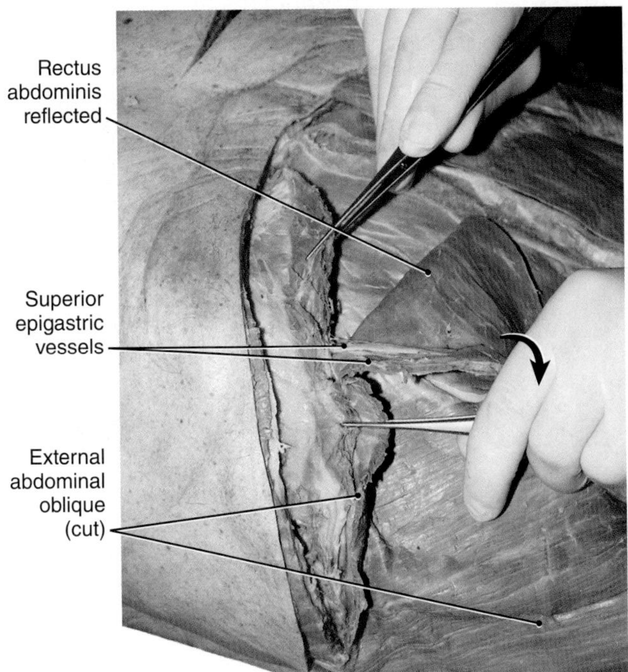

Fig. 11.4 Rectus abdominis and abdominal oblique muscles reflected inferiorly.

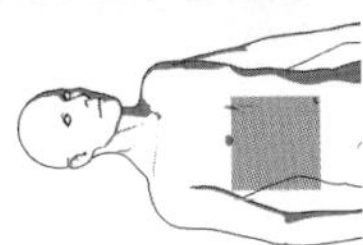

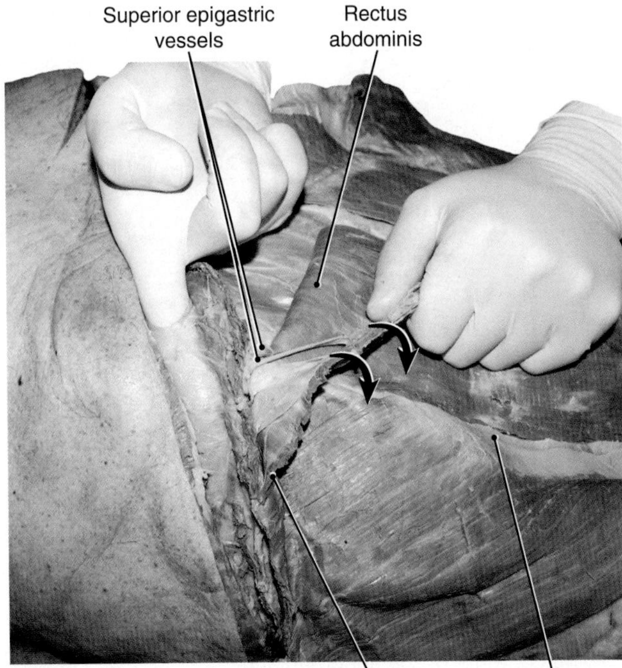

Fig. 11.5 Blunt dissection to expose the peritoneal cavity.

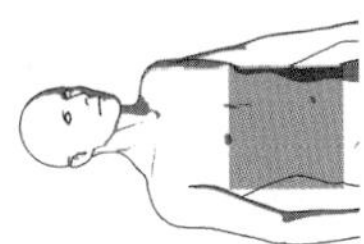

- When necessary, use blunt dissection to expose the peritoneal cavity (Fig. 11.5).
- Cut the attachments of the diaphragm, falciform ligament, and ligamentum teres (round ligament) of the liver to the abdominal wall.
- Reflect the anterolateral abdominal wall toward the pubic symphysis and observe the contents of the abdominal cavity (Figs. 11.6 and 11.7).

Technique 2

- Reflect the rectus sheath and expose the rectus abdominis muscle and the posterior lamina of the rectus sheath (Figs. 11.8 and 11.9).
- Make a midline vertical incision at the linea alba from the xiphoid process to the pubic symphysis.
- Make a second horizontal incision from the xiphoid process to the midaxillary line and reflect the muscle flap laterally (Fig. 11.10).
- Use the same technique on the contralateral side and expose the peritoneal cavity (Fig. 11.11).

Technique 3

- Make a midline vertical incision on the linea alba from the xiphoid process to the pubic symphysis.
- Make a second horizontal incision from the right to the left midaxillary lines, passing through the umbilicus, and laterally reflect the four muscle flaps (Fig. 11.12).
- Identify and cut the falciform and round ligaments on the anterior surface of the liver.

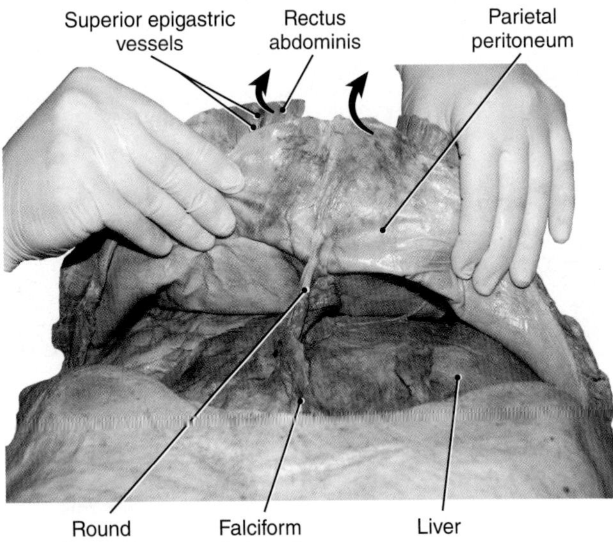

Fig. 11.6 Attachments of the diaphragm, falciform ligament, and round ligament of the liver incised at the abdominal wall, with the anterolateral abdominal wall reflected toward the pubic symphysis.

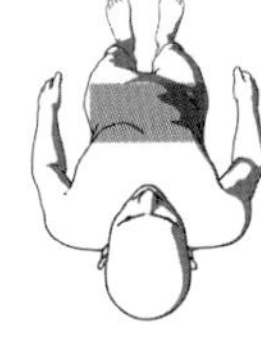

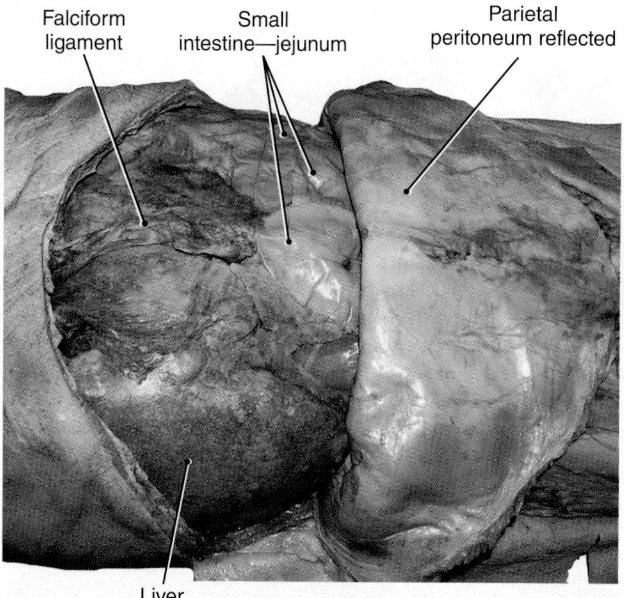

Fig. 11.7 Parietal peritoneum reflected, showing contents of the abdomen and anterolateral abdominal wall.

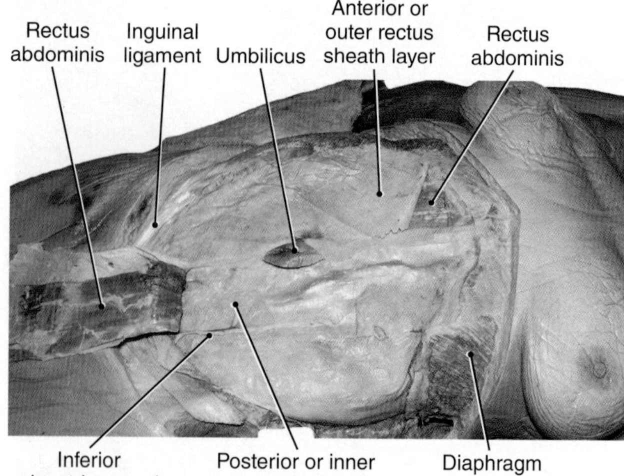

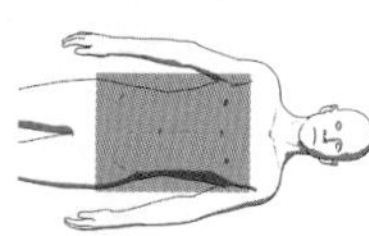

Fig. 11.9 Observe the exposed rectus abdominis muscles and posterior lamina of the rectus sheath.

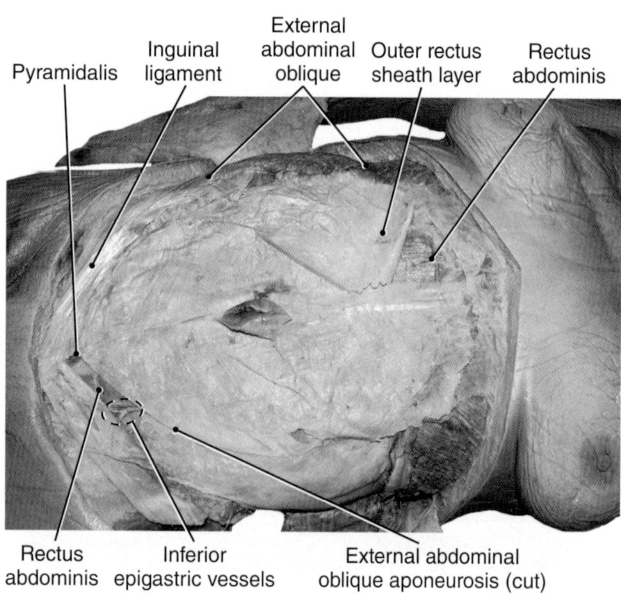

Fig. 11.8 Rectus sheath reflected.

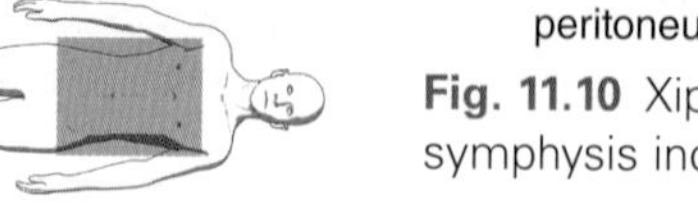

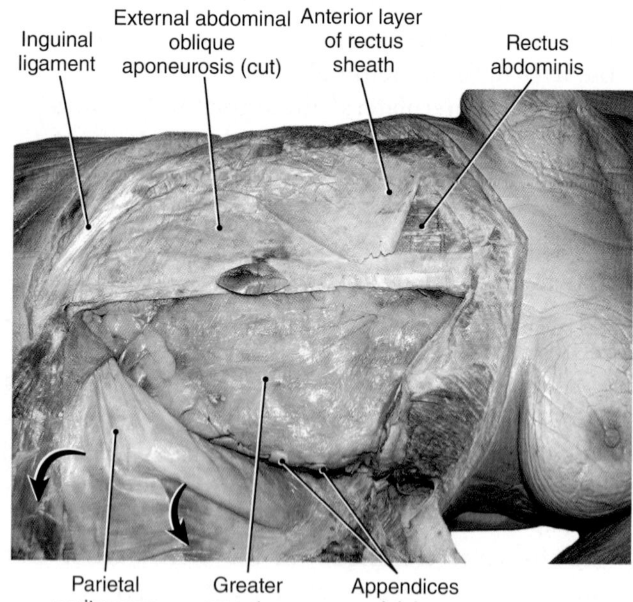

Fig. 11.10 Xiphoid process to pubic symphysis incision.

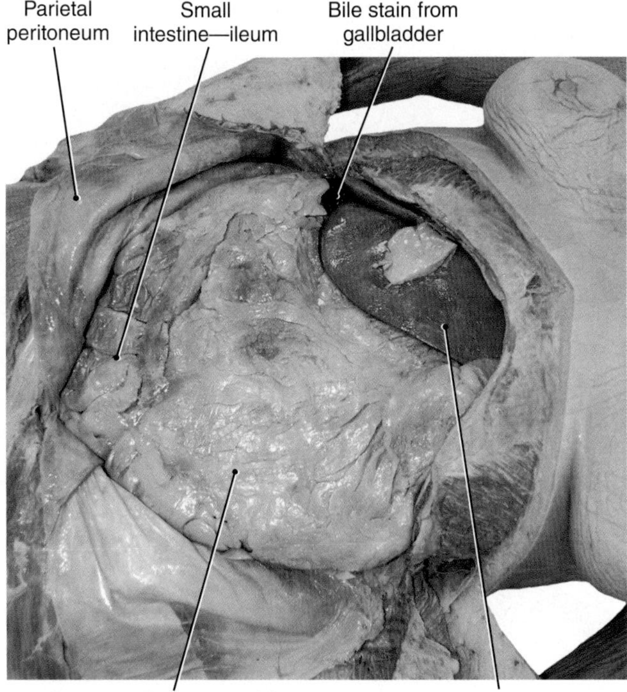

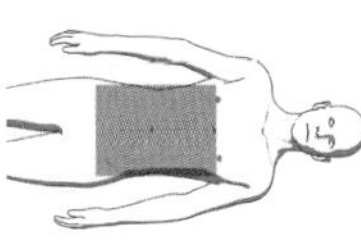

Fig. 11.11 Second horizontal incision from the xiphoid process to the midaxillary line on both sides with the laterally reflected muscle flap.

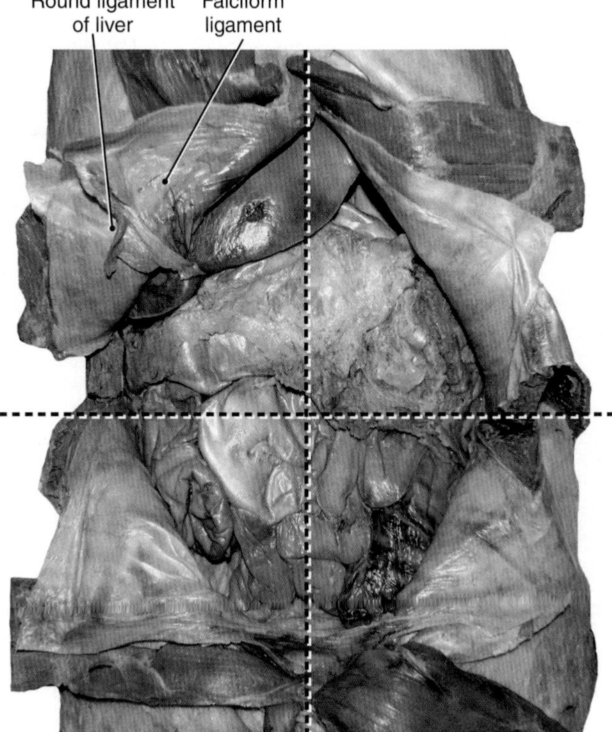

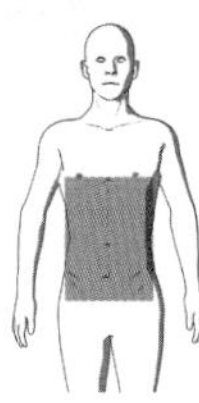

Fig. 11.12 Midline vertical incision at the linea alba from the xiphoid process to pubic symphysis, with the second horizontal incision from right to left midaxillary lines through the umbilicus, with four muscle flaps reflected laterally.

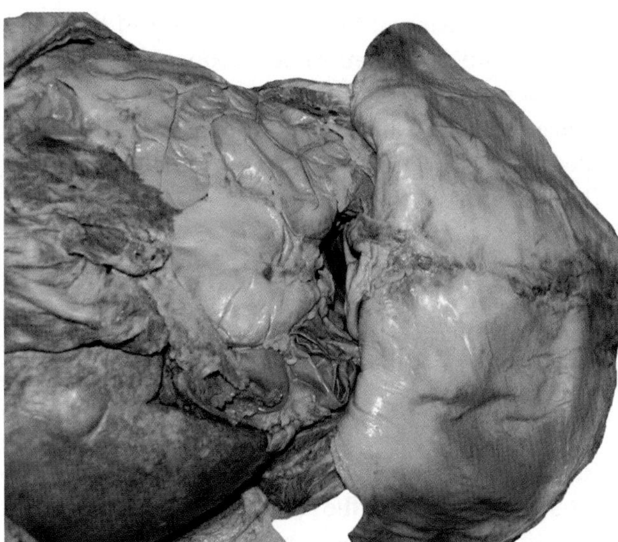

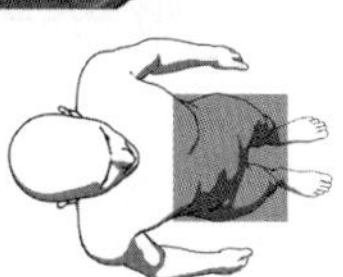

Fig. 11.13 Five peritoneal folds at the internal surface of the anterior abdominal wall: two lateral folds, two medial folds, and one median umbilical fold.

DISSECTION **TIP**

In some specimens the peritoneal cavity is small. To expose it further, with a saw, cut the ribs in the midaxillary line on both sides of the cadaver. You also may extend the cuts with those made previously to expose the thoracic cavity.

In some cadavers, you will be able to separate the parietal peritoneum from the transversalis fascia. In most, however, these two layers are tightly adherent.

PERITONEAL STRUCTURES

- **Trace the round ligament of the liver along its pathway from the anterior surface of the liver to the median aspect of the anterolateral abdominal wall to the umbilicus.**
- **At the internal (posterior) surface of the anterior abdominal wall, identify five notable peritoneal folds: the lateral (right and left), the medial (right and left), and the single median umbilical folds (Fig. 11.13).**

ANATOMY **NOTE**

The peritoneal fold covering the inferior epigastric artery and vein is the lateral umbilical peritoneal fold. The medial umbilical folds are formed by an elevation of the peritoneum over the obliterated umbilical arteries. Similarly, the median umbilical fold is an elevation of the peritoneum over the remnants of the urachus (intraabdominal part of allantois). The space between the medial umbilical fold and the median umbilical fold is termed the *supravesical fossa.* The depressed region between the medial umbilical fold and the lateral umbilical fold is termed the *medial inguinal fossa.* The lateral inguinal fossa is the area lateral to the lateral inguinal fold.

- Make an incision at the posterior layer of the rectus sheath (and peritoneum) and expose the rectus abdominis muscle (Fig. 11.14).
- Trace the course of the inferior epigastric artery and identify its origin from the external iliac artery (Figs. 11.15–11.17).

DISSECTION TIP

In approximately 30% of cadavers, the inferior epigastric artery will give rise to the obturator artery, which travels medially over the pelvic brim.

- Remove the peritoneum covering the inferior epigastric artery and the base of the rectus abdominis muscle, and identify the inguinal ligament (Fig. 11.18).

ANATOMY NOTE

Notice the triangle of Hesselbach formed by the lateral border of the rectus abdominis muscle, the inguinal ligament, and the inferior epigastric vessels.

- Laterally to the inferior epigastric artery and vein, identify the deep inguinal ring and the ductus deferens (round ligament of the uterus in females) passing within it.

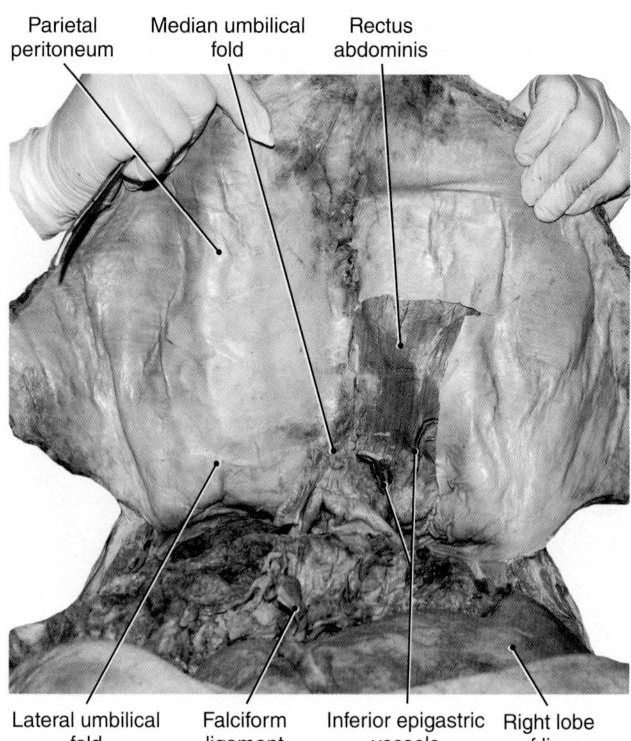

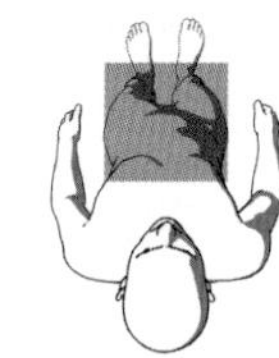

Fig. 11.15 Appreciate the inferior epigastric artery and vein, as well as the medial and lateral umbilical peritoneal folds.

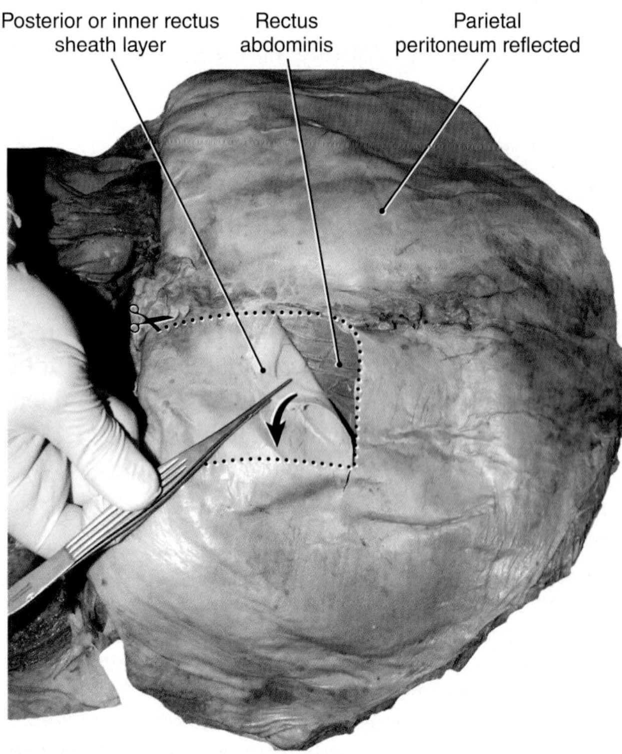

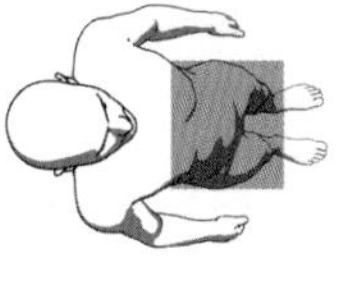

Fig. 11.14 Posterior layer of the rectus sheath cut exposing the rectus abdominis muscle.

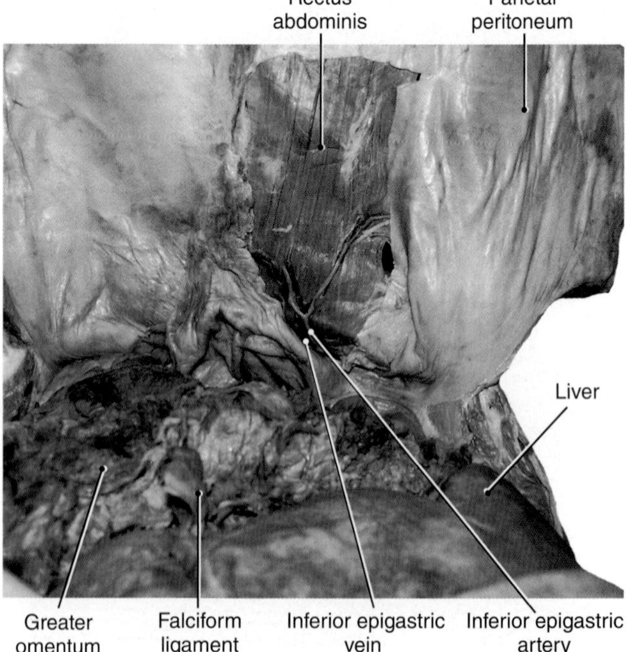

Fig. 11.16 Dissect the inferior epigastric artery and vein.

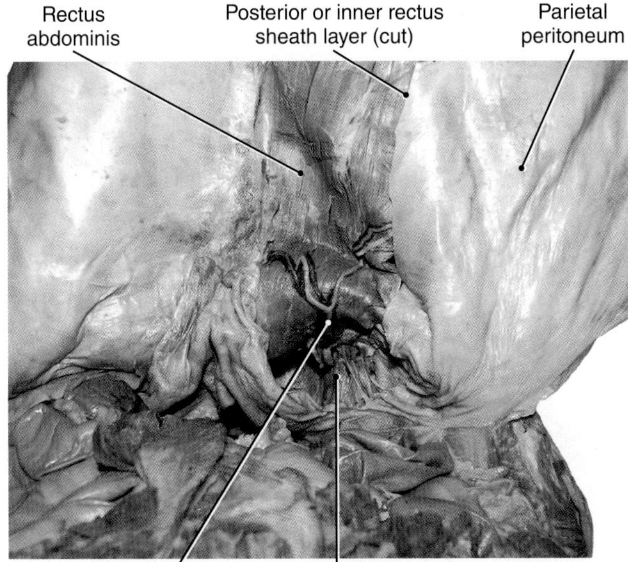

Fig. 11.17 Dissect the inferior epigastric artery where it arises from the external iliac artery.

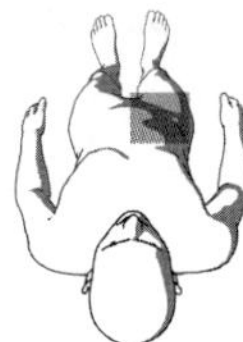

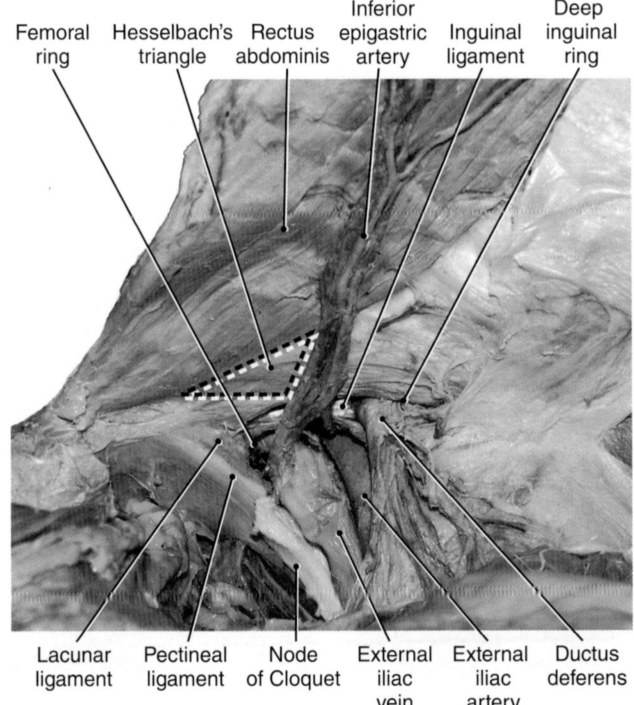

Fig. 11.18 Dissect the peritoneum covering the inferior epigastric artery and base of the rectus abdominis muscle and identify the inguinal ligament. Continue the dissection by locating the pubic tubercle, and lateral to it, identify the pectineal ligament.

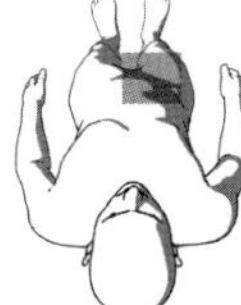

- **Continue the dissection by identifying the pubic tubercle and, lateral to it, a strong ligamentous band running over the periosteum of the pectineal line, the *pectineal ligament* (Cooper's ligament) (see Fig. 11.18).**
- **Note the medial one-third of the inguinal ligament forming an aponeurotic expansion attaching to the pectineal line of the pubis and pectineal ligament, the *lacunar ligament* (Gimbernat's ligament) (see Fig. 11.18).**
- **Lateral to the lacunar ligament, expose the femoral vessels and identify the *femoral ring* (lying medial to the femoral vein), the opening to the femoral canal.**

DISSECTION **TIP**

Clean the adipose tissue at the proximal femoral canal and look for a large lymph node, the *node of Cloquet.*

- **Retract the femoral vein medially and note a fascial partition under the inguinal ligament between the femoral vein and the iliopsoas muscle. This partition between the vascular portion (lacuna vasorum) and the muscular portion (lacuna musculorum) is called the *iliopectineal ligament* (see Fig. 11.18).**
- **Inspect the contents of the peritoneal cavity and identify the liver, stomach (with its greater and lesser curvatures), small and large intestines, and greater omentum (Fig. 11.19).**

ANATOMY **NOTE**

The peritoneal cavity is traditionally divided into two parts, the greater and lesser sacs, or into supracolic and infracolic compartments. The *greater sac* is the entire area of the peritoneal cavity with the exception of the area extending behind the stomach to the diaphragm at the left side, which is the *lesser sac* (omental bursa). Similarly, the *supracolic compartment* is the area of the peritoneal cavity that extends from the transverse mesocolon to the diaphragm. The *infracolic compartment* is the area of the peritoneal cavity extending from the transverse mesocolon below to the pelvic brim.

- **Identify the greater curvature of the stomach and lift the greater omentum (Fig. 11.20).**
- **Expose the transverse colon with its transverse mesocolon and identify the ileum, jejunum, cecum, and ascending, transverse, descending, and sigmoid colons (Fig. 11.21).**
- **Observe the space between the liver and the stomach and identify the gallbladder and lesser omentum (Fig. 11.22).**
- **With blunt dissection using your fingertips, separate any adhesions between the stomach and the liver (Fig. 11.23).**

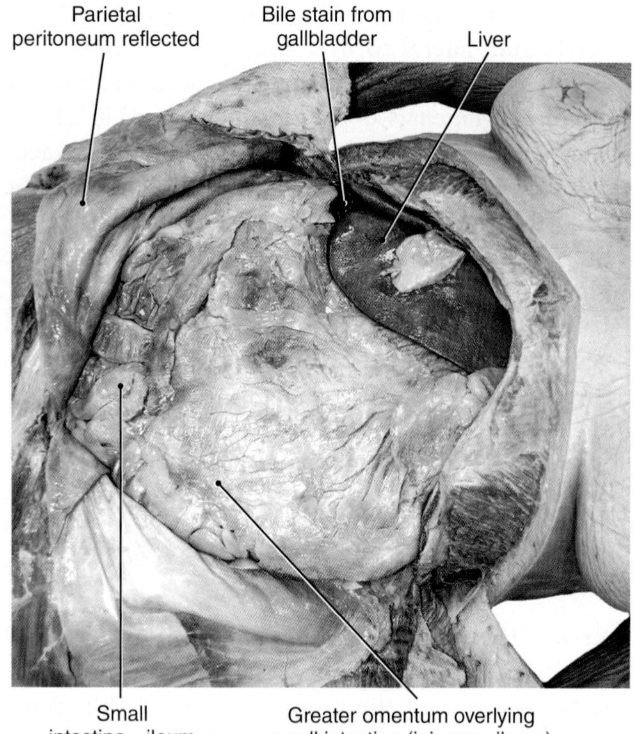

Fig. 11.19 Appreciate the liver, stomach, small and large intestines, and greater omentum.

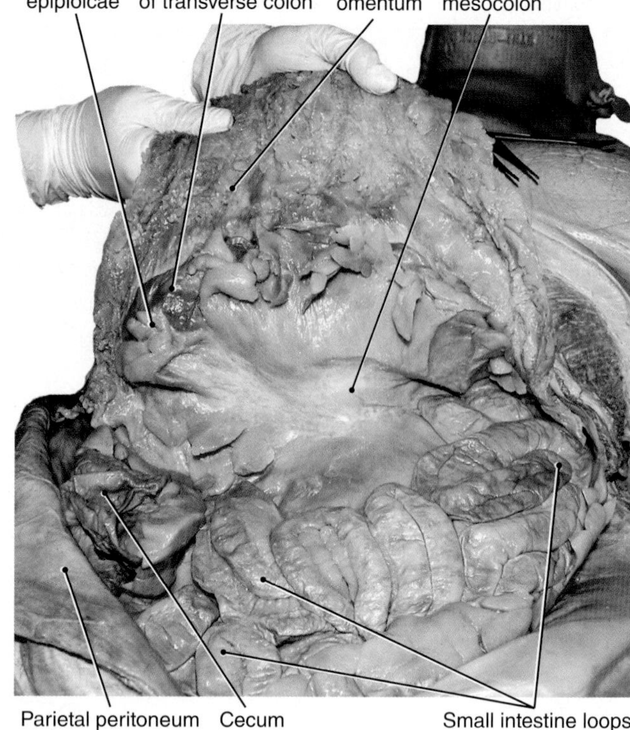

Fig. 11.21 Expose and locate the transverse colon and mesocolon.

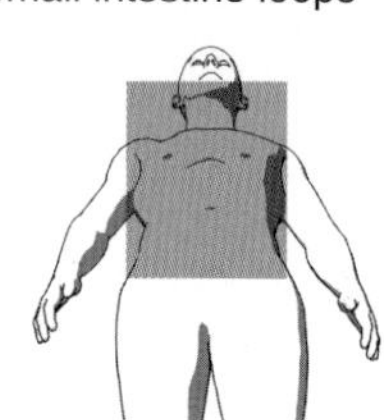

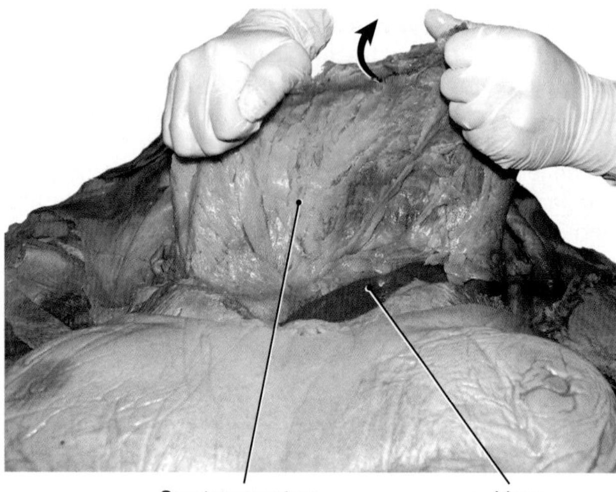

Fig. 11.20 Lift the greater omentum at the greater curvature of stomach.

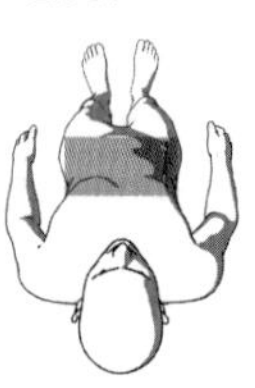

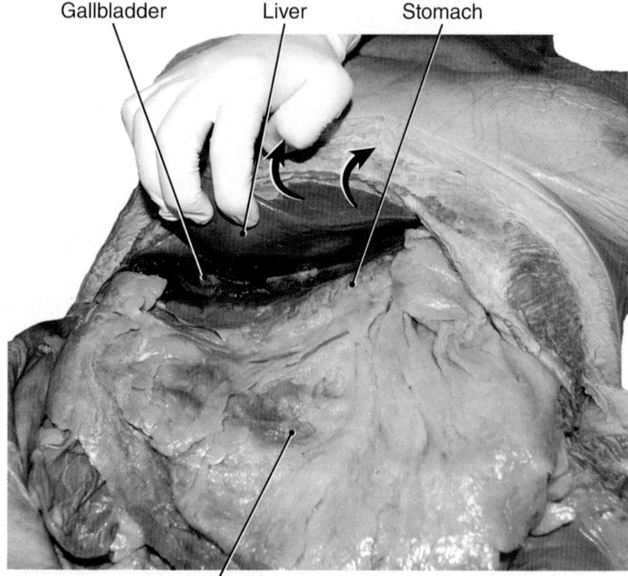

Fig. 11.22 Locate the space between the liver and stomach and identify the gallbladder and lesser omentum.

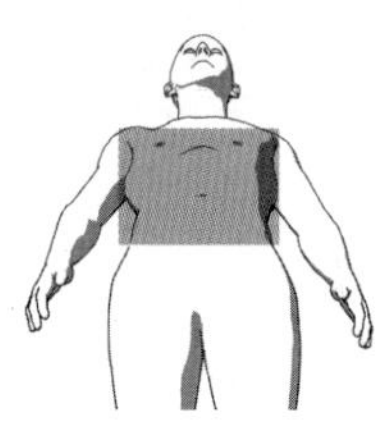

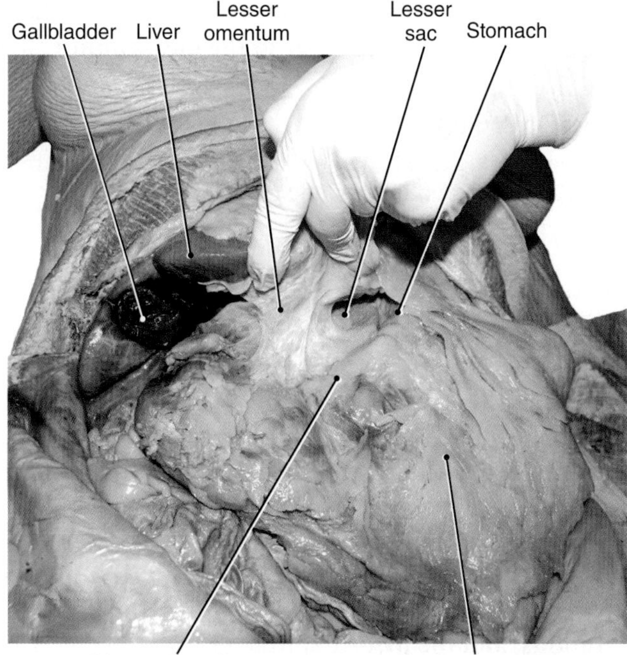

Fig. 11.23 Continue the blunt dissection with your fingers.

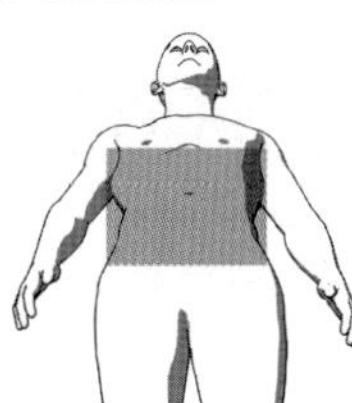

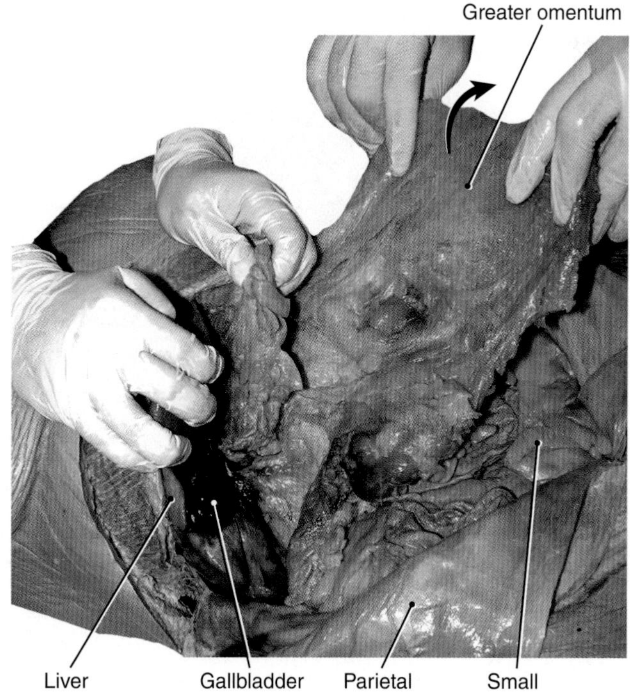

Fig. 11.24 Cut the greater omentum approximately 3 cm from the greater curvature of the stomach but do *not* cut its connection with the transverse colon.

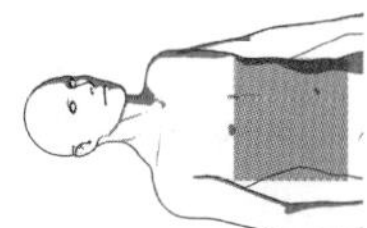

DISSECTION TIP

Often, you will find several adhesions between the contents of the peritoneal cavity. Take some time and separate these adhesions to restore the normal anatomy and position of the organs.

- **Cut the greater omentum 3 to 4 cm away from the greater curvature and leave its attachments to the transverse colon (Fig. 11.24).**
- **Pull the stomach away from the transverse colon and note the area of the lesser sac. Also notice the pancreas lying directly behind the stomach (Fig. 11.25).**
- **Continue the dissection by pulling the stomach inferiorly from the liver and note the omental (*epiploic*) *foramen* (of Winslow) (Fig. 11.26).**
- **Pass a probe or scissors underneath the lesser omentum through the epiploic foramen (Fig. 11.27 and Plate 11.1).**

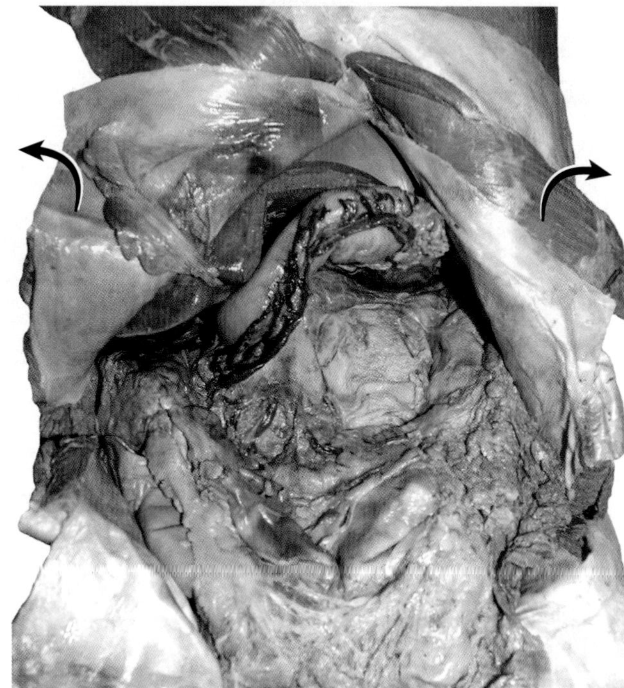

Fig. 11.25 Pull the stomach from the transverse colon to appreciate the lesser sac and pancreas.

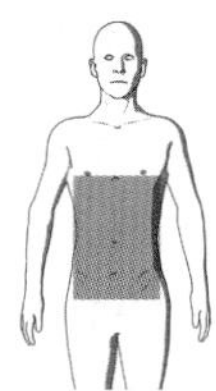

PALPATION AND IDENTIFICATION OF STRUCTURES (WITHOUT DISSECTION)

1. Lesser omentum
2. Omental (epiploic) foramen
3. Stomach
4. Gallbladder

Fig. 11.26 Pull the stomach inferiorly from the liver and locate the omental (epiploic) foramen.

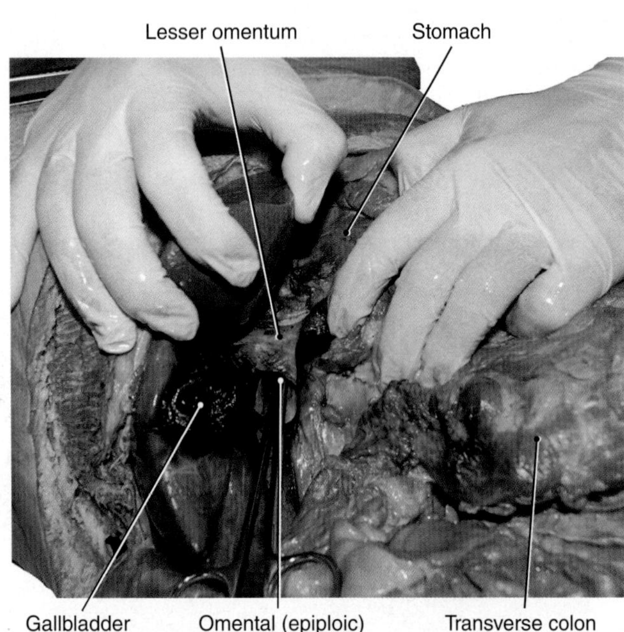

Fig. 11.27 Pass a probe or scissors posterior to the lesser omentum via the omental (epiploic) foramen.

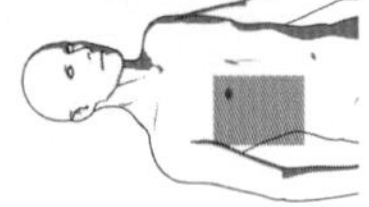

5. Spleen
6. Liver
7. Small intestine
8. Large intestine

Lesser Omentum

- **The *lesser omentum* includes the hepatogastric and hepatoduodenal ligaments. To distinguish them, note that the *hepatogastric* ligament connects the liver to the stomach, whereas the *hepatoduodenal* ligament connects the liver to the duodenum.**

ANATOMY **NOTE**

The hepatoduodenal ligament contains the bile duct, the hepatic artery, and the hepatic portal vein.

Omental Foramen

- **Place your thumb at the *omental foramen* and index finger on top of the hepatoduodenal ligament and feel for these structures. This is called the *Pringle maneuver* and is useful for controlling hemorrhage from the hepatic artery when accidentally injured.**

Stomach

- **Palpate the anterior surface of the *stomach* and notice the greater and lesser curvatures, the body, the fundus, and the pyloric sphincter.**

DISSECTION **TIP**

Note on neighboring cadavers the variable stomach shapes and sizes, which are normal features.

Gallbladder

- **Identify the *gallbladder* (if present) on the inferior surface of the liver.**

DISSECTION **TIP**

A surgical landmark to identify the gallbladder is the point of intersection between the ninth costal cartilage and the linea semilunaris.

Spleen

- **Lift the stomach and pass your fingers posterior to it to reach the spleen. Feel the *gastrosplenic ligament* connecting the greater curvature of the stomach to the spleen.**
- **Palpate the *spleen,* and with your palm, try to feel the posterior surface of the spleen up against the body wall.**

DISSECTION **TIP**

While attempting this maneuver, your palm will come up against the *splenorenal ligament,* which connects the spleen to the body wall. Similarly, if you try to reach the diaphragm, moving your fingertips upward from the spleen, you will feel the *phrenicocolic ligament* connecting the spleen to the diaphragm.

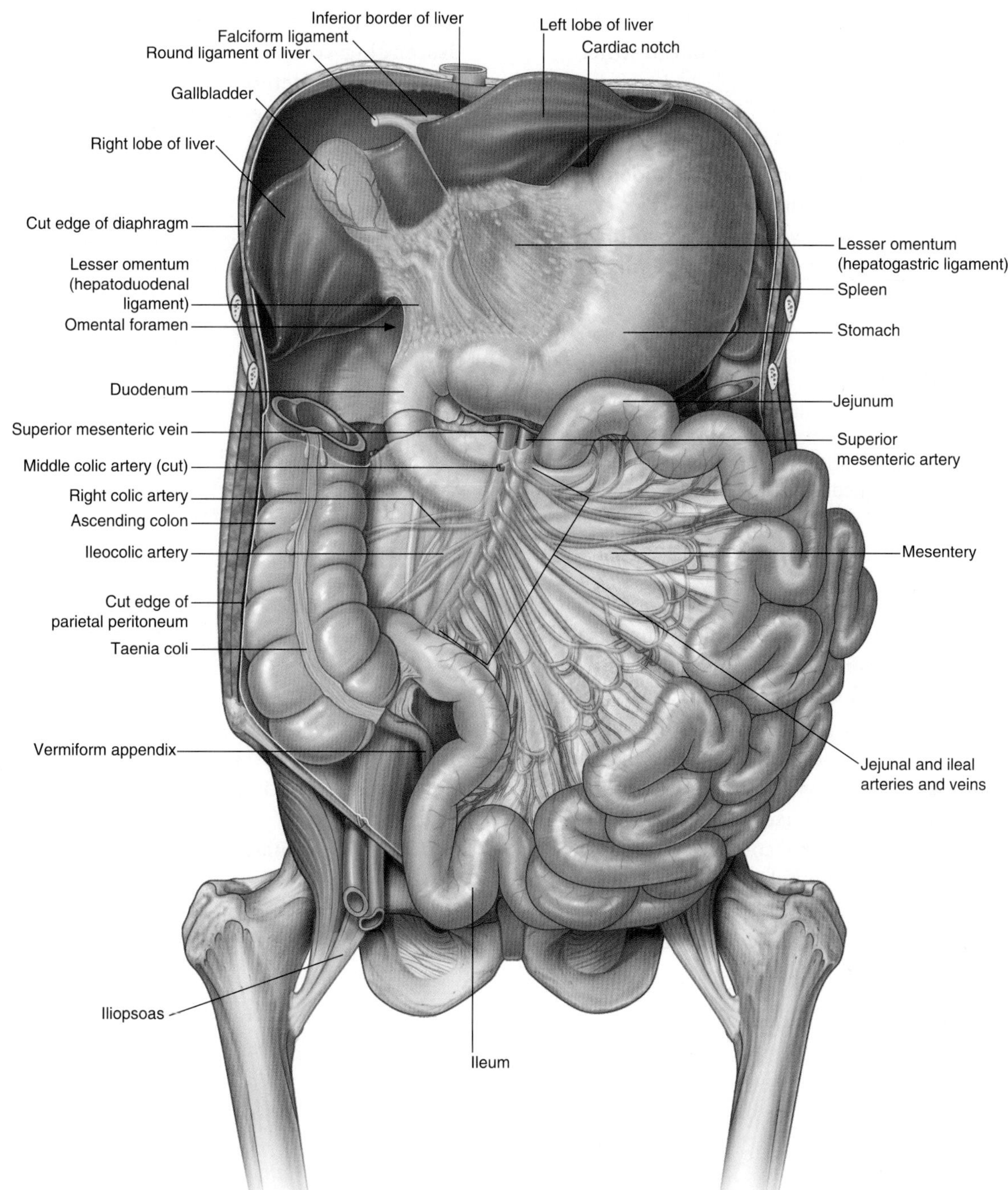

Plate 11.1 Lesser omentum. (From Drake RL et al. *Gray's Atlas of Anatomy*, 3rd edition, Philadelphia, Elsevier, 2021, p. 166.)

Liver

- **With your fingertips, palpate the *liver* and identify the falciform, round, and coronary ligaments.**

Small Intestine

- **Palpate the pyloric sphincter and, distal to it, feel for the much softer, first portion of the duodenum.**
- **Lift the greater omentum and identify the transverse colon with its mesentery, the *transverse mesocolon.***
- **Just behind the transverse mesocolon, the second part of the duodenum passes vertically on the right side of the cadaver.**
- **Identify the mesentery of the ileum and jejunum.**
- **The mesentery of the ileum and jejunum covers the third (horizontal) part of the duodenum.**
- **Identify the final, fourth part, of the duodenum, the *duodenojejunal flexure.***
- **At the duodenojejunal flexure feel for a connective tissue band, the "suspensory ligament of the duodenum" (ligament of Treitz).**

- **Continue palpating the *jejunum,* which makes up approximately two-fifths of the small intestine.**

Large Intestine

- **Palpate the distal part of the *ileum* and, in the right lower quadrant of the abdominal cavity, identify the *cecum* and the ileocecal junction.**
- **Explore the cecum for an attached vermiform *appendix.* Notice that the vermiform appendix has its own mesentery, the *mesoappendix.***

DISSECTION **TIP**

In most cadavers the vermiform appendix originates from the posterior part of the cecum. This is termed a *retrocecal appendix.* In addition, the vermiform appendix often has been surgically removed; look for the original location of the vermiform appendix from the cecum, if possible.

- **Continue identifying the ascending, transverse, descending, and sigmoid colon. The rectum and anus will not be identified during this part of dissection.**
- **Palpate the proximal part of the ascending colon, the *ileocecal junction,* as well as its distal part the right colic or hepatic flexure at the level of the liver.**
- **At the hepatic flexure, the ascending colon turns left and becomes the transverse colon.**
- **Similarly, the transverse colon reaches the splenic flexure or left colic flexure, which turns to the right (inferiorly) to become the descending colon.**
- **At the lower level of the left lower quadrant, the descending colon becomes the sigmoid colon, exhibiting a characteristic S shape. Notice its mesentery, the *sigmoid mesocolon.***

DISSECTION **TIP**

It is difficult to appreciate the entire length of the sigmoid mesocolon and sigmoid colon because most of it is located within the pelvic cavity. This portion will be identified during a later dissection.

- **With your hands, lift and medially pull up the ascending colon and descending colon and identify the longitudinal depressions; they rest in the right and left paracolic gutters.**

DISSECTION **TIP**

The large intestine exhibits some characteristic morphologic features:

- ***Teniae coli* are three narrow muscular bands of the external longitudinal muscle layer of the large intestine.**
- ***Haustra,* or sacculations, are pouches produced by the teniae coli.**
- ***Appendices epiploicae* are peritoneum-covered fat-filled sacs, attached in rows along the teniae coli.**

LABORATORY IDENTIFICATION CHECKLIST

LIGAMENTS

- ☐ Gastrosplenic
- ☐ Hepatogastric
- ☐ Hepatoduodenal
- ☐ Inguinal (Poupart's)
- ☐ Lacunar (Gimbernat's)
- ☐ Pectineal (Cooper's)
- ☐ Median arcuate
- ☐ Medial arcuate
- ☐ Lateral arcuate
- ☐ Median umbilical (urachus)
- ☐ Medial umbilical

LIVER

- ☐ Falciform
- ☐ Round (ligamentum teres)
- ☐ Right triangular
- ☐ Left triangular
- ☐ Coronary
- ☐ Suspensory of duodenum (of Treitz)

OTHER CONNECTIVE TISSUES

- ☐ Greater omentum
- ☐ Lesser omentum
- ☐ External oblique aponeurosis
- ☐ Linea alba
- ☐ Anterior sheath of rectus abdominis
- ☐ Posterior sheath of rectus abdominis
- ☐ Greater omentum
- ☐ Lesser omentum
- ☐ Transverse mesocolon
- ☐ Sigmoid mesentery
- ☐ Appendicular mesentery
- ☐ Mesentery
- ☐ Appendices epiploicae
- ☐ Teniae coli

ORGANS

- ☐ Esophagus
- ☐ Liver
  - ☐ Left lobe
  - ☐ Right lobe
  - ☐ Caudate
  - ☐ Quadrate
- ☐ Gallbladder
  - ☐ Fundus
  - ☐ Body
  - ☐ Neck
- ☐ Pancreas
- ☐ Spleen
- ☐ Stomach
  - ☐ Fundus
  - ☐ Body
  - ☐ Cardia
  - ☐ Pylorus
  - ☐ Greater curvature
  - ☐ Lesser curvature
- ☐ Small intestine
  - ☐ Duodenum
  - ☐ Jejunum
  - ☐ Ileum
- ☐ Large intestine
  - ☐ Cecum
  - ☐ Vermiform appendix
  - ☐ Ileocecal junction
    - ☐ Ascending colon
    - ☐ Transverse colon
    - ☐ Descending colon
    - ☐ Sigmoid colon
- ☐ Right colic flexure
- ☐ Left colic flexure

MUSCLES

- ☐ External abdominal oblique
- ☐ Internal abdominal oblique
- ☐ Transversus abdominis
- ☐ Rectus abdominis
- ☐ Pyramidalis
- ☐ Psoas major
- ☐ Psoas minor (variant)

BONES

- ☐ Lower ribs 9 to 11
- ☐ Xiphoid process of sternum
- ☐ Sacrum
- ☐ Iliac crest

SPACES

- ☐ Omental (epiploic) foramen (of Winslow)
- ☐ Omental bursa
- ☐ Peritoneal cavity

VESSELS

- ☐ Inferior epigastric artery
- ☐ Inferior epigastric vein
- ☐ Superior epigastric artery
- ☐ Superior epigastric vein
- ☐ External iliac vein
- ☐ External iliac artery

In most cadavers, the liver occupies a significant portion of the peritoneal cavity. The gallbladder may be difficult to see at this point but look for its fundus.

DISSECTION TIP

The gallbladder, if not surgically removed, will become visible as the dissection proceeds.

DISSECTION STEPS

- **With a scalpel, make a horizontal incision at the lower edge of the liver, removing 3 to 4 cm (1½ inches) of liver parenchyma (Fig. 12.1).**
- **Pull the stomach downward and fully expose the gallbladder and the hepatoduodenal ligament (Figs. 12.2 and 12.3).**

DISSECTION TIP

Stripping away the hepatoduodenal ligament, you will see several nerves running along the bile duct and proper hepatic artery. These nerves are part of the autonomic nervous system and are primarily sympathetic fibers (Fig. 12.4).

- **With scissors or a probe, carefully strip away the hepatoduodenal ligament and expose the bile duct, proper hepatic artery, and hepatic portal vein (see Figs. 12.4 and 12.5).**
- **Note the relationships among these three structures: within the hepatoduodenal ligament, the hepatic**

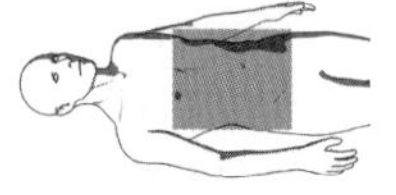

Fig. 12.1 Horizontal incision at the lower edge of the liver.

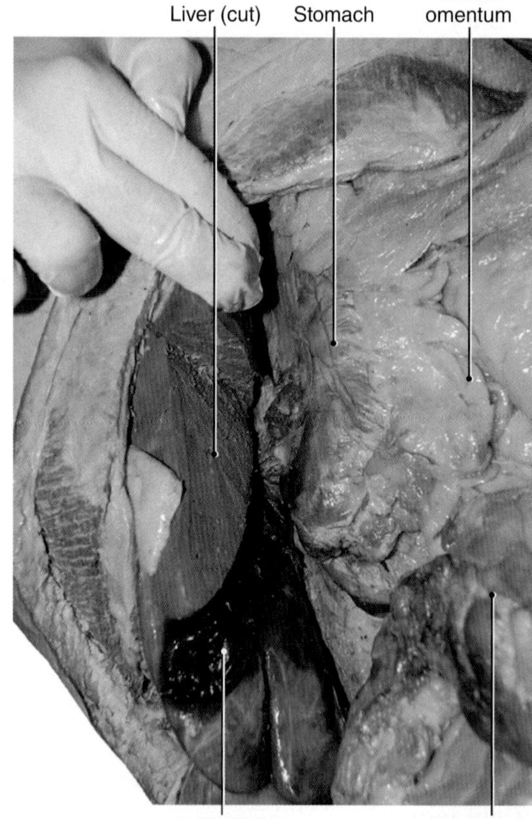

Fig. 12.2 Identify the gallbladder.

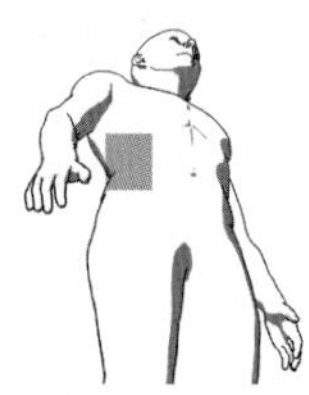

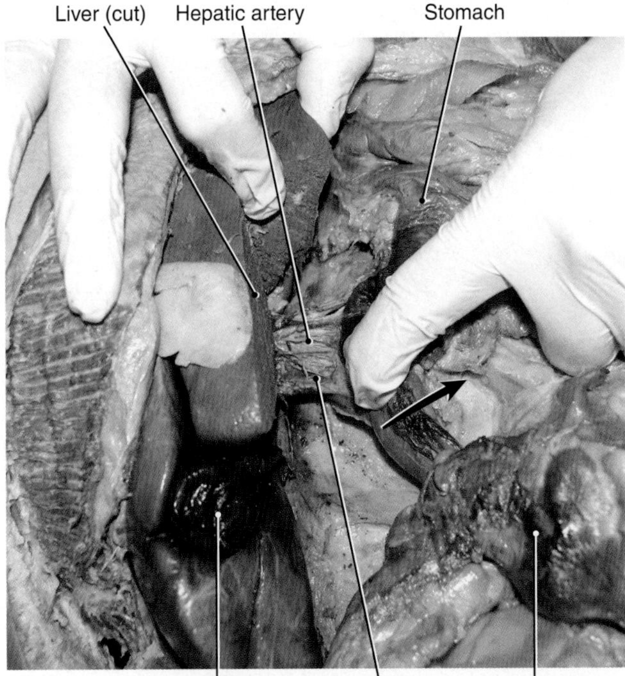

Fig. 12.3 Pull the stomach downward to expose the gallbladder and hepatoduodenal ligament.

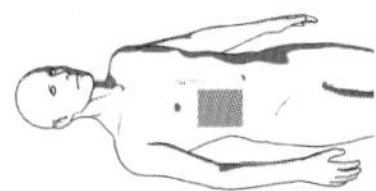

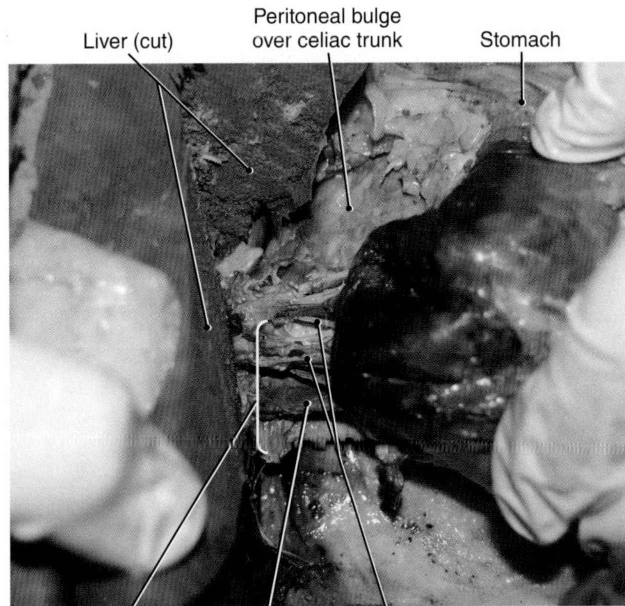

Fig. 12.4 Cut the hepatoduodenal ligament to expose the bile duct, proper hepatic artery, hepatic portal vein, hepatic portal triad, and autonomic nerve fibers.

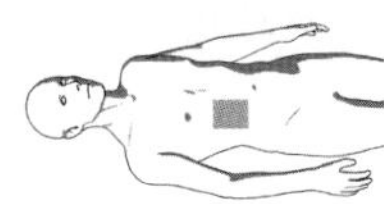

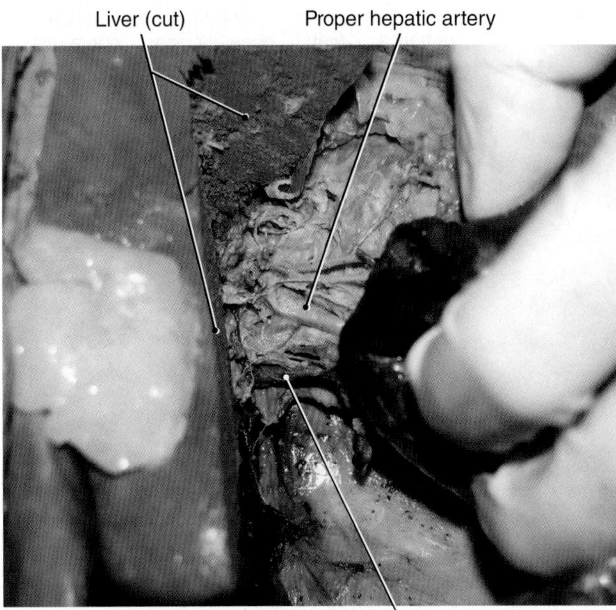

Fig. 12.5 View shows the relationship between the proper hepatic artery and bile duct.

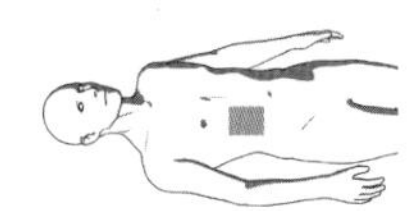

portal vein is located posteriorly, deep to the bile duct and proper hepatic artery (Fig. 12.6).

- **Clean the proper hepatic artery toward the liver and identify the right and left hepatic arteries.**
- **Look for the *cystic artery* supplying the gallbladder.**
- **The cystic artery usually arises from the right hepatic artery or the proper hepatic artery.**
- **Dissect out the cystic duct from the gallbladder toward its junction with the common hepatic duct to form the bile duct (Fig. 12.7).**
- **Once these structures are cleaned and identified, observe the *hepatocystic triangle* formed by the common hepatic duct, the cystic duct, and the liver.**
- **In most cases, the cystic artery is identified within this triangular region (Plate 12.1).**

DISSECTION **TIP**

In about 65% of cases, the cystic artery arises from the right hepatic artery. If you are not able to identify the cystic artery in its typical location, lift the cystic duct and look deep to it.

- **To expose the celiac trunk and its branches, with blunt dissection, release the transverse and the descending colons from the gastrocolic ligament (Figs. 12.8 and 12.9).**
- **With scissors, cut the gastrocolic ligament at the superior border of the transverse colon and release it from the stomach (Fig. 12.10).**

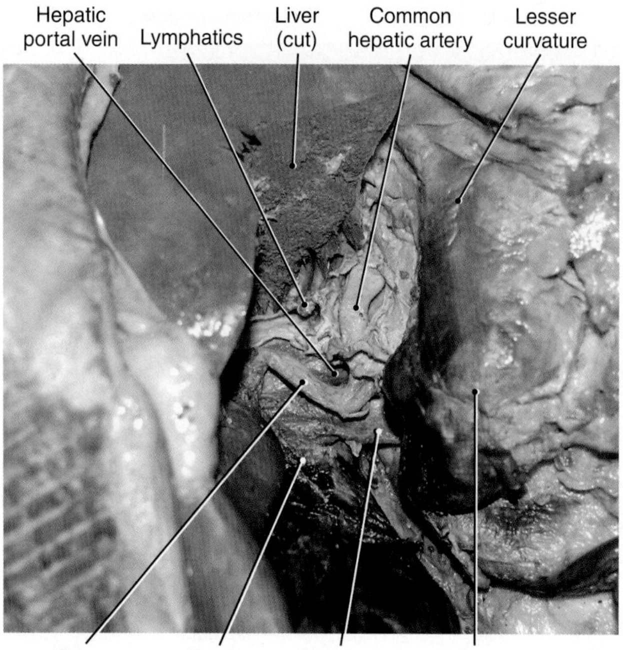

Hepatic portal vein
Lymphatics
Liver (cut)
Common hepatic artery
Lesser curvature
Proper hepatic artery
Cystic duct
Bile duct
Pylorus

Fig. 12.6 View demonstrates the relationship of proper hepatic artery, bile duct, and hepatic portal vein.

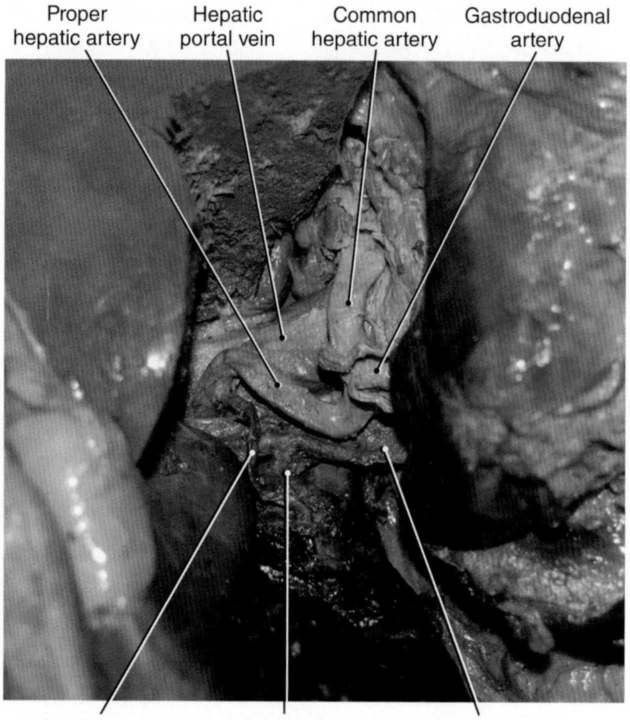

Proper hepatic artery
Hepatic portal vein
Common hepatic artery
Gastroduodenal artery
Cystic artery
Cystic duct
Bile duct

Fig. 12.7 View shows the dissected cystic duct from the gallbladder to the junction with the common hepatic duct.

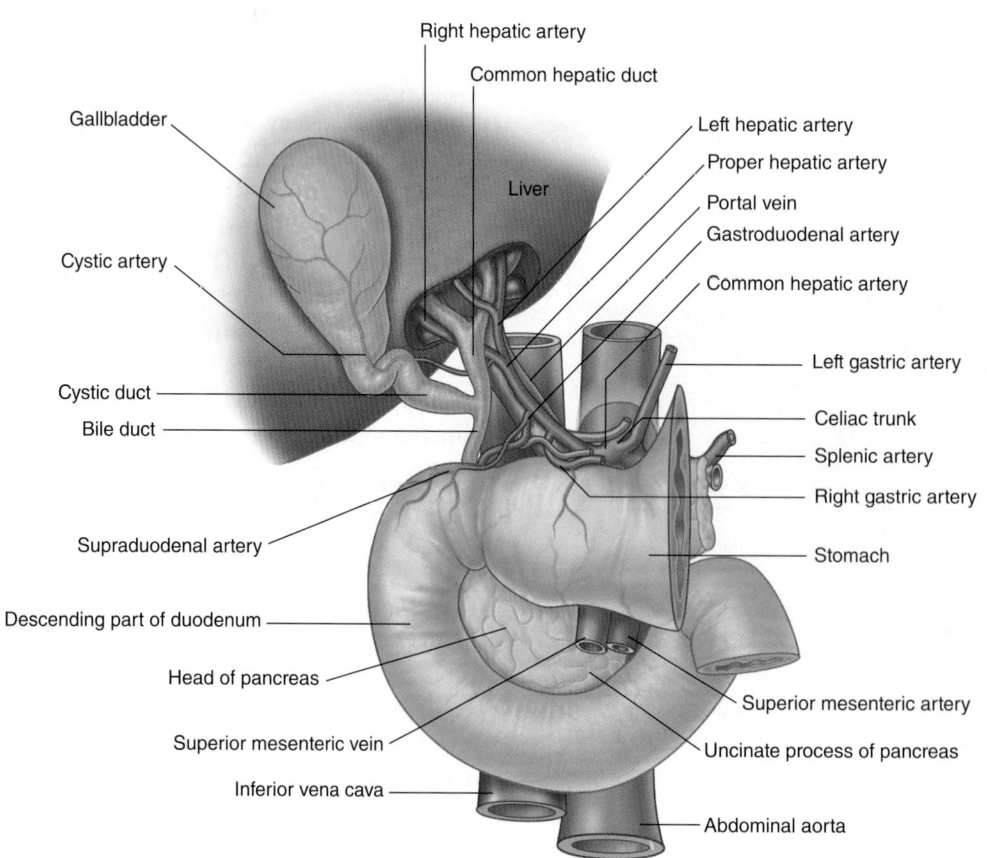

Plate 12.1 Distribution of common hepatic artery. (From Drake RL et al. *Gray's Anatomy for Students*, 5th edition, Philadelphia, Elsevier, 2015, Figure 4.126, p. 346.)

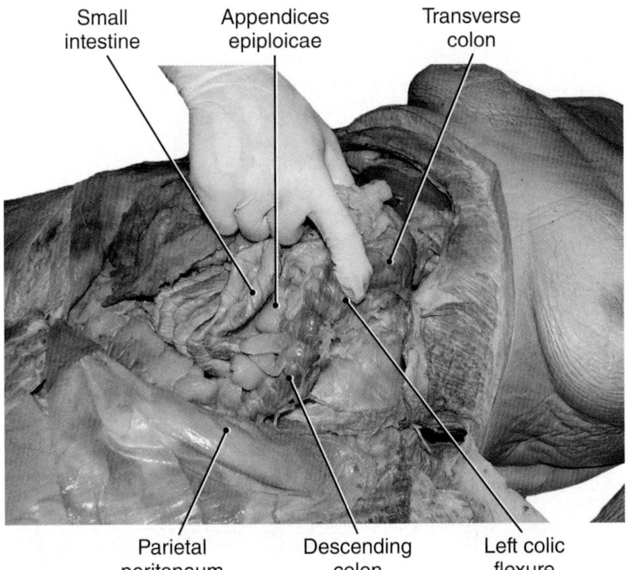

Fig. 12.8 Identify the transverse and descending colons.

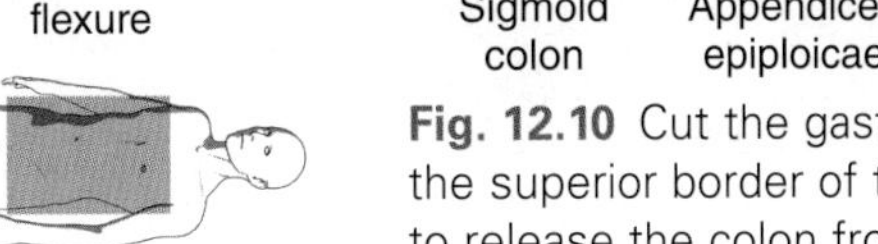

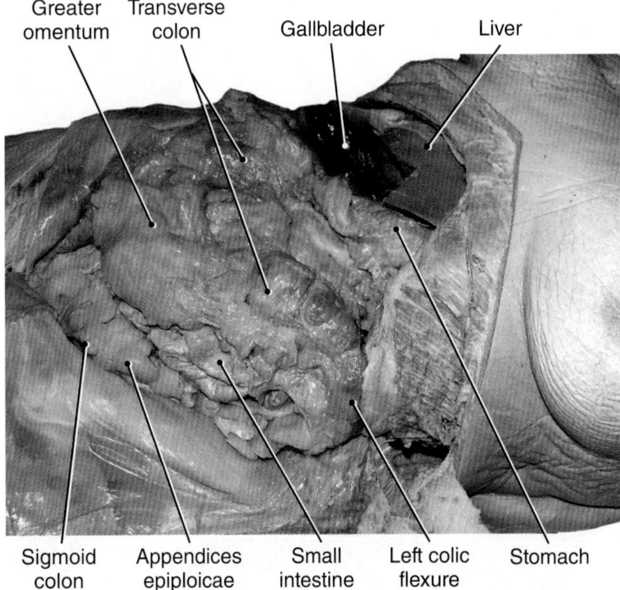

Fig. 12.10 Cut the gastrocolic ligament at the superior border of the transverse colon to release the colon from the stomach.

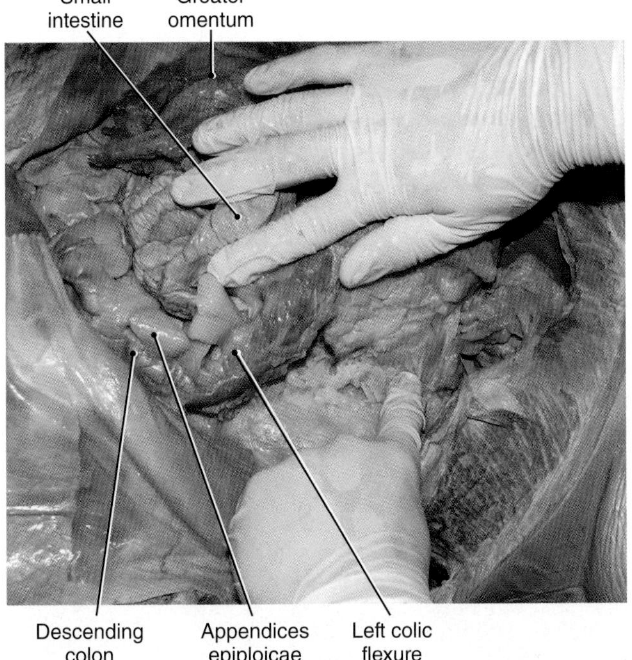

Fig. 12.9 Blunt dissection of the transverse and descending colons from the gastrocolic ligament.

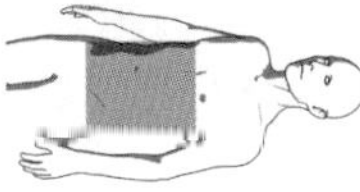

- **To expose the splenic artery and spleen, cut the inferior edge of the costal cartilages with a saw to expose fully the area anterior to the spleen. Place paper towels underneath the costal cartilages (Fig. 12.11).**
- **Identify the inferior border of the spleen, hidden by the gastrosplenic and splenorenal ligaments and, usually, abundant adipose tissue (Fig. 12.12).**

DISSECTION **TIP**

The spleen rests on an abundance of adipose tissue. Once the adipose tissue is cleaned away, the spleen will drop inferiorly and posteriorly, and its vessels will be stressed and possibly broken. Place some folded paper towels posterior to the spleen to keep it at the same level as the pancreas. In addition, the paper towels will absorb any embalming fluid that accumulates in this space.

- **Clean the fat and the gastrosplenic and splenorenal ligaments and expose the splenic pedicle receiving the splenic artery and vein (Fig. 12.13).**
- **Continue the exposure of the splenic artery and vein and identify the splenic hilum (Fig. 12.14).**
- **Identify the short gastric arteries, which pass to the greater curvature of the stomach.**
- **Note the relationship of the spleen with the stomach and the pancreas.**
- **Identify the left gastroomental (gastroepiploic) artery, which typically derives from the most inferior splenic artery hilar branch (Fig. 12.15).**
- **Pull the stomach upward and expose the tail of the pancreas (see Fig. 12.15).**
- **Continue the dissection of the splenic artery and vein from the hilum of the spleen toward the celiac trunk.**
- **The splenic artery is tortuous and lies hidden at the upper border of the tail and body of the pancreas (Fig. 12.16).**
- **Lift the stomach upward and expose the body and tail of the pancreas (Fig. 12.17).**
- **Clean out the splenic artery and vein from the adjacent pancreas (Fig. 12.18).**

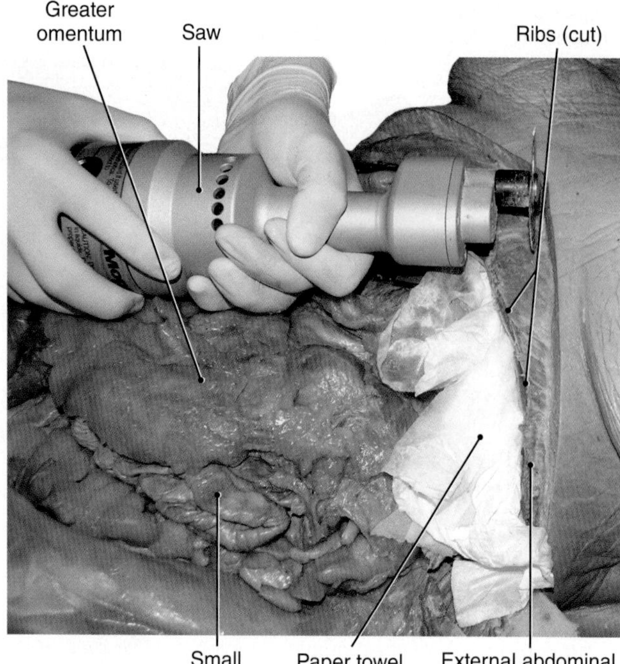

Fig. 12.11 Saw the inferior edge of the costal cartilages.

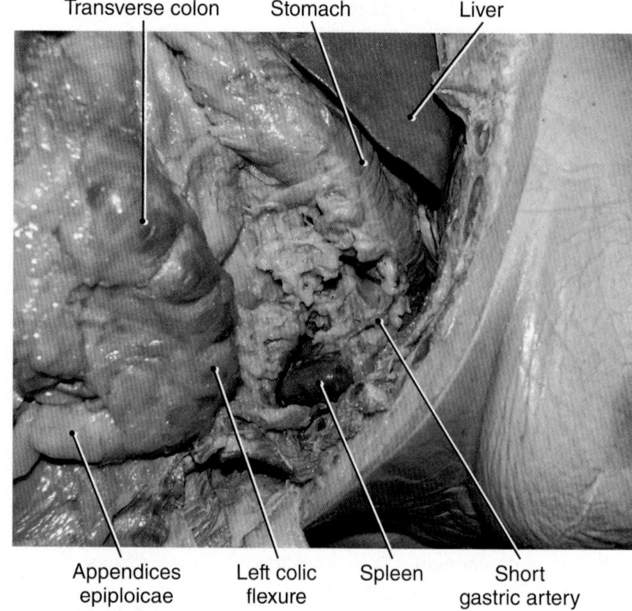

Fig. 12.13 Clean away the fat to expose the splenic pedicle.

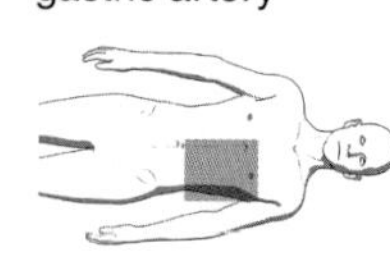

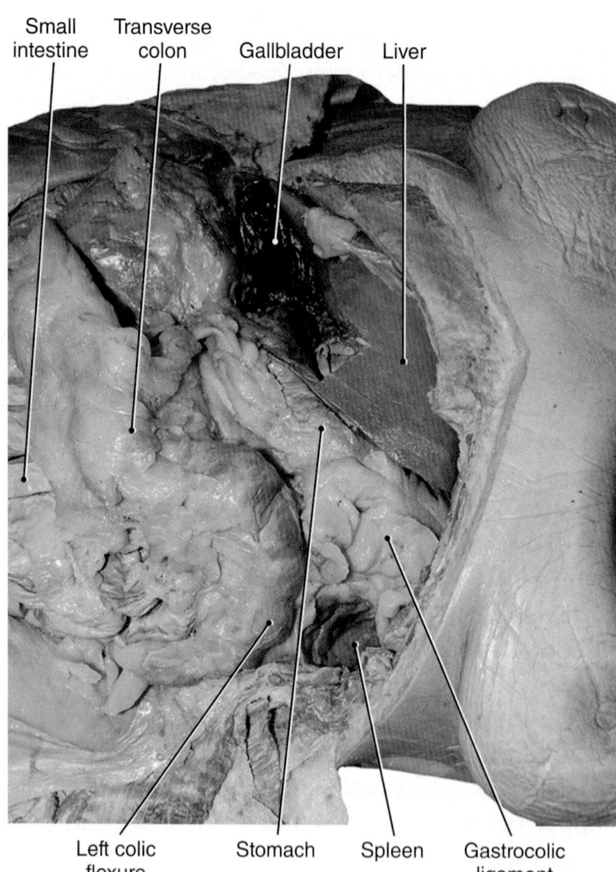

Fig. 12.12 Identify the inferior borders of the spleen.

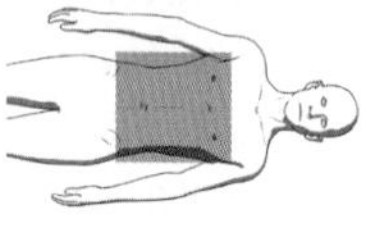

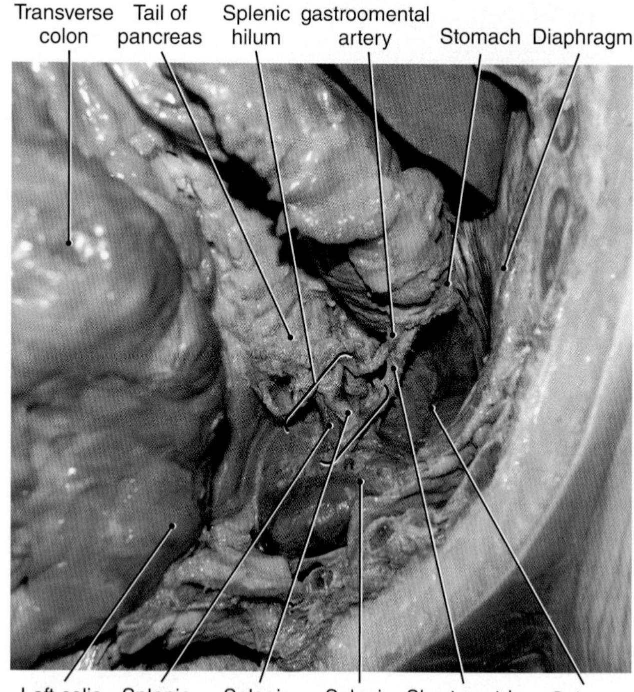

Fig. 12.14 Expose the splenic artery and vein and identify the splenic hilum.

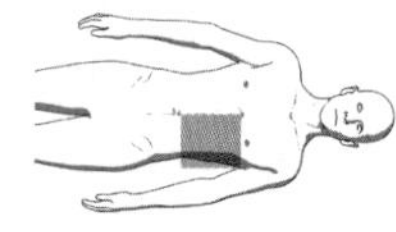

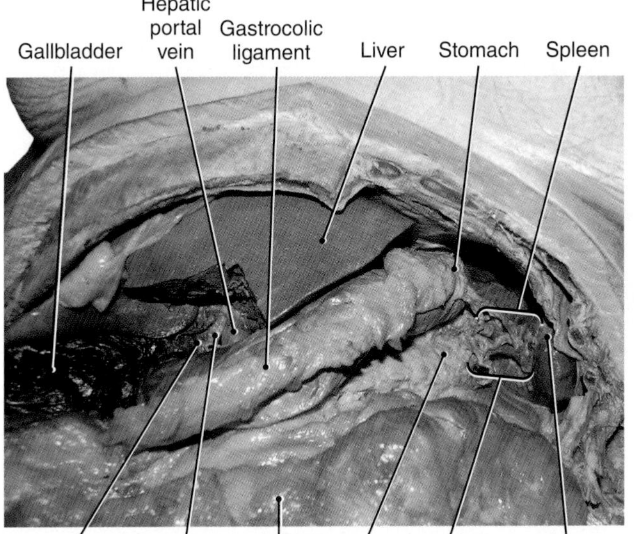

Fig. 12.15 Identify the left gastroomental (gastroepiploic) artery and pull the stomach upward to expose the tail of the pancreas.

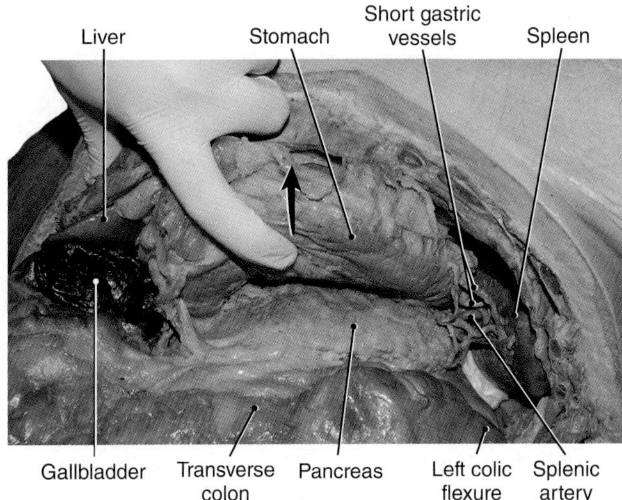

Fig. 12.17 Lift the stomach upward to expose the body and tail of the pancreas.

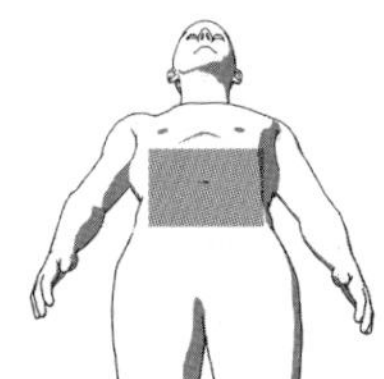

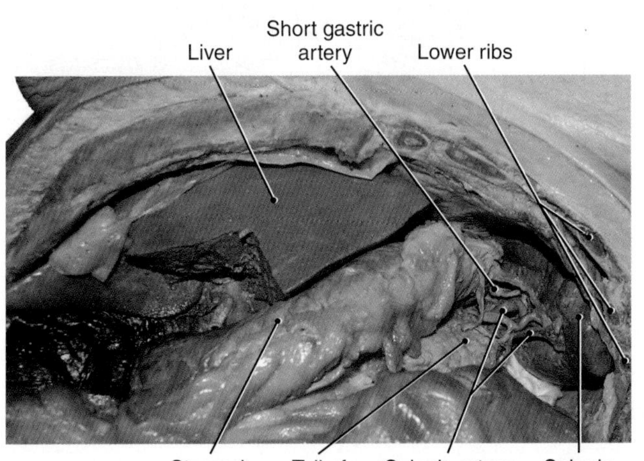

Fig. 12.16 Identify the splenic artery.

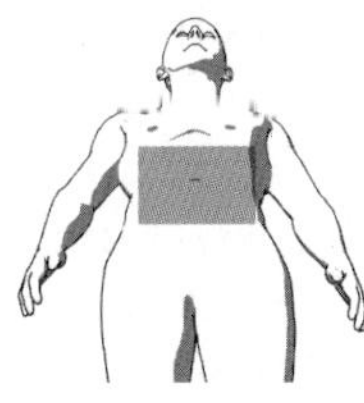

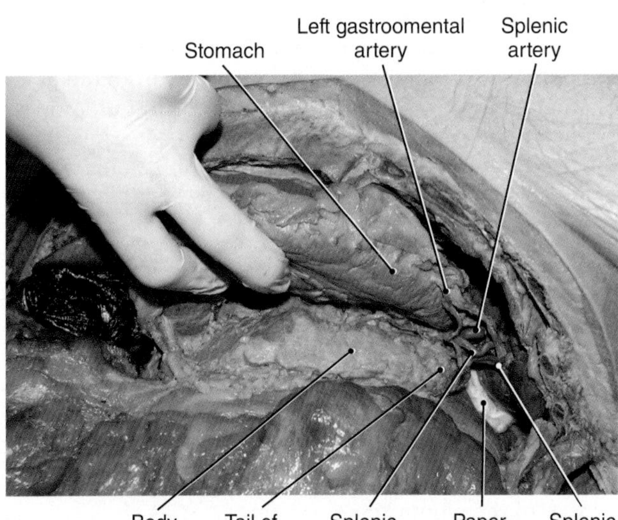

Fig. 12.18 Dissect out the splenic artery and vein from the adjacent pancreas.

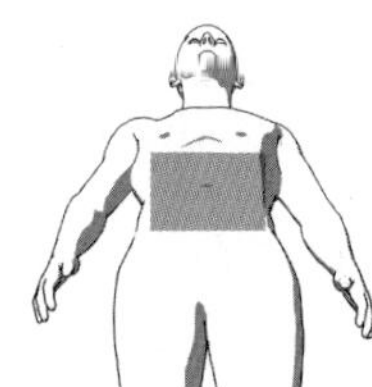

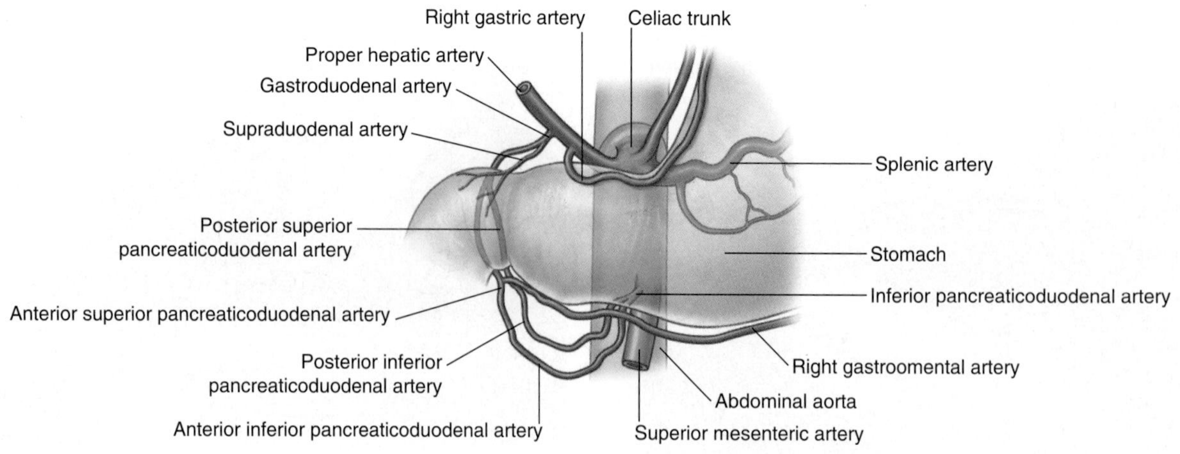

Plate 12.2 Branches of celiac trunk and gastroduodenal artery. (From Drake RL et al. *Gray's Atlas of Anatomy*, 3rd edition, Philadelphia, Elsevier, 2021, p. 162).

- **Do *not* pull the splenic artery away from the pancreas, because most of its branches are short and can be injured easily.**
- **To visualize the area of the celiac trunk, it is necessary to lift the stomach upward and expose the pancreas. Palpate the upper border of the pancreas, and with your fingers, feel the celiac trunk as a prominent bulge covered by the overlying peritoneum (Plate 12.2).**

DISSECTION **TIP**

The reason for not dissecting the entire celiac trunk from the right side, at this time, is that the view from the gallbladder offers only limited exposure of the area. It is simpler to release the stomach from the gastrocolic ligament and greater omentum, identify the splenic artery at the splenic hilum, and then dissect the middle portion of the celiac trunk.

IDENTIFICATION OF DIFFERENT PARTS OF THE STOMACH

ANATOMY **NOTE**

The stomach is divided into four main regions: the cardia, fundus, body, and pylorus.

- Identify the *lesser curvature* and the *greater curvature* of the stomach.
- Identify the *angular notch*, found between the body and pyloric part of the stomach.
- Look for the cardia and the *cardiac notch* between the esophagus and fundus.

ANATOMY **NOTE**

The *fundus* is the portion of the stomach above the cardiac notch. The pylorus is divided further into the pyloric antrum and pyloric canal.

- **Return to the exposed proper hepatic artery and dissect backward toward its origin from the common hepatic artery (Figs. 12.19 and 12.20).**

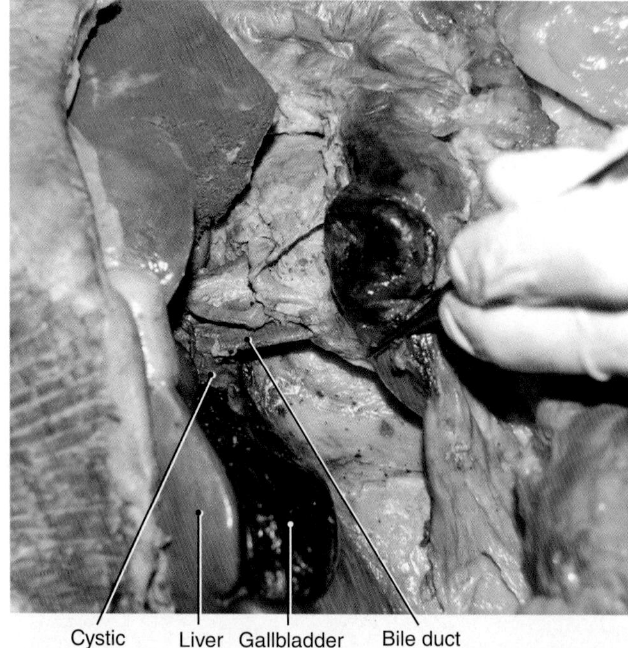

Fig. 12.19 Identify the bile and cystic ducts.

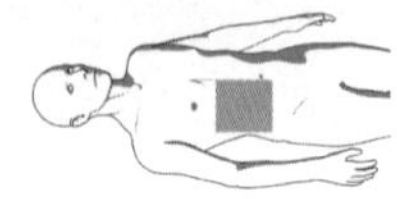

- **Identify and expose the other branch of the common hepatic artery, the gastroduodenal artery (see Fig. 12.20).**
- **Dissect out the right side of the lesser curvature of the stomach and identify the *right gastric artery*, a branch of the proper hepatic artery.**
- **Next to the right gastric artery, identify the right gastric vein and its connection to the right gastroomental (gastroepiploic) vein via the prepyloric vein of Mayo.**
- **On the left side of the lesser curvature of the stomach, identify and clean the left gastric artery; then trace it back from its origin from the celiac trunk (Fig. 12.21).**

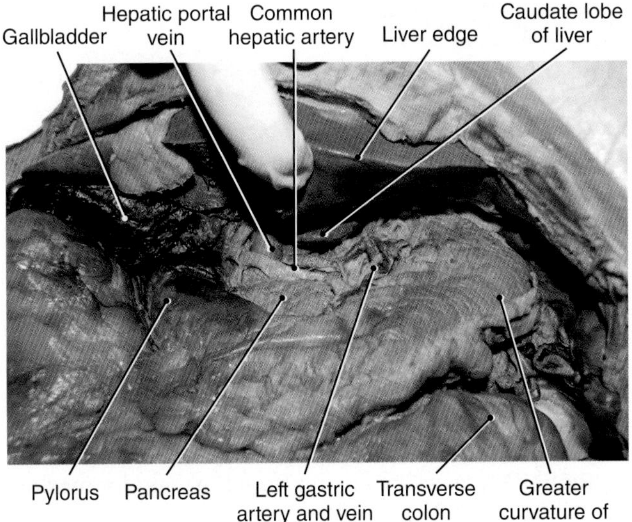

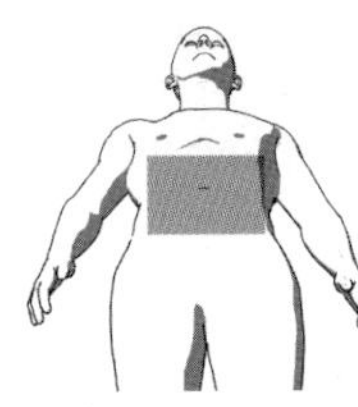

Fig. 12.20 Dissect the proper hepatic artery backward, toward its origin from the common hepatic artery.

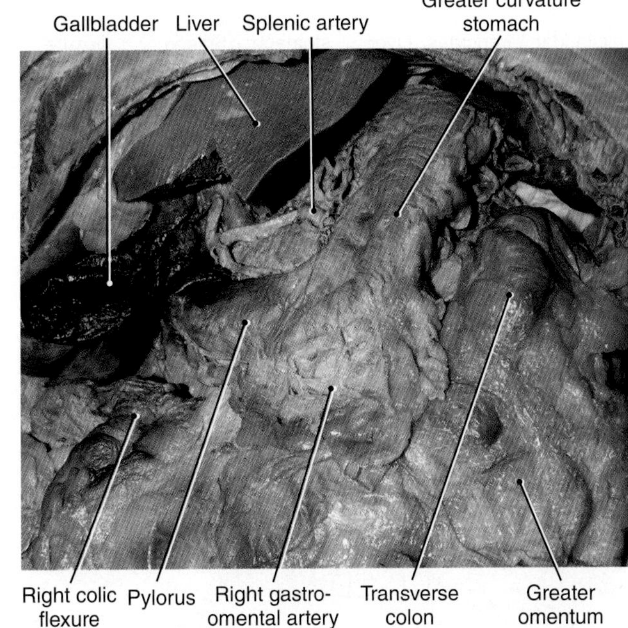

Fig. 12.22 Identify the greater curvature of the stomach.

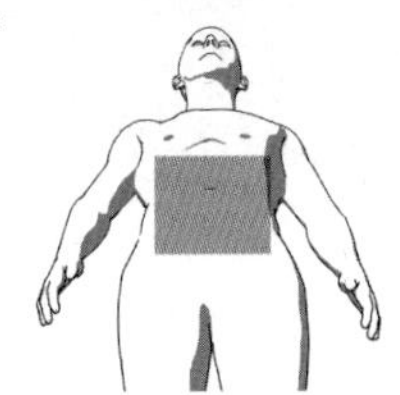

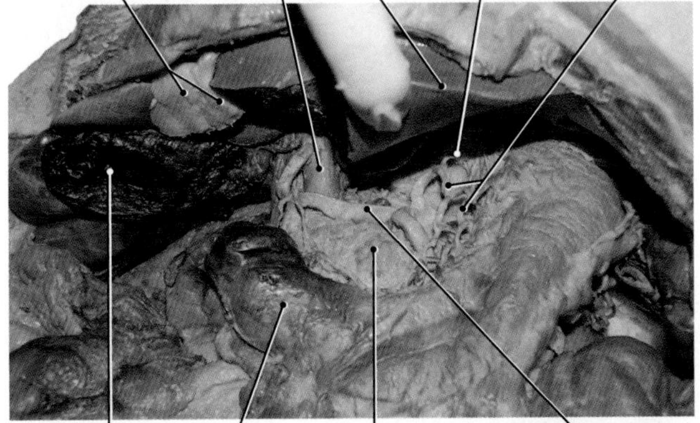

Fig. 12.21 Identify and clean the left gastric artery.

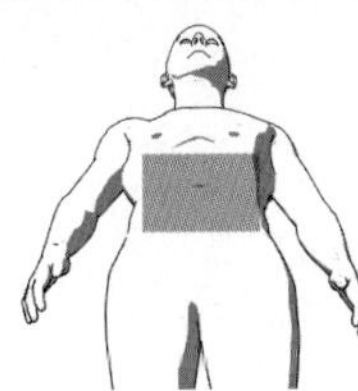

- Note the esophageal arterial branches of the left gastric artery ascending toward the esophagus.
- The left gastric artery is accompanied by the left gastric vein. Trace out any esophageal tributaries to the left gastric vein.
- In the area between the greater curvature of the stomach and the pylorus, dissect out the fat within the gastrocolic ligament and greater omentum and identify the right gastroomental (gastroepiploic) artery (Figs. 12.22 and 12.23).
- Similarly, dissect between the left side of the greater curvature of the stomach and spleen and identify the left gastroomental (gastroepiploic) artery.
- After identifying the right and left gastroomental (gastroepiploic) arteries, with scissors, cut along the line marking the junction between the body of the stomach and the pyloric antrum, 4 to 5 cm (~2 inches) proximal to the pylorus (Fig. 12.24).
- Retract the two parts of the transected stomach laterally and expose the celiac trunk and pancreas (Fig. 12.25).
- Lift the splenic artery from the upper border of the pancreas and dissect it out (Fig. 12.26).
- Once the splenic artery is fully exposed, notice its tortuosity (Fig. 12.27).
- Place the left side of the stomach in such a position that you can visualize all the branches of the celiac trunk and identify the origins and distributions of these branches (Figs. 12.28 and 12.29).

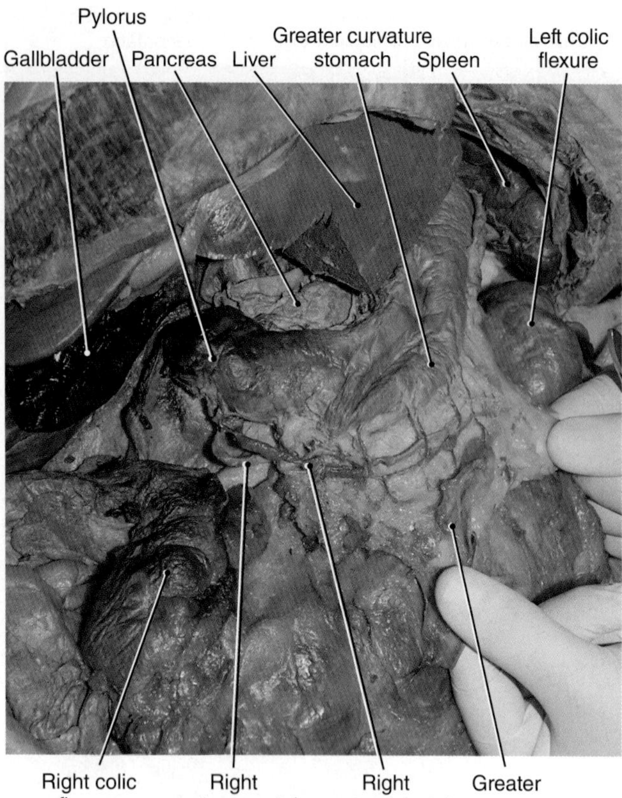

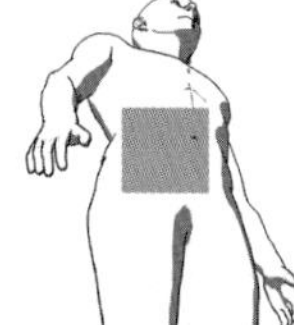

Fig. 12.23 Dissect out the fat within the gastrocolic ligament and greater omentum and identify the right gastroomental (gastroepiploic) artery.

DISSECTION TIP

Note the following common arterial variations of the celiac trunk:

- Celiac trunk and superior mesenteric artery arising as a common trunk (celiomesenteric trunk, 2.5% of cases)
- Proper hepatic and superior mesenteric arteries arising as a common trunk (hepatomesenteric trunk)
- Splenic artery and left gastric artery arising as a common trunk (lienogastric [splenogastric] trunk, 5.5%)
- Left gastric and common hepatic artery arising as a common trunk (gastrohepatic or hepatogastric trunk, 1.5%)
- Left gastric artery arising from the left hepatic artery (25%)
- Right hepatic artery arising from the superior mesenteric artery (18%)
- Cystic artery arising from proper hepatic artery or left hepatic artery
- Aberrant left hepatic artery arising from the left hepatic artery (25%)

ANATOMY NOTE

The pancreas typically is subdivided into the following parts: head, neck, body, and tail. The head is encircled by the first three parts of the duodenum and contains the *uncinate process*, which is located posteroinferiorly to the superior mesenteric artery and vein. Its terminal part, the tail, is related to the hilum of the spleen and left.

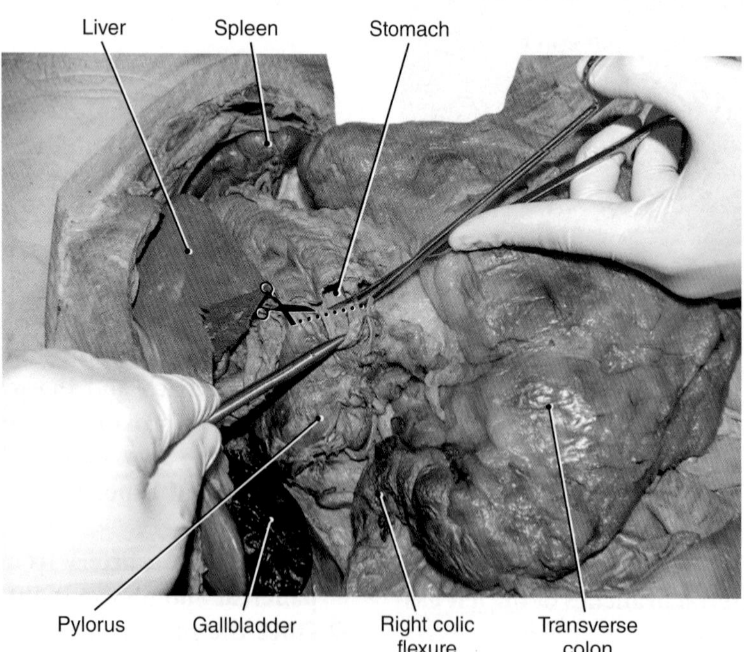

Fig. 12.24 With scissors, cut along the junction between the body of the stomach and the pyloric antrum.

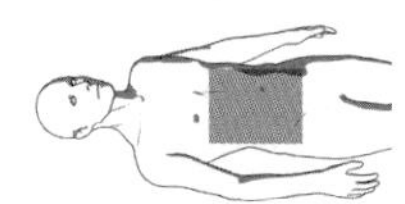

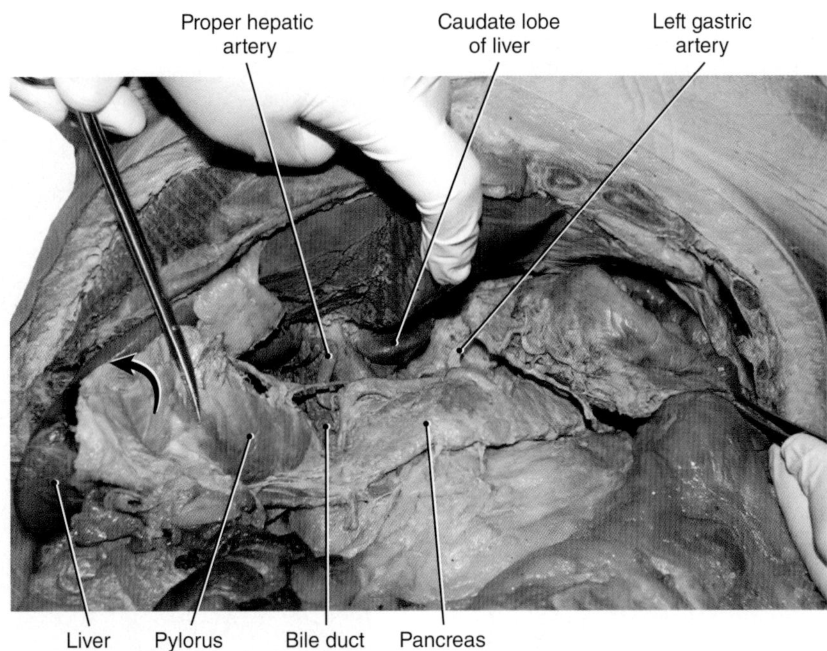

Fig. 12.25 Expose the celiac trunk and pancreas.

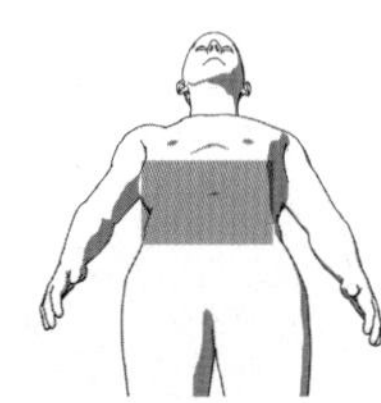

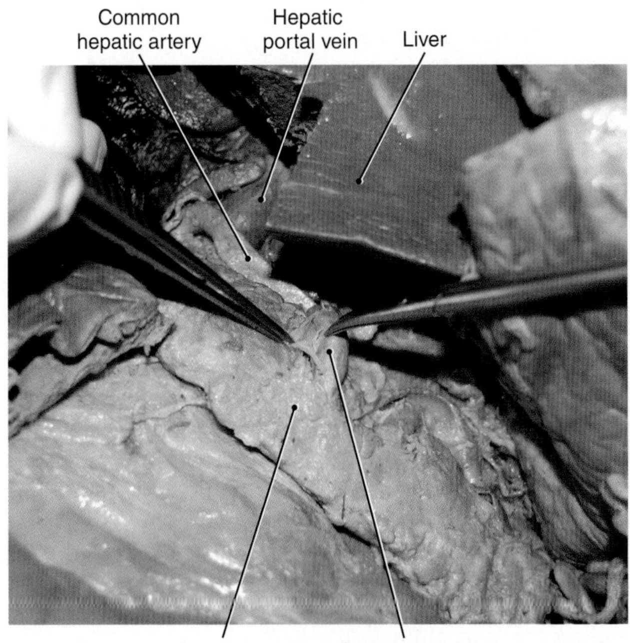

Fig. 12.26 Dissect the splenic artery from the upper border of the pancreas.

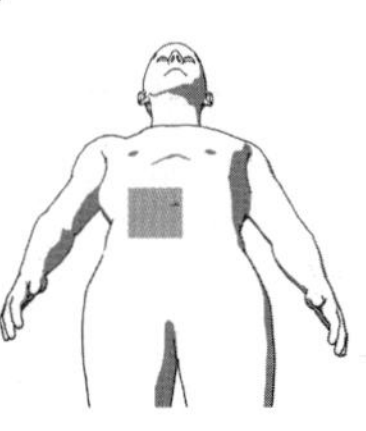

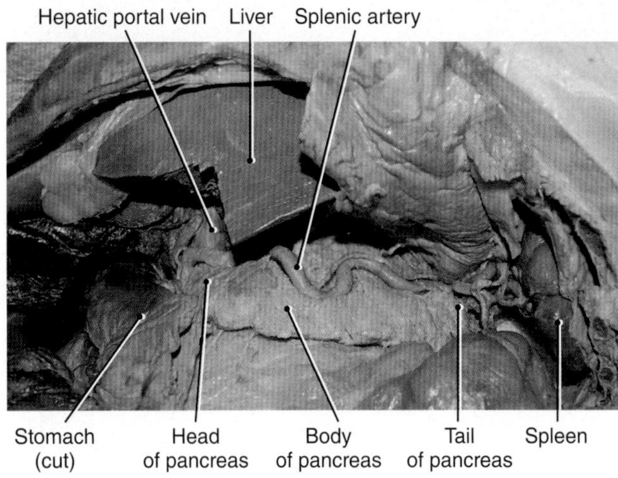

Fig. 12.27 Note the tortuous route of the splenic artery.

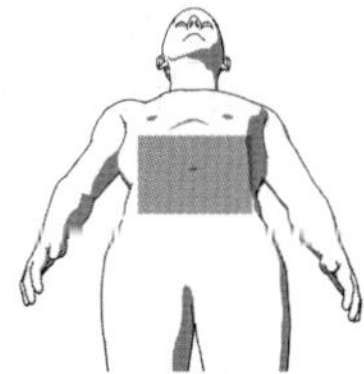

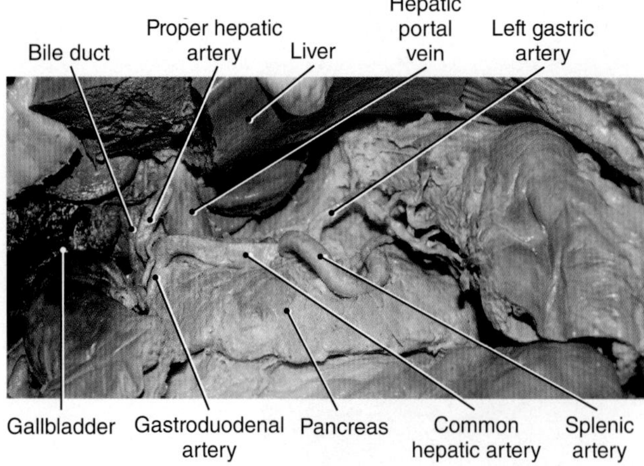

Fig. 12.28 Displace the stomach to visualize the branches of the celiac trunk.

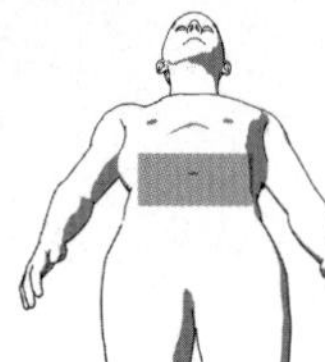

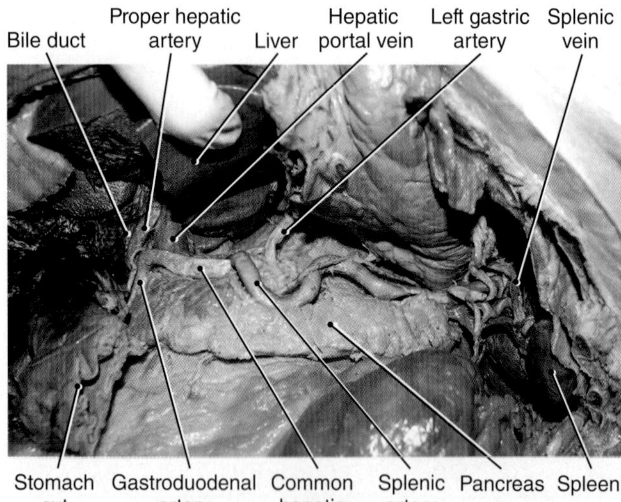

Fig. 12.29 Identify the origins and distributions of the branches of the celiac trunk.

- On the right side of the cadaver, dissect out the branches of the gastroduodenal artery anteriorly.
- Around the head of the pancreas, look for the origin of the two terminal branches of the gastroduodenal artery, the right gastroomental (gastroepiploic) and superior pancreaticoduodenal arteries (Fig. 12.30).
- The right gastroomental (gastroepiploic) artery is typically found around the right side of the greater curvature of the stomach.
- The superior pancreaticoduodenal artery divides into the posterior superior and anterior superior pancreaticoduodenal arteries supplying the head of the pancreas (see Fig. 12.30).

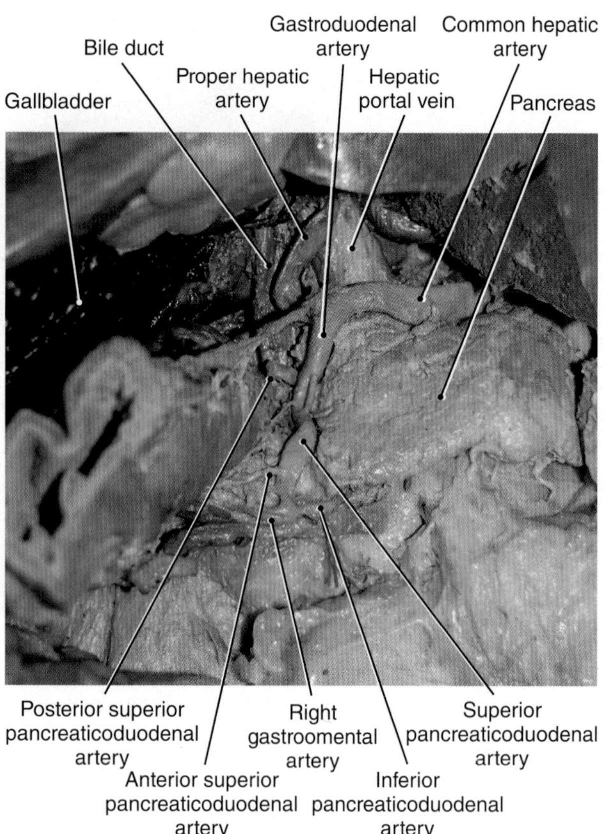

Fig. 12.30 Identify the origin of the two terminal branches of the gastroduodenal artery, the right gastroomental (gastroepiploic) artery and the superior pancreaticoduodenal artery.

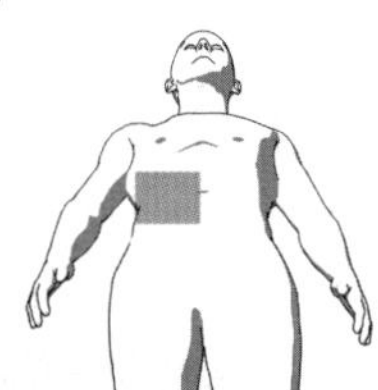

DISSECTION TIP

To expose the arterial branches, as well as the course of the bile duct down to the duodenum, reflect the stomach and duodenum to the left. Use your fingers to dissect the area underneath the duodenum and inferior vena cava; this is an avascular plane that is easily reflected to the left. This is called the *Kocher maneuver*, or "kocherizing" (Fig. 12.31).

DISSECTION TIP

A good way to trace and expose the posterior superior pancreaticoduodenal (PSPD) artery is to dissect out the bile duct from the lateral side (see Fig. 12.31). The artery that crosses over the bile duct is the PSPD. Furthermore, this artery passes behind the head of the pancreas and the second part of the duodenum.

- Follow the gastroduodenal artery posteriorly toward the 1st part of the duodenum and expose the origin of the PSPD artery (Figs. 12.32 and 12.33).
- Trace the course of the anterior superior pancreaticoduodenal artery (see Figs. 12.33 and 12.34) and expose its anastomosis with the inferior pancreaticoduodenal artery, a branch of the superior mesenteric artery.

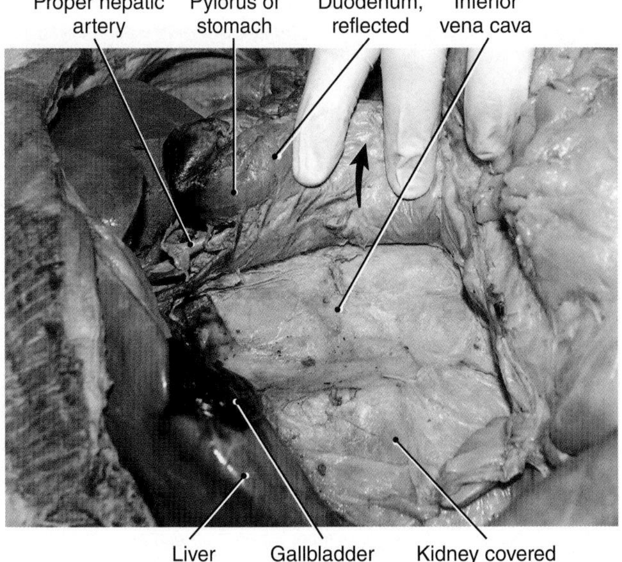

Fig. 12.31 Reflect the stomach and duodenum to the left, and bluntly dissect the area underneath the duodenum and inferior vena cava using the Kocher maneuver.

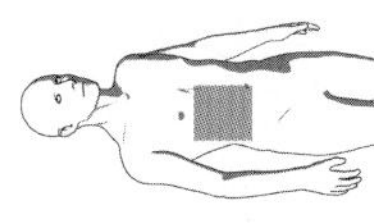

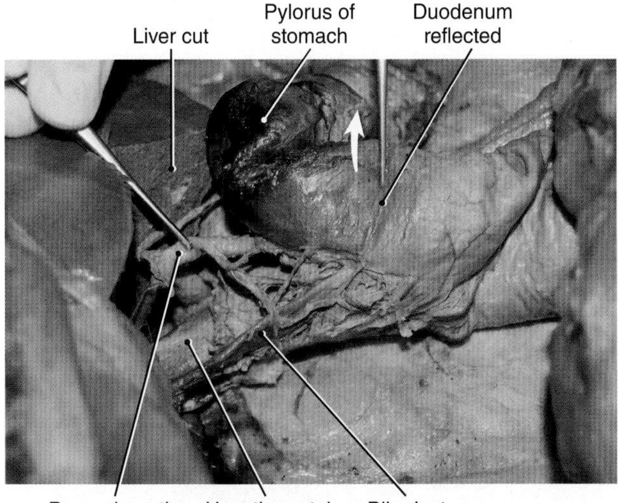

Fig. 12.32 Follow the gastroduodenal artery posteriorly toward the 1st part of the duodenum and expose the origin of the posterior superior pancreaticoduodenal artery.

OPTIONAL DISSECTION OF BRANCHES OF SPLENIC ARTERY

- **Lift the splenic artery up and look for the origin of several branches. The following landmarks help identify these branches:**
  1. Lift the pancreas and look for the point where the portal vein crosses the pancreas posteriorly (neck of the pancreas). At this point, look for a branch from the splenic artery, the *dorsal pancreatic artery.*

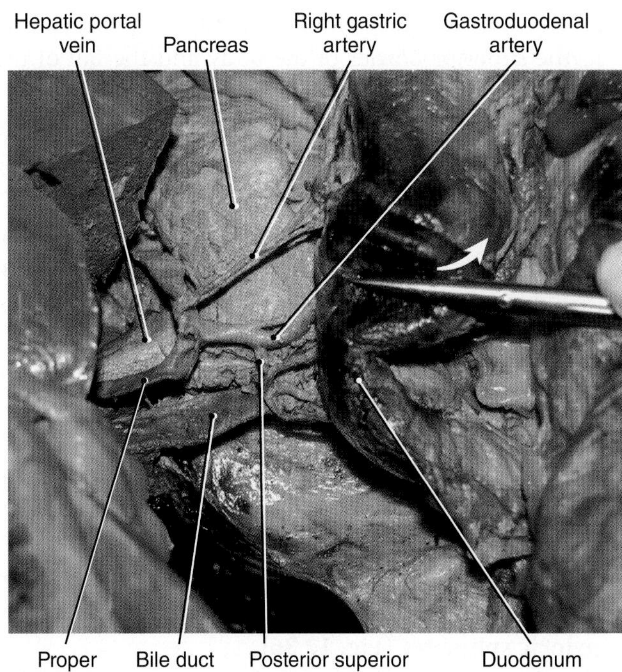

Fig. 12.33 Trace the course of the anterior superior pancreaticoduodenal artery.

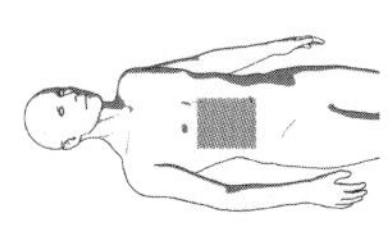

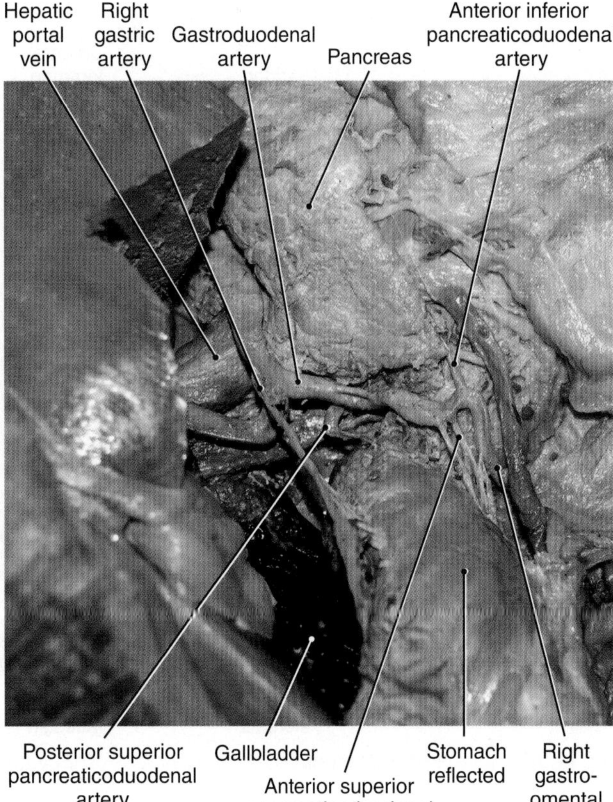

Fig. 12.34 Expose the anterior superior pancreaticoduodenal artery's anastomosis with the inferior pancreaticoduodenal artery.

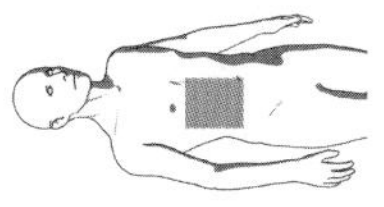

2. The splenic artery often gives off small branches at the superior border of the body and the tail of the pancreas, the *short pancreatic branches.*
3. The largest of these short pancreatic branches is the *great pancreatic artery*, which is often found at the distal one-third of the pancreas near its tail.
4. At the same point of the great pancreatic artery, look for a branch of the splenic artery traveling to the posterior part of the stomach supplying the gastric fundus, the *posterior gastric artery.*
5. Look 1 to 2 cm superior to the inferior border of the pancreas; embedded in its substance is the *transverse pancreatic artery*.

- **Make a horizontal incision at the pyloric antrum, pylorus, and duodenum and observe the inner surface of these structures (Fig. 12.35).**
- **Appreciate the gastric folds at the inner surface of the pyloric antrum and the circular muscle of the pyloric sphincter (Fig. 12.36).**
- **Continue the incision at the first, second, and third parts of the duodenum and note the circular folds of Kerckring (Figs. 12.37 and 12.38).**
- **Cut the gastroduodenal artery and expose the course of the bile duct toward the duodenum (Fig. 12.39).**

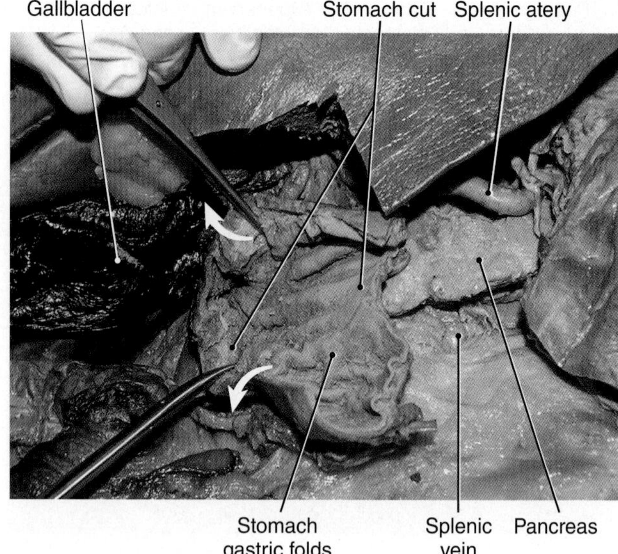

Fig. 12.36 Note gastric rugae on the internal surface of the pyloric antrum and circular muscle of the pyloric sphincter.

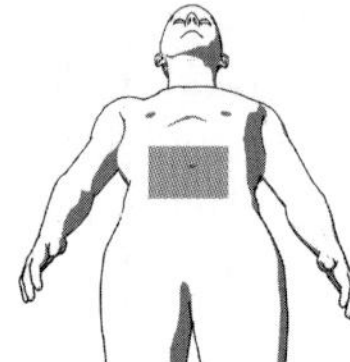

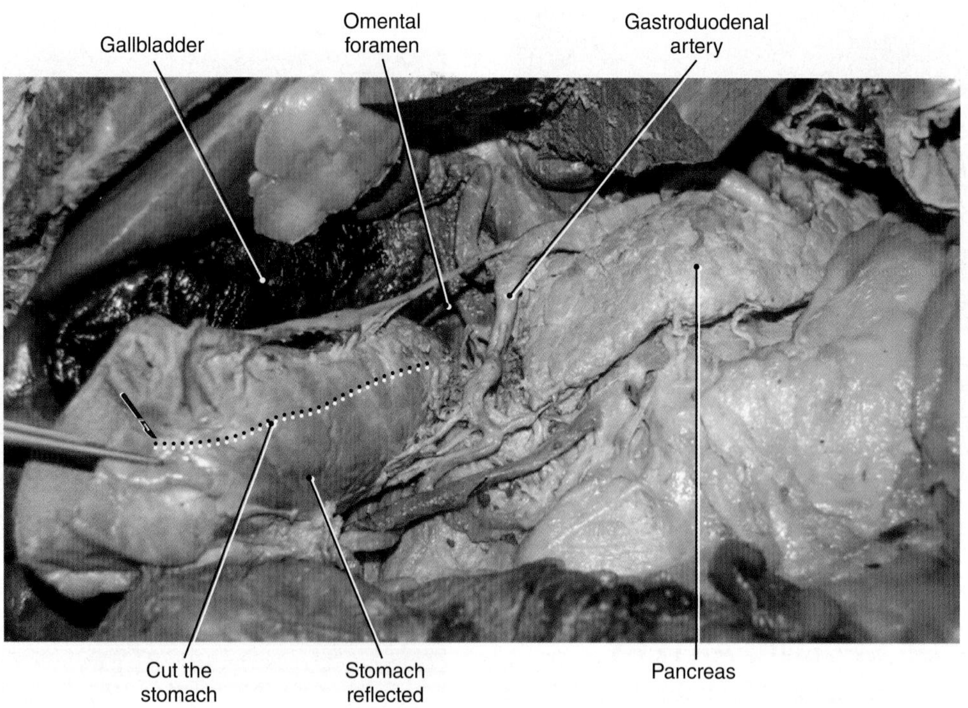

Fig. 12.35 Make a horizontal cut at the pyloric antrum, pylorus, and duodenum.

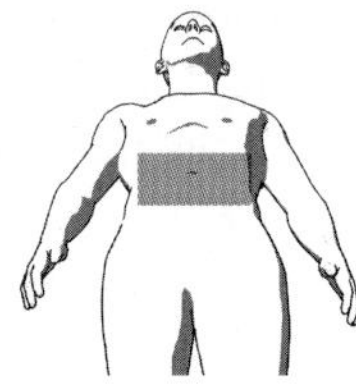

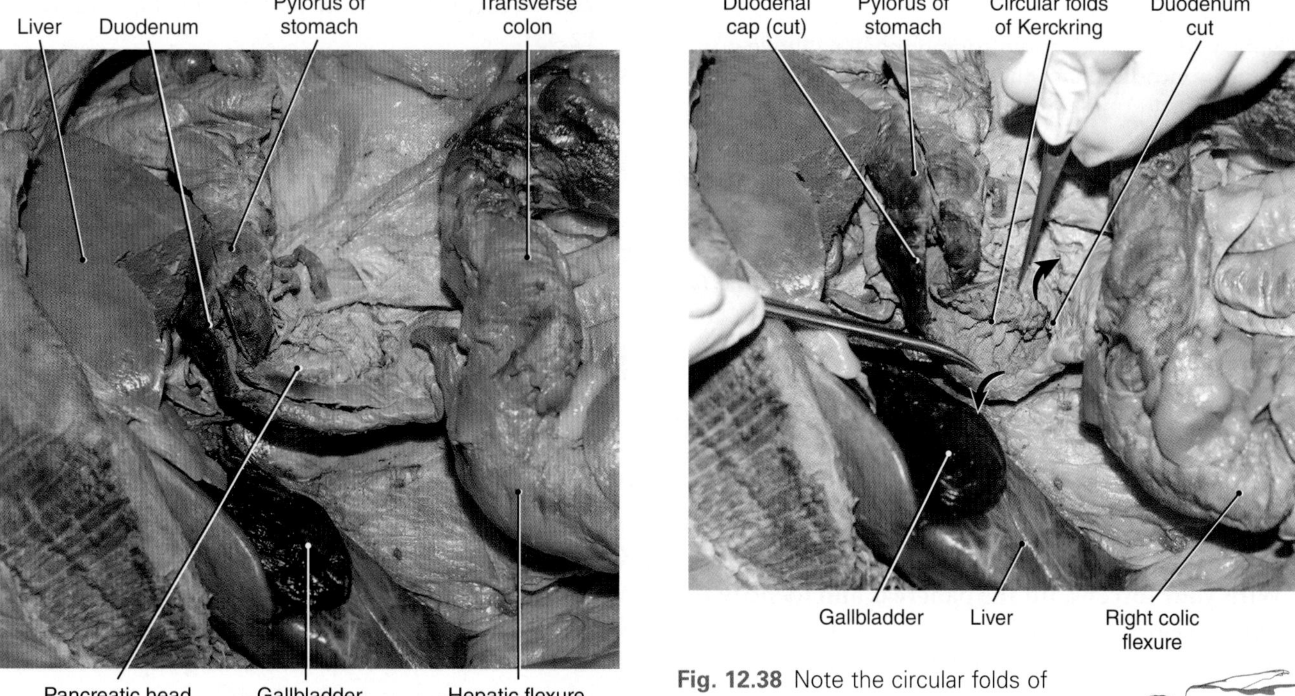

Fig. 12.37 Continue an incision through the first, second, and third parts of duodenum.

Fig. 12.38 Note the circular folds of Kerckring.

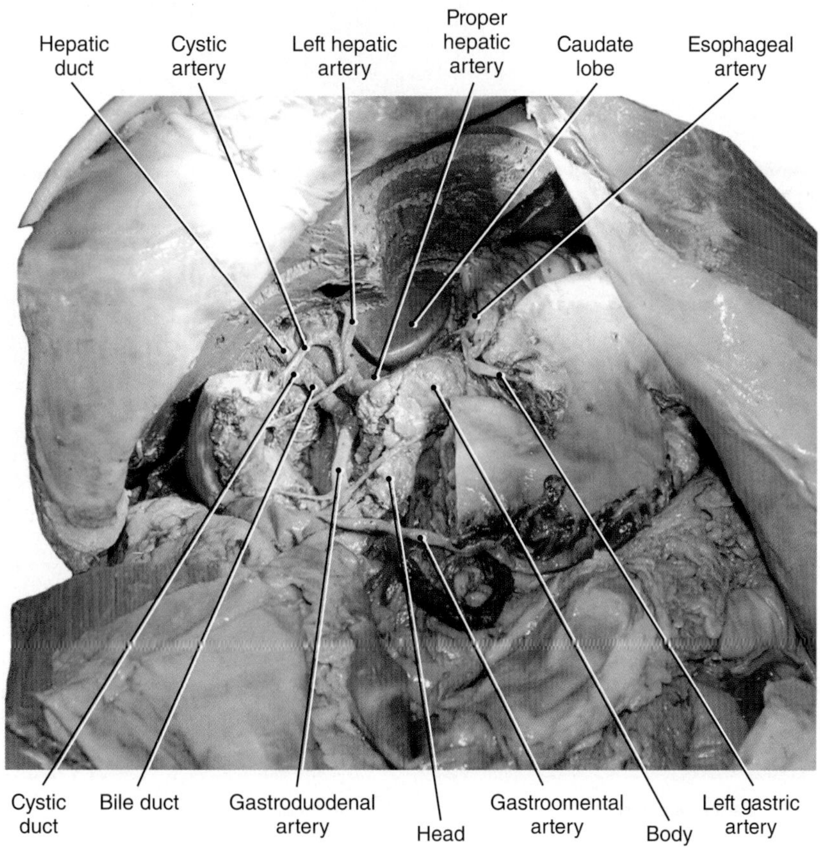

Fig. 12.39 Cut the gastroduodenal artery and expose the course of the bile duct.

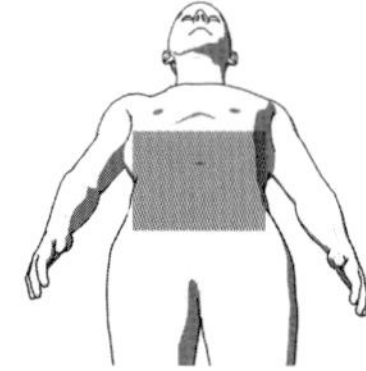

ANATOMY **NOTE**

The bile duct is divided into supraduodenal (above duodenum), retroduodenal (behind duodenum), and pancreatic parts (terminal part) (Fig. 12.40).

- **Open up the descending part of the duodenum and identify the intraduodenal portion of the bile duct; find its connection with the pancreatic duct (of Wirsung), forming the hepatopancreatic ampulla (of Vater).**
- **Identify the duodenal papilla, which contains the hepatopancreatic ampulla.**
- **Expose the pancreatic duct into the substance of the pancreas by removing pancreatic tissue with your forceps (see Fig. 12.40).**
- **Look for an accessory pancreatic duct (of Santorini), if present.**
- **With your forceps, lift the pancreas and identify the *splenic vein* (Fig. 12.41).**
- **Expose the splenic vein along its entire length and trace out its junction with the superior mesenteric vein to form the *hepatic portal vein* (Figs. 12.42 and 12.43).**
- **Next to the superior mesenteric vein, look for the inferior mesenteric vein, usually draining into the splenic vein (Plate 12.3).**
- **Continue exposing the tributaries of the superior mesenteric vein.**
- **Next to its tributaries, expose the arterial branches of the *superior mesenteric artery* (Fig. 12.44).**

DISSECTION **TIP**

The vast majority of tissue that must be removed to expose the branches of the superior mesenteric artery and vein is fat and dense autonomic nerve tissue.

- **Lift the transverse colon and observe the transverse *mesocolon* (Fig. 12.45).**
- **With your fingertips, penetrate the transverse mesocolon and expose the underlying superior mesenteric artery and vein (Fig. 12.46).**

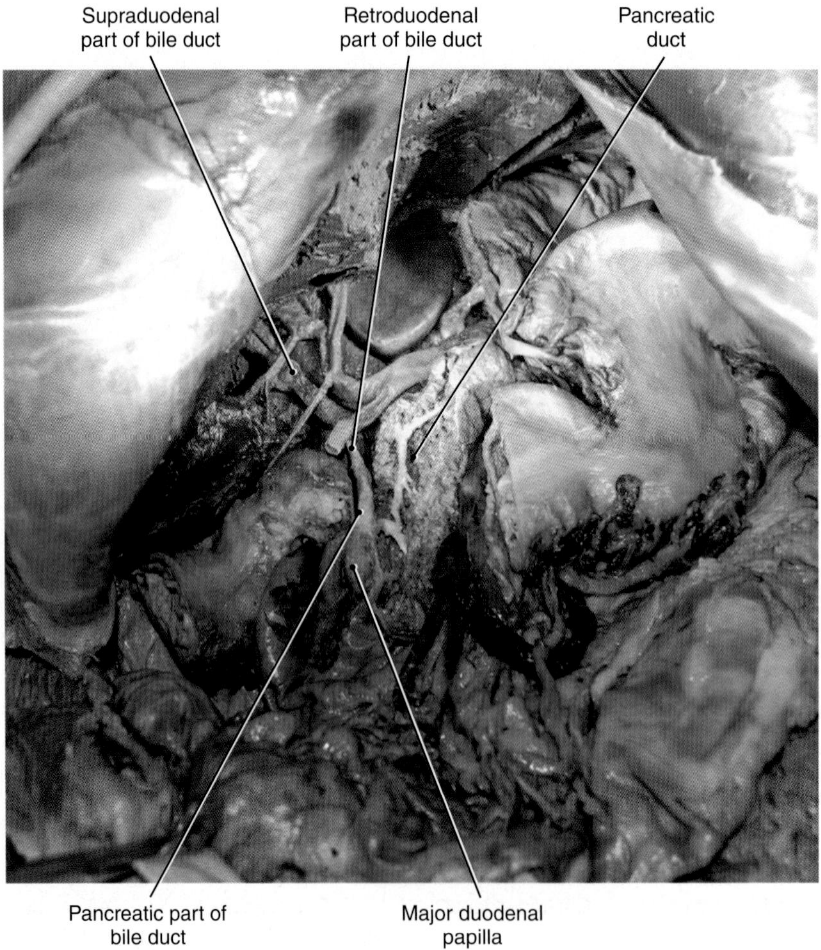

Fig. 12.40 Note divisions of the bile duct: supraduodenal, retroduodenal, and pancreatic parts.

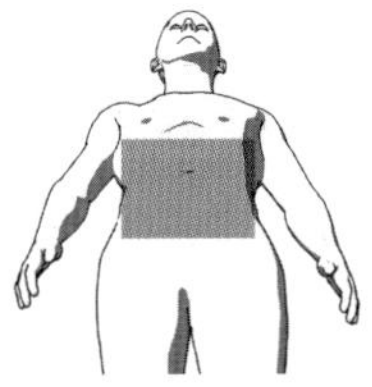

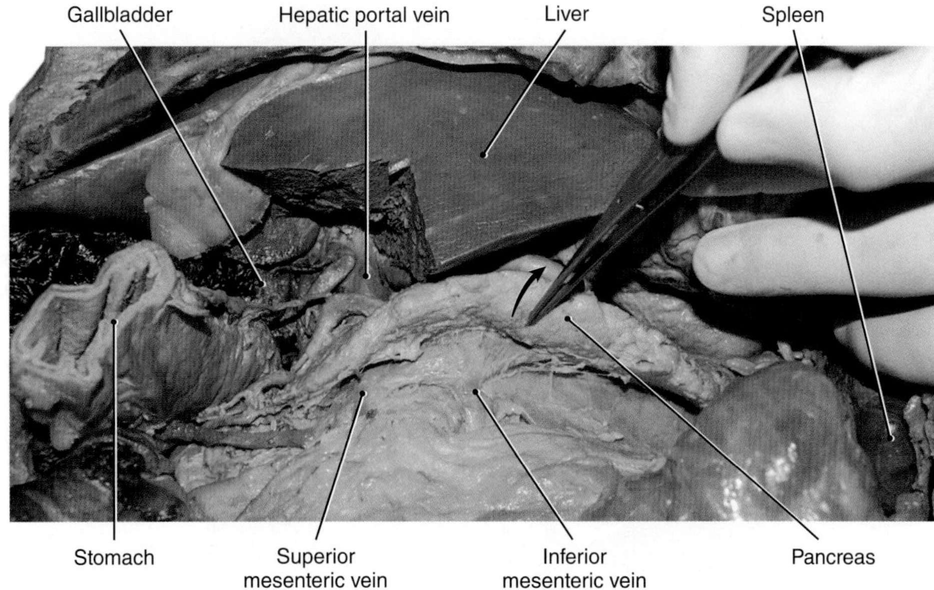

Fig. 12.41 With forceps, lift up the pancreas and identify the splenic vein.

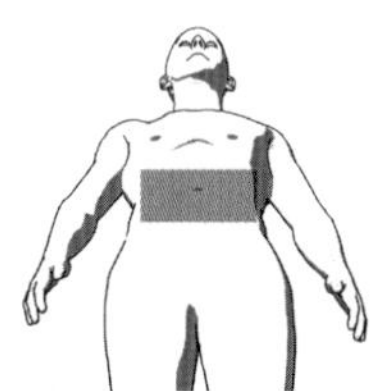

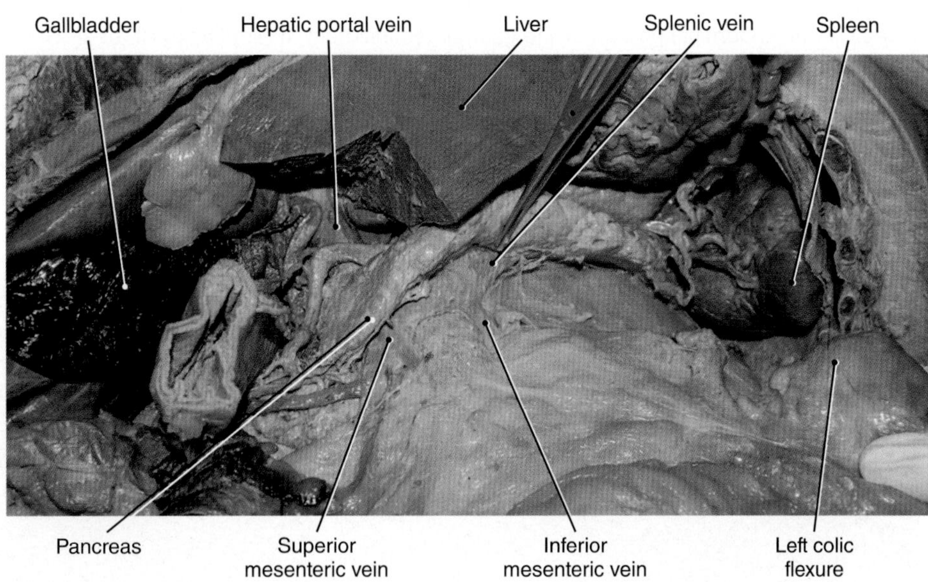

Fig. 12.42 Expose the splenic vein along its entire length.

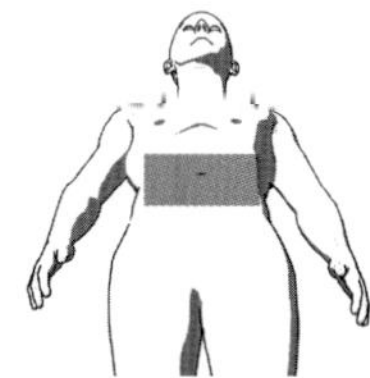

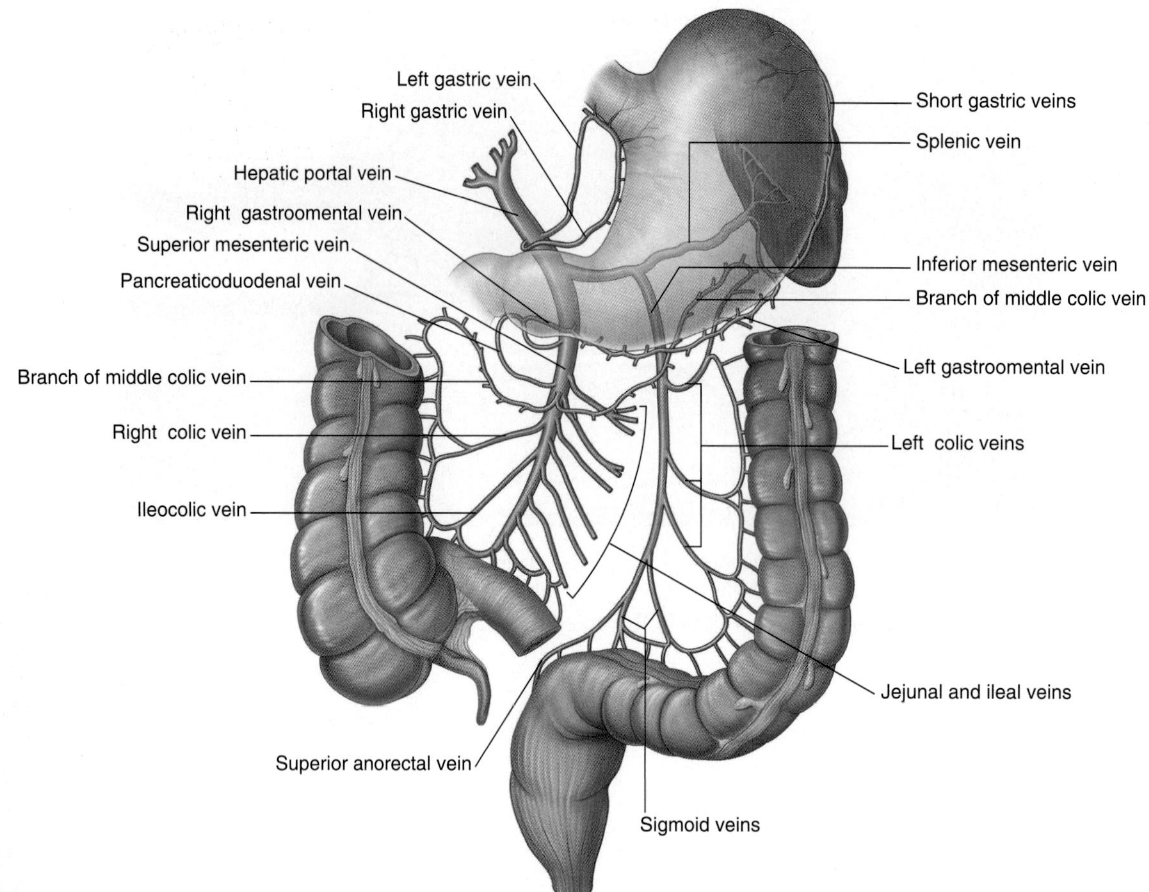

Plate 12.3 Venous drainage of the abdominal portion of the gastrointestinal tract. (From Drake RL et al. *Gray's Atlas of Anatomy*, 3rd edition, Philadelphia, Elsevier, 2021, p. 183).

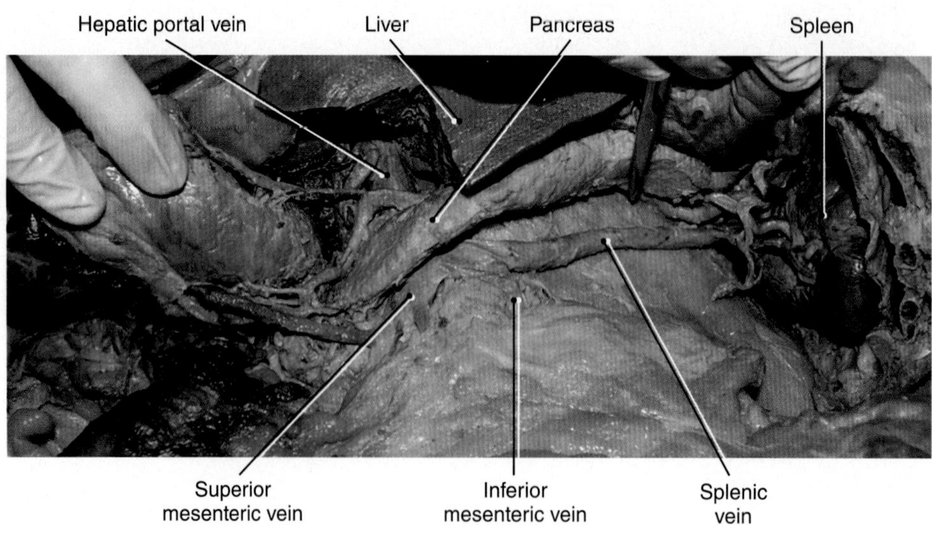

Fig. 12.43 Trace the splenic vein to its junction with the superior mesenteric vein to form the hepatic portal vein.

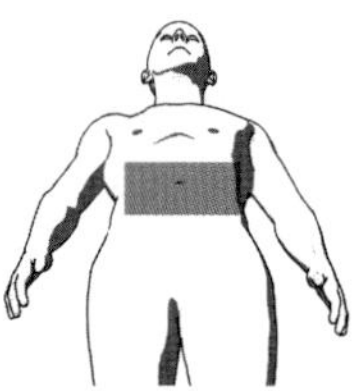

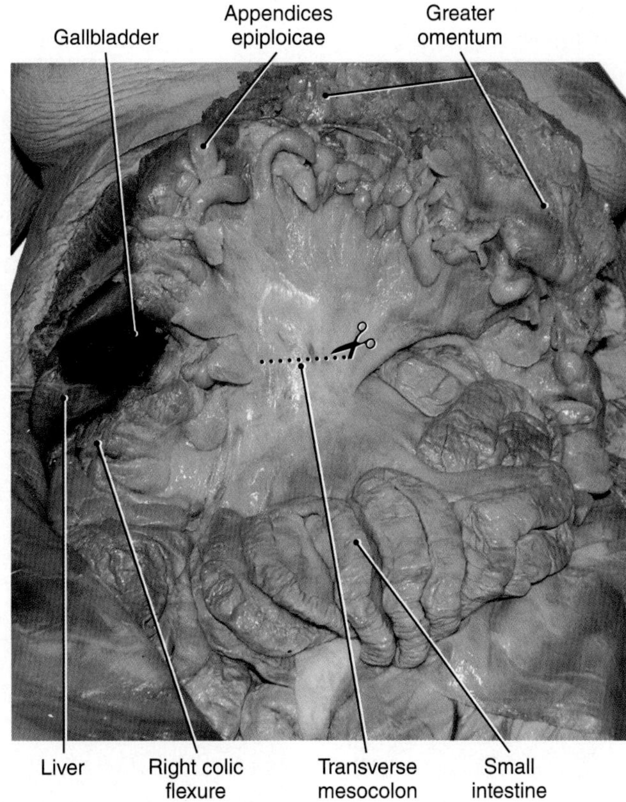

Fig. 12.45 Lift the transverse colon to see the transverse mesocolon.

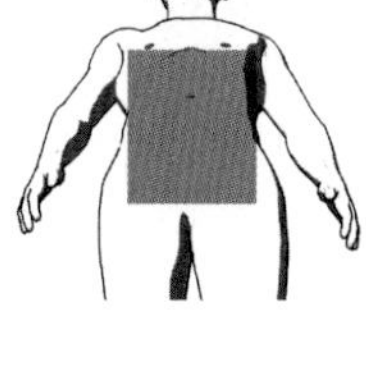

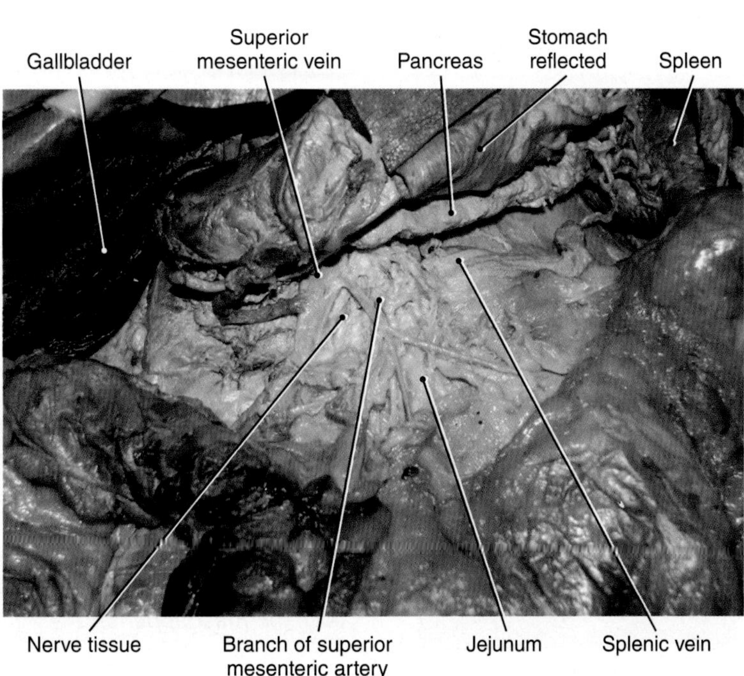

Fig. 12.44 Expose the tributaries of the superior mesenteric vein and arterial branches of the superior mesenteric artery.

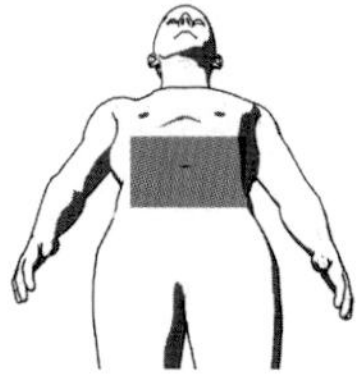

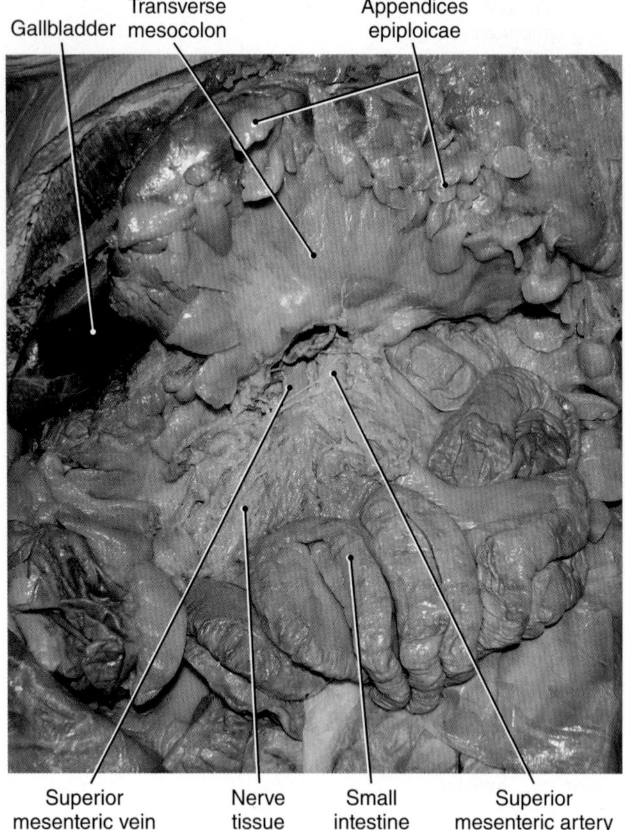

Fig. 12.46 With your fingertips, penetrate the transverse mesocolon and expose the underlying superior mesenteric artery and vein.

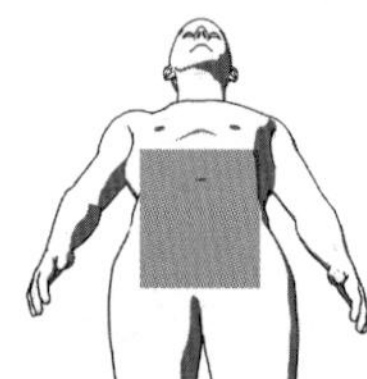

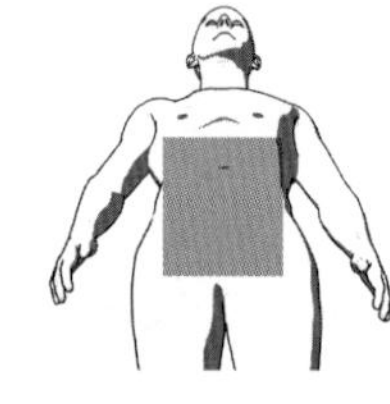

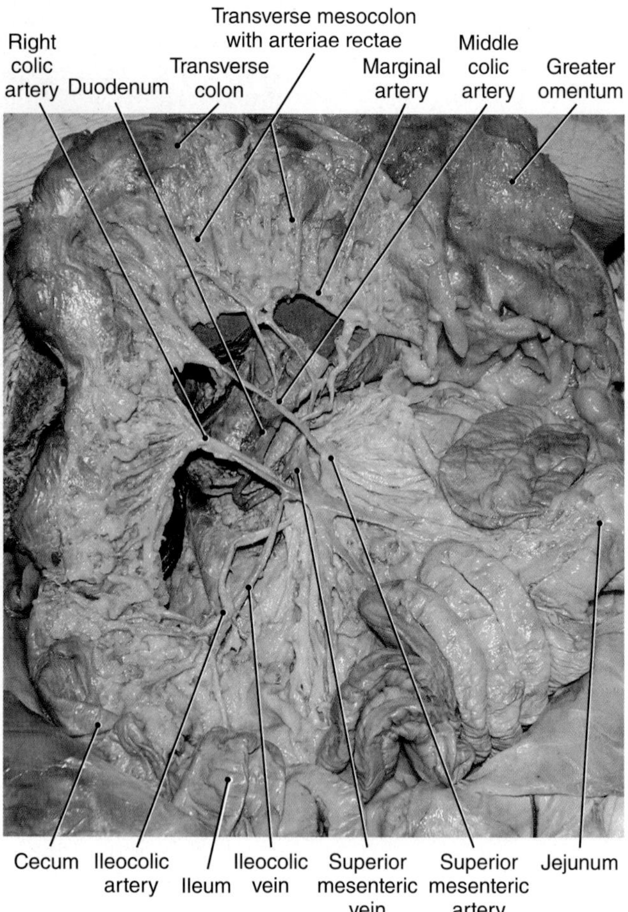

Fig. 12.48 Identify the ileocolic artery and trace it to the ileocecal junction.

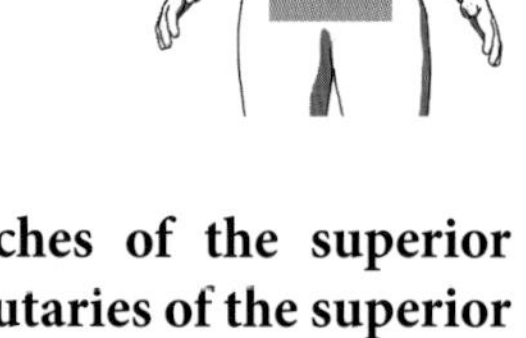

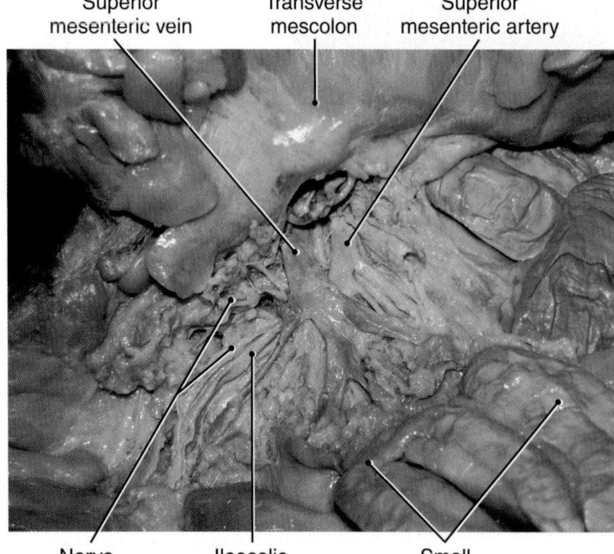

Fig. 12.47 Continue separating tributaries of the superior mesenteric vein and branches of the superior mesenteric artery from the fat and nerve tissue.

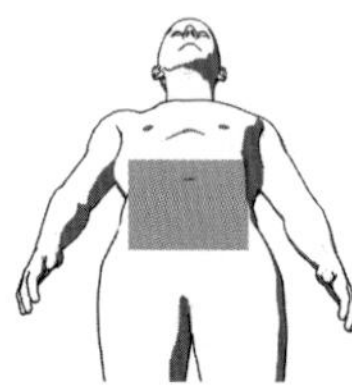

- **Continue cleaning the branches of the superior mesenteric artery and the tributaries of the superior mesenteric vein from the fat and nerve tissue (Fig. 12.47).**

DISSECTION **TIP**

The ileocolic artery is fairly constant and provides a good landmark for this dissection (Fig. 12.48).

ANATOMY **NOTE**

The ileocolic artery gives rise to the appendicular artery supplying the vermiform appendix in its own mesentery, the *mesoappendix.*

- **Identify the ileocolic artery and trace it to the *ileocecal junction,* between the ileum and the cecum.**
- **Identify the middle and right colic arteries that supply the transverse and the ascending colon, respectively (see Fig. 12.48).**
- **Look for a branch of the middle colic artery, the marginal artery (of Drummond), that supplies the**

ascending, transverse, and descending colons and anastomose with the left colic artery, a branch of the inferior mesenteric artery (see Fig. 12.52).

- Once the main three arterial branches of the *superior mesenteric artery* (middle colic, right colic, and ileocolic) are identified, expose the ileal and jejunal arteries from their origin from the superior mesenteric artery to the margin of the ileum and jejunum.

DISSECTION TIP

Realize that the mesenteric fat is much more abundant in the ileal mesentery than in the jejunal mesentery.

- Dissect out the vascular arcades, appreciating their greater number in the ileum than in the jejunum (Fig. 12.49).
- Similarly, the vasa recti are shorter and more numerous in the ileum (Figs. 12.50 and 12.51).
- Once the dissection of the superior mesenteric vessels is concluded, lift the transverse colon and review all dissected structures (Figs. 12.52 and 12.53).
- Retract the small intestine to the right and expose the transverse, descending, and sigmoid colons (Fig. 12.54).

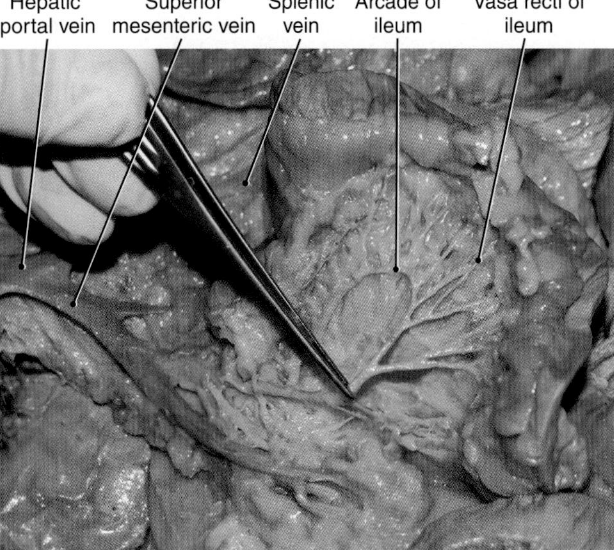

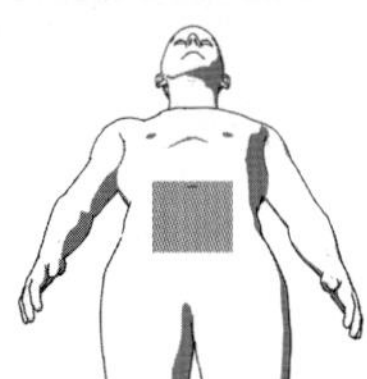

Fig. 12.50 Notice that the vasa recti are shorter and more numerous in the ileum than in the jejunum. Note the increased number of arcades in the ileum compared with the jejunum.

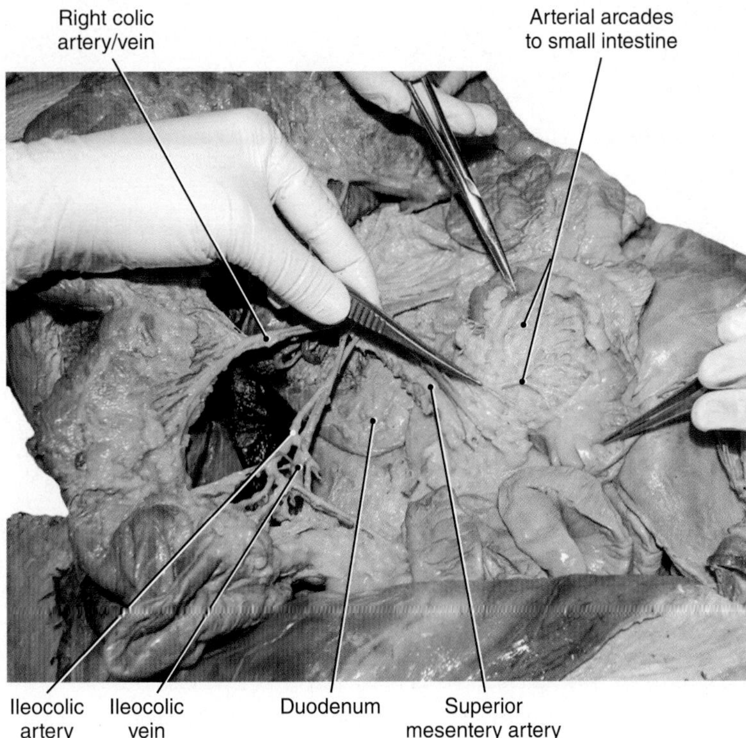

Fig. 12.49 Dissect out the vascular arcades.

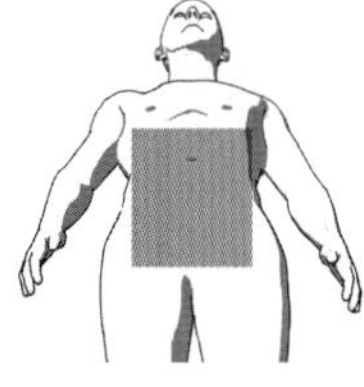

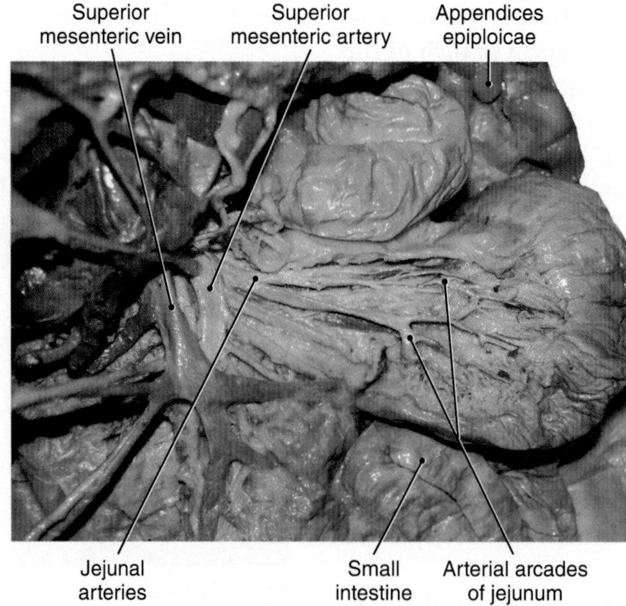

Fig. 12.51 Note the increased number of arcades in the ileum compared to the jejunum.

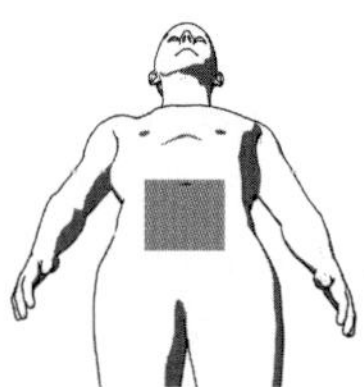

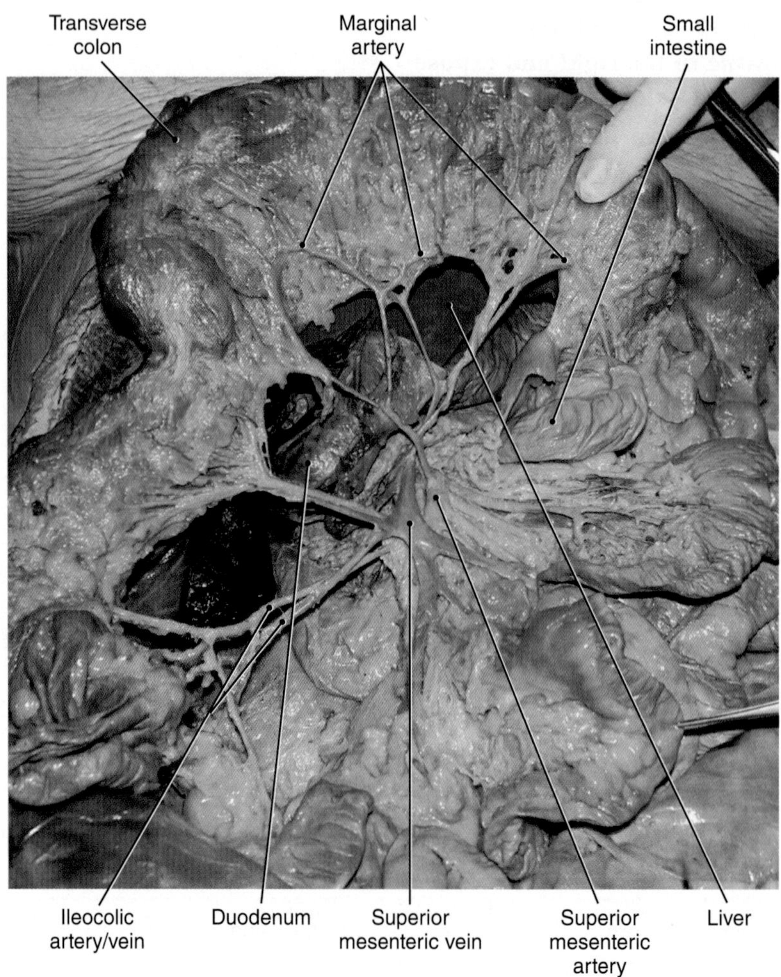

Fig. 12.52 Concluded dissection of the superior mesenteric vessels.

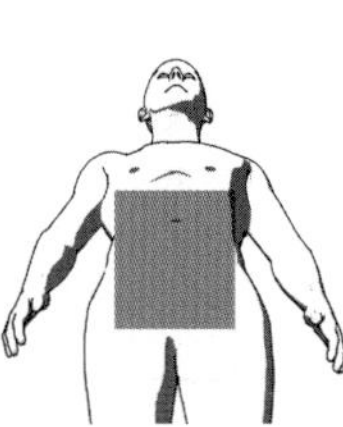

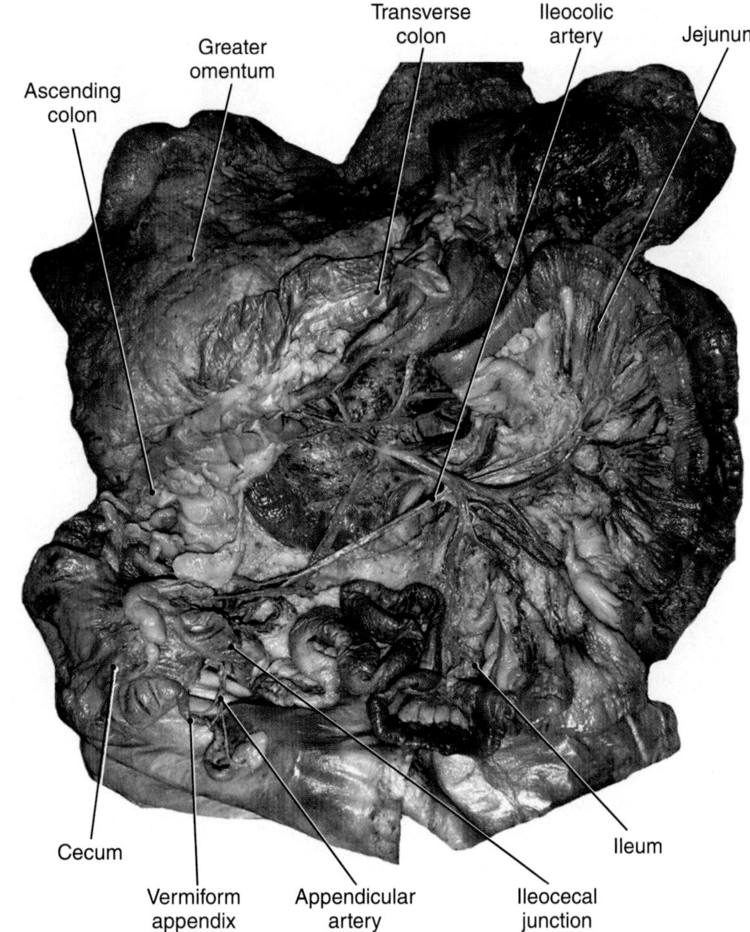

Fig. 12.53 Lift the transverse colon and review its related structures.

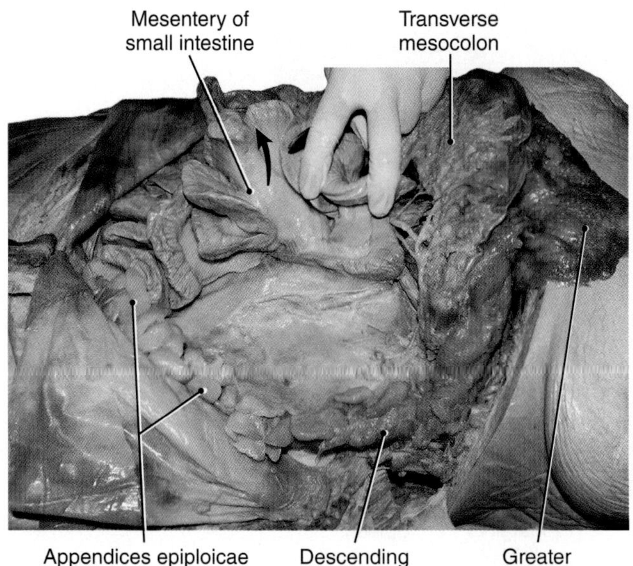

Fig. 12.54 Retract the small intestine to the right and expose the transverse, descending, and sigmoid colons.

- **With scissors, continue the exposure of the inferior mesenteric vein (Fig. 12.55) toward the margins of the colon.**
- **To the right or medial to the inferior mesenteric vein, identify the *inferior mesenteric artery* (Plate 12.4).**

DISSECTION TIP

Both the inferior mesenteric artery and the inferior mesenteric vein require additional effort to expose because of the dense nerve plexuses covering them. To facilitate the dissection of the branches of the inferior mesenteric artery, make a shallow incision between the lateral wall of the descending colon and the body of the white line of Toldt (left paracolic gutter), and release the descending colon from the peritoneum. In addition, do *not* remove the nerve plexus when you expose the inferior mesenteric vessels. This nerve tissue will be examined in a later dissection of the posterior abdominal wall.

- **Identify the branches of the inferior mesenteric artery, the left artery, and the sigmoid arteries and fully expose them (Fig. 12.56).**

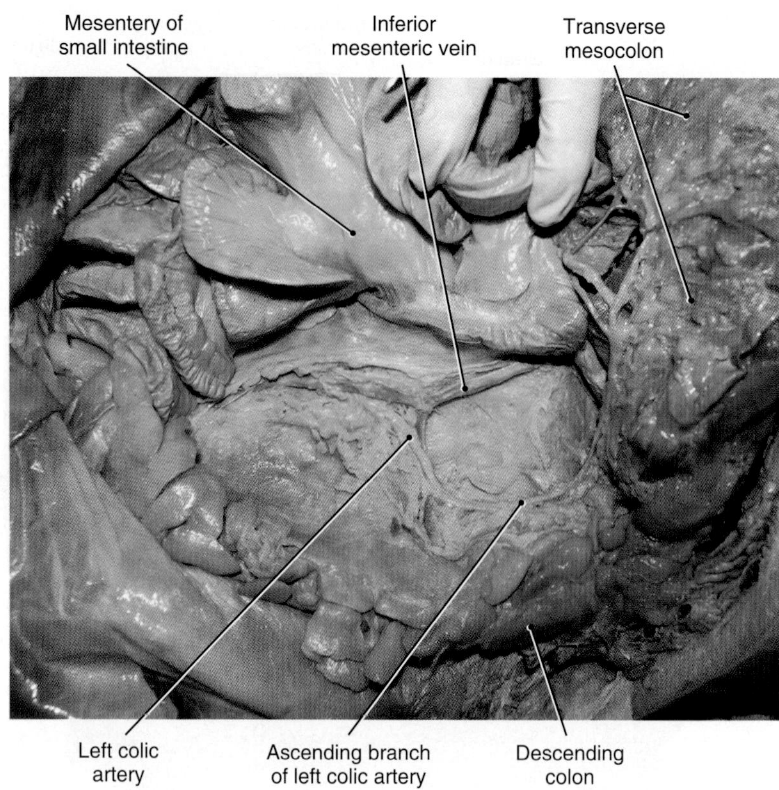

Fig. 12.55 With scissors, continue exposure of the inferior mesenteric vein.

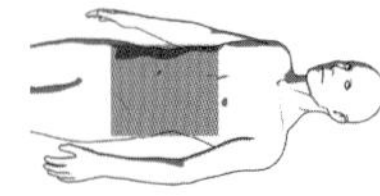

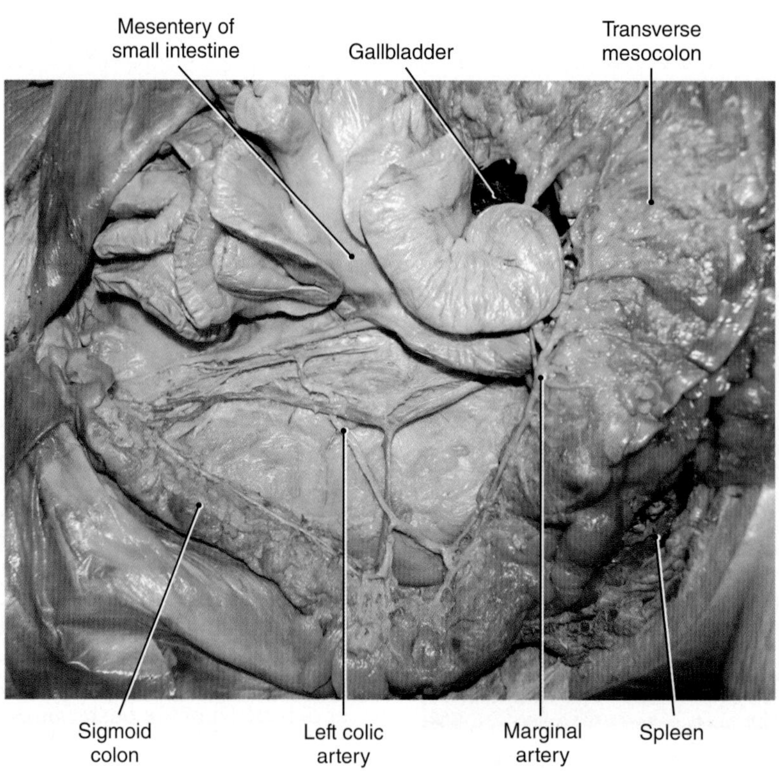

Fig. 12.56 Identify and fully expose the branches of the inferior mesenteric artery, and left colic and sigmoid arteries.

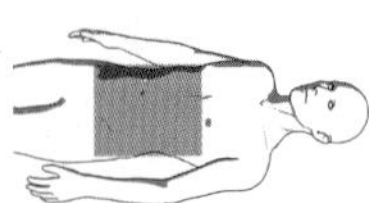

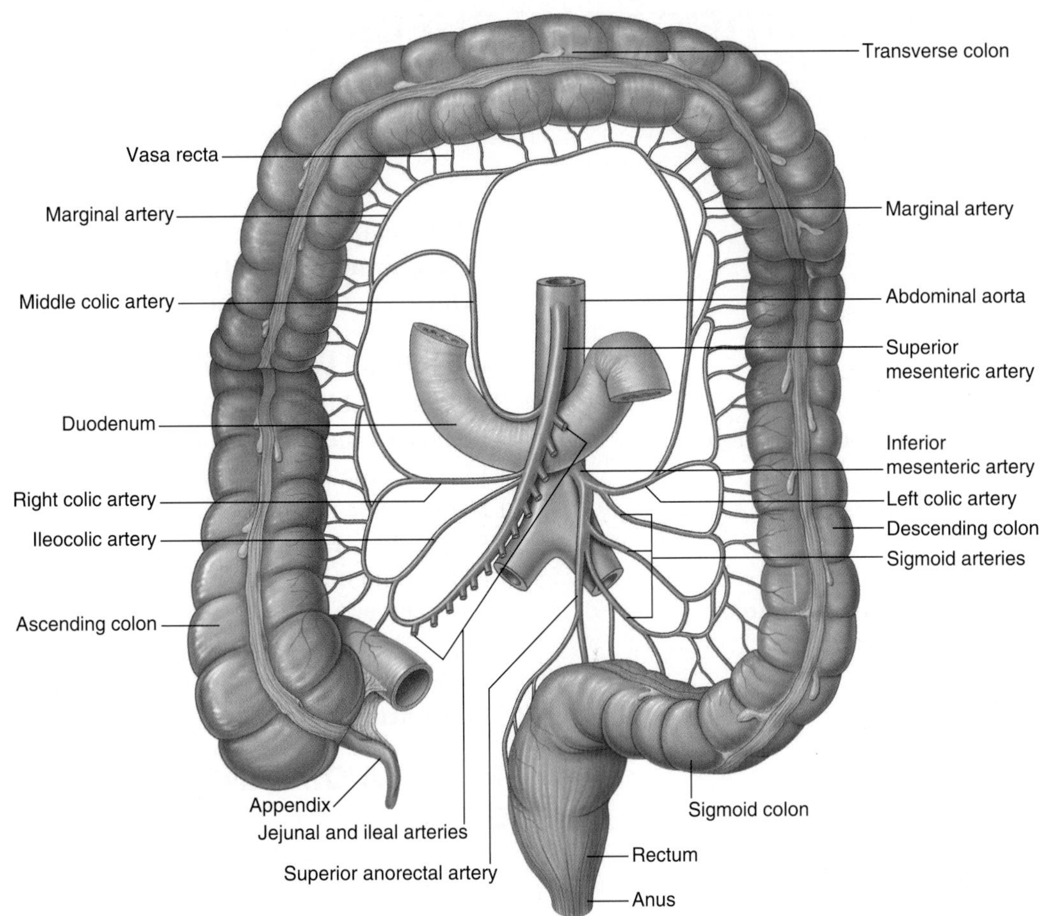

Plate 12.4 Superior and inferior mesenteric arteries. (From Drake RL et al. *Gray's Atlas of Anatomy*, 3rd edition, Philadelphia, Elsevier, 2021, p. 172).

IF TIME PERMITS

- Tie two strings close together around the proximal segment of the jejunum and cut between them.
- Perform the same technique along a distal portion of the ileum.
- Clean the two segments and observe their internal morphology.
- Note the increased number of plicae circulares and villi, as well as increased wall thickness in the jejunum compared to the ileum.
- Similarly, place a ligature at the ileocecal junction and another ligature at the midportion of the ascending colon.
- Remove this segment and examine its internal morphology.
- Identify the ileocecal valve.

LABORATORY IDENTIFICATION CHECKLIST

ARTERIES

- ☐ Abdominal aorta
- ☐ Celiac trunk
  - ☐ Common hepatic
  - ☐ Proper hepatic
  - ☐ Gastroduodenal
  - ☐ Right gastroomental (gastroepiploic)
  - ☐ Right gastric
  - ☐ Splenic
  - ☐ Short gastrics
  - ☐ Left gastric
  - ☐ Left gastroomental (gastroepiploic)
- ☐ Superior mesenteric artery
  - ☐ Ileocolic
  - ☐ Appendicular
  - ☐ Right colic
  - ☐ Middle colic
- ☐ Inferior mesenteric
  - ☐ Left colic
  - ☐ Sigmoid
  - ☐ Superior anorectal
- ☐ Marginal (formed between ileocolic [right, middle] and left colic arteries)
- ☐ Jejunal and ileal arteries (arcades) and recti branches

VEINS

- ☐ Inferior vena cava
  - ☐ Hepatic
- ☐ Hepatic portal
  - ☐ Superior mesenteric
  - ☐ Splenic
  - ☐ Inferior mesenteric

LYMPH NODES

- ☐ Mesenteric

MUSCLES

- ☐ External abdominal oblique
- ☐ Internal abdominal oblique
  - ☐ Cremaster
- ☐ Transversus abdominis
- ☐ Rectus abdominis
- ☐ Pyramidalis
- ☐ Crus (right and left) of diaphragm
- ☐ Psoas major
- ☐ Psoas minor (variant)
- ☐ Quadratus lumborum

CONNECTIVE TISSUE

- ☐ External oblique aponeurosis
- ☐ Greater omentum
- ☐ Lesser omentum
- ☐ Transverse mesocolon
- ☐ Sigmoid mesentery
- ☐ Mesoappendix
- ☐ Mesentery

Liver

- ☐ Falciform ligament
- ☐ Ligamentum teres

VISCERA/ORGANS

Esophagus

- ☐ Abdominal esophagus

Stomach

- ☐ Fundus
- ☐ Body
- ☐ Cardia
- ☐ Pylorus
- ☐ Greater curvature
- ☐ Lesser curvature

Small Intestine

- ☐ Duodenum
- ☐ Jejunum
- ☐ Ileum

Large Intestine

- ☐ Cecum
- ☐ Vermiform appendix
- ☐ Ascending colon
- ☐ Transverse colon
- ☐ Descending colon
- ☐ Sigmoid colon
- ☐ Appendices epiploicae
- ☐ Teniae coli

Liver

- ☐ Left lobe
- ☐ Right lobe
- ☐ Caudate
- ☐ Quadrate

Gallbladder

☐ Fundus
☐ Body
☐ Neck

Pancreas

☐ Head
☐ Neck
☐ Body
☐ Tail
☐ Uncinate process

Spleen

☐ Splenic notch
☐ Hilum

EXPOSING THE KIDNEYS

- Cut the white lines of Toldt (paracolic gutters) along the edges of the ascending and descending colons and reflect the large and small intestines to the left of the abdominal cavity (Fig. 13.1).
- With your fingers, retract the duodenum and pancreas to the left, without disrupting their vascular supply (Fig. 13.2).
- Palpate the abdominal aorta on the left and the *inferior vena cava* (IVC) on the right.
- With scissors, cut the peritoneum of the posterior abdominal wall and expose the IVC (Fig. 13.3).
- To the right of the IVC, dissect out the perirenal (renal) fascia (of Gerota), which is filled predominantly with abundant perirenal fat (Fig. 13.4).
- Trace the right ureter; expose its course from the kidney to the pelvic brim and as it crosses over the iliac arteries.
- Remove the fat posterior to the kidney, known as the *pararenal* fat (Fig. 13.5).

DISSECTION TIP

For the removal of the perirenal and pararenal fat, use scissors or a probe and scrape it from the kidney capsule.

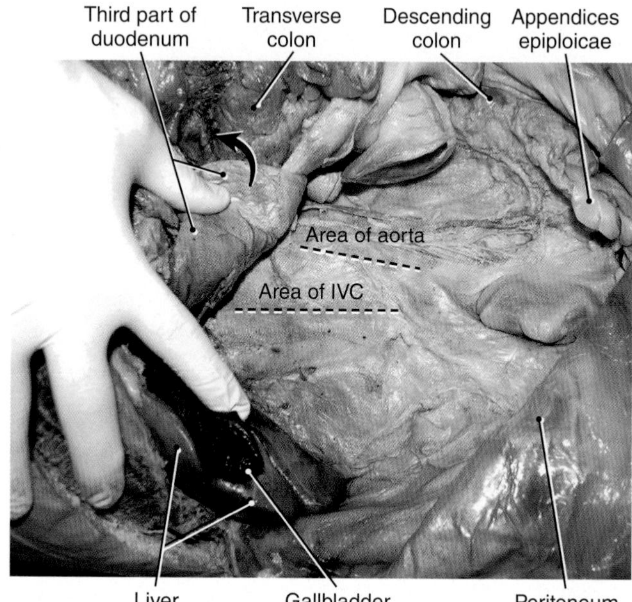

Fig. 13.2 Retract the duodenum and pancreas. *IVC*, Inferior vena cava.

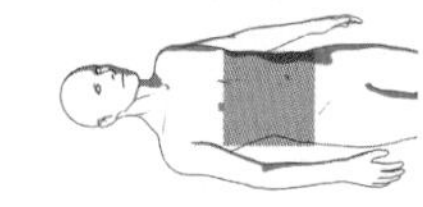

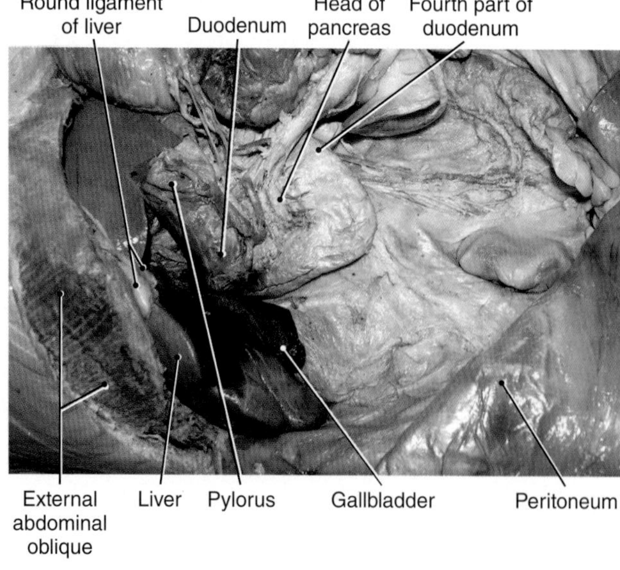

Fig. 13.1 Cut along the edges of ascending and descending colons (lines of Toldt) with large and small intestines reflected to the left of the abdominal cavity.

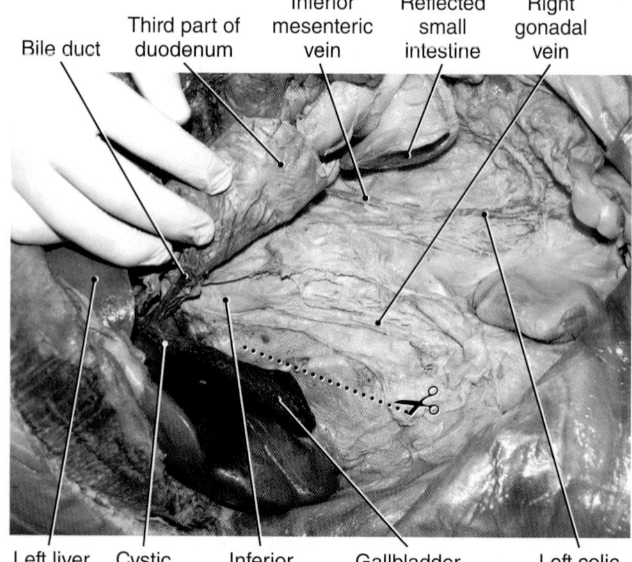

Fig. 13.3 Peritoneum of the posterior abdominal wall incised to expose the inferior vena cava.

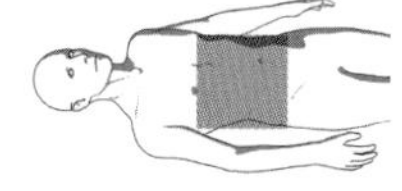

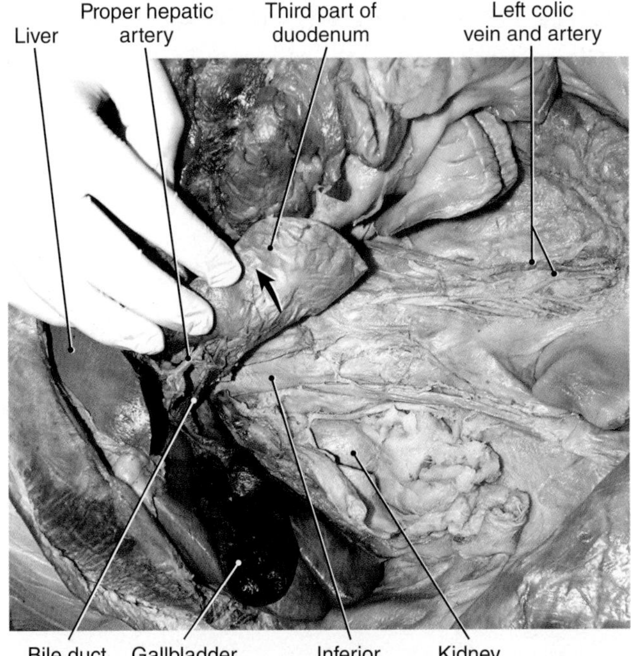

Fig. 13.4 Perirenal fascia (of Gerota) dissected to the right of the inferior vena cava.

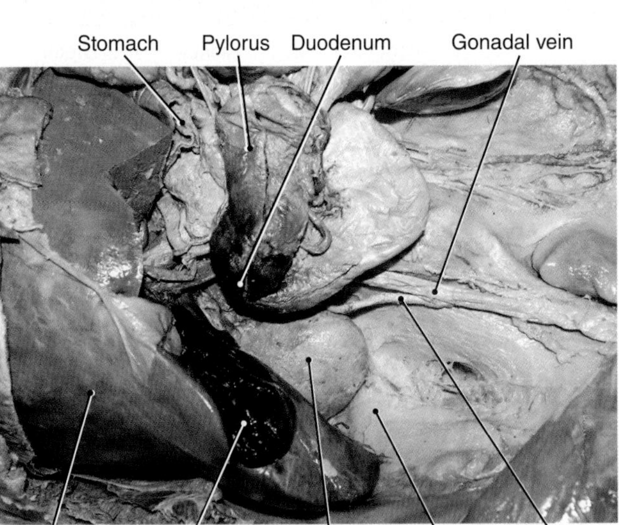

Fig. 13.5 Right ureter exposed as it leaves the right kidney, toward the pelvic brim and over the iliac arteries. Pararenal fat has been removed posterior to the kidney.

- Remove enough fascia and adipose tissue to clearly expose the kidneys and suprarenal glands. Free up the margins of the suprarenal glands, taking care to preserve their blood vessels, especially along their medial borders.
- Remove all fat from the posterior part of the kidney capsule.

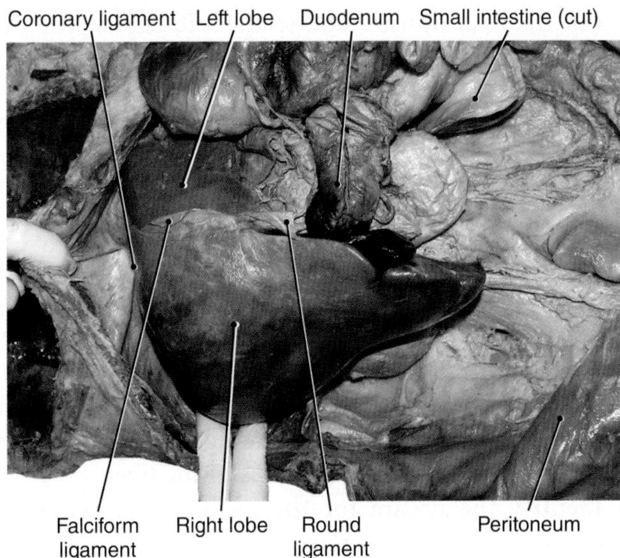

Fig. 13.6 Falciform, left triangular, and coronary ligaments cut and right triangular ligament incised on lifting liver.

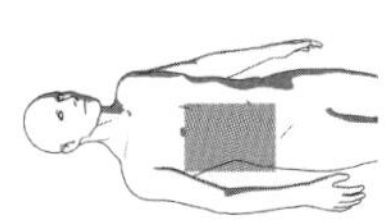

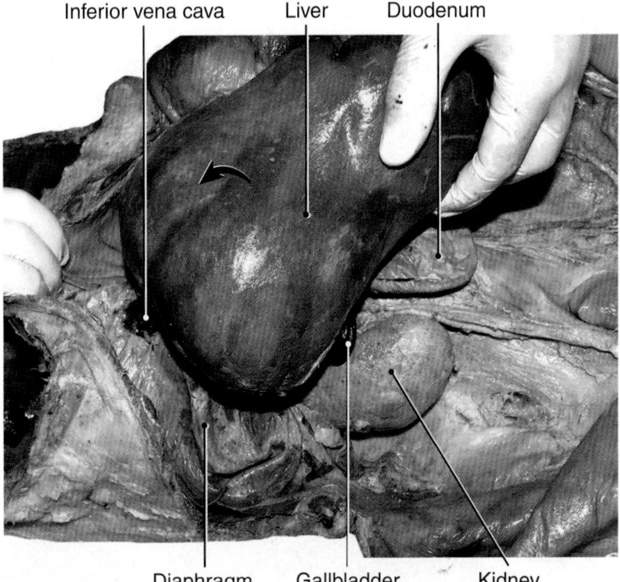

Fig. 13.7 With liver pulled inferiorly, cut the inferior vena cava in the space between the superior aspect of the liver and the undersurface of the diaphragm.

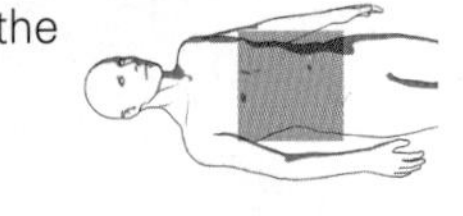

LIVER

- **Reflect the liver medially and expose the entire posterior abdominal wall.**
- **Cut the falciform, left triangular, and coronary ligaments.**
- **Place your fingertips underneath the lateral side of the liver, lift it up slightly, and cut the right triangular ligament (Fig. 13.6).**
- **Pull the liver inferiorly, and in the space between the diaphragm and the liver, cut the IVC (Fig. 13.7).**

- Lift the liver upward and to the left; expose the infrahepatic portion of the IVC away from the body wall (Fig. 13.8).
- Gently pull the liver to the left; otherwise, you will damage the right suprarenal vein as it enters the IVC.
- With a scalpel, make an incision through the IVC superior to the level of the renal veins and reflect the liver to the left (Fig. 13.9).
- The liver is attached to the abdominal cavity only by the hepatic portal vein, hepatic artery, and bile duct.
- On the reflected liver, identify the right and left lobes (divided by the falciform ligament), as well as the quadrate and caudate lobes of the liver.
- Identify the fissure for the ligamentum venosum and the ligamentum teres (round ligament) of the liver.
- Identify the round, left triangular, and coronary ligaments (Fig. 13.10).
- To identify the ligamentum venosum, reflect the caudate lobe and clean the fissure for the ligament (Fig. 13.11).
- Reflect the inferior vena cava slightly inferiorly and expose the suprarenal gland and the bare area of the liver (Fig. 13.12).

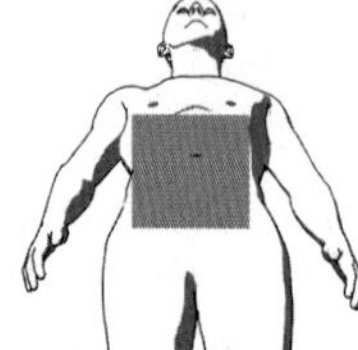

Fig. 13.8 Liver lifted upward and to the left exposing the infrahepatic portion of the inferior vena cava.

KIDNEYS AND SUPRARENAL GLANDS

- Clean out the connective tissue and fat over the IVC and expose the right gonadal vein and right and left renal veins (Figs. 13.13 and 13.14).
- Continue the exposure of the left renal vein to the left and clean away the fat and connective tissue over the abdominal aorta (Fig. 13.15).

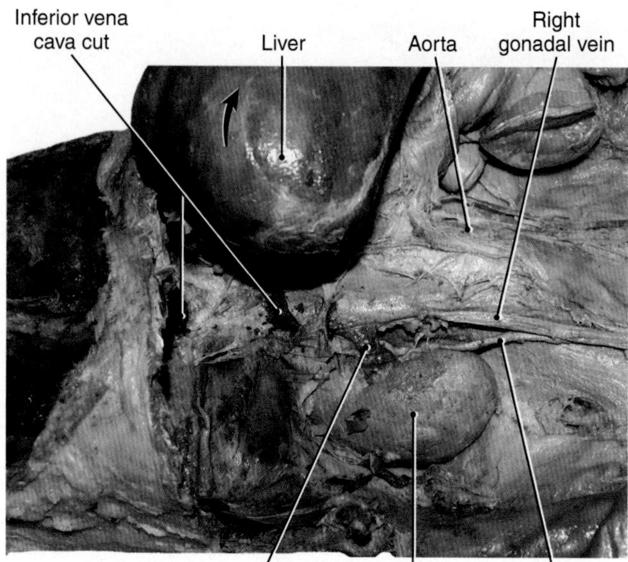

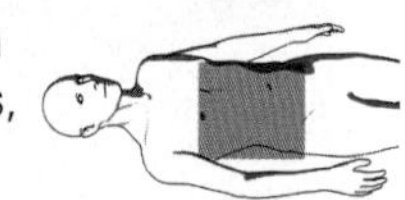

Fig. 13.9 Incision through the inferior vena cava superior to the level of the renal veins, with the liver reflected.

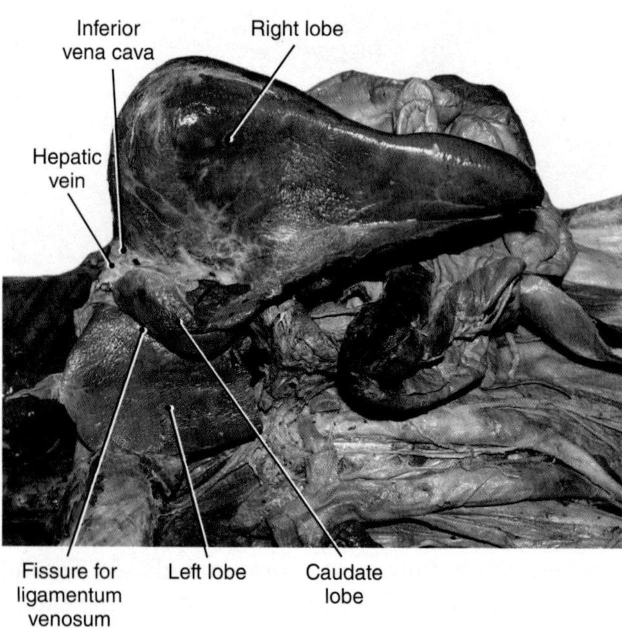

Fig. 13.10 Identify the right and left lobes of the liver. Trace the inferior vena cava and the hepatic vein. Identify the fissure for the ligamentum venosum between the left lobe of the liver and the caudate lobe.

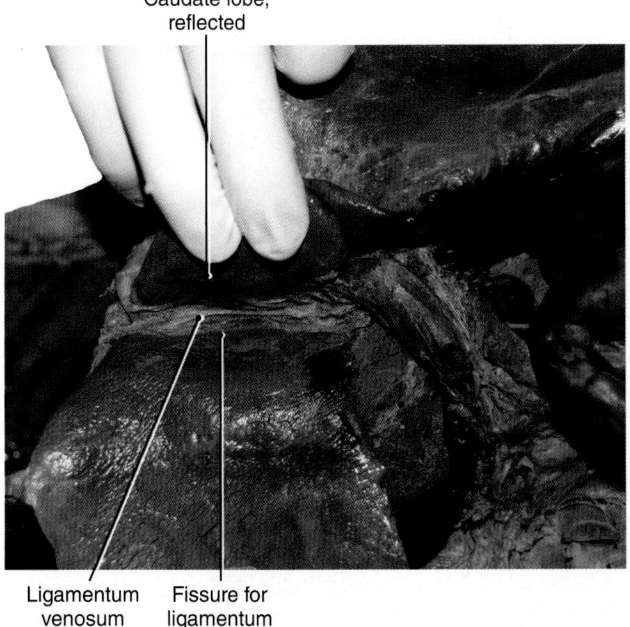

Fig. 13.11 Caudate lobe reflected and fissure cleaned to identify the ligamentum venosum.

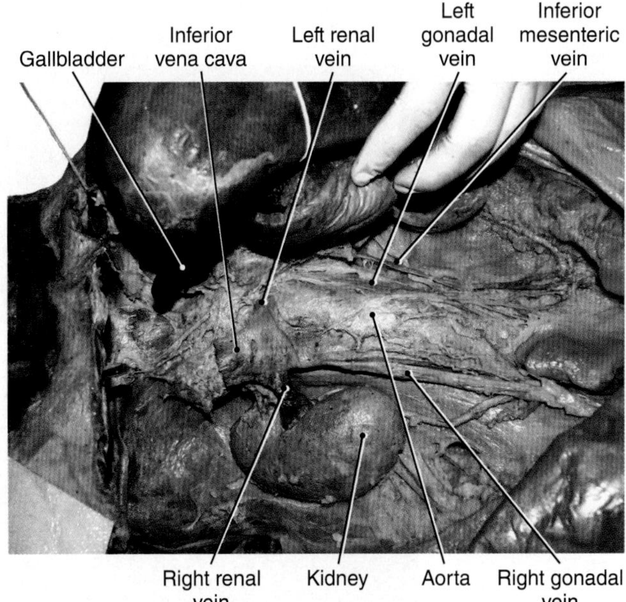

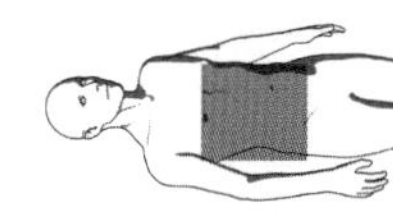

Fig. 13.13 Fat and connective tissue cleaned over the inferior vena cava, exposing the right gonadal and right renal veins.

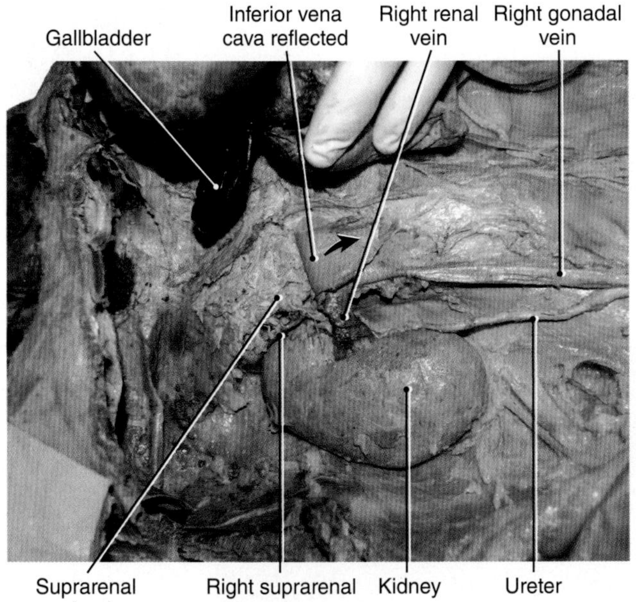

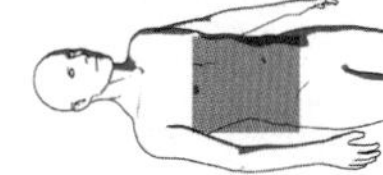

Fig. 13.12 Suprarenal gland and bare area of the liver exposed by reflecting the inferior vena cava slightly inferiorly.

- **Paying special attention, identify the gonadal artery arising from the aorta just inferior to the level of the right renal vein.**
- **In the space between the IVC and aorta, identify the right lymphatic trunk and the sympathetic fibers ascending from the superior hypogastric plexus. This plexus is located just anterior to the promontory of the sacrum (Fig. 13.16).**
- **Complete the dissection by exposing the branches of the *inferior mesenteric artery* (Figs. 13.17 and 13.18).**
- **Identify and expose the renal arteries and veins.**

ANATOMY **NOTE**

The left renal vein crosses over the aorta, inferior to the origin of the superior mesenteric artery, to reach the IVC. In contrast, the right renal artery passes posterior to the IVC (Fig. 13.19).

DISSECTION **TIP**

Additional renal arteries are often seen arising from the aorta; these are normal variations.

- **Identify the right suprarenal gland with its connection between the right suprarenal vein and the IVC (see Fig. 13.12). This vein is very short.**
- **Dissect out the right superior, middle, and inferior suprarenal arteries, typically arising from the inferior phrenic artery, aorta, and renal artery, respectively (Fig. 13.20).**
- **Notice the drainage of the right gonadal vein directly into the IVC (Plate 13.1).**
- **Identify the left suprarenal gland and expose the left suprarenal vein and left gonadal vein draining into the left renal vein.**
- **With a scalpel, make a coronal incision and expose the outer cortex, as well as the inner medulla, of the suprarenal gland.**

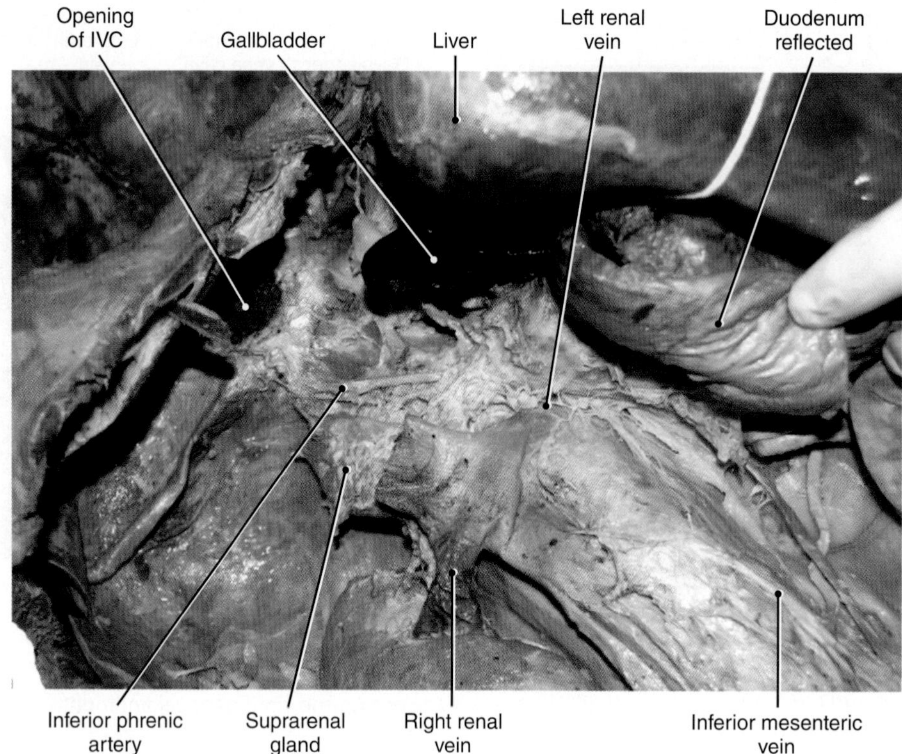

Fig. 13.14 Left renal vein exposed. *IVC*, Inferior vena cava.

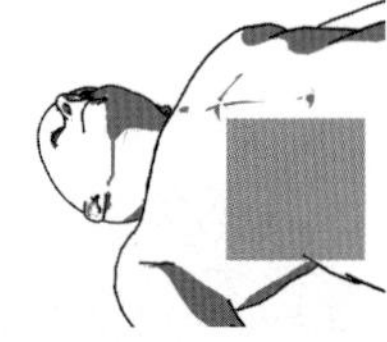

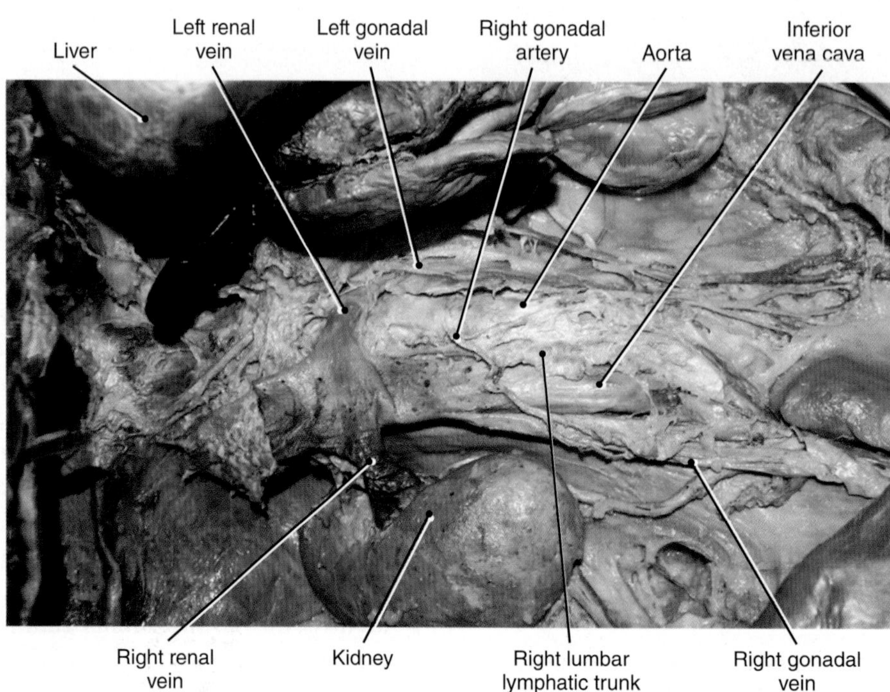

Fig. 13.15 Left renal vein exposed, showing the left gonadal vein, with the gonadal artery arising from the aorta just inferior to the right renal vein.

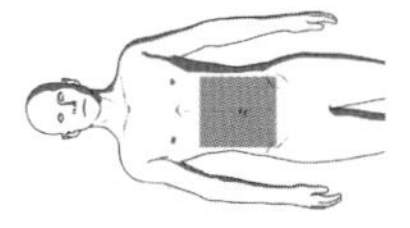

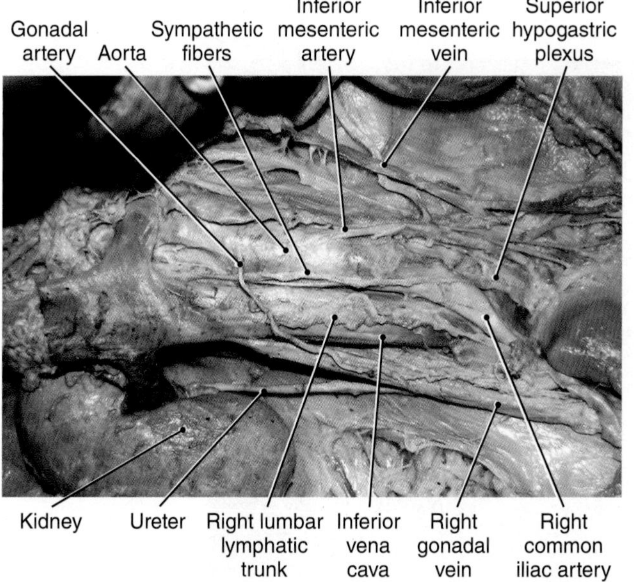

Fig. 13.16 Right lymphatic trunk and sympathetic fibers ascending from the superior hypogastric plexus.

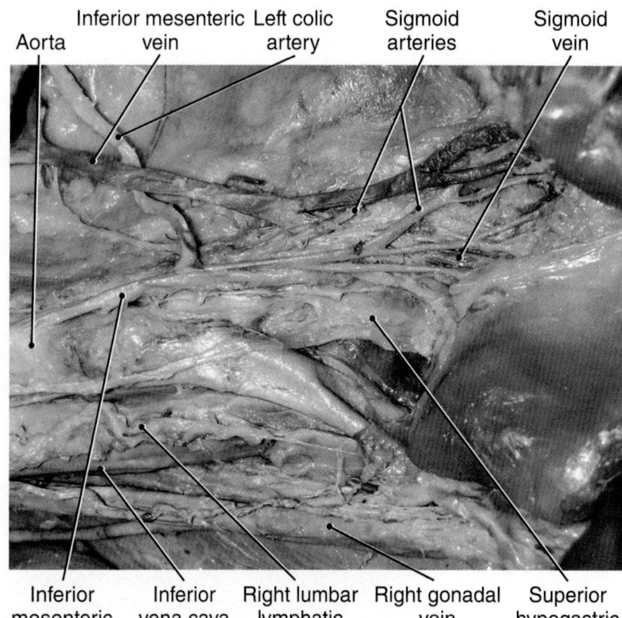

Fig. 13.17 Dissection completed by exposing the inferior mesenteric artery.

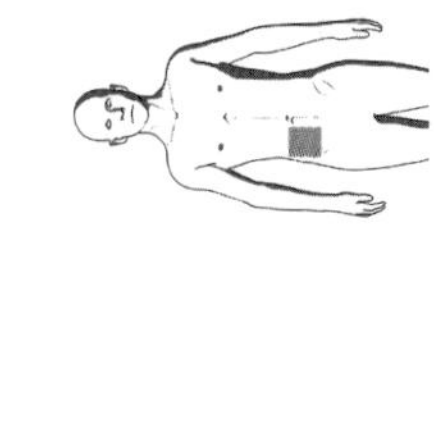

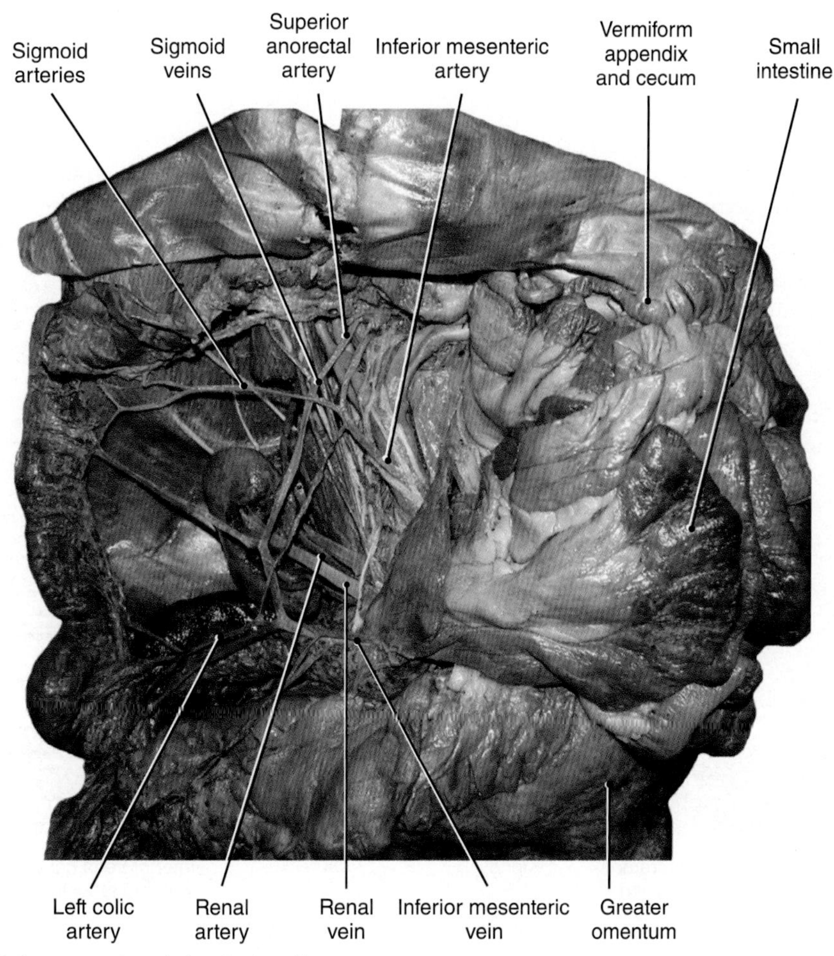

Fig. 13.18 Structures of the posterior abdominal wall.

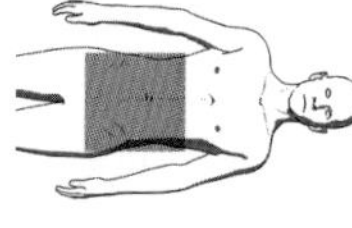

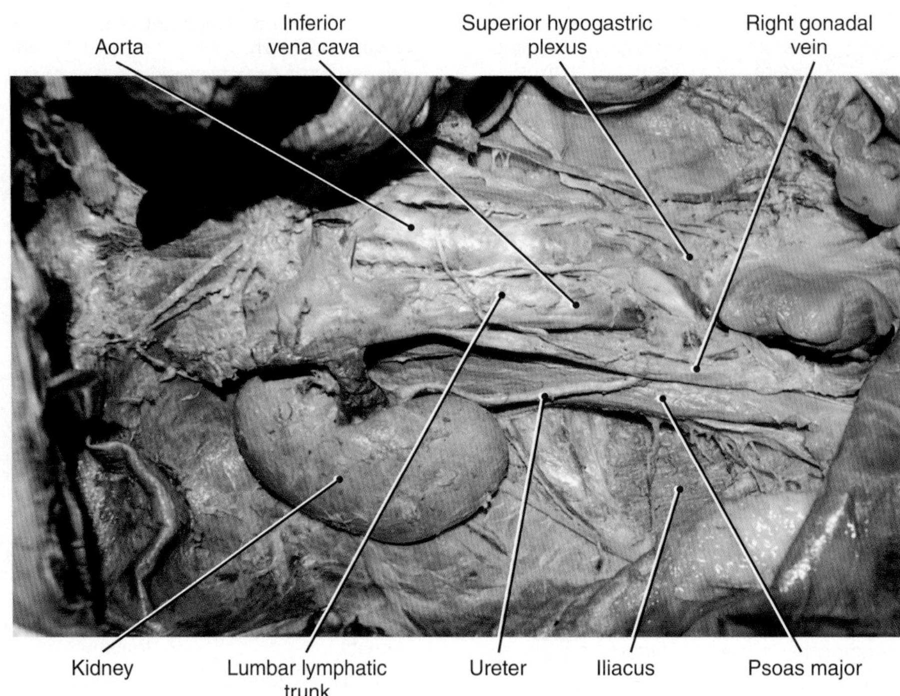

Fig. 13.19 Locate and expose the renal arteries and veins.

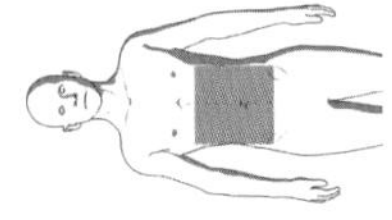

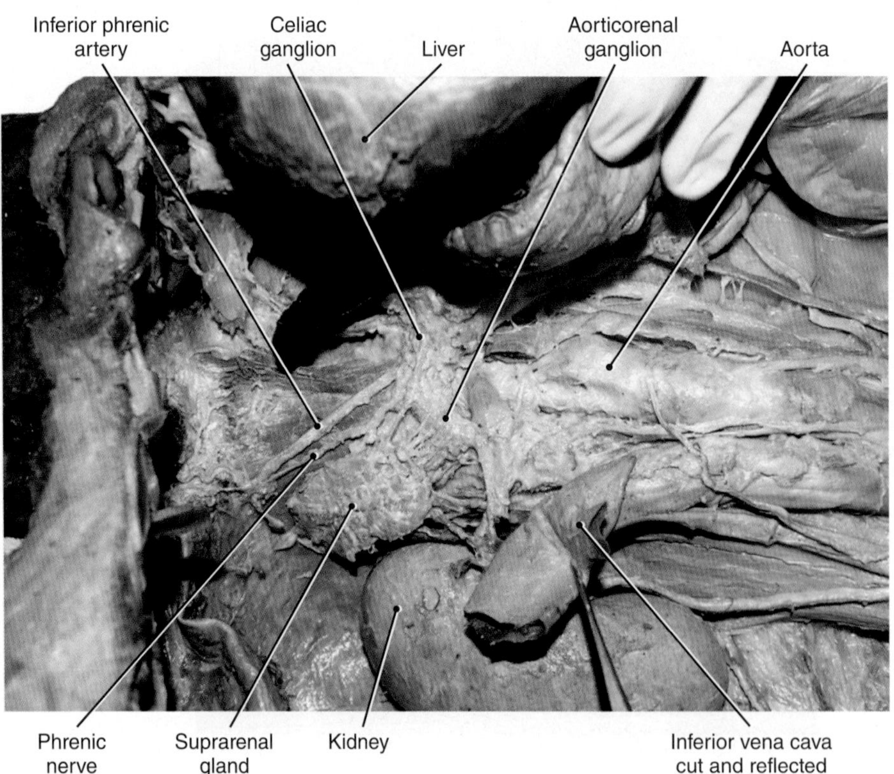

Fig. 13.20 Dissect the right superior, middle, and inferior suprarenal arteries typically arising from the inferior phrenic artery, aorta, and renal artery, respectively.

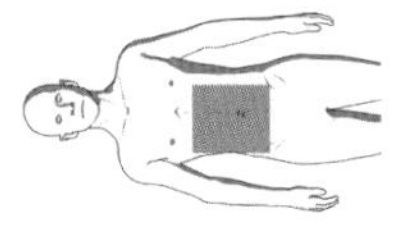

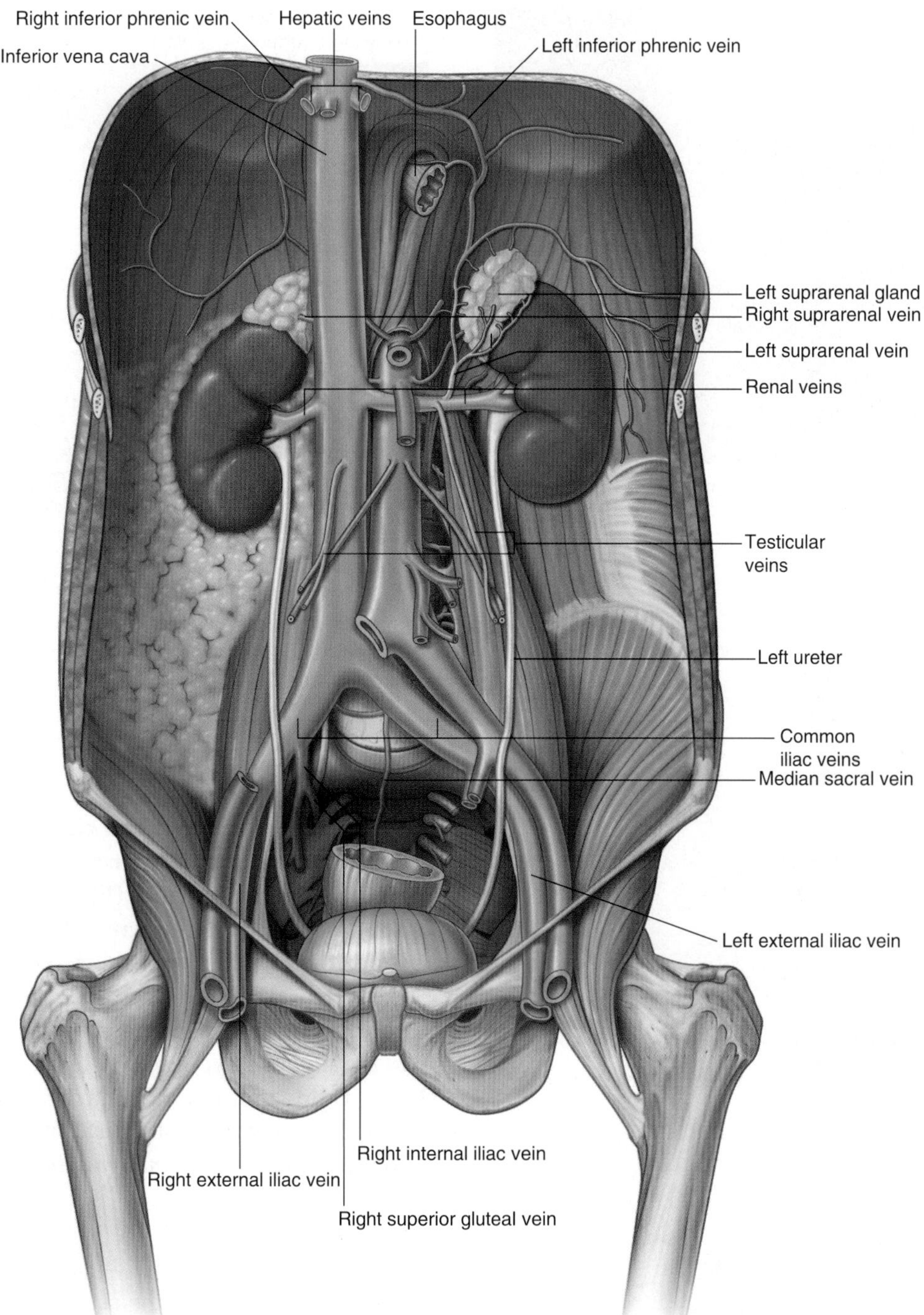

Plate 13.1 Inferior vena cava and tributaries. (From Drake RL et al. *Gray's Anatomy for Students*, 3rd edition, Philadelphia, Elsevier, 2015, Figure 4.141, p. 377.)

- **Hold one of the two kidneys in your hand. Make a vertical incision along its lateral border and transect the kidney into two parts (Fig. 13.21).**
- **Open and inspect the inner part of the kidney.**
- **Identify the outer layer, the renal cortex, and the inner layer, the *renal medulla* (Plate 13.2).**

ANATOMY **NOTE**

Realize that the cortex sends extensions into the medulla, the *renal columns.* The renal medulla is composed of *pyramids,* projections of the renal *papillae,* which contain collecting ducts that drain urine into the minor *calyces.* About 10 minor calyces combine to form 3 major calyces; all major calyces combine to form the *renal pelvis,* located at the hilum of the kidney (Plate 13.2).

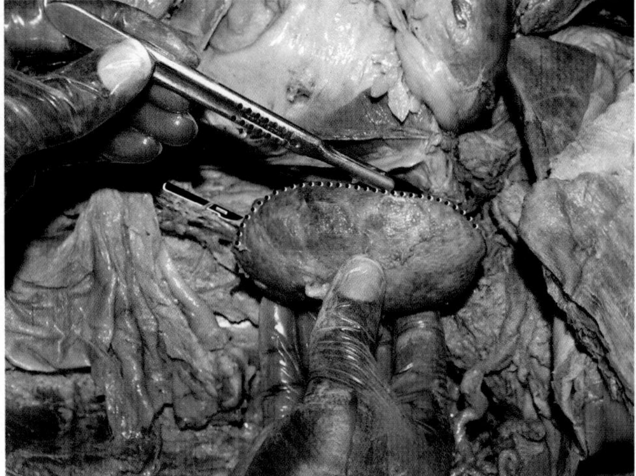

Fig. 13.21 An incision into the kidney along its border allows access to its internal structures.

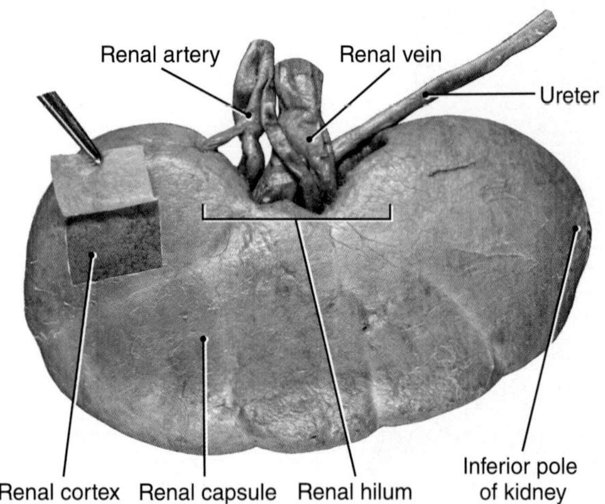

Fig. 13.22 The external anatomy of the anterior surface of the kidney.

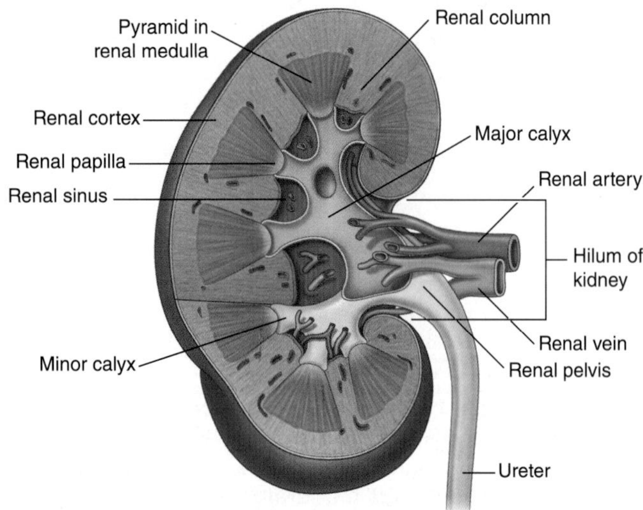

Plate 13.2 Internal structure of the kidney. (From Drake RL et al. *Gray's Atlas of Anatomy*, 3rd edition, Philadelphia, Elsevier, 2015, p. 190.)

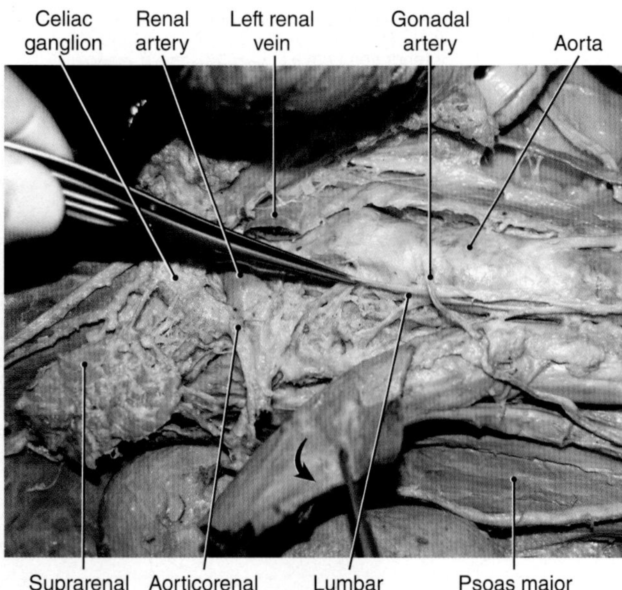

Fig. 13.23 Right sympathetic trunk between the inferior vena cava (IVC) and abdominal aorta.

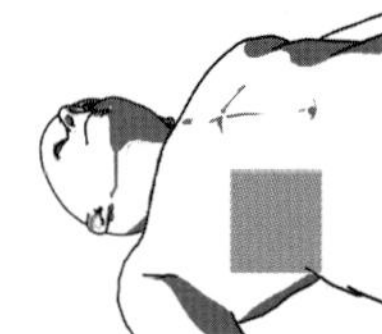

- **Between the inferior vena cava and the abdominal aorta, at the level of the right renal vein, locate the right sympathetic trunk (Fig. 13.23).**
- **You also can trace the sympathetic trunk just underneath the IVC, between the psoas major muscle and the vertebral column (Figs. 13.24 and 13.25). The sympathetic trunk contributes lumbar splanchnic nerves to the superior hypogastric plexus (see Fig. 13.24).**
- **The right and left renal arteries are surrounded by a dense network of neural fibers (see Fig. 13.22). Identify the *aorticorenal ganglion.***

ANATOMY **NOTE**

This ganglion further connects with the celiac ganglion, occupying the area over the celiac trunk (see Fig. 13.22). Preganglionic sympathetic fibers reach the celiac, aorticorenal, and superior mesenteric ganglia by way of the greater, lesser, and least thoracic splanchnic nerves, respectively. These fibers synapse in the ganglia, and postganglionic fibers travel along the arteries of the abdomen.

- **Lift the kidney upward and clean out the posterior surface of the renal hilum (Fig. 13.26).**
- **Identify the psoas major muscle and remove the fascia over the right crus of the diaphragm and psoas major muscle (Fig. 13.27).**

NERVES

- **At the opening of the IVC, look for the inferior phrenic artery and trace it to its origin from the aorta.**

DISSECTION **TIP**

In some cases, the inferior phrenic artery originates from the celiac trunk.

- **Next to the inferior phrenic artery, dissect out the continuation of the phrenic nerve into the abdominal cavity (see Fig. 13.27). The phrenic nerve accompanies the inferior phrenic artery and is related to the phrenic ganglion.**

Inferior phrenic artery
Aorta
Lumbar splanchnic nerve
Lumbar sympathetic ganglion
Phrenic nerve
Suprarenal gland
Inferior vena cava
Lumbar sympathetic trunk
Ureter
Superior hypogastric plexus

Fig. 13.24 The sympathetic trunk is shown giving rise to lumbar splanchnic nerves that contribute to the superior hypogastric plexuses.

- **Lift the kidney upward and look between the superomedial border of the psoas major and the right crus of the diaphragm for the greater, lesser, and least thoracic splanchnic nerves (Figs. 13.28 and 13.29).**

DISSECTION **TIP**

You also may pull the celiac ganglion upward and look for the greater thoracic splanchnic nerve underneath.

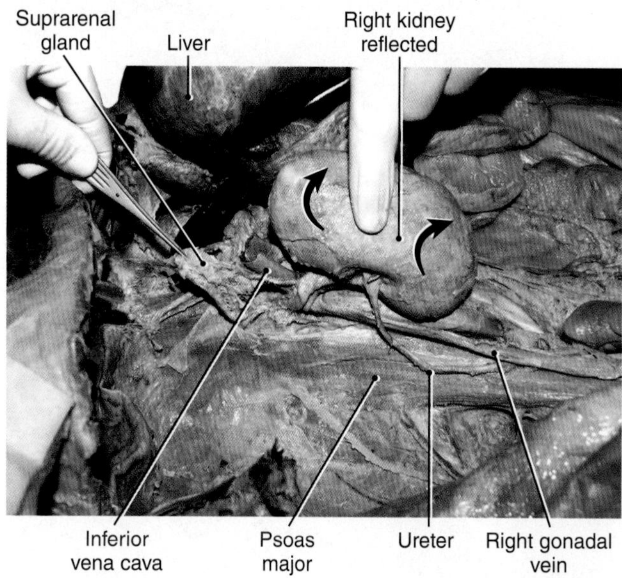

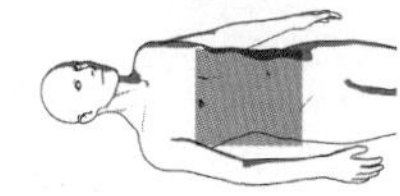

Fig. 13.26 Right kidney lifted upward in order to clean out the posterior surface of the renal hilum.

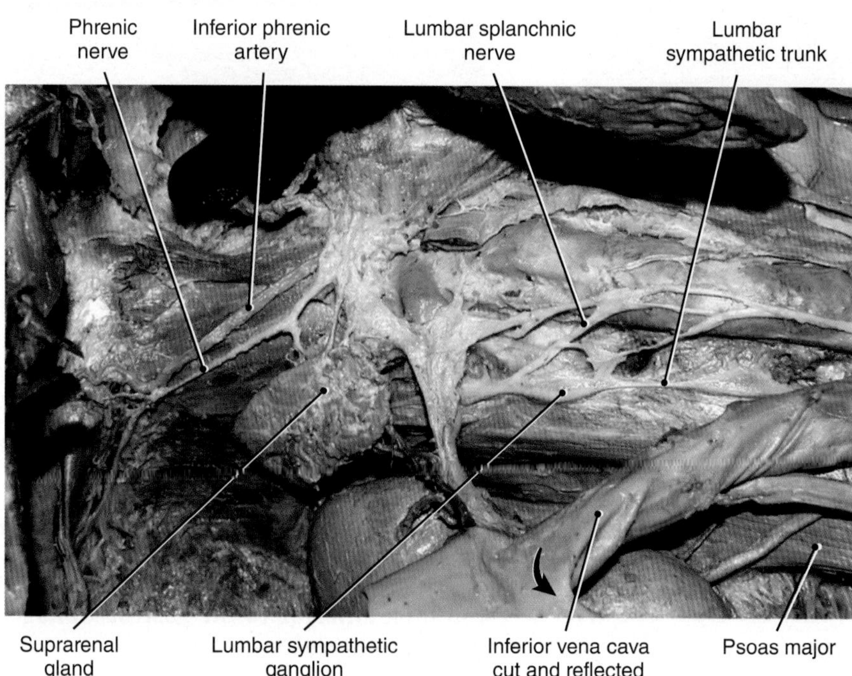

Fig. 13.25 The sympathetic trunk courses underneath the inferior vena cava between the psoas major muscle and vertebral column.

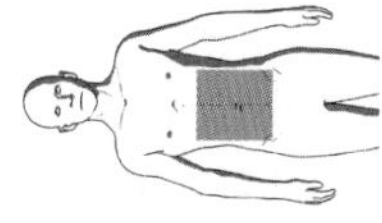

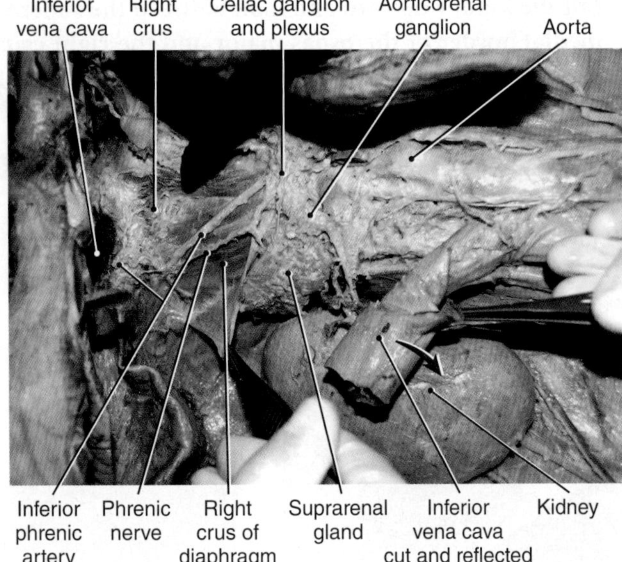

Fig. 13.27 Fascia removed over the right crus of the diaphragm and psoas major muscle.

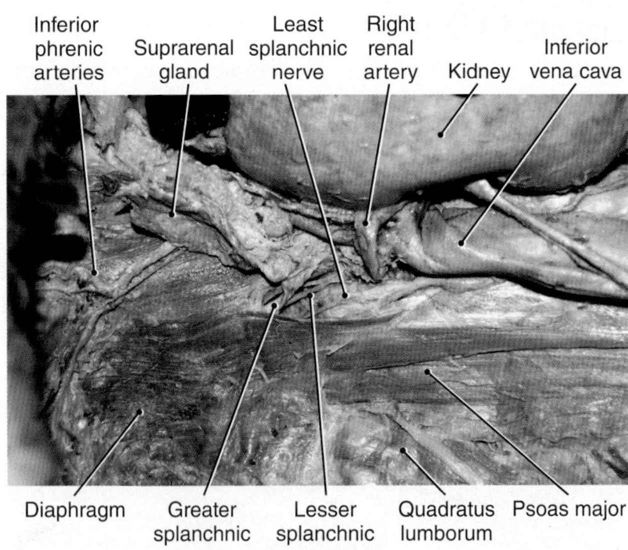

Fig. 13.29 Greater, lesser, and least splanchnic nerves coursing between thoracic the superomedial border of the psoas major muscle and the right crus of the diaphragm.

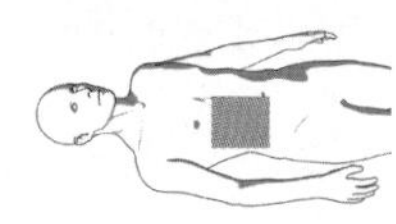

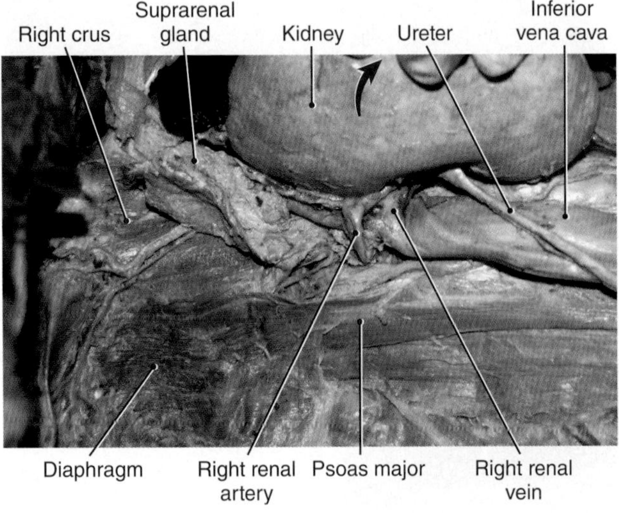

Fig. 13.28 Appreciate the underlying structures with the kidney lifted.

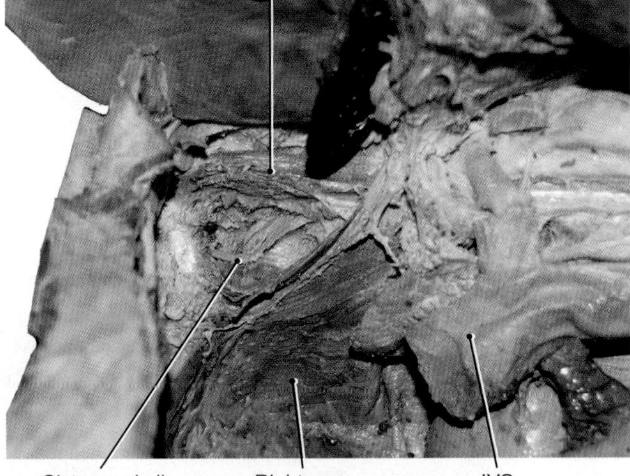

Fig. 13.30 A vertical incision at the right crus of the diaphragm exposes cisterna chyli. *IVC*, Inferior vena cava.

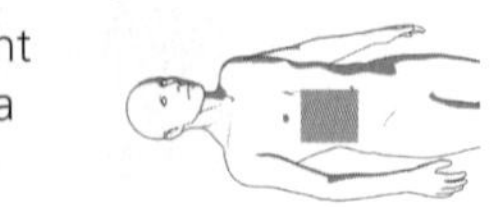

- **Trace these nerves to their terminations at the celiac ganglion (for the greater), aorticorenal ganglion (for the lesser), and superior mesenteric ganglion (for the least).**
- **Between the abdominal aorta and the IVC and at the left side of the aorta, identify the right and left lumbar lymph trunks, respectively.**
- **These lymph trunks eventually join the intestinal lymph trunk and form the *cisterna chyli*. Make a vertical incision at the right crus of the diaphragm and expose the cisterna chyli (Fig. 13.30).**
- **Open up the thoracic cavity and identify the anterior and posterior vagal trunks around the lower part of the esophagus.**
- **Place slight traction on the anterior vagal trunk, which originates primarily from the left vagus nerve, and look anterior to the gastroesophageal junction for a mobile structure.**
- **Locate the anterior vagal trunk and expose its branches.**
- **Similarly, place slight traction on the posterior vagal trunk in the thorax (primarily right vagus nerve) and find the medial side of the *esophageal hiatus*, or the**

right side of the esophagus, for identification of the posterior vagal trunk (Fig. 13.31).

INSPECTION OF POSTERIOR ABDOMINAL STRUCTURES

- Observe the thoracic and abdominal surfaces of the diaphragm. Note the central tendinous portion of the diaphragm, the *central tendon.*
- Lateral to the esophagus, identify the *right and left crura,* the two muscular extensions of the diaphragm arising from the central tendon and inserting onto the 2nd or 3rd lumbar (L2 or L3) vertebrae.
- Fibers from the right and left crura intermix to encircle the esophagus as it passes through the diaphragm. Just superior to the celiac trunk, the right and left crura are united by a midline tendon, the *median arcuate ligament.*
- Laterally, the diaphragm attaches to the ribs and inferolaterally it attaches to the psoas major forming a thickened connective tissue band, the *medial arcuate ligament.*
- More laterally, the diaphragm arches over the quadratus lumborum to attach to the 12th rib, forming another thickened connective tissue band over the quadratus lumborum, the *lateral arcuate ligament* (see Fig. 13.31).

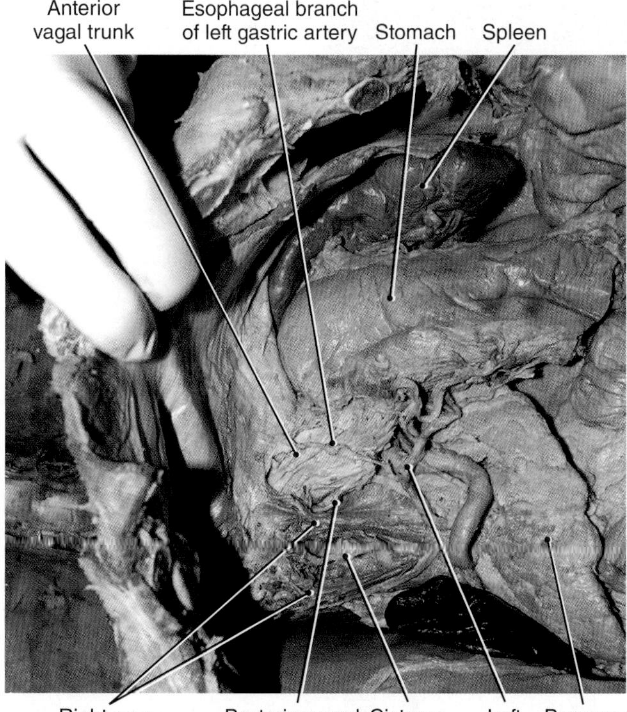

Fig. 13.31 Thoracic cavity opened and anterior and posterior vagal trunks around the lower esophagus.

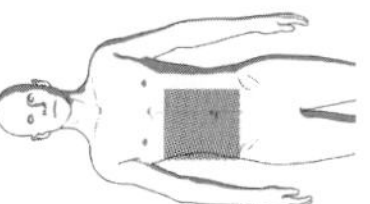

- Remove any remaining fat inferior to the right and left kidneys to expose the lumbar plexus and the underlying muscles (Fig. 13.32).
- Identify the psoas major muscle and, lateral to it, the quadratus lumborum muscle.

DISSECTION TIP

In about 50% of cadaveric donors, the psoas minor muscle is evident on the anterior surface of the psoas major.

- Inferior to the quadratus lumborum, identify the iliacus muscle, which lies in the iliac fossa. Palpate the 12th rib and, at its inferior border, expose the *subcostal nerve.*
- On the lateral side of the psoas major muscle, identify the *genitofemoral nerve* as it travels on its anterior surface.
- A few centimeters below the origin of the *iliohypogastric nerve,* identify the *ilioinguinal nerve,* which travels from the lateral side of the psoas major muscle toward the anterior superior iliac spine.
- At the lateral side of the distal end of the psoas major muscle in the abdominal cavity, identify the *femoral nerve* and, lateral to it, the much smaller *lateral femoral cutaneous nerve.*
- Medial to the psoas major muscle, place a probe or a pair of scissors and separate the psoas major

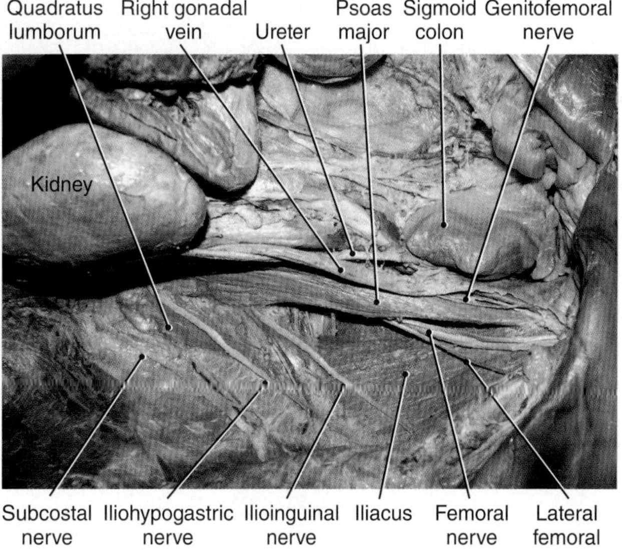

Fig. 13.32 Removal of fat inferior to the right and left kidneys exposes branches of the lumbar plexus and underlying muscles.

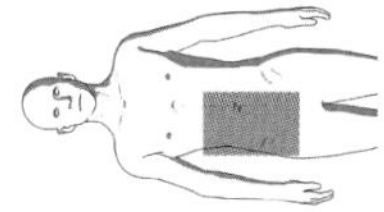

from the adjacent external iliac artery and vein (Fig. 13.33).

- **Deep and medial to the psoas major muscle, identify the *obturator nerve* (Fig. 13.34).**
- **Once all branches of the lumbar plexus are identified, on one side of the cadaver, carefully remove the psoas major muscle in a piecemeal fashion and expose the origin of the nerves of the lumbar plexus (Fig. 13.35 and Plate 13.3).**

DISSECTION **TIP**

In most cadavers, the lumbar plexus exhibits great variation.

- The most common variation is that the ilioinguinal and iliohypogastric nerves fuse and split into their terminal branches just proximal to the *anterior superior iliac spine*.
- Similarly, the subcostal and iliohypogastric nerves can be fused and split more distally.

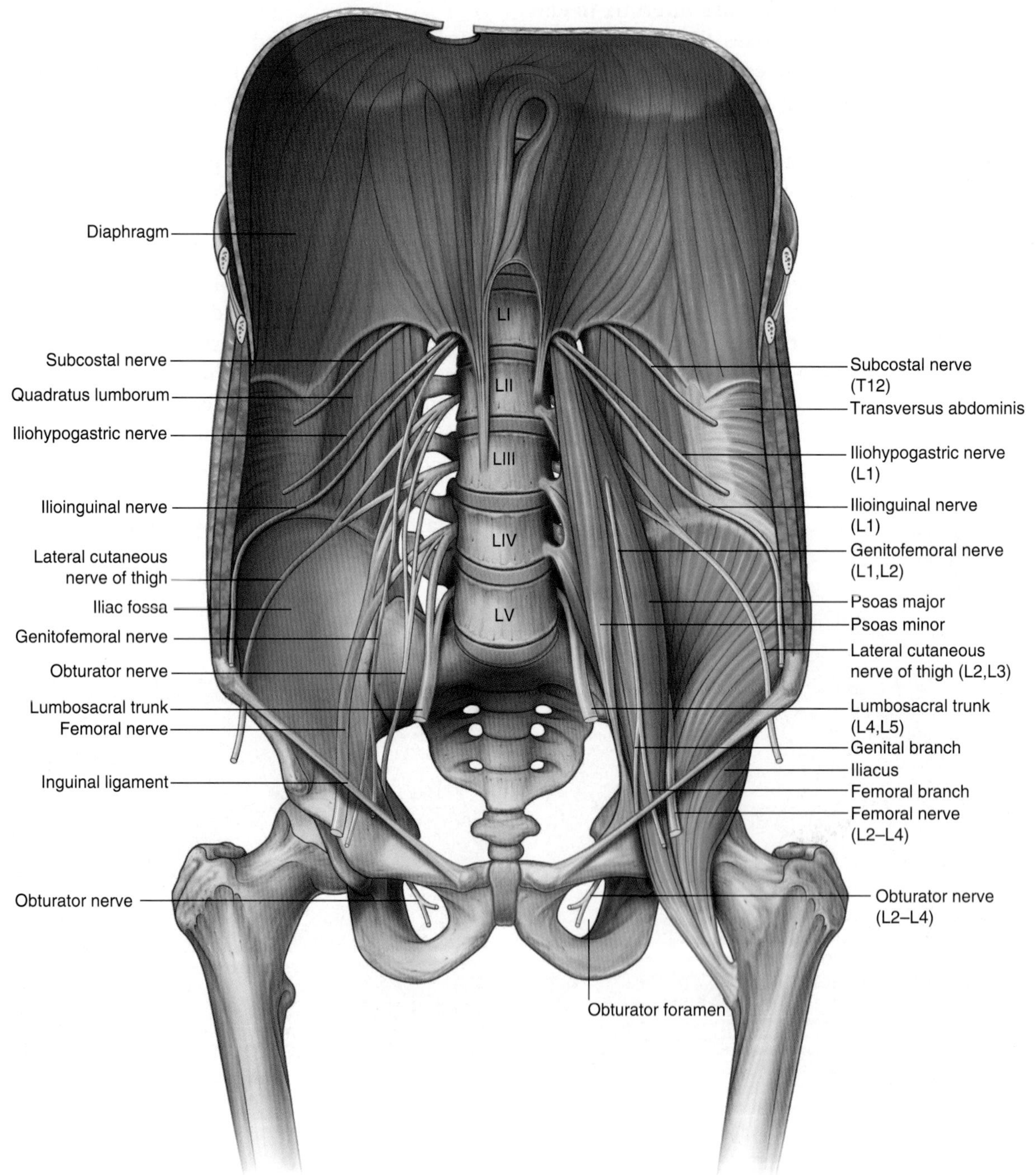

Plate 13.3 The lumbar plexus. (From Drake RL et al. *Gray's Atlas of Anatomy*, 3rd edition, Philadelphia, Elsevier, 2021, p. 198.)

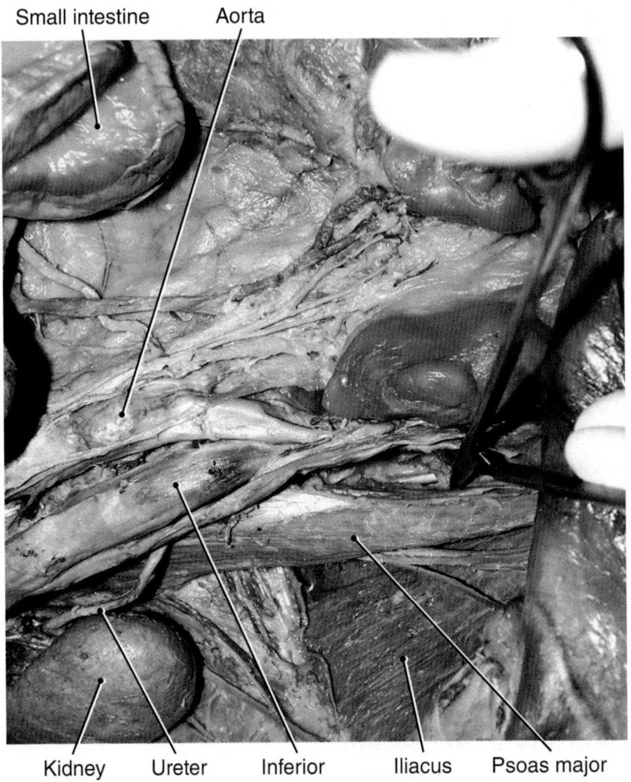

Fig. 13.33 Psoas major muscle separated from the adjacent external iliac artery and vein.

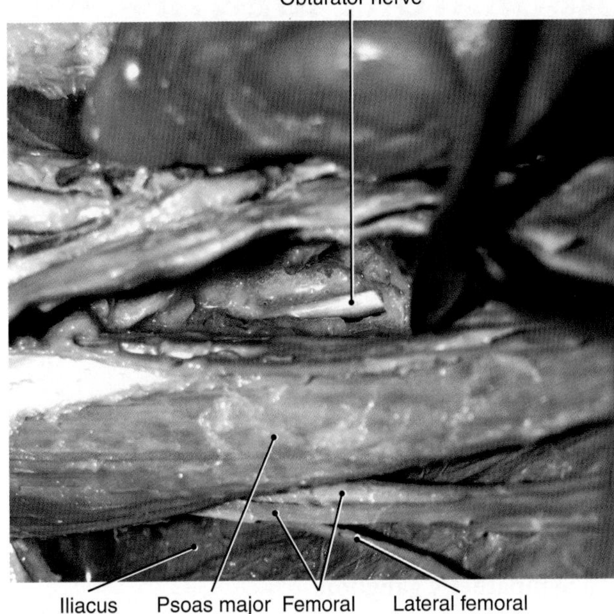

Fig. 13.34 The obturator nerve lies deep and medial to the psoas major muscle.

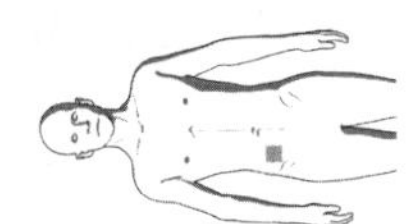

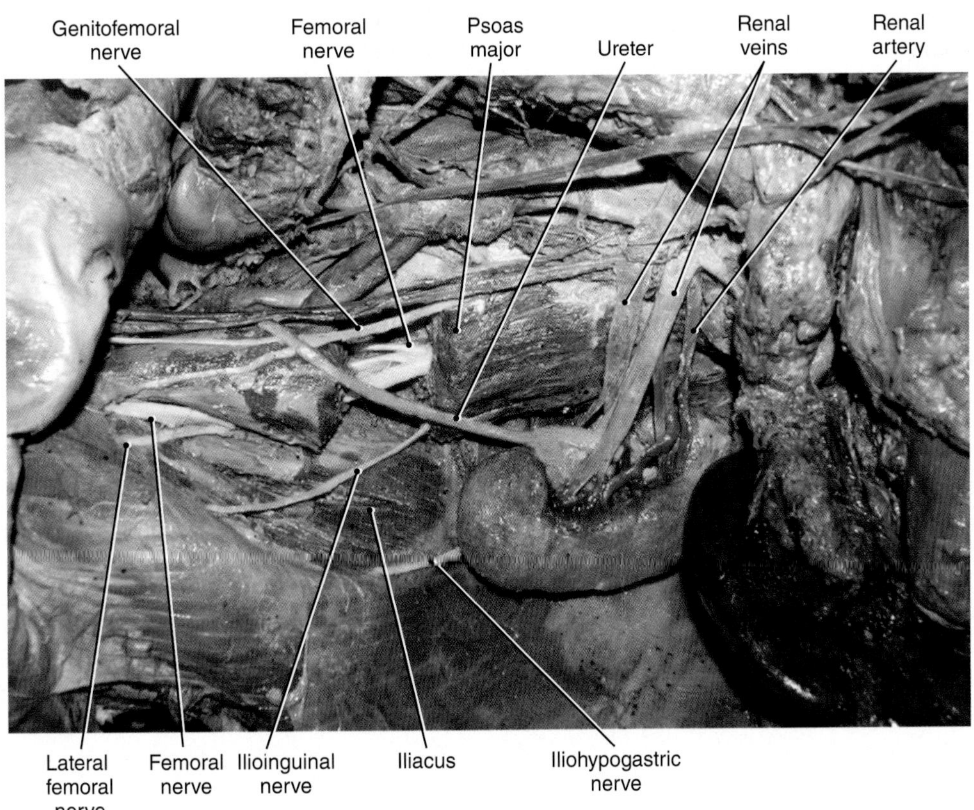

Fig. 13.35 Psoas major muscle removed exposing the origin of the lumbar plexus branches.

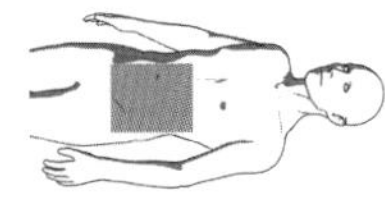

LABORATORY IDENTIFICATION CHECKLIST

NERVES/CONNECTIVE TISSUE

- ☐ Iliohypogastric
- ☐ Ilioinguinal
- ☐ Genitofemoral
- ☐ Lateral femoral cutaneous
- ☐ Femoral
- ☐ Obturator
- ☐ Accessory obturator (variation)
- ☐ Lumbosacral trunk
- ☐ Sympathetic trunk
  - ☐ Gray/white rami communicantes
  - ☐ Sympathetic ganglion
  - ☐ Lumbar splanchnic
- ☐ Celiac ganglia
- ☐ Celiac plexus
- ☐ Suprarenal plexus
- ☐ Aorticorenal ganglion
- ☐ Superior mesenteric plexus
- ☐ Intermesenteric (aortic) plexus

ARTERIES

- ☐ Right and left inferior phrenic
- ☐ Superior suprarenal
- ☐ Middle suprarenal
- ☐ Inferior suprarenal
- ☐ Renal
- ☐ Gonadal
- ☐ Lumbar
- ☐ Subcostal
- ☐ Iliolumbar

VEINS

- ☐ Inferior vena cava (IVC)
- ☐ Inferior phrenic
- ☐ Suprarenal
- ☐ Renal
- ☐ Gonadal
- ☐ Lumbar
- ☐ Iliolumbar

LYMPH

- ☐ Cisterna chyli

MUSCLES/CONNECTIVE TISSUE

- ☐ Right crus
  - ☐ Ligament of Treitz
- ☐ Left crus
- ☐ Psoas major
- ☐ Psoas minor (variant)
- ☐ Quadratus lumborum
- ☐ Transversus abdominis
- ☐ Median arcuate ligament
- ☐ Medial arcuate ligament
- ☐ Lateral arcuate ligament

ORGANS

- ☐ Kidney
- ☐ Ureter
- ☐ Suprarenal gland

BONES

- ☐ Coxal (hip), right and left
- ☐ Sacrum
- ☐ Vertebrae
  - ☐ 12th thoracic (T12)
  - ☐ 1st to 5th lumbar (L1–L5)

CLINICAL APPLICATIONS

PERITONEAL ASPIRATION/LAVAGE

Clinical Application

Procedure introduces a trocar to withdraw fluid or to introduce saline into the peritoneal cavity for irrigation.

Anatomical Landmarks (Figs. V.1 and V.2)

- Infraumbilical region
- Skin
- Subcutaneous tissue
- Linea alba/rectus abdominis muscle
- Transversalis fascia
- Extraperitoneal fat
- Parietal peritoneum

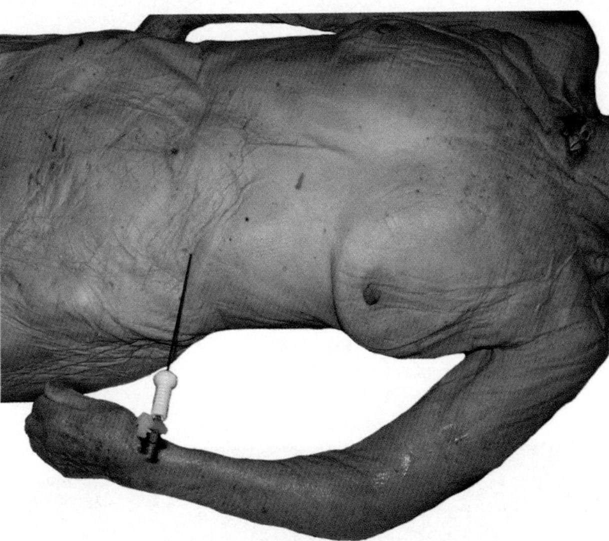

Fig. V.1

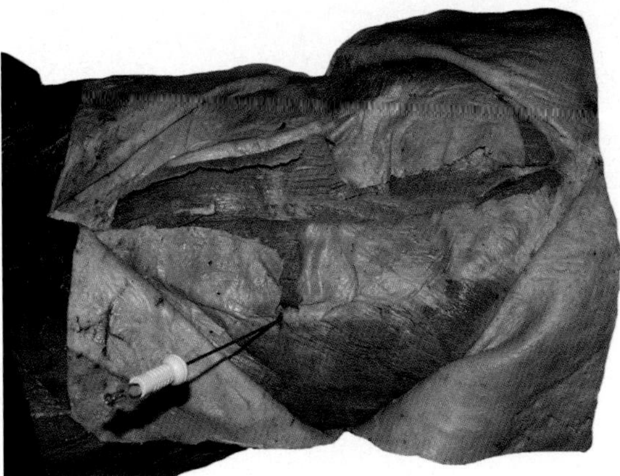

Fig. V.2

- Umbilicus
- Anterior superior iliac spine (ASIS)

PARACENTESIS

Clinical Application

Procedure withdraws fluid (e.g., ascites) from the peritoneal cavity.

Anatomical Landmarks

Infraumbilical Region

- Skin
- Subcutaneous tissue
- Linea alba
- Median umbilical fold/ligament
- Medial umbilical fold/ligament
- Transversalis fascia
- Extraperitoneal fat/space
- Greater peritoneal sac

About 5 cm Superior to ASIS

Layers traversed:

- Skin (lateral to rectus abdominis)
- Subcutaneous tissue
- External abdominal oblique aponeurosis
- Internal abdominal oblique muscle
- Transversus abdominis muscle
- Transversalis fascia
- Extraperitoneal fat/space
- Peritoneum

PUDENDAL NERVE BLOCK

Clinical Application

Procedure places a bolus of local anesthetic into the pudendal canal, anesthetizing the pudendal nerve and its branches.

Anatomical Landmarks (Figs. V.3 and V.4)

- Vaginal orifice
- Lateral vagina wall and mucosa
- Vaginal mucosa
- Ischial spine
- Coccygeus
- Sacrospinous ligament (resistance)
- Pudendal canal (Alcock's canal)
- Pudendal nerve
- Internal pudendal artery
- Internal pudendal vein

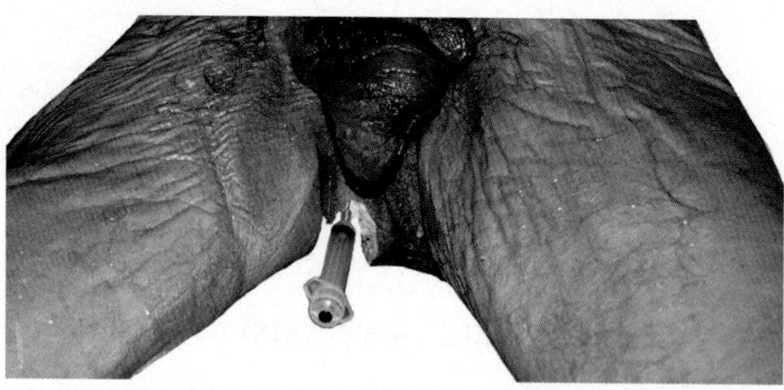

Fig. V.3

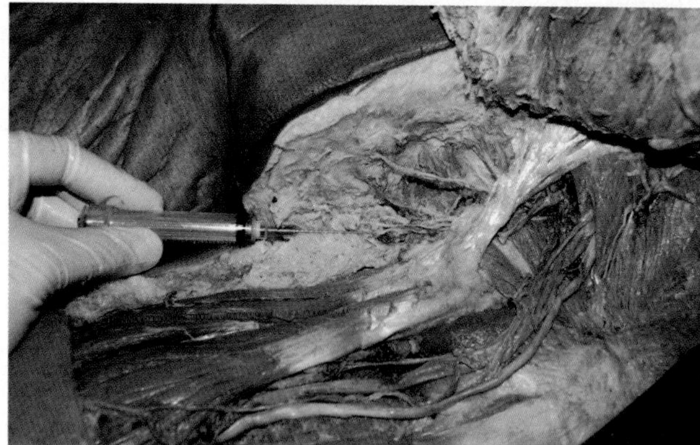
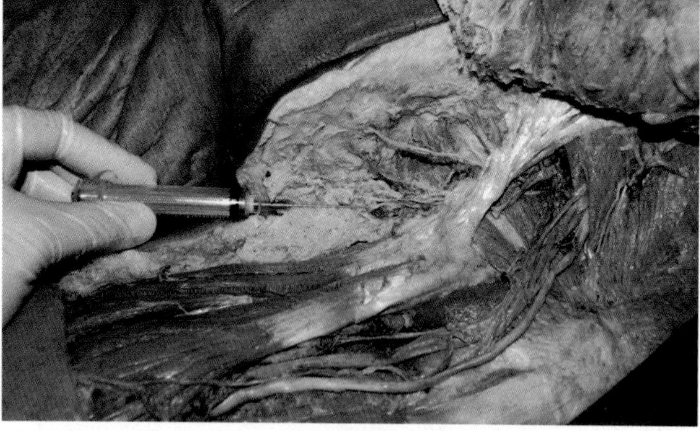

Fig. V.4

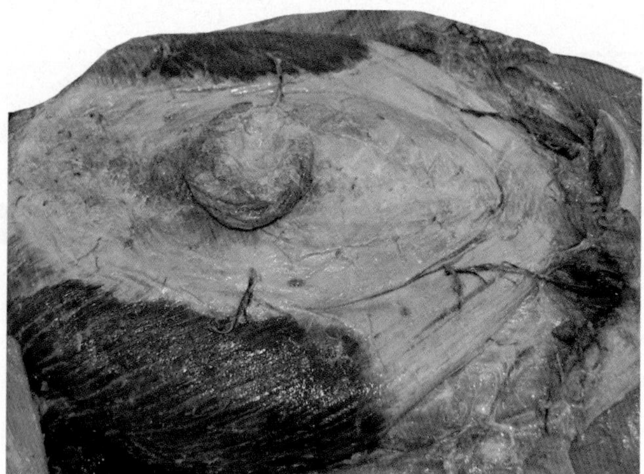

Fig. V.5

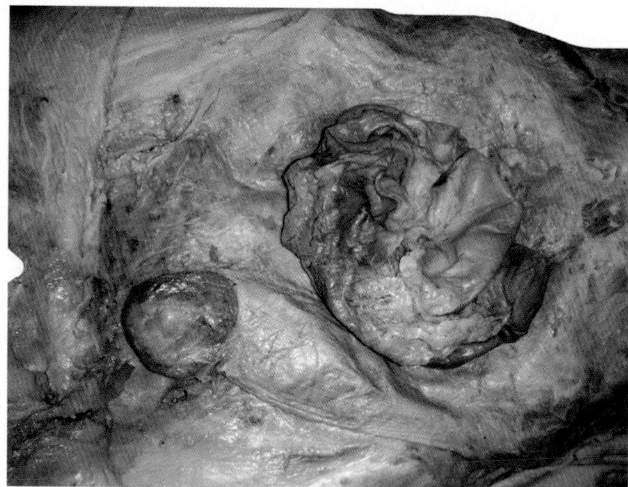

Fig. V.6

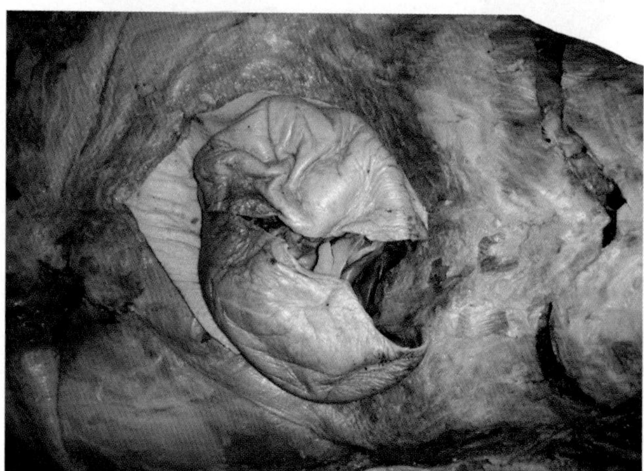

Fig. V.7

HERNIATIONS AND OTHER PATHOLOGIES

The following cadavers exhibited marked herniations and other examples of abdominal and vascular abnormalities, including life-threatening aortic aneurysm.

- Umbilical hernia (Fig. V.5)
- Umbilical hernia and an indirect inguinal hernia (Figs. V.6 and V.7)
- Massive malignancies in the abdominal cavity and the liver (Fig. V.8)
- Multiple malignant nodules in a sagittal section of the liver (Fig. V.9)
- Example of hepatomegaly (Fig. V.10)
- Dissected liver with evident hepatic arteries and veins (Fig. V.11)
- Example of splenomegaly (Fig. V.12)
- Examples of kidneys with cysts (Figs. V.13–V.15)
- Abdominal aortic aneurysm; large Gore-Tex tube placed at site is visible (Fig. V.16)
- Large abdominal aortic aneurysm (Fig. V.17)

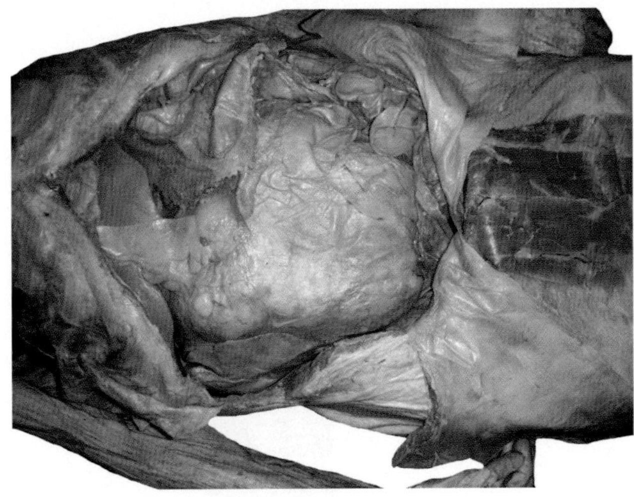

Fig. V.8

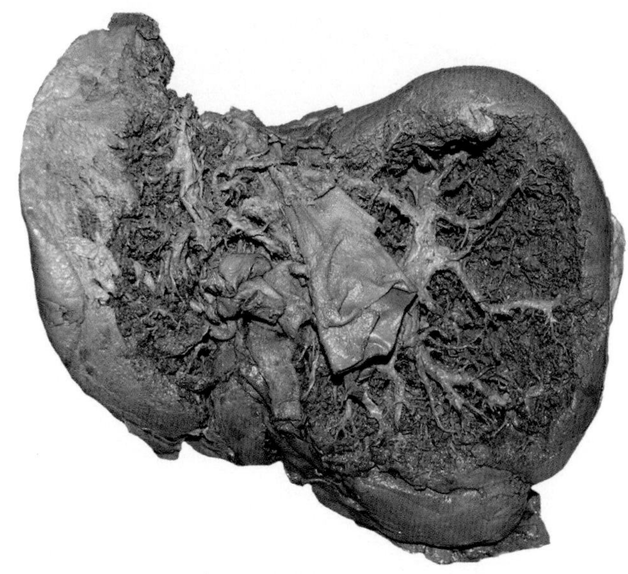

Fig. V.11

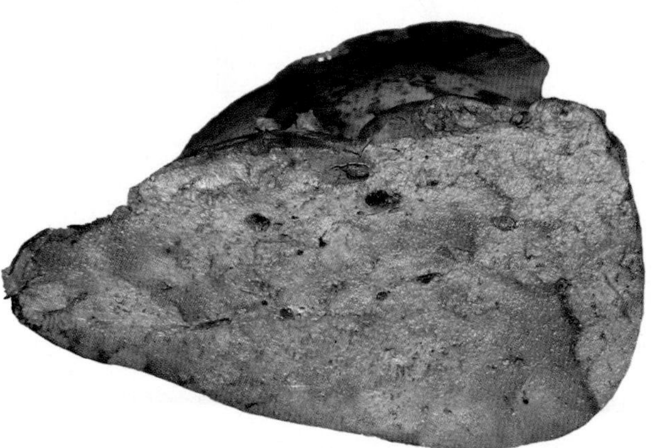

Fig. V.9

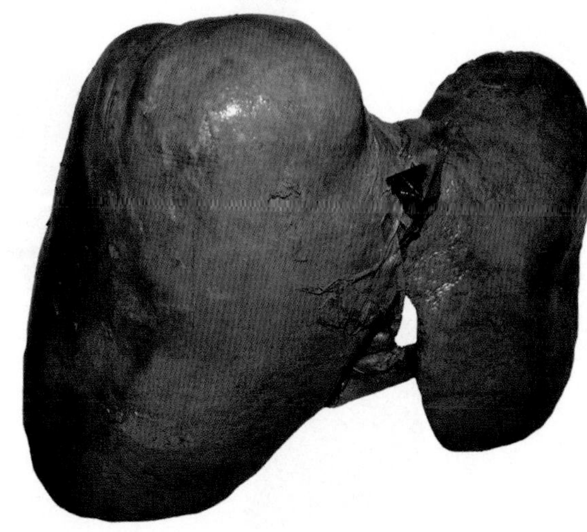

Fig. V.10

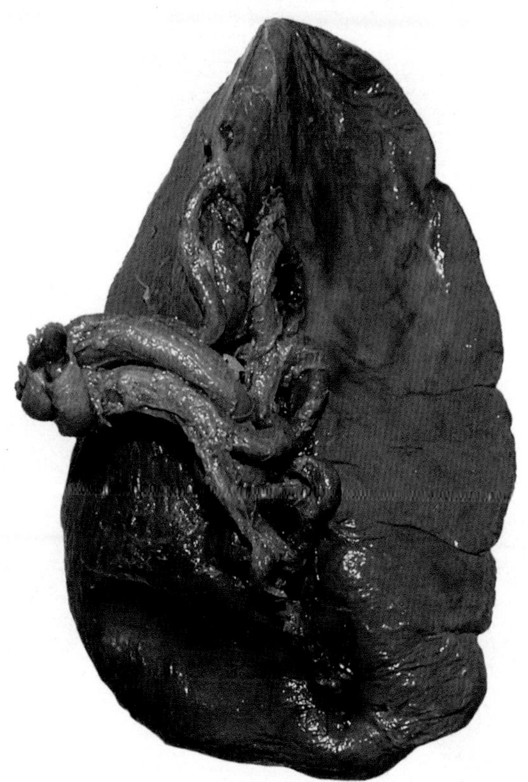

Fig. V.12

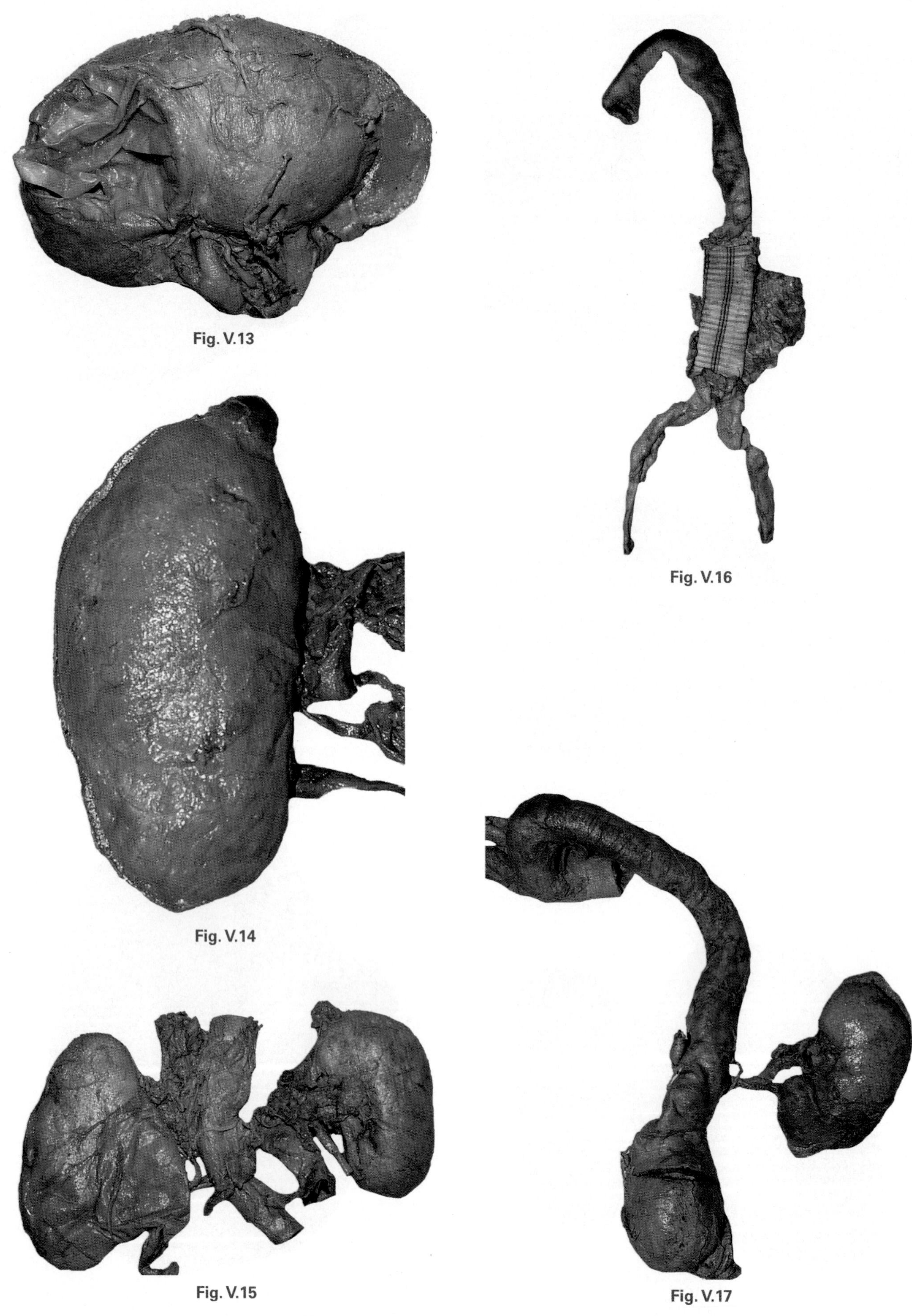
Fig. V.13

Fig. V.14

Fig. V.15

Fig. V.16

Fig. V.17

SECTION VI

PELVIS AND PERINEUM

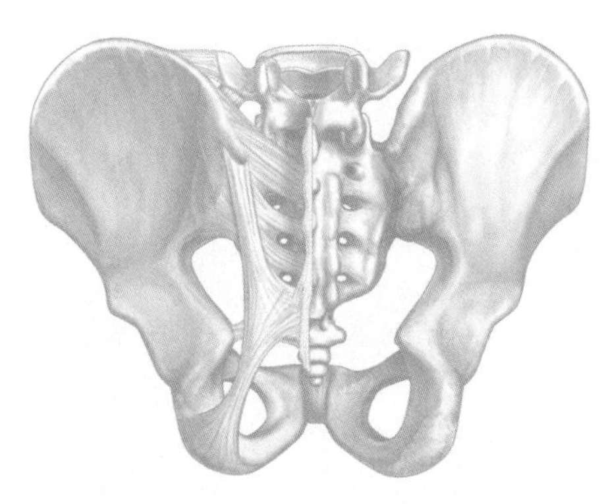

CHAPTER 14 PELVIS

Several techniques are used for dissection of the pelvis. This chapter describes the traditional midline hemipelvectomy as technique 1. Subsequently, a second technique is described, involving the removal of the male urethra with the penis, prostate and seminal glands, and urinary bladder en bloc for further examination. Finally, a third technique is employed to demonstrate a variation of techniques 1 and 2.

MIDLINE HEMIPELVECTOMY (MALE)

Technique 1

- **Identify the rectosigmoid junction and expose the rectum (Fig. 14.1). Posterior to the pubic symphysis, palpate the urinary bladder.**
- **With a probe or scissors, dissect out and reflect the peritoneum from the posterior surface of the urinary bladder (Figs. 14.2 and 14.3). Notice the median umbilical ligament connecting to the urinary bladder (urachus).**

ANATOMY **NOTE**

The adipose tissue between the posterior surface of the urinary bladder and the peritoneum is termed *preperitoneal fat*.

- **Place your fingertips, using blunt dissection, between the urinary bladder and the pubic symphysis into the retropubic space of Retzius (Fig. 14.4).**
- **Pull on the fascia attached to the lateral sides of the median umbilical ligament and at the superior part of the urinary bladder, the *vesicoumbilical fascia*, and reflect it posteriorly. With this maneuver, observe the expansion of the retropubic space of Retzius.**
- **Mobilize the rectum and the bladder. With a saw, cut the pubic symphysis vertically 2 to 3 cm lateral to the midline (Fig. 14.5).**
- **Mobilize the rectum laterally, and with a scalpel, extend the incision from the pubic symphysis backward toward the sacrum and pelvis (Fig. 14.6). Cut**

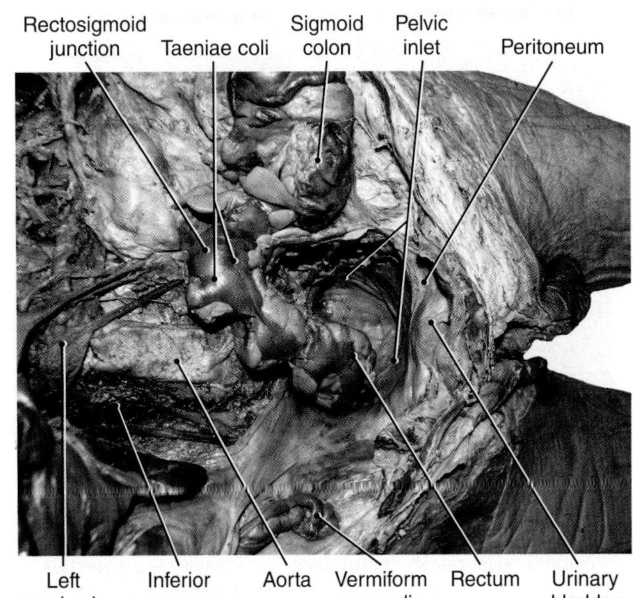

Fig. 14.1 Identification of the rectosigmoid junction and exposure of the rectum within the pelvic inlet.

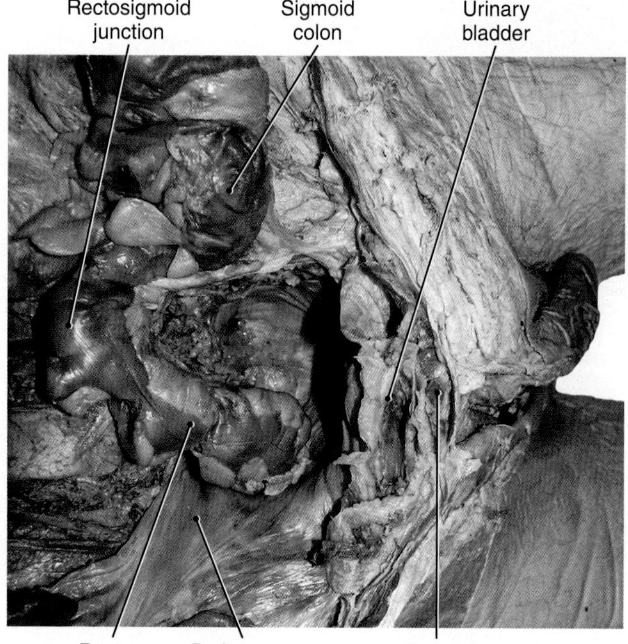

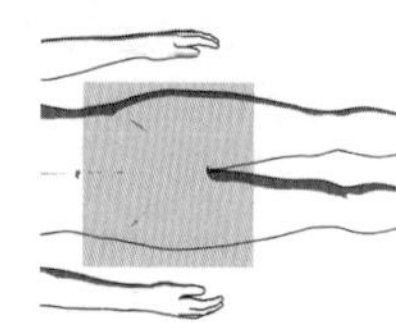

Fig. 14.2 Exposure of the urinary bladder posterior to pubic symphysis from the overlying peritoneum.

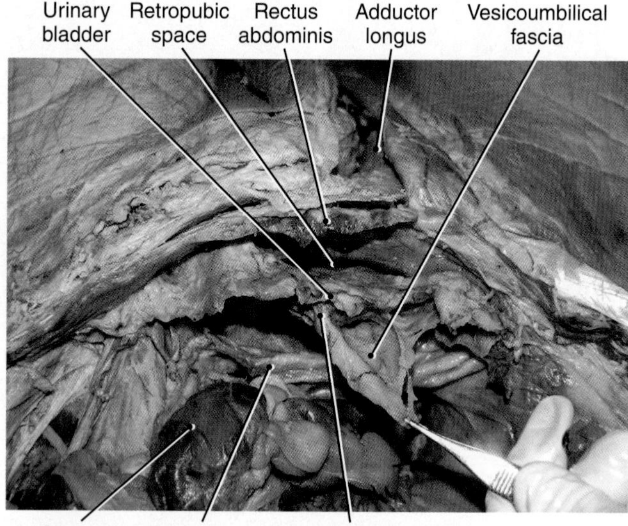

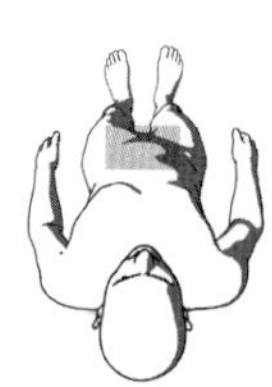

Fig. 14.4 Blunt dissection between the urinary bladder and the pubic symphysis into the retropubic space (of Retzius).

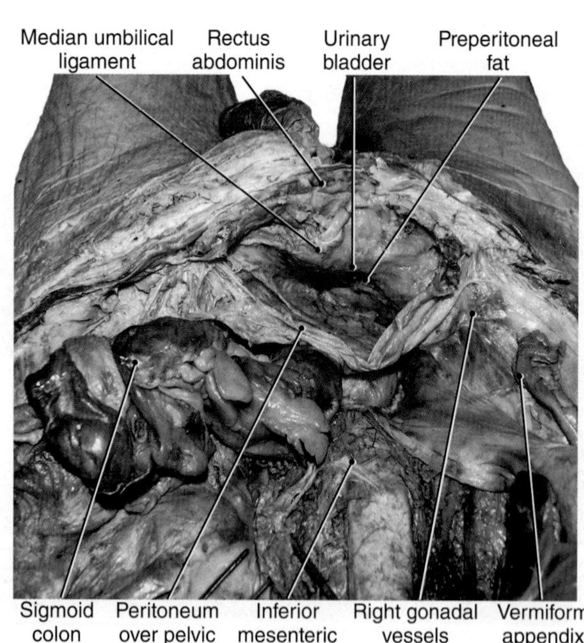

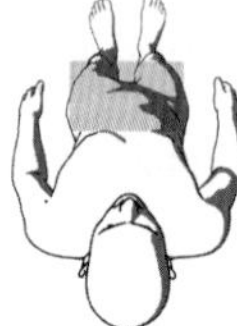

Fig. 14.3 Peritoneum reflection from posterior surface of urinary bladder.

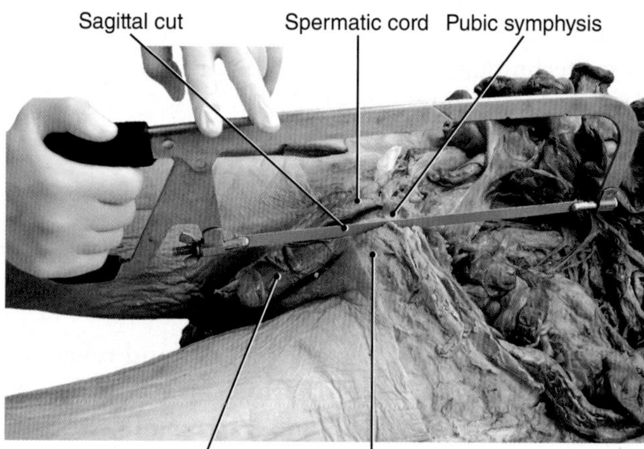

Fig. 14.5 The pubic symphysis is cut vertically about 2–3 cm (1 inch) lateral to midline.

the peritoneum, urinary bladder, aorta, and all soft tissues.

- **With a scalpel, make a second horizontal incision starting from the aorta, at the level of the kidneys, and extending laterally along the borders of the iliac crest (Fig. 14.7).**
- **With the cadaver on its side, and using a saw, cut the sacrum through its promontory, up through the 4th lumbar vertebra. Saw through the pubic symphysis and make a horizontal incision along the iliac crest (as previously described) and detach this portion of the body (Figs. 14.7 and 14.8).**

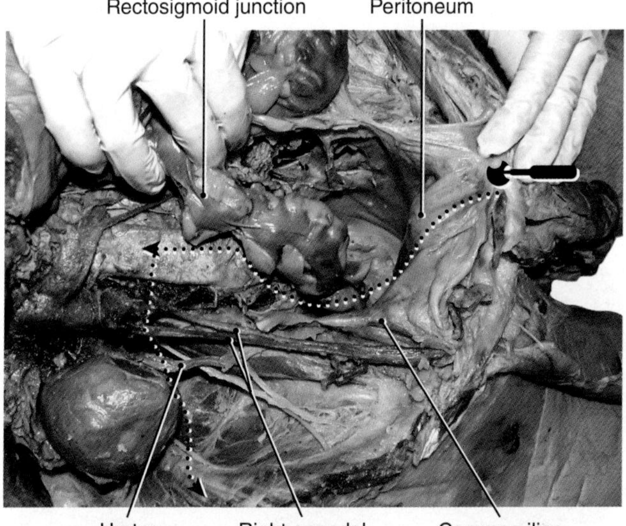

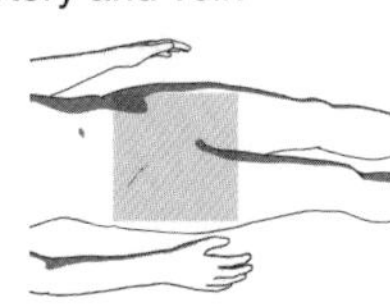

Fig. 14.6 An incision is extended from the pubic symphysis posteriorly and inferiorly toward the sacrum and pelvis *(dashed line with arrowheads).*

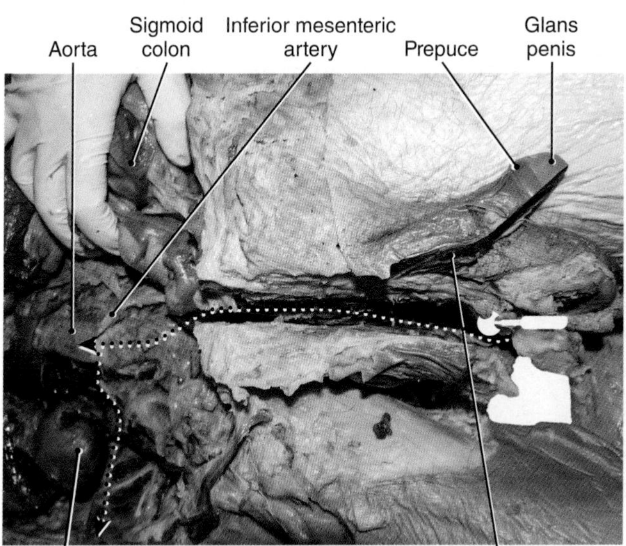

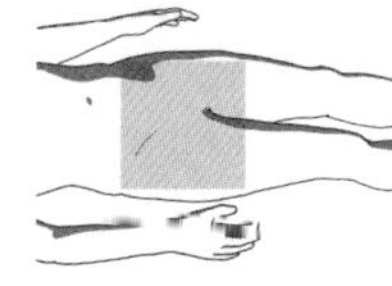

Fig. 14.7 A second horizontal incision is extended from the aorta laterally toward the iliac crest.

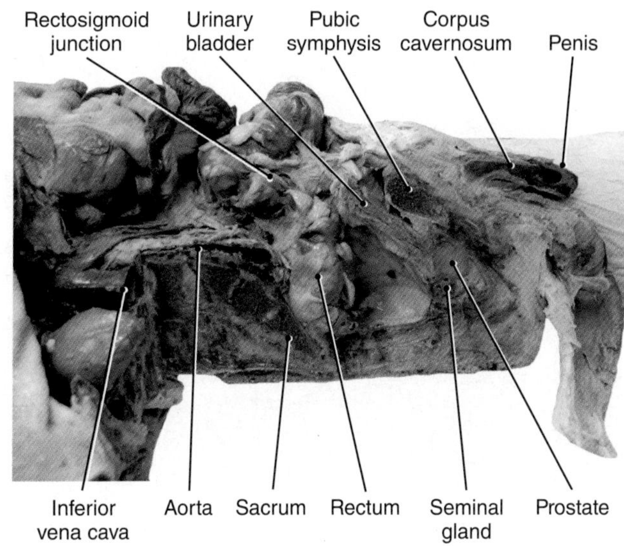

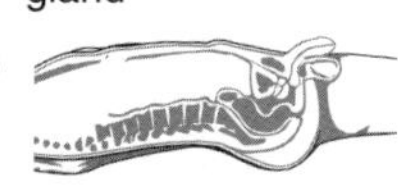

Fig. 14.8 After the cadaver is turned on its side, the saw is passed through the cut-open pubic symphysis. A horizontal cut is made along the iliac crest, and this portion is detached.

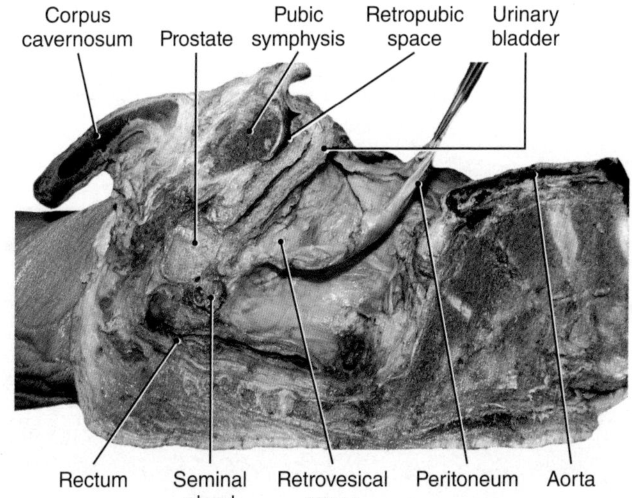

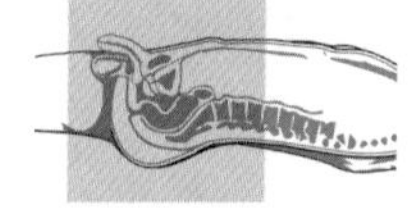

Fig. 14.9 The peritoneum posterior to the urinary bladder is reflected upwardly.

DISSECTION TIP

For the hemipelvectomy, you will need the help of your colleagues to lift and turn the cadaver on its side.

- **With scissors, reflect the parietal peritoneum upward (Fig. 14.9).**
- **Start cleaning the soft tissues and adipose tissue around larger structures (Fig. 14.10).**
- **Identify the aorta and expose the external iliac artery (Fig. 14.11).**
- **Trace the ductus deferens and expose it toward the prostate. On surface of the external iliac artery, identify the ureter. Trace and expose the ureter to its entrance to the urinary bladder (Fig. 14.12).**
- **Inferior to the external iliac artery, expose the external iliac vein. Retract the external iliac vein inferiorly and clean the adipose tissue superior to it. Just inferior to the course of the external iliac vein, identify the obturator nerve and trace it to the obturator foramen (Fig. 14.13).**
- **Identify the internal iliac artery and expose its anterior and posterior divisions.**

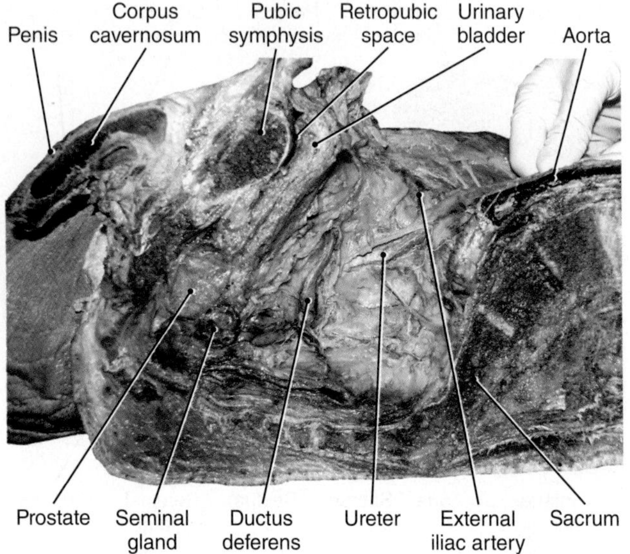

Fig. 14.10 The soft tissues and the adipose tissue are cleaned around large structures.

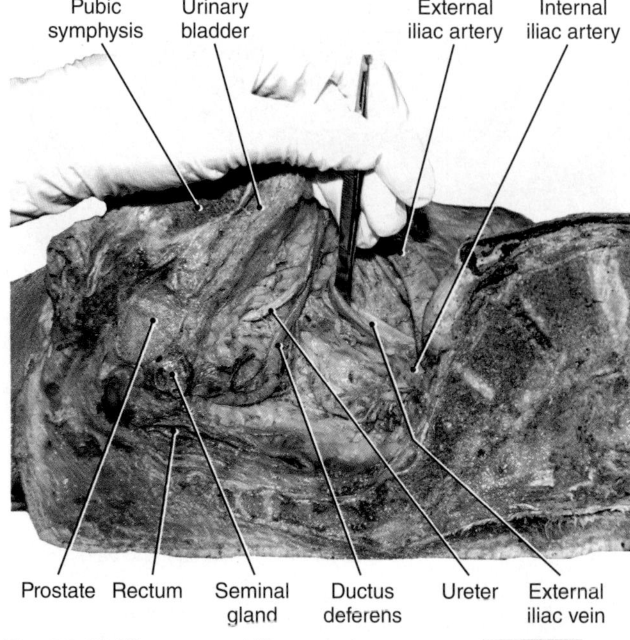

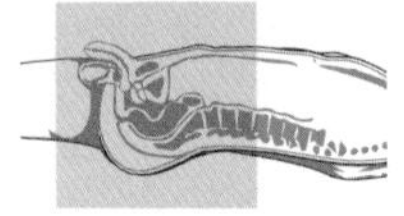

Fig. 14.12 The external iliac vein is retracted inferiorly. The ductus deferens and ureter are exposed.

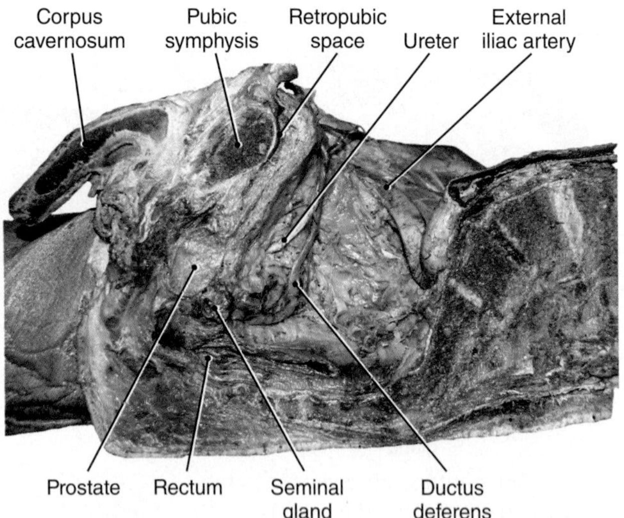

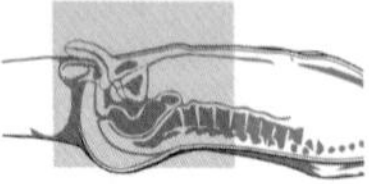

Fig. 14.11 Exposure of the external iliac artery, with the ductus deferens exposed toward the prostate and the ureter to its entrance.

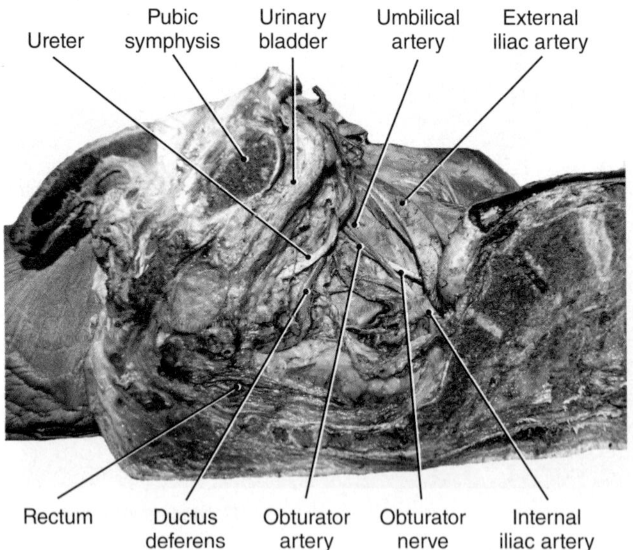

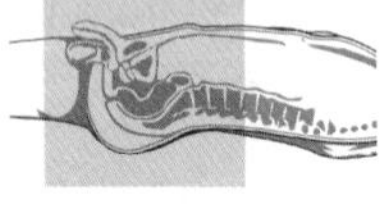

Fig. 14.13 The obturator nerve is traced to the obturator foramen.

DISSECTION **TIP**

The branches of the internal iliac artery are very variable. An easy way to avoid confusion is to rely on landmarks (discussed in later dissection tips) and always name the artery based on its distribution, not its origin.

- **Identify the internal iliac artery and expose its anterior and posterior divisions. Expose the branches of the anterior division of the internal iliac artery. These branches are the umbilical, obturator, inferior gluteal, internal pudendal, middle anorectal, inferior vesical, and uterine arteries (Figs. 14.14–14.23). These arteries are discussed in the following dissection tips and figures.**

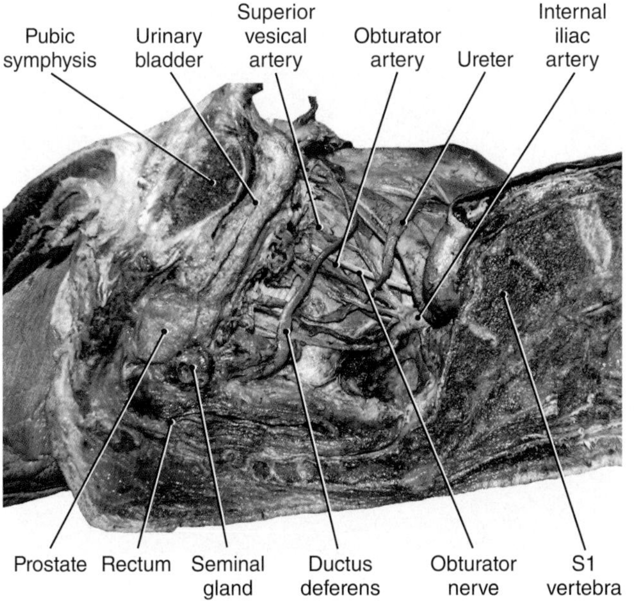

Fig. 14.14 The internal iliac artery is exposed with its anterior and posterior divisions.

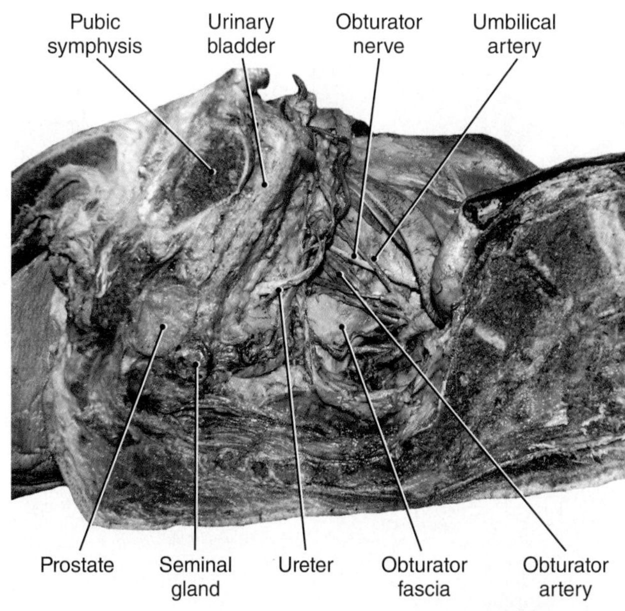

Fig. 14.16 Appreciate the major landmarks of the pelvis in relation to the branches of the internal iliac artery.

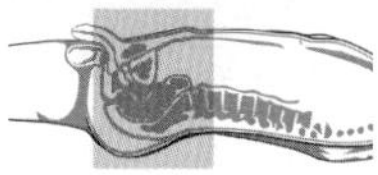

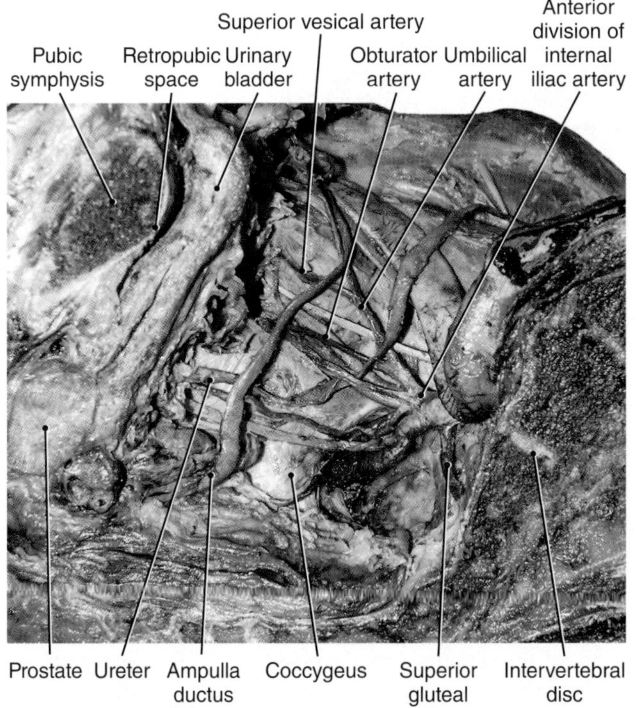

Fig. 14.15 The branches of the anterior division of the internal iliac artery are dissected out.

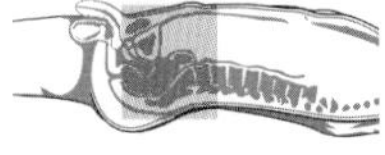

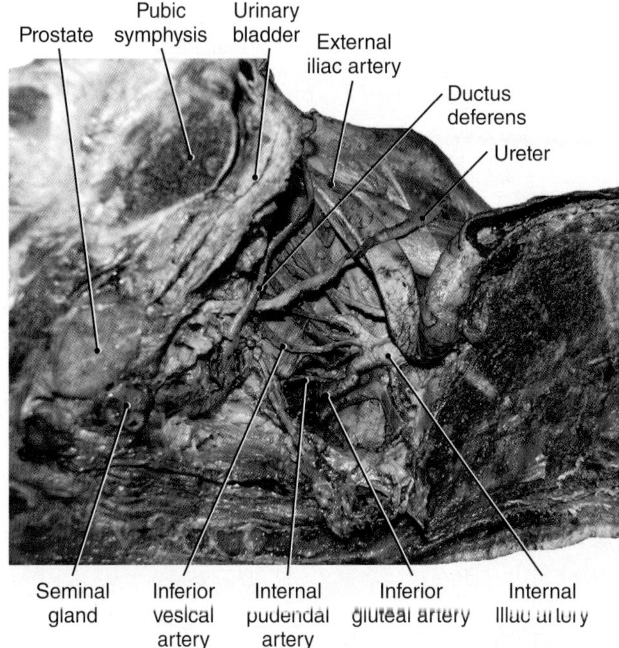

Fig. 14.17 Appreciate the branches of the anterior division of the internal iliac artery.

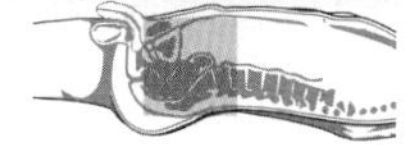

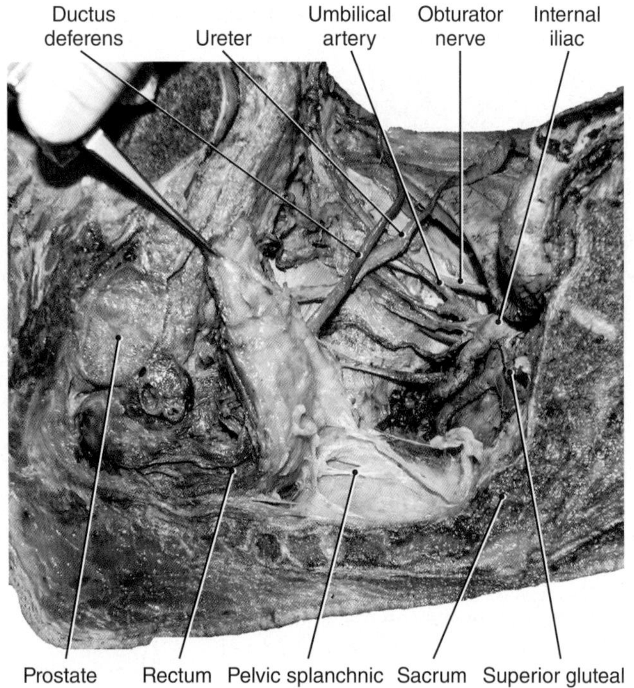

Fig. 14.18 The sympathetic trunk is exposed in the pelvis with the gray communicating rami passing lateral to the nerves of the sacral plexus.

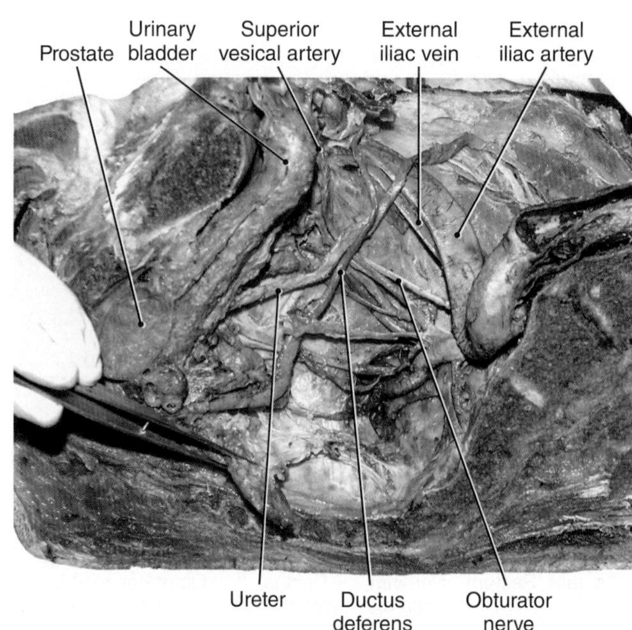

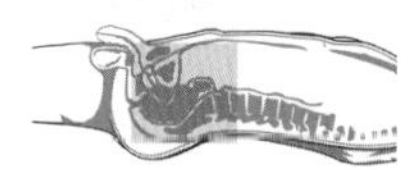
Fig. 14.20 To expose the pubococcygeus and iliococcygeus muscles, clean all the pelvic fascia and adipose tissue over the levator ani inferior to the prostate.

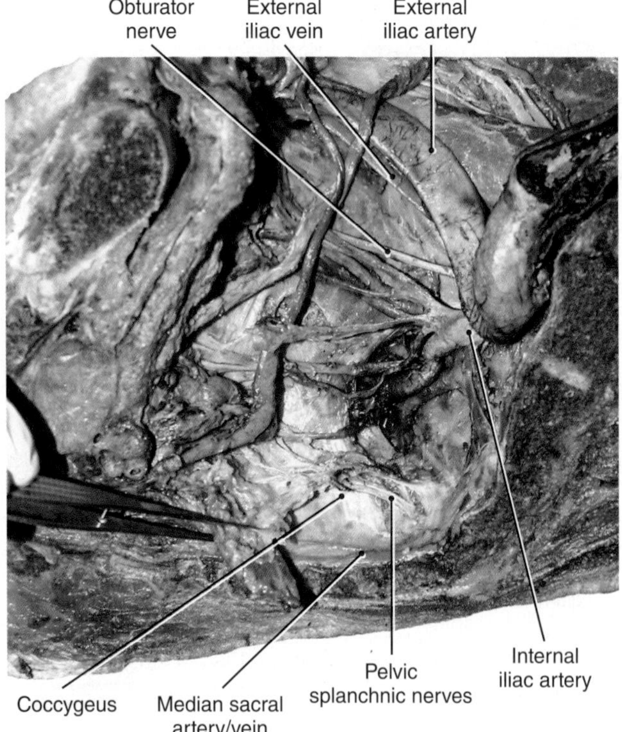

Fig. 14.19 To expose the pelvic splanchnic nerves fully, lift the rectum and anal canal superiorly.

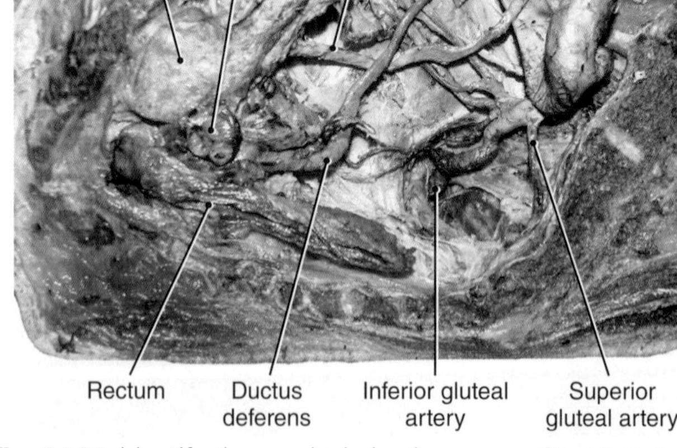

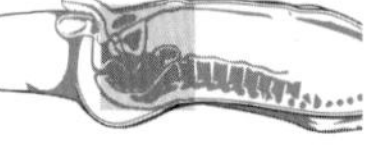
Fig. 14.21 Identify the seminal gland (vesicle) and locate where the ductus deferens enters seminal gland (vesicles).

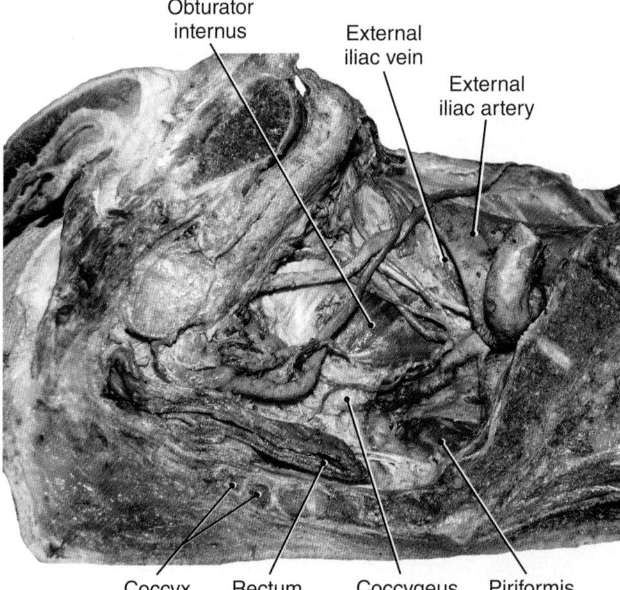

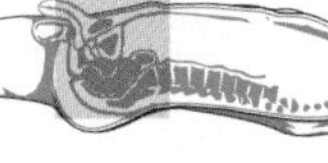

Fig. 14.22 Locate the coccygeus muscle that arises from the ischial spine and sacrospinous ligament and attaches to the coccyx and lower part of the sacrum.

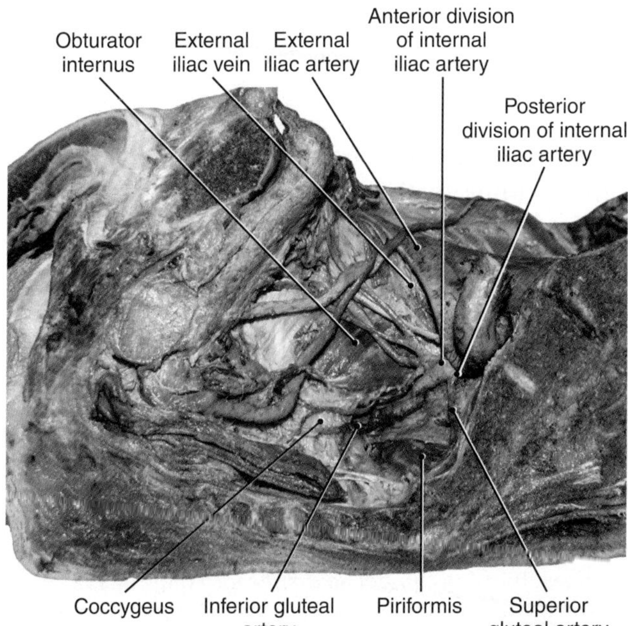

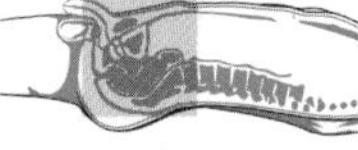

Fig. 14.23 The obturator internus fascia is cleaned, exposing the obturator internus muscle.

DISSECTION TIPS

Branches of Internal Iliac Artery: Anterior Division (Plate 14.1)

Umbilical artery: Usually the first branch of the anterior division. The umbilical artery courses upward and superior to the urinary bladder to become the median umbilical ligament (Figs. 14.13, 14.15, and 14.16). The umbilical artery often gives off the superior vesical branches that supply the superior portion of the urinary bladder; in 75% of cases, there are two or three superior vesical arteries.

Obturator artery: Usually arises parallel to the origin of the umbilical artery; travels with the obturator nerve to split into anterior and posterior branches in the obturator foramen (Figs. 14.14 and 14.15). The obturator artery travels anterior to the obturator internus and its fascia and is crossed medially by the ureter and the ductus deferens. It gives rise to small branches: iliac, vesical, and pubic.

The main variation of the obturator artery is that in 30% of cases, it arises from the inferior epigastric artery.

Inferior gluteal artery: Arises at the posterior side of the anterior division and is mainly distributed to the buttocks. The landmark for identifying the inferior gluteal artery is to look for the artery passing between the 1st and 2nd sacral nerves and between the piriformis and coccygeus muscles (Fig. 14.17).

Internal pudendal artery: The artery is more anterior in position than the inferior gluteal artery as these arteries leave the pelvis. The internal pudendal artery does not pass between S1 and S2 nerves but typically courses lower between the piriformis and coccygeus muscles (Fig. 14.17). It also accompanies the pudendal nerve to Alcock's canal. Several small branches arise from the internal pudendal artery: inferior rectal, perineal, artery of the bulb, urethral artery, deep artery of the penis or clitoris, and dorsal artery of the penis or clitoris.

Middle anorectal: It arises with or from the internal pudendal, inferior vesical, or inferior gluteal arteries; mainly supplies the rectum.

Inferior vesical (vaginal in females): Usually arises from the internal pudendal artery. The inferior vesical artery supplies the fundus of the urinary bladder, the prostate, and the seminal glands.

Uterine: Usually arises from the medial surface of the anterior trunk. It runs medially on the levator ani and the broad ligament, and at about 2 cm at the cervix of the uterus, it crosses in front of the ureter to anastomose with the ovarian artery. The uterine artery typically gives off a *superior* branch, supplying the body and fundus of the uterus, and a *vaginal* branch, supplying the cervix and vagina.

○ **Expose the branches of the posterior division of the internal iliac artery: These branches are the iliolumbar, lateral sacral, and the superior gluteal arteries.**

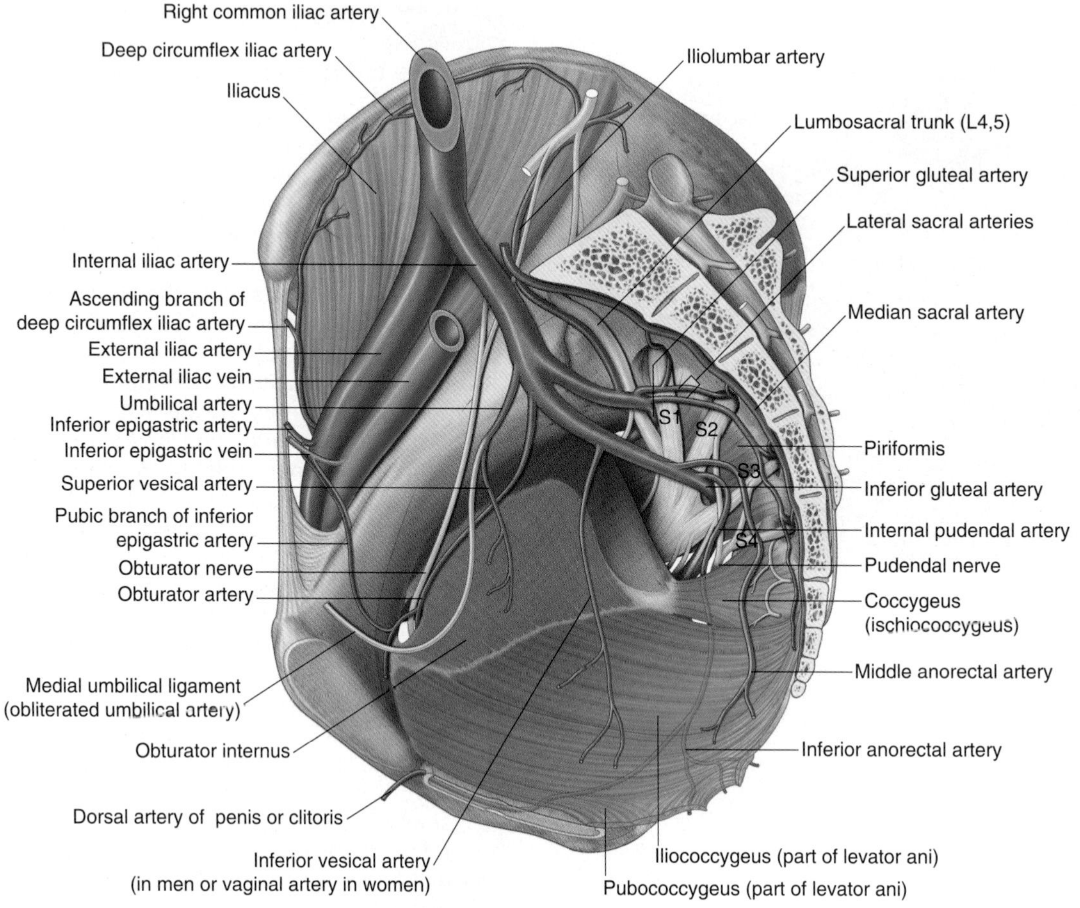

Plate 14.1 Arteries of the pelvis. (From Drake RL et al. *Gray's Atlas of Anatomy*, 3rd edition, Philadelphia, Elsevier, 2021, p. 248.)

DISSECTION TIPS

Branches of Internal Iliac Artery: Posterior Division (See Plate 14.1)

Iliolumbar: This artery typically is found between the lumbosacral trunk and the obturator nerve. It then ascends superolaterally to the iliac fossa, finally to reach the psoas major muscle. The iliolumbar artery gives off an iliac and a lumbar branch.

Lateral sacral: Usually, two lateral sacral arteries are present, superior and inferior. The *superior* lateral sacral artery usually enters the 1st or 2nd sacral foramina. The *inferior* lateral sacral artery runs obliquely across the piriformis muscle to the medial side of the sacral foramina. It anastomoses with the middle sacral artery.

Superior gluteal: Largest branch of the posterior trunk and a direct continuation of its posterior trunk. The superior gluteal artery runs backward between the lumbosacral trunk and the 1st sacral nerve (Figs. 14.15 and 14.18). It divides into superficial and deep branches in the buttocks.

- **Behind the internal and external iliac arteries, identify the obturator internus muscle covered with the obturator fascia (a part of the endopelvic fascia).**
- **Expose the inferior part of the obturator fascia and note its white, thickened band of fibers, the *tendinous arch of the levator ani* (arcus tendineus levator ani).**

ANATOMY NOTE

The tendinous arch runs from the obturator internus to the posterior part of the pubic bone and serves as an attachment site for the fibers of the levator ani muscle (Fig. 14.29). The tendinous arch is continuous with the obturator internus fascia.

The floor of the pelvis is mainly composed of the levator ani (anteriorly) and the coccygeus (posteriorly) muscles, forming the *pelvic diaphragm* (Fig. 14.19).

The levator ani consists mainly of the pubococcygeus muscle arising from the anterior/middle portion of the tendinous arch of levator ani and the iliococcygeus. It further divides into the puborectalis and pubovaginalis (in females) muscles and the levator prostatae (in males) muscles.

The iliococcygeus muscle arises mainly from the tendinous arch of the levator ani and attaches to the coccyx. The coccygeus muscle arises from the ischial spine and sacrospinous ligament and attaches to the coccyx and lower part of the sacrum (Fig. 14.22).

DISSECTION **TIP**

To expose the pubococcygeus and the iliococcygeus muscles, clean all the pelvic fascia and adipose tissue over the levator ani muscle inferior to the prostate (see Figs. 14.20 and 14.21). These muscles are often atrophied, and clear borders may be difficult to identify.

- **Clean the superior fascia of the pelvic diaphragm, which covers the levator ani. Note the continuity of the tendinous arch of the levator ani and the obturator internus fascia.**
- **Clean the obturator internus fascia and expose the obturator internus muscle (Figs. 14.22 and 14.23).**
- **Expose the sympathetic trunk in the pelvis and observe the pelvic gray communicating rami passing lateral to nerves of the sacral plexus (there are no white communicating rami below the level of L2 or L3) and the origins of the pelvic splanchnic nerves (see Figs. 14.18 and 14.19; Plate 14.2).**
- **To expose the pelvic splanchnic nerves completely, lift the rectum and anal canal superiorly. Note the pelvic splanchnic nerves penetrating the piriformis and coccygeus muscles to reach the lateral wall of the rectum. Trace the obturator nerve through the obturator foramen and expose the lumbosacral trunk and the sacral nerves.**
- **Expose the ductus deferens to the seminal gland. Expose the dilation of the ductus deferens near the seminal gland, the *ampulla*. Expose the seminal gland and identify the ejaculatory duct formed by the union of the ductus deferens and the seminal gland.**
- **Identify the prostate and expose its superior portion, the base, which is in contact with the urinary bladder. On either side of the prostate, palpate, if possible, the lateral lobes. Look for the wedge-shaped median lobe, located anterior to the ejaculatory ducts. Palpate the posterior lobe.**

Dissection of the Female Pelvis

- **Identify the broad ligament with its different portions—the mesosalpinx, mesovarium, and mesometrium.**
- **Identify the ovaries and the peritoneal fold covering the ovarian vessels, the suspensory ligament (infundibulopelvic) (Fig. 14.24).**
- **Identify the proper ligament of the ovary.**

DISSECTION **TIP**

This ovarian ligament connects to the body of the uterus and the round ligament of the uterus.

- **At the base of the broad ligament, look for a thickening of the endopelvic fascia, the cardinal ligament (ligament of Mackenrodt). Inferiorly, identify the uterosacral ligament connecting the uterus to the sacrum.**

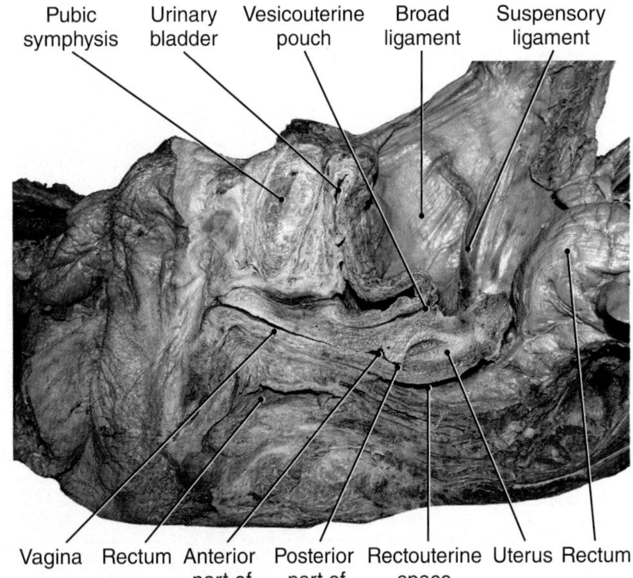

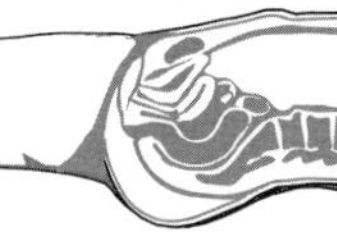

Fig. 14.24 Identify the broad ligament of the uterus and suspensory ligament of the ovary; appreciate the relationship between the rectum and the uterus forming the pouch of Douglas (retrovesical space).

DISSECTION **TIP**

The cardinal and uterosacral ligaments may be difficult to identify in the cadaver. However, by pulling the uterus anteriorly toward the pubic symphysis and to the right, you may feel the left uterosacral ligament.

- **On the hemisected uterus, identify the fundus, body, and cervix. Anterior to the cervix, identify the vagina. The deepest portion of the vagina behind the cervix is the posterior part of the fornix (Figs. 14.24 and 14.25).**
- **On the hemisected pelvis, observe the most inferior portion of the abdomen, the pouch of Douglas (rectouterine space) (Fig. 14.24).**

ANATOMY **NOTE**

A connective tissue septum extends inferiorly from the pouch of Douglas (retrovesical space) between the rectum and the vagina/uterus to attach to the perineal body, the rectovaginal septum (fascia of Denonvilliers). Its counterpart in the male is the rectoprostatic septum.

Ongoing Dissection of Male Pelvis

- **With a paper towel, clean the contents of the rectum and anal canal. Internally, identify the transverse folds of the rectum (valves of Houston), the anal columns (of Morgagni), and the pectinate line (Fig. 14.26).**
- **Make a midsagittal incision through the prostate and identify the three portions of the urethra: prostatic, membranous, and spongy (Fig. 14.27). Within the prostatic urethra, identify an elevation, the *urethral crest*, and in the midline, the opening of**

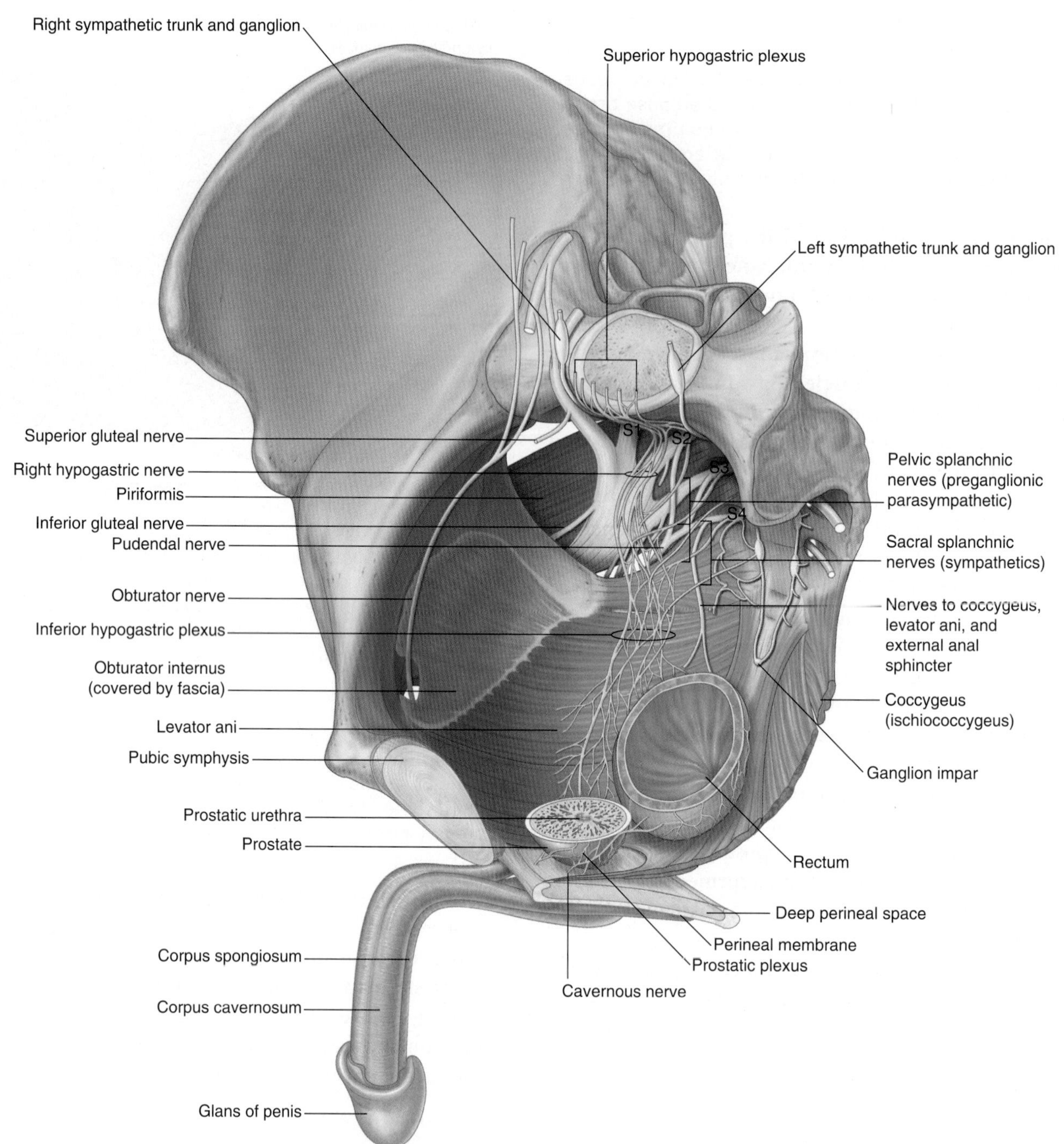

Plate 14.2 Nerves of the pelvis. (From Drake RL et al. *Gray's Atlas of Anatomy*, 3rd edition, Philadelphia, Elsevier, 2021, p. 256.)

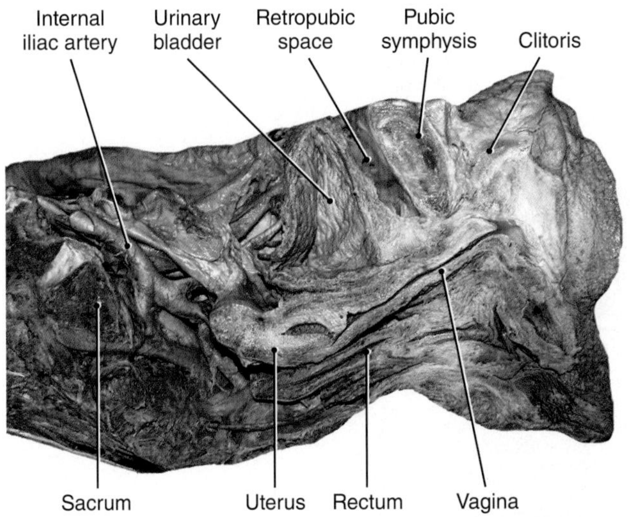

Fig. 14.25 Identify the vaginal canal with its anterior and posterior parts of the fornix.

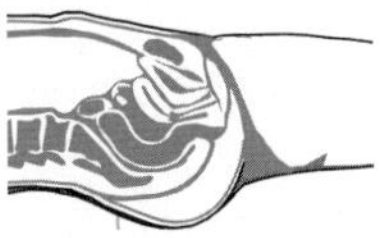

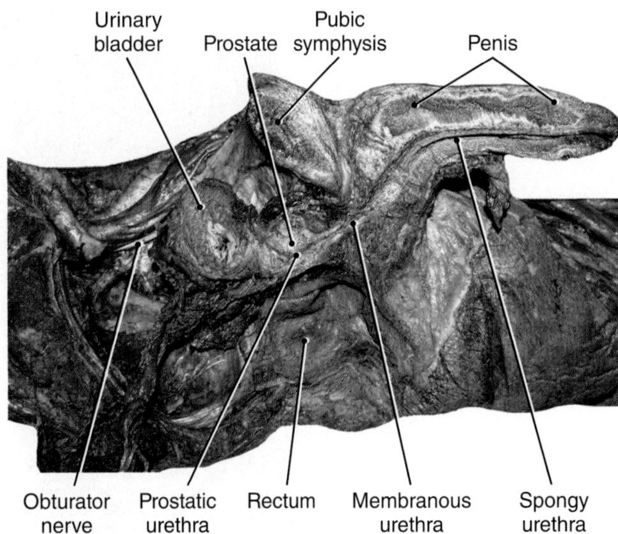

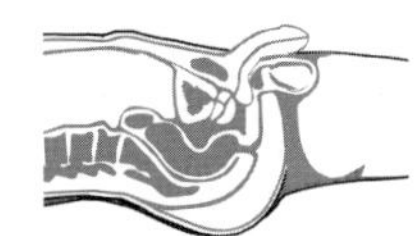

Fig. 14.27 In this hemisected pelvis, appreciate the anatomic components of the urethra (prostatic, membranous, and spongy parts).

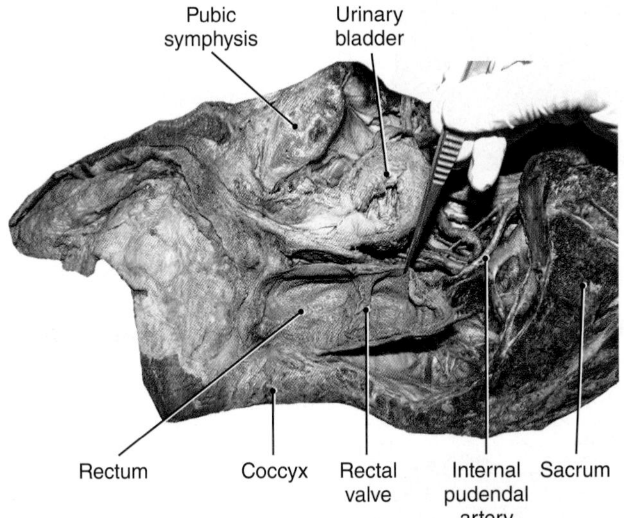

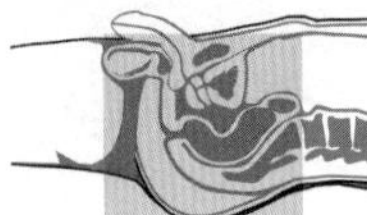

Fig. 14.26 In this specimen, note internal structures of the rectum and anal canal (transverse folds, valves of Houston).

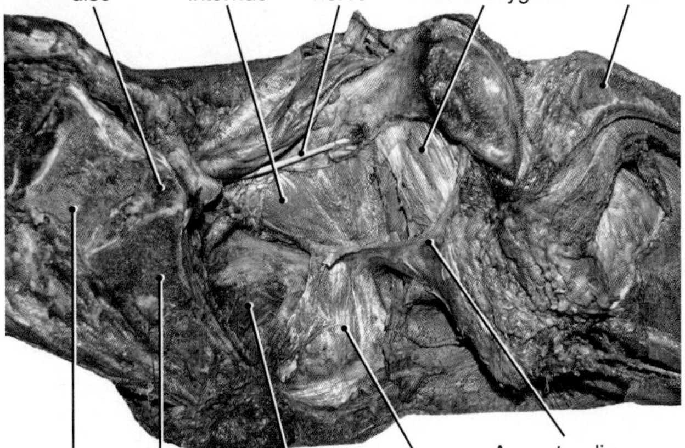

Fig. 14.28 The arteries and veins are removed and musculature is exposed. *L5*, 5th lumbar; *S1*, 1st sacral.

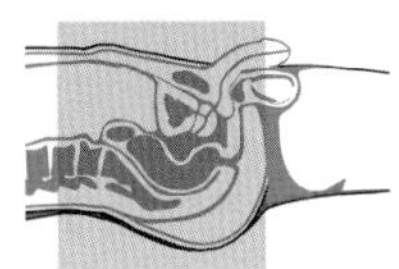

the prostatic utricle. Lateral and distal to the prostatic utricle, identify the ejaculatory ducts. Lateral to the urethral crest, identify the openings of the prostatic ducts.

- In Fig. 14.28 the arteries and veins have been removed and the underlying musculature has been exposed.
- Pull the hemisected urinary bladder medially and posteriorly and identify the puboprostatic ligaments (pubovesical in females) lying laterally between the pubic symphysis and the bladder (Fig. 14.29).
- Identify the trigone of the urinary bladder.

DISSECTION TIP

Trigone identification is difficult in the hemisected specimen because the incision plane usually transects it.

- Identify the ureteric orifice and the interureteric ridge or crest created by a muscular fold between the two ureteric orifices. The orifice of the urethra forms a muscular elevation, the *uvula.*
- Lift the rectum upward and expose the pelvic splanchnic nerves (Fig. 14.30).

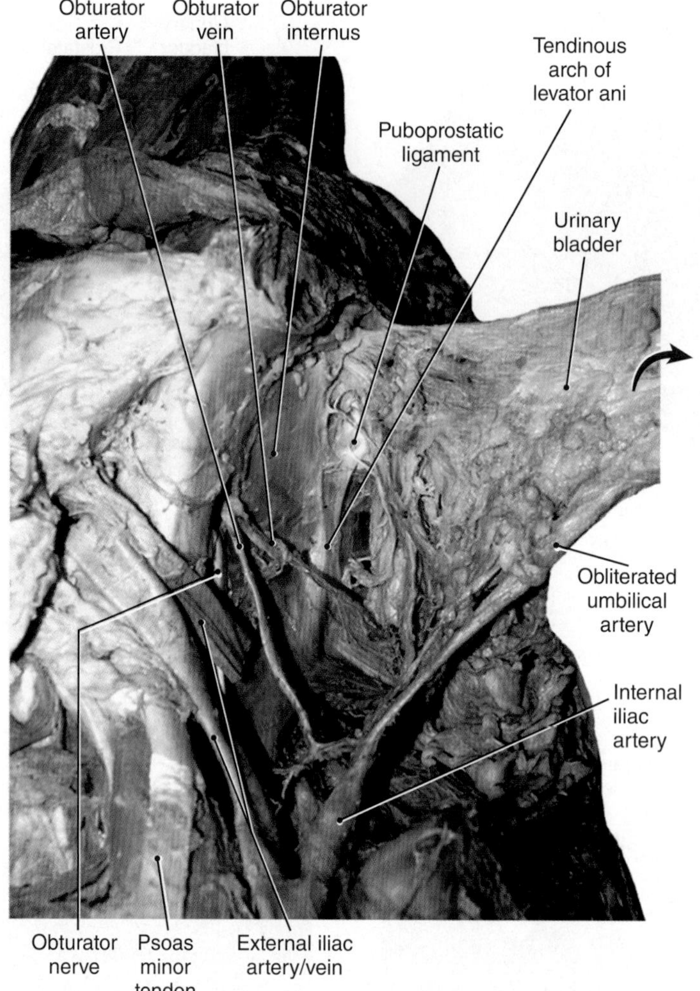

Fig. 14.29 The urinary bladder is retracted medially and the puboprostatic ligaments are identified in the space between the obturator internus muscle and the urinary bladder, just behind the pubic symphysis.

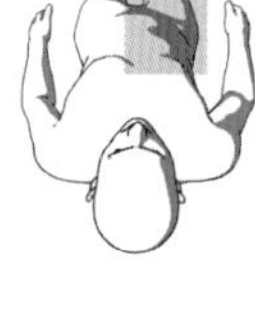

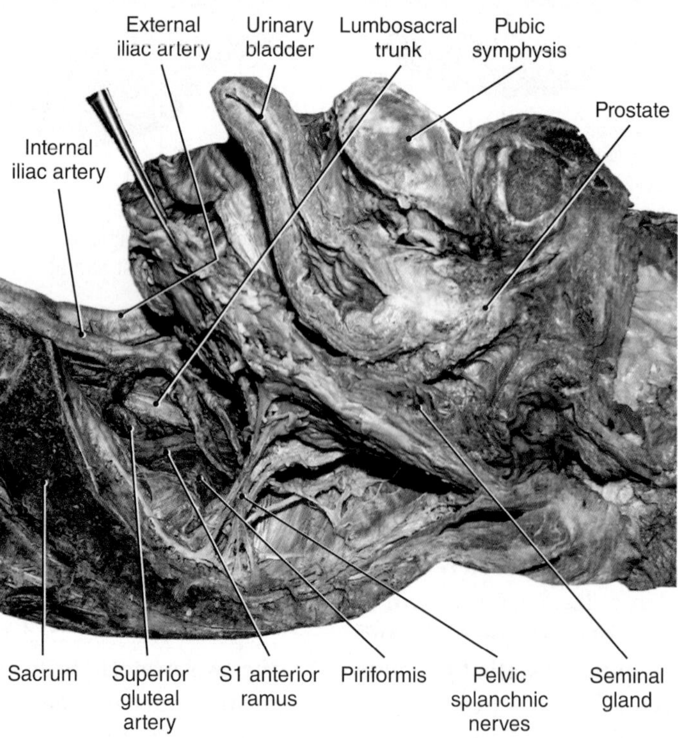

Fig. 14.30 The rectum is lifted upwardly to expose the pelvic splanchnic nerves. *S1,* 1st sacral vertebra.

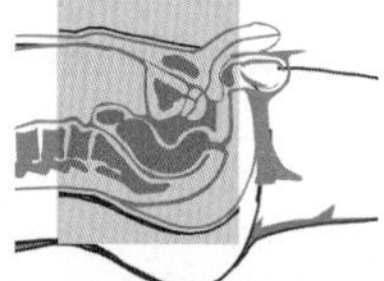

PARAMEDIAN HEMIPELVECTOMY (MALE)

Technique 2

- Identify the rectosigmoid junction and expose the rectum. Posterior to the pubic symphysis, palpate the urinary bladder.
- With a probe or scissors, dissect out and reflect the peritoneum from the posterior surface of the urinary bladder. Notice the median umbilical ligament connecting to the urinary bladder (urachus).
- Place your fingertips, using blunt dissection, between the urinary bladder and the pubic symphysis into the retropubic space of Retzius.
- Pull on the fascia attached to the lateral sides of the median umbilical ligament and at the superior part of the urinary bladder, the *vesicoumbilical fascia*, and reflect it posteriorly. With this maneuver, observe the expansion of the retropubic space of Retzius.
- Mobilize the rectum and the bladder. With a saw, cut 5 to 7 cm lateral to the pubic symphysis at the midpoint of the superior pubic ramus (Fig. 14.31).
- With a scalpel, make a second horizontal incision starting from the aorta, at the level of the kidneys, and extending laterally along the borders of the iliac crest (Fig. 14.31).
- With the cadaver on its side, and using a saw, cut the sacrum through its promontory, up through the 4th lumbar vertebra. Detach this portion of the body (Fig. 14.32).

DISSECTION TIP

For the hemipelvectomy, you will need the help of your colleagues to lift and turn the cadaver on its side.

- With a scalpel, expose the superior and inferior pubic rami. Identify the obturator internus muscle (Fig. 14.32).
- Begin cleaning the soft tissues and adipose tissue around the superior and inferior pubic rami (Fig. 14.33).
- Identify the lateral edge of the urinary bladder and trace the ductus deferens inferiorly to the seminal gland (Fig. 14.34).
- Trace and expose the rectum and clean the adipose tissue from the area between the rectum and the seminal gland (Fig. 14.35).
- Transect the lateral margin of the superior and inferior pubic rami close to the pubic symphysis (Fig. 14.36).

DISSECTION TIP

Place your index finger in the space between the bladder and the pubic symphysis (retropubic space of Retzius) and, using blunt dissection, separate the pubic symphysis from the urinary bladder (Fig. 14.37). Try to reach as deep as possible toward the membranous urethra.

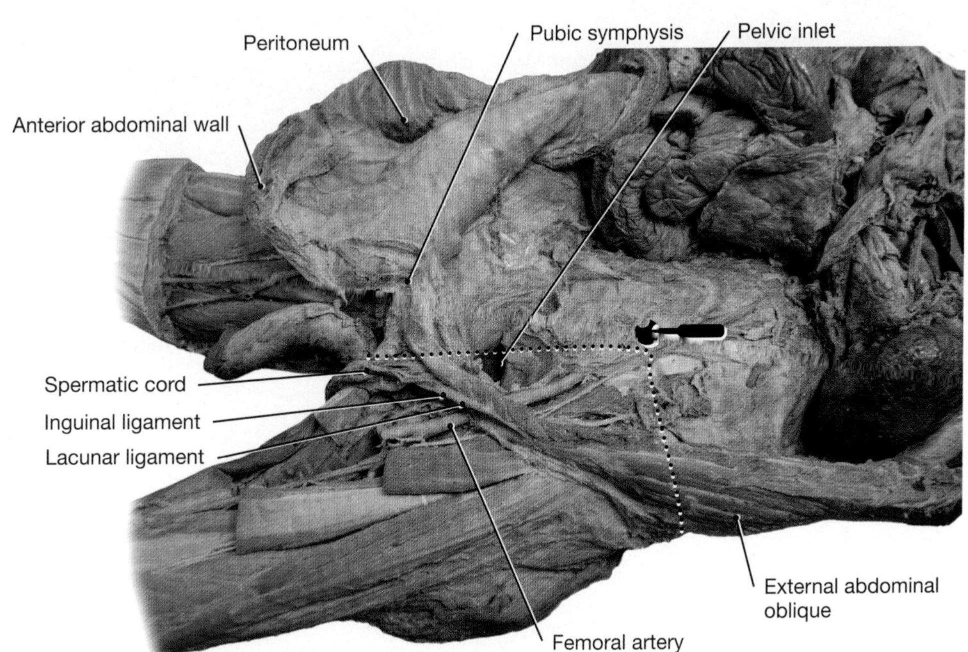

Fig. 14.31 Male pelvis showing the drawing lines for a paramedian hemipelvectomy.

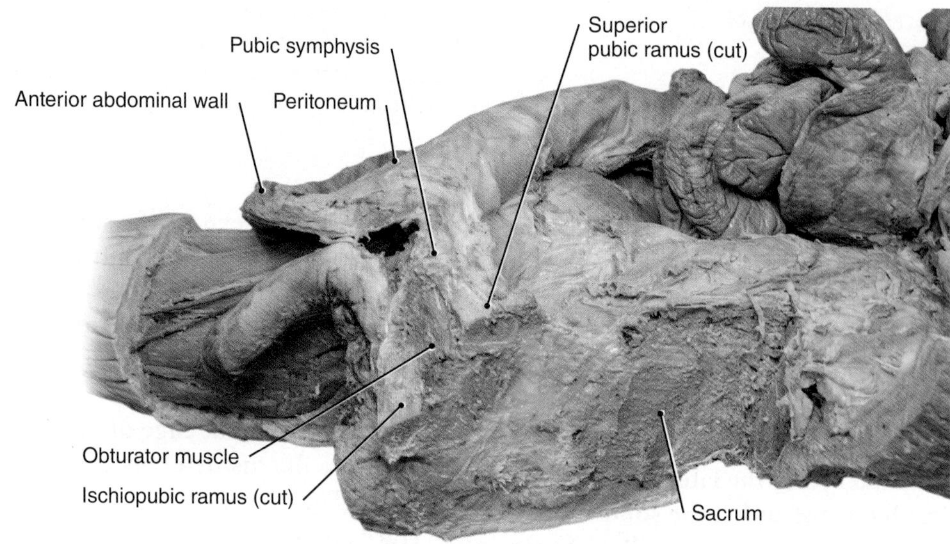

Fig. 14.32 A completed paramedian hemipelvectomy with the superior and inferior pubic rami exposed.

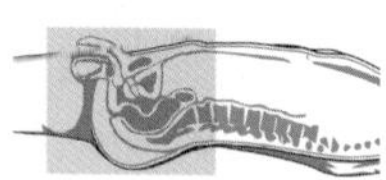

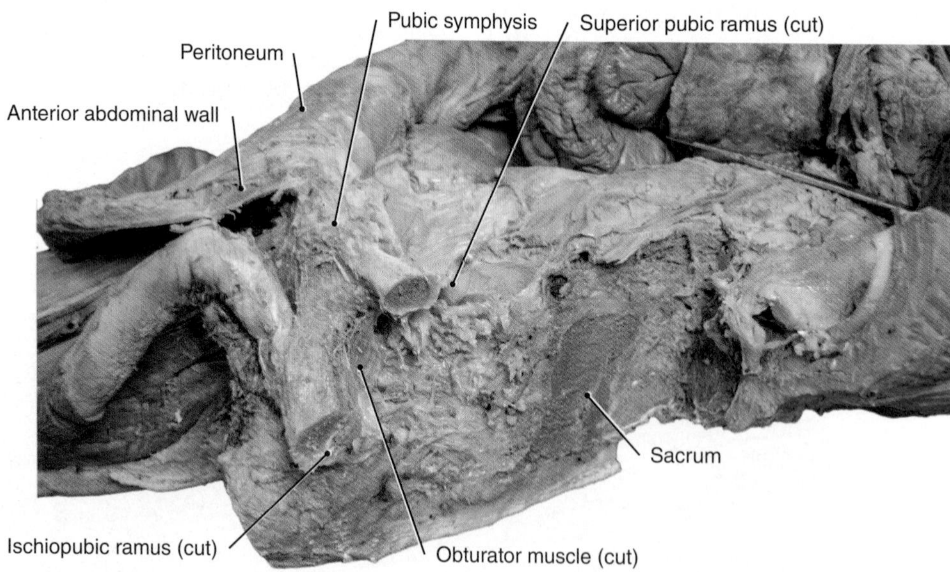

Fig. 14.33 A completed paramedian hemipelvectomy with the superior and inferior pubic rami fully exposed and the obturator internus muscle removed.

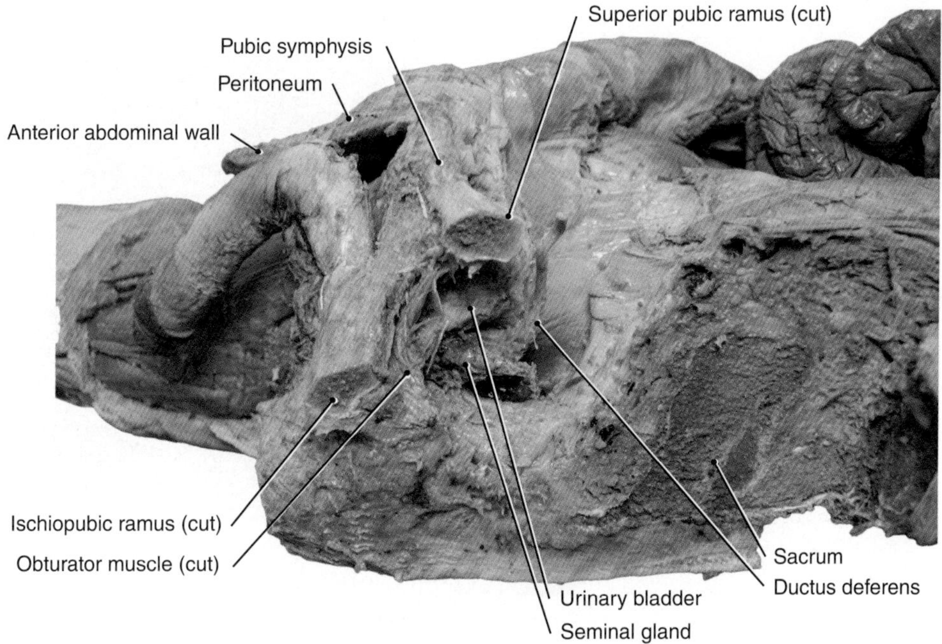

Fig. 14.34 The lateral edge of the seminal gland and urinary bladder are exposed.

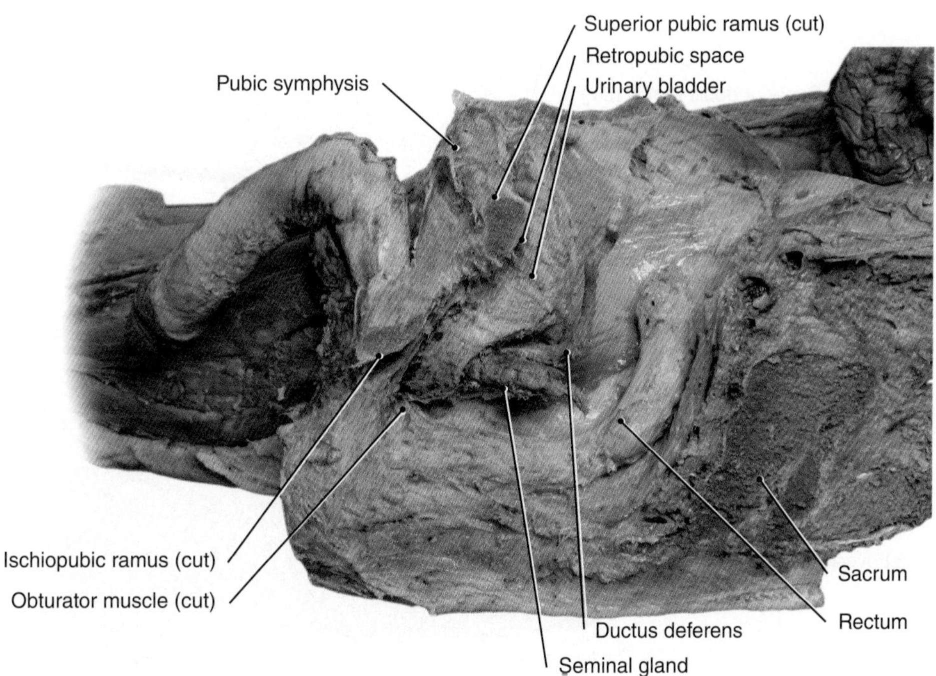

Fig. 14.35 A portion of the superior and inferior pubic rami has been transected and the rectum has been exposed.

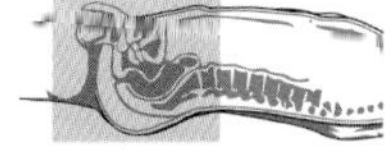

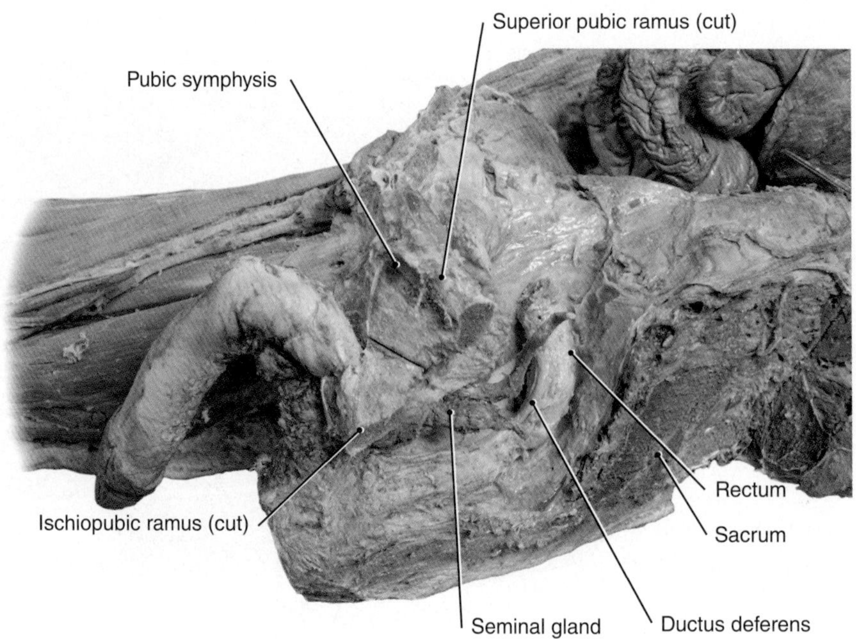

Fig. 14.36 A further portion of the superior and inferior pubic rami have been transected and the rectum has been exposed.

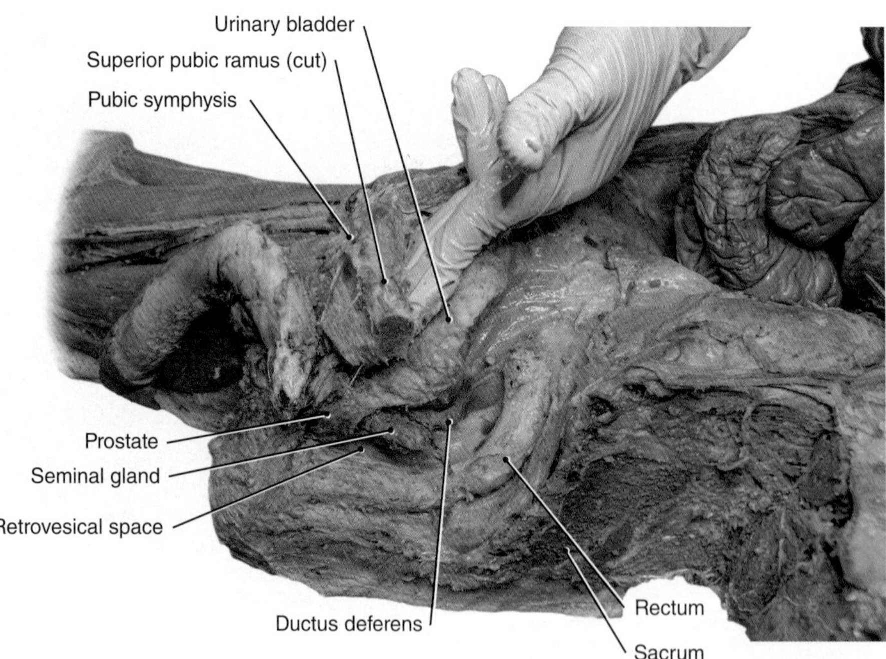

Fig. 14.37 The inferior pubic ramus has been transected and the index and middle fingers are separating the pubic symphysis from the urinary bladder.

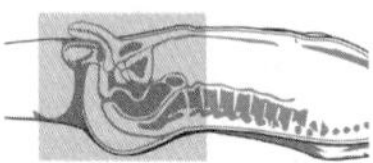

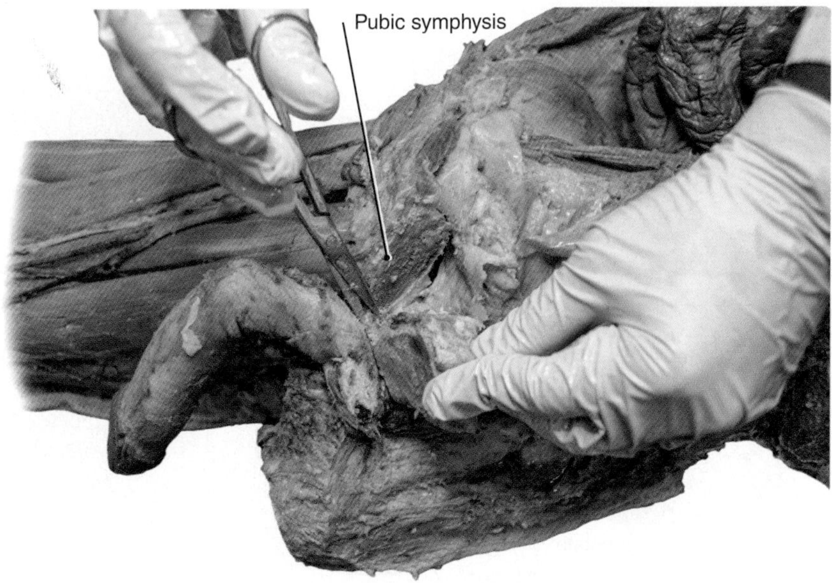

Fig. 14.38 With a pair of scissors the pubic symphysis is fully separated from the underlying structures.

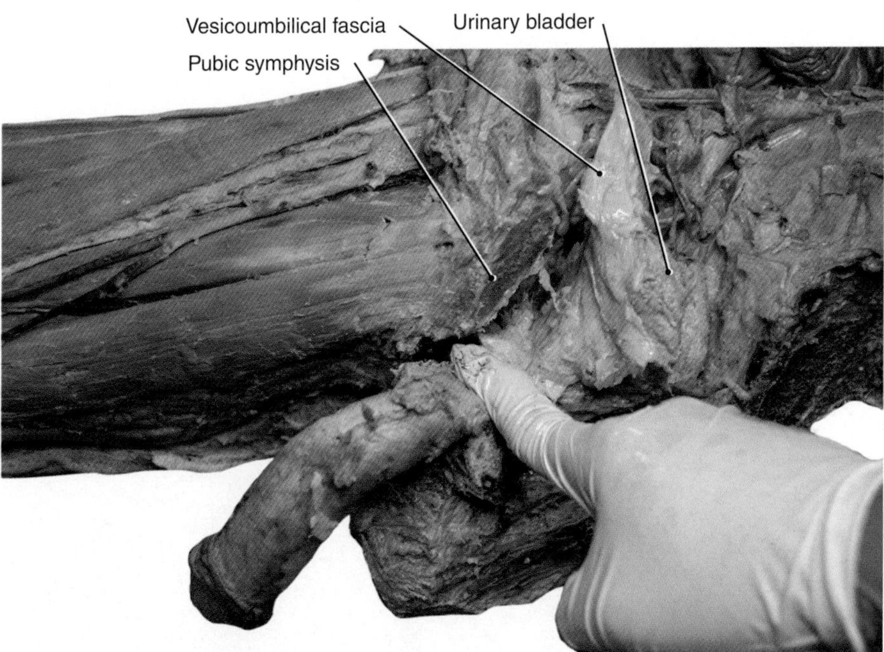

Fig. 14.39 The pubic symphysis has been removed and the index finger is pushing downward the prostate and the urinary bladder.

○ **Make a midline cut at the pubic symphysis (Fig. 14.38).**

DISSECTION TIP

The inferior surface of the pubic symphysis is difficult to detach after the midline incision from the penis and prostate. Use scissors to separate the connective tissue from the pubic symphysis and the underlying structures (Fig. 14.39).

○ **Once the pubic symphysis is removed, apply pressure over the prostate ensuring that there are no attachments left on the lateral side of the pubic symphysis that remain intact laterally (Fig. 14.40).**

○ **With the use of scissors detach all remaining soft tissues from the area between the inferior surface of the prostate and seminal gland and the rectum (Fig. 14.41). Then remove en bloc from the cadaver the penis-prostate-seminal gland-urinary bladder structure (Figs. 14.42 and 14.43).**

○ **Clean the penis-prostate-seminal gland-urinary bladder structures from all soft and adipose tissues (Fig. 14.44).**

○ **With a scalpel transect the penis at its midportion (Fig. 14.45). Identify the corpus cavernosum, corpus spongiosum, spongy urethra, deep dorsal vein of penis, deep artery of penis, and the fascia of penis (Buck's fascia).**

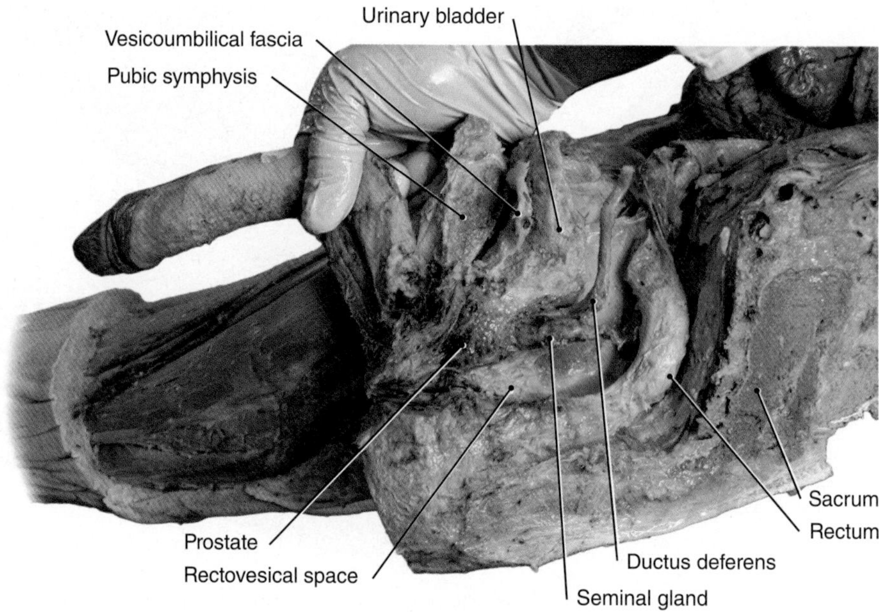

Fig. 14.40 The penis-prostate-seminal gland-urinary bladder is dissected away from the attachments of the surrounding structures.

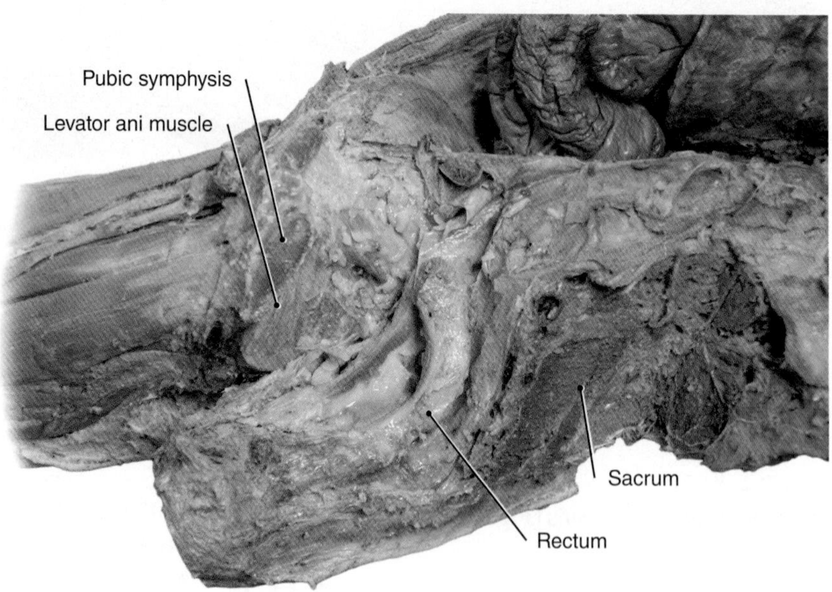

Fig. 14.41 A complete en bloc removal of the penis-prostate-seminal gland-urinary bladder from the cadaver.

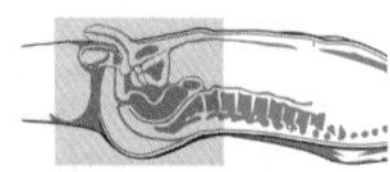

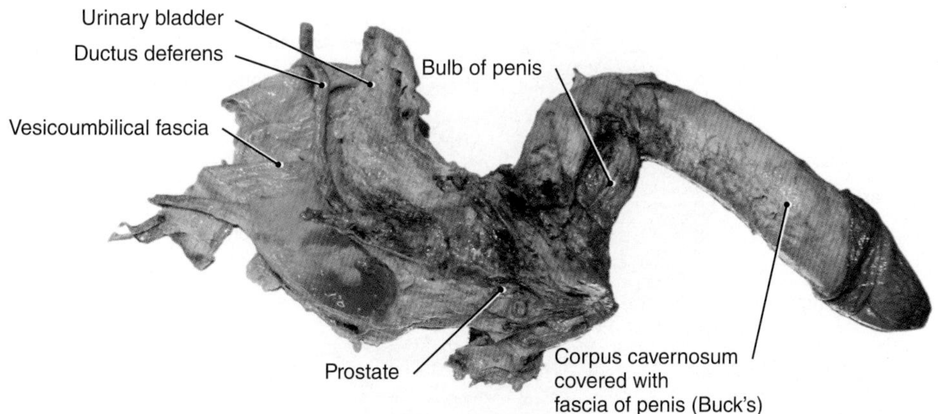

Fig. 14.42 The penis-prostate-seminal gland-urinary bladder is placed on a tray for further dissection.

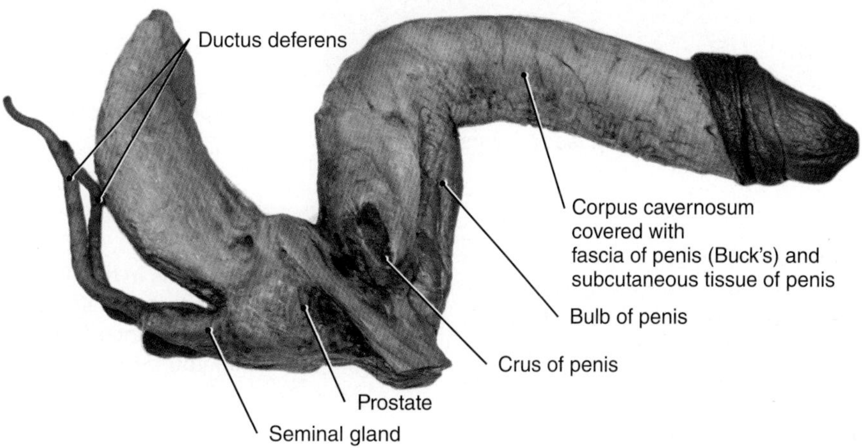

Fig. 14.43 The penis-prostate-seminal gland-urinary bladder is dissected out from all soft and adipose tissues, exposing the ductus deferens.

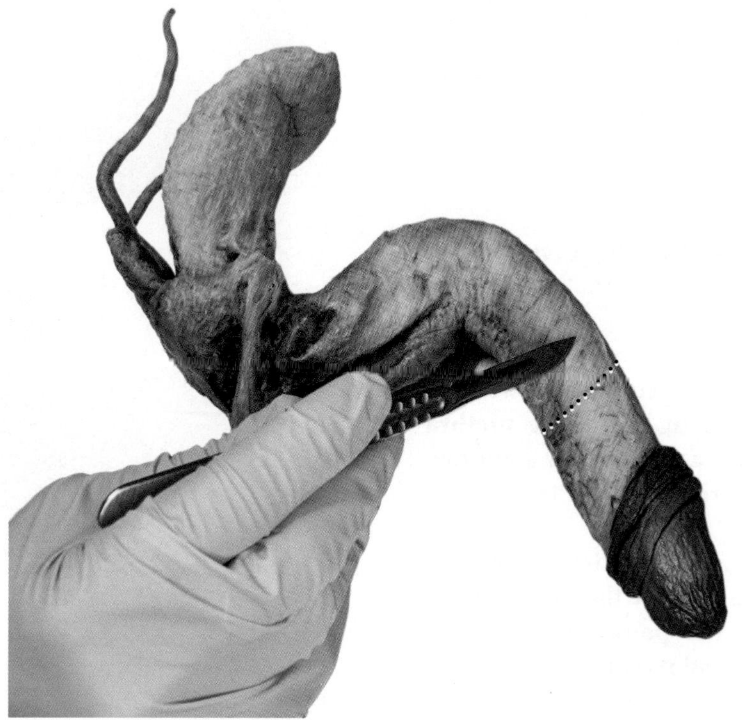

Fig. 14.44 A transection of the penis at its midportion.

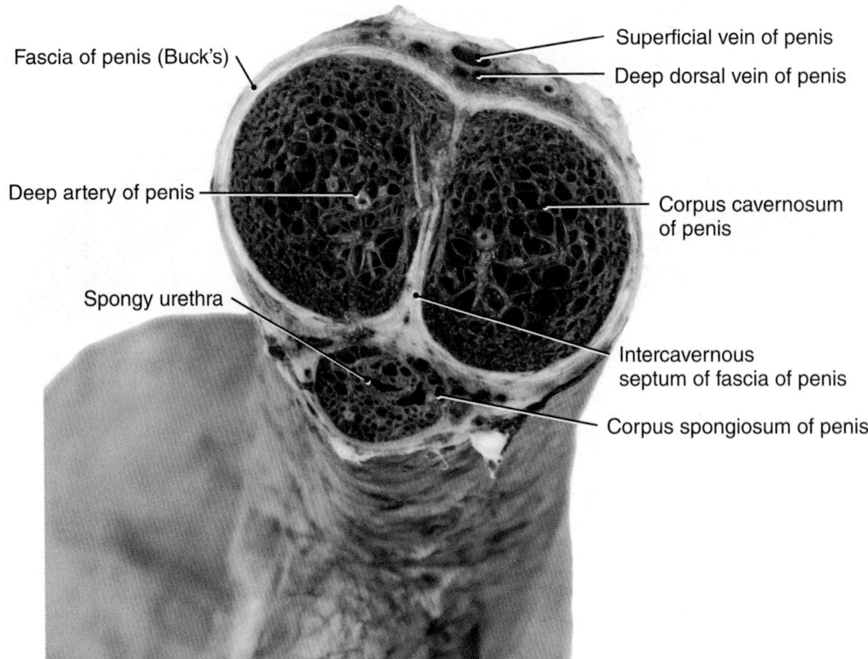

Fig. 14.45 A view of the transected penis, exposing the corpus cavernosum and corpus spongiosum, dorsal vein of the penis, deep artery of the penis, and the accompanying fascia layers.

ANATOMY NOTE

The penis serves as the common outlet for both urine and semen. It comprises three main parts: the root, body, and glans. The erectile tissue consists of three cylindrical bodies: the paired corpora cavernosa on the dorsal side and the single corpus spongiosum on the ventral side. Each cavernous body is enveloped by a fibrous capsule called the tunica albuginea, and the deep fascia of the penis (Buck's fascia) lies superficial to this outer covering. This fascia, an extension of the deep perineal fascia, forms a robust membranous layer that binds together the corpora cavernosa and corpus spongiosum. The corpus spongiosum houses the spongy portion of the urethra. The corpora cavernosa are fused in the median plane, with a posterior separation to form the crura of the penis. Internally, the cavernous tissue is divided by the intercavernous septum penis.

DISSECTION TIP

If you have not had another specimen removed en bloc, you can use superglue to reattach the two pieces of the penis (Fig. 14.46).

- **After the reattachment is complete, insert a wooden stick into the spongy part of the penile urethra (Fig. 14.47). This will serve as a guide for a midline incision of the penis, ensuring accurate transection of the urethra.**
- **With a scalpel begin a midline incision from the external urethral orifice alongside the wooden stick indicating the pathway of the spongy urethra. Identify the glans of the penis and its corona, the corpus cavernosum, and the fascia of the penis (Fig. 14.48).**

DISSECTION TIP

Transecting the penis in the midline, even with the aid of a wooden stick, can be challenging in an embalmed cadaver. Request assistance from your colleagues to hold the penis while you perform the midline incision.

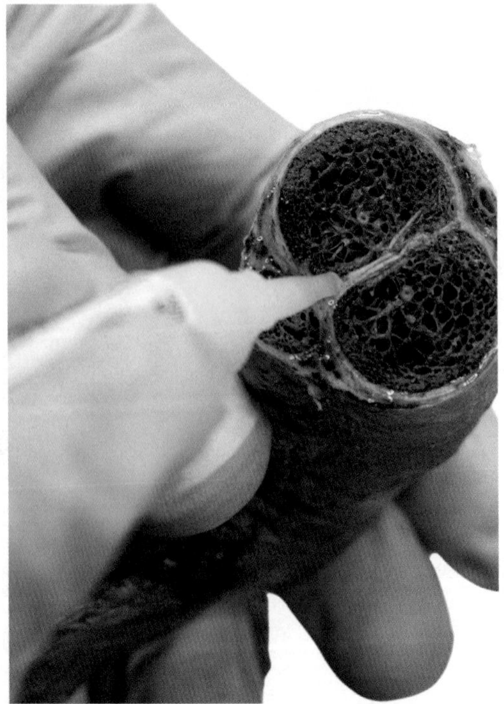

Fig. 14.46 Reattachment of the transected specimen with a superglue.

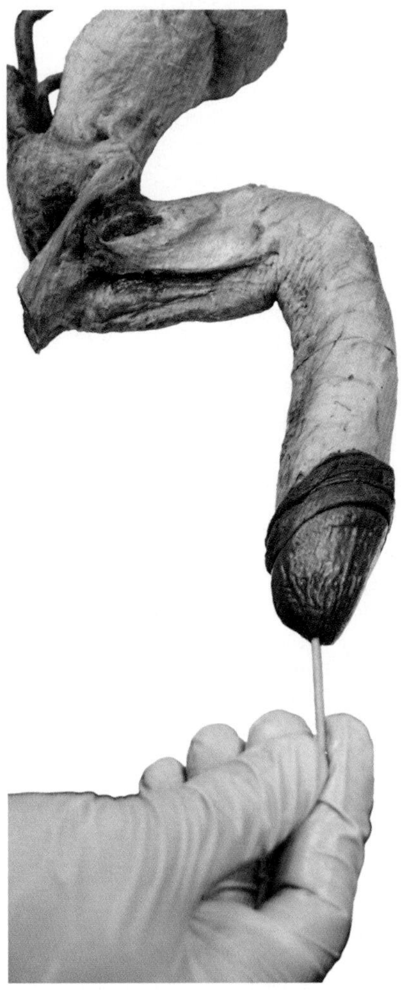

Fig. 14.47 Insertion of a wooden stick at the external urethral orifice to aid the midline incision of the penis.

- **Continue the incision from the spongy urethra to the membranous and prostatic portions. Once the urethra is exposed, vertically transect the urinary bladder fully exposing the structure of the penis-prostate-seminal gland-urinary bladder (Fig. 14.49).**

Technique 3

- **Insert a wooden stick into the spongy part of the penile urethra through the external urethral orifice. This will serve, later in the dissection, as a guide for a midline incision of the penis, ensuring accurate transection of the urethra (Fig. 14.50).**
- **With the use of scissors or scalpel cut the fundiform ligament of the penis and clean the pubic symphysis anteriorly and superiorly from any soft tissues (Fig. 14.51).**

DISSECTION **TIP**

Use your index finger to push the penis inferiorly in order to expose more of the area between the pubic symphysis and the penis.

- **Transect the pubic symphysis bilaterally, 3 cm from the midline on each side (Fig. 14.52).**
- **Remove the pubic symphysis to expose the entire length of the penis, prostate, and urinary bladder (Fig. 14.53).**

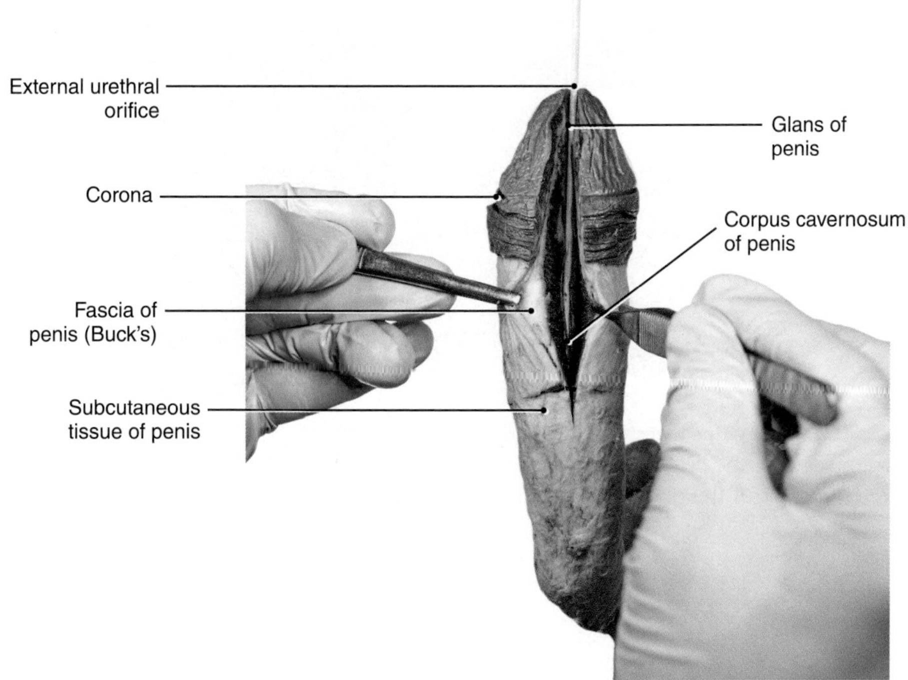

Fig. 14.48 Midline incision of the penis following the wooden stick as a guide.

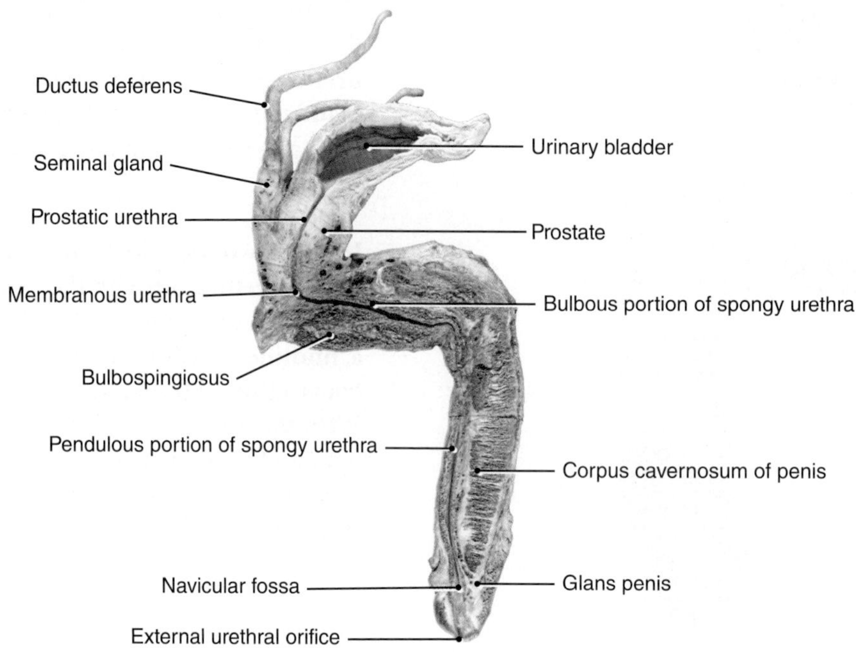

Fig. 14.49 A completed midline incision of the penis-prostate-seminal gland-urinary bladder.

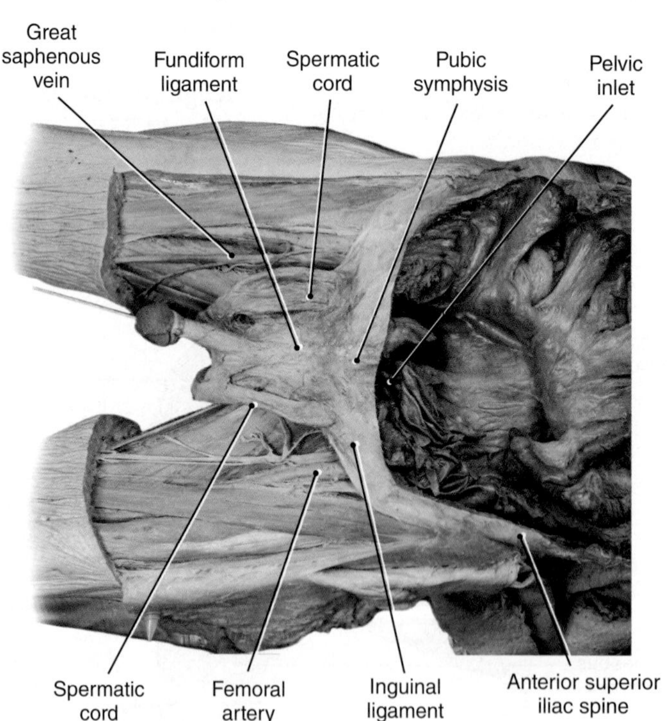

Fig. 14.50 Insertion of a wooden stick at the external urethral orifice to aid the midline incision of the penis.

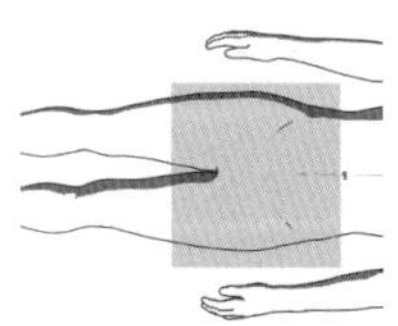

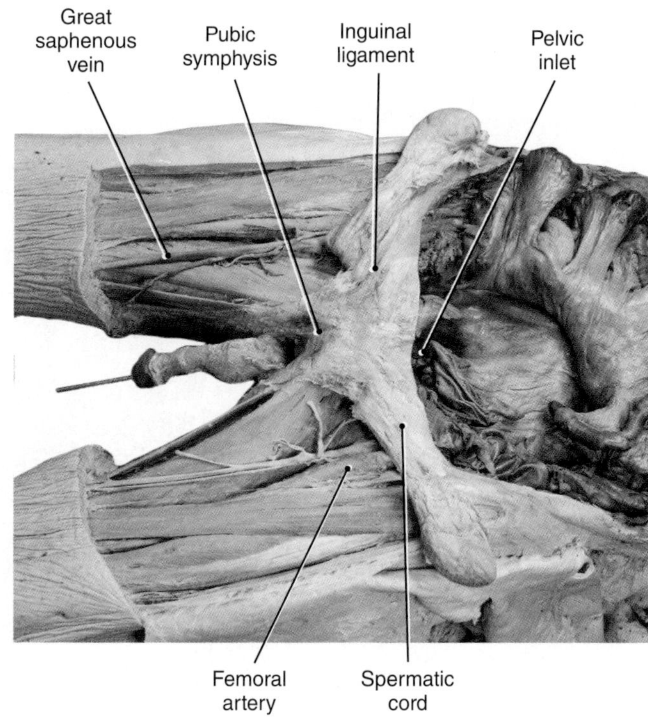

Fig. 14.51 Complete detachment of the penis from the fundiform ligament.

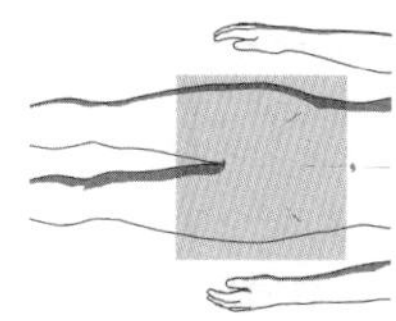

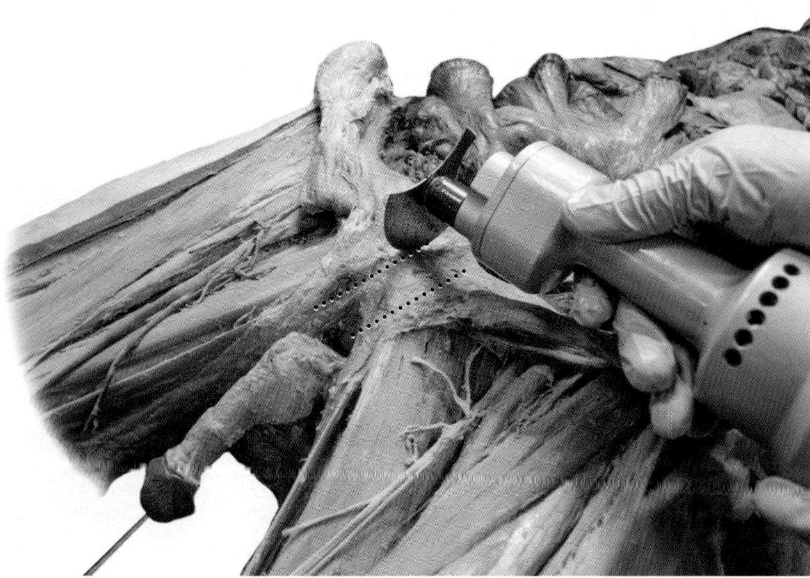

Fig. 14.52 Transection of the pubic symphysis.

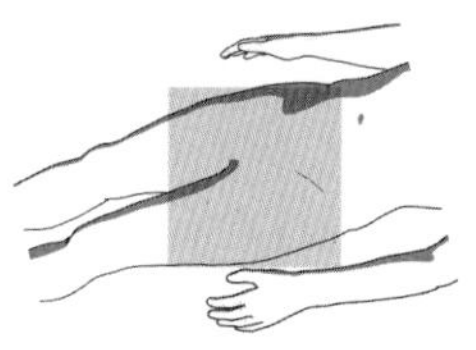

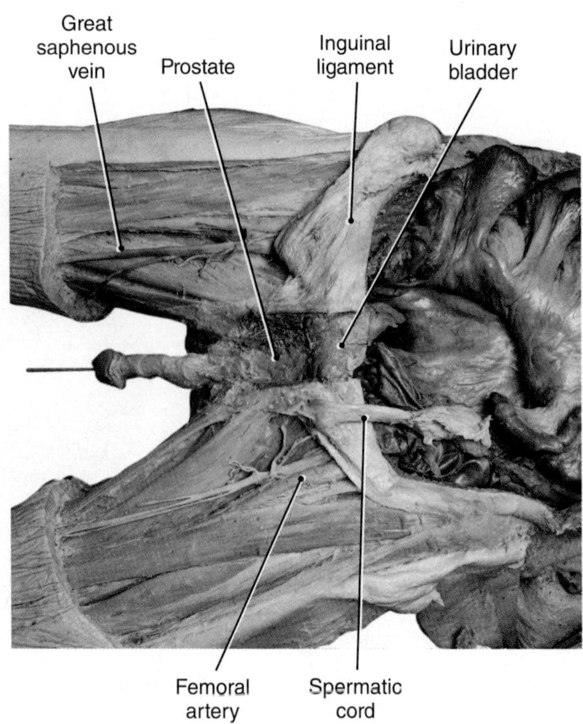

Fig. 14.53 Transection of the pubic symphysis and exposure of the underlying penis-prostate and urinary bladder.

- **With your index finger use blunt dissection to further separate the structures attached to the prostate, seminal glands, and urinary bladder laterally and inferiorly (Fig. 14.54).**
- **With a scalpel begin a midline incision from the external urethral orifice alongside the wooden stick indicating the pathway of the spongy urethra. Identify the glans of the penis and its corona, the corpus cavernosum, and the fascia of the penis (Fig. 14.55).**
- **Continue the incision from the spongy urethra to the membranous and prostatic portions (Fig. 14.56). Once the urethra is exposed, vertically transect the urinary bladder fully exposing the structure of the penis-prostate-seminal gland-urinary bladder (Fig. 14.57).**

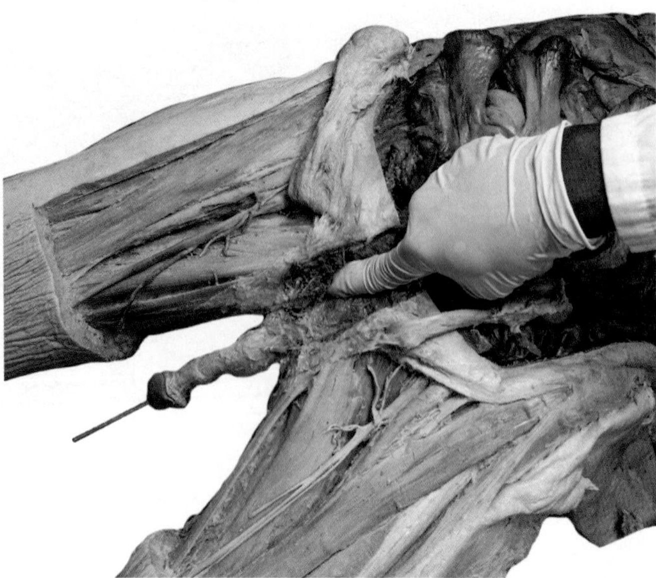

Fig. 14.54 The pubic symphysis has been removed and the index finger is separating the lateral border of the pubic symphysis from the urinary bladder.

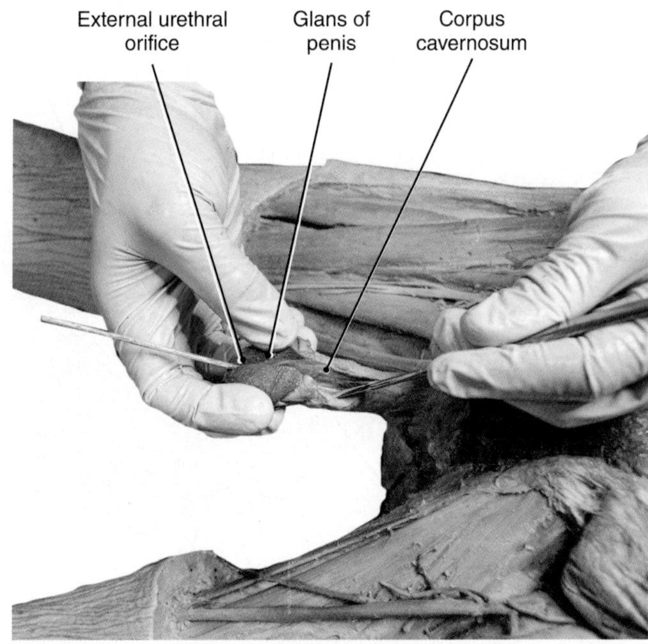

Fig. 14.55 A midline incision of the penis using the wooden stick at the external urethral orifice as a guide.

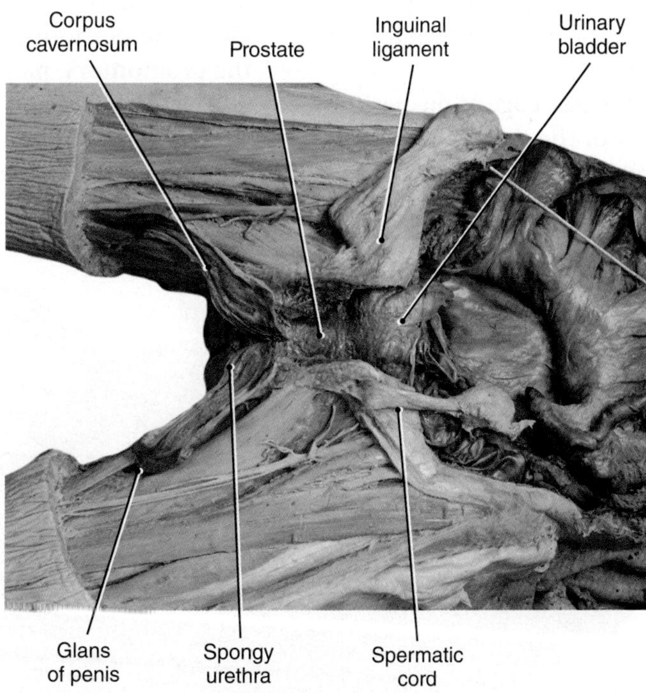

Fig. 14.56 Partial midline incision of the penis, involving the spongy urethra.

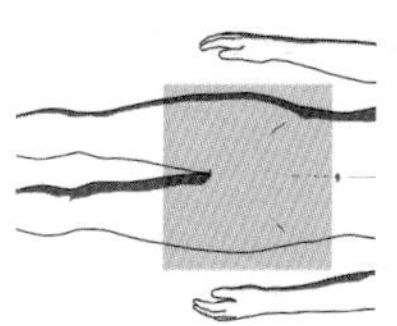

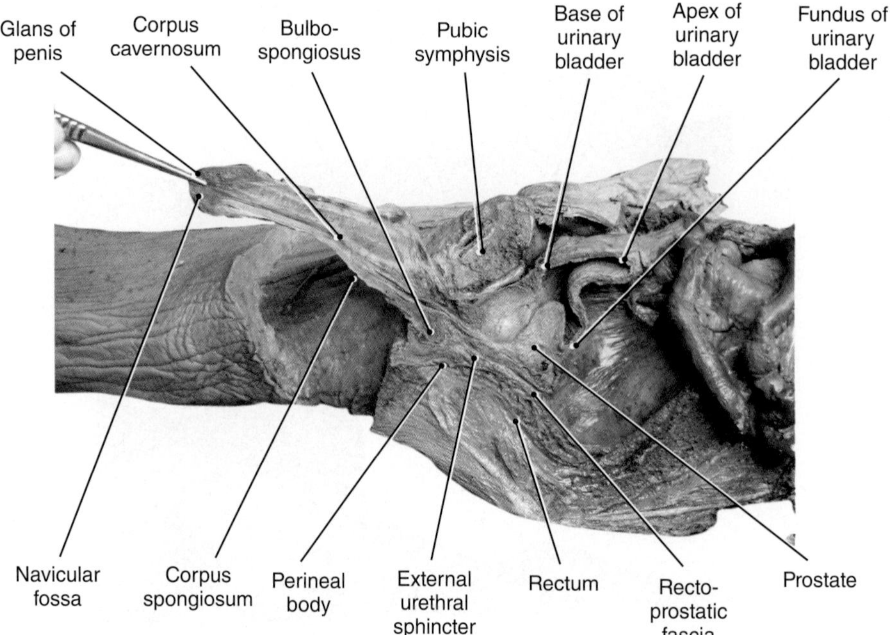

Fig. 14.57 A complete midline exposed of the hemipelvectomy showing the penis, prostate, rectum, seminal glands, and urinary bladder.

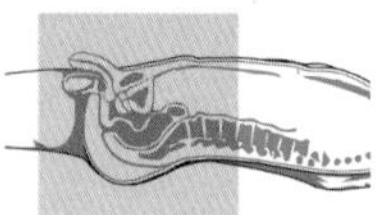

- **Use the steps as described in techniques 1 and 2 to complete the hemipelvectomy. Identify the different portions of the male urethra and appreciate the anatomic relationships.**
- **With a pair of forceps, lift the free edge of the peritoneum over the promontory of the sacrum and raise it upward, detaching it from the underlying adipose tissue (Fig. 14.58). Continue the detachment of the peritoneum over the urinary bladder (Fig. 14.59).**
- **Once the peritoneum is fully detached laterally to the promontory, palpate for the external iliac artery and vein (Fig. 14.60). With your scissors, separate the overlying soft tissues to start exposing the external iliac artery and vein.**

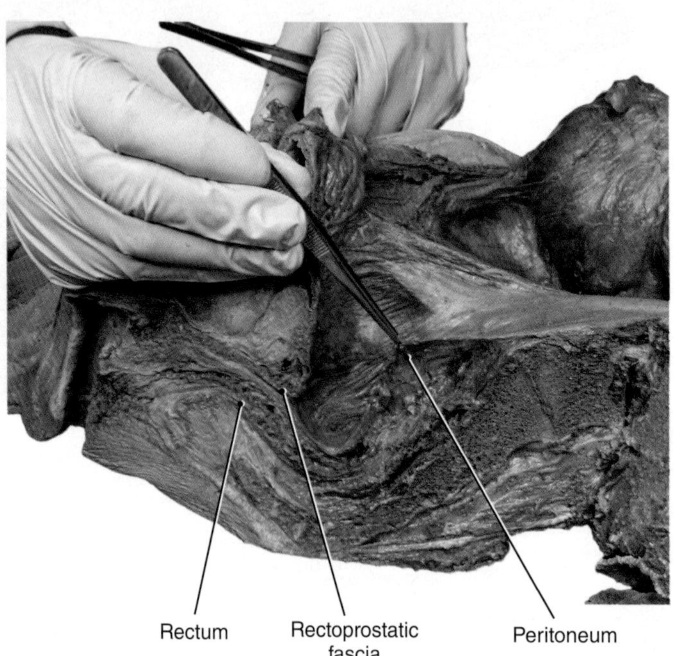

Fig. 14.58 Lift and separate of the peritoneum from the free edge of the hemipelvectomy.

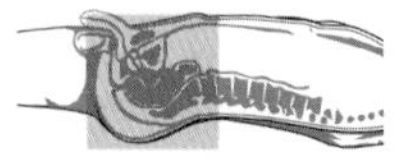

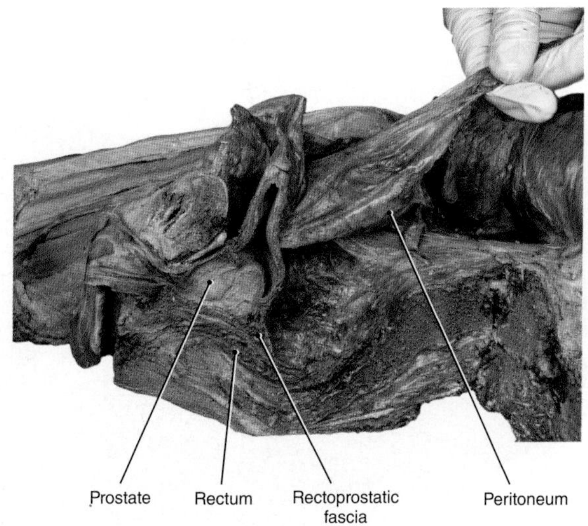

Fig. 14.59 Lift and separate of the peritoneum from the remainder of the pelvic inlet and urinary bladder.

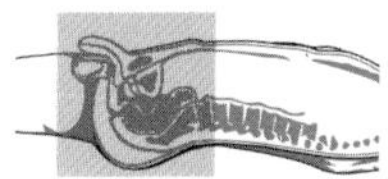

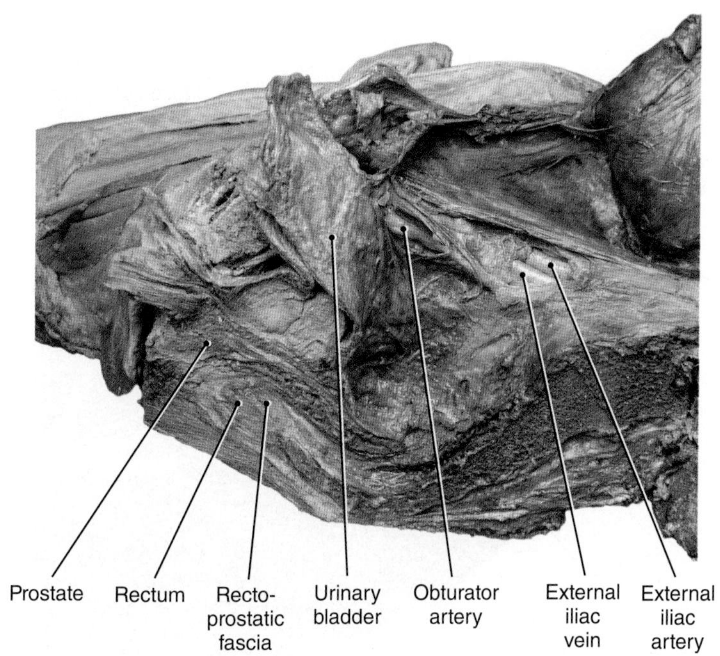

Fig. 14.60 Complete removal of the peritoneum from pelvic inlet and exposure of the proximal part of the external iliac artery and vein.

- **As the exposure of the external iliac artery and vein continues, trace the obturator nerve and artery running parallel to the external iliac artery and vein toward the obturator foramen (Fig. 14.61). Continue the exposure of all the branches of the external iliac artery and vein. Inferiorly identify the internal iliac artery and vein.**
- **Once the exposure of all the branches of the external and internal iliac arteries is complete, lift the urinary bladder upward and forward to create enough space to trace the entire length of the arterial branches of the external iliac artery and vein (Fig. 14.62). Similarly, you can pull the urinary bladder medially and again trace all the arterial branches (Fig. 14.63).**

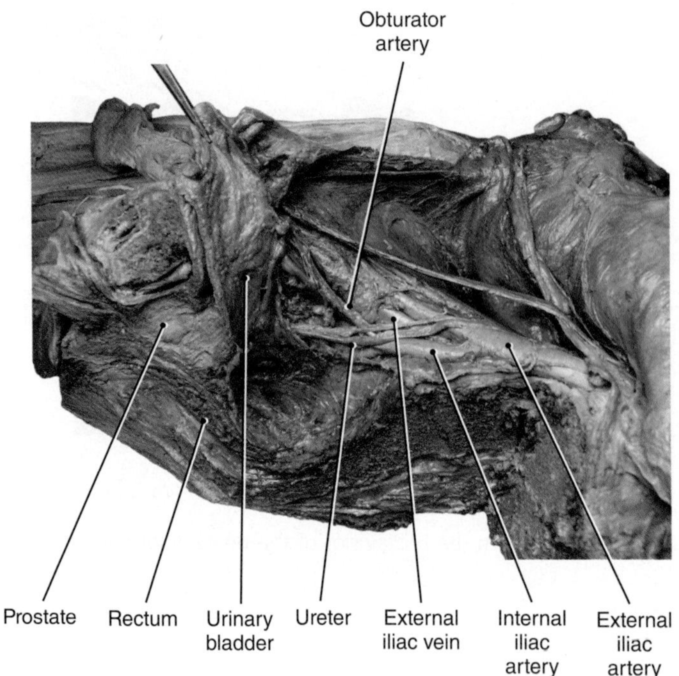

Fig. 14.61 Exposure of the proximal part of the external iliac artery and vein, ureter, and obturator artery.

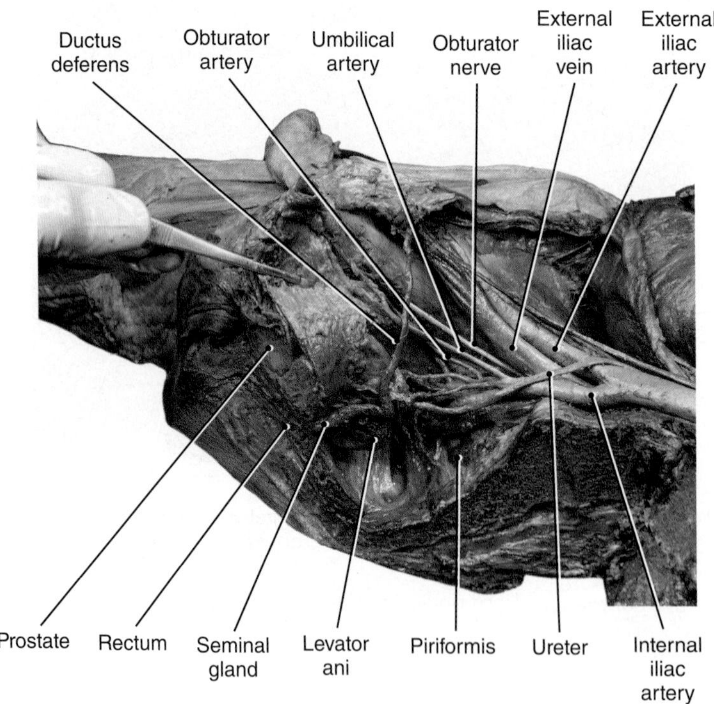

Fig. 14.62 Exposure of the branches of the external iliac artery and vein, ureter, and obturator artery and nerve and internal iliac artery and vein.

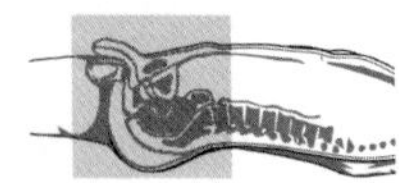

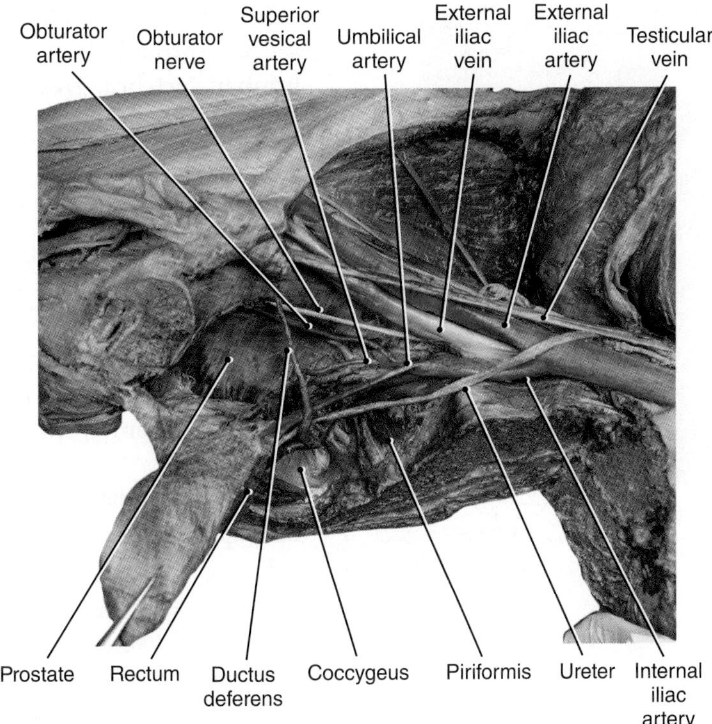

Fig. 14.63 Retraction of the urinary bladder laterally to expose the branches of the external iliac artery and vein, ureter, and obturator artery and nerve and internal iliac artery and vein.

PARAMEDIAN HEMIPELVECTOMY (FEMALE)

Technique 2

The dissection of the female pelvis has already been described. However, in this portion of the chapter, we will describe a modified approach to the midline hemipelvectomy.

- **Before the paramedian hemipelvectomy begins, identify the broad ligament of the uterus, the suspensory ligament of the ovary, the round ligament of the uterus, and the uterine body. Appreciate the relationship between the rectum and the uterus forming the pouch of Douglas (retrovesical space) (Fig. 14.64, Plate 14.3).**
- **Identify the rectosigmoid junction and expose the rectum. Posterior to the pubic symphysis, palpate the urinary bladder.**
- **Place your fingertips, using blunt dissection, between the urinary bladder and the pubic symphysis into the retropubic space of Retzius.**
- **Mobilize the rectum and the bladder. With a saw, cut 5 to 7 cm lateral to the pubic symphysis at the midpoint of the superior pubic ramus (Figs. 14.65 and 14.66).**

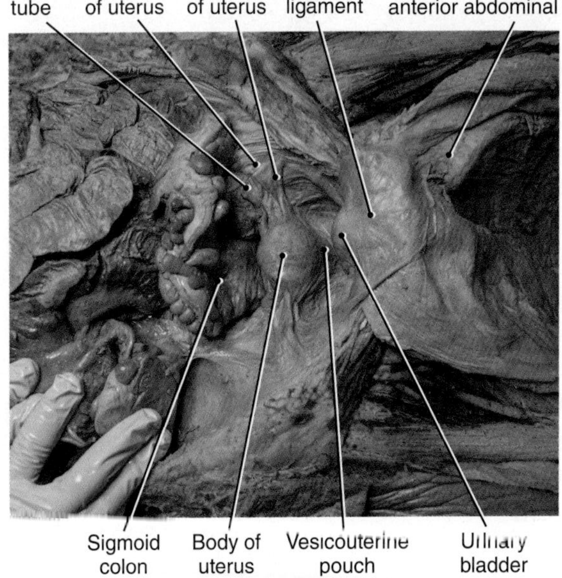

Fig. 14.64 Identify the broad ligament of the uterus, the suspensory ligament of the ovary, the round ligament of the uterus, the uterine body, and the pouch of Douglas (retrovesical space) between the rectum and the uterus.

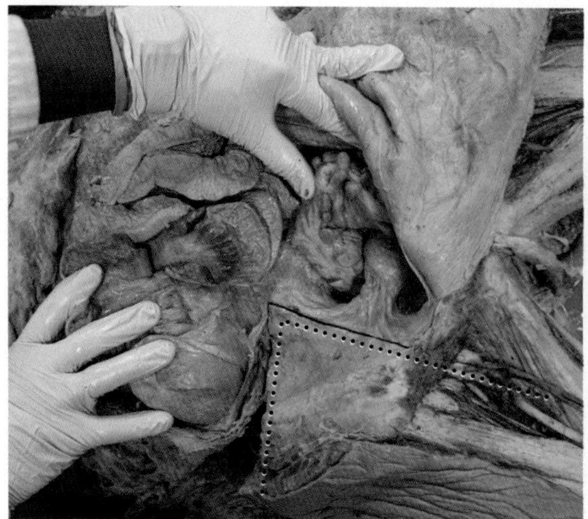

Fig. 14.65 Female pelvis showing the lines for a paramedian hemipelvectomy.

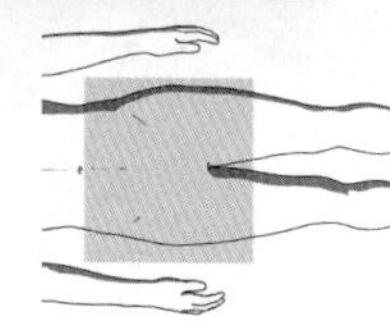

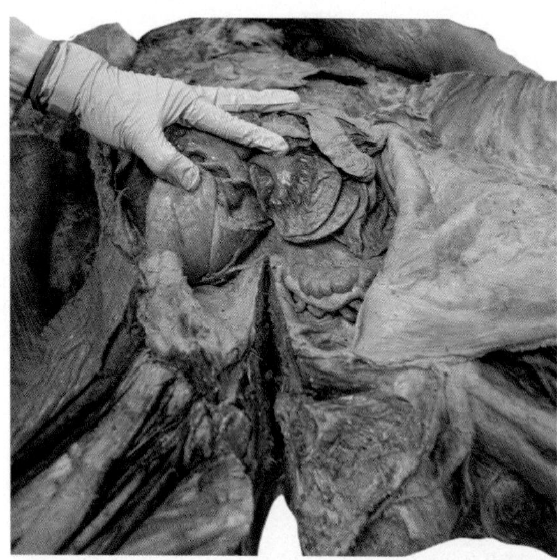

Fig. 14.66 A partly separated lower limb with the corresponding part of the pelvis.

- With a scalpel, make a second horizontal incision starting from the aorta, at the level of the kidneys, and extending laterally along the borders of the iliac crest.
- With the cadaver on its side, and using a saw, cut the sacrum through its promontory, up through the 4th lumbar vertebra. Detach this portion of the body (Fig. 14.67).

DISSECTION **TIP**

For the hemipelvectomy, you will need the help of your colleagues to lift and turn the cadaver on its side.

- With a scalpel, expose the superior and inferior pubic rami. Identify the obturator internus muscle (Fig. 14.68).
- Begin cleaning the soft tissues and adipose tissue around the superior and inferior pubic rami (Fig. 14.68).

DISSECTION **TIP**

Place your paper towels lateral to the rectum. In most of the cadavers there is a significant accumulation of fluid that will leak toward your dissection field (Fig. 14.68).

- Transect the lateral margin of the superior and inferior pubic rami close to the pubic symphysis. Identify the lateral edge of the urinary bladder and trace the ureter. Appreciate the anatomical relationships of the uterus with surrounding structures (Fig. 14.69).
- Transect the lateral margin of the superior and inferior pubic rami close to the pubic symphysis. Make a midline cut at the pubic symphysis alongside the accompanying structures (urinary bladder, rectum, vagina, and uterus) (Fig. 14.70).
- Once the pubic symphysis and the accompanying structures are transected, detach the peritoneum from the free edge of the hemipelvectomy and remove it (Fig. 14.71).
- Expose the vessels as described in the previous section of this chapter (Fig. 14.72).
- Pull the urinary bladder and uterus laterally to expose further the arterial branches of the external iliac artery (Fig. 14.73).

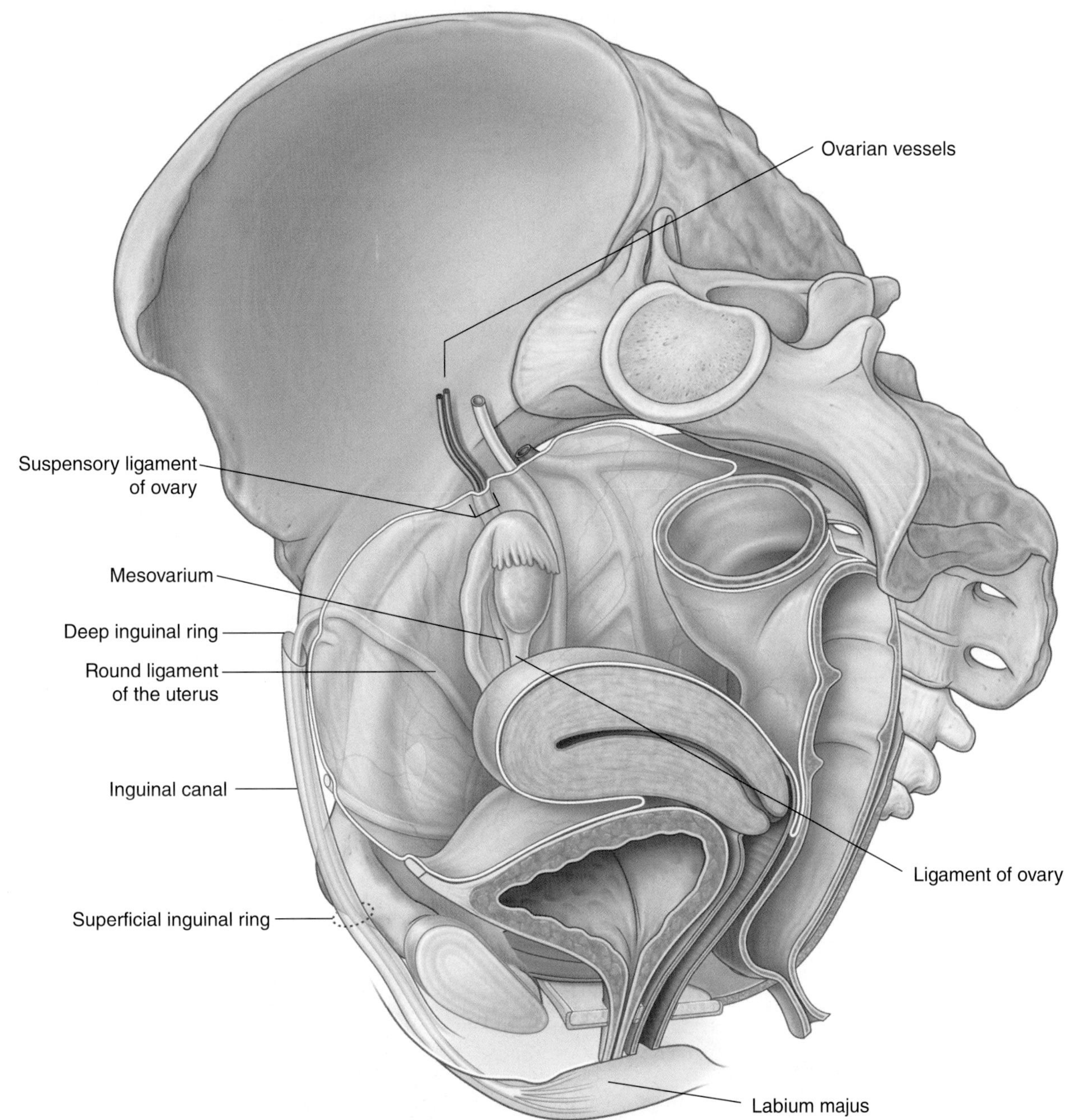

Plate 14.3 Peritoneal relationships of the urinary bladder, uterus, and rectum. (From Drake RL et al., *Gray's Anatomy for Students*, 5th edition, Philadelphia, Elsevier, 2024, Figure 5.51, p. 468.)

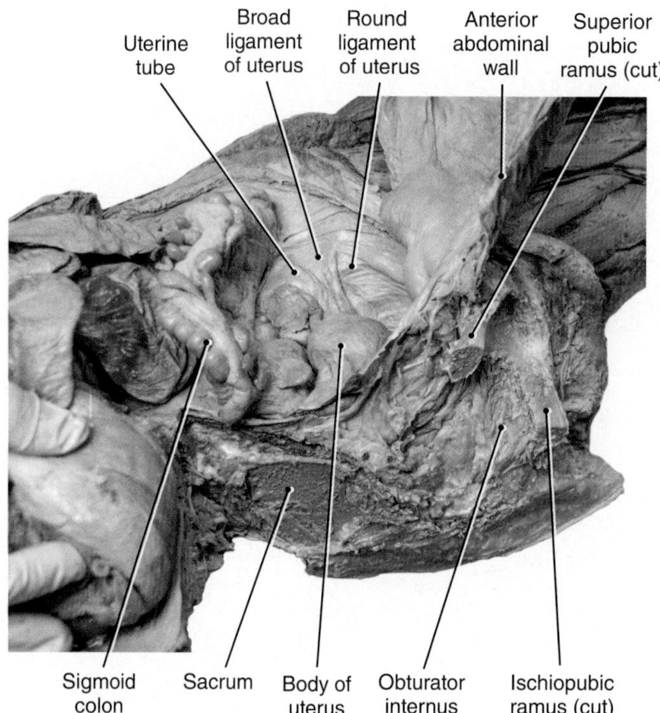

Fig. 14.67 A completed paramedian hemipelvectomy with the superior and inferior pubic rami exposed.

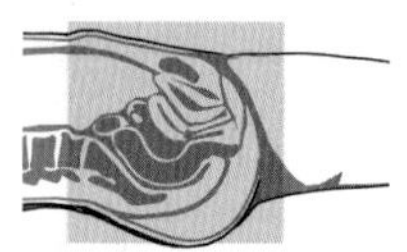

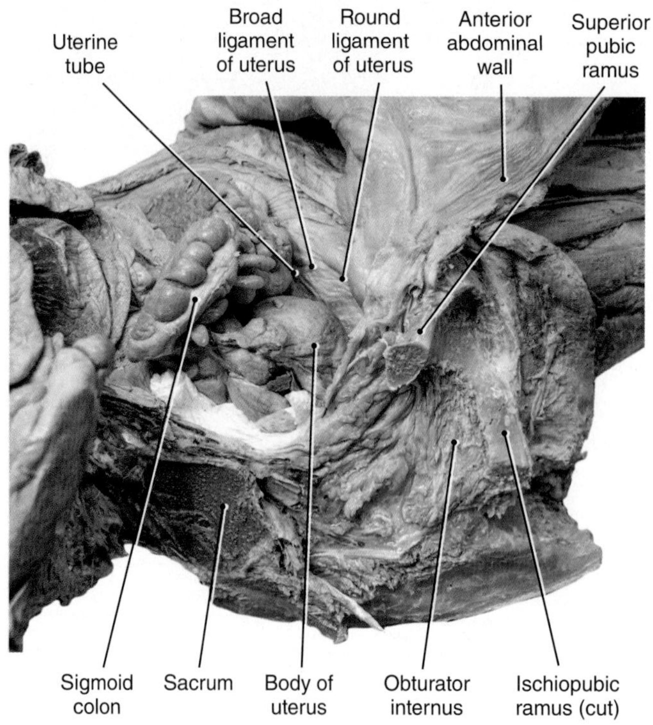

Fig. 14.68 A completed paramedian hemipelvectomy with the superior and inferior pubic rami fully exposed and the obturator internus muscle removed. Paper towel is placed around the rectum.

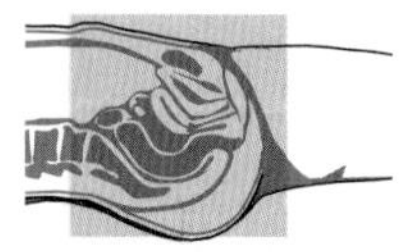

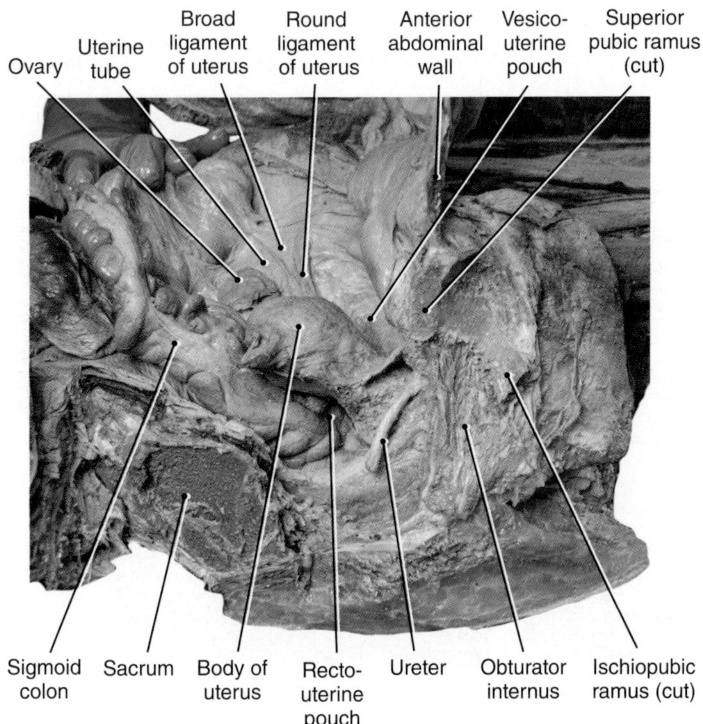

Fig. 14.69 The superior and inferior pubic rami have been transected and the ureter and uterus are exposed.

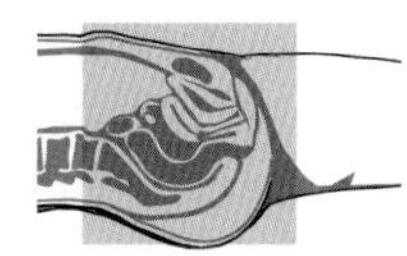

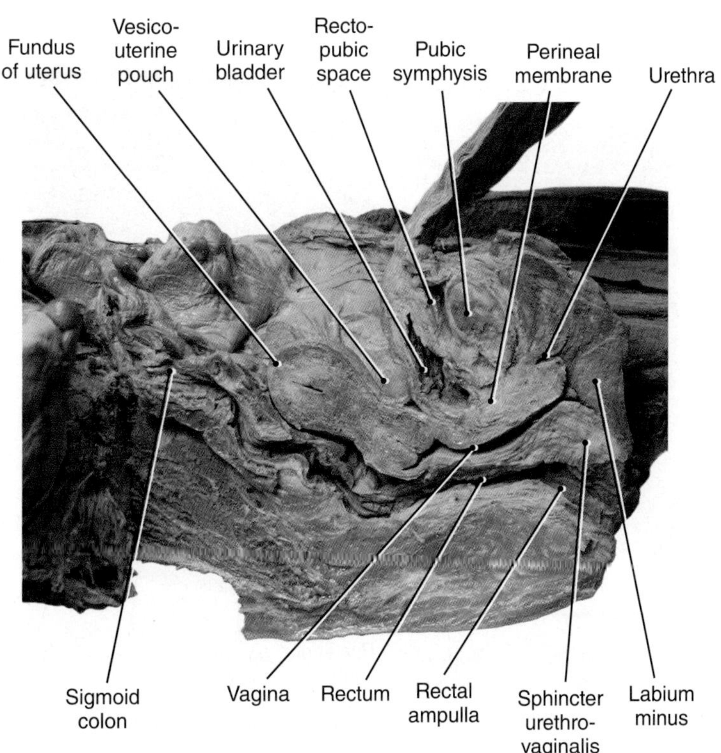

Fig. 14.70 Complete the midline incision of the female pelvis and expose the vagina and uterus.

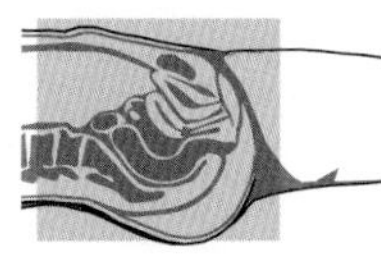

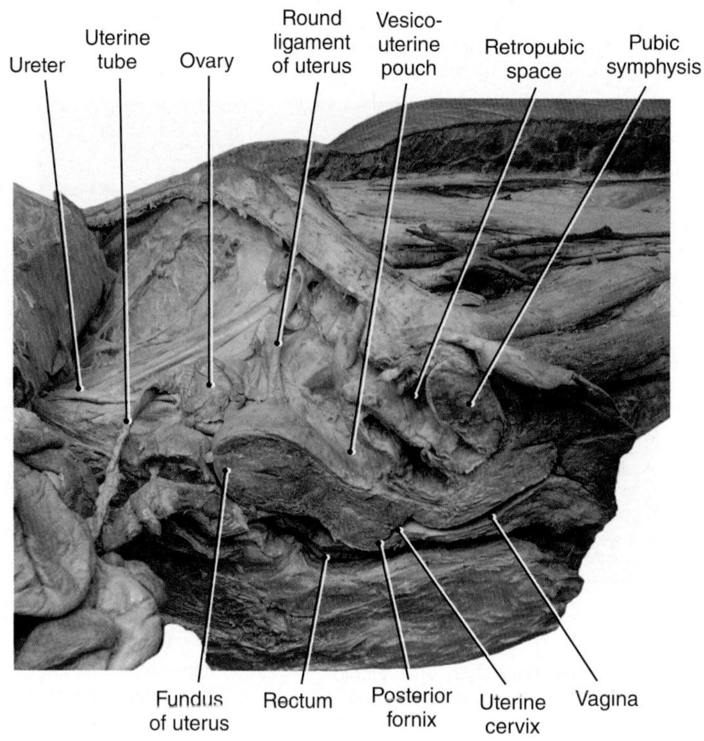

Fig. 14.71 Removal of the peritoneum from pelvic inlet and exposure of the proximal part of the external iliac artery and vein.

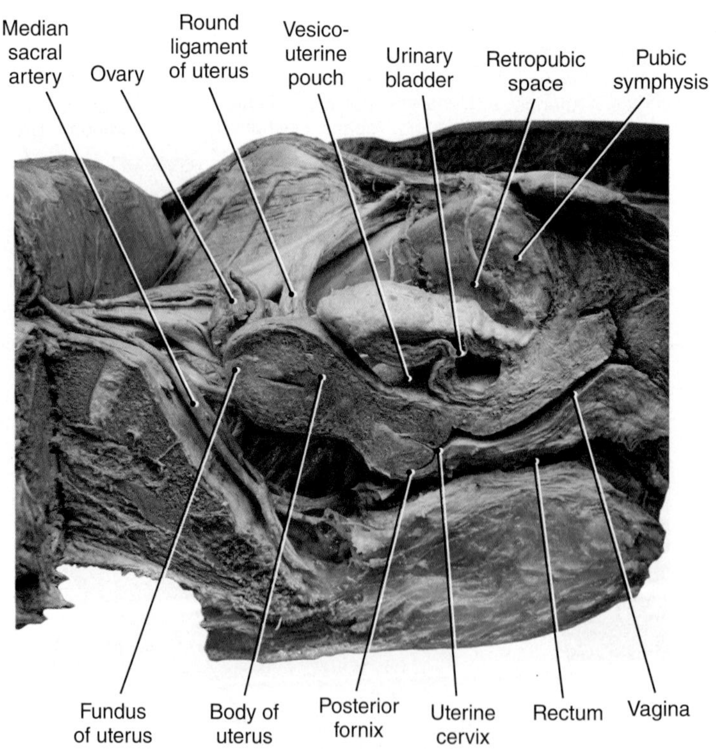

Fig. 14.72 Exposure of the branches of the external iliac artery and vein, ureter, and obturator artery and nerve and internal iliac artery and vein.

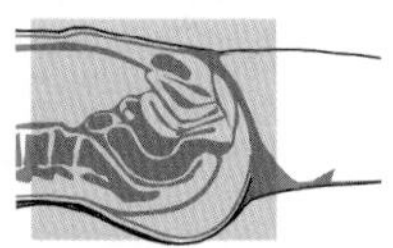

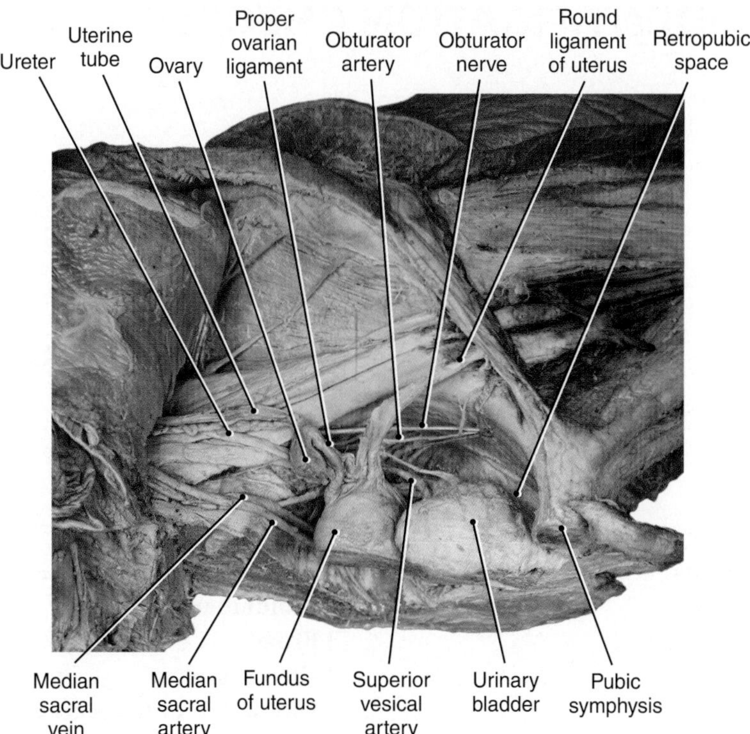

Fig. 14.73 Retraction of the urinary bladder and body of the uterus laterally to expose the branches of the external iliac artery and vein, ureter, and obturator artery and nerve and internal iliac artery and vein.

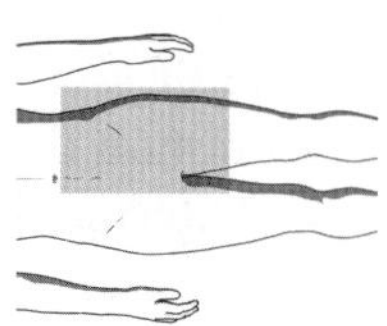

LABORATORY IDENTIFICATION CHECKLIST

NERVES

- ☐ Pudendal
- ☐ Obturator
- ☐ Lumbosacral trunk
- ☐ S1 anterior rami
- ☐ S2 anterior rami
- ☐ S3 anterior rami
- ☐ S4 anterior rami
- ☐ Pelvic splanchnic
- ☐ Sacral sympathetic trunk/ganglia
- ☐ Superior hypogastric plexus
- ☐ Inferior hypogastric plexus
- ☐ Sacral splanchnic nerves

ARTERIES

- ☐ Aorta
- ☐ Middle sacral
- ☐ Common iliac
  - ☐ External iliac
  - ☐ Internal iliac
    - ☐ *Anterior division*
    - ☐ Umbilical
    - ☐ Superior vesical
    - ☐ Obturator
    - ☐ Uterine
    - ☐ Vaginal
    - ☐ Inferior gluteal
    - ☐ *Posterior division*
    - ☐ Lateral sacral
    - ☐ Iliolumbar
    - ☐ Superior gluteal
- ☐ Gonadal (testicular/ovarian)
- ☐ Internal pudendal
- ☐ Superior anorectal

VEINS

- ☐ Inferior vena cava
- ☐ Common iliac
  - ☐ External iliac
  - ☐ Internal iliac

MUSCLES

- ☐ Piriformis
- ☐ Obturator internus
- ☐ Levator ani
- ☐ Coccygeus
- ☐ Pubococcygeus
- ☐ Iliococcygeus

CONNECTIVE TISSUE

- ☐ Pelvic fascia
- ☐ Obturator fascia

LIGAMENTS

- ☐ Sacrotuberous
- ☐ Sacrospinous
- ☐ Iliolumbar
- ☐ Broad
- ☐ Uterosacral
- ☐ Lateral (cardinal, Mackenrodt)

ORGANS/URINARY/REPRODUCTIVE

- ☐ Urinary bladder
- ☐ Ureter
- ☐ Sigmoid colon
- ☐ Rectosigmoid junction
- ☐ Rectum
- ☐ Anal canal

Male

- ☐ Prostate
- ☐ Seminal gland
- ☐ Ductus deferens

Female

- ☐ Uterus
- ☐ Uterine tube
- ☐ Ovary

SPACES

- ☐ Retropubic
- ☐ Retrovesical (pouch of Douglas)
- ☐ Retrouterine

BONES

- ☐ Sacrum
- ☐ Coccyx
- ☐ Hip bone
  - ☐ Ilium
  - ☐ Ischium
  - ☐ Pubic

BEFORE YOU BEGIN

Dissection of the male and female perineum is discussed separately in this chapter.

DISSECTION TIP

To best dissect the perineum, there are two techniques: (1) start with dissection of the lower part of the anterior wall, extending to the midthigh and then expose the structures of the perineum; (2) perform the gluteal region dissection first, including the ischioanal fossae and thighs. This makes it much easier to expose and dissect the structures of the perineum.

DISSECTION OF THE MALE CADAVER

Technique 1

- **Place the cadaver in the supine position. Place a block under the sacrum and abduct the thighs as much as possible.**
- **Draw a horizontal line between the anterior superior iliac spines, a second vertical line bilaterally from the anterior superior iliac spine to the midthigh, and a third horizontal line from the lateral side of the thigh to its medial surface as shown in Fig. 15.1.**
- **Remove the skin and the underlying subcutaneous tissues underneath the area covered by the lines drawn on the cadaver. Expose the fundiform ligament of the penis, the anterior superior iliac spine, the lateral part of the inguinal ligament, the spermatic cord, the femoral artery and vein at the saphenous hiatus, and the great saphenous vein (Fig. 15.2). Lift the penis upward and remove the skin leaving intact the glans of the penis. Similarly, remove the scrotum exposing the full length of the spermatic cord with the adjacent testis.**
- **With a pair of forceps lift the fascia lata covering the thigh muscle and remove it to expose the muscles and the vasculature from the inguinal ligament distally to the midthigh (Fig. 15.3).**
- **Once the fascia lata is removed identify the muscles of the thigh such as vastus lateralis, vastus medialis, rectus femoris, sartorius, adductor longus, gracilis, femoral artery, vein, and nerve, and great saphenous vein (Fig. 15.4). The detailed dissection of the remainder of the thigh is shown in the chapter of the lower limb.**
- **Lift the penis upwardly and identify the superficial perineal fascia (Colles' fascia) rich in adipose tissue and blood vessels (Fig. 15.5). From here onward the dissection becomes identical to later steps of technique 2.**

Fig. 15.1 Skin incision tracing for dissecting the perineal region.

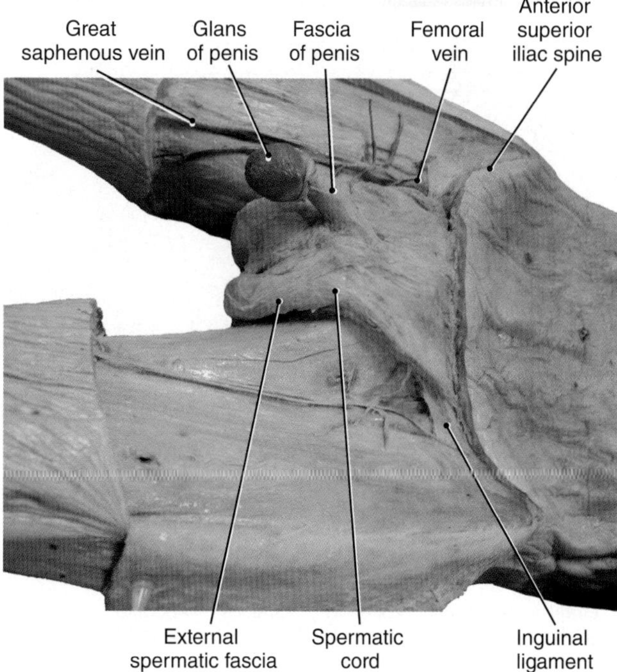

Fig. 15.2 Removal of the skin and subcutaneous tissue over the perineal, lower anterior abdominal, and midthigh areas.

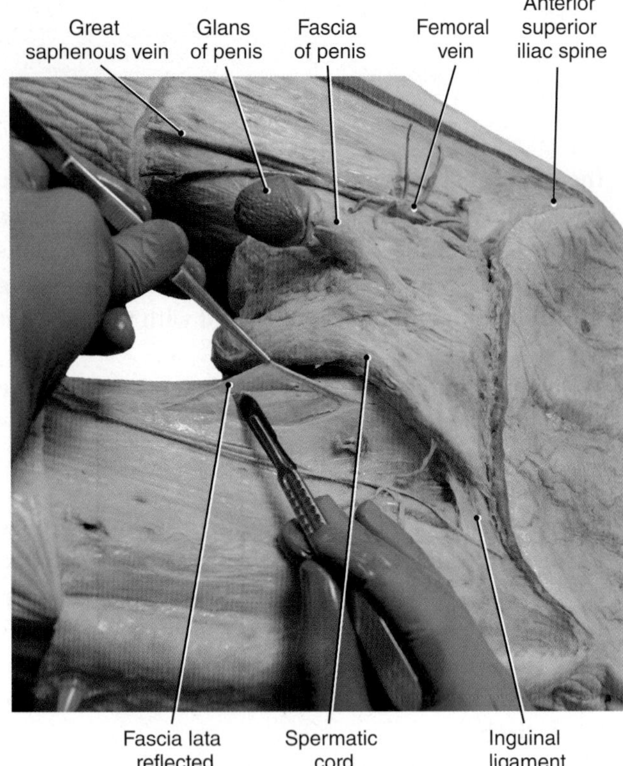

Fig. 15.3 Removal of the fascia lata over the midthigh area.

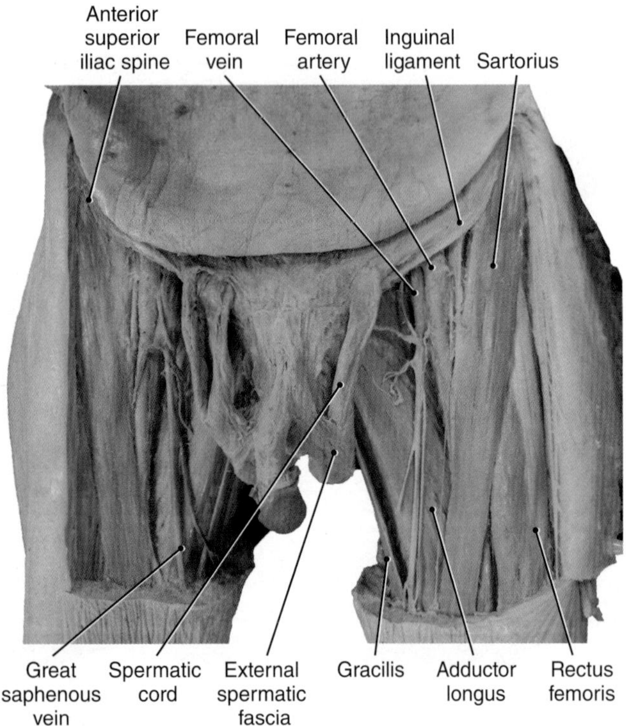

Fig. 15.4 Complete removal of the fascia lata over the midthigh areas bilaterally exposing the muscles of the midthigh.

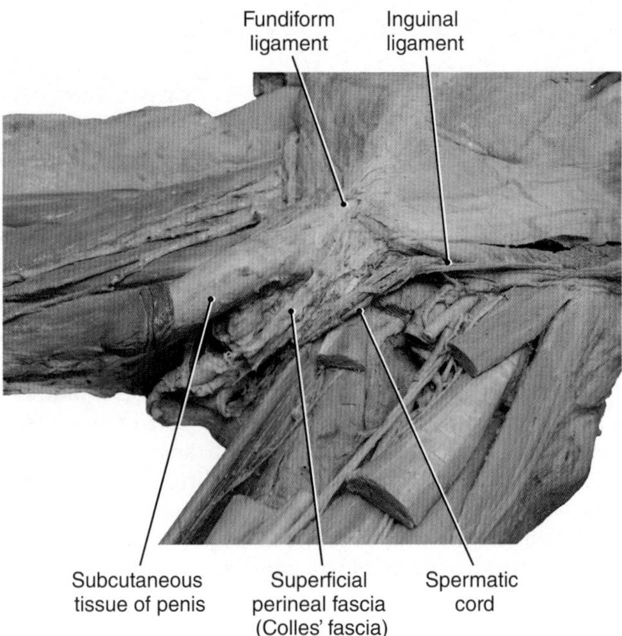

Fig. 15.5 Exposure of the superficial perineal fascia (Colles' fascia) embedded in the adipose tissue.

DISSECTION OF THE MALE CADAVER

Technique 2

- **Place the cadaver in the supine position. Place a block under the sacrum and abduct the thighs as far as possible. A wooden block or rod is placed between the thighs at the level of the femoral condyles to maintain them in abduction (Fig. 15.6).**
- **Identify the adductor longus and gracilis muscles. These muscles can be transected so that the thighs can be abducted more easily. In this specimen, it was not necessary to transect these muscles (Fig. 15.7).**
- **Draw imaginary lines outlining the borders of the *urogenital triangle:* a line between the ischial tuberosities and two lines along the ischiopubic rami to the pubic symphysis (Fig. 15.8). At the midpoint of a line connecting the two ischial tuberosities, palpate a fibromuscular mass of tissue, the *perineal body.***

ANATOMY **NOTE**

The perineal body is an important structure because the superficial and deep transverse perineal muscles, the bulbospongiosus muscle, the levator ani muscle, and the external anal sphincter muscle are attached to it.

- **Remove the skin of the urogenital region, including the scrotum. Reflect the testis toward the inguinal ligament and expose the urogenital triangle. Lift the penis upwardly and remove the adipose tissue and the rich venous network (Fig. 15.9).**
- **Continue from here if you used technique 1.**

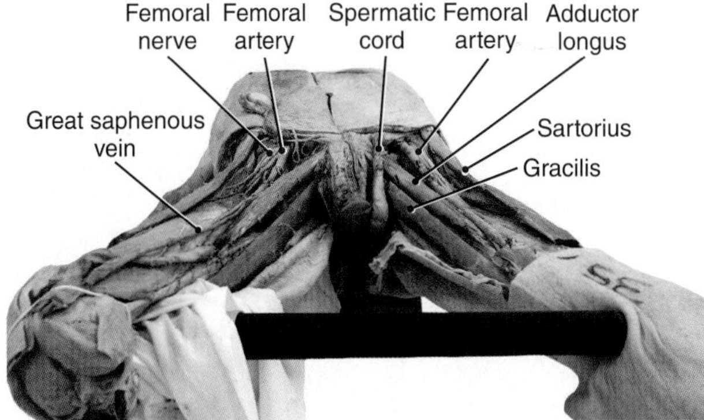

Fig. 15.6 Male cadaver in supine position with block under sacrum with thighs abducted.

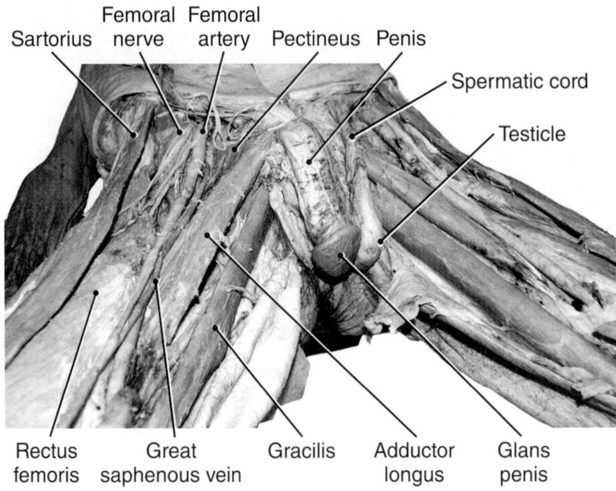

Fig. 15.7 Transecting the adductor longus and gracilis muscles to abduct the thighs more easily was not necessary in this cadaver.

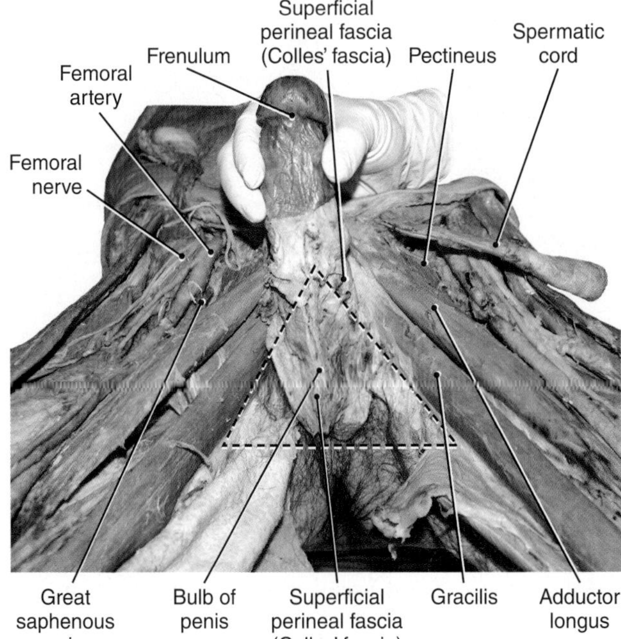

Fig. 15.8 Urogenital triangle *(dashed outline)*, with the line between the ischial tuberosities and two lines along the ischiopubic rami to the pubic symphysis.

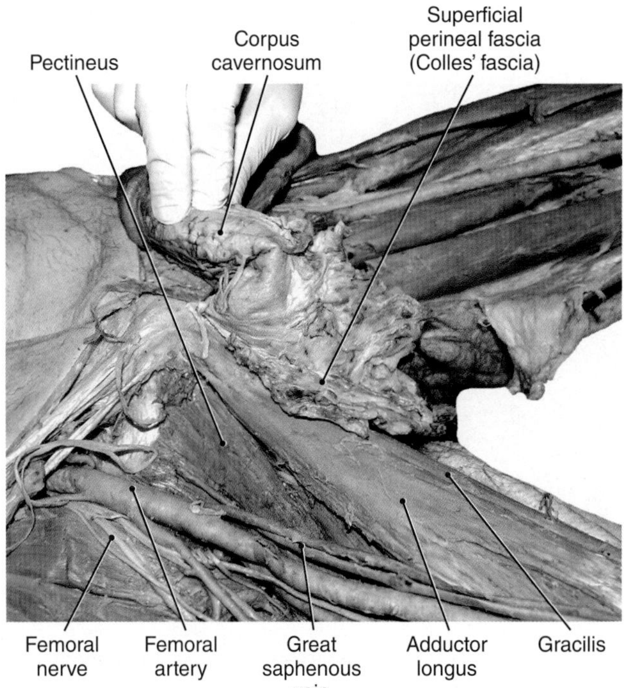

Fig. 15.9 The skin of the urogenital region is removed and the testis is reflected toward the inguinal ligament, exposing the urogenital triangle.

ANATOMY NOTE

The fat that is removed here is located in the superficial perineal fascia (of Colles). This fascia is the continuation of Scarpa's fascia (membranous layer of anterior abdominal wall) into the perineum (Figs. 15.10 and 15.11). Camper's fascia (fatty layer of anterior abdominal wall) continues into the perineum (Plate 15.1).

DISSECTION TIP

The superficial perineal fascia is fairly thick and intermingled with the adipose tissue of the urogenital triangle. This fascia attaches laterally to the ischiopubic rami.

- **Remove Colles' fascia and identify the corpus cavernosum laterally and the corpus spongiosum medially (see Fig. 15.11).**
- **Expose the bulbospongiosus muscle covered with a fascial layer, the *deep perineal fascia* (Gallaudet's fascia).**

ANATOMY NOTE

The deep perineal fascia invests the bulbospongiosus muscle, superficial transverse perineal muscles, and ischiocavernosus muscles.

- **Continue the exposure of the bulbospongiosus inferiorly, exposing the deep perineal fascia. The potential space between the superficial perineal fascia and deep perineal fascia is called the *superficial perineal cleft* (space between Colles' and Gallaudet's fasciae) (Figs. 15.12 and 15.13).**

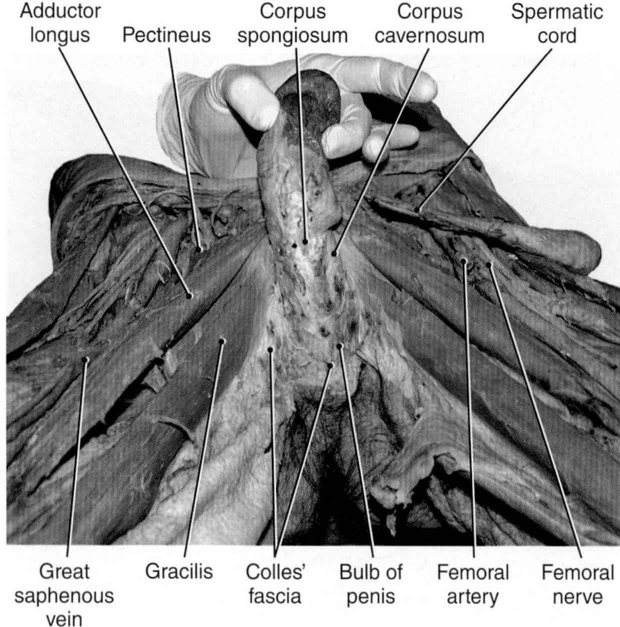

Fig. 15.10 Lift the penis upward and remove the adipose tissue and the rich venous network.

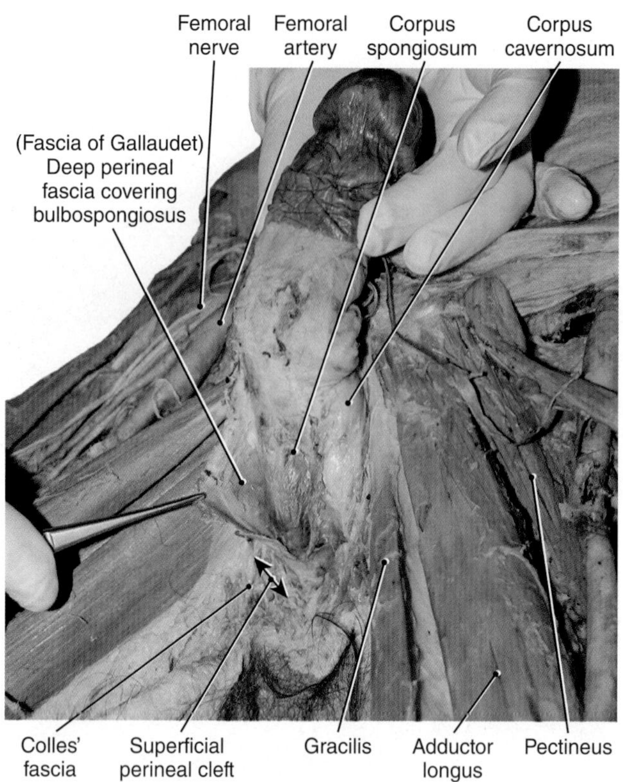

Fig. 15.12 Exposure of the bulbospongiosus muscle is continued inferiorly, further revealing the deep perineal fascia.

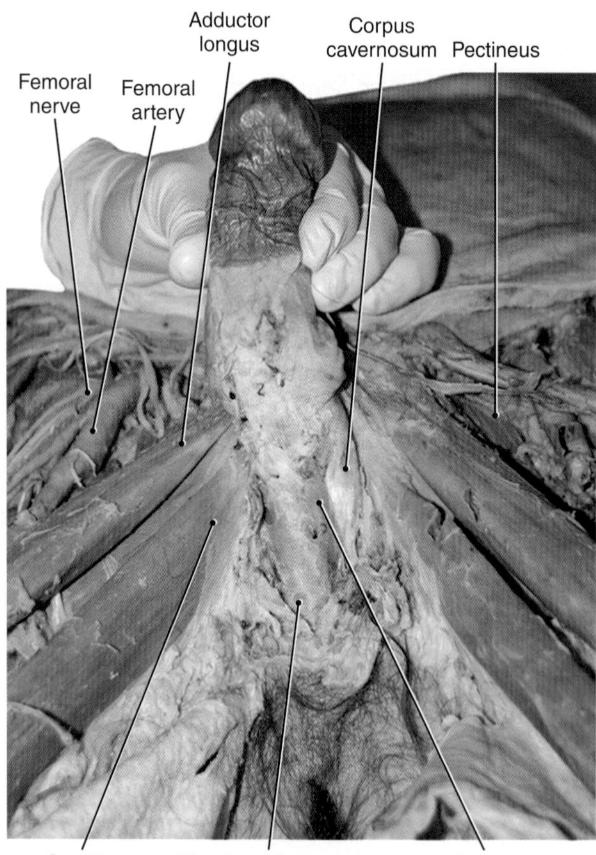

Fig. 15.11 Colles' fascia is removed to identify the corpus cavernosum laterally and the corpus spongiosum medially. The bulbospongiosus muscle is covered with the deep perineal fascia.

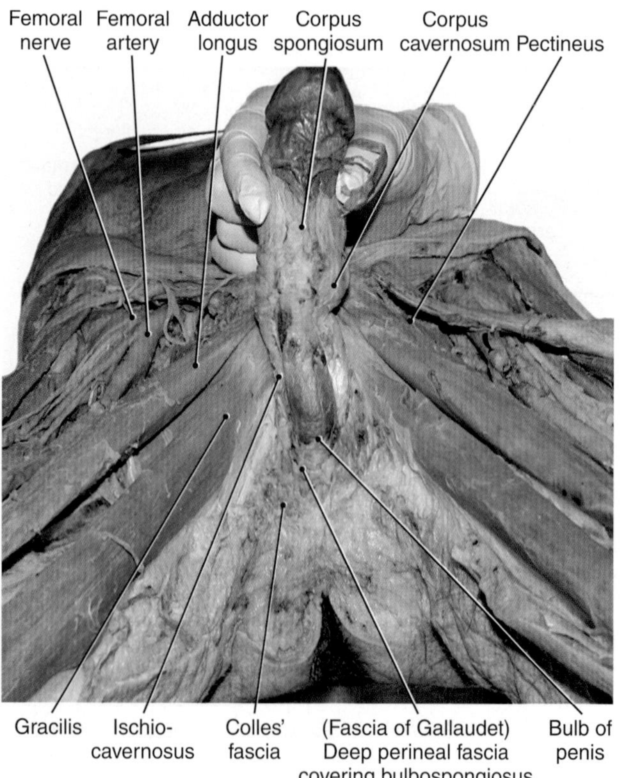

Fig. 15.13 The ischiocavernosus muscle arises from the ischiopubic ramus.

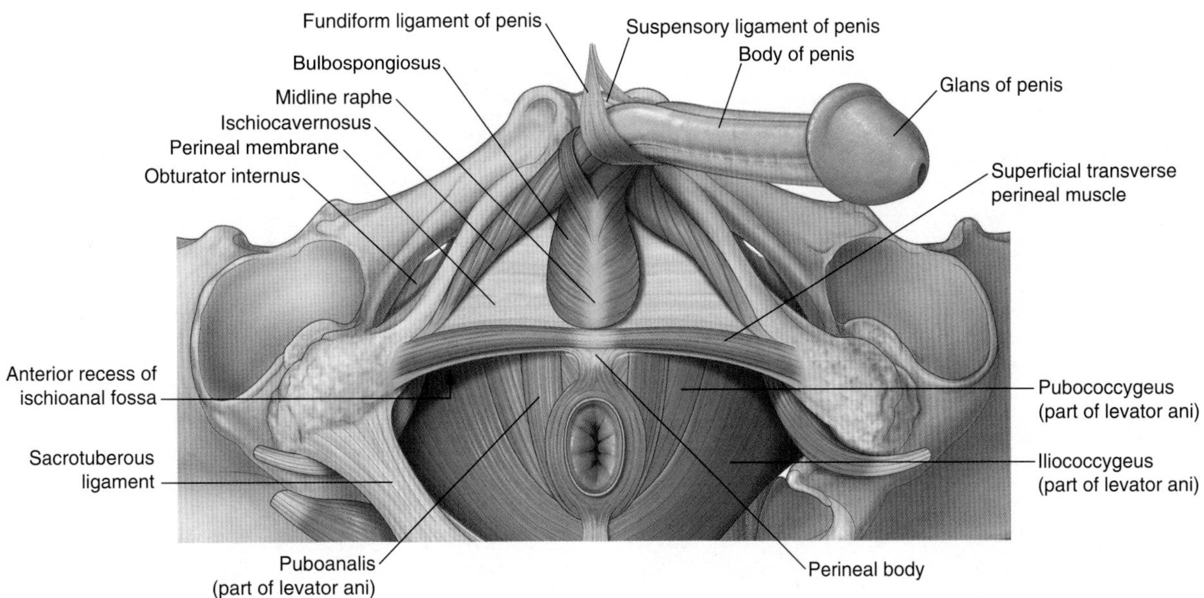

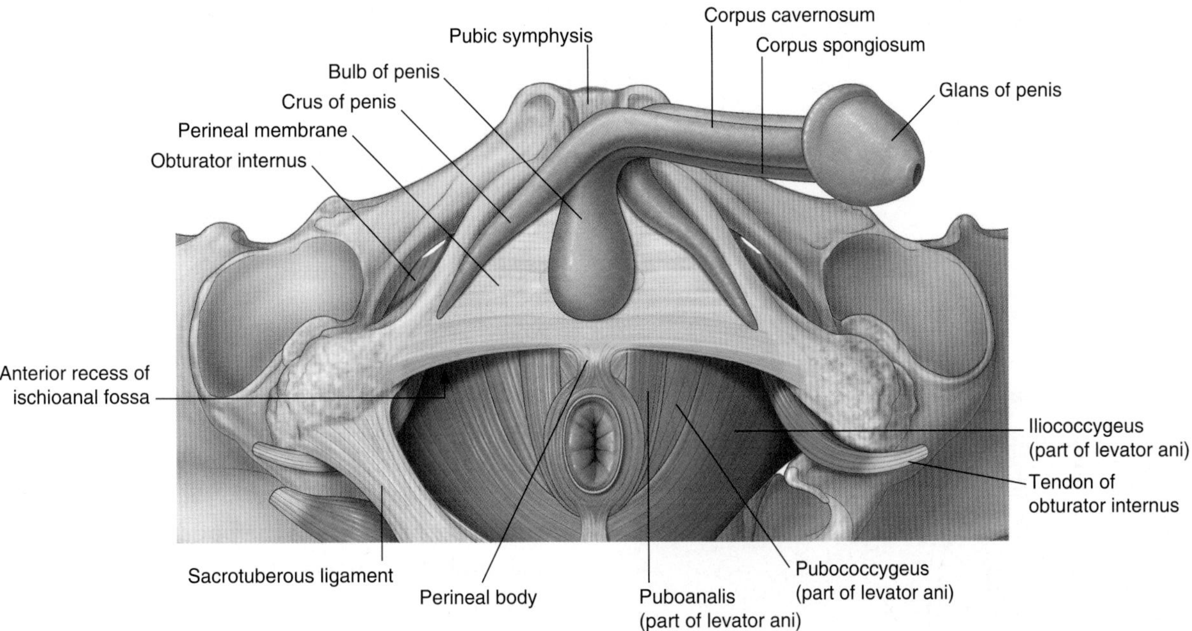

Plate 15.1 Muscles of the superficial perineal space in males. (From Drake RL et al. *Gray's Atlas of Anatomy*, 3rd edition, Philadelphia, Elsevier, 2021, p. 262.)

DISSECTION TIP

During the removal of the superficial perineal cleft, you may encounter branches of the posterior femoral cutaneous nerve, as well as scrotal vessels and nerves.

- **Dissect lateral to the bulbospongiosus muscle and identify the ischiocavernosus muscle arising from the ischiopubic ramus (see Fig. 15.13). The ischiocavernosus surrounds the crus of the penis (corpora cavernosa), a bilateral collection of erectile tissue (Fig. 15.14).**

- **The inferior portion of the corpus spongiosum becomes dilated, forming the bulb of the penis. At the level of the bulb, remove the superficial perineal fascia and identify the superficial perineal muscle laterally (Figs. 15.15 and 15.16).**

DISSECTION TIP

The superficial transverse perineal muscle is absent in some cadavers. It also has been shown that these muscles atrophy with age.

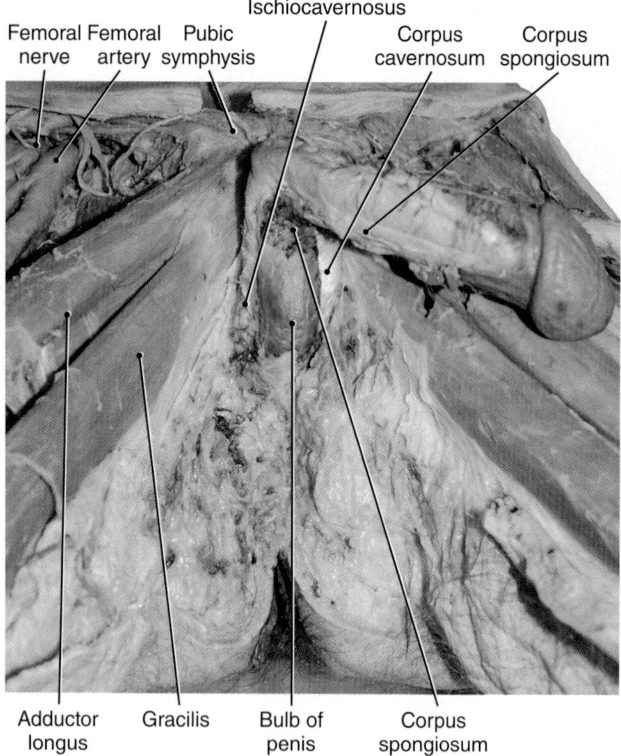

Fig. 15.14 The crus of the penis is surrounded by the ischiocavernosus muscle.

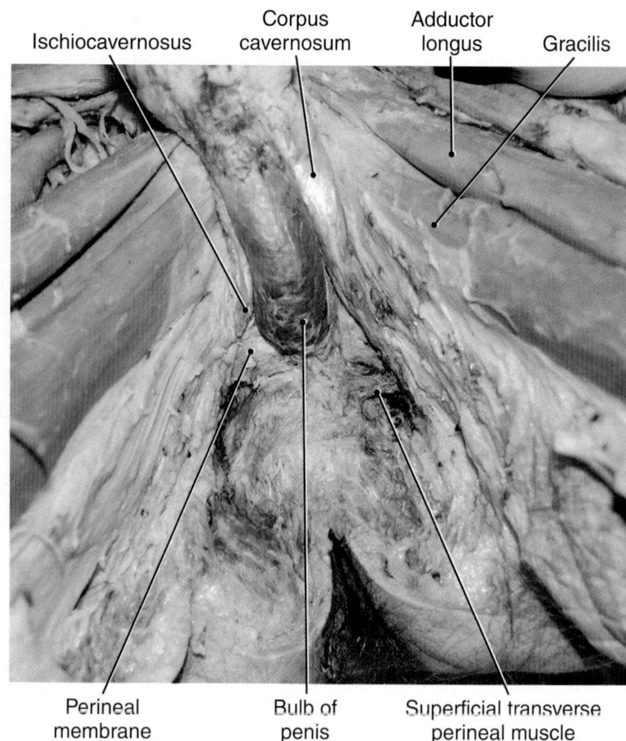

Fig. 15.16 The superficial fascia is removed at the level of the penile bulb to identify the superficial perineal muscle laterally.

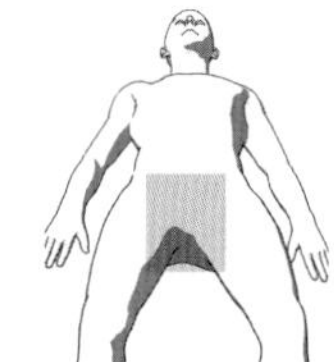

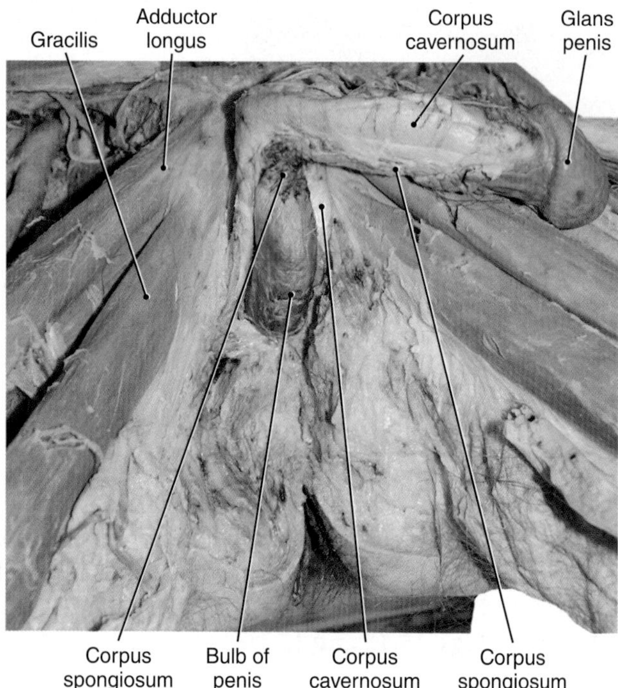

Fig. 15.15 The dilated corpus spongiosum forms the bulb of the penis.

- **Clean the superficial transverse perineal muscles, and superior to them, expose the perineal membrane (Fig. 15.17).**
- **Inferior and lateral to the transverse perineal muscles, expose the perineal nerve and perineal artery, which are branches of the pudendal nerve and internal pudendal artery, respectively (see Figs. 15.16 and 15.17).**
- **Expose the ischiocavernosus muscle along the ischiopubic ramus (Fig. 15.18).**
- **Lift the penis and expose the crus. Make an incision into the crus and expose its spongy matrix and its *tunica albuginea*, the outer covering of the corpus (Fig. 15.19). Observe the pubic symphysis for the *suspensory ligament* of the penis, arising from deep fascia of the anterior abdominal wall, and the *fundiform ligament*, arising from the membranous layer of the superficial fascia of the abdomen.**
- **Cut the ischiocavernosus muscle and reflect it anteriorly to expose the perineal membrane (Fig. 15.20).**

DISSECTION **TIP**

The bulbourethral gland in males may be difficult to find in the deep perineal space.

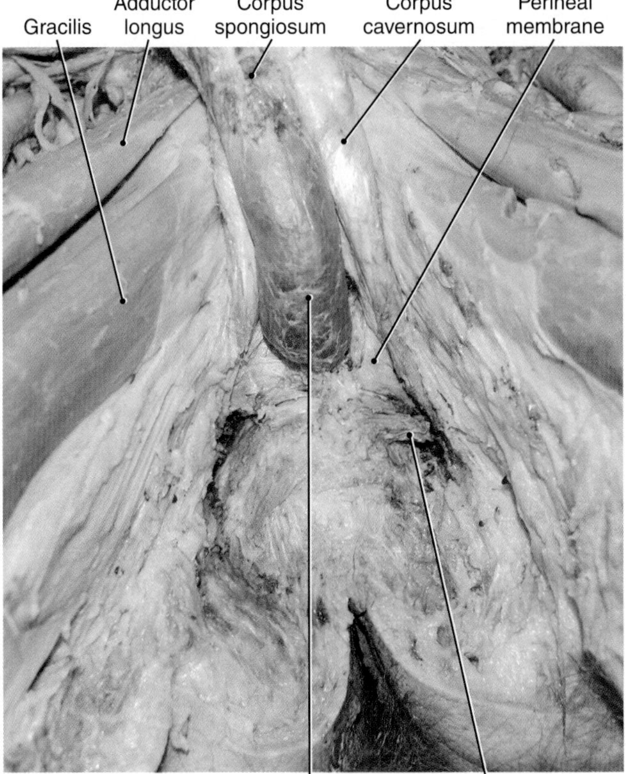

Fig. 15.17 The superficial transverse perineal muscles are cleaned and the perineal membrane is exposed. The perineal nerve and artery are inferior and lateral to the transverse perineal muscle.

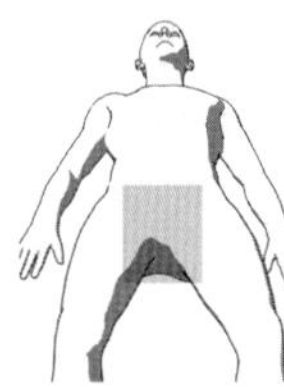

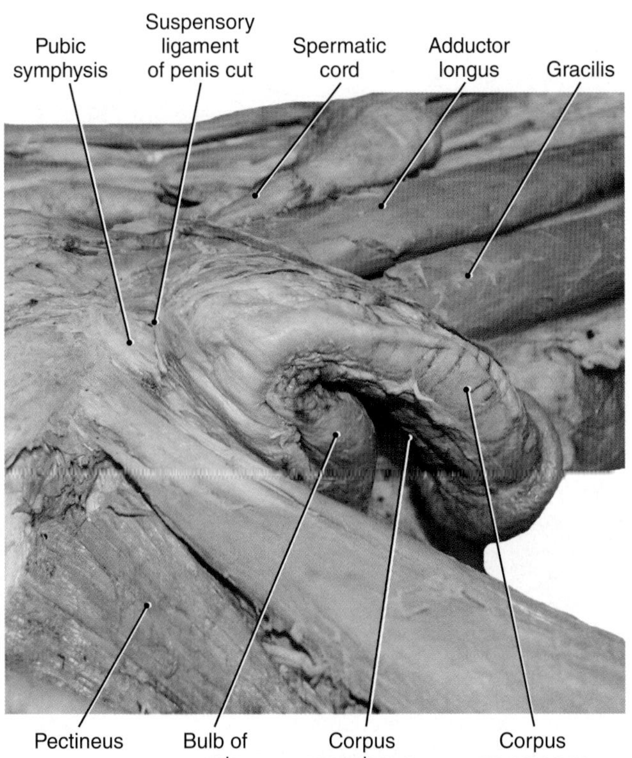

Fig. 15.18 The ischiocavernosus muscle is exposed along the ischiopubic ramus.

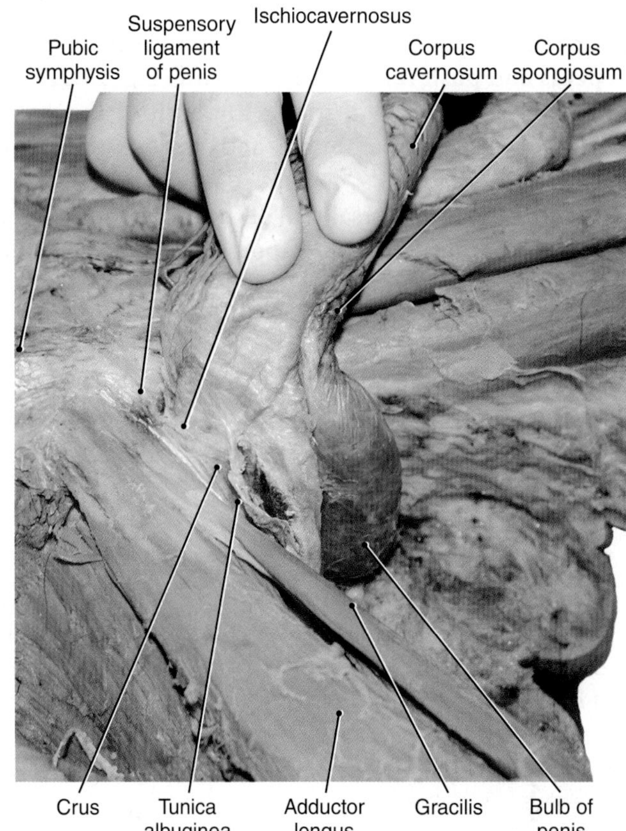

Fig. 15.19 The penis is lifted to expose the crus with an incision revealing the spongy matrix and the tunica albuginea.

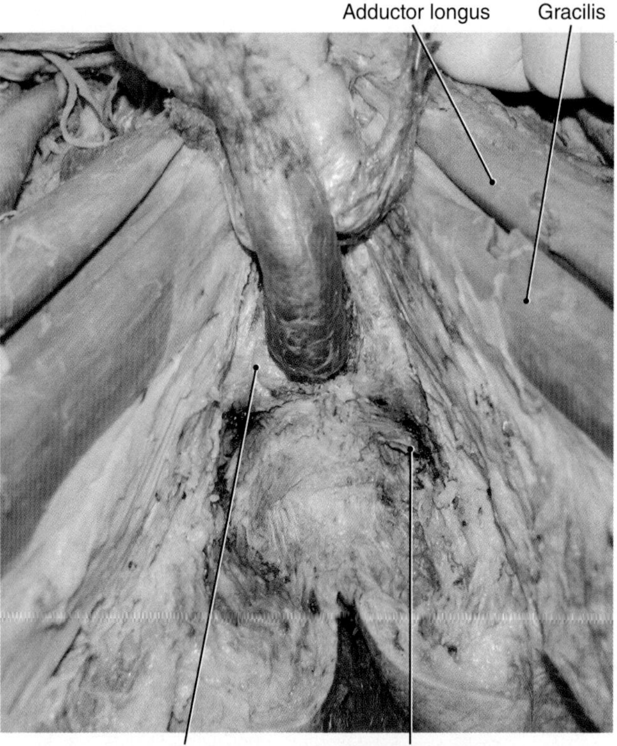

Fig. 15.20 The ischiocavernosus muscle is reflected anteriorly to expose the perineal membrane.

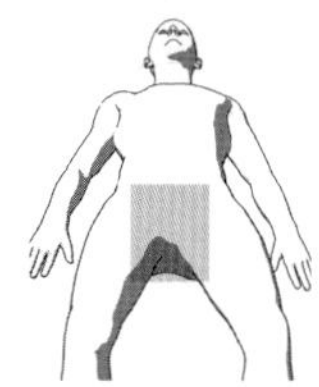

- Cut the suspensory and fundiform ligaments of the penis and push the penis downward (Fig. 15.21).
- With a scalpel, cut through the bulb of the penis at the perineal membrane and remove the penis (Fig. 15.22).
- Identify the deep dorsal vein of the penis, the urethra, and the perineal body and appreciate the dimensions of the perineal membrane.

ANATOMY **NOTE**

The deep dorsal vein of the penis is a large vein located deep to Buck's fascia (of the penis) just inferior to the arcuate pubic ligament. The deep dorsal vein anastomoses with the internal pudendal veins through the prostatic venous plexus.

- Palpate the perineal membrane between the deep dorsal vein of the penis and the urethra and note its thickening, the *transverse perineal ligament* (see Fig. 15.22).

DISSECTION **TIP**

Inferior and lateral to the superficial transverse perineal muscle, locate the perineal nerve and the perineal artery, tracing these toward the ischioanal fossa if time permits.

- Reflect the deep perineal membrane and expose the underlying musculature, the deep transverse perineal muscle, and the sphincter urethrae (Fig. 15.23).

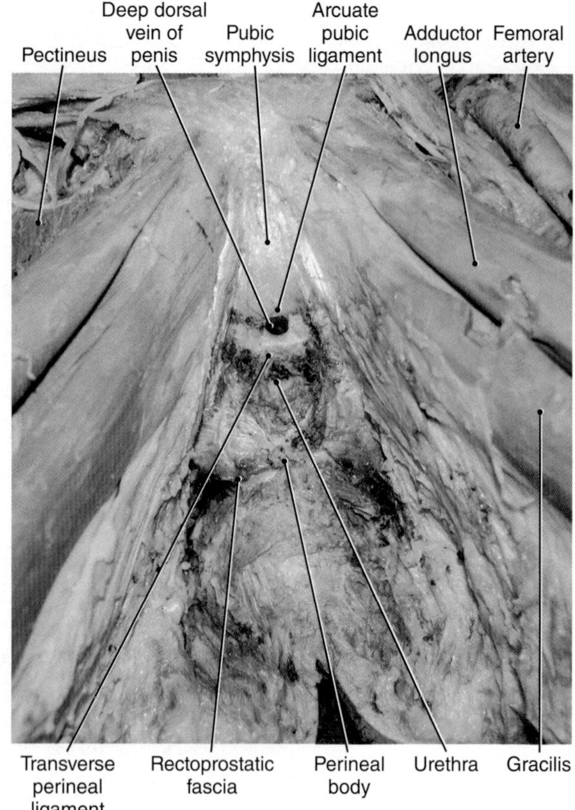

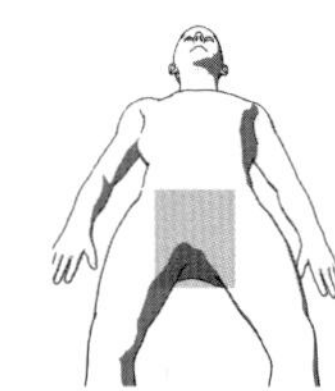

Fig. 15.22 The bulb of the penis is cut from perineal membrane and the penis is removed revealing the deep dorsal vein, urethra, and perineal body.

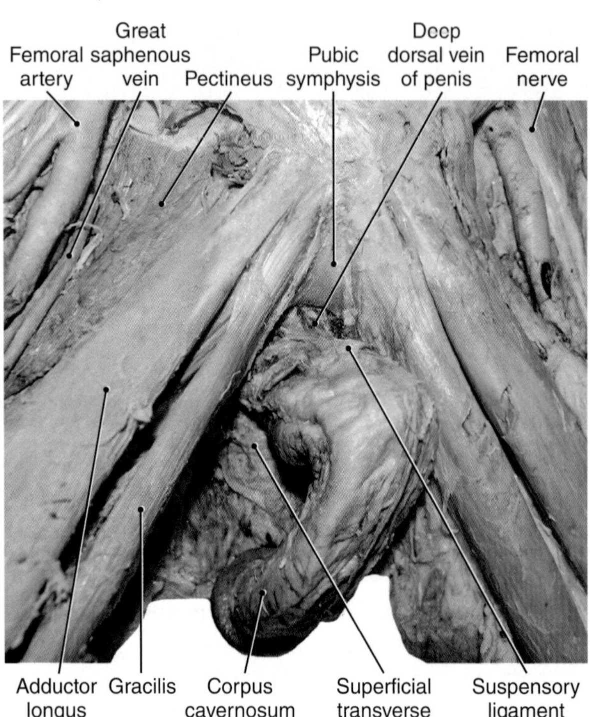

Fig. 15.21 The suspensory and fundiform ligaments are cut and the penis is pushed downward.

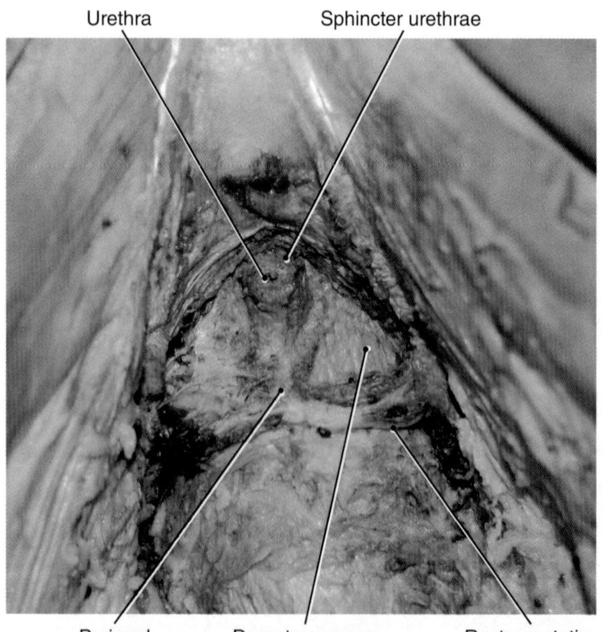

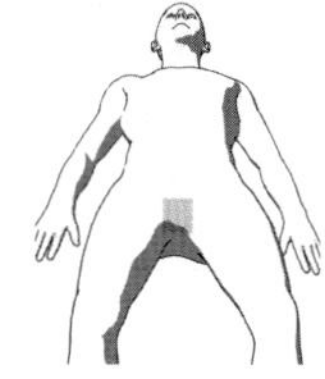

Fig. 15.23 The deep perineal membrane is reflected, exposing the underlying musculature, the deep transverse perineal muscle, and the sphincter urethrae.

DISSECTION **TIP**

If time permits, cut the external urethral orifice of the penis and open the corpus spongiosum to expose the urethra. Extend the incision throughout the entire course of the urethra.

DISSECTION OF THE FEMALE CADAVER

With the female cadaver in the supine position, identify the following structures (Figs. 15.24 and 15.25):

- **Anterior commissure of labia majora**
- **Labia majora**
- **Labia minora**
- **Glans of clitoris**
- **Vaginal orifice**
- **Vestibular fossa**
- **Posterior commissure of labia majora**
- **Make an incision into the skin around the vaginal orifice, leaving the labia minora and clitoris intact. Incise the skin following the medial surface of the labia majora to the anterior commissure of the labia majora. Reflect the skin laterally and detach along the medial thigh (Figs. 15.26 and 15.27; Plate 15.2).**
- **Draw a horizontal line between the anterior superior iliac spines, a second vertical line bilaterally from the anterior superior iliac spine to the midthigh, and a third horizontal line from the lateral side of the thigh to its medial surface (identical to technique 1 for the male perineum).**
- **Remove the skin and the underlying subcutaneous tissues underneath the area covered by the lines drawn on the cadaver. Expose the anterior superior**

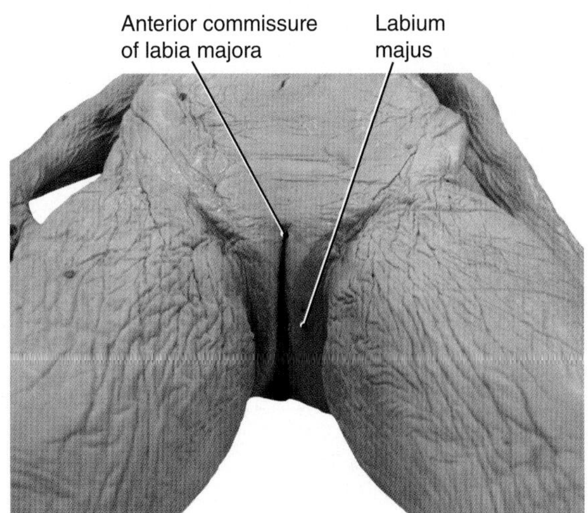

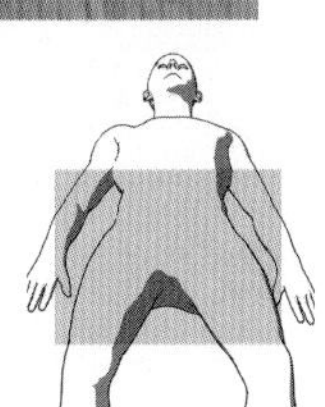

Fig. 15.24 Female cadaver placed in the supine position.

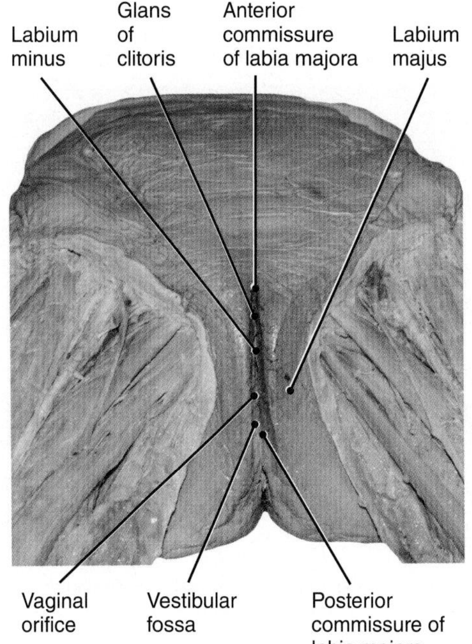

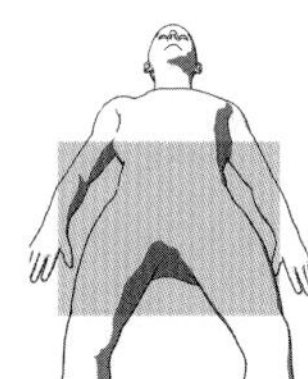

Fig. 15.25 Female cadaver placed in the supine position with the skin from the inguinal ligament to the midthigh removed.

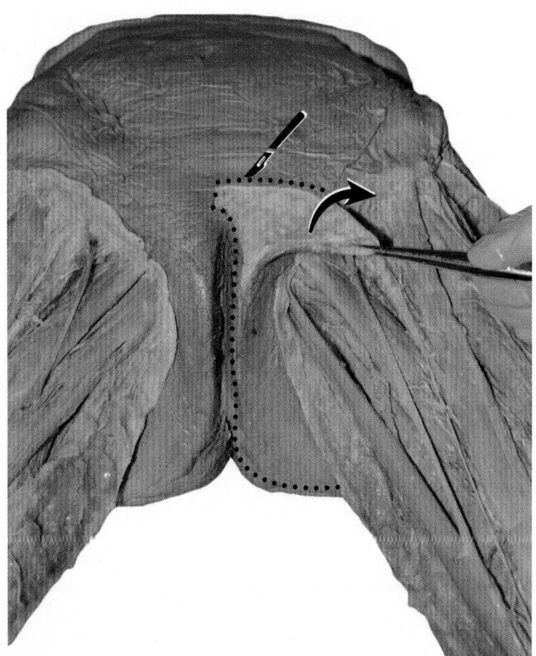

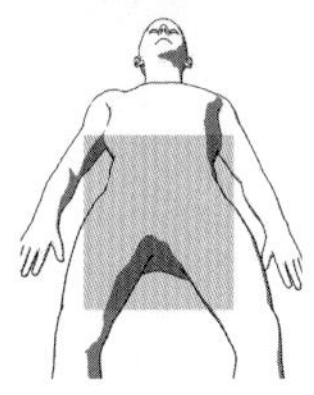

Fig. 15.26 The *dotted lines* demarcate the incision points and reflection of the skin laterally.

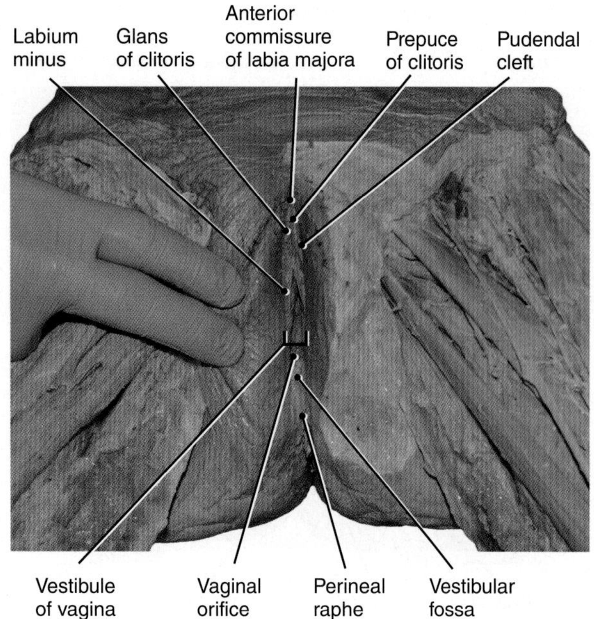

Fig. 15.27 Female cadaver in the supine position, exposing the external genitalia.

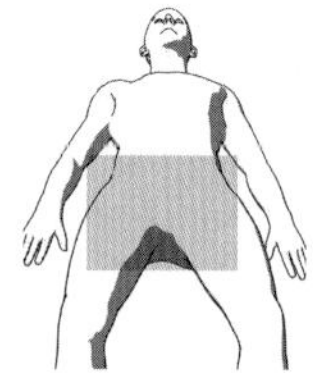

iliac spine, the lateral part of the inguinal ligament, the round ligament of the uterus, the femoral artery and vein at the saphenous hiatus, and the great saphenous vein. With a pair of forceps lift the fascia lata covering the thigh muscles and remove it to expose the muscles and the vasculature from the inguinal ligament distally to the midthigh.

- **Once the fascia lata is removed identify the muscles of the thigh such as vastus lateralis, vastus medialis, rectus femoris, sartorius, adductor longus, gracilis, femoral artery, vein, and nerve, and great saphenous vein (Fig. 15.28). The detailed dissection of the remainder of the thigh is shown in the chapter on the lower limb.**

ANATOMY **NOTE**

There are two layers that make up the superficial perineal fascia: a fatty superficial layer and a membranous deep layer (Colles' fascia). The fatty layer gives shape to the labia majora. The membranous layer of the superficial perineal fascia is attached to the ischiopubic rami and the perineal membrane.

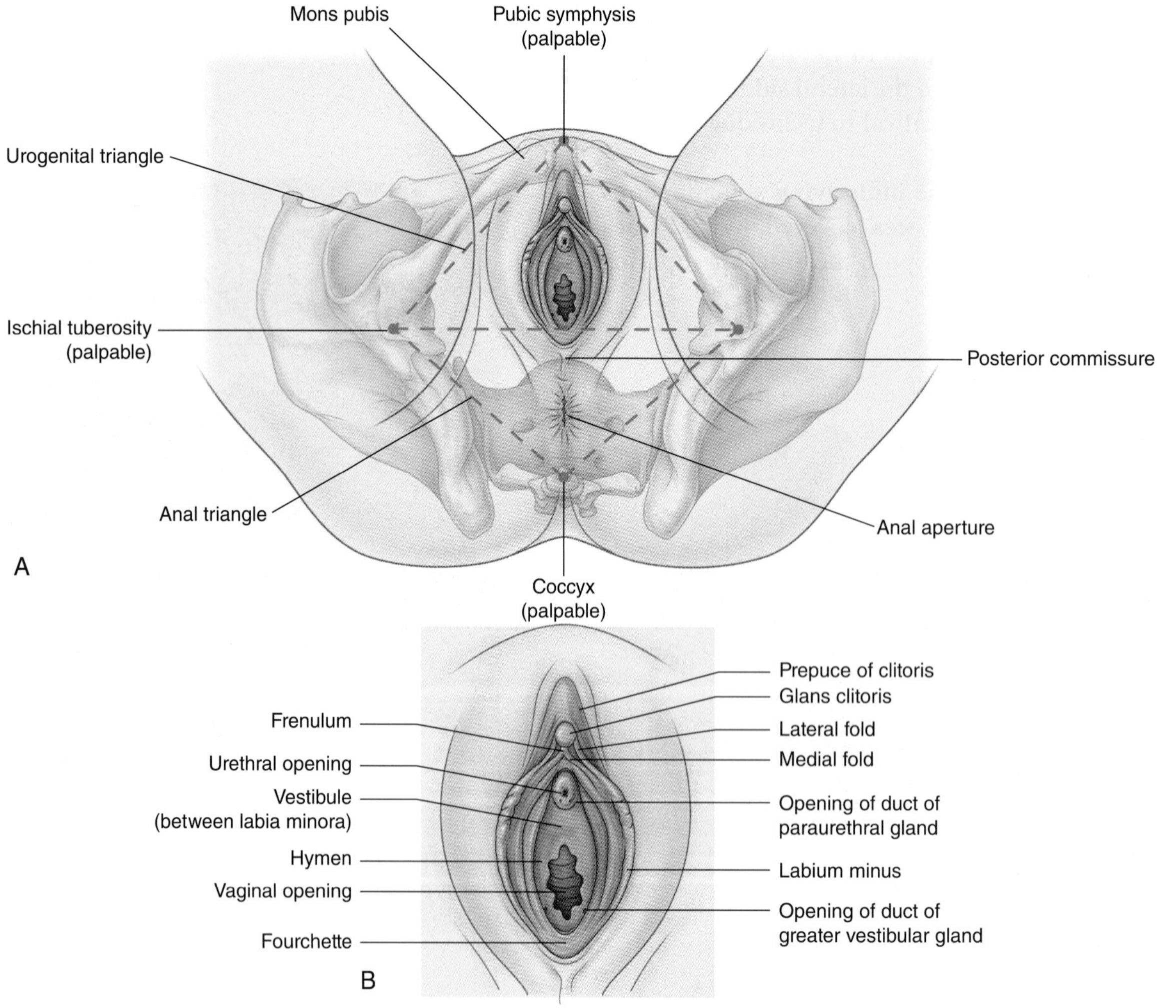

Plate 15.2 A, Urogenital triangle in female. B, External genitalia. (From Drake RL et al. *Gray's Anatomy for Students*, 5th edition, Philadelphia, Elsevier, 2024, Figure 5.74, p. 504.)

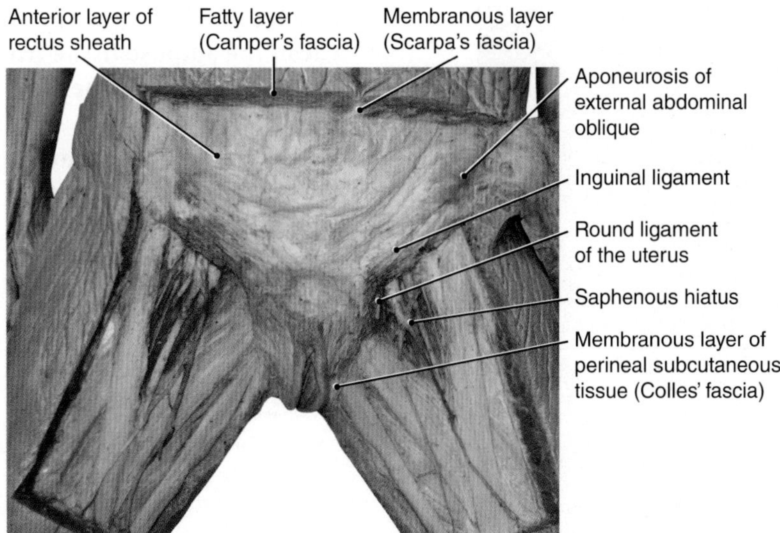

Fig. 15.28 Removal of the skin and subcutaneous tissues over the lower anterior abdominal wall, perineum, and midthighs, exposing the underlying structures.

DISSECTION TIP

Remnants of the round ligament of the uterus may be found as the removal of the superficial fascia is taking place.

- **Remove the superficial fatty layer of the superficial perineal fascia to expose the superficial perineal (Colles') fascia and the fat of the ischioanal fossa (Fig. 15.29).**
- **Cut open the superficial perineal fascia to reveal the deep perineal (investing or Gallaudet's) fascia. This fascia covers the bulbospongiosus muscle located lateral to the labia minora (Fig. 15.30 and Plate 15.3).**
- **Identify the bulbospongiosus muscle. Dissect lateral to the bulbospongiosus muscle to identify the ischiocavernosus muscle running along the ischiopubic ramus. Use blunt dissection to locate the deep and superficial branches of the perineal artery, vein, and nerve (Fig. 15.31).**

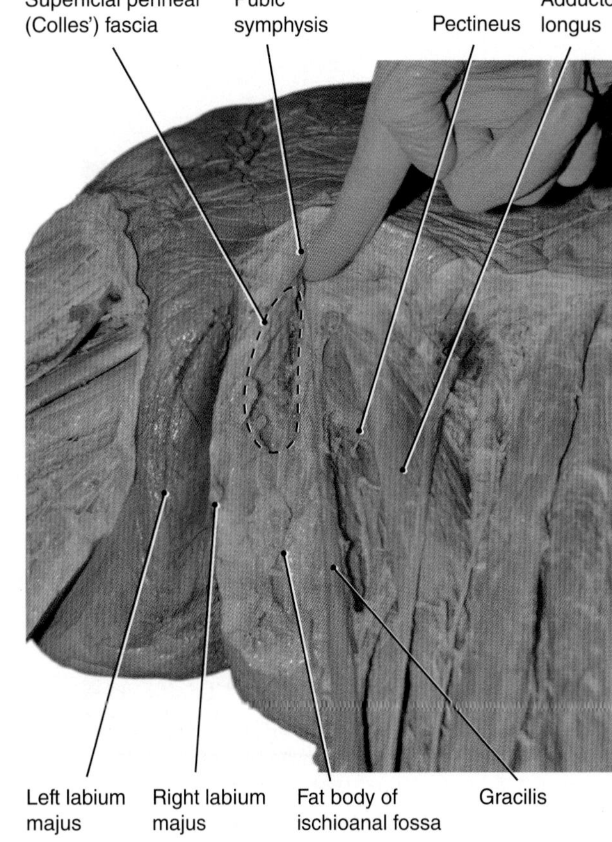

Fig. 15.29 The superficial perineal (Colles') fascia is exposed, as well as the musculature of the left thigh.

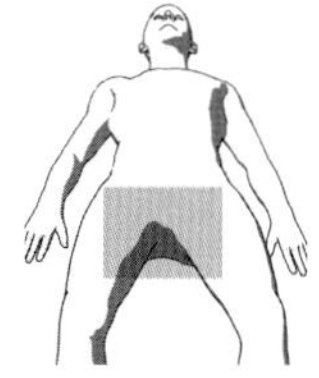

ANATOMY NOTE

The bulbospongiosus muscle attaches anteriorly to the corpus cavernosus clitoris and posteriorly to the perineal body. The bulbospongiosus muscle in the female is separate and does not attach in the midline as in males. The ischiocavernosus muscle covers the surface of the crus of the clitoris.

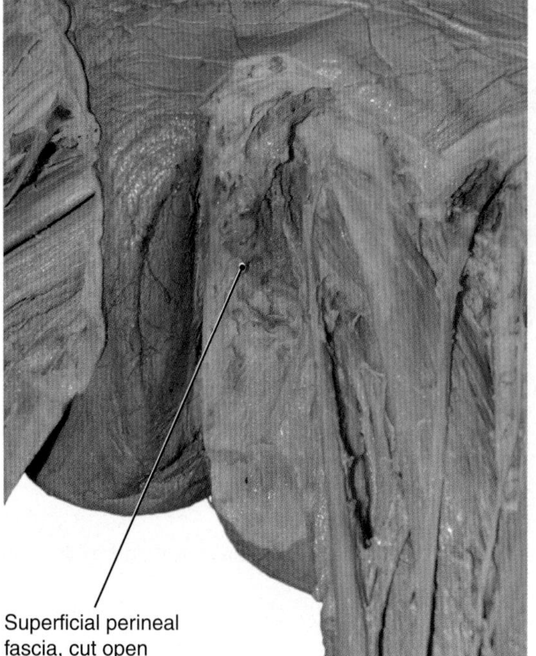

Fig. 15.30 The superficial perineal (Colles') fascia is cut open.

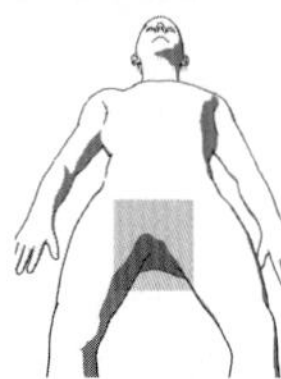

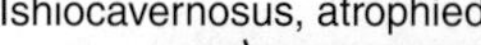

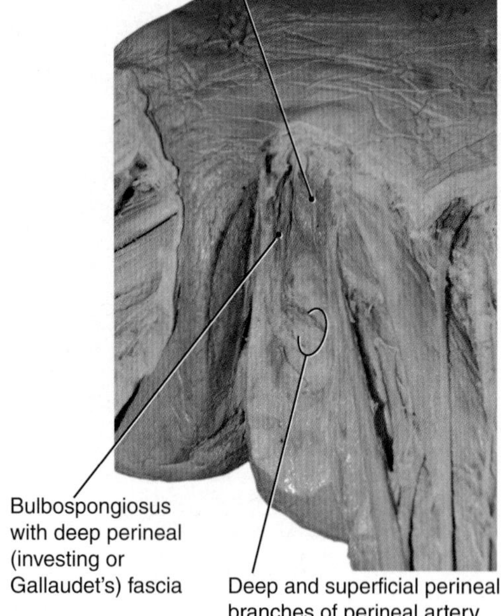

Fig. 15.31 The bulbospongiosus and deep perineal fascia are exposed, as well as the superficial and deep branches of perineal artery, vein, and nerve.

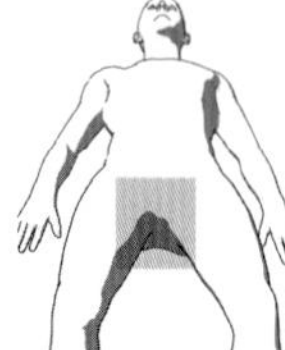

- **Dissect further to reveal the crus of the clitoris. Clean the adipose tissue from the deep and superficial branches of the perineal artery, vein, and nerve (Fig. 15.32).**
- **Reflect the bulbospongiosus muscle laterally to reveal the bulb of the vestibule (Fig. 15.33).**
- **Cut the crus of the clitoris and reflect it laterally (Fig. 15.34).**
- **Identify the perineal membrane (Fig. 15.35).**

DISSECTION TIP

In some female cadavers the musculature of the perineum can be severely atrophied because of age. However, the branches of the superficial perineal nerve and accompanying vasculature remain intact.

- **Reflect the superficial perineal fascia (Colles' fascia) inferiorly over the area of the crus of clitoris and the ischiocavernosus (Fig. 15.36).**

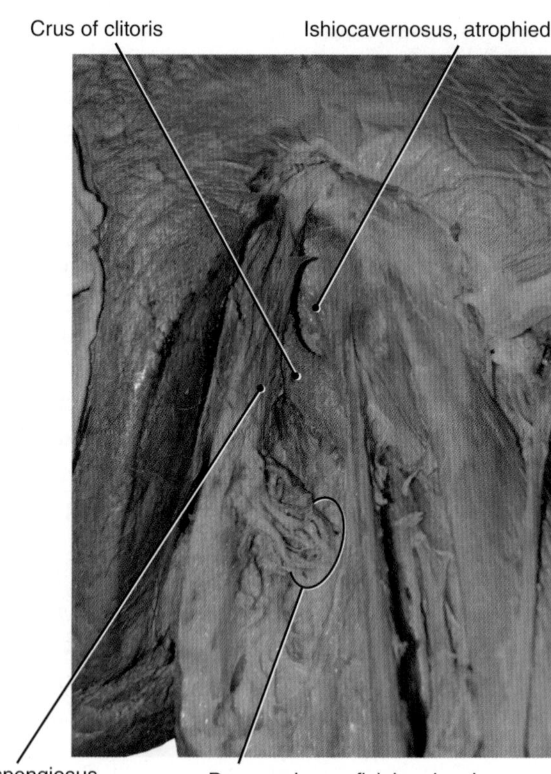

Fig. 15.32 The crus of the clitoris is exposed.

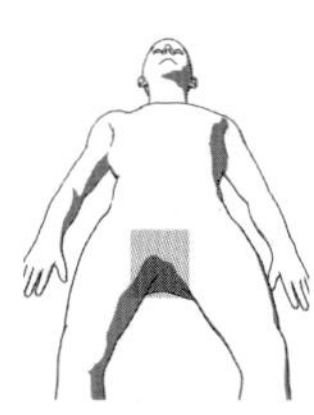

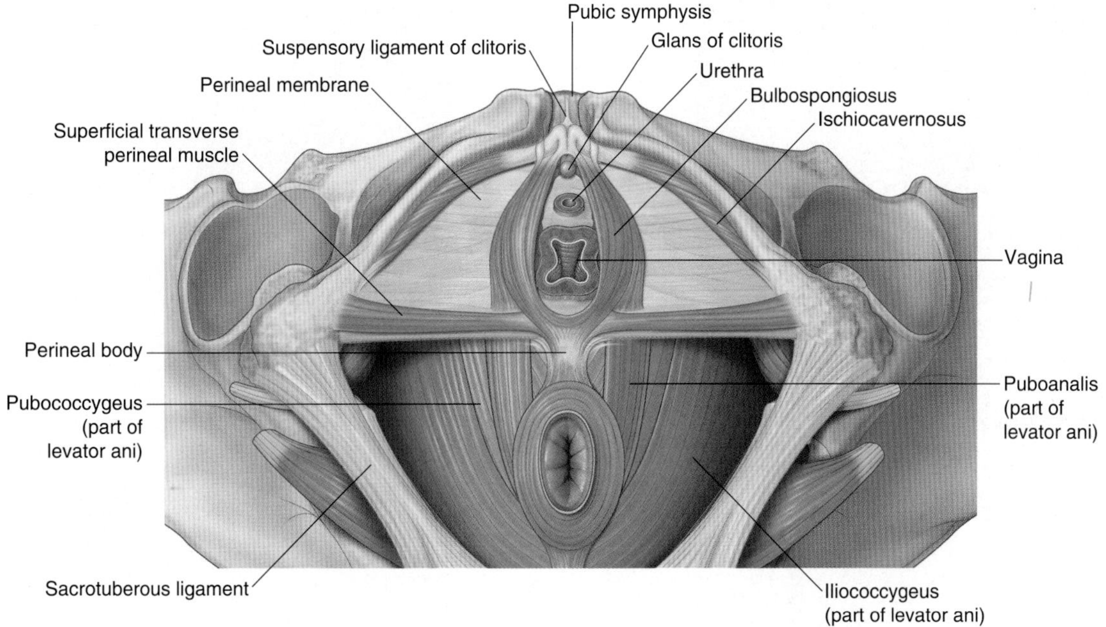

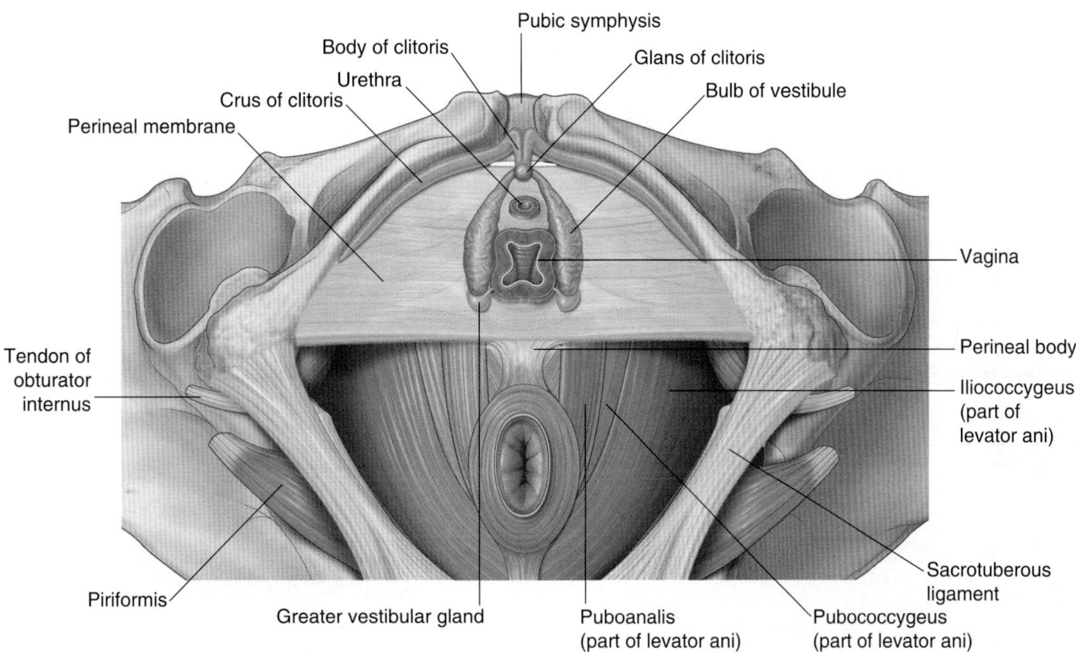

Plate 15.3 Muscles (top) and erectile tissues (bottom) of the superficial perineal space in females. (From Drake RL et al. *Gray's Atlas of Anatomy*, 3rd edition, Philadelphia, Elsevier, 2021, p. 264.)

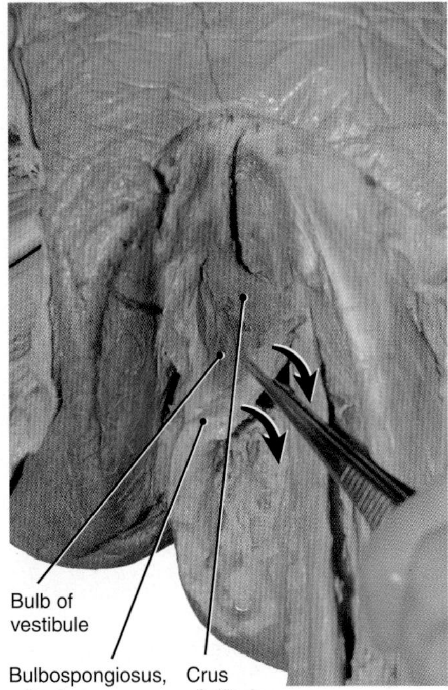

Fig. 15.33 The bulbospongiosus is reflected, exposing the bulb of the vestibule.

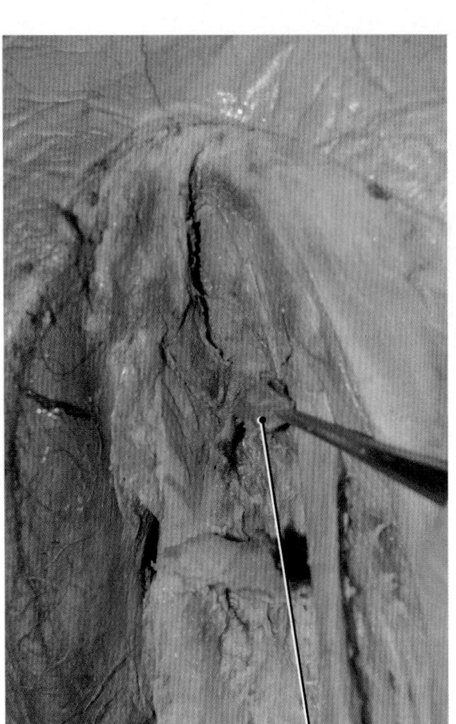

Fig. 15.34 The crus of the clitoris is cut and reflected.

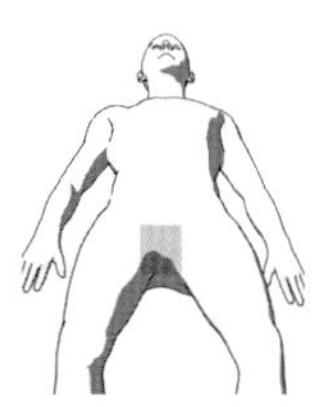

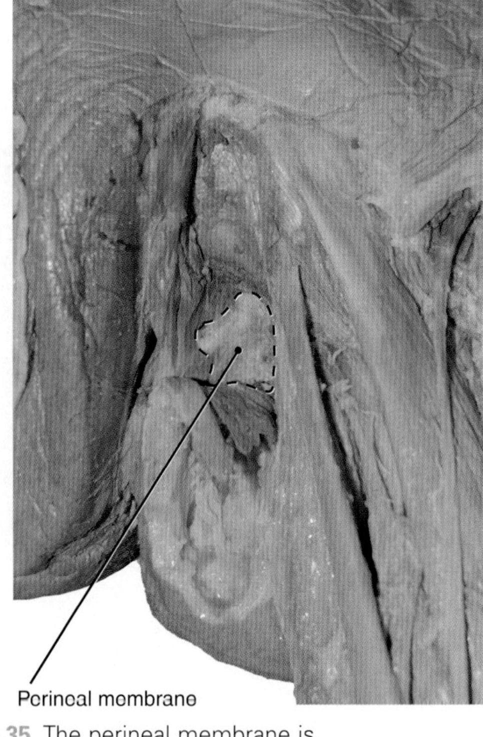

Fig. 15.35 The perineal membrane is exposed.

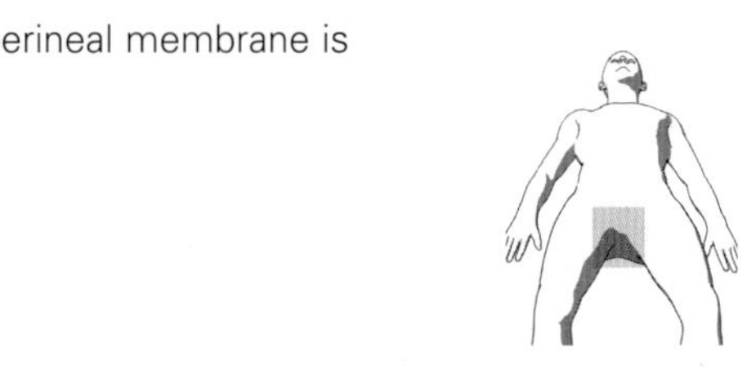

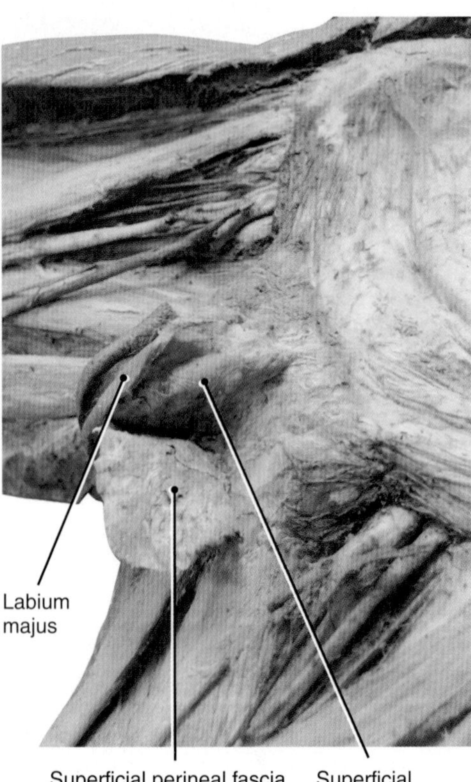

Fig. 15.36 Reflected part of the superficial perineal fascia (Colles' fascia) and adipose tissue from the ischioanal fossa.

- Identify a branch of the superficial perineal nerve underneath the superficial perineal fascia (Fig. 15.37).
- Expose all branches of the superficial perineal nerve underneath the superficial perineal fascia (Fig. 15.38).
- Expose all branches of the superficial perineal nerve underneath the superficial perineal fascia and trace them in the ischioanal fossa (Fig. 15.39).

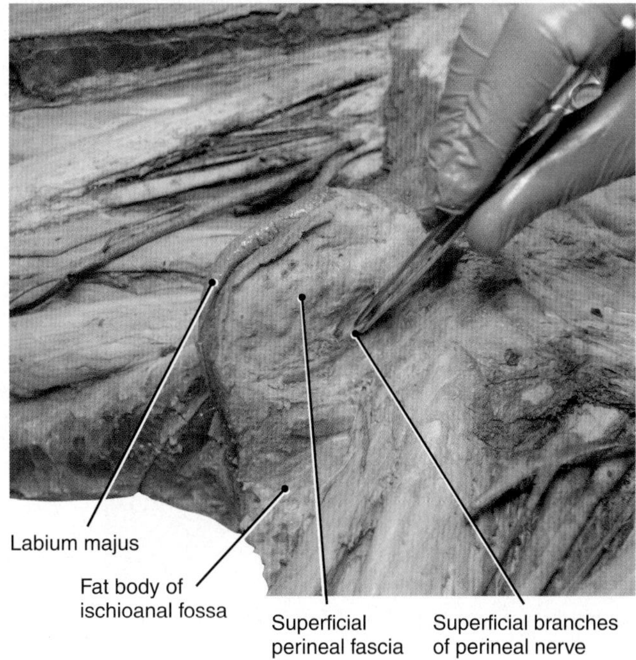

Fig. 15.37 Superficial perineal nerve identified underneath the superficial perineal fascia.

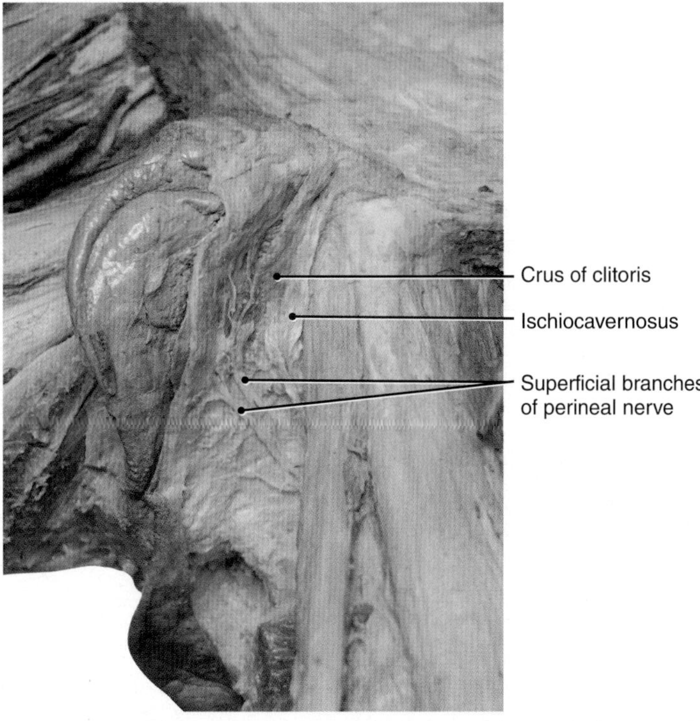

Fig. 15.38 Exposure of multiple branches of the superficial perineal nerve underneath the superficial perineal fascia.

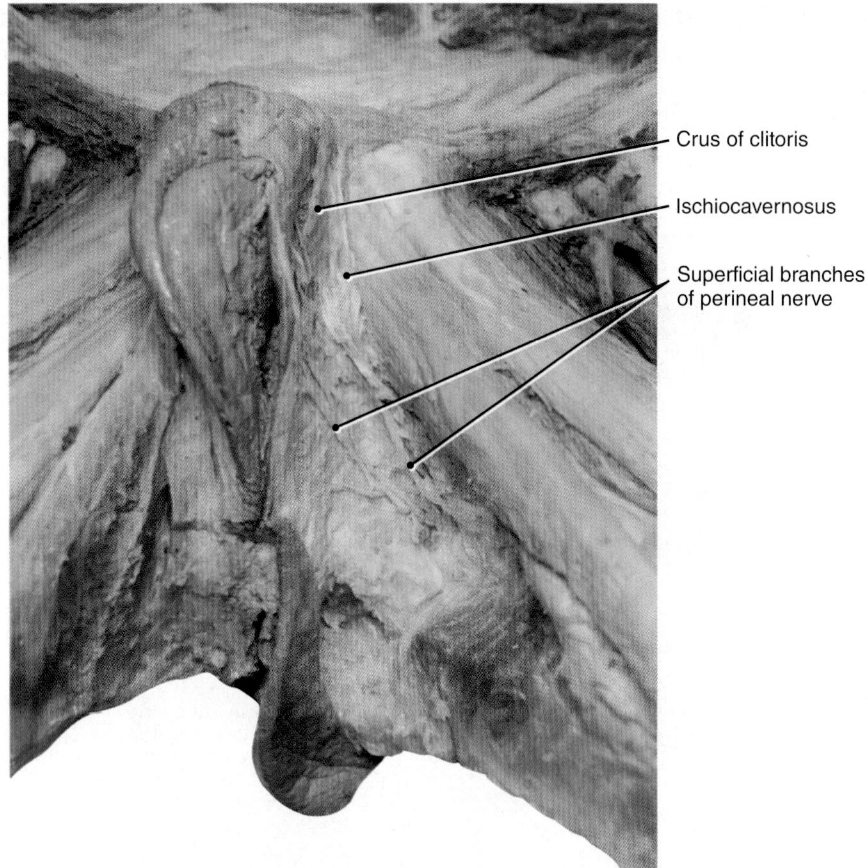

Fig. 15.39 Exposure of all superficial perineal nerve branches underneath the superficial perineal fascia.

LABORATORY IDENTIFICATION CHECKLIST

NERVES

- ☐ Femoral
  - ☐ Muscular branches
  - ☐ Cutaneous branches
- ☐ Obturator
  - ☐ Anterior branch
  - ☐ Posterior branch
- ☐ Ilioinguinal
- ☐ Perineal
  - ☐ Superficial branch

ARTERIES

- ☐ Femoral
- ☐ Obturator
- ☐ Deferential
- ☐ Perineal

VEINS

- ☐ Great saphenous
- ☐ Femoral
- ☐ Deep dorsal of penis
- ☐ Perineal

MUSCLES

- ☐ Sartorius
- ☐ Gracilis
- ☐ Adductor longus
- ☐ Pectineus
- ☐ Iliopsoas
- ☐ Bulbospongiosus
- ☐ Ischiocavernosus
- ☐ Superficial transverse perineal
- ☐ Deep transverse perineal
- ☐ Sphincter urethrae

CONNECTIVE TISSUE

- ☐ Superficial perineal fascia
- ☐ Corpora cavernosa
- ☐ Bulb of penis
- ☐ Bulb of vestibule
- ☐ Corpus spongiosum
- ☐ Crus of penis/clitoris
- ☐ Perineal membrane
- ☐ Perineal body
- ☐ Suspensory ligament of penis/clitoris
- ☐ Prepuce of penis/clitoris
- ☐ Glans of penis/clitoris
- ☐ Spermatic cord
- ☐ Scrotum
- ☐ Labia majora
- ☐ Labia minora
- ☐ Rectoprostatic fascia
- ☐ Pubic symphysis
- ☐ Anterior commissure of labia majora
- ☐ Glans of clitoris
- ☐ Vaginal orifice
- ☐ Vestibular fossa
- ☐ Posterior commissure of labia majora

BONES

- ☐ Right/left pubic bone
- ☐ Ischial spine

Clinical Application

Figs. VI.1 and VI.2 depict the pelvic cavity with viscera removed. Note the superior and inferior hypogastric plexuses.

Figs. VI.3 and VI.4 show large tumors in the uterus.

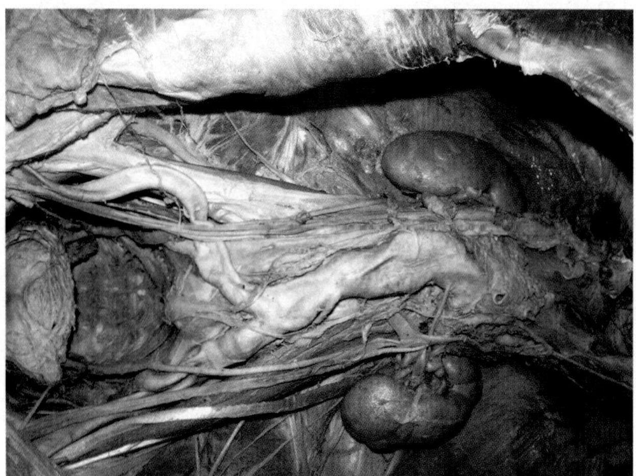

Fig. VI.1

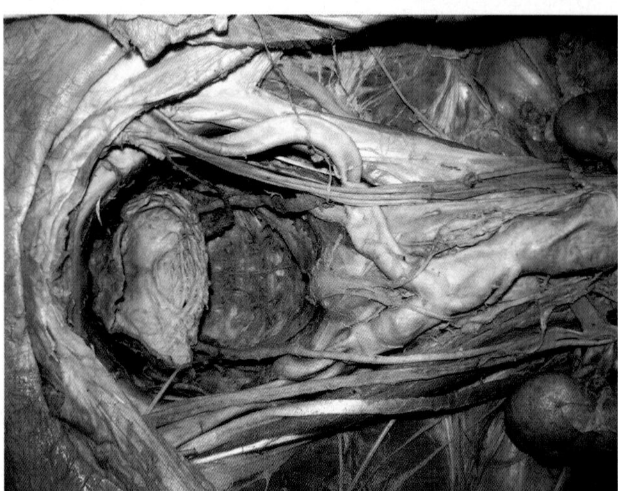

Fig. VI.2

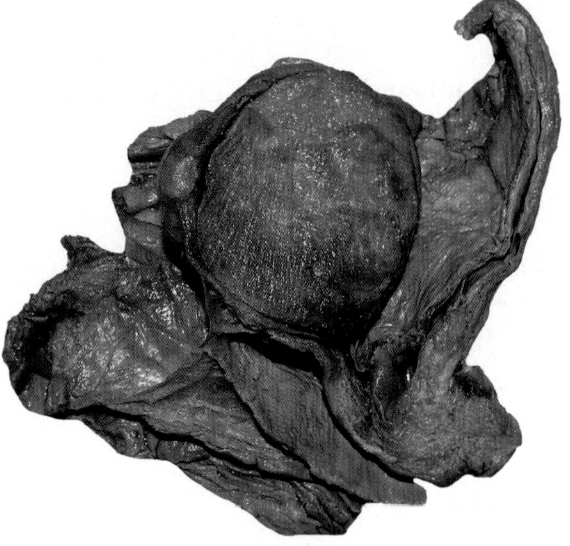

Fig. VI.3

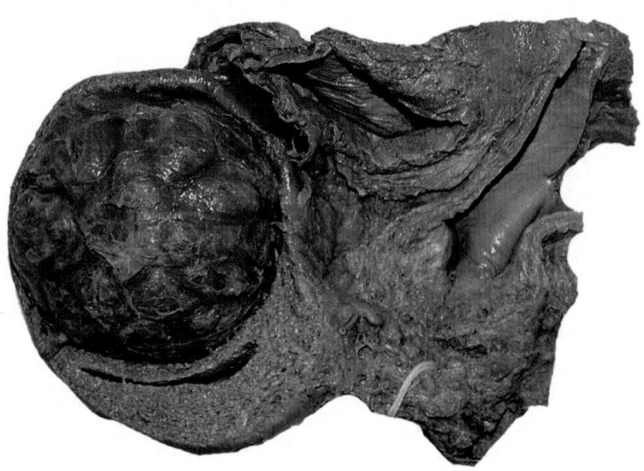

Fig. VI.4

SECTION VII

LOWER LIMB

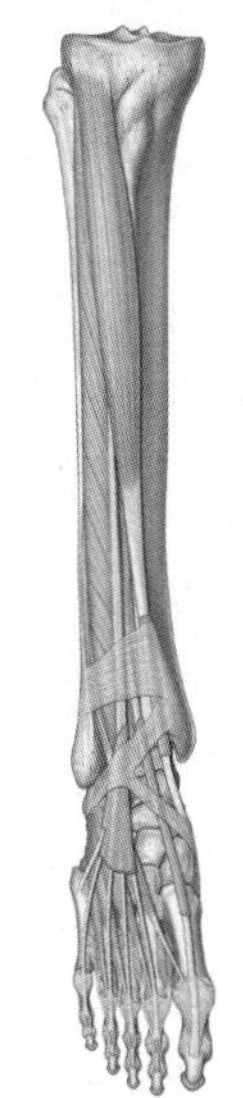

CHAPTER 16 GLUTEAL REGION

BEFORE YOU BEGIN

Typically, you will not need to make additional skin incisions if you continue the dissection on the same cadaver on which you performed the dissection of the back in Chapter 2 (Fig. 16.1).

If not, place the cadaver in the prone position and incise the skin and subcutaneous tissues along the iliac crest to the posterior superior iliac spine (Figs. 16.2 and 16.3).

Extend this incision medially to the intergluteal cleft, anterior to the area covering the perineum.

SKIN AND SUPERFICIAL FASCIA

- **Reflect the skin and superficial fascia from the gluteal region and posterior thigh by making a longitudinal midline skin incision distally to the knee. Make a circumferential incision through the skin of the leg, just distal to the knee (see Figs. 16.2 and 16.3).**
- **There is typically a large amount of adipose tissue over the gluteus maximus muscle. Remove the adipose tissue and deep fascia in the gluteal region, exposing the gluteus maximus muscle (Figs. 16.4–16.6).**

DISSECTION TIP

In many atlases, you will find the gluteus maximus muscle shown with no fat. To create a clean specimen, remove the fat between the fibers of the gluteus maximus muscle (see Fig. 16.6).

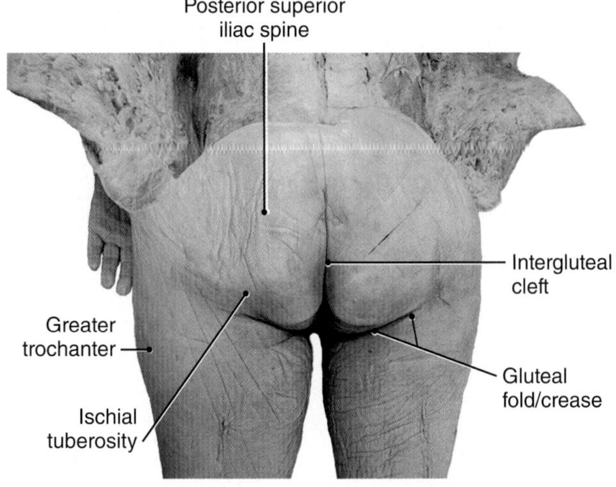

Fig. 16.1 Surface anatomy of the gluteal region.

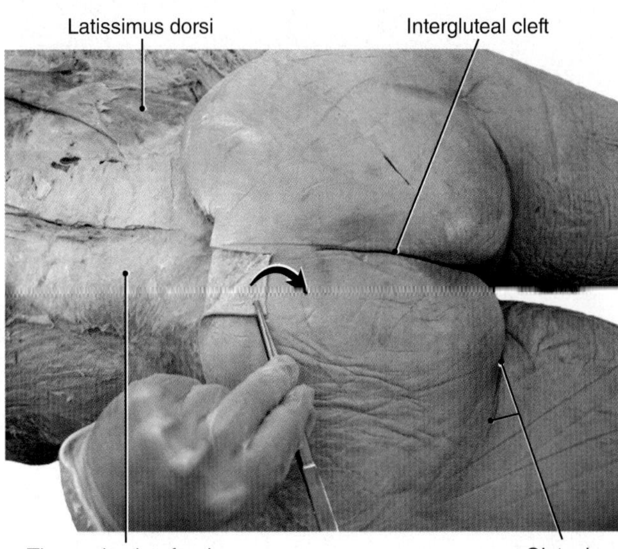

Fig. 16.2 Gluteal region with reflected skin, demonstrating dissection from the midline.

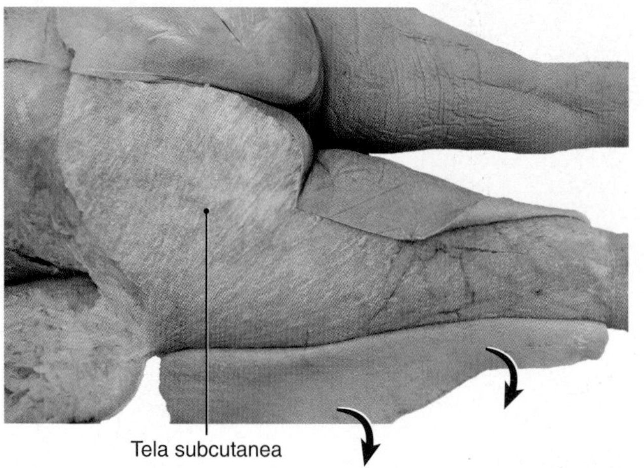

Fig. 16.3 Gluteal and posterior thigh regions with skin reflected, revealing membranous layer of subcutaneous tissue (tela subcutanea).

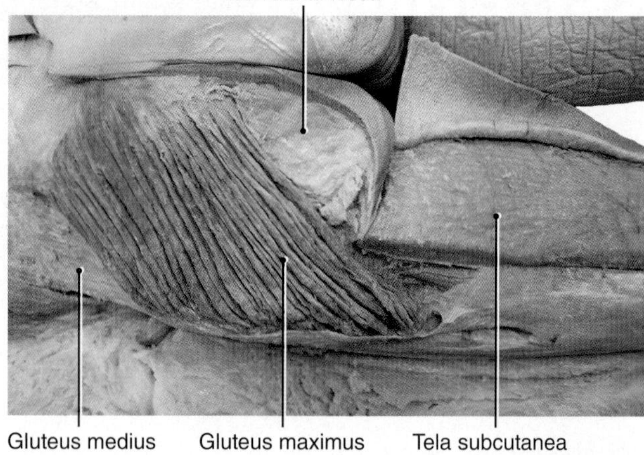

Fig. 16.5 Further gluteal region dissection, revealing the gluteus medius (covered with fascia) muscle superiorly, the gluteus maximus muscle inferiorly, and the ischioanal fossa and tela subcutanea medially.

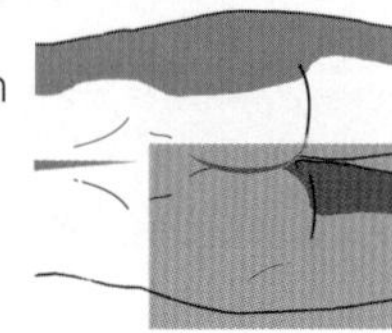

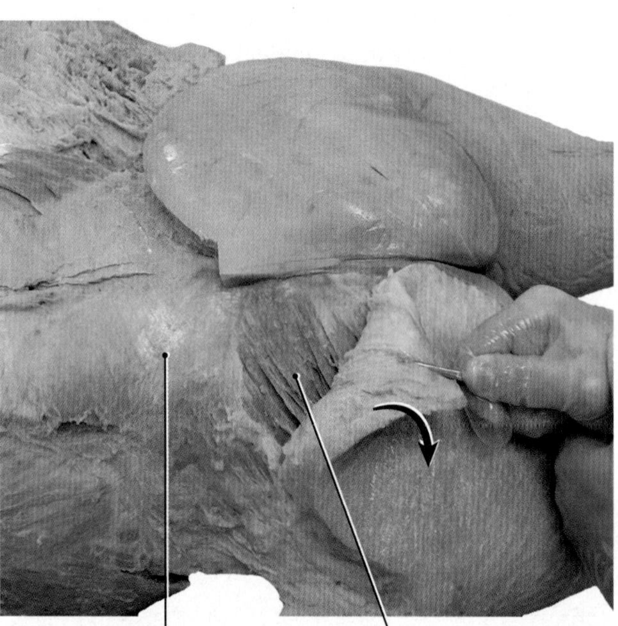

Fig. 16.4 Gluteal region with thoracolumbar fascia superiorly and reflected subcutaneous tissue, revealing the gluteus maximus muscle inferiorly.

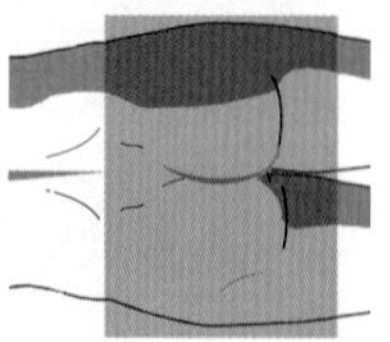

Ischioanal fossa

Gluteus medius

Gluteus maximus

Fig. 16.6 Closer view highlighting the gluteus medius (covered with fascia) muscle superiorly, the gluteus maximus muscle inferiorly, and the ischioanal fossa medially.

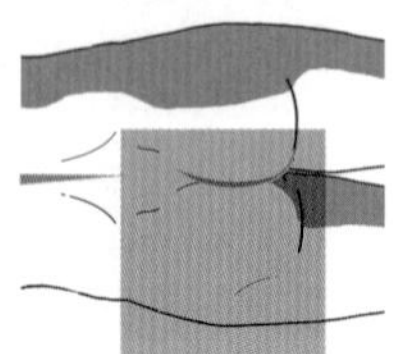

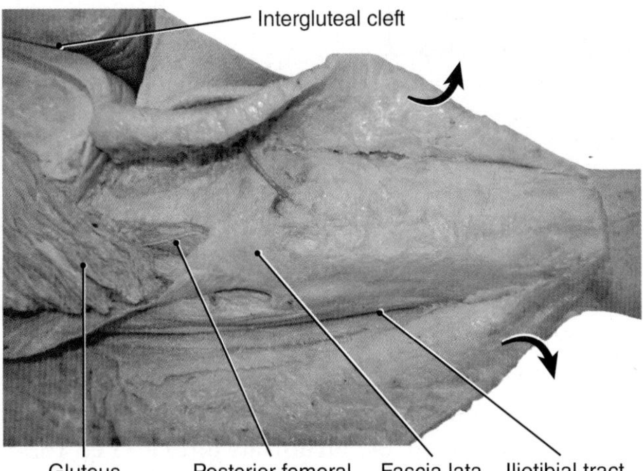

Fig. 16.7 Posterior thigh region with skin and subcutaneous tissue reflected, revealing the posterior femoral cutaneous nerve, fascia lata, and iliotibial tract.

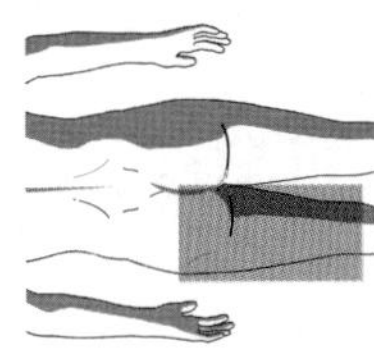

- **Reflect the skin over the posterior portion of the thigh. The adipose tissue and deep fascia will be removed later during the dissection (Fig. 16.7).**

DISSECTION **TIP**

As you delineate the superior and inferior borders of the gluteus maximus muscle, protect the posterior femoral cutaneous nerve from damage by being cautious along the inferior border of the gluteus maximus muscle.

SUPERFICIAL MUSCLES

- **Palpate the sacrotuberous ligament at the medial border of the gluteus maximus muscle by placing your fingertips into the ischioanal fossa (Fig. 16.8).**
- **Palpate the superior border of the gluteus maximus and insert your fingertips into the space between the gluteus maximus muscle and fascia over the gluteus medius muscle (Fig. 16.9).**
- **Using your fingertips, lift the upper portion of the gluteus maximus muscle from the underlying gluteus medius muscle.**

DISSECTION **TIP**

In most cadavers, the deep fascia and aponeurotic tissues along the superior border of the gluteus maximus muscle blend with those of the gluteus medius muscle. However, the muscular fibers of the gluteus medius muscle run almost perpendicular to the orientation of the gluteus maximus muscle, and the two muscles can be separated readily once you have clearly exposed their fibers.

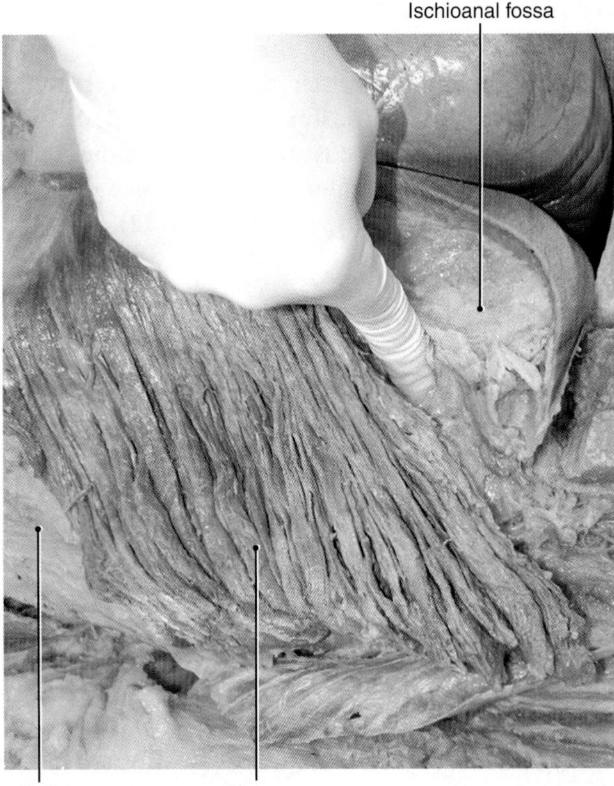

Fig. 16.8 Fingertips in gluteal region highlight gluteus medius superiorly, gluteus maximus inferiorly, and ischioanal fossa medially (palpation of lateral wall of fossa–obturator internus).

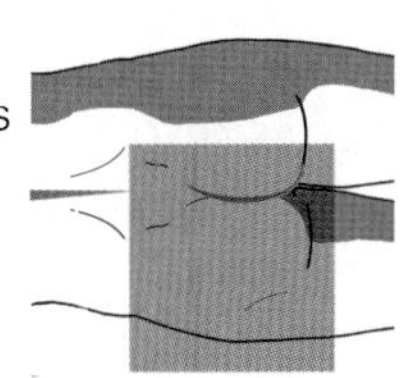

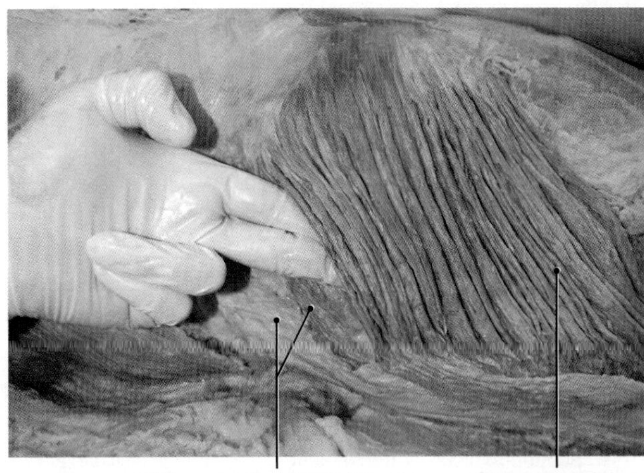

Fig. 16.9 Gluteal region after dissecting the superior border of the gluteus maximus muscle superficially, revealing the deeper gluteus medius fascia and muscle.

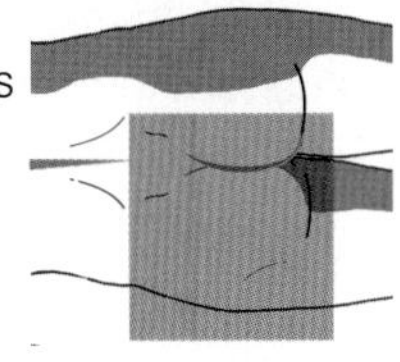

DEEP DISSECTION

- Make an incision along the lateral border of the gluteus maximus muscle, separating it from its connection to the iliotibial tract (Fig. 16.10).
- Lift the gluteus maximus medially toward the sacrum and identify the greater trochanter and overlying trochanteric bursa (Figs. 16.11 and 16.12).

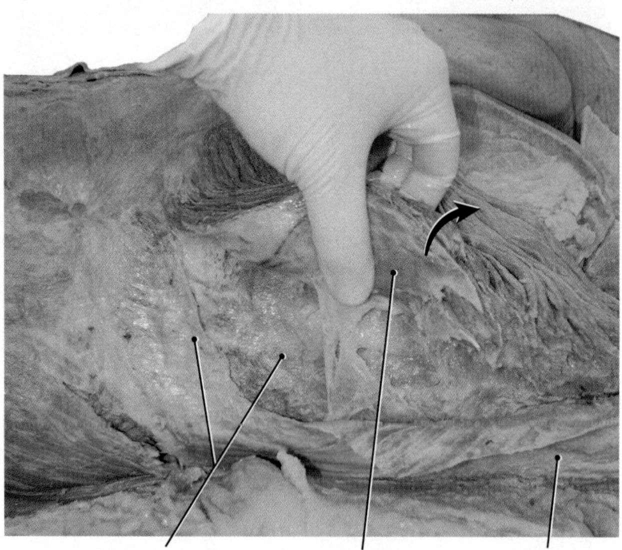

Fig. 16.10 Reflecting the gluteus maximus muscle demonstrates the deeper lying muscle fibers of the gluteus medius muscle.

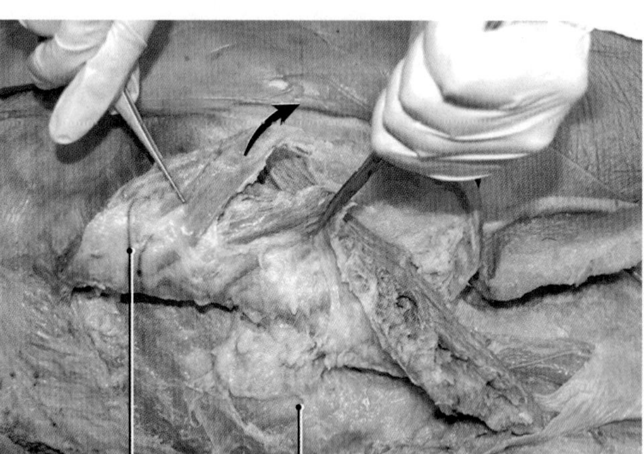

Fig. 16.11 Reflection of the superolateral border of the gluteus maximus muscle, revealing the superior gluteal artery and vein and trochanteric bursa.

DISSECTION TIP

The trochanteric bursa appears as loose connective tissue over the greater trochanter, intermingled with adipose tissue. It often is cleaned away during routine dissection.

- Reflect the gluteus maximus muscle medially from the gluteal tuberosity of the femur; remove the deep fascia and adipose tissue along its inferior border (Fig. 16.13).
- Clean the sciatic and the posterior femoral cutaneous nerves from the adipose tissue and trace them proximally from under the piriformis muscle (Fig. 16.14). Once you identify the posterior femoral cutaneous nerve, identify its perineal branch traveling medially.

DISSECTION TIP

To identify the posterior femoral cutaneous nerve, make a small opening through the fascia lata on the posterior aspect of the thigh and identify the sciatic nerve. Medial to the sciatic nerve, you will be able to identify the posterior femoral cutaneous nerve. In some specimens, the sciatic nerve may split in the gluteal region, with one part traveling above or through and the other part below the piriformis muscle.

- The gluteus maximus muscle is partially attached to the sacrotuberous ligament. Palpate the sacrotuberous

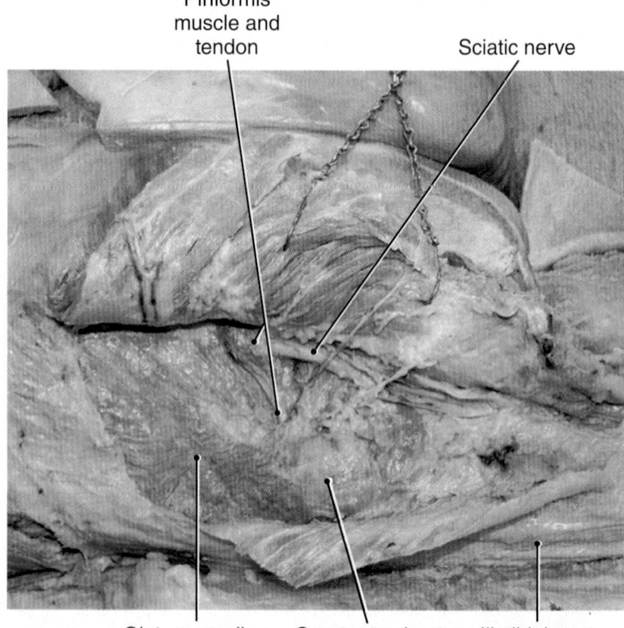

Fig. 16.12 Gluteal region with reflected gluteus maximus muscle, revealing the gluteus medius and piriformis muscles and sciatic nerve.

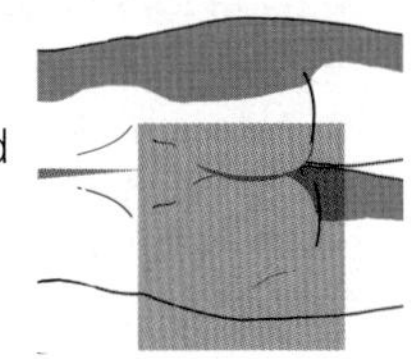

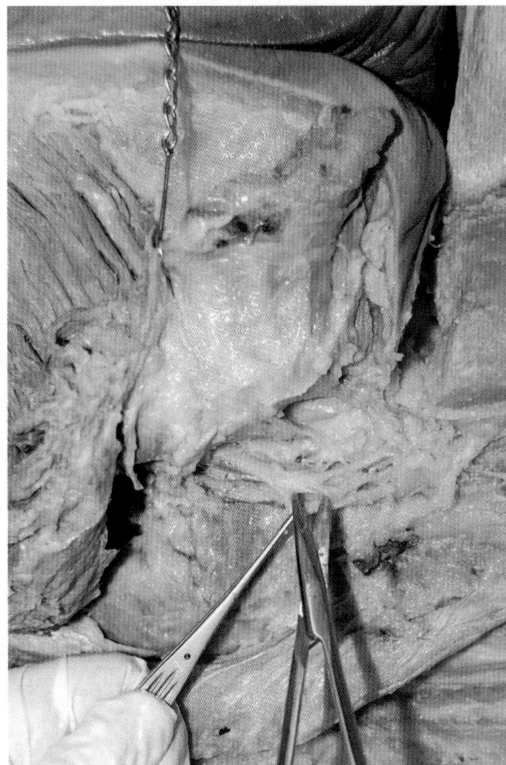

Fig. 16.13 Connective tissue cleaned around the posterior femoral cutaneous and sciatic nerves.

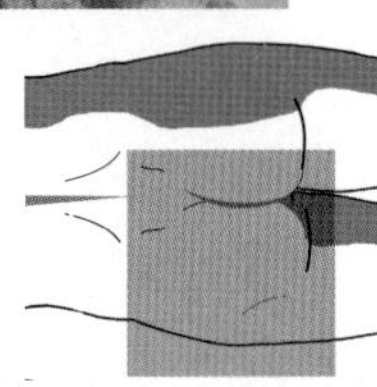

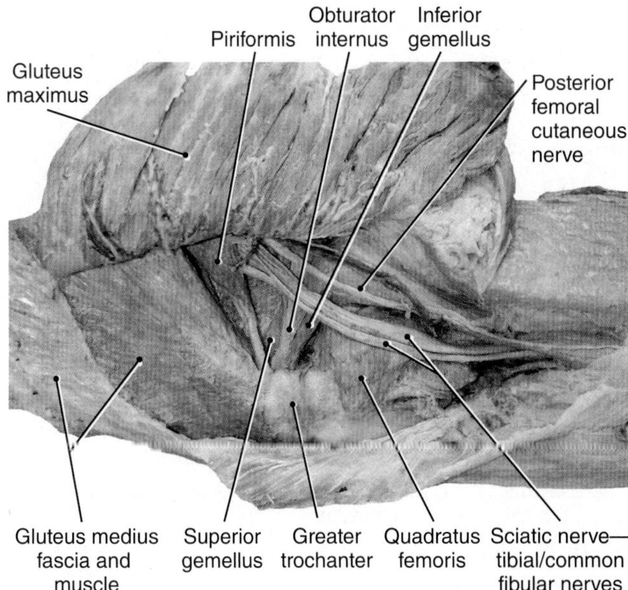

Fig. 16.14 Reflected gluteus maximus muscle, revealing gluteus medius, rotator muscles (piriformis, superior/inferior gemelli, obturator internus, quadratus femoris), sciatic nerve, and posterior femoral cutaneous nerve.

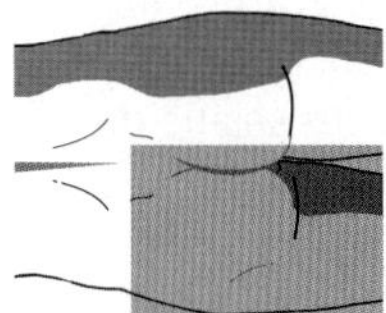

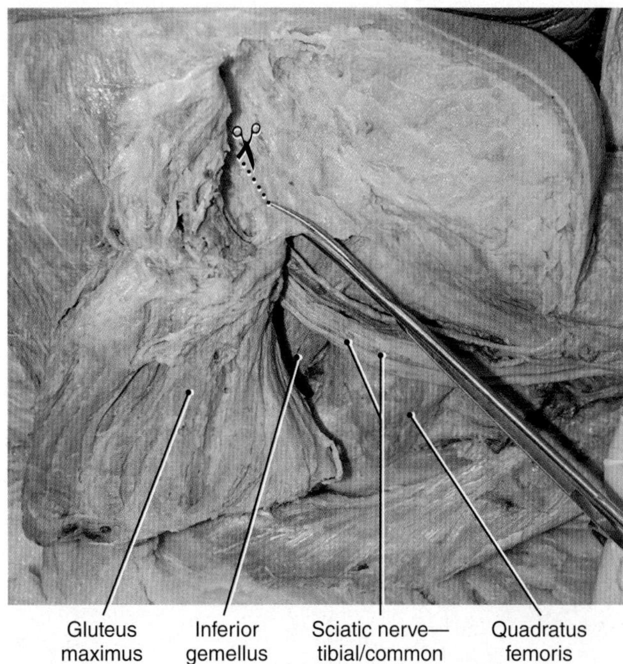

Fig. 16.15 Reflected gluteus maximus muscle revealing the quadratus femoris muscle and tibial and common fibular nerves.

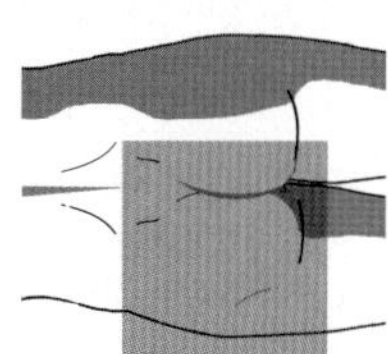

ligament as you did earlier (see Fig. 16.8); reflect the gluteus maximus muscle medially toward the sacrum and expose the sacrotuberous ligament.

- **Use a scalpel to cut the attachment of the gluteus maximus muscle from the sacrotuberous ligament. With scissors, cut the lateral portion of the sacrotuberous ligament and free the gluteus maximus muscle (Fig. 16.15).**
- **Clean and expose the inferior gluteal vessels and nerve from the deep surface of the gluteus maximus muscle (Figs. 16.16 and 16.17).**
- **Lift the posterior femoral cutaneous and sciatic nerves and clean the adipose and connective tissues from the structures that lie deep to the gluteus maximus muscle, such as the piriformis, obturator internus, and superior and inferior gemellus muscles (Figs. 16.18 and 16.19).**
- **Inferior to the obturator internus and gemelli muscles, identify the quadratus femoris muscle.**

DISSECTION **TIP**

The obturator internus, superior gemellus, and inferior gemellus muscles often are seen as a combined tripartite tendon with indistinguishable borders. With scissors or a probe, separate these three muscles at the margin of the lesser sciatic foramen.

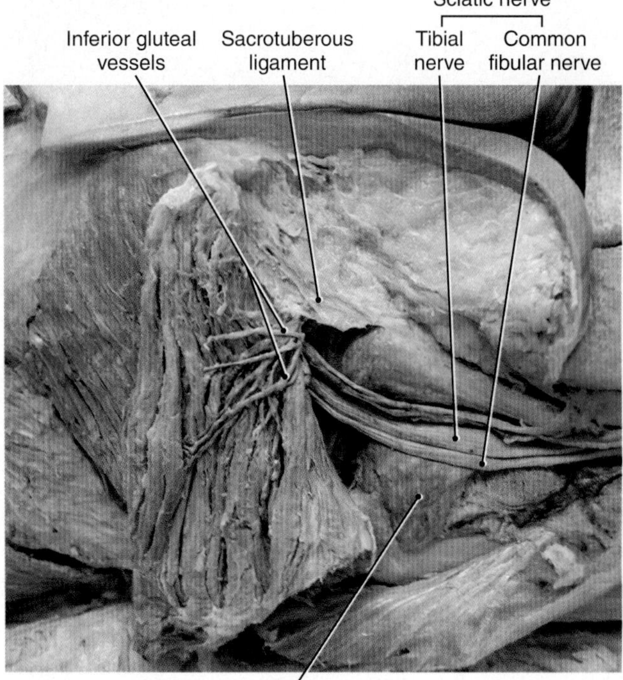

Fig. 16.16 Gluteus maximus muscle reflected superiorly, revealing the inferior gluteal vessels, quadratus femoris muscle, and tibial and common fibular nerves.

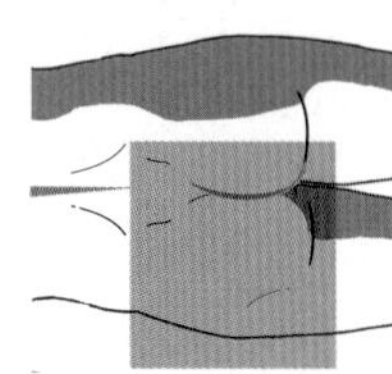

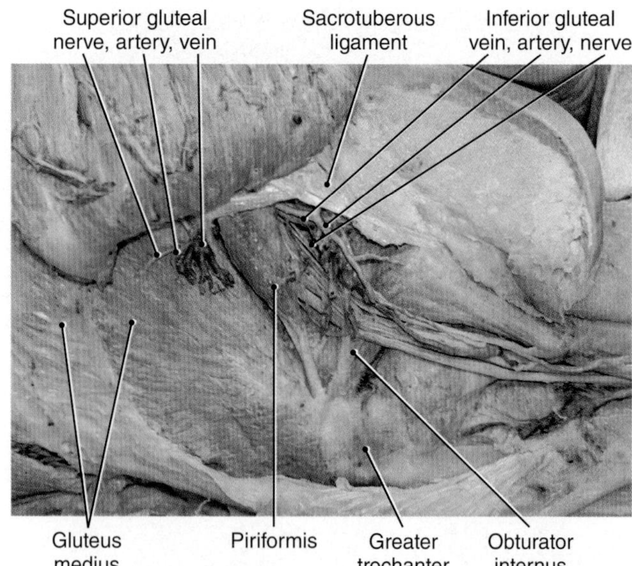

Fig. 16.18 Gluteal region with gluteus maximus reflected, revealing the superior and inferior gluteal arteries and veins oriented around the piriformis muscle.

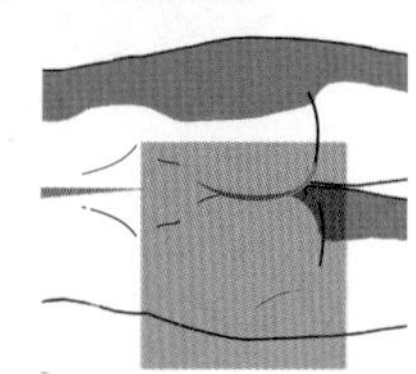

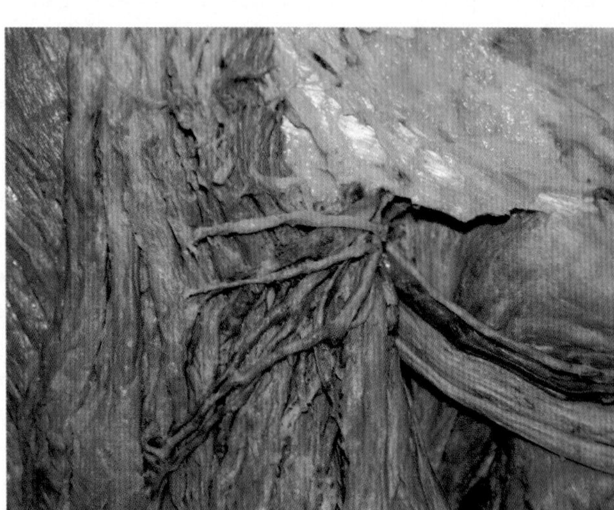

Fig. 16.17 Closer view of Fig. 16.16 showing the gluteal region with the gluteus maximus reflected, revealing the inferior gluteal artery and vein and sacrotuberous ligament.

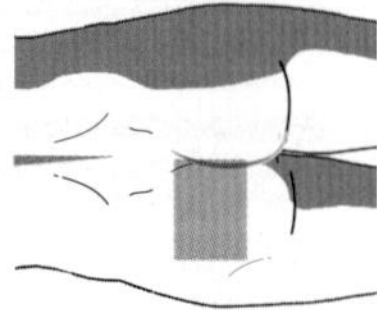

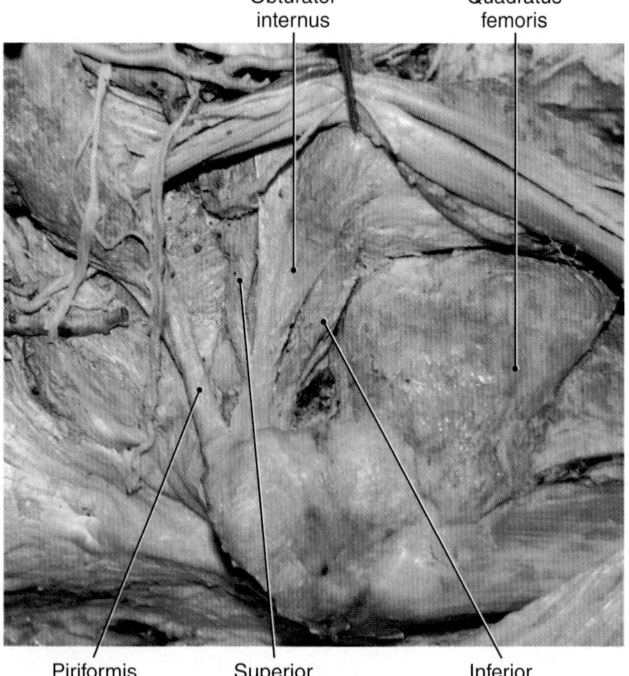

Fig. 16.19 Gluteal region close-up view highlighting the lateral rotator muscles (piriformis, superior/inferior gemelli, obturator internus, and quadratus femoris) with sciatic nerve reflected medially.

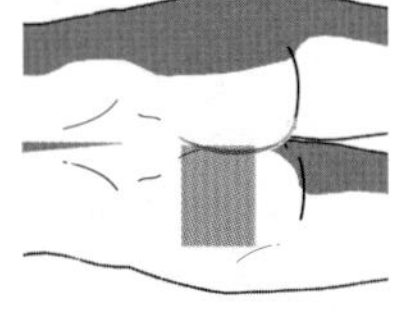

- **Identify the borders of the gluteus medius and tensor fasciae latae muscles. The tensor fasciae latae muscle arises from the anterior portion of the iliac crest. Its tendon is covered by the fascia lata and continues distally as the iliotibial tract. Place your fingertips at the inferior border of the gluteus medius muscle and lift it upward (Fig. 16.20).**
- **At the superior space between the gluteus maximus and gluteus medius muscles, identify the superficial branch of the superior gluteal artery (Figs. 16.21 and 16.22).**
- **Cut the attachment of the gluteus medius from the greater trochanter and reflect it superiorly. On its deep surface, identify the deep branch of the superior gluteal artery (see Fig. 16.22).**
- **The muscle exposed underneath the reflected gluteus medius is the gluteus minimus muscle. Deep and inferior to the sacrotuberous ligament, identify the nerve to the obturator internus, internal pudendal artery, its venae comitantes, and the pudendal nerve (Fig. 16.23). The venae comitantes are the pair of veins that accompany the internal pudendal artery.**

DISSECTION TIP

The nerve to the quadratus femoris and inferior gemellus muscles is a small branch that may be found by retracting the sciatic nerve posteromedially; observe this small nerve traveling deep to the gemelli and obturator internus muscles.

PUDENDAL CANAL AND ISCHIOANAL FOSSA

Note: This part of the dissection involves opening the pudendal canal and dissecting the ischioanal fossa; it also may be performed separately with the dissection of the perineum.

- **Dissect and clean away the adipose tissue of the structures inferior to the sacrotuberous ligament and identify the internal pudendal artery, internal pudendal vein, and the pudendal nerve (Fig. 16.24).**
- **Identify the continuation of the obturator fascia at the ischioanal fossa, the *lunate fascia*. This fascia encircles the internal pudendal artery and vein and pudendal nerve branches (Figs. 16.25 and 16.26).**

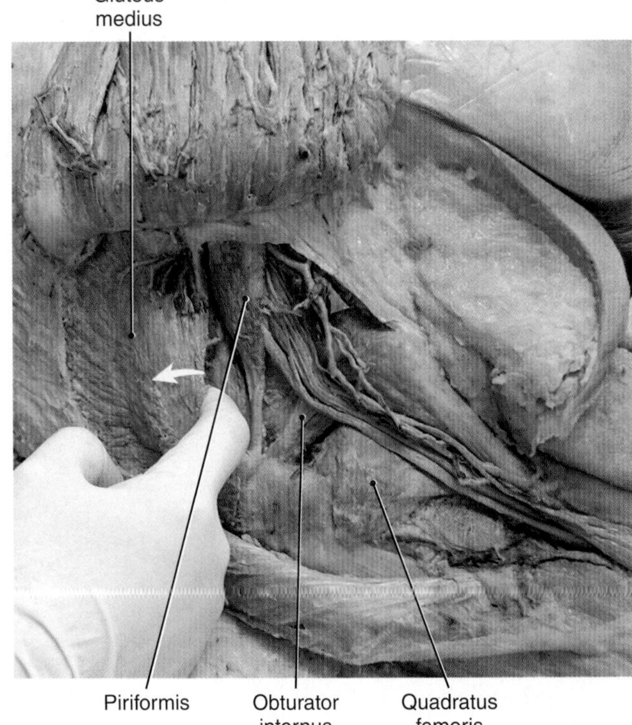

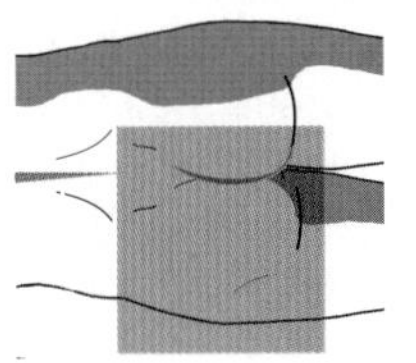

Fig. 16.20 Reflected gluteus maximus muscle reveals gluteus medius muscle, "lateral rotators" (piriformis, obturator internus, quadratus femoris muscles), and the sciatic nerve.

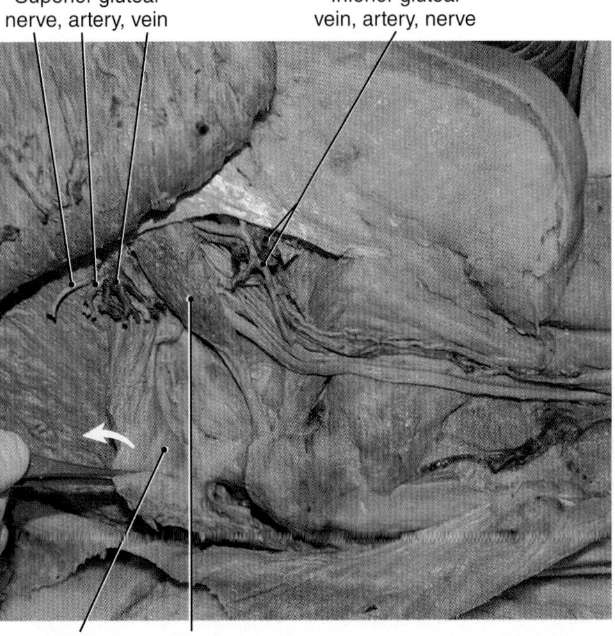

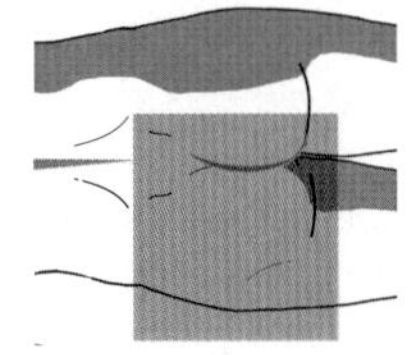

Fig. 16.21 Gluteus maximus reflected, revealing piriformis muscle and superior and inferior gluteal neurovascular bundles.

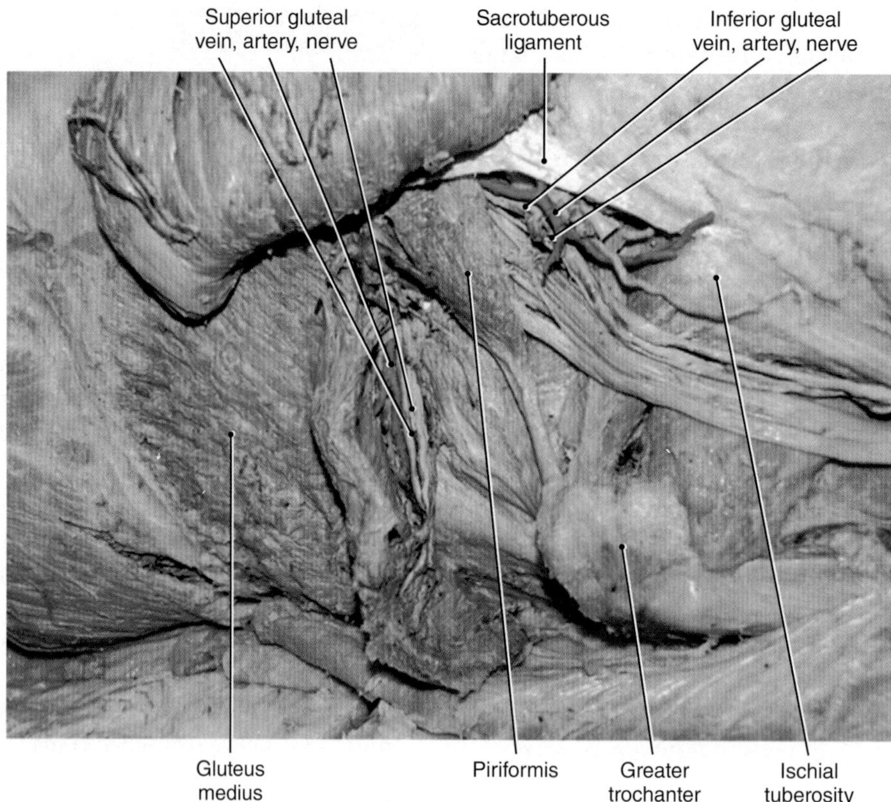

Fig. 16.22 The gluteus maximus muscle is reflected, highlighting the piriformis muscle and superior and inferior gluteal neurovascular bundles.

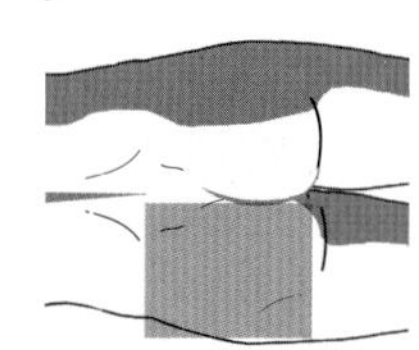

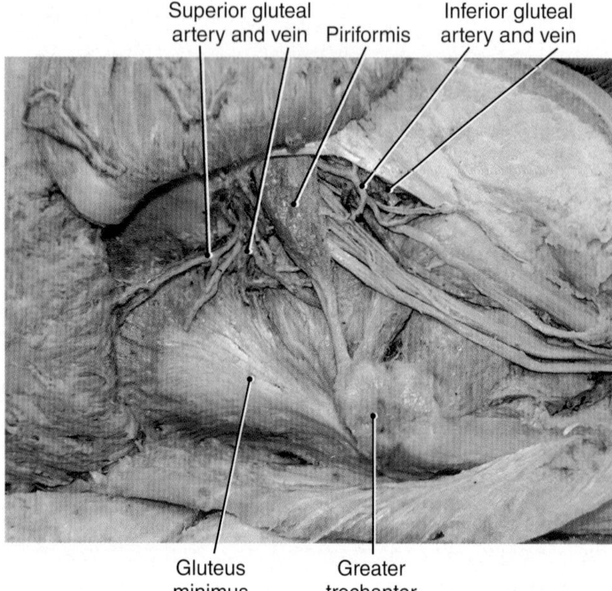

Fig. 16.23 Gluteal region with reflection of the gluteus maximus muscle medially and the gluteus medius muscle superiorly, revealing the gluteus minimus muscle and the superior gluteal neurovascular bundle lying superficial to the gluteus minimus muscle.

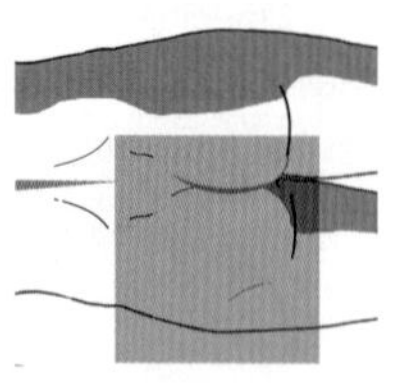

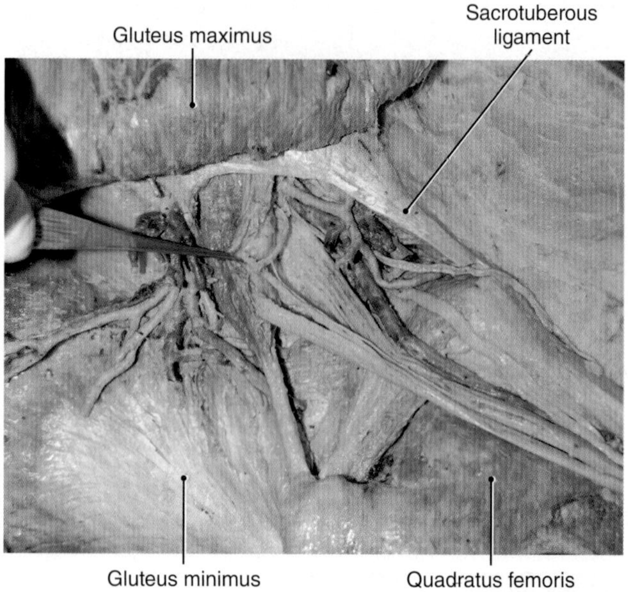

Fig. 16.24 Gluteal region with reflection of the gluteus maximus muscle medially and gluteus medius muscle superiorly, revealing the gluteus minimus muscle and the superior gluteal neurovascular bundle lying superficial to the gluteus minimus muscle.

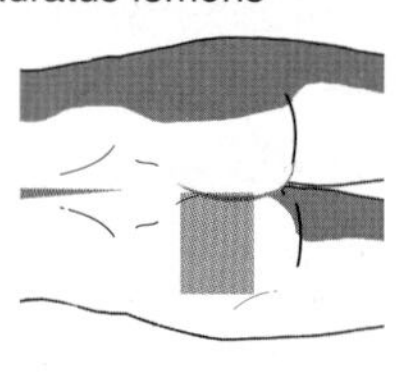

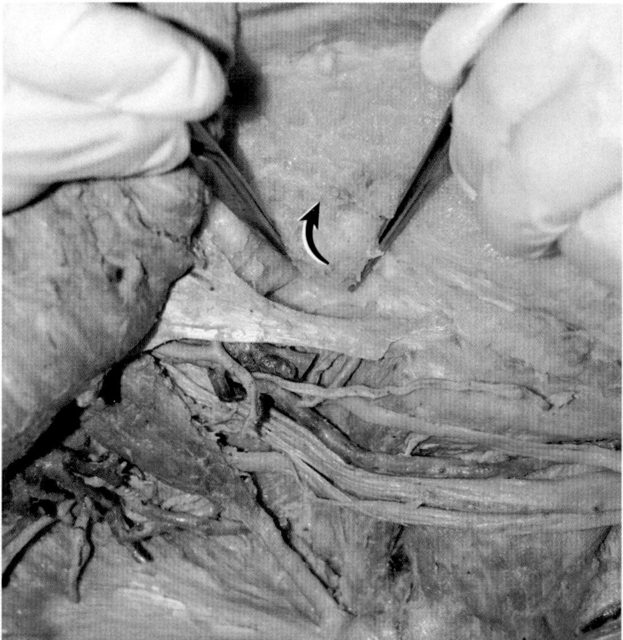

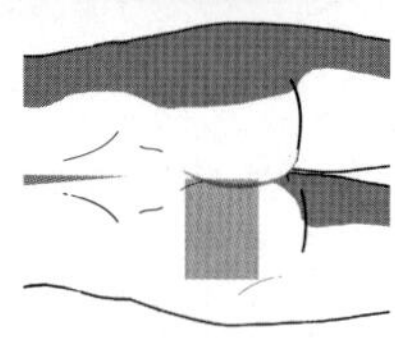

Fig. 16.25 Gluteal region with reflection of gluteus maximus, highlighting piriformis muscle, sacrotuberous ligament, and superior/inferior gluteal neurovascular bundles.

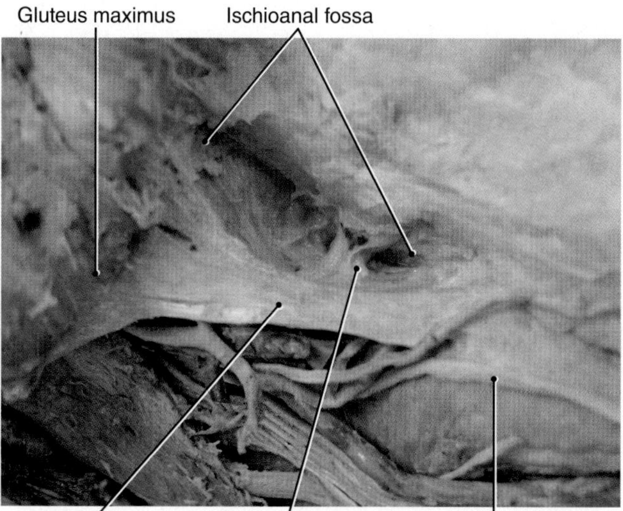

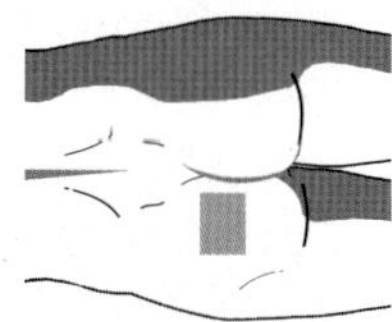

Fig. 16.26 Gluteus maximus reflected, revealing the ischioanal fossa, sacrotuberous ligament, pudendal neurovascular bundle, and posterior femoral cutaneous nerve.

DISSECTION TIP

Identifying the lunate fascia and the point of entrance of the internal pudendal artery and vein and the pudendal nerve into the gluteal region is useful for exposing these structures when a large amount of adipose tissue is present.

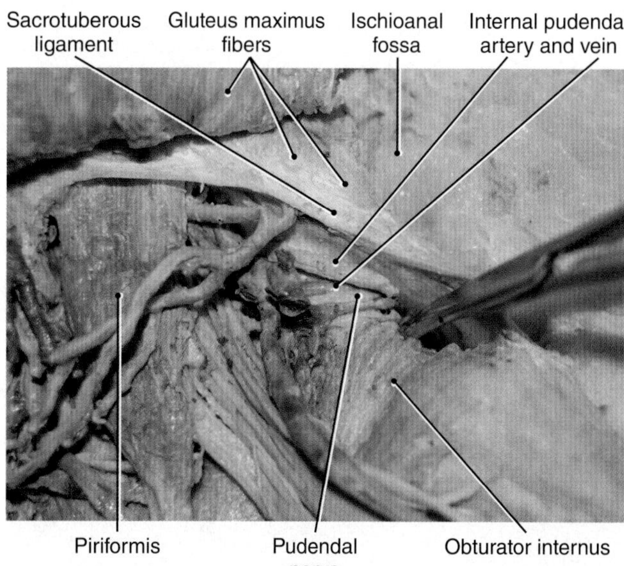

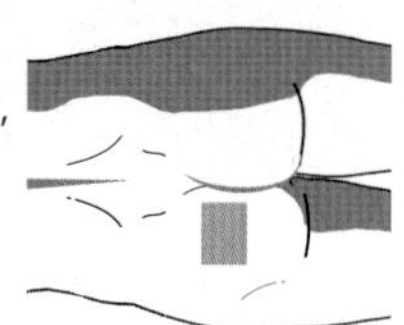

Fig. 16.27 Gluteus maximus muscle reflected, revealing sacrotuberous ligament, gluteus maximus fibers, ischioanal fossa border, obturator internus muscle, and pudendal neurovascular bundle.

- **Separate the inferior border of the sacrotuberous ligament with scissors and cut its inferior attachment from the ischial tuberosity (Fig. 16.27).**
- **Reflect the sacrotuberous ligament upward toward the reflected gluteus maximus muscle and expose the contents of the pudendal canal (Alcock's canal) (Figs. 16.28 and 16.29).**
- **Expose the pudendal, inferior anal, and perineal nerves (Fig. 16.30).**
- **Remove all the adipose tissue from the ischioanal fossa thoroughly so that the branches of the pudendal nerve and internal pudendal artery are fully identified (Figs. 16.31 and 16.32, Plate 16.1).**
- **Expose the levator ani muscle and the fascia of the obturator internus muscle as well as the external anal sphincter (Figs. 16.33 and 16.34, Plate 16.2).**

POSTERIOR THIGH

- **Palpate the iliotibial tract, the band into which the tensor fasciae latae and the gluteus maximus muscles (partially) insert.**
- **Note the lateral intermuscular septum, which begins from the deep surface of the fascia lata and attaches to the *linea aspera* (rough line) of the femur.**
- **Identify the space between the quadratus femoris and adductor magnus (adductor minimus) muscles and find the medial circumflex femoral artery (Fig. 16.35).**

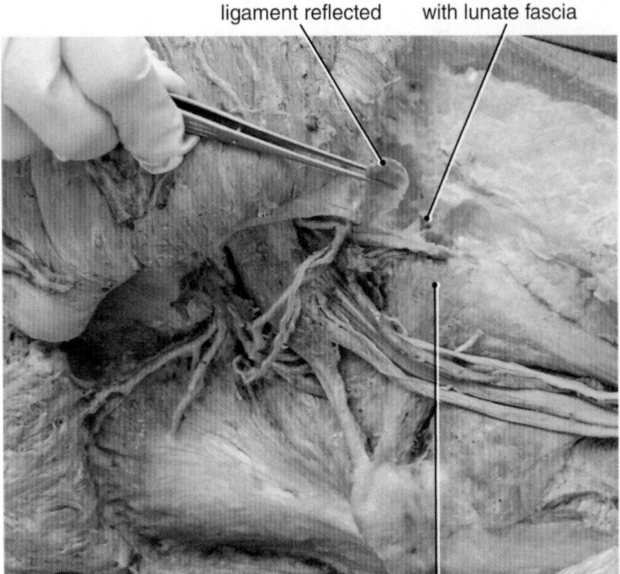

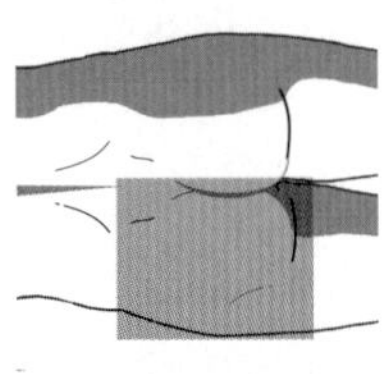

Fig. 16.28 The sacrotuberous ligament held between forceps with gluteus maximus muscle reflected, revealing the ischioanal fossa border, obturator internus muscle, and pudendal neurovascular bundle within the lunate fascia.

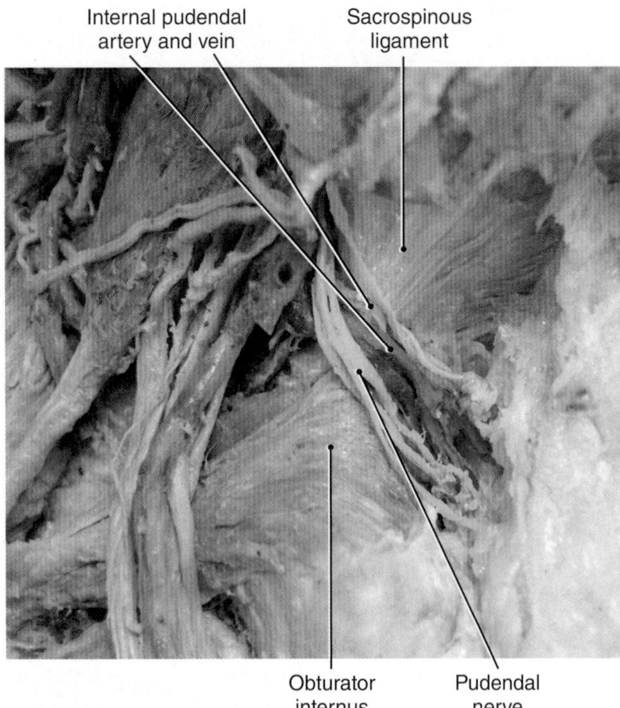

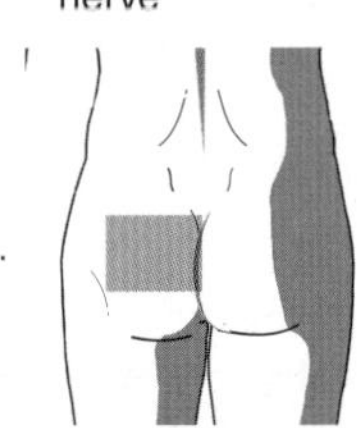

Fig. 16.30 The sacrotuberous ligament is reflected, revealing the obturator internus muscle, pudendal nerve, internal pudendal artery and vein, and sacrospinous ligament.

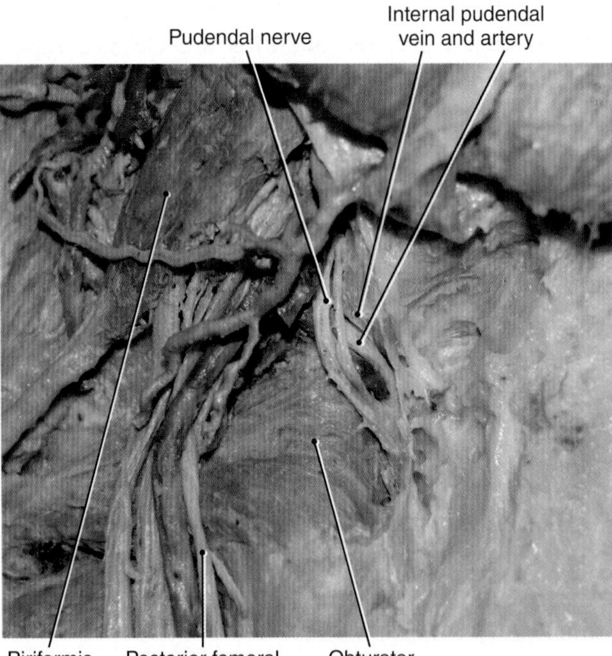

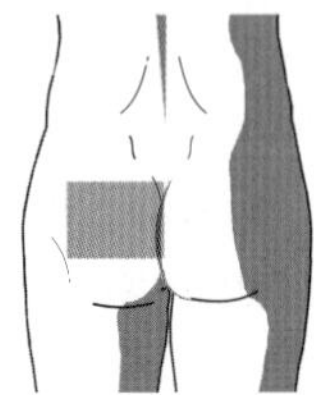

Fig. 16.29 Gluteus maximus muscle reflected, revealing the piriformis muscle, posterior femoral cutaneous nerve, obturator internus muscle, ischioanal fossa, pudendal nerve, and internal pudendal artery and vein.

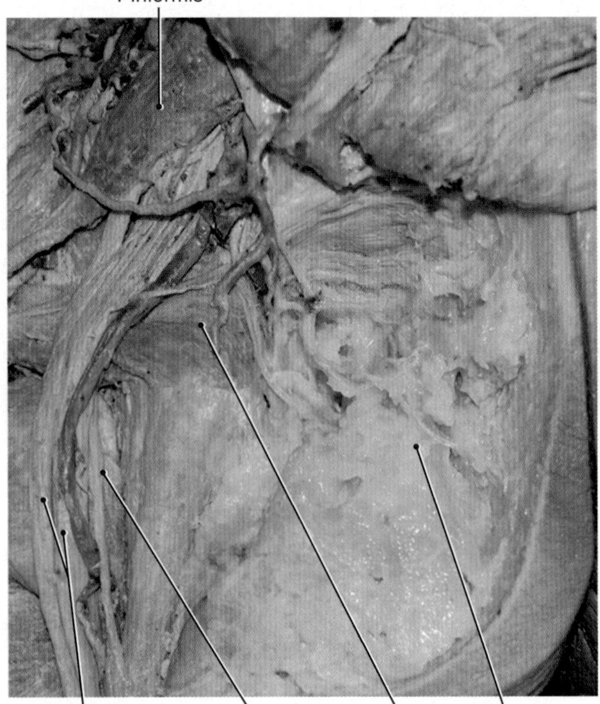

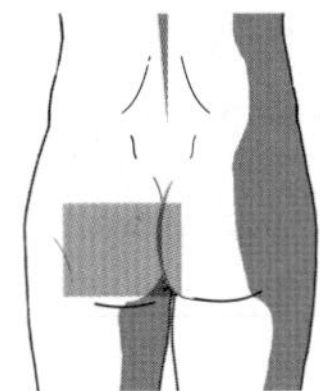

Fig. 16.31 Reflected gluteus maximus muscle reveals the piriformis and obturator internus muscles, tibial and common fibular nerves of sciatic nerve, posterior femoral cutaneous nerve, and ischioanal fossa.

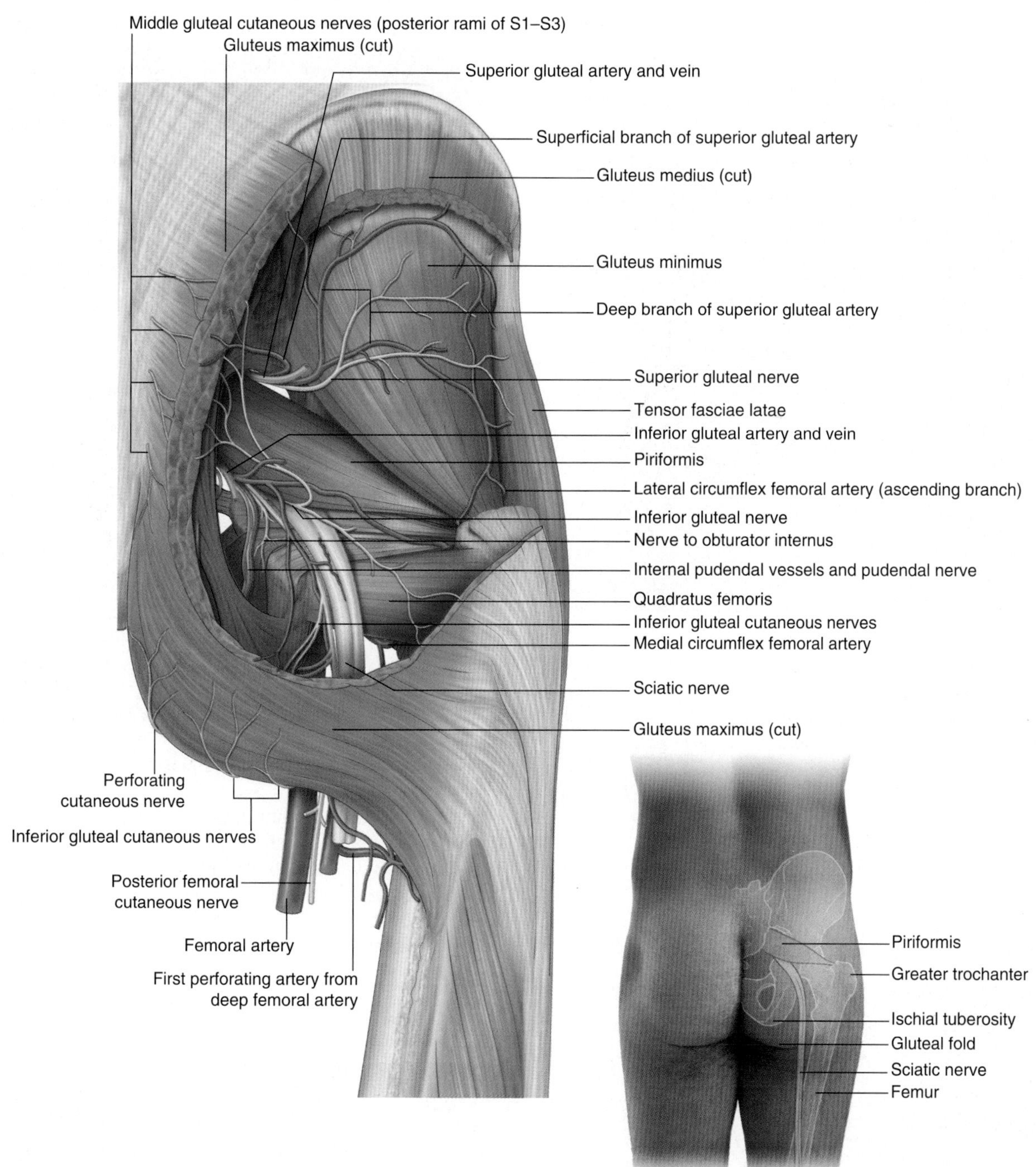

Plate 16.1 Arteries and nerves of the gluteal region and sciatic nerve in the gluteal region as it relates to the surface (posterior view). (From Drake RL et al. *Gray's Atlas of Anatomy*, 3rd edition, Philadelphia, Elsevier, 2021.)

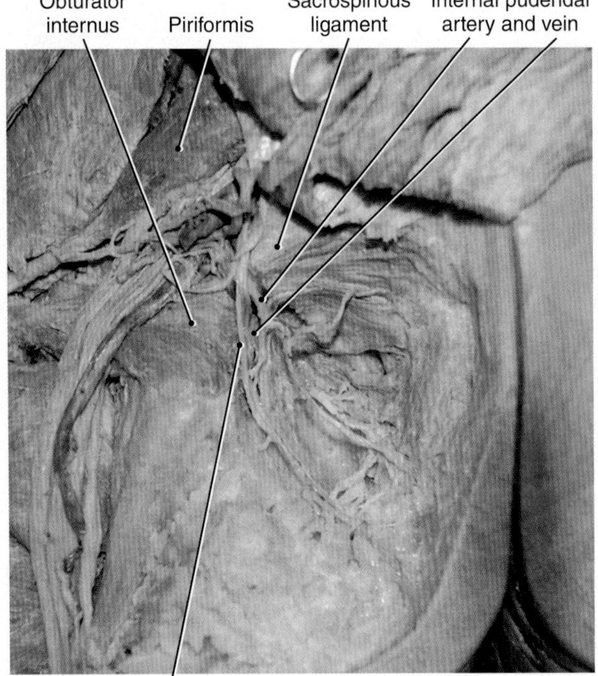

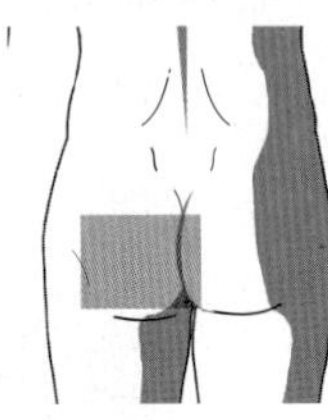

Fig. 16.32 Sacrotuberous ligament reflected, revealing obturator internus, pudendal nerve, internal pudendal artery and vein, and sacrospinous ligament.

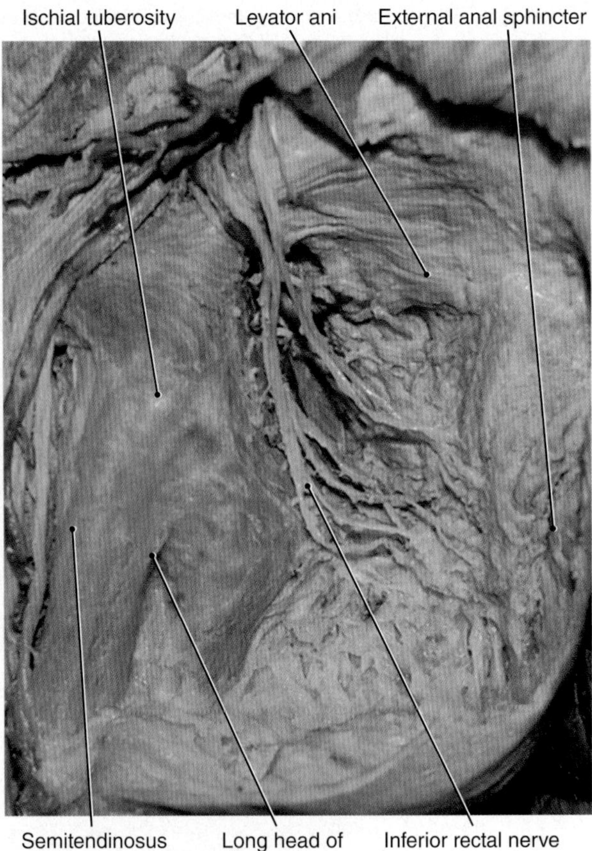

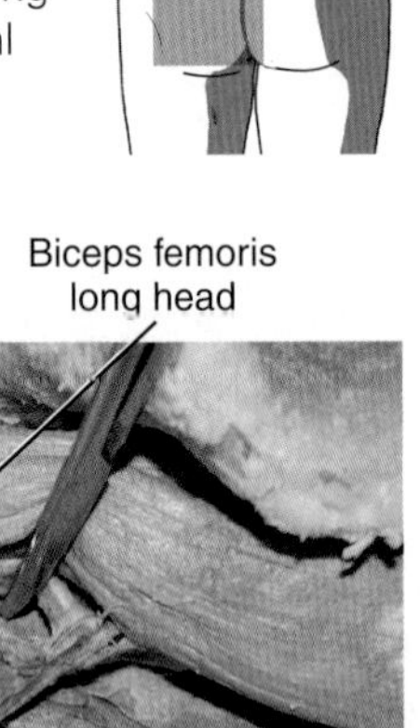

Fig. 16.33 Superior aspect of posterior thigh and ischioanal fossa, highlighting ischial tuberosity, "hamstring" muscles (semitendinosus, semimembranosus, long head of biceps femoris), and inferior anal nerve branches.

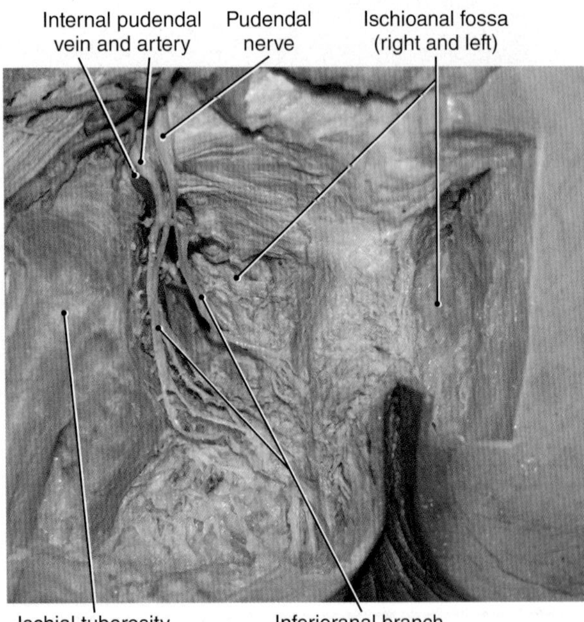

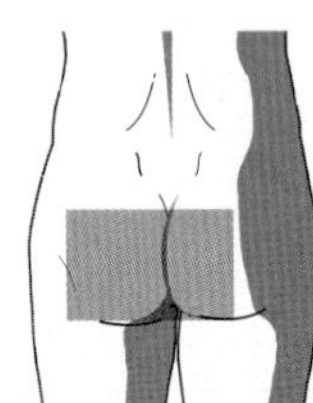

Fig. 16.34 Bilateral ischioanal fossae highlighting subcutaneous fat, the pudendal nerve, internal pudendal artery and vein, and the inferior anal nerve branches.

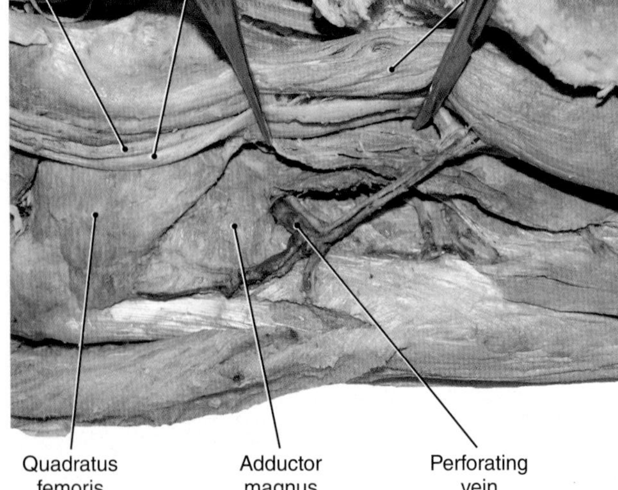

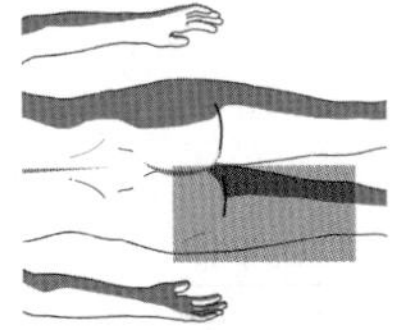

Fig. 16.35 Superior posterior thigh with retracted tibial and common fibular nerves and long head of biceps femoris muscle, highlighting the quadratus femoris and adductor longus muscles and perforating vein.

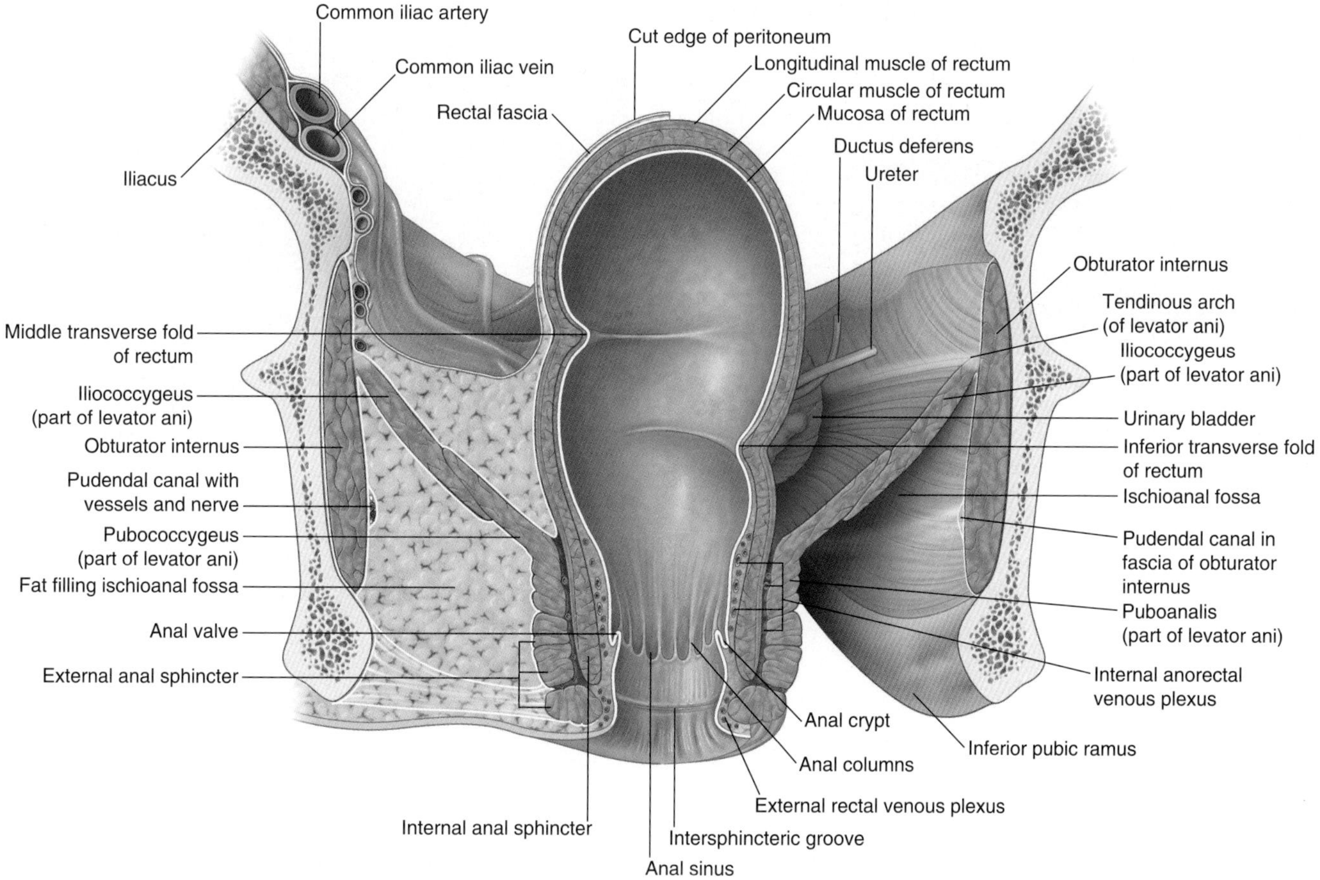

Plate 16.2 Coronal section through rectum and anal canal depicting the contents of ischioanal fossa. (From Drake RL et al. *Gray's Atlas of Anatomy*, 3rd edition, Philadelphia, Elsevier, 2021.)

- **With blunt dissection, separate the muscles of the posterior thigh ("hamstrings") and identify the long and short heads of the biceps femoris muscle as well as the semitendinosus and semimembranous muscles (Fig. 16.36).**
- **Dissect out their origins from the ischial tuberosity.**
- **Retract the long head of the biceps femoris laterally to expose the sciatic nerve.**
- **Note the division of the sciatic nerve into the tibial and common fibular (peroneal) nerves as it approaches the popliteal fossa (Fig. 16.37).**

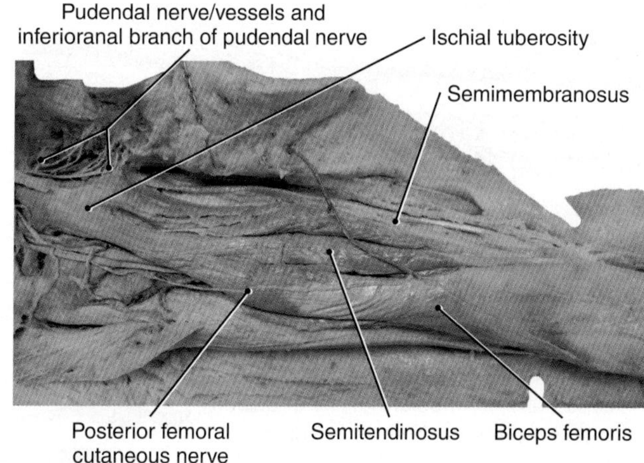

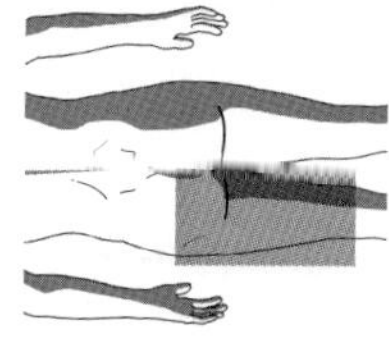

Fig. 16.36 Reflected skin and subcutaneous tissue of the posterior thigh and ischioanal fossa, revealing the pudendal nerve superiorly and inferior anal nerve inferiorly, internal pudendal artery and vein, ischial tuberosity, and biceps femoris, semitendinosus, and semimembranosus muscles.

DISSECTION **TIP**

Typically, the division of the sciatic nerve into the tibial and common fibular nerves occurs near the popliteal fossa. However, some cadavers may have a high split of the sciatic nerve, or two nerves may exit from the inferior border of the piriformis muscle, with a lateral nerve (common fibular) and a medial nerve (tibial).

- **Look at the lateral aspect of the sciatic nerve. The only branches to arise from its lateral surface innervate the short head of the biceps femoris muscle (Fig. 16.38).**
- **Clean the perforating arteries and veins, which provide the arterial supply and venous drainage of the posterior thigh (Figs. 16.39–16.41, Plate 16.3).**

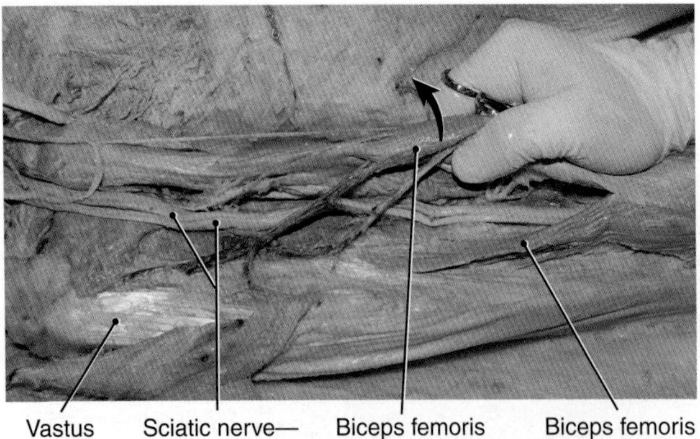

Fig. 16.37 Posterior thigh, highlighting the sciatic nerve (tibial/common fibular nerves) and biceps femoris muscle (long and short heads).

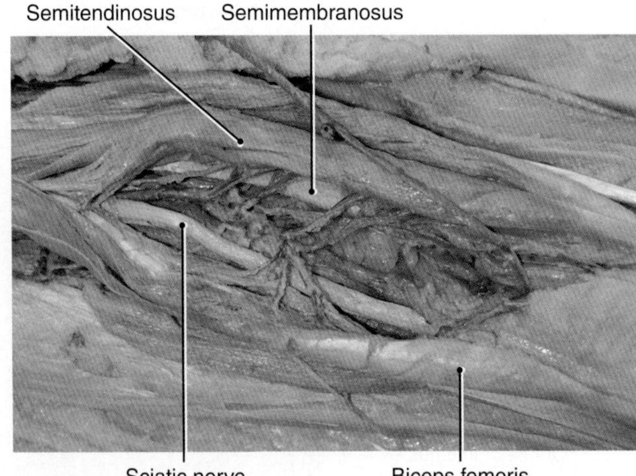

Fig. 16.39 Posterior thigh, highlighting sciatic nerve between the "hamstrings": biceps femoris lateral, semitendinosus medial and superficial, and semimembranosus muscle medial and deep.

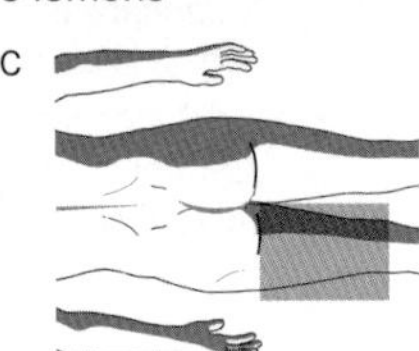

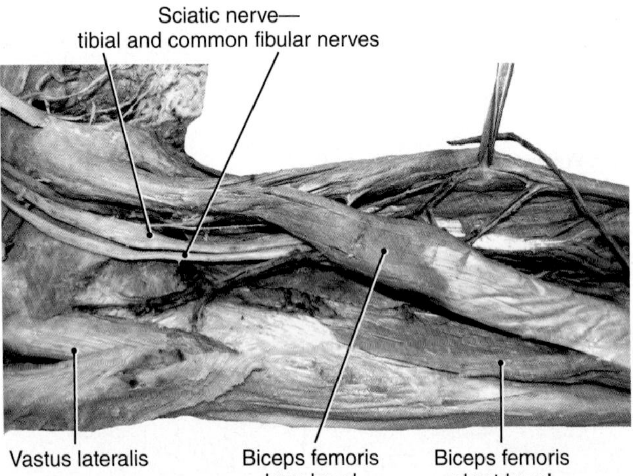

Fig. 16.38 Posterior thigh, showing the tibial and common fibular nerves of sciatic nerve and the long and short heads of biceps femoris muscle.

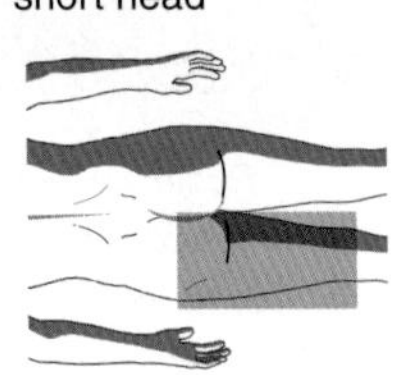

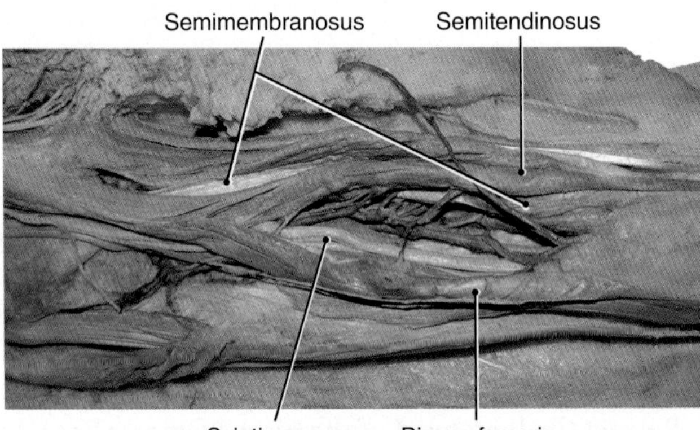

Fig. 16.40 Posterior thigh, showing the sciatic nerve between the hamstring muscles (biceps femoris, semitendinosus, semimembranosus).

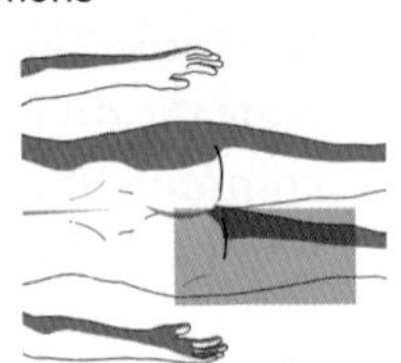

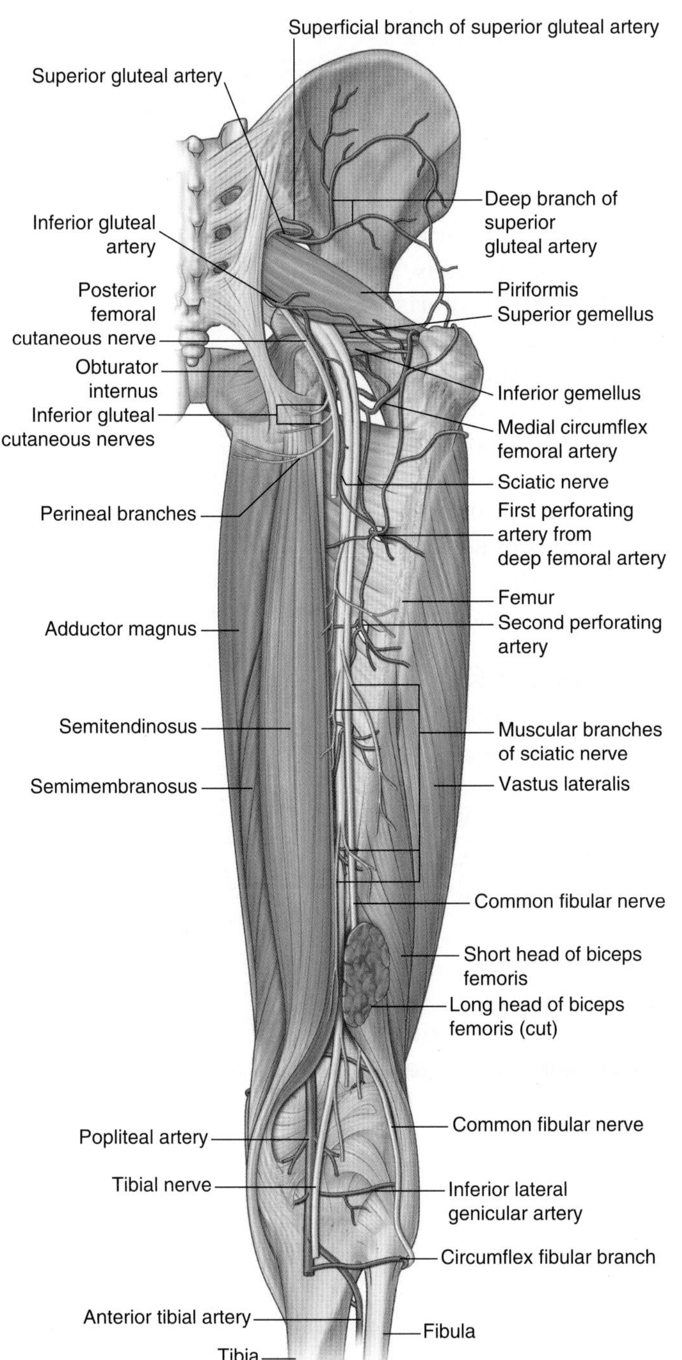

Plate 16.3 Arteries and nerves of the posterior thigh. (From Drake RL et al. *Gray's Atlas of Anatomy,* 3rd edition, Philadelphia, Elsevier, 2021.)

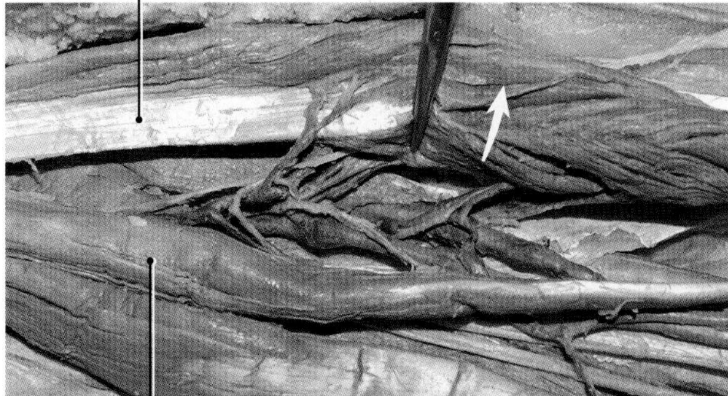

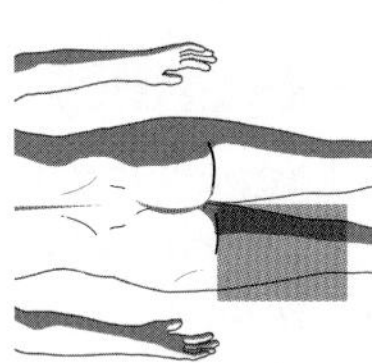

Fig. 16.41 Posterior thigh revealing musculature: biceps femoris laterally, semitendinosus reflected laterally, and semimembranosus medially.

LABORATORY IDENTIFICATION CHECKLIST

NERVES

- ☐ Superior gluteal
- ☐ Inferior gluteal
- ☐ Pudendal
  - ☐ Inferior anal
- ☐ Posterior femoral cutaneous
  - ☐ Sciatic
    - ☐ Tibial
    - ☐ Common fibular

ARTERIES

- ☐ Superior gluteal
- ☐ Inferior gluteal
- ☐ Internal pudendal
  - ☐ Inferior anorectal
- ☐ Medial circumflex femoral
- ☐ Perforating arteries

VEINS

- ☐ Superior gluteal
- ☐ Inferior gluteal
- ☐ Internal pudendal
- ☐ Perforating veins

MUSCLES

- ☐ Gluteus maximus
- ☐ Gluteus medius
- ☐ Gluteus minimus
- ☐ Piriformis
- ☐ Superior gemellus
- ☐ Obturator internus
- ☐ Inferior gemellus
- ☐ Quadratus femoris
- ☐ Semimembranosus
- ☐ Semitendinosus
- ☐ Biceps femoris
  - ☐ Long head
  - ☐ Short head
- ☐ Adductor minimus
- ☐ Tensor fasciae latae
- ☐ Levator ani
- ☐ External anal sphincter

LIGAMENTS

- ☐ Sacrotuberous
- ☐ Sacrospinous

FOSSA/CANAL

- ☐ Ischioanal fossa
- ☐ Alcock's canal

FASCIA

- ☐ Gluteal
- ☐ Obturator internus
- ☐ Lunate
- ☐ Fascia lata
- ☐ Iliotibial tract

BURSA

- ☐ Trochanteric bursa

BEFORE YOU BEGIN

Palpate the following bony landmarks on the cadaver or on yourself:

- Anterior superior iliac spine
- Pubic tubercle
- Pubic symphysis
- Greater trochanter of femur
- Medial and lateral femoral condyles
- Patella
- Tibial tuberosity
- Head and neck of fibula
- Medial and lateral malleoli of tibia and fibula, respectively

DISSECTION STEPS

- **Make a horizontal skin incision on the thigh 2 to 3 cm (~1 inch) inferior and parallel to the inguinal ligament.**
- **Leave the skin intact over the external genitalia.**
- **At the midpoint of this horizontal incision, make a vertical incision to the anterior portion of the patella.**
- **Make an encircling incision around the knee (Fig. 17.1).**
- **Reflect the skin medially over the thigh and identify the superficial veins (Fig. 17.2).**
- **Continue the dissection by making a vertical incision from the knee toward the ankle (Fig. 17.3).**
- **Make a transverse incision between the malleoli.**
- **Reflect the skin of the leg laterally (Fig. 17.4).**
- **Start exposing the superficial veins of the leg and thigh (Fig. 17.5).**
- **Identify the great saphenous vein and saphenous nerve (Fig. 17.6).**
- **Clean the superficial fascia over the *great saphenous vein*, starting from the ankle toward the knee (Fig. 17.7).**

ANATOMY NOTE

Around the knee, the saphenous nerve is located deep to the great saphenous vein. In the leg medial to the tibia, however, the great saphenous vein runs parallel with the saphenous nerve (Fig. 17.8). The great saphenous vein arises from the medial side of the dorsal venous arch of the foot and ascends anterior to the medial malleolus, along the medial side of the leg and thigh, finally draining into the femoral vein.

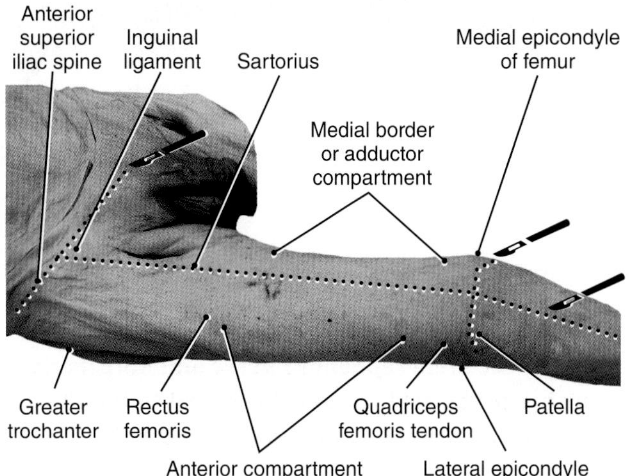

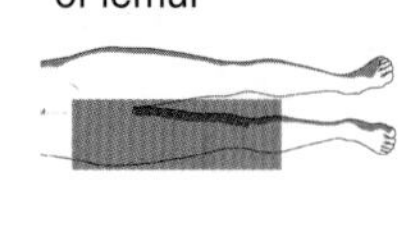

Fig. 17.1 Three thigh dissection incisions: horizontal cut inferior and parallel to inguinal ligament, vertical cut to anterior patella at midpoint of horizontal incision, and encircling cut around the knee.

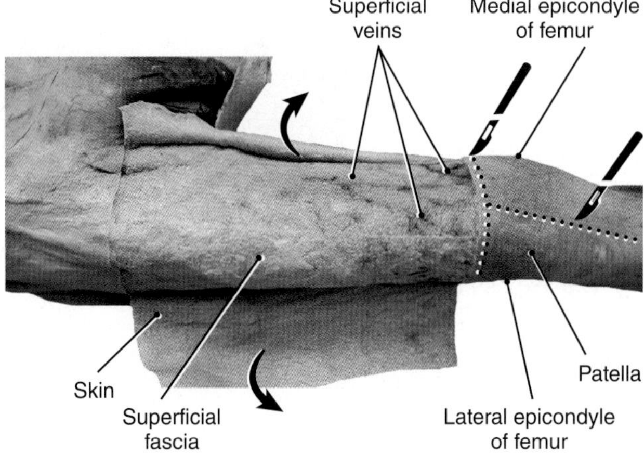

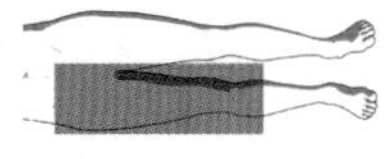

Fig. 17.2 Skin reflected medially over thigh, revealing superficial veins.

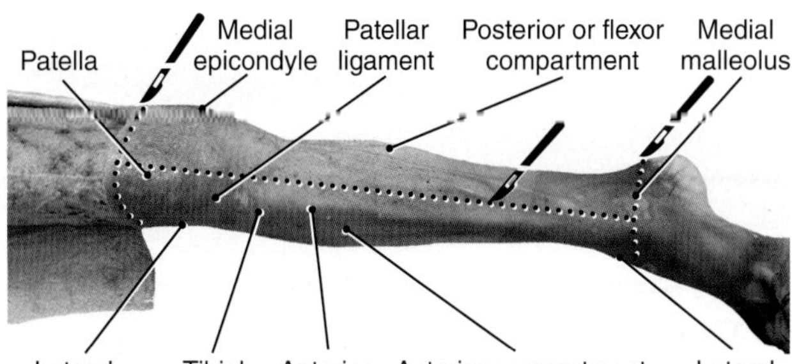

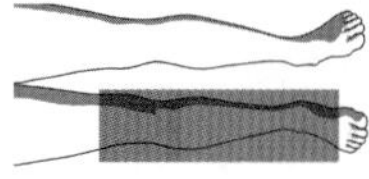

Fig. 17.3 Vertical incision from the knee toward the ankle and transverse incision between the malleoli.

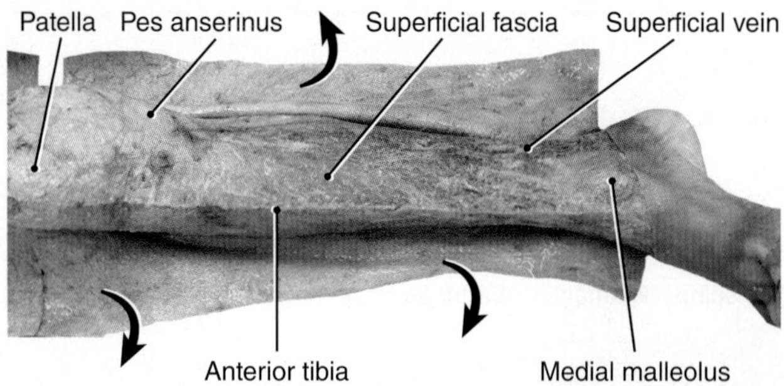

Fig. 17.4 Transverse cut between the malleoli, with skin of leg reflected.

- Identify the great saphenous nerve and note its relationship to the saphenous vein medial to the tibia.
- Remove the skin from the posterior aspect of the leg to the ankle (Fig. 17.9).
- Leave the superficial and deep fasciae (crural fascia) intact.
- Identify the *small* (lesser) *saphenous vein*, which begins from the lateral aspect of the dorsal venous arch of the foot.

ANATOMY **NOTE**

The small saphenous vein ascends just inferior to the lateral malleolus, accompanying the sural nerve, and finally drains into the popliteal vein (Fig. 17.10).

- Identify the sural nerve.
- Observe the sural nerve and the small saphenous vein as they penetrate the deep crural fascia to travel to the popliteal fossa (Fig. 17.11).
- On the anterior part of the leg, on its medial side over the patellar ligament, expose the infrapatellar branch of the saphenous nerve (Fig. 17.12).
- Follow the great saphenous vein toward the thigh and clean the fat off the superficial fascia around the vein (Fig. 17.13).

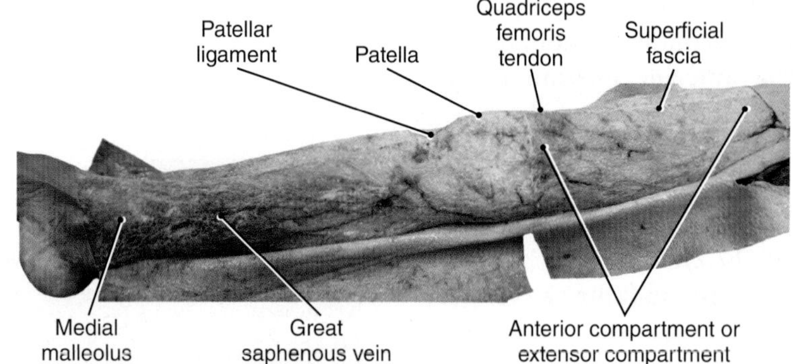

Fig. 17.5 Exposure of superficial veins of the leg and thigh.

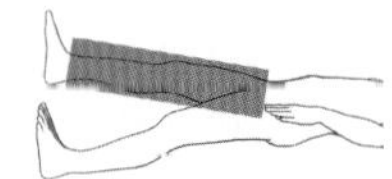

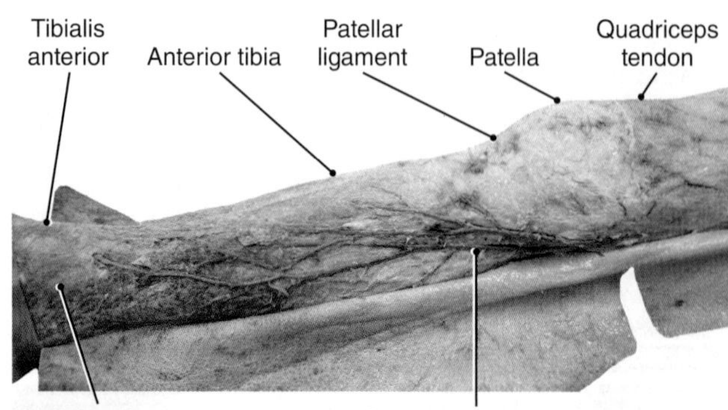

Fig. 17.6 Skin of leg reflected, showing great saphenous vein and tibialis anterior muscle.

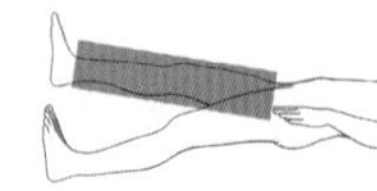

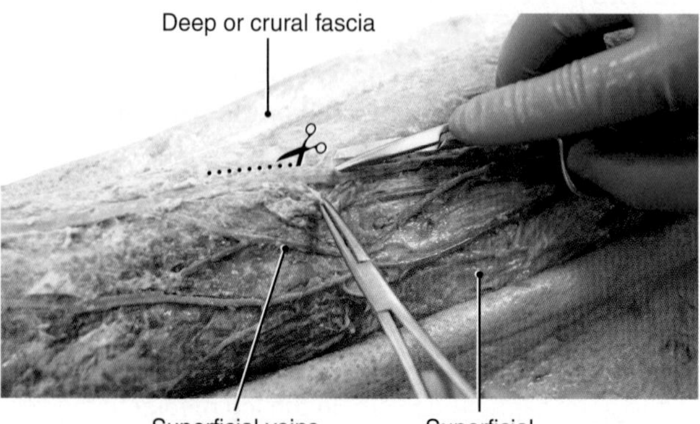

Fig. 17.7 Superficial fascia cleaned away over great saphenous vein.

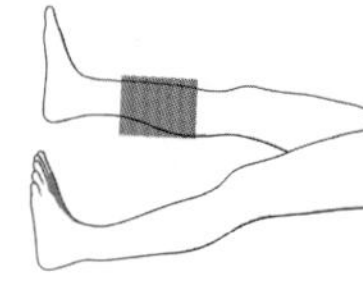

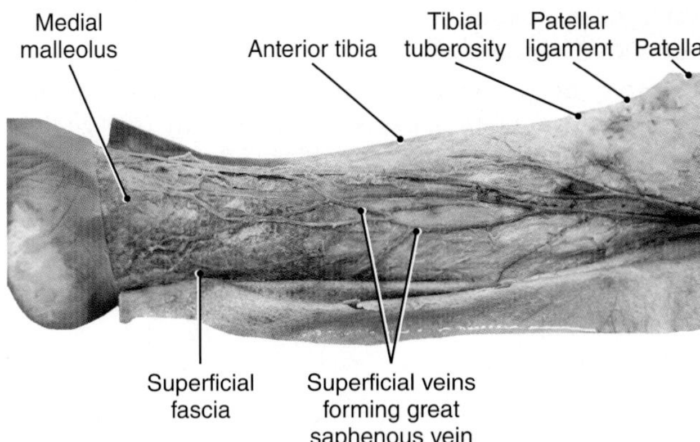

Fig. 17.8 In the leg medial to the tibia, note how the great saphenous vein runs parallel with the saphenous nerve.

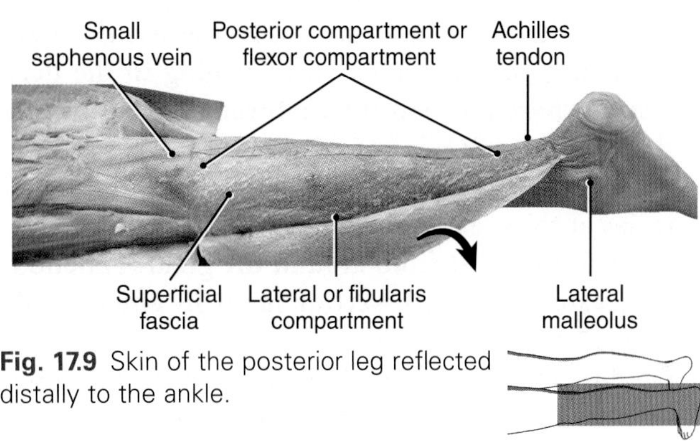

Fig. 17.9 Skin of the posterior leg reflected distally to the ankle.

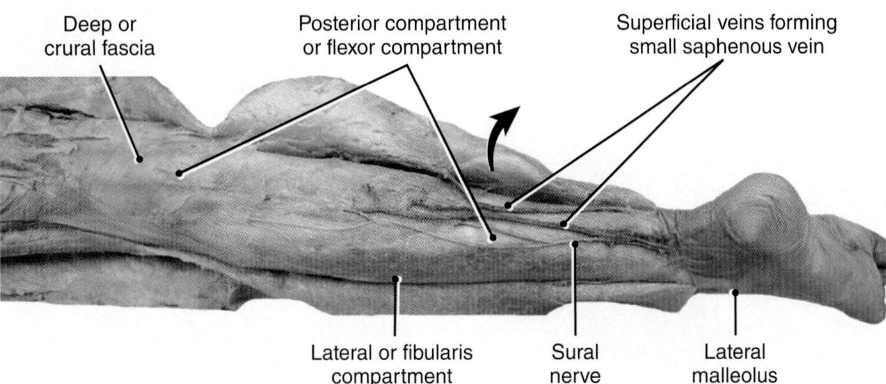

Fig. 17.10 Skin of leg reflected, revealing the posterior and lateral compartments of the leg, deep fascia, and small saphenous vein.

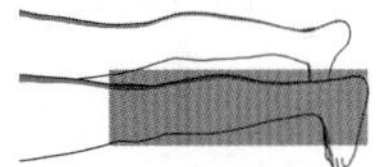

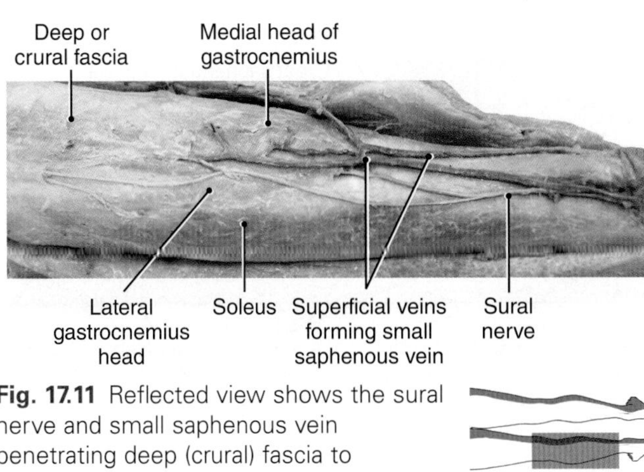

Fig. 17.11 Reflected view shows the sural nerve and small saphenous vein penetrating deep (crural) fascia to travel to popliteal fossa.

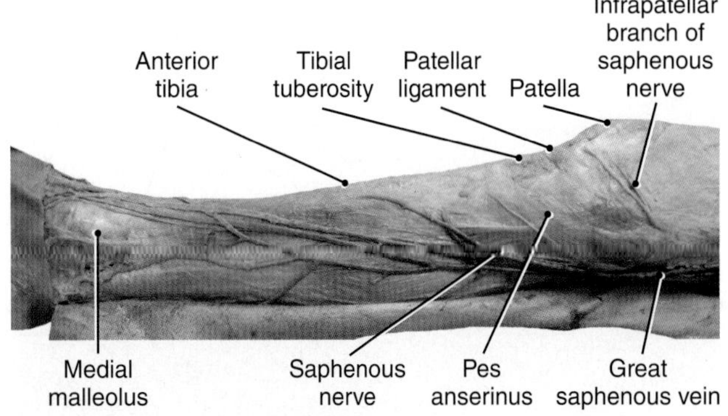

Fig. 17.12 Infrapatellar branch of saphenous nerve exposed on the medial side of the anterior leg over the patellar ligament.

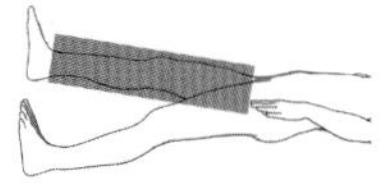

- Expose the great saphenous vein toward the *fossa ovalis* (saphenous hiatus), the opening in the deep fascia, where the vein travels through to drain into the femoral vein.
- Expose the superficial and deep perforating tributaries of the great saphenous vein (Fig. 17.14).
- Start cleaning fat from around the great saphenous vein, extending the dissection medially and laterally (Fig. 17.15).
- Do not cut through the deep fascia of the thigh but identify the anterior cutaneous branches of the femoral nerve intermingled with the tributaries of the great saphenous vein.
- Lateral to the vein, identify the rectus femoris muscle.
- On top of and lateral to the muscle, identify the lateral femoral cutaneous nerves (Fig. 17.16).

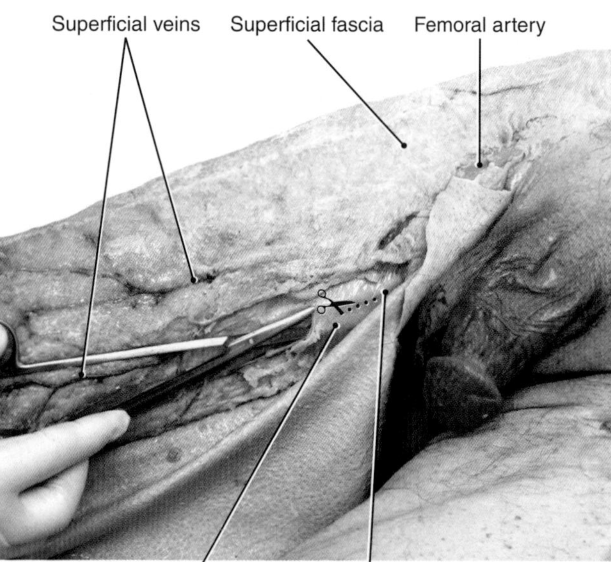

Fig. 17.13 Fat of superficial fascia cleaned away from around the great saphenous vein.

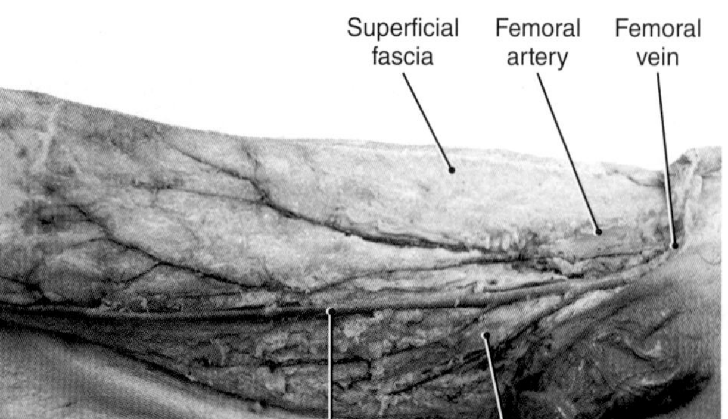

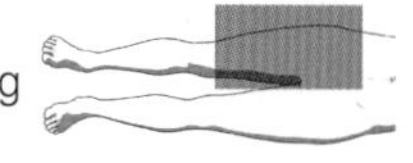

Fig. 17.14 View of the great saphenous vein and its superficial and deep perforating tributaries.

DISSECTION TIP

Observe the lymphatics in the area of the fossa ovalis, but do not spend time exposing all of them. Realize that the inguinal nodes are so named based on their position relative to the deep fascia lata. The deep inguinal nodes are located deep to it, whereas the superficial nodes are superficial to the deep fascia.

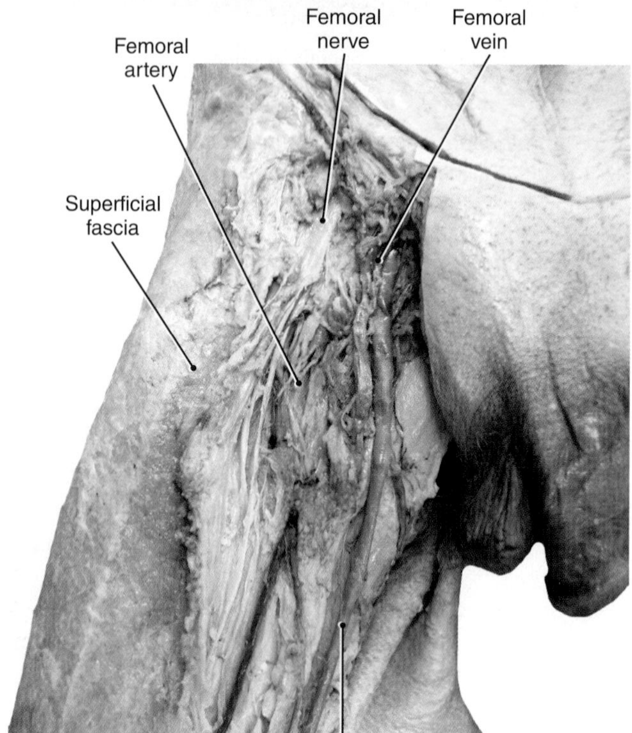

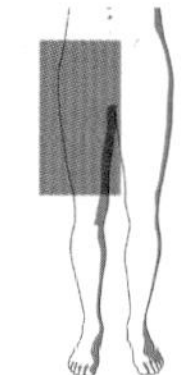

Fig. 17.15 Fat cleaned away from around the great saphenous vein, with dissection extended medially and laterally.

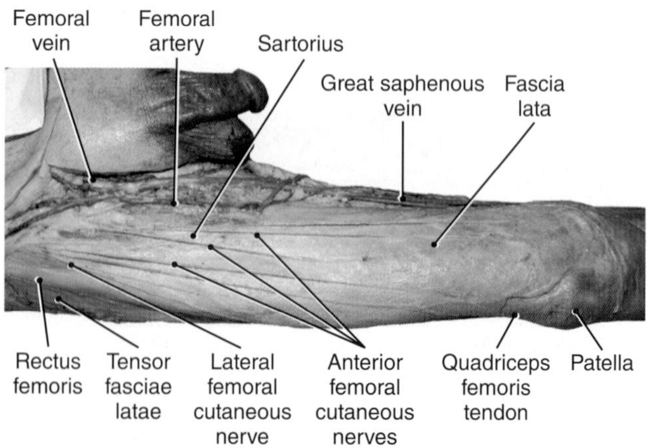

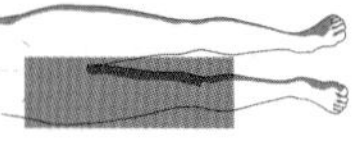

Fig. 17.16 Appreciate the anterior cutaneous branches of the femoral nerve intermingled with tributaries of the great saphenous vein and rectus femoris muscle with lateral femoral cutaneous nerve.

- Cut the distal ends of the cutaneous nerves you previously dissected.
- Reflect the nerves medially and preserve them.
- Cut the deep fascia of the thigh, *fascia lata,* and expose the sartorius muscle (Fig. 17.17).
- Continue reflecting the fascia lata over the vastus medialis muscle (Fig. 17.18).
- Expose the quadriceps femoris muscles of the extensor compartment of the thigh; the vastus medialis, lateralis, and intermedius muscles; and the rectus femoris muscle and their tendons attaching to the patella.
- Continue the exposure by noting the fascia lata laterally and its thickened distal part, the *iliotibial tract,* attaching to the lateral condyle of the tibia (Fig. 17.19).
- Reflect the rectus femoris muscle medially and expose the vastus intermedius muscle underneath (Fig. 17.20).
- Place the cutaneous nerves back in their original position over the dissected muscles and appreciate their location (Fig. 17.21).

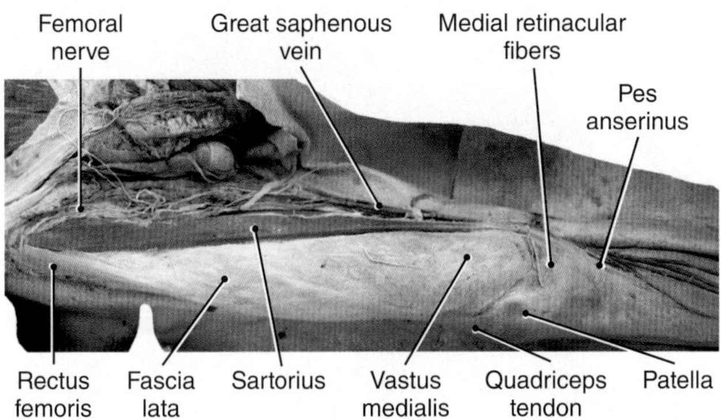

Fig. 17.17 Distal ends of dissected cutaneous nerve reflected, with deep fascia (fascia lata) cut, exposing the sartorius muscle.

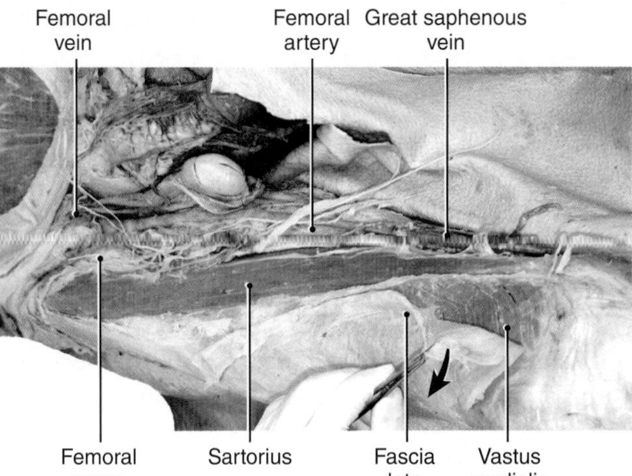

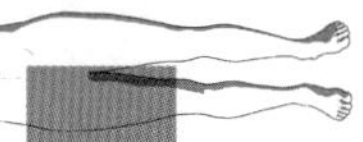

Fig. 17.18 View of fascia lata reflected over vastus medialis muscle.

- Expose the femoral vein and dissect out the *cribriform fascia,* which fills the saphenous hiatus (Fig. 17.22).
- Cut the femoral sheath around the femoral artery and vein.
- Note the relationship between the femoral artery and vein; the femoral artery is located lateral to the femoral vein. The femoral nerve lies lateral to the femoral artery (Fig. 17.23).

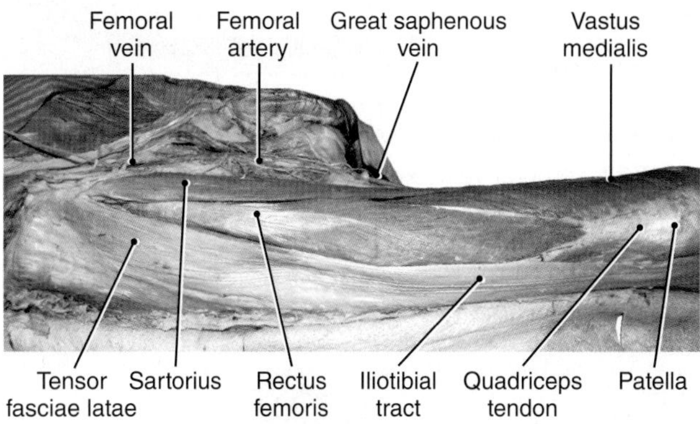

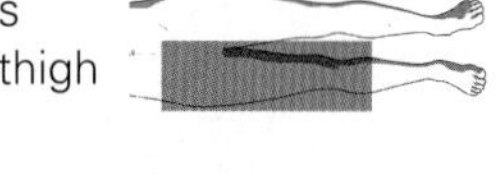

Fig. 17.19 Exposed quadriceps femoris muscles of extensor compartment of thigh with tendon attaching to the patella.

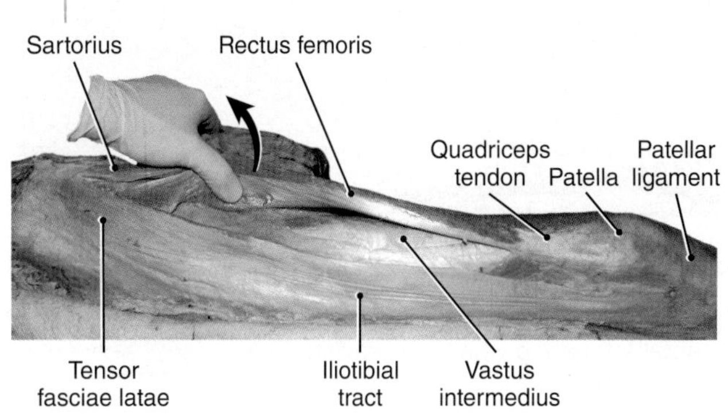

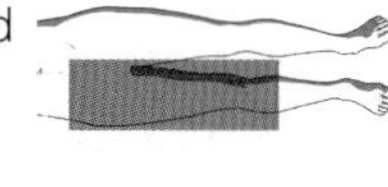

Fig. 17.20 Rectus femoris muscle reflected medially, exposing the vastus intermedius muscle.

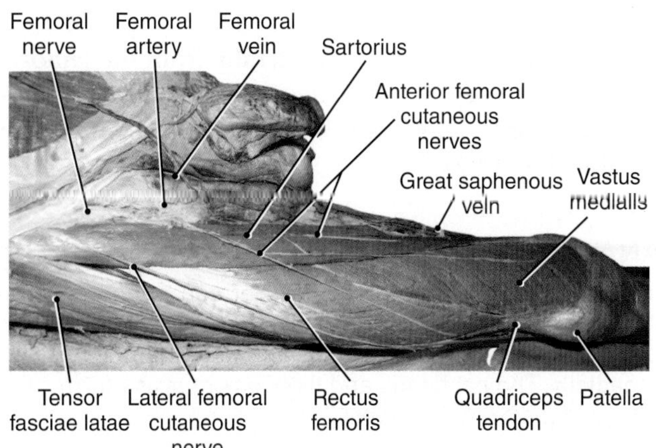

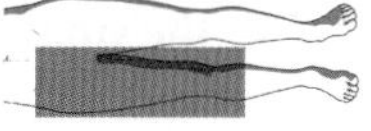

Fig. 17.21 Appreciate the position of the cutaneous nerves of the anterior thigh.

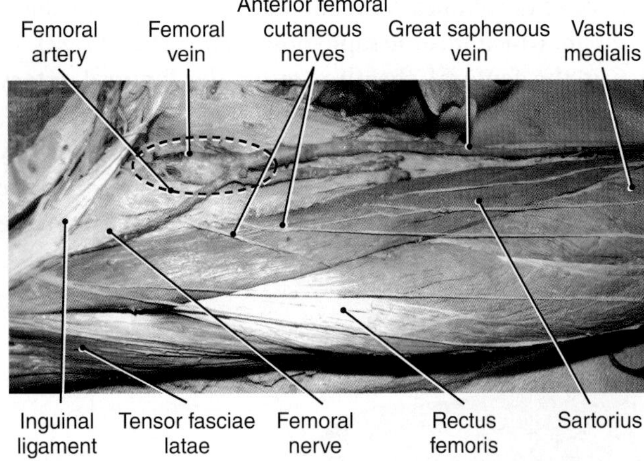

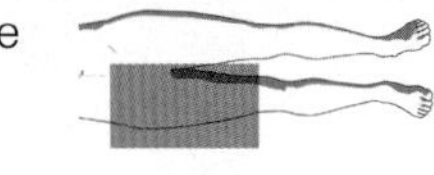

Fig. 17.22 Femoral vein exposed, and the cribriform fascia that fills the saphenous hiatus *(dashed line)* is dissected.

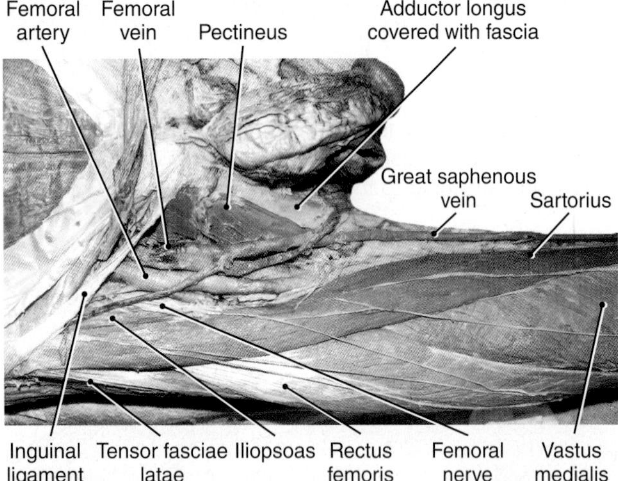

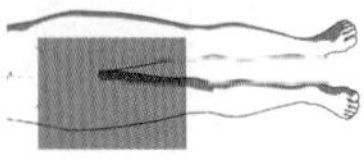

Fig. 17.23 Femoral sheath incised around femoral artery and vein to appreciate their relationship.

- Clean the fascia covering the femoral artery and vein and trace these vessels underneath the inguinal ligament to the femoral triangle.
- Continue removing fat and expose the adductor longus and gracilis muscles medially (Fig. 17.24).
- Retract the femoral artery laterally from the femoral vein, and deep between these vessels, note the iliopsoas muscle lying over the anterior aspect of the hip joint (Fig. 17.25).

ANATOMY **NOTE**

The area you just dissected is called the *femoral triangle*, formed by the inguinal ligament superiorly, the sartorius muscle laterally, and the adductor longus muscle medially. The pectineus and iliopsoas muscles form the floor of the triangle (Plate 17.1).

- Cut the smaller venous tributaries draining to the femoral vein for better exposure of the femoral triangle.

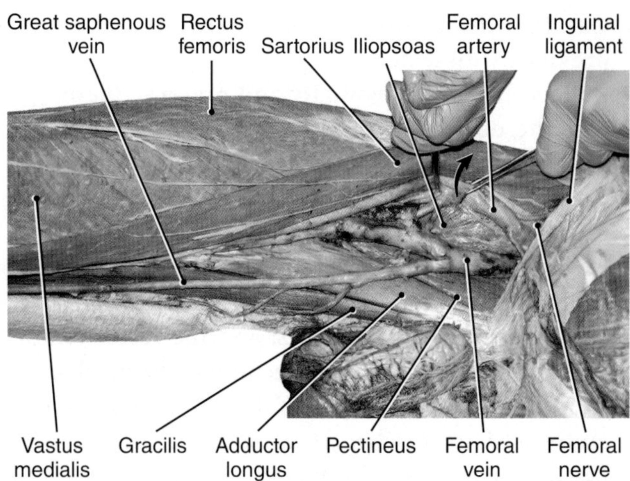

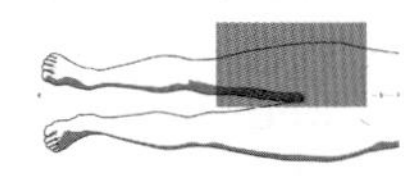

Fig. 17.24 View of femoral artery and vein underneath inguinal ligament showing adductor longus and gracilis muscles.

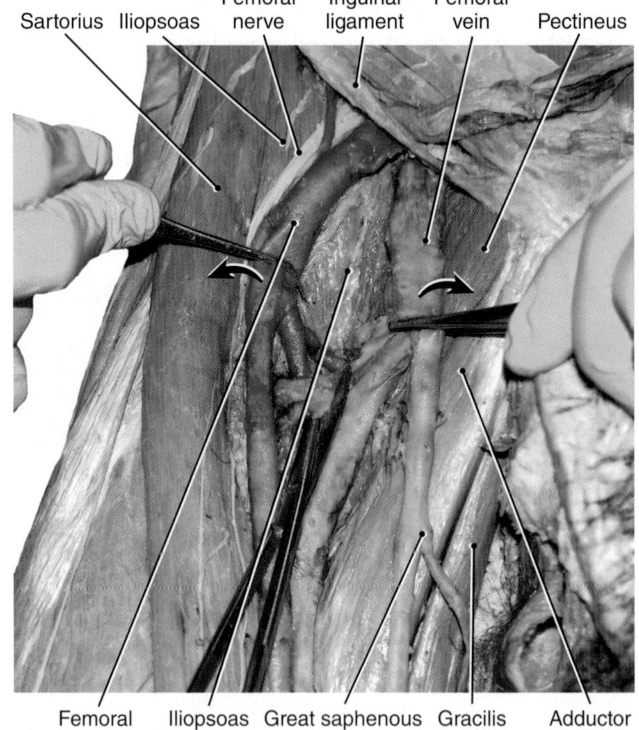

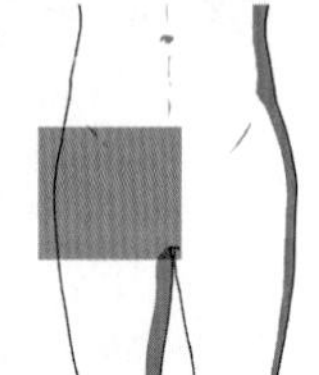

Fig. 17.25 Femoral artery retracted laterally from the femoral vein, highlighting deep-lying iliopsoas muscle over anterior aspect of capsule of hip joint.

- Medial to the iliopsoas muscle, note the pectineus muscle, and more medially, the adductor longus muscle.
- Clean the femoral artery and vein proximal to the femoral canal and trace the lateral femoral cutaneous nerve underneath the inguinal ligament, just medial to the anterior superior iliac spine (Fig. 17.26).

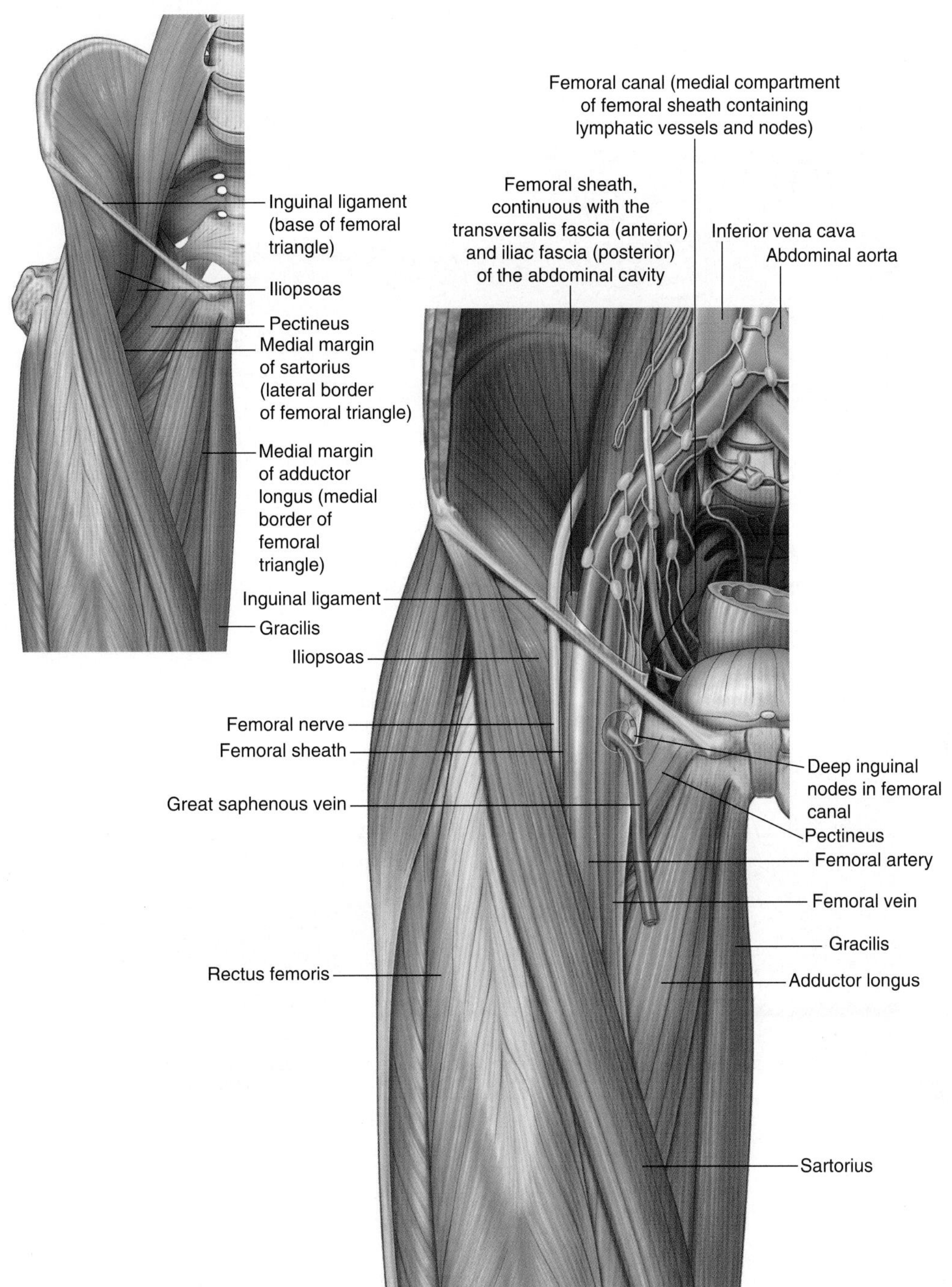

Plate 17.1 Borders and contents of the femoral triangle. (From Drake RL et al. *Gray's Atlas of Anatomy*, 3rd edition, Philadelphia, Elsevier, 2021.)

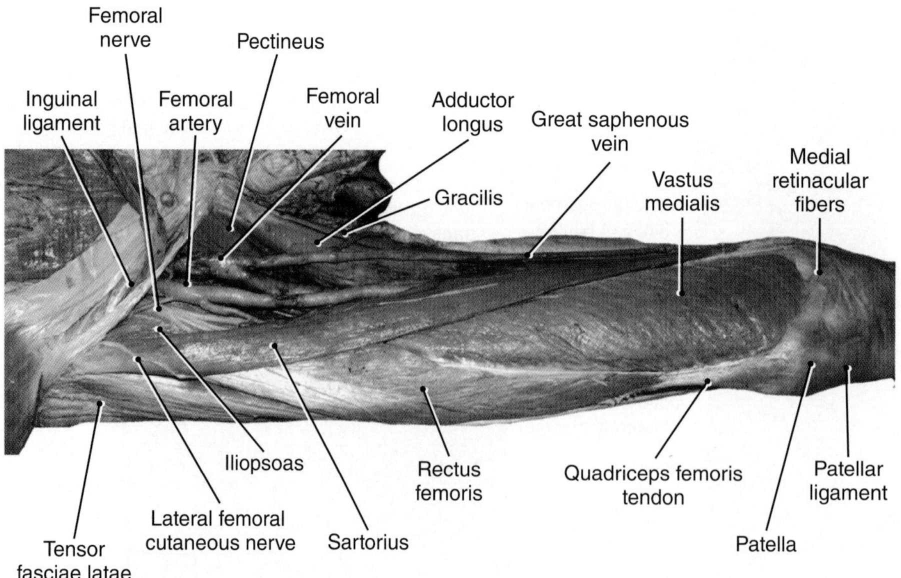

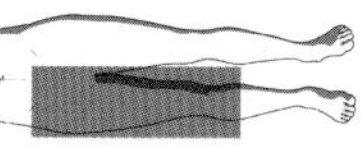

Fig. 17.26 Femoral artery and vein cleaned proximal to femoral canal, showing the lateral femoral cutaneous nerve.

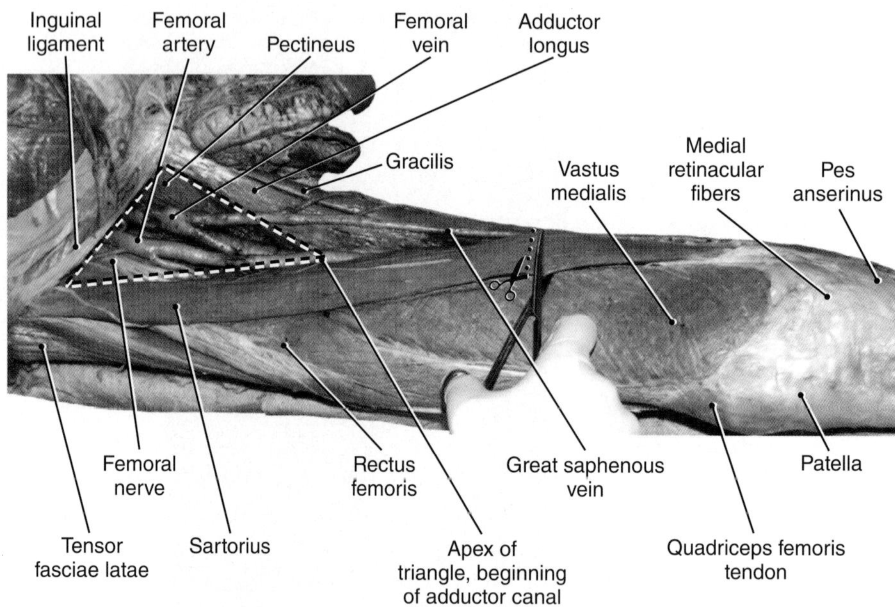

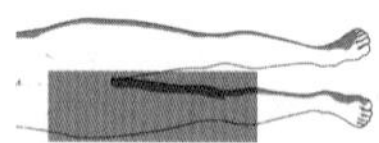

Fig. 17.27 Smaller tributaries draining the femoral vein cut to expose the femoral triangle *(outline)* and appreciate the pectineus and adductor longus muscles.

- **Cut the sartorius muscle at its distal quarter and expose the adductor canal (Figs. 17.27 and 17.28).**

ANATOMY **NOTE**

The adductor canal is formed by the adductor magnus, adductor longus, and vastus medialis muscles. The canal begins at the apex of the femoral triangle and ends at the adductor hiatus, which is the canal formed by the adductor magnus tendon at the posterior knee. After passing through the adductor hiatus and reaching the posterior part of the knee, the femoral artery and femoral vein are termed the *popliteal artery* and *popliteal vein* (Fig. 17.29).

- **Within the adductor canal, expose and identify the femoral artery, femoral vein, saphenous nerve, nerve to the vastus medialis muscle, and the descending genicular artery (see Fig. 17.29).**
- **Expose the aperture in the tendon of insertion of the adductor magnus, the adductor hiatus (Fig. 17.30).**
- **Identify the nerve to the vastus medialis muscle and trace the nerve to its termination on the muscle.**
- **Distal to the level of the adductor hiatus, trace the saphenous nerve and expose it at the posteromedial aspect of the knee where it meets the great saphenous vein.**

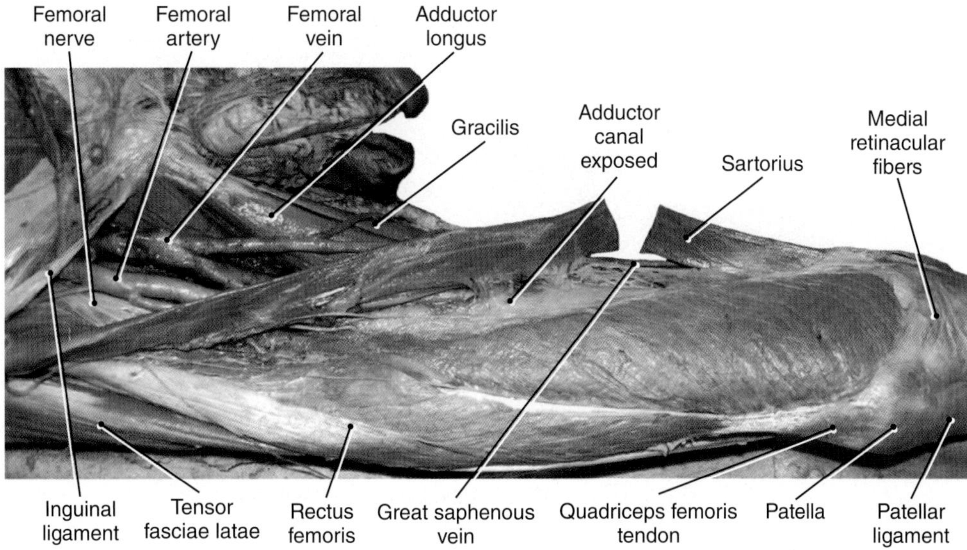

Fig. 17.28 View of cut sartorius muscle, exposing the adductor canal.

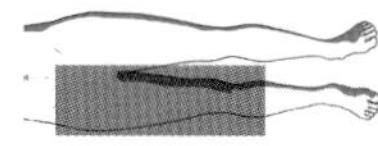

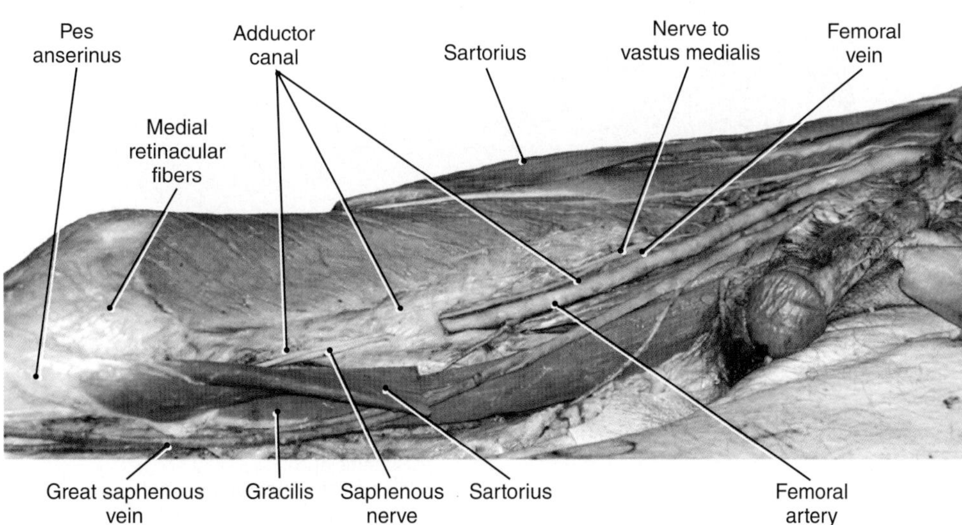

Fig. 17.29 View of the femoral artery and vein, saphenous nerve, nerve to vastus medialis muscle, and descending genicular artery within the adductor canal.

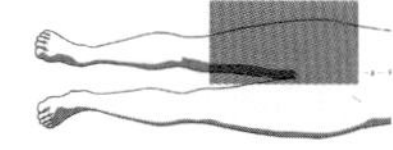

- **With scissors, cut the femoral vein a few centimeters inferior to the femoral canal and reflect it inferiorly (Figs. 17.31 and 17.32).**
- **Fully expose the pectineus, adductor longus, and gracilis muscles.**
- **Pull the femoral artery medially and dissect out its branches (Figs. 17.33 and 17.34).**
- **Identify the lateral circumflex femoral artery and expose its descending branch supplying the vastus lateralis, which travels in the muscle between the vastus lateralis and vastus intermedius (this is a fairly constant dissection landmark).**

ANATOMY **NOTE**

The lateral circumflex femoral artery also gives off several perforating branches to the vastus intermedius.

- **Continue the dissection by exposing the deep femoral artery *(profunda femoris)* deep to the adductor longus muscle (see Figs. 17.33 and 17.34, Plate 17.2).**
- **Expose several of the perforating branches mainly supplying the posterior compartment of the thigh.**
- **Identify the medial circumflex femoral artery and expose it between the iliopsoas and pectineus muscles.**

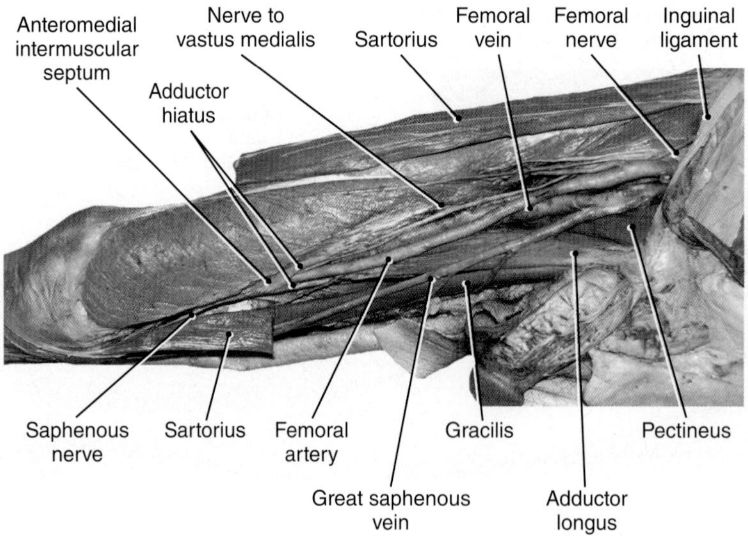

Fig. 17.30 View of the adductor hiatus, the aperture in the tendon of insertion of the adductor magnus muscle.

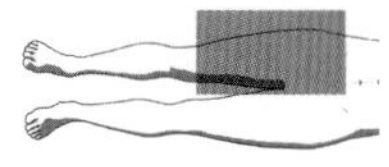

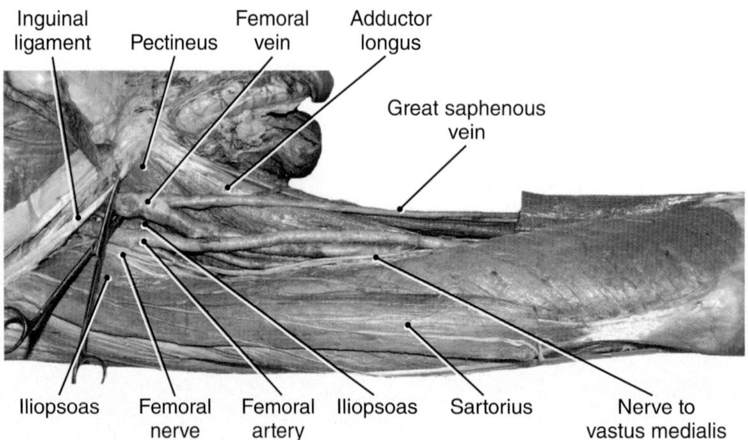

Fig. 17.31 View of the musculature with the femoral vein incised inferior to the femoral canal.

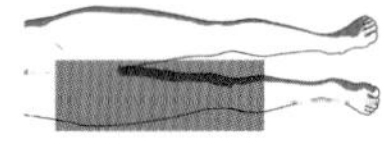

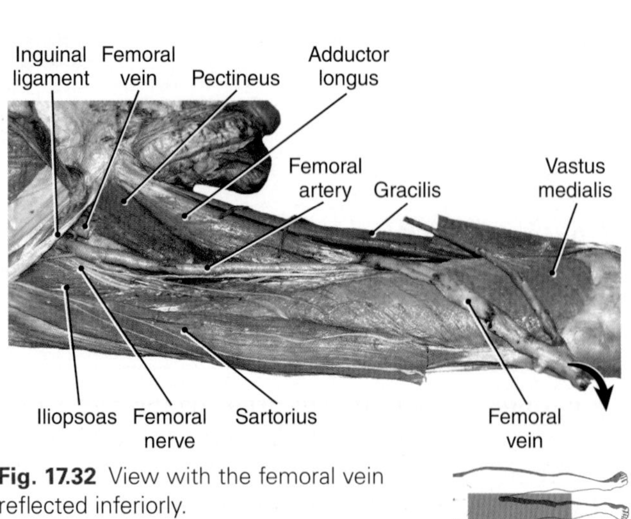

Fig. 17.32 View with the femoral vein reflected inferiorly.

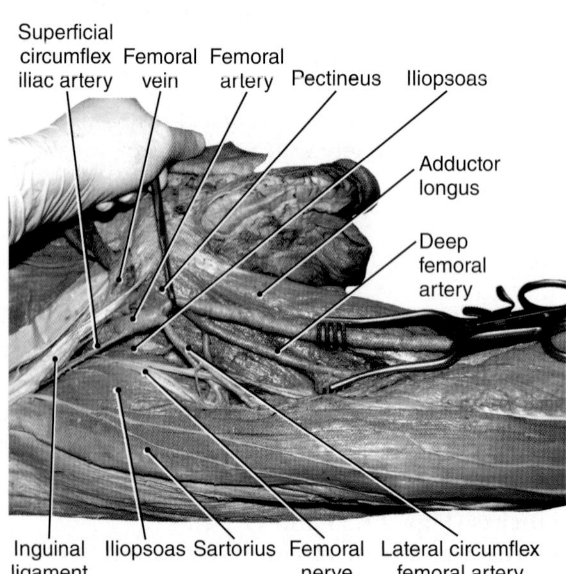

Fig. 17.33 Femoral artery pulled medially and its branches dissected.

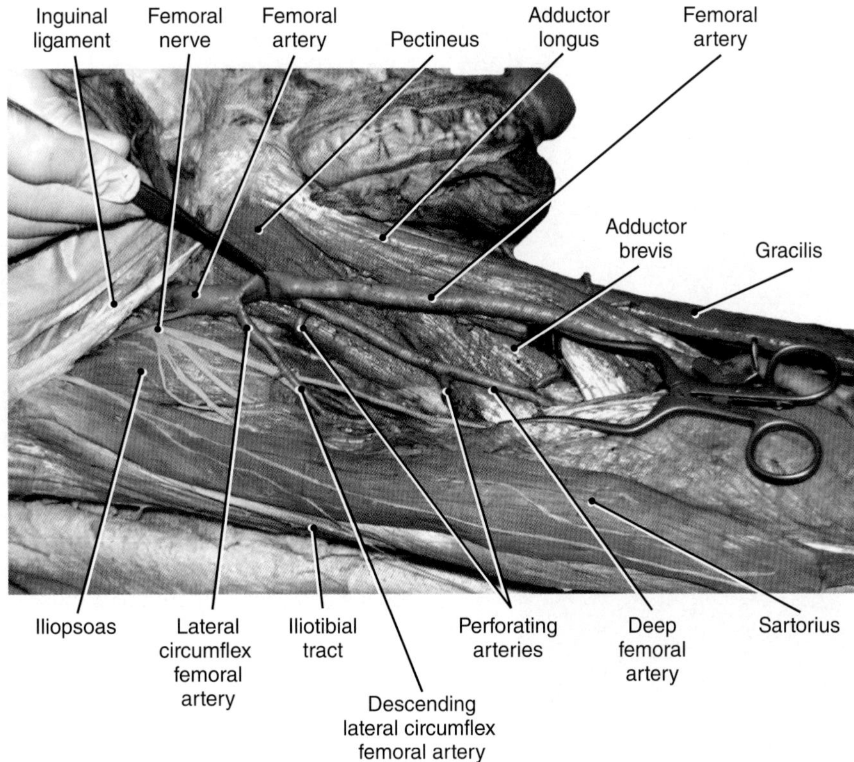

Fig. 17.34 Appreciate the lateral circumflex femoral artery and its descending branch.

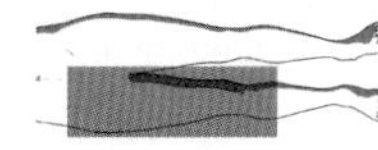

DISSECTION **TIP**

If it is large enough, dissect out the transverse branch of the lateral circumflex femoral artery running to the posterior surface of the femur below the greater trochanter and contributing to the so-called cruciate anastomosis. Look for an ascending branch from the lateral circumflex femoral artery that runs upward to anastomose with the deep circumflex iliac and superior gluteal arteries. In some specimens, a retractor is useful to retract the tissues between the adductor longus and vastus intermedius muscles.

DISSECTION **TIP**

Remember that an artery's name is based on its distribution, not its origin. The lateral circumflex femoral, medial circumflex femoral, and deep femoral arteries commonly originate from a common trunk.

If time permits, from the exposed femoral artery, look for the following arteries:

- **Superficial circumflex iliac artery, which travels toward the anterior superior iliac spine.**
- **Superficial epigastric artery, which travels upward toward the anterolateral abdominal wall, crossing over the inguinal canal.**
- **Superficial and deep external pudendal vessels typically are small arteries that anastomose with branches of the internal pudendal artery. Do not attempt to identify these two vessels.**

ANATOMY **NOTE**

The so-called cruciate anastomosis classically involves the confluence of four arteries posterior to the proximal part of the femur: (1) the transverse branch of the lateral circumflex femoral artery, (2) the medial circumflex femoral artery, (3) the descending branch of the inferior gluteal artery, and (4) the ascending branch of the first perforating artery.

DISSECTION **TIP**

From personal observations, the *transverse* branch of the lateral circumflex femoral artery is only rarely significant in this anastomosis, although the *ascending* branch does participate. Actually, the transverse branch of the lateral circumflex femoral artery may be very small or absent.

ANATOMY **NOTE**

Anastomoses around the hip also involve other vessels such as the superior gluteal, iliolumbar, deep circumflex iliac, ascending branch of the lateral circumflex femoral, and the obturator arteries. Therefore with occlusion of the femoral artery, many possible routes can form a collateral circulation between the iliac arteries and the lower limb.

- **In the space between the adductor longus and vastus intermedius muscles, identify the adductor brevis muscle (Fig. 17.35).**
- **With scissors, cut the pectineus muscle just inferior to the inguinal ligament and reflect it laterally (Fig. 17.36).**

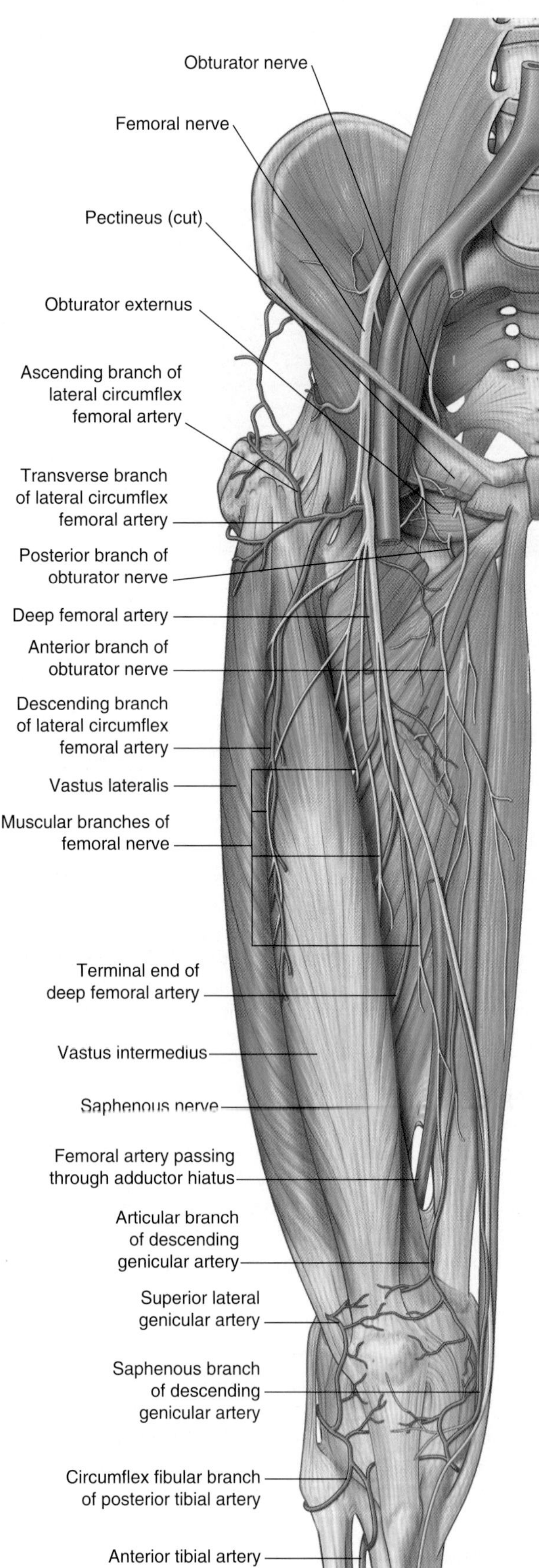

Plate 17.2 Deep arteries and nerves of the thigh. (From Drake RL et al. *Gray's Atlas of Anatomy*, 3rd edition, Philadelphia, Elsevier, 2021.)

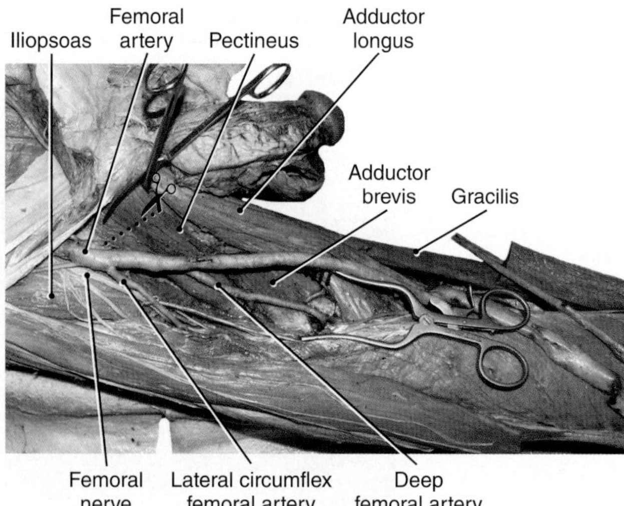

Fig. 17.35 Appreciate the adductor brevis muscle in the space between the adductor longus and vastus intermedius muscles.

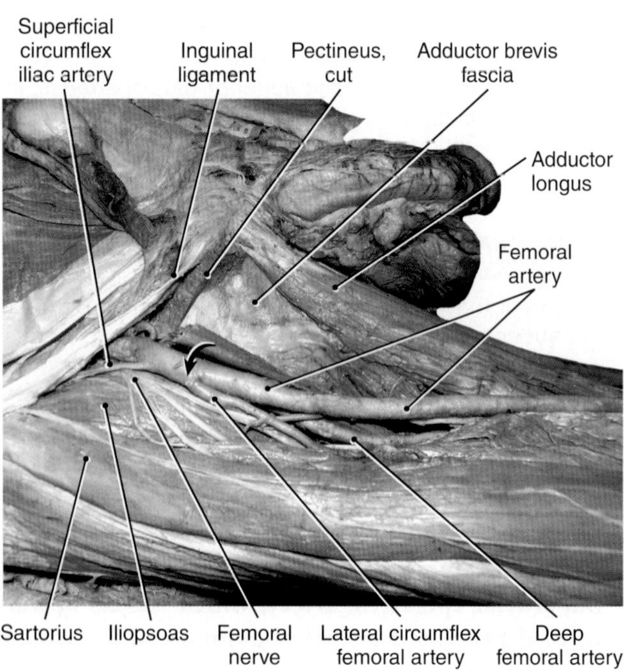

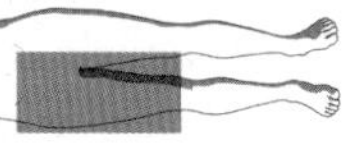

Fig. 17.36 View the pectineus muscle incised inferior to the inguinal ligament and reflected laterally.

- Note the adductor brevis fascia over the proximal part of the adductor brevis muscle. Remove the fascia carefully and expose the obturator artery and nerve (Figs. 17.37 and 17.38).

ANATOMY **NOTE**

The *obturator nerve* splits into two divisions: anterior and posterior. The *anterior division* courses anterior to the adductor brevis to innervate the adductor longus and brevis muscles.

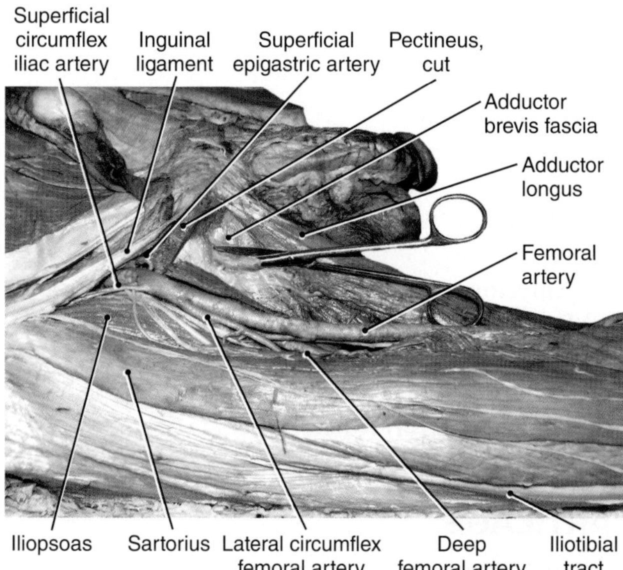

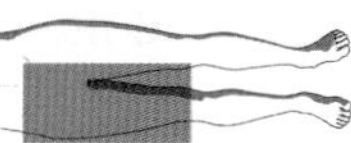

Fig. 17.37 Adductor brevis fascia removed, exposing the obturator artery and nerve.

- Reflect the adductor brevis muscle laterally and identify the *posterior division* of the obturator nerve innervating the adductor magnus.

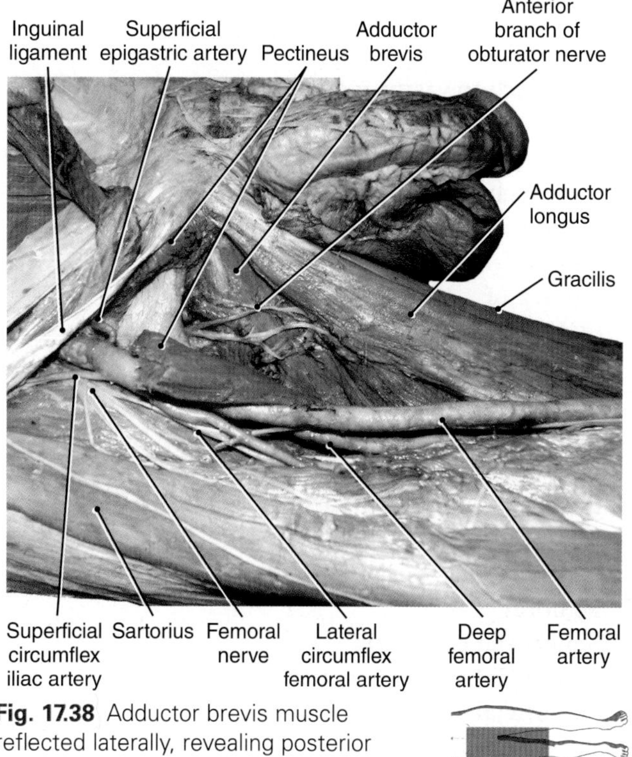

Fig. 17.38 Adductor brevis muscle reflected laterally, revealing posterior division of obturator nerve.

LABORATORY IDENTIFICATION CHECKLIST

NERVES

- ☐ Femoral
  - ☐ Branch to vastus medialis
  - ☐ Branch to rectus femoris
  - ☐ Branch to vastus lateralis
  - ☐ Branch to vastus intermedius
  - ☐ Saphenous
- ☐ Lateral femoral cutaneous
- ☐ Obturator
  - ☐ Anterior division
  - ☐ Posterior division
- ☐ Sciatic
  - ☐ Tibial
  - ☐ Common fibular
- ☐ Posterior femoral cutaneous

ARTERIES

- ☐ Femoral
- ☐ Superficial epigastric
- ☐ Superficial circumflex iliac
- ☐ Superficial external pudendal
- ☐ Deep external pudendal
- ☐ Deep femoral (profunda femoris)
- ☐ Medial circumflex femoral
- ☐ Lateral circumflex femoral
- ☐ Perforating
- ☐ Descending genicular
- ☐ Popliteal
- ☐ Superior genicular
- ☐ Middle genicular
- ☐ Inferior genicular
- ☐ Obturator
  - ☐ Acetabular branch

VEINS

- ☐ Great saphenous
- ☐ Small (lesser) saphenous
- ☐ Superficial epigastric
- ☐ Superficial circumflex iliac
- ☐ External pudendal
- ☐ Popliteal
- ☐ Deep femoral (profunda femoris)
- ☐ Femoral

CONNECTIVE TISSUE

- ☐ Fascia lata
- ☐ Anteromedial intermuscular septum
- ☐ Medial intermuscular septum
- ☐ Lateral intermuscular septum
- ☐ Posterior intermuscular septum
- ☐ Vastoadductor membrane

LIGAMENTS

- ☐ *Hip*
  - ☐ Iliofemoral
  - ☐ Pubofemoral
  - ☐ Ischiofemoral
  - ☐ Ligament of head of femur
  - ☐ Acetabular labrum/transverse acetabular
- ☐ *Knee*
  - ☐ Anterior cruciate
  - ☐ Posterior cruciate
  - ☐ Transverse (genicular)
  - ☐ Tibial (medial) collateral
  - ☐ Fibular (lateral) collateral
  - ☐ Oblique popliteal

CARTILAGE

- ☐ Medial meniscus
- ☐ Lateral meniscus

MUSCLES

Anterior Compartment (Extensor Compartment)

- ☐ Sartorius
- ☐ Iliopsoas
- ☐ Iliacus
- ☐ Rectus femoris
- ☐ Vastus medialis
- ☐ Vastus lateralis
- ☐ Vastus intermedius
- ☐ Articularis genus

Femoral Triangle

- ☐ Borders
  - ☐ Inguinal ligament, superior border
  - ☐ Adductor longus, medial border
  - ☐ Sartorius, lateral border
- ☐ Floor
  - ☐ Iliopsoas
  - ☐ Pectineus
- ☐ Contents (medial to lateral)
  - ☐ Femoral canal with lymphatics
  - ☐ Femoral vein
  - ☐ Femoral artery
  - ☐ Femoral nerve

Adductor Canal (Subsartorial, or Hunter's Canal)

Extends from femoral triangle apex to adductor hiatus

- ☐ **Contents**
  - ☐ **Femoral artery**
  - ☐ **Femoral vein**
  - ☐ **Nerve to vastus medialis**
  - ☐ **Saphenous nerve**
  - ☐ **Descending genicular**

Tendons/Retinacula

- ☐ **Quadriceps femoris tendon**
- ☐ **Patellar ligament**
- ☐ **Medial retinaculum**
- ☐ **Lateral retinaculum**

Medial Compartment (Adductor Compartment)

- ☐ **Gracilis**
- ☐ **Pectineus**
- ☐ **Obturator externus**
- ☐ **Adductor longus**
- ☐ **Adductor brevis**
- ☐ **Adductor magnus**
- ☐ **Femoral head**
- ☐ **Ischial or hamstring head**
- ☐ **Adductor minimus**

POSTERIOR COMPARTMENT (FLEXOR COMPARTMENT)

- ☐ **Biceps femoris**
  - ☐ **Long head**
  - ☐ **Short head**
- ☐ **Semitendinosus muscle**
- ☐ **Semimembranosus muscle**

Pes anserinus

- ☐ **Sartorius**
- ☐ **Gracilis**
- ☐ **Semitendinosus**

BURSAE

- ☐ **Suprapatellar**
- ☐ **Prepatellar**
- ☐ **Infrapatellar**

BONES

- ☐ **Hip**
- ☐ **Femur**
- ☐ **Patella**
- ☐ **Proximal tibia**
- ☐ **Proximal fibula**

BEFORE YOU BEGIN

Identify the great and small (lesser) saphenous veins and the saphenous and sural nerves from the previous dissection of the thigh and leg in Chapter 17.

POSTERIOR LEG

- **Insert scissors or a probe between the semitendinosus and biceps femoris muscles into the popliteal fossa and remove the superficial adipose tissue (Fig. 18.1).**
- **Insert scissors or a probe underneath the crural fascia (Fig. 18.2) and divide the fascia into two parts.**
- **Reflect the semitendinosus and biceps femoris muscles and expose the contents of the popliteal fossa (Fig. 18.3). Note the sciatic nerve dividing into the tibial and common fibular nerves.**

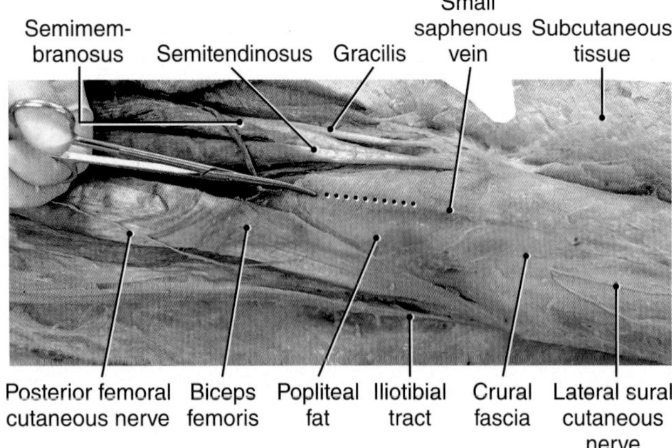

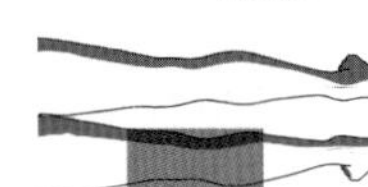

Fig. 18.1 Scissors inserted between semitendinosus and biceps femoris muscles, into popliteal fossa, with superficial adipose tissue removed.

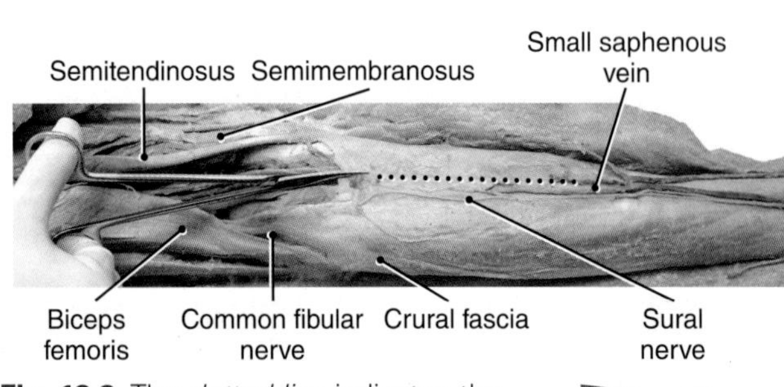

Fig. 18.2 The *dotted line* indicates the crural fascia cut into two parts.

- **Clean the fat and the lymphatics within the popliteal fossa and identify the following structures (Plate 18.1):**
  - **Posterior femoral cutaneous nerve**
  - **Small saphenous vein**
  - **Tibial nerve**
  - **Common fibular nerve**
  - **Popliteal vein**
  - **Popliteal artery**

DISSECTION TIP

Identify the following landmarks (see also Chapter 17):

- The ***great saphenous vein*** and the saphenous nerve accompany each other along the medial aspect of the leg and thigh.
- The ***small saphenous vein*** and the sural nerve accompany each other along the posterior aspect of the leg. The small saphenous vein usually drains into the popliteal vein and often exhibits anastomoses with the great saphenous vein.
- The ***sural nerve*** is formed by the union of the medial sural cutaneous nerve, a branch of the tibial nerve, and a communicating branch of the lateral sural cutaneous nerve arising from the common fibular nerve. The sural nerve terminates as the ***lateral dorsal cutaneous nerve*** on the lateral foot.
- Clean the popliteal artery and identify its division into **anterior and posterior tibial arteries**. Look for the popliteal artery's genicular branches, the superior lateral, superior medial, inferior lateral, inferior medial, and middle genicular arteries.
- To find the **superior lateral and superior medial genicular arteries**, remove the fat just superior to the lateral and medial condyles of the femur at the origin of the medial and lateral heads of the gastrocnemius muscle, respectively.
- The **middle genicular artery** is usually found arising from the anterior surface of the popliteal artery (deep from your view) just posterior to the knee joint.
- The **inferior lateral genicular artery** is usually found underneath the lateral head of the gastrocnemius muscle.
- The **inferior medial genicular artery** is usually found underneath the medial head of the gastrocnemius muscle.

DISSECTION TIP

Do not try to identify all branches of the genicular arteries; some are too small. Similarly, exposing the anastomoses around the knee requires special preparation of the specimen (e.g., filling arteries with red latex).

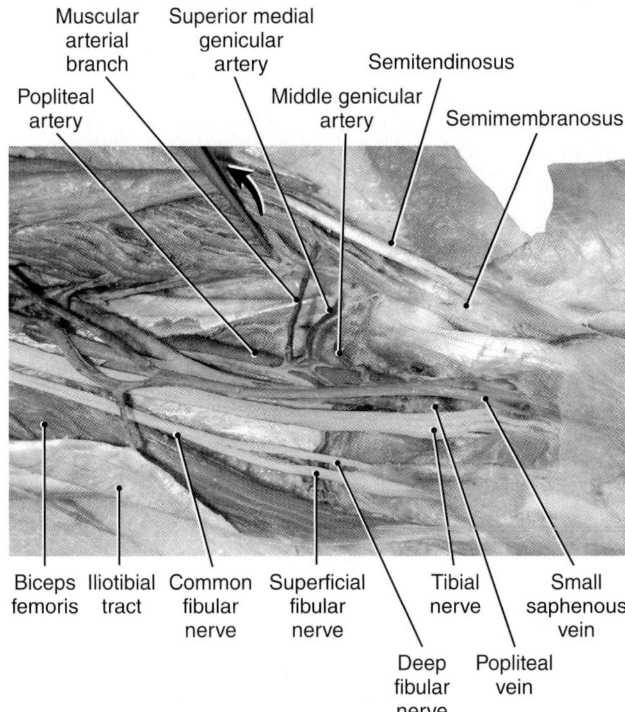

Fig. 18.3 Semitendinosus and biceps femoris muscles reflected laterally, exposing the contents of the popliteal fossa.

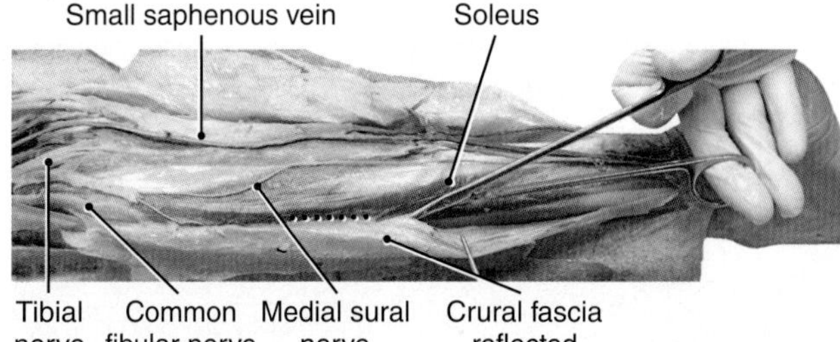

Fig. 18.4 Removing fascia, being careful not to disturb superficial veins and cutaneous nerves.

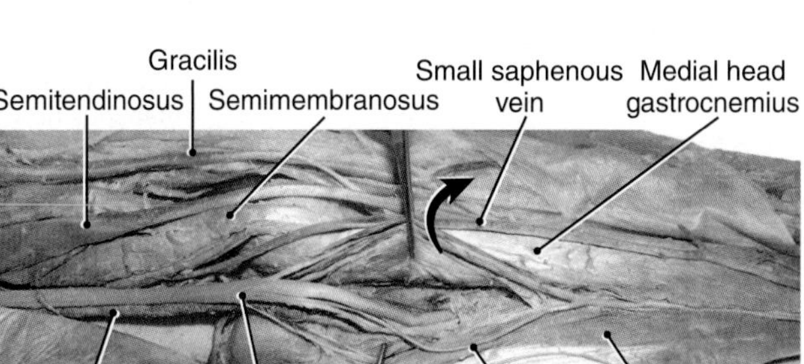

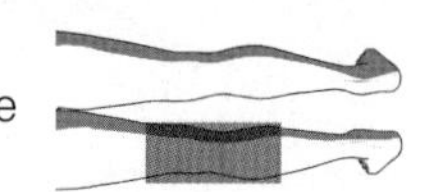

Fig. 18.5 Close-up view with medial and lateral heads of the gastrocnemius muscle retracted laterally.

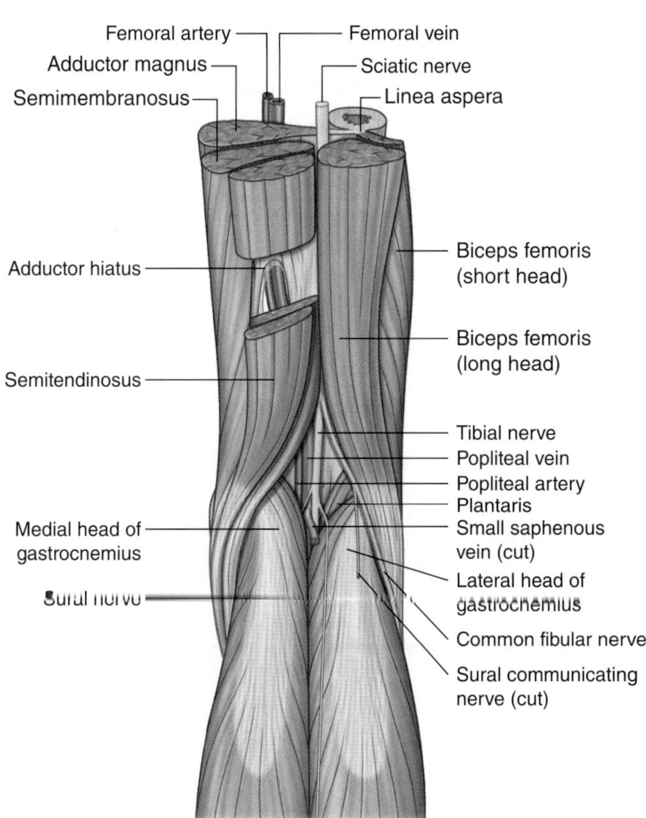

Plate 18.1 Structures in the popliteal fossa. (From Drake RL et al. *Gray's Anatomy for Students*, 5th edition, Philadelphia, Elsevier, 2024.)

- **Completely remove the crural fascia from the underlying muscles of the posterior compartment of the leg, without disturbing the superficial veins and cutaneous nerves (Fig. 18.4).**
- **Identify the medial and lateral heads of the gastrocnemius muscle and retract them laterally (Fig. 18.5).**
- **Trace the tibial nerve and identify its medial sural cutaneous branch (Fig. 18.6).**
- **Expose all the muscles of the posterior and lateral compartments of the leg.**
- **Identify the common fibular nerve and trace its course from the thigh to the neck of the fibula (see Fig. 18.6).**
- **Separate the lateral head of the gastrocnemius muscle from the underlying soleus muscle (Fig. 18.7). Look for the *Achilles tendon*, the common tendon of the gastrocnemius and soleus muscles inserting onto the calcaneus.**
- **Preserve the lateral sural cutaneous nerve as you reflect the lateral head of the gastrocnemius muscle. Similarly, preserve the medial sural cutaneous nerve and the tibial nerve as you reflect the medial head of the gastrocnemius muscle.**
- **Expose the underlying soleus muscle and identify the tendon of the plantaris muscle on the posterior surface of the soleus.**

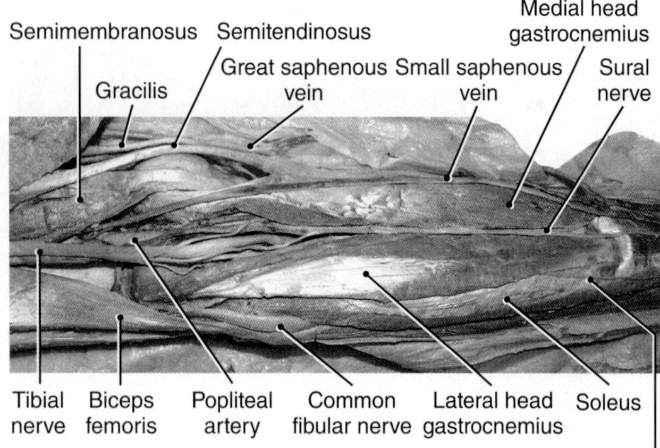

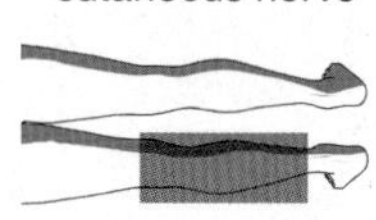

Fig. 18.6 Appreciate the tibial nerve and medial sural cutaneous branch as well as muscles of the posterior and lateral compartments of the leg.

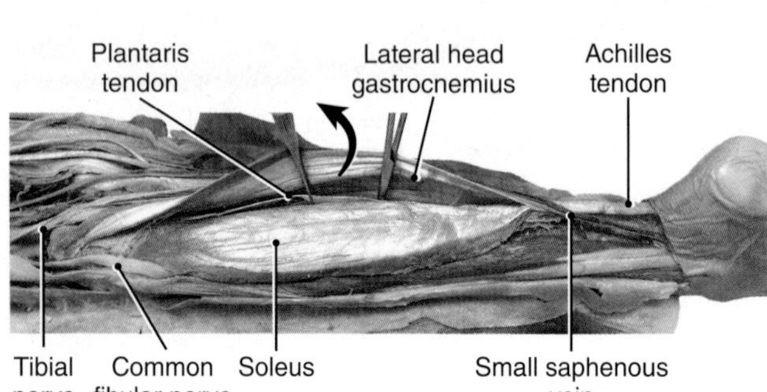

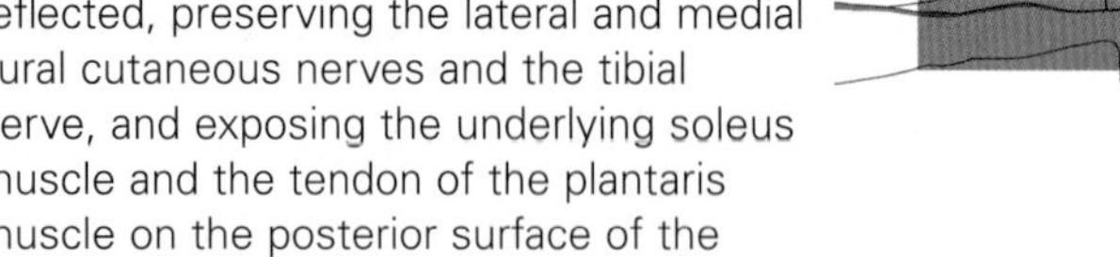

Fig. 18.7 The gastrocnemius muscle reflected, preserving the lateral and medial sural cutaneous nerves and the tibial nerve, and exposing the underlying soleus muscle and the tendon of the plantaris muscle on the posterior surface of the soleus muscle.

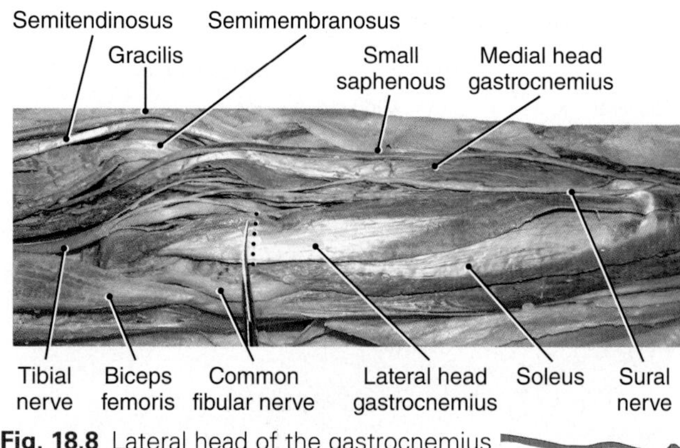

Fig. 18.8 Lateral head of the gastrocnemius muscle cut at the level of the femoral condyle.

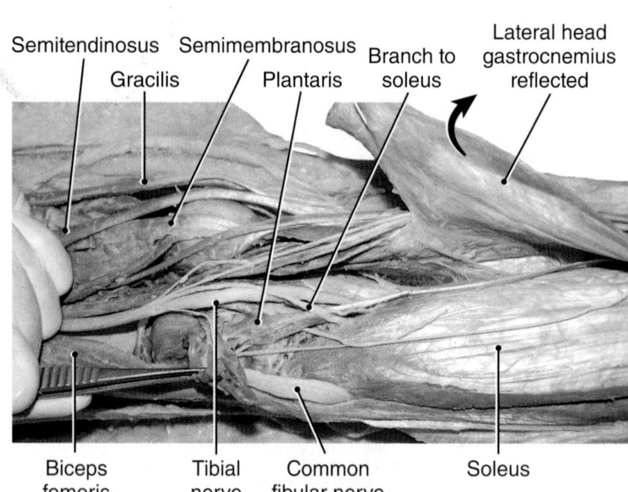

Fig. 18.9 Close-up view highlights the muscle belly of the plantaris muscle.

- **Cut the lateral head of the gastrocnemius muscle at the level of the femoral condyle (Fig. 18.8).**
- **Reflect the lateral head of the gastrocnemius muscle medially and expose the tendon of the plantaris muscle. Identify the muscle belly of the plantaris muscle (Fig. 18.9).**
- **Identify the branch from the tibial nerve, the nerve to the soleus muscle.**
- **With forceps, lift the lateral border of the soleus muscle and separate it from the underlying fascia over the flexor hallucis longus and flexor digitorum longus muscles (Fig. 18.10).**
- **With scissors, cut the soleus muscle close to its attachment to the tibia and fibula and reflect it medially (Fig. 18.11).**
- **Clean the fascia and expose the flexor hallucis longus and flexor digitorum longus muscles as well as**

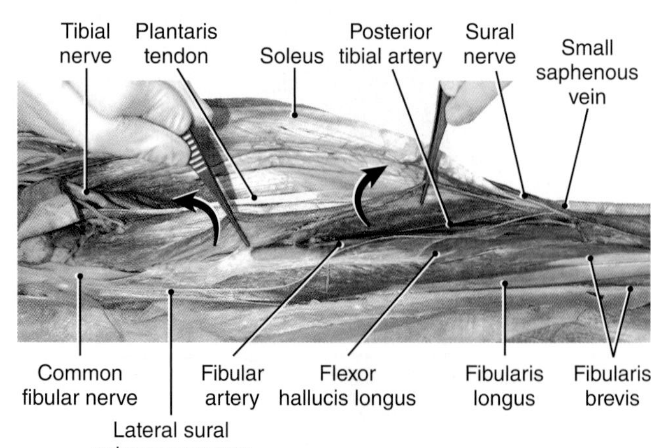

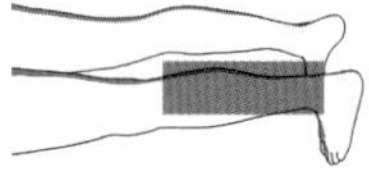

Fig. 18.10 Lateral border of the soleus muscle detached from the underlying fascia over the flexor hallucis longus and flexor digitorum longus muscles.

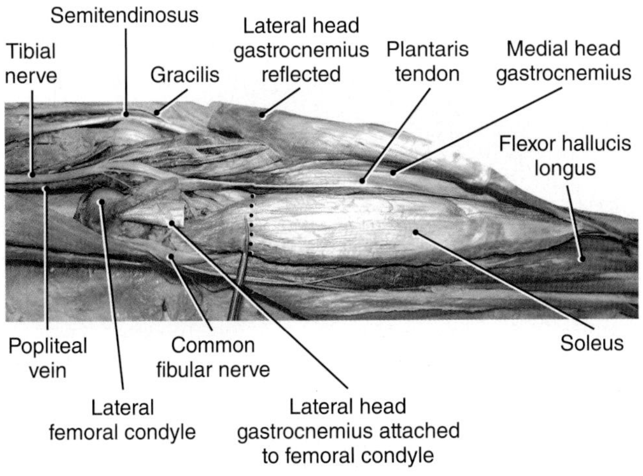

Fig. 18.11 Soleus muscle cut proximal to its tibiofibular attachment and reflected medially.

the muscles of the lateral compartment of the leg, the fibularis longus and fibularis brevis (Fig. 18.12).

- **Expose the tibialis posterior muscle as it travels along the posterior surface of the interosseous membrane to reach the foot (Fig. 18.13). Trace the division of the common fibular nerve into deep and superficial fibular nerves (Plate 18.2).**

ANATOMY **NOTE**

The anterior tibial artery travels anterior to the interosseous membrane, whereas the posterior tibial artery gives rise to a fibular branch that travels to the lateral compartment and deep to the flexor hallucis longus muscle. Soon after arising from the common fibular nerve, the superficial fibular nerve enters the lateral compartment of the leg.

KNEE

- **Place the cadaver in the supine position and observe the knee joint. Identify the tendon of the quadriceps femoris muscle attaching to the patella.**
- **Identify the patellar ligament and the strong, thick fascia on the medial and lateral sides of the knee joint, the *medial and lateral retinacula* of the knee (Fig. 18.14).**
- **Cut the medial and lateral retinacula and expose the patellar ligament and the tendon of the quadriceps femoris muscle (Fig. 18.15).**

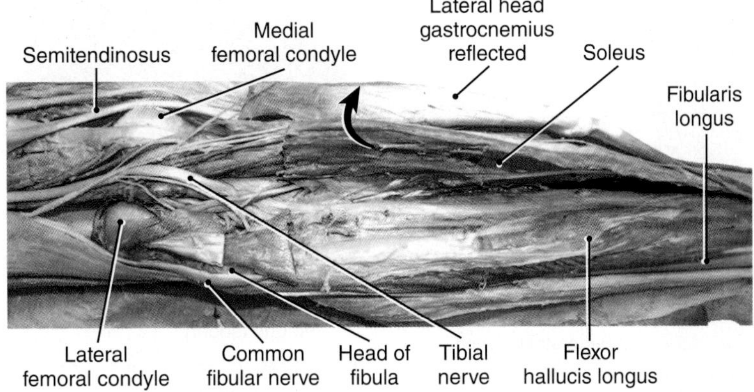

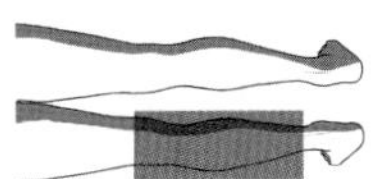

Fig. 18.12 Fascia cleaned, exposing flexor hallucis longus, flexor digitorum longus, and lateral compartment muscles.

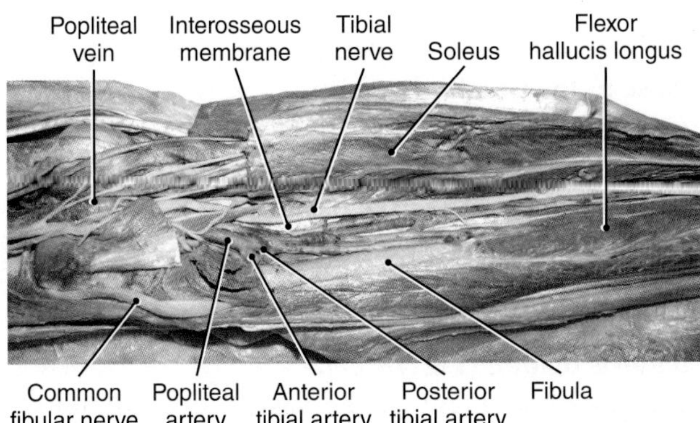

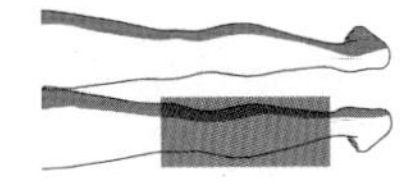

Fig. 18.13 Tibialis posterior muscle exposed along the posterior surface of interosseous membrane.

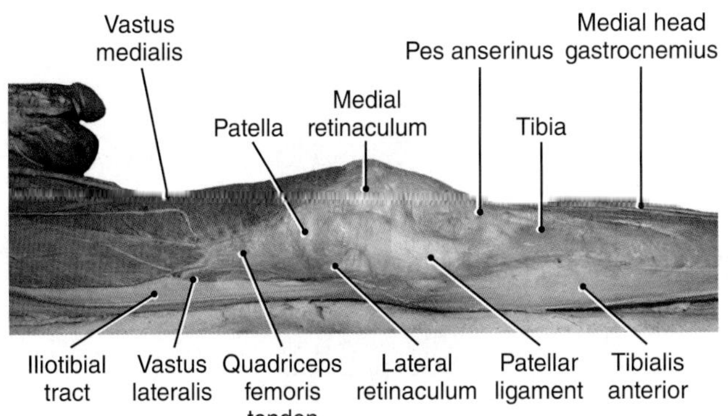

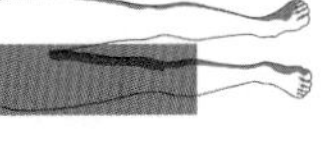

Fig. 18.14 Supine position, highlighting the tendon of quadriceps femoris muscle, patellar ligament, and thick fascia on the sides of the knee joint (medial/lateral retinacula).

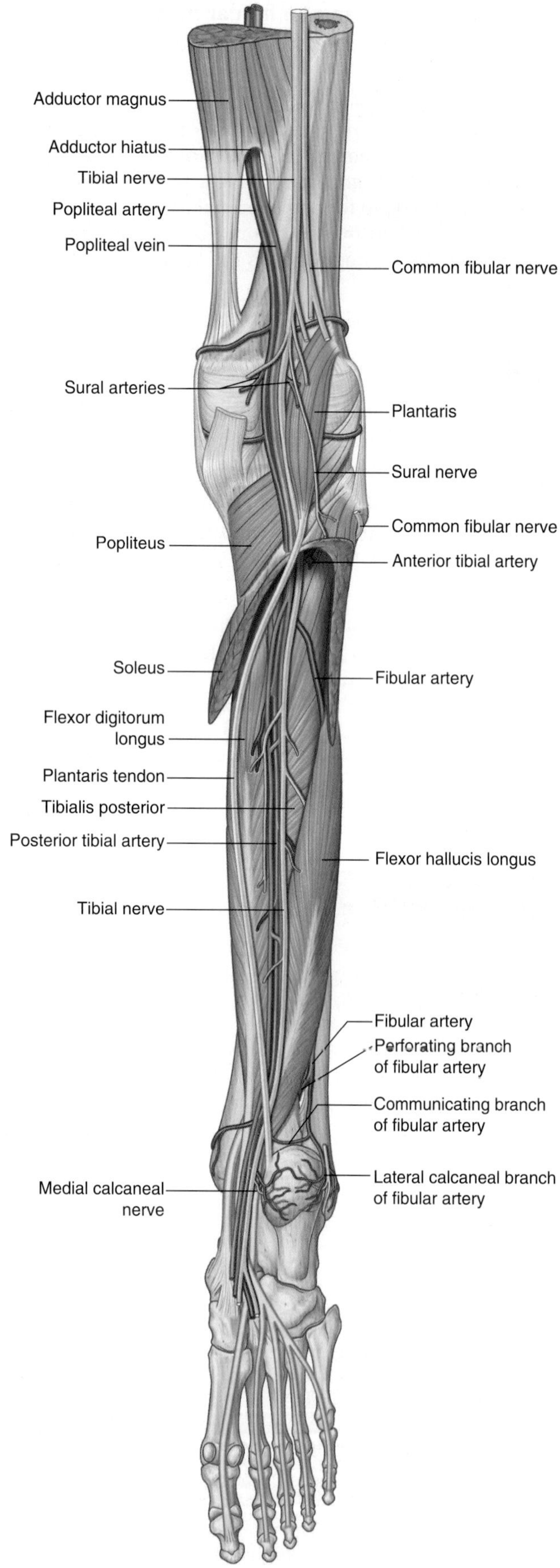

Adductor magnus
Adductor hiatus
Tibial nerve
Popliteal artery
Popliteal vein
Common fibular nerve
Sural arteries
Plantaris
Sural nerve
Common fibular nerve
Popliteus
Anterior tibial artery
Soleus
Fibular artery
Flexor digitorum longus
Plantaris tendon
Tibialis posterior
Posterior tibial artery
Flexor hallucis longus
Tibial nerve
Fibular artery
Perforating branch of fibular artery
Communicating branch of fibular artery
Medial calcaneal nerve
Lateral calcaneal branch of fibular artery

Plate 18.2 Arteries and nerves of the posterior leg. (From Drake RL et al. *Gray's Atlas of Anatomy*, 3rd edition, Philadelphia, Elsevier, 2021.)

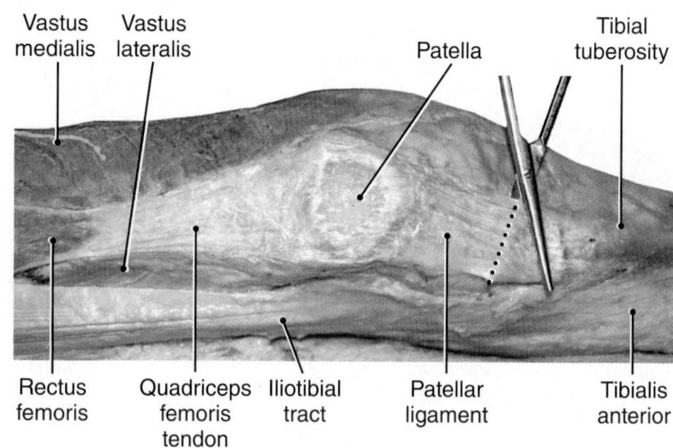

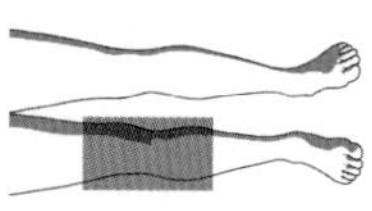

Fig. 18.15 Medial and lateral retinacula cut, exposing patellar ligament and quadriceps femoris tendon. Patellar ligament scissors cut *(dotted line)* close to tibial tuberosity.

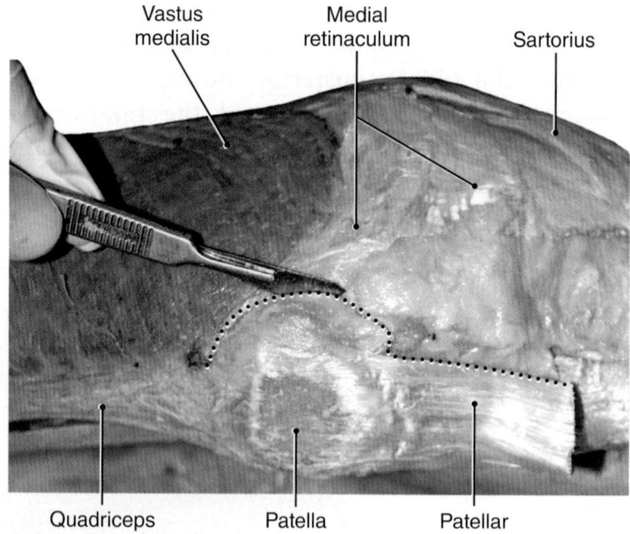

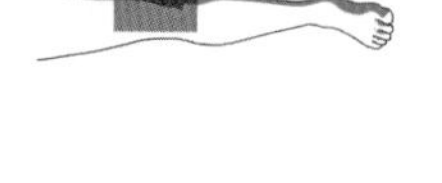

Fig. 18.16 Incision continued with scalpel lateral and medial to patella.

- **With scissors or a scalpel, cut the patellar ligament close to the tibial tuberosity.**
- **Continue the incision with a scalpel lateral and medial to the patella to separate the patella from surrounding connective tissue (Fig. 18.16).**
- **Detach the patella from its subcutaneous prepatellar and infrapatellar bursae and fat and reflect it superiorly, preserving its attachment to the quadriceps femoris tendon (Fig. 18.17).**
- **Cut the attachment of the vastus medialis muscle from the medial side of the knee and expose this area (Fig. 18.18).**
- **Similarly, cut the tendon of the biceps femoris muscle from the head of the fibula (Fig. 18.19).**

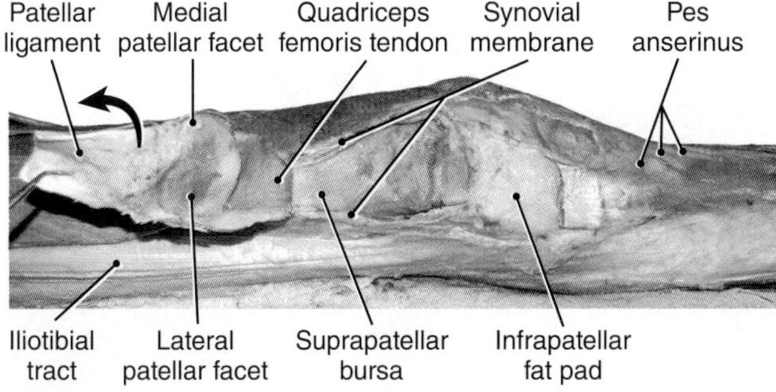

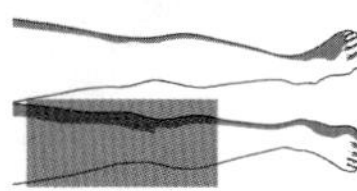

Fig. 18.17 Patella detached from bursae and fat and reflected superiorly, retaining quadriceps femoris muscle attachment.

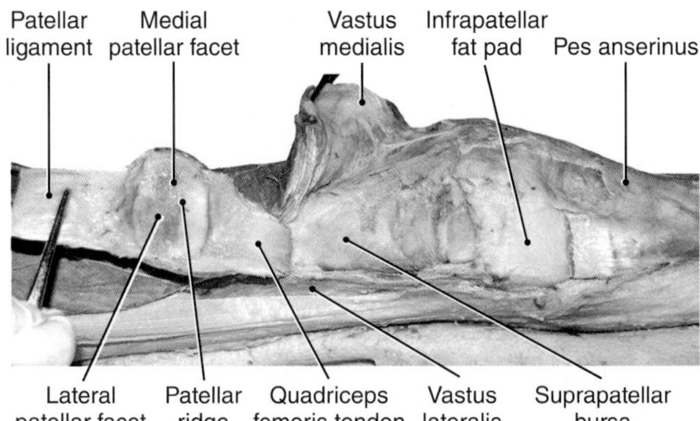

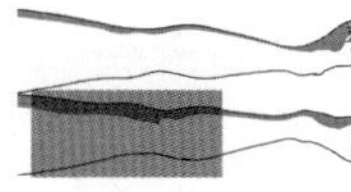

Fig. 18.18 Vastus medialis muscle reflected from the medial side of knee.

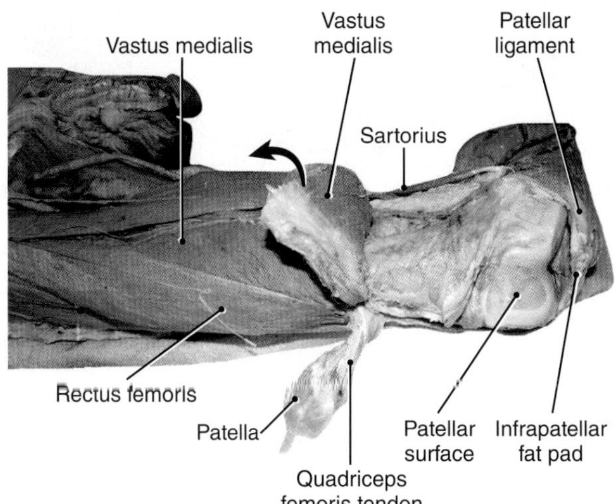

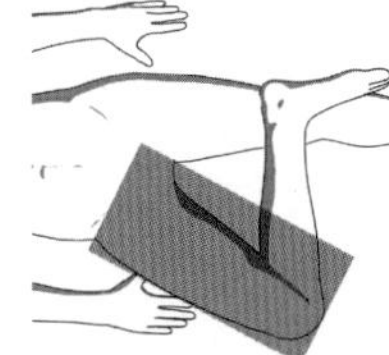

Fig. 18.19 Tendon of the biceps femoris muscle incised from the head of fibula.

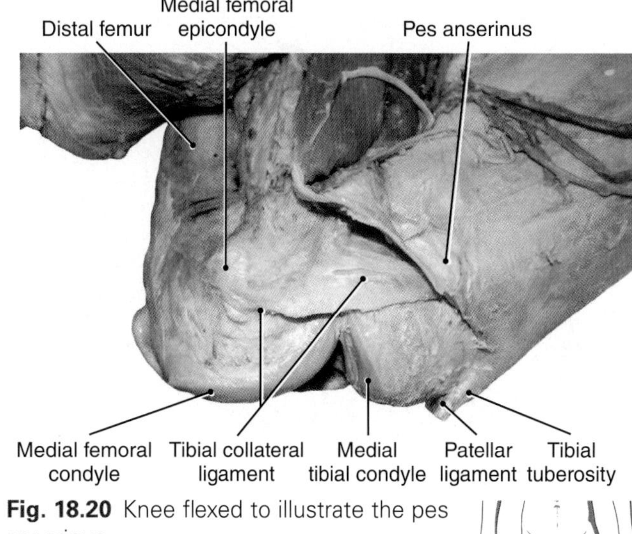

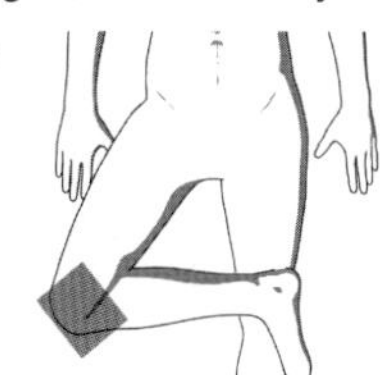

Fig. 18.20 Knee flexed to illustrate the pes anserinus.

- **After releasing these attachments, flex the knee joint (Fig. 18.20).**
- **On the medial side of the knee joint, inferior and medial to the tuberosity of the tibia, trace the common insertion of the tendons of the sartorius, gracilis, and semitendinosus muscles, the *pes anserinus*.**
- **Just superior to the pes anserinus, identify the *tibial* (medial) collateral ligament.**

ANATOMY **NOTE**

The **tibial collateral ligament** is a thick band of connective tissue that extends from the medial femoral epicondyle to the medial tibial condyle; it also attaches to the medial meniscus.

- **Using scissors, cut the tibial collateral ligament (Fig. 18.21). Similarly, cut the biceps femoris tendon and identify a thick band of connective tissue extending from the lateral femoral condyle to the head of the fibula, the *fibular* collateral ligament.**
- **Remove the infrapatellar fat pad and infrapatellar synovial fold to expose the anterior cruciate ligament and the medial and lateral menisci between the femur and tibia (Fig. 18.22).**
- **Further expose the anterior cruciate ligament. With scissors, cut the anterior cruciate ligament (Fig. 18.23).**
- **Expose the posterior cruciate ligament by flexing the knee joint farther and observe the ligament as it is stretched (Fig. 18.24 and Plate 18.3).**

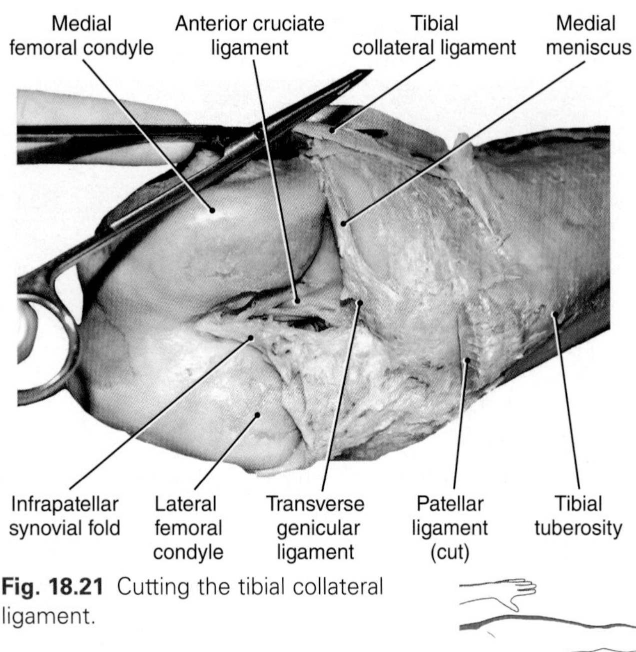

Fig. 18.21 Cutting the tibial collateral ligament.

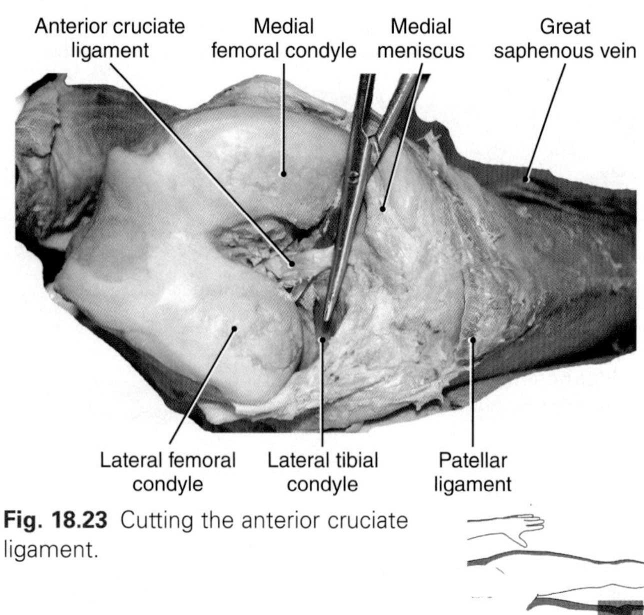

Fig. 18.23 Cutting the anterior cruciate ligament.

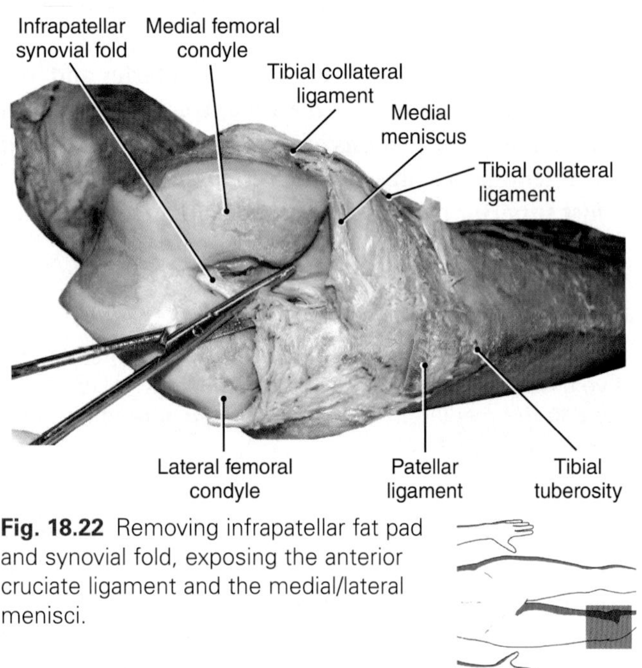

Fig. 18.22 Removing infrapatellar fat pad and synovial fold, exposing the anterior cruciate ligament and the medial/lateral menisci.

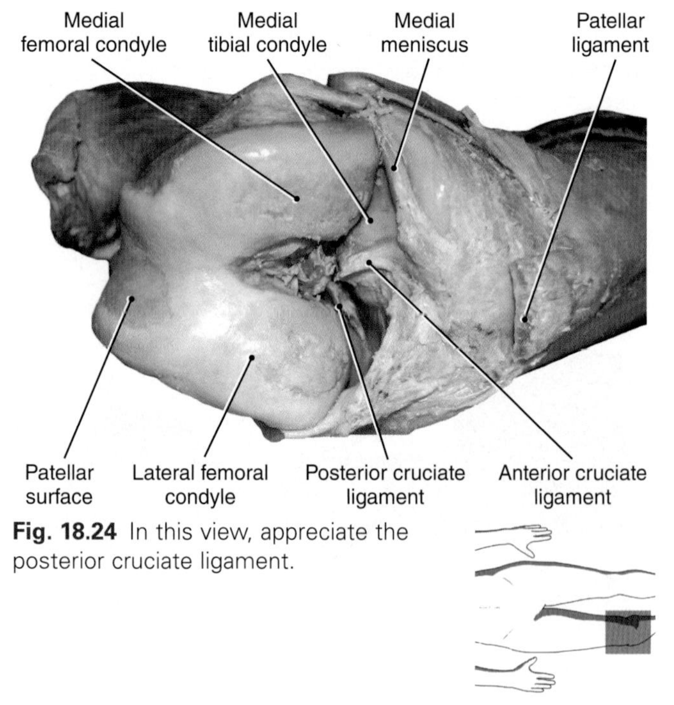

Fig. 18.24 In this view, appreciate the posterior cruciate ligament.

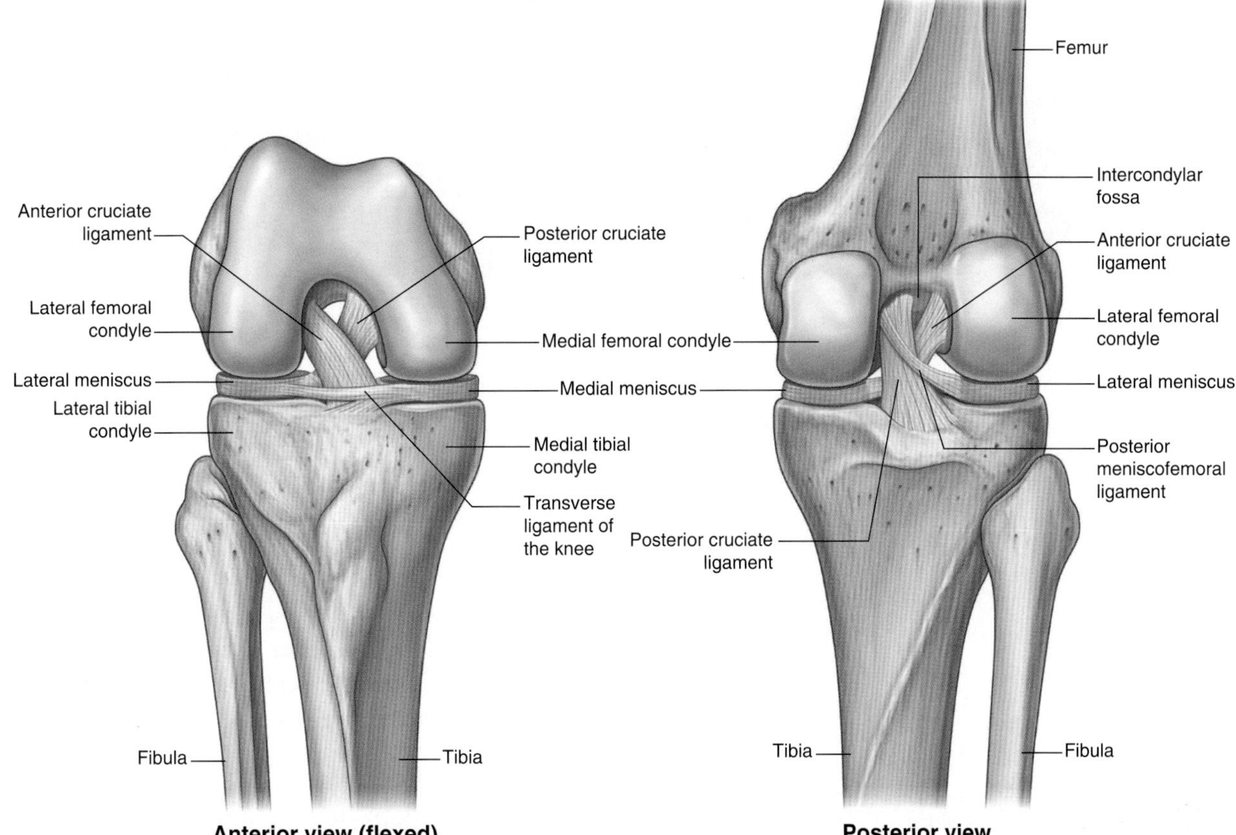

Plate 18.3 Anterior and posterior views of the knee. (From Drake RL et al. *Gray's Atlas of Anatomy*, 3rd edition, Philadelphia, Elsevier, 2021.)

DISSECTION **TIP**

If time permits, cut the posterior part of the fibrous capsule of the knee joint. Again, identify the lateral and medial menisci and the posterior cruciate ligament. Find a thick connective tissue band between the lateral meniscus and the posterior cruciate ligament, the posterior meniscofemoral ligament.

ANTERIOR LEG

- **With the cadaver supine, remove the remaining skin over the leg and expose the *crural fascia* (deep fascia) over the anterior compartment of the leg (Fig. 18.25).**
- **Make a midline longitudinal incision along the lateral side of the anterior border of the tibia, reflecting the crural fascia laterally (Fig. 18.26).**
- **Identify the *superior extensor retinaculum,* a flat, broad part of the deep fascia extending from the tibia to the fibula above the lateral malleolus (Fig. 18.27).**
- **Identify the *tibialis anterior* muscle. Place your fingertip on its inferior border, and with blunt dissection, expose the extensor digitorum longus muscle (Fig. 18.28).**

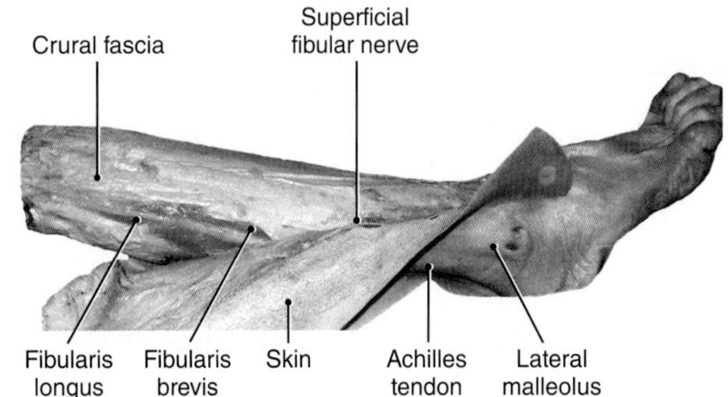

Fig. 18.25 Remaining skin over leg removed, exposing crural fascia over the anterior compartment.

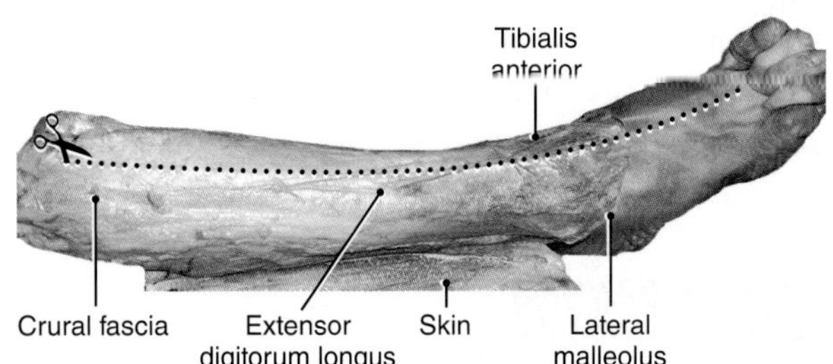

Fig. 18.26 *Dotted line* shows a midline longitudinal incision along the lateral side of the anterior border of the tibia.

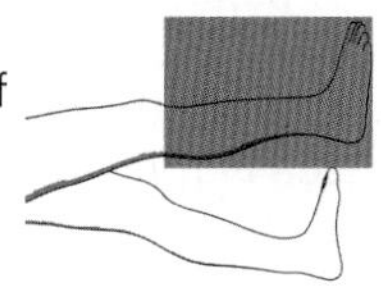

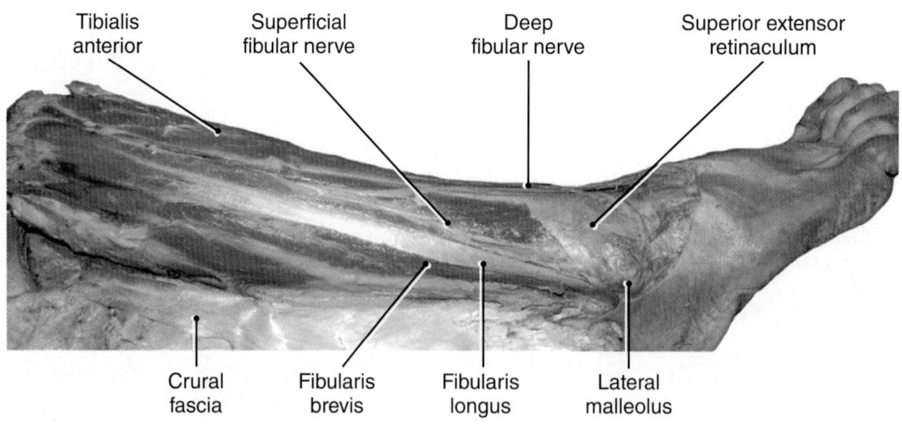

Fig. 18.27 In this view, appreciate the superior extensor retinaculum.

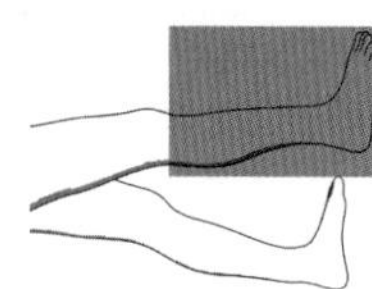

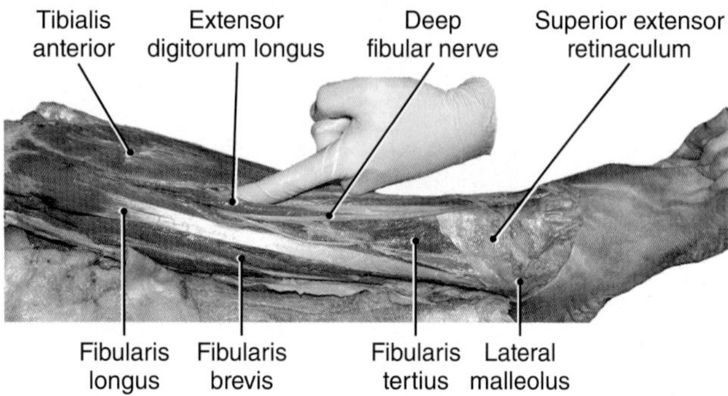

Fig. 18.28 Extensor digitorum longus tendons on dorsum of foot toward lateral four digits.

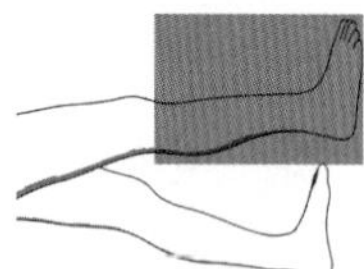

- **Trace its tendons toward the dorsum of the foot, where they run to the lateral four digits.**
- **Find the fibularis tertius muscle (if present), which is best seen distally lateral to the extensor digitorum longus muscle.**
- **Appreciate the extensor hallucis longus muscle in the space between the tibialis anterior and extensor digitorum longus muscles (Fig. 18.29). Note that the tendon of the extensor hallucis longus inserts onto the base of the distal phalanx of the 1st digit.**

DISSECTION **TIP**

To better visualize the deep part of the anterior compartment, place two retractors (one proximal and one distal) between the **tibialis anterior** and **fibularis longus** muscles (see Fig. 18.44).

- **Identify the *interosseous membrane* and the area between the extensor digitorum longus and tibialis anterior muscles (Fig. 18.30).**

LATERAL LEG

- **Reflect the fibularis longus muscle inferiorly and expose the fibularis brevis muscle as well as the superficial fibular nerve (Fig. 18.31).**

ANATOMY **NOTE**

The fibularis longus is located superficially to the fibularis brevis muscle. Trace the insertion of the tendon of the fibularis brevis onto the tuberosity of the 5th metatarsal bone.

DISSECTION **TIP**

To highlight dissection landmarks, clean the fascia over the anteromedial surface of the tibia and expose the periosteum (Fig. 18.32).

ANKLE

- **Using a scalpel, make a shallow, circumferential incision on the dorsum of the foot (Fig. 18.33).**

DISSECTION **TIP**

The skin of the dorsum of the foot is thin; therefore the incision must be shallow. Do not spend too much time exposing the entire dorsal venous arch.

- **Reflect the skin over the dorsum of the foot and expose the tendons of the extensor hallucis and extensor digitorum muscles.**
- **Identify and expose the dorsal venous arch, then trace the small saphenous vein at the lateral aspect of the**

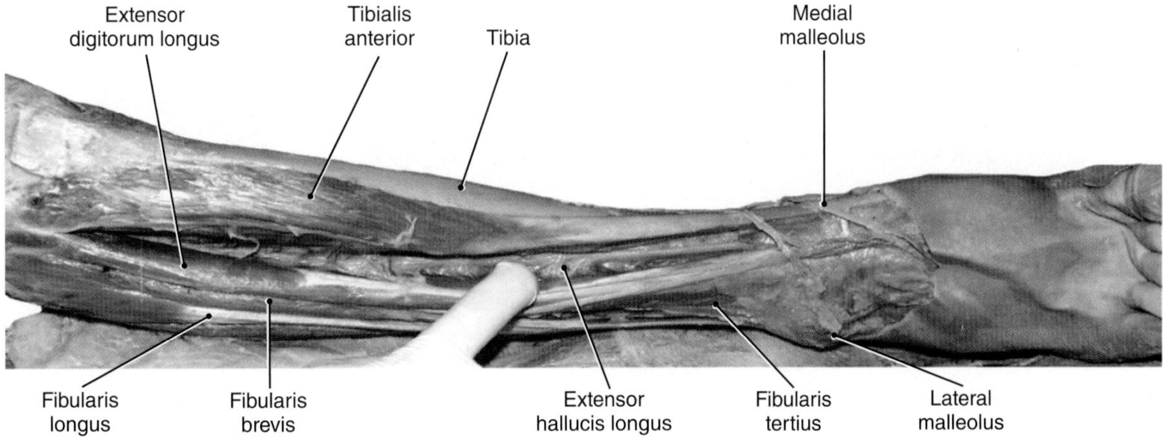

Fig. 18.29 View the highlighting fibularis tertius, longus, and brevis muscles; anterior intermuscular septum; and extensor hallucis longus muscle.

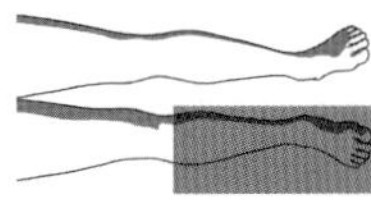

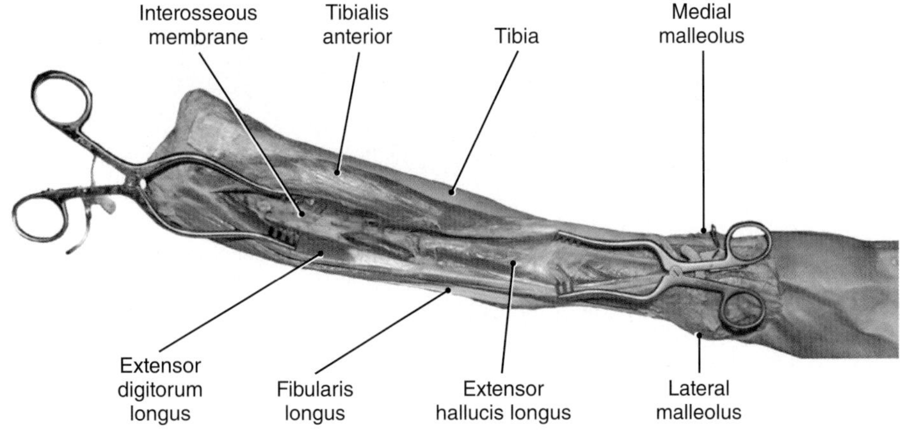

Fig. 18.30 Retractors placed between the tibialis anterior and fibularis longus muscles, highlighting the deep part of the anterior compartment of the leg.

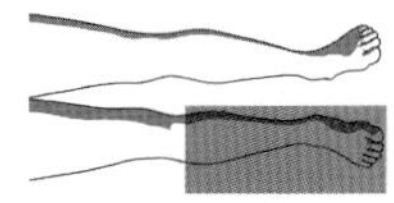

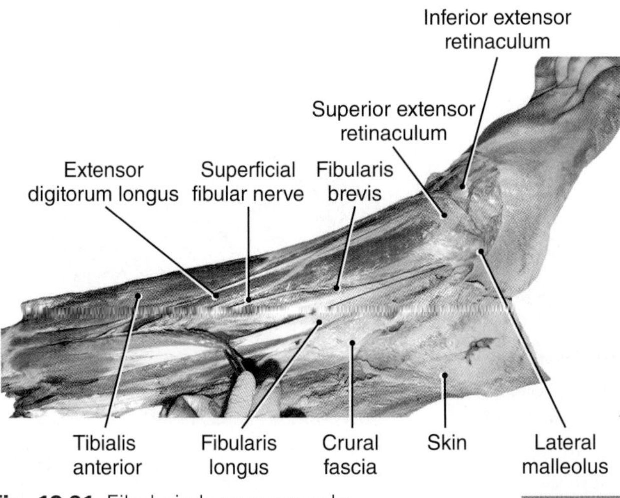

Fig. 18.31 Fibularis longus muscle reflected inferiorly, exposing fibularis brevis muscle as well as superficial fibular nerve.

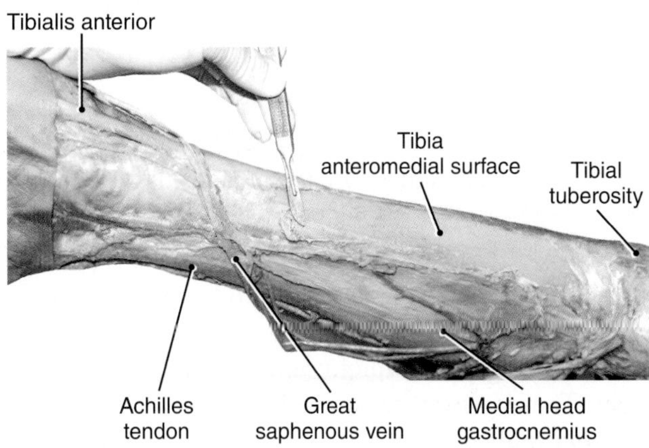

Fig. 18.32 Cleaning fascia over anteromedial tibial surface, exposing the periosteum.

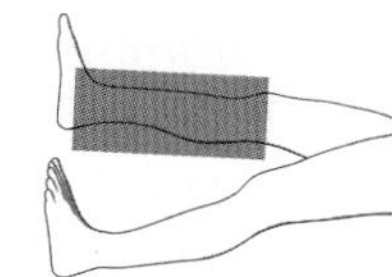

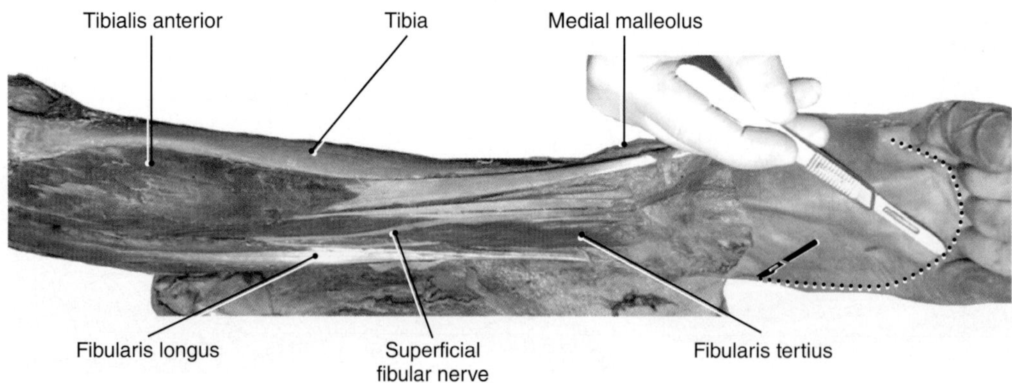

Fig. 18.33 Shallow circumferential incision *(dotted line)* on the dorsum of foot.

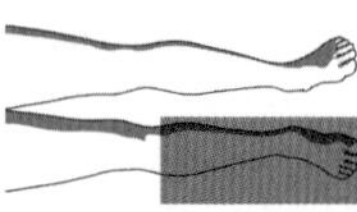

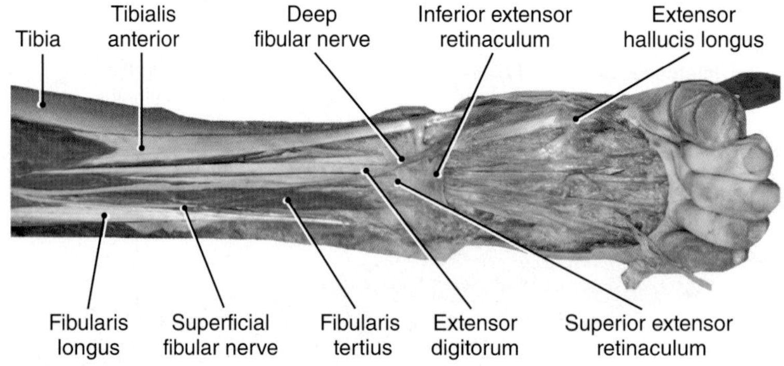

Fig. 18.34 Appreciate the superior and inferior parts of the extensor retinaculum.

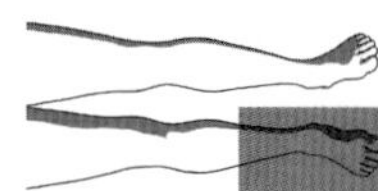

arch and the great saphenous vein at the medial portion of the dorsal venous arch traveling superiorly, anterior to the medial malleolus.

- **Identify the extensor retinaculum, divided into the superior and inferior parts.**

ANATOMY **NOTE**

The superior extensor retinaculum extends from the tibia to the fibula above the lateral malleolus as a broad, flat part of the deep fascia (Fig. 18.34).

- **The inferior extensor retinaculum is a Y-shaped band of deep fascia forming a passage for the tendons of the extensor digitorum longus and fibularis tertius muscles. The inferior extensor retinaculum attaches to the *medial malleolus* (proximal part) and to the *plantar aponeurosis* (distal band) (see Figs. 18.34 and 18.35).**
- **Cut the superior and inferior portions of the extensor retinaculum over the tendons of the extensor digitorum muscle (Fig. 18.36).**
- **Free the tendons of the extensor digitorum, extensor hallucis longus, tibialis anterior, and fibularis tertius**

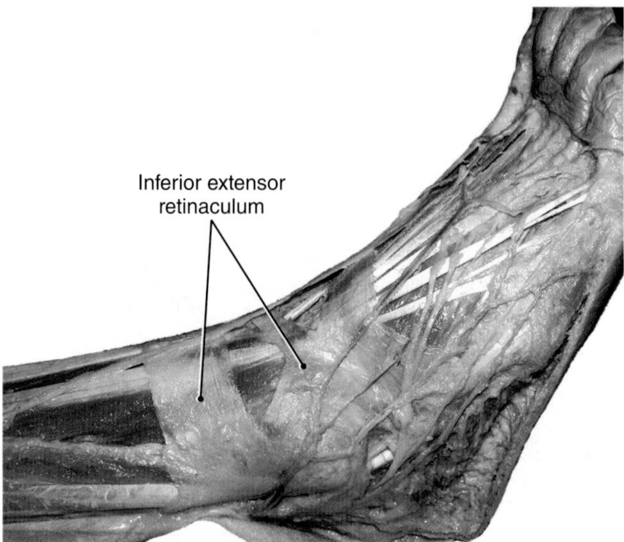

Fig. 18.35 Note the inferior extensor retinaculum as a Y-shaped band of deep fascia forming a passage for the tendons of the extensor digitorum longus and fibularis tertius muscles.

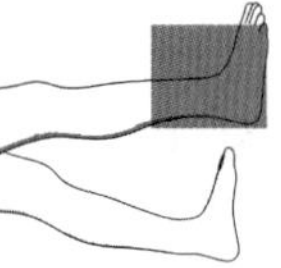

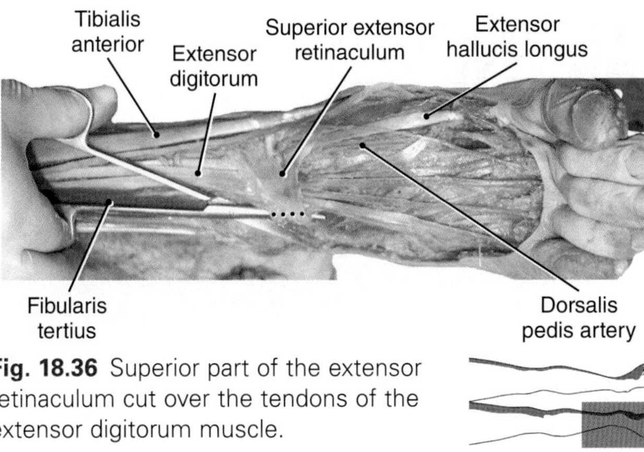

Fig. 18.36 Superior part of the extensor retinaculum cut over the tendons of the extensor digitorum muscle.

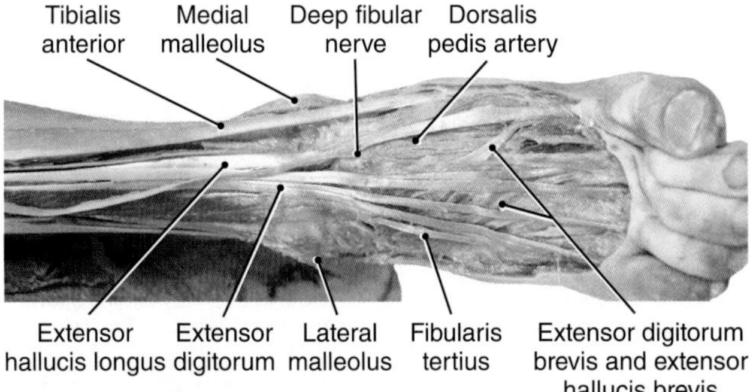

Fig. 18.37 Tendons of extensor digitorum, extensor hallucis longus, tibialis anterior, and fibularis tertius separated from the underlying bursae and soft tissue.

muscles from the underlying bursae and soft tissues, toward their insertions (Fig. 18.37).

- **Identify the extensor digitorum brevis and its medial part, the extensor hallucis brevis, inserting onto the base of the proximal phalanx of the 1st digit.**
- **Follow the anterior tibial artery to the level of the ankle joint between the extensor halluces and extensor digitorum longus muscles, where the anterior tibial artery becomes the dorsalis pedis artery (see Fig. 18.37 and Plate 18.4).**

DISSECTION **TIP**

The dorsalis pedis artery is absent in approximately 20% of the population.

DISSECTION **TIP**

If time permits, continue the dissection as follows:

- Trace out the tendon of the extensor hallucis longus muscle to the distal phalanx of the 1st digit.
- Compare the extensor hallucis longus with the extensor digitorum longus muscle inserting onto the middle and distal phalanges.
- Follow the terminal branches of the dorsalis pedis artery: deep plantar branch and 1st metatarsal branch.

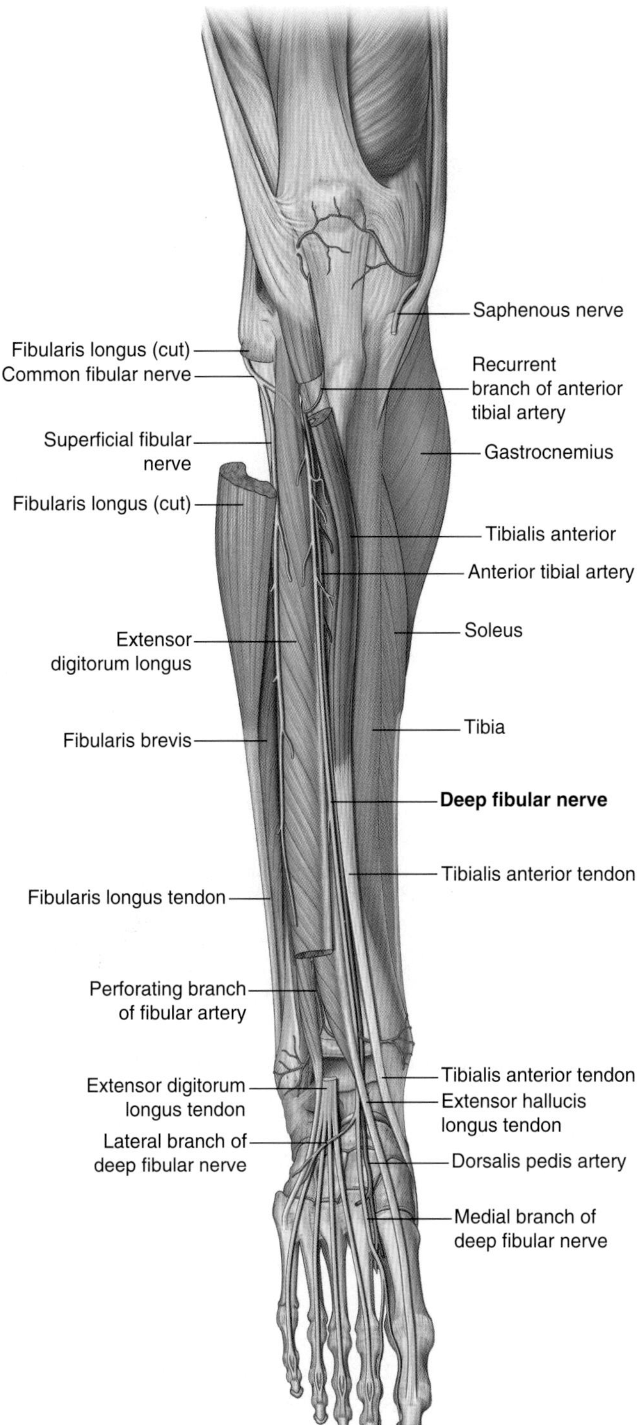

Plate 18.4 Arteries and nerves of the anterolateral leg. (From Drake RL et al. *Gray's Atlas of Anatomy*, 3rd edition, Philadelphia, Elsevier, 2021.)

- **Continue the dissection along the lateral aspect of ankle joint at the level of the *lateral malleolus* (Fig. 18.38).**
- **Expose the tendons of the fibularis brevis and fibularis longus muscles (see Fig. 18.38).**
- **Clean the fat around the lateral malleolus and expose the structures of this region (see Fig. 18.38).**

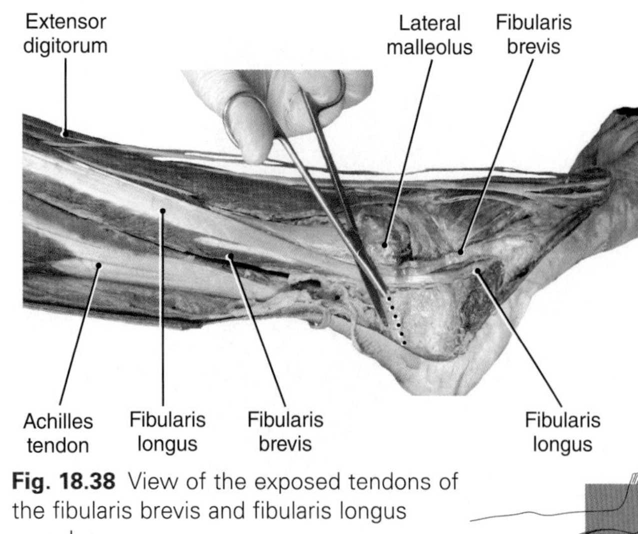

Fig. 18.38 View of the exposed tendons of the fibularis brevis and fibularis longus muscles.

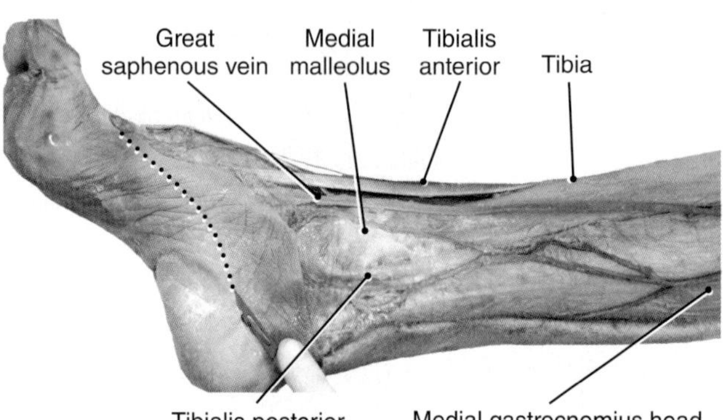

Fig. 18.39 View of the skin incision over the medial malleolus.

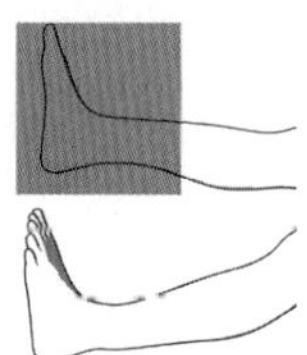

- Cut the skin over the medial malleolus and expose the crural fascia (Fig. 18.39).
- With scissors, cut the crural fascia over the medial malleolus (Fig. 18.40).
- Identify the flexor retinaculum attaching between the medial malleolus and the medial surface of the calcaneus. This flexor retinaculum forms the tarsal tunnel.
- Cut the flexor retinaculum and expose the tibial nerve, the posterior tibial artery, the tibialis posterior muscle, the flexor digitorum longus muscle, and the Achilles tendon.
- If time permits, expose the tendon of the tibialis posterior muscle to the navicular bone, one of its many insertion sites.

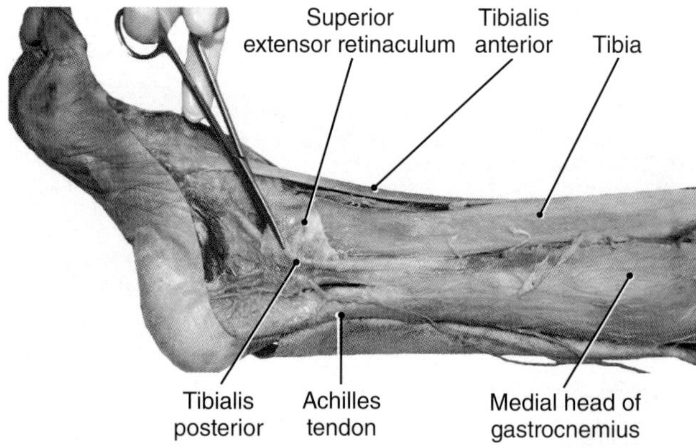

Fig. 18.40 Crural (deep) fascia cut over the medial malleolus.

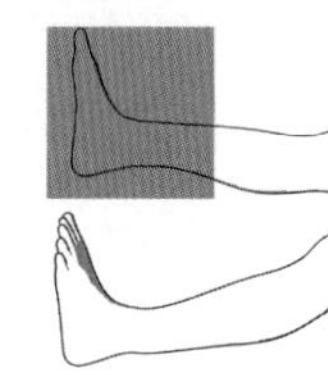

Flexor digitorum longus
Tibialis posterior
Tibialis anterior
Tibia
Flexor digitorum longus
Tibial nerve
Posterior tibial artery
Posterior tibial vein
Flexor hallucis longus
Achilles tendon

Fig. 18.41 Note the relationship of the structures passing through the tarsal tunnel.

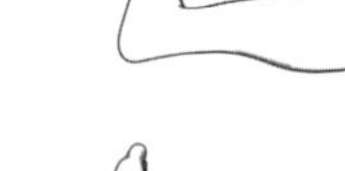

ANATOMY **NOTE**

The relationship of these structures to the medial malleolus is important for their recognition (Figs. 18.41 and 18.42). From anterior to posterior, the structures are arranged as follows (Plate 18.5):

- Tendon of tibialis posterior muscle
- Tendon of flexor digitorum longus muscle
- Posterior tibial artery and vein
- Tibial nerve
- Flexor hallucis longus muscle

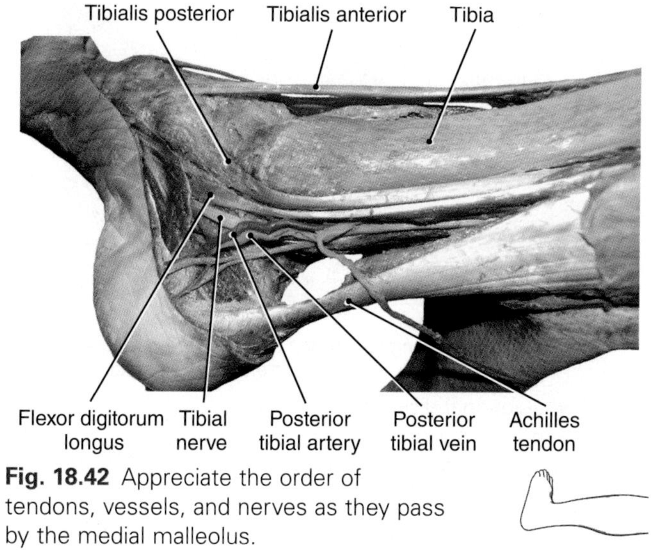

Fig. 18.42 Appreciate the order of tendons, vessels, and nerves as they pass by the medial malleolus.

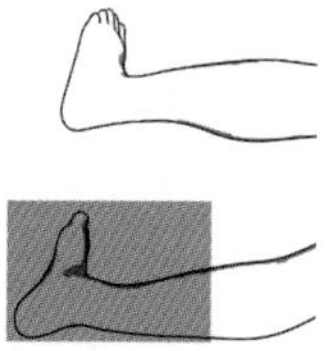

OPTIONAL DISSECTION OF LIGAMENTS OF FOOT AND ANKLE

- **Identify the lateral ligament of the ankle, formed by the anterior and posterior talofibular ligaments and the calcaneofibular ligament.**
- **Identify the interosseous talocalcaneal ligament on the lateral side of the foot (Fig. 18.43).**
- **Expose and cut the tendons of the tibialis anterior and tibialis posterior muscles at their insertion points.**
- **Just underneath, identify the deltoid ligament (medial side of ankle), formed by the anterior tibiotalar, tibionavicular, tibiocalcaneal, and posterior tibiotalar parts (Fig. 18.44).**
- **Look lateral and underneath the tendon of the tibialis posterior muscle for the plantar calcaneonavicular *(spring)* ligament connecting the calcaneus to the navicular bones.**
- **Lateral to the calcaneonavicular ligament, expose the long and short plantar ligaments (Fig. 18.45). See also Chapter 19.**

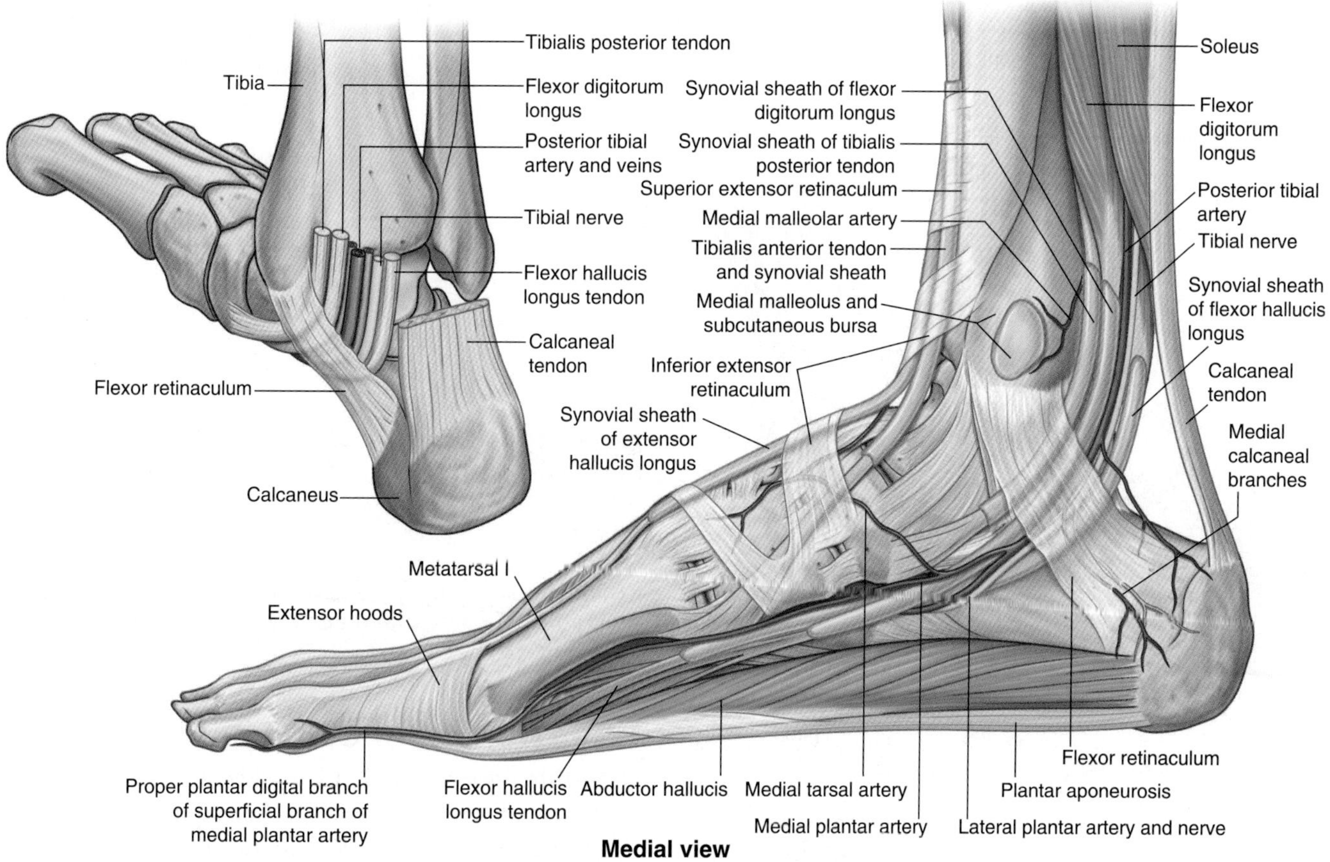

Plate 18.5 Structures of the medial foot and ankle. (From Drake RL et al. *Gray's Atlas of Anatomy*, 3rd edition, Philadelphia, Elsevier, 2021.)

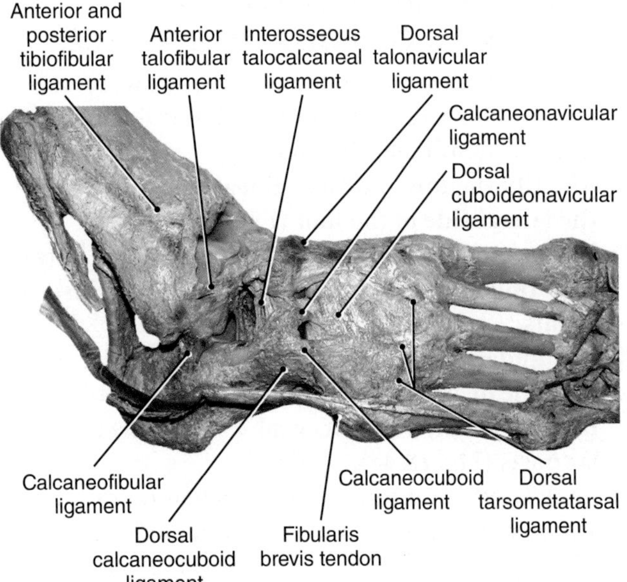

Fig. 18.43 Optional dissection: lateral view of the ankle and foot, highlighting the ligaments.

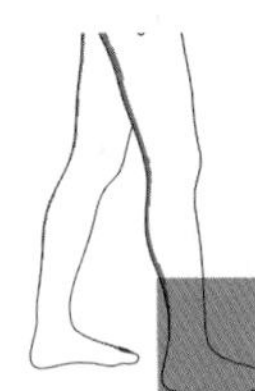

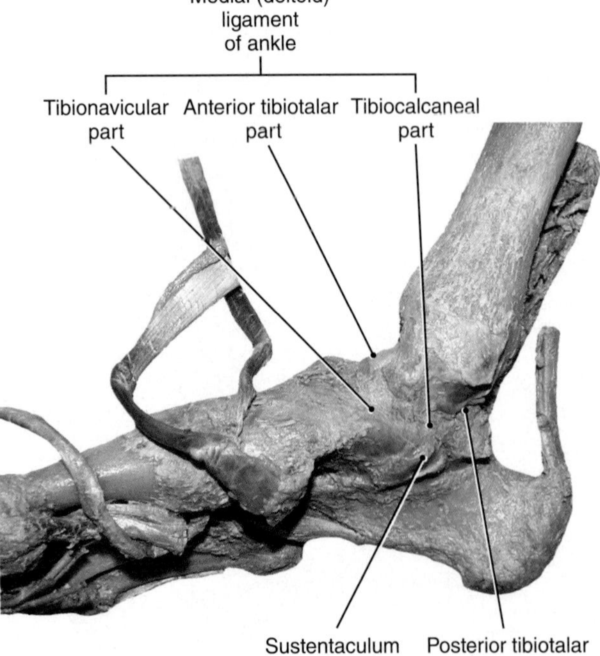

Fig. 18.44 Optional dissection: medial view of the ankle, demonstrating the deltoid (medial) ligament.

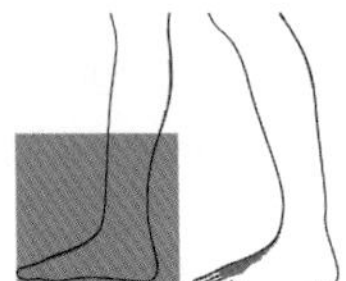

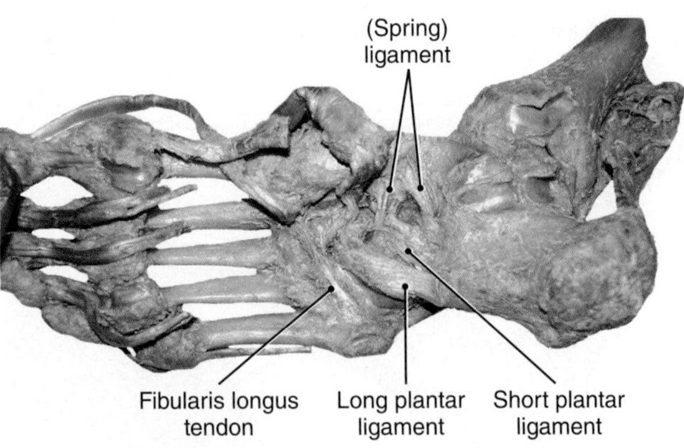

Fig. 18.45 Optional dissection: plantar view of the foot, highlighting plantar calcaneonavicular (spring) ligament and long and short plantar ligaments.

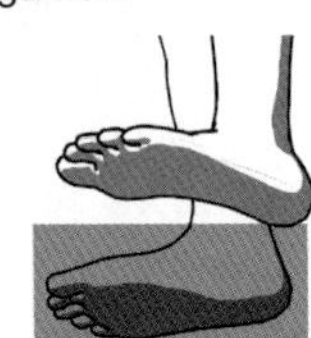

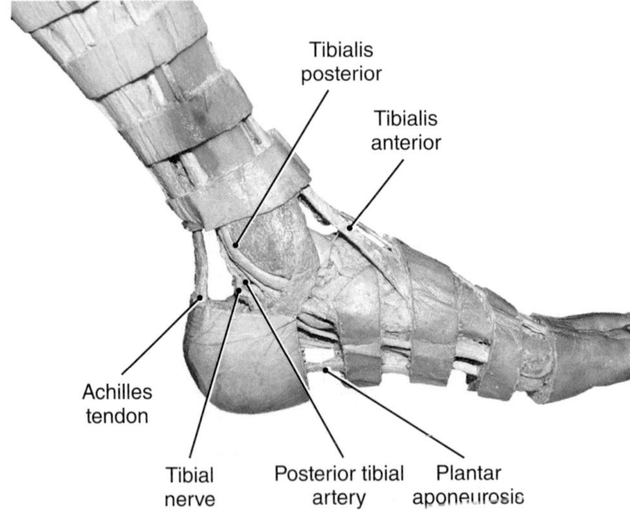

Fig. 18.46 Special dissection: lateral view, demonstrating the depth from the skin to various layers of the foot, ankle, and leg, from superficial to deep.

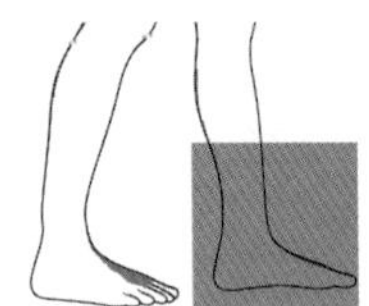

DISSECTION TIP

The long plantar ligament crosses over the tendon of the fibularis longus muscle. The short plantar (plantar calcaneocuboid) ligament attaches to the cuboid bone. Sometimes, the long plantar ligament may be confused with the spring ligament attached to the navicular bone (see Fig. 18.45).

CREATIVE DISSECTION

- **In this dissection, strips of skin are left intact. We dissected the intervals in between to appreciate the depth from the skin to the different layers of the foot, ankle, and leg, from superficial to deep (Figs. 18.46–18.48).**

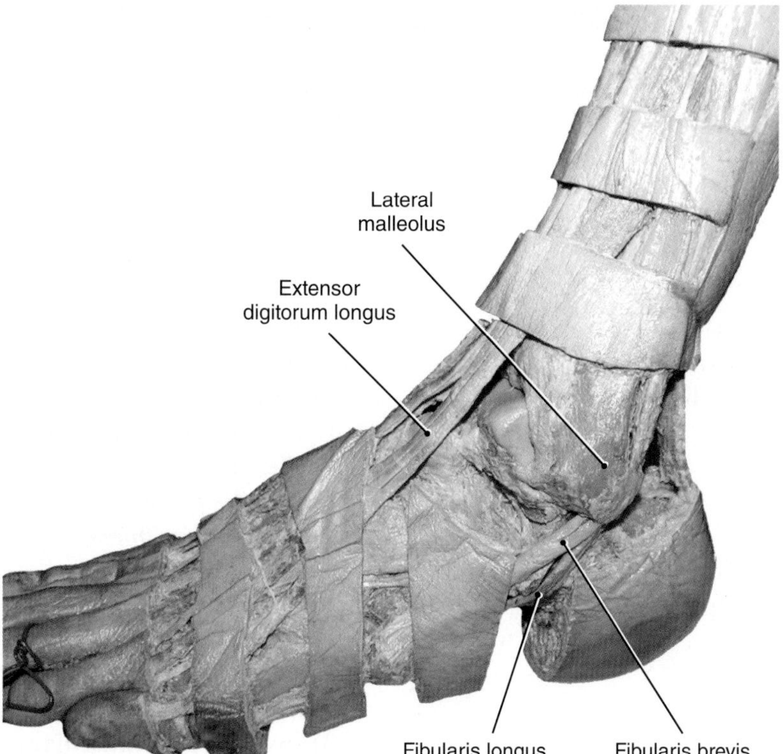

Fig. 18.47 Special dissection: medial view; appreciate the depth from the skin (superficial to deep) to the different layers of the foot, ankle, and leg.

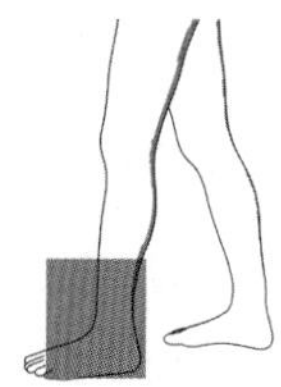

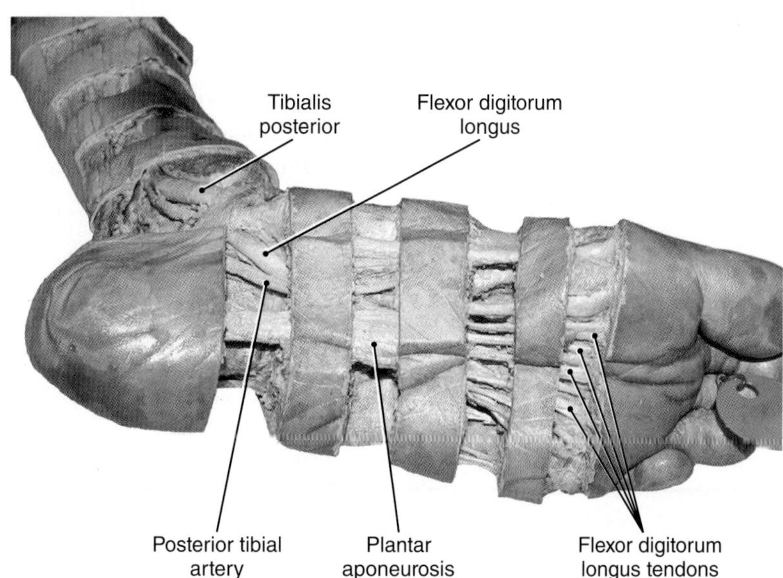

Fig. 18.48 Special dissection: plantar view, highlighting differing layers of the foot and ankle, from superficial to deep.

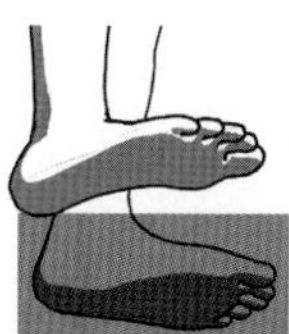

LABORATORY IDENTIFICATION CHECKLIST

NERVES

- ☐ Common fibular
  - ☐ Superficial fibular
  - ☐ Lateral sural cutaneous
- ☐ Sural communicating (normally formed from tibial and common fibular, but can form independently)
- ☐ Deep fibular
- ☐ Tibial
  - ☐ Medial sural cutaneous
- ☐ Sural (normally formed from tibial and common fibular, but can form independently)

ARTERIES

- ☐ Popliteal
- ☐ Anterior tibial
- ☐ Posterior tibial
- ☐ Circumflex fibular
- ☐ Fibular

VEINS

- ☐ *Superficial*
  - ☐ Great (long) saphenous
  - ☐ Small (lesser) saphenous
- ☐ Deep
  - ☐ Popliteal
  - ☐ Posterior tibial
  - ☐ Fibular
  - ☐ Anterior tibial
  - ☐ Sural

MUSCLES

- ☐ *Anterior compartment*
  - ☐ Tibialis anterior
  - ☐ Extensor hallucis longus
  - ☐ Extensor digitorum longus
  - ☐ Fibularis tertius
- ☐ *Posterior compartment*
- ☐ Superficial
  - ☐ Gastrocnemius
  - ☐ Soleus
  - ☐ Plantaris
- ☐ Deep
  - ☐ Popliteus
  - ☐ Flexor hallucis longus
  - ☐ Flexor digitorum longus
  - ☐ Tibialis posterior
- ☐ *Lateral compartment*
- ☐ Fibularis longus
- ☐ Fibularis brevis

CONNECTIVE TISSUE

- ☐ Anterior intermuscular septum
- ☐ Transverse intermuscular septum
- ☐ Posterior intermuscular septum
- ☐ Interosseous membrane of the leg
- ☐ Superior extensor retinaculum

LIGAMENTS

- ☐ *Lateral ankle complex*
  - ☐ Anterior talofibular ligament
  - ☐ Calcaneofibular ligament
  - ☐ Posterior talofibular ligament
- ☐ *Medial ankle complex*
  - • Deltoid
  - • Anterior tibiotalar part
  - • Tibionavicular part
  - • Tibiocalcaneal part
  - • Posterior tibiotalar part
  - • Long
  - • Short
  - • Spring

BONES

- ☐ Fibula
- ☐ Tibia

BEFORE YOU BEGIN

Identify and palpate the **calcaneus**, the **lateral longitudinal arch**, and the five **metatarsal heads** (**Fig. 19.1**).

SKIN AND SUBCUTANEOUS TISSUE

- **Make a longitudinal incision starting from the lateral side of the calcaneus and following the lateral side of the lateral longitudinal arch, terminating at the 1st metatarsal head (Fig. 19.2).**

DISSECTION TIP

You also could begin the incision from the plantar surface of the 1st metatarsal head and then end at the calcaneus.

DISSECTION TIP

An alternate incision involves making a longitudinal cut from the calcaneus to the 1st digit and a second, transverse incision from the 1st digit to the lateral longitudinal arch, then removing the skin laterally from the foot.

- **Reflect the skin medially while maintaining its attachment to the calcaneus (Fig. 19.3). Observe the**

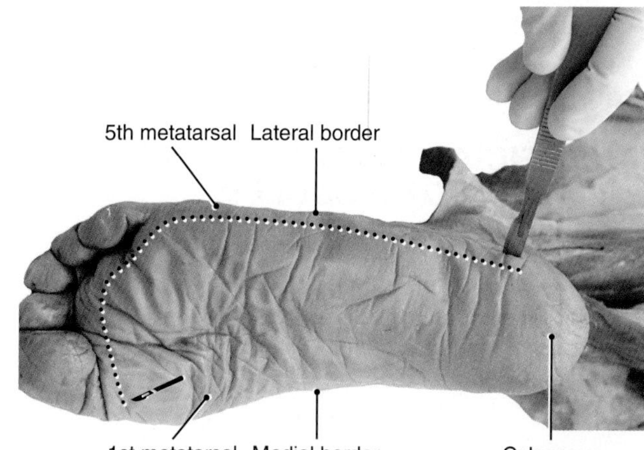

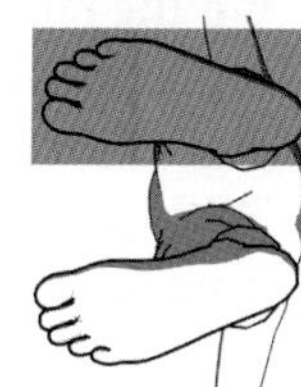

Fig. 19.2 Longitudinal incision starts from lateral side of the calcaneus and follows the lateral longitudinal arch.

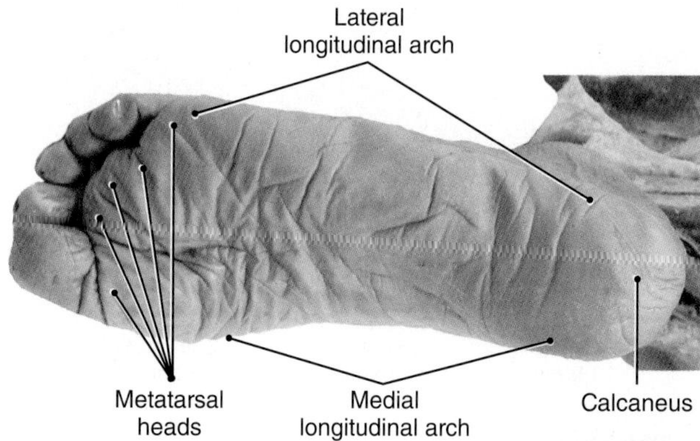

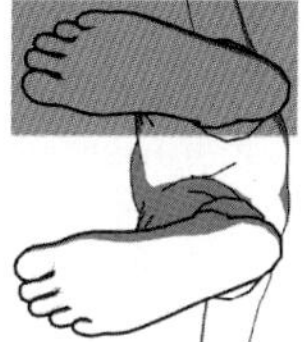

Fig. 19.1 View of the plantar surface of the foot for identifying the calcaneus, lateral longitudinal arch, and five metatarsal heads.

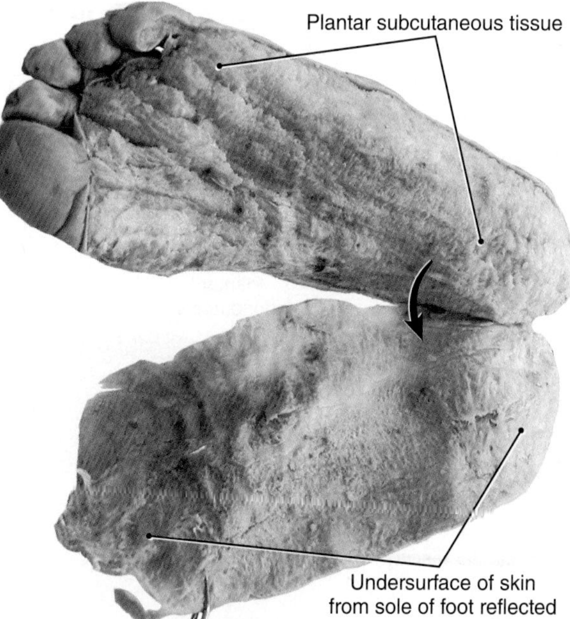

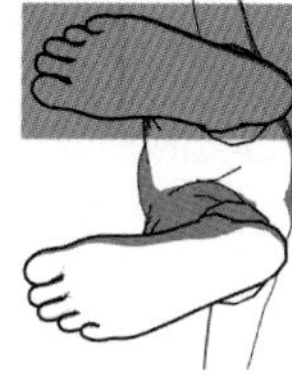

Fig. 19.3 Skin completely reflected over the plantar portion of the foot, maintaining attachment to the calcaneus.

fatty, plantar subcutaneous tissue and the thick layer of connective tissue, the plantar aponeurosis.

- With a scalpel, make an incision from the lateral side of the calcaneus, reflecting the plantar subcutaneous tissue over the plantar aponeurosis medially (Fig. 19.4).
- Remove the fat and expose the plantar aponeurosis with its fibrous slips to the digits.

(SUPERFICIAL) FIRST LAYER OF PLANTAR FOOT MUSCLES

ANATOMY **NOTE**

The three muscles that make up the first and most superficial layer of muscles of the plantar surface of the foot are the abductor hallucis, flexor digitorum brevis, and abductor digiti minimi.

- On the lateral side of the foot, identify the abductor digiti minimi muscle and the underlying flexor digiti minimi muscle (Fig. 19.5).
- With a scalpel, cut the plantar aponeurosis at its junction with the flexor digiti minimi muscle and reflect it toward the calcaneus (see Figs. 19.5 and 19.6).
- Just underneath the plantar aponeurosis, separate the flexor digitorum brevis muscle, which arises from the deep surface of the aponeurosis (see Fig. 19.6).
- Carefully dissect out the fibrous attachments between the plantar aponeurosis and the digits (Fig. 19.7).
- Identify and clean the abductor hallucis muscle located on the medial side of the foot (see Fig. 19.7).
- Lateral to the abductor hallucis muscle, clean and expose the tendons of the flexor digitorum brevis muscle (see Fig. 19.7)

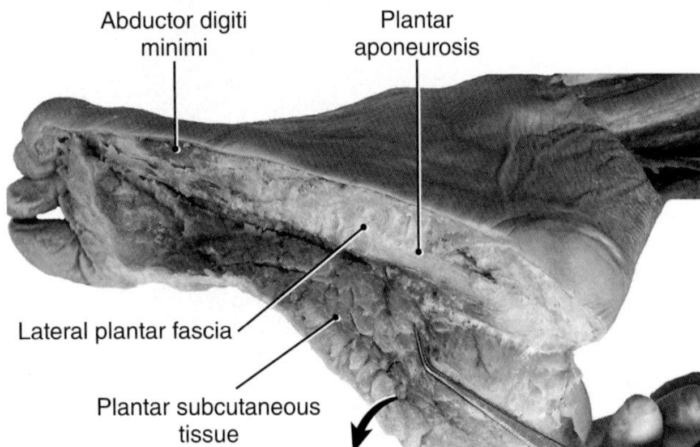

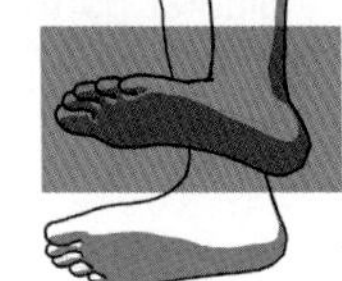

Fig. 19.4 Lateral side of the calcaneus dissected, reflecting fat over the plantar aponeurosis medially.

- Lateral to the flexor digitorum brevis, identify and clean the abductor digiti minimi muscle (see Fig. 19.7).
- Between the abductor hallucis and flexor digitorum brevis muscles, identify and expose the medial plantar nerve (see Fig. 19.7).
- Identify the digital branches of the medial plantar nerve (see Fig. 19.7).

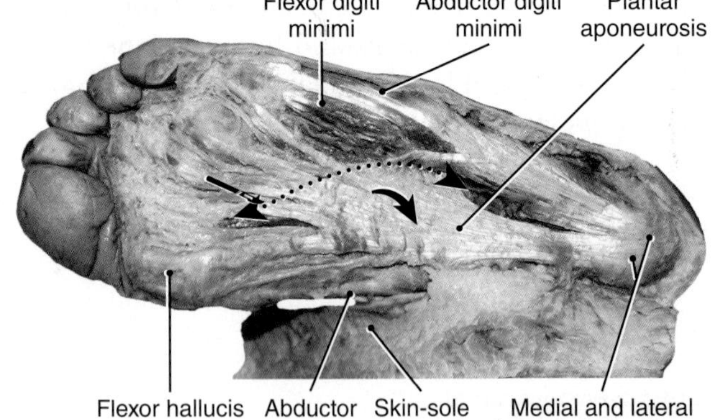

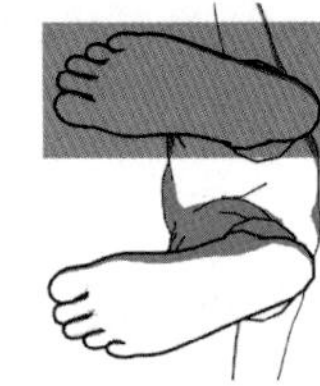

Fig. 19.5 Fat removal exposes the plantar aponeurosis and fibrous slips to the digits.

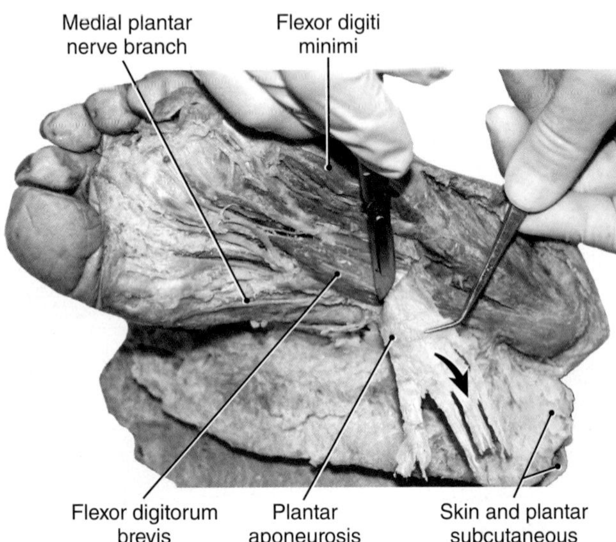

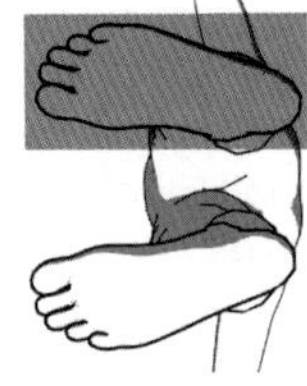

Fig. 19.6 Abductor digiti minimi muscle and the underlying flexor digiti minimi on the lateral side of the foot, with plantar aponeurosis reflected toward the calcaneus, and the flexor digitorum brevis muscle separated.

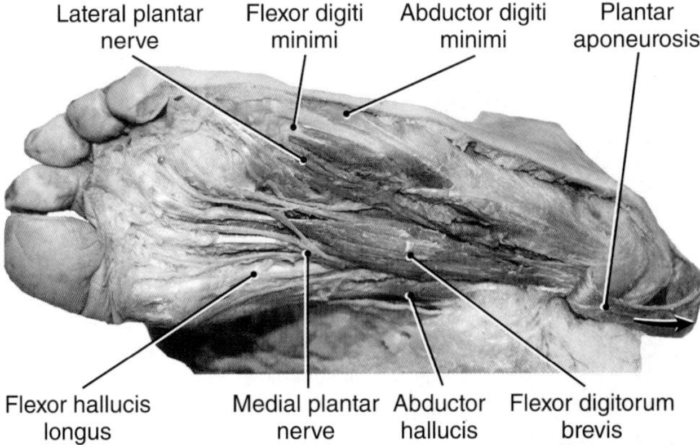

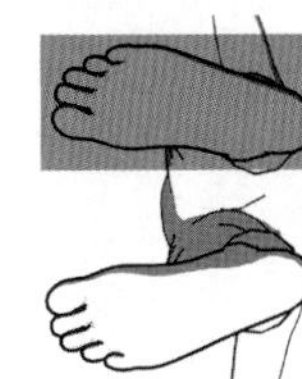

Fig. 19.7 Dissected view between plantar aponeurosis and digits reveals digital branches of medial plantar nerve, abductor hallucis muscle, and tendons of flexor digitorum brevis and abductor digiti minimi muscles.

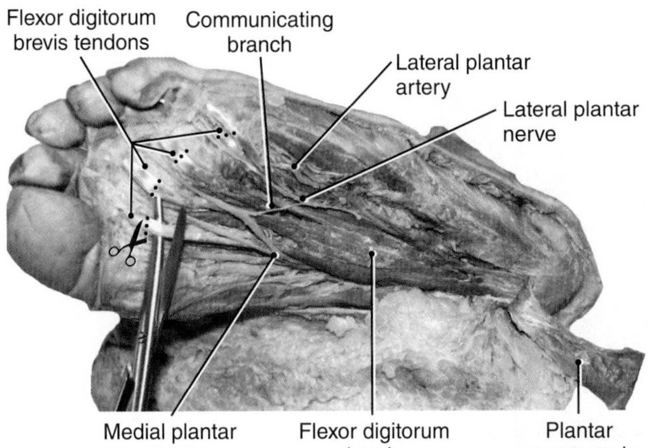

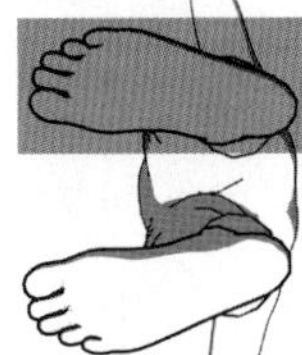

Fig. 19.8 Medial plantar nerve exposed between the abductor hallucis and flexor digitorum brevis muscles, with the distal parts of the flexor digitorum brevis tendons incised.

SECOND LAYER OF PLANTAR FOOT MUSCLES

ANATOMY **NOTE**

The muscles that make up the second layer of muscles of the plantar region of the foot are the flexor hallucis longus, flexor digitorum longus, lumbricals, and quadratus plantae.

- **Identify the distal part of the tendons of the flexor digitorum brevis muscle and cut them using scissors (Fig. 19.8).**

DISSECTION **TIP**

Be careful not to cut the medial plantar nerve.

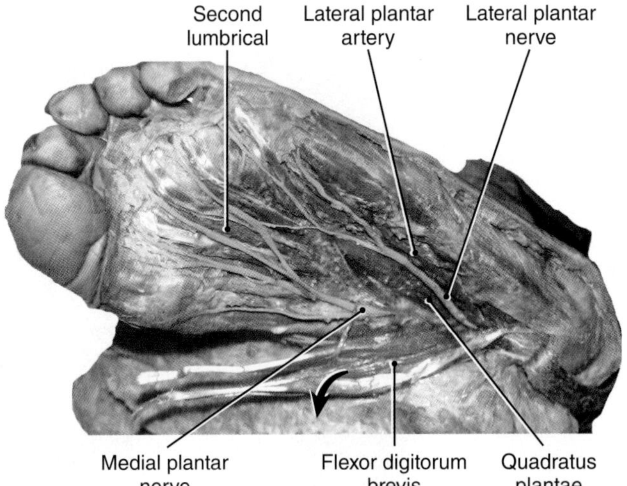

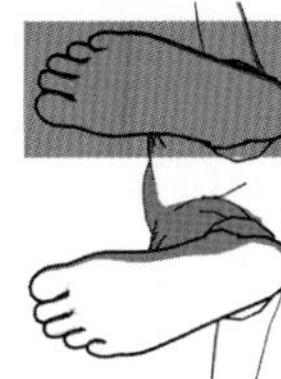

Fig. 19.9 View of the lateral plantar nerve and artery underneath the flexor digitorum brevis muscle.

- **Reflect the tendons (with the belly of the flexor digitorum brevis) posteriorly (Fig. 19.9).**
- **Just underneath the flexor digitorum brevis, clean and expose the lateral plantar nerve and lateral plantar artery as they travel to the lateral side of the foot (see Fig. 19.9 and Plate 19.1).**
- **Identify and clean the tendon of the flexor hallucis longus muscle located on the medial side of the foot and inserting onto the base of the distal phalanx of the 1st digit (Fig. 19.10).**
- **Lateral to the flexor hallucis longus muscle, identify the tendons of the flexor digitorum longus muscle inserting onto the distal phalanges of the remaining four digits (see Fig. 19.10).**
- **Arising from the tendons of the flexor digitorum longus, identify the four lumbrical muscles (see Fig. 19.10).**
- **Lateral to the main belly of the flexor digitorum longus, identify a small muscle arising from the calcaneus and inserting onto the flexor digitorum, the quadratus plantae muscle (see Fig. 19.10).**

THIRD LAYER OF PLANTAR FOOT MUSCLES

ANATOMY **NOTE**

The muscles that occupy the third layer of muscles of the plantar aspect of the foot are the adductor hallucis, flexor hallucis brevis, abductor digiti minimi, and flexor digiti minimi brevis.

- **With scissors, cut the tendon of the flexor digitorum longus at the posterior aspect of the foot near the calcaneus (Fig. 19.11).**

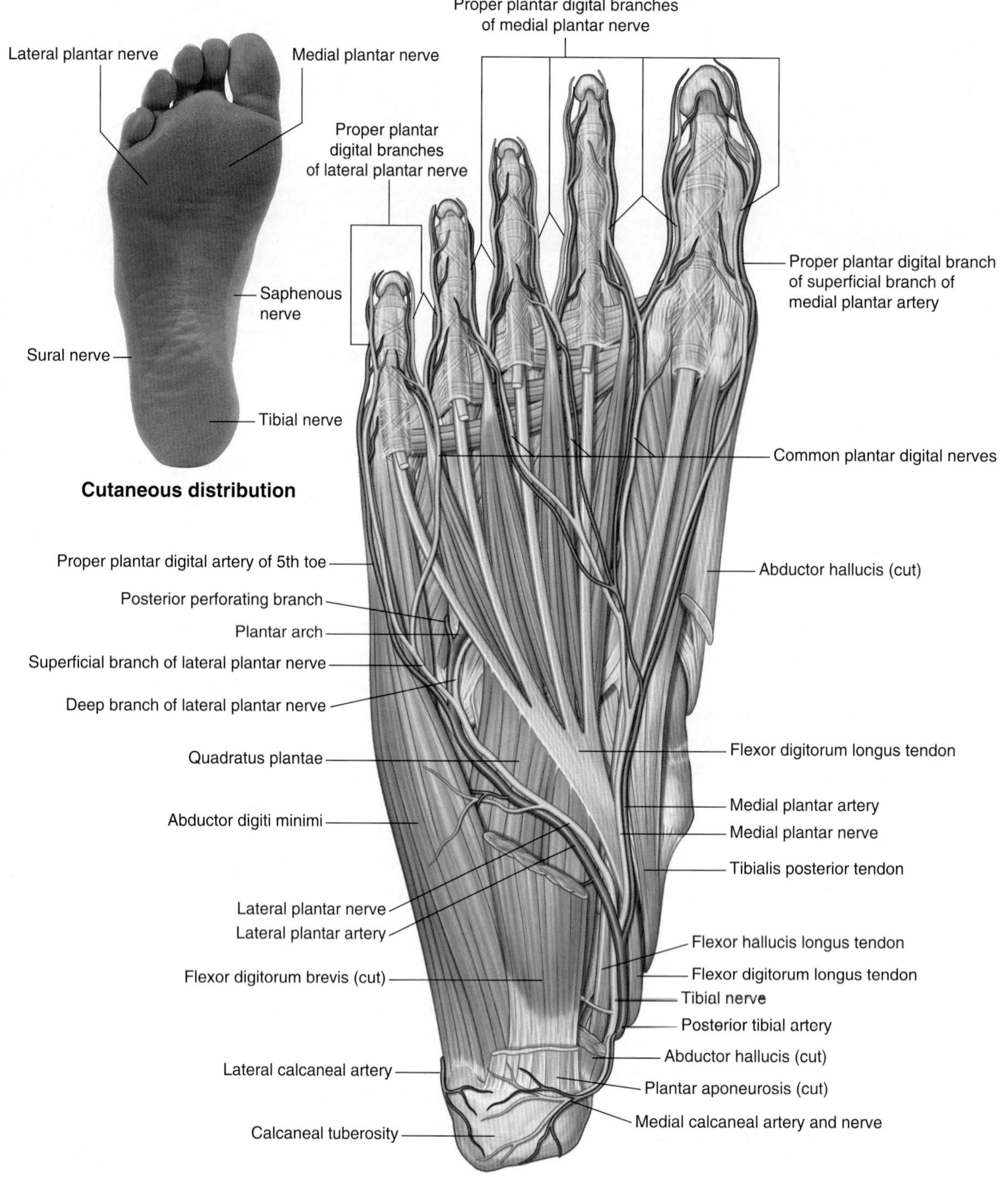

Plate 19.1 Arteries and nerves of the sole of the foot. (From Drake RL et al. *Gray's Atlas of Anatomy*, 3rd edition, Philadelphia, Elsevier, 2021.)

- **Continue the dissection by transecting the quadratus plantae muscle close to its calcaneal origin (Fig. 19.12).**
- **Reflect the transected muscle toward the toes (Fig. 19.13).**
- **Clean the small amounts of fascia and fat (Fig. 19.14).**
- **Identify the two heads of the adductor hallucis muscle, the oblique head and transverse head (see Fig. 19.14).**
- **Posterior to the two heads of the adductor hallucis muscle, identify the fibularis longus tendon and its attachments (see Fig. 19.14).**
- **Cut the tendon of the flexor hallucis longus muscle and reflect it toward the great toe, exposing the flexor hallucis brevis muscle underneath.**
- **On the lateral side of the foot, retract the tendon of the abductor digiti minimi muscle, and medially and deep to it, identify the flexor digiti minimi brevis muscle.**

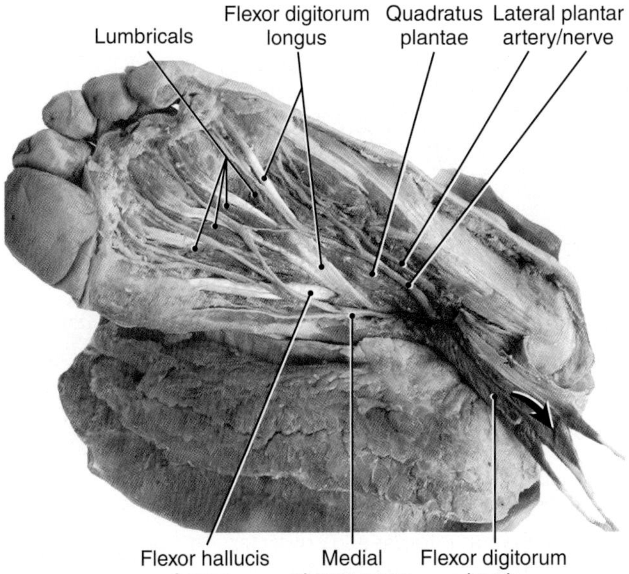

Fig. 19.10 View highlighting the tendon of the flexor hallucis longus muscle on the medial side of the foot.

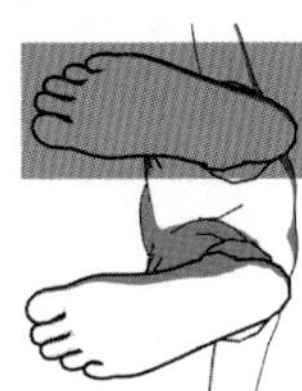

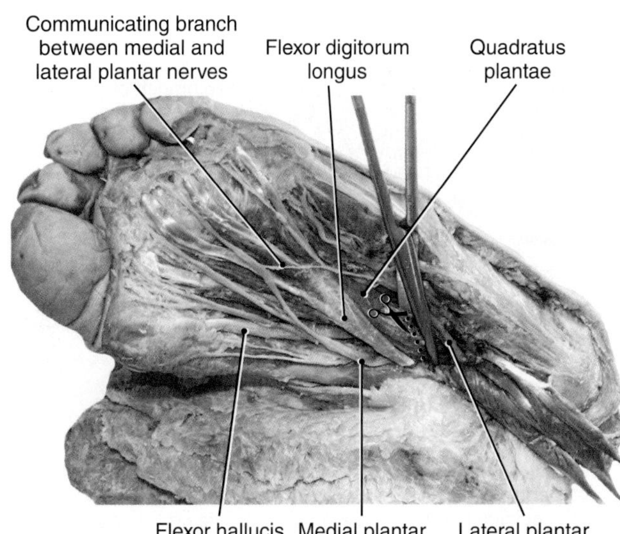

Fig. 19.12 Quadratus plantae muscle transected.

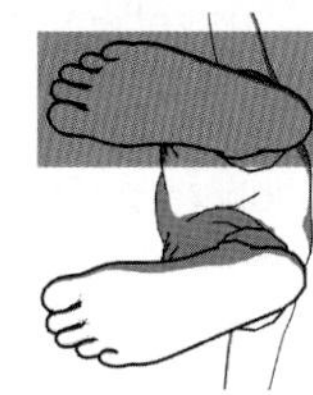

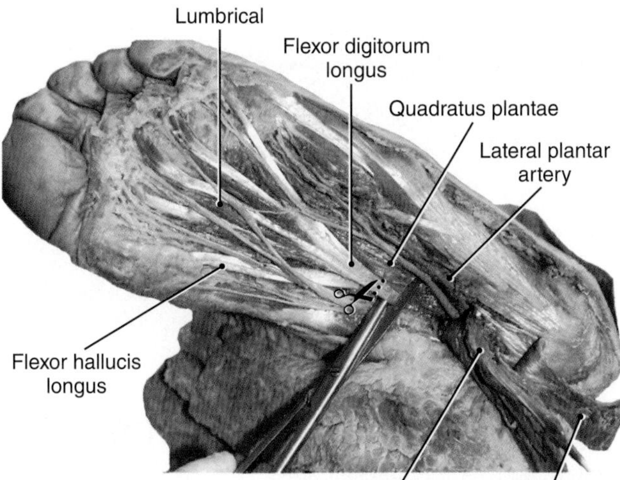

Fig. 19.11 Tendon of the flexor digitorum longus incised at the posterior aspect of the foot near the calcaneus.

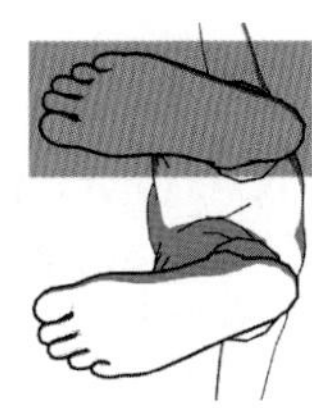

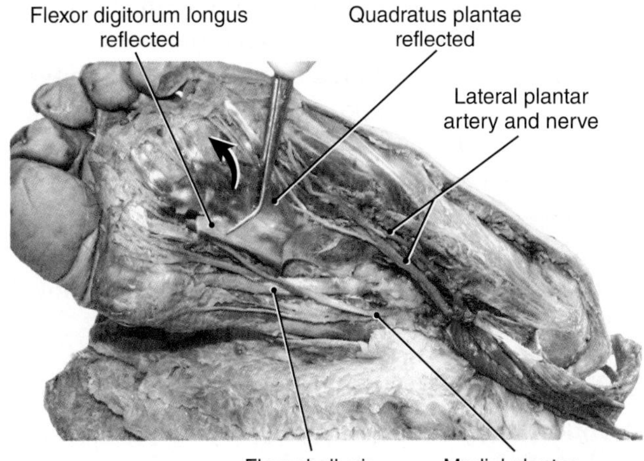

Fig. 19.13 Quadratus plantae muscle reflected toward the toes

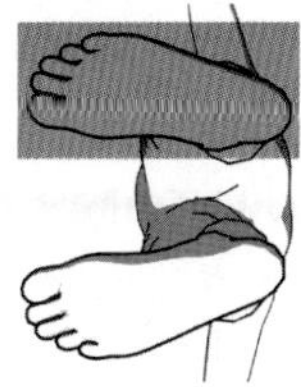

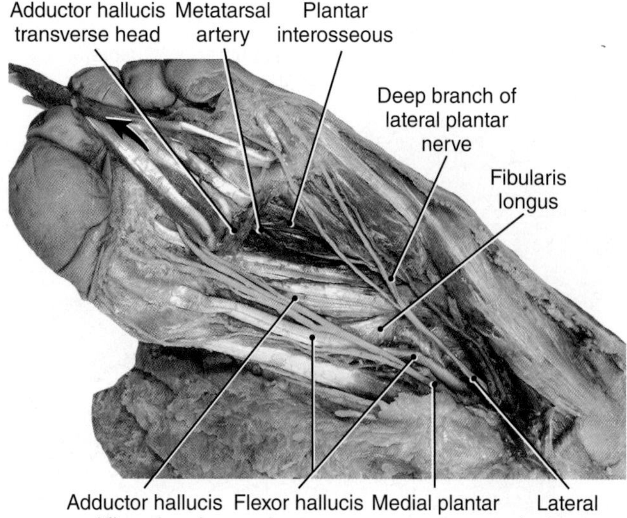

Fig. 19.14 Tendon of the flexor hallucis longus reflected toward the great toe, exposing the flexor hallucis brevis muscle; tendon of abductor digiti minimi reflected to locate the flexor digiti minimi brevis muscle.

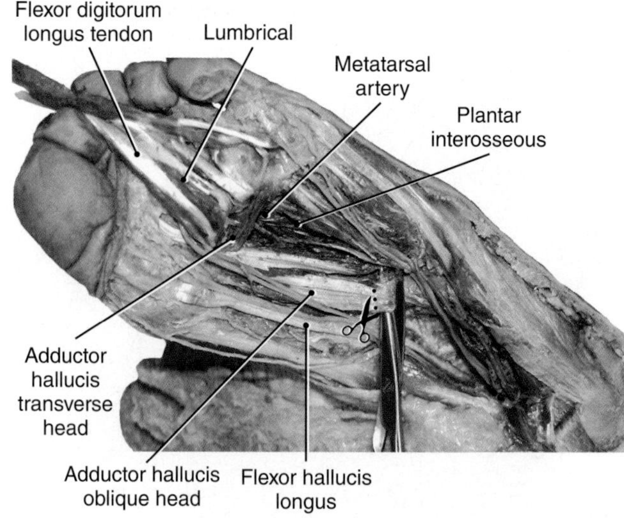

Fig. 19.15 Plantar interosseous muscles exposed in the space between the two heads of the adductor hallucis muscle, with the oblique head cut.

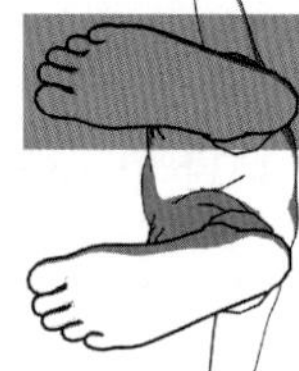

(DEEP) FOURTH LAYER OF PLANTAR FOOT MUSCLES

- **Trace the lateral plantar nerve from its origin to its final distribution and identify its superficial and deep branches (see Fig. 19.1 and Plate 19.2).**
- **In the space between the two heads of the adductor hallucis muscle, expose the interosseous muscles (see Fig. 19.14).**
- **With scissors, cut the oblique head of the adductor hallucis muscle (Fig. 19.15).**
- **Fully expose and trace the fibularis longus tendon to its insertion onto the medial cuneiform and 1st metatarsal bones (Fig. 19.16).**

OPTIONAL DISSECTION

- **Follow the lateral plantar artery along the lateral plantar nerve and identify the deep branch of the lateral plantar nerve at the lateral side of the oblique head of the adductor hallucis muscle (see Plate 19.1).**

ANATOMY **NOTE**

At this point, the lateral plantar artery gives off a branch to form the plantar arch, just underneath the oblique head of the adductor hallucis muscle.

- **Identify the plantar arch and trace its branches, the metatarsal branches, which provide plantar digital vessels to the digits (see Plate 19.1).**

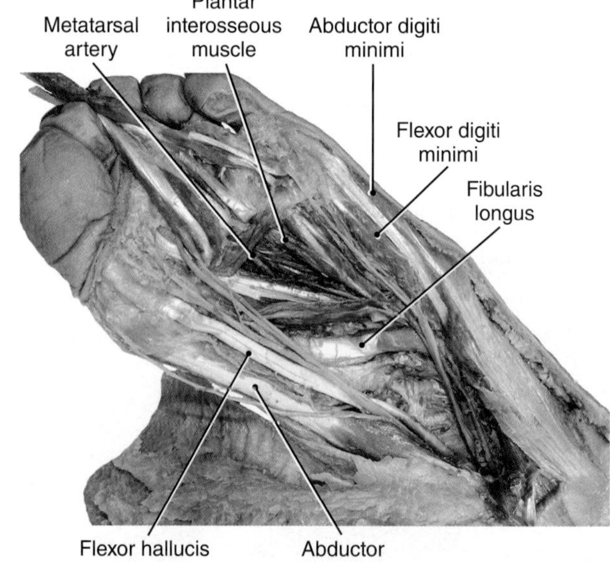

Fig. 19.16 Identify the fibularis longus tendon and insertion onto the medial cuneiform and 1st metatarsal bones.

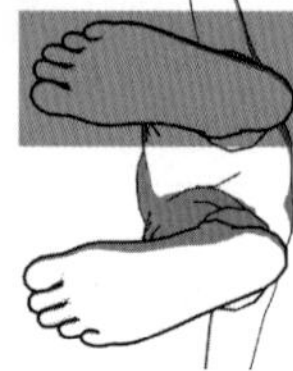

ANATOMY **NOTE**

In the space between the 1st and 2nd metatarsals, the deep plantar arch joins the plantar branch of the dorsalis pedis artery.

- **Follow the plantar arch to the base of the 1st metatarsal and identify the plantar branch to the dorsalis pedis artery (see Plate 19.1).**

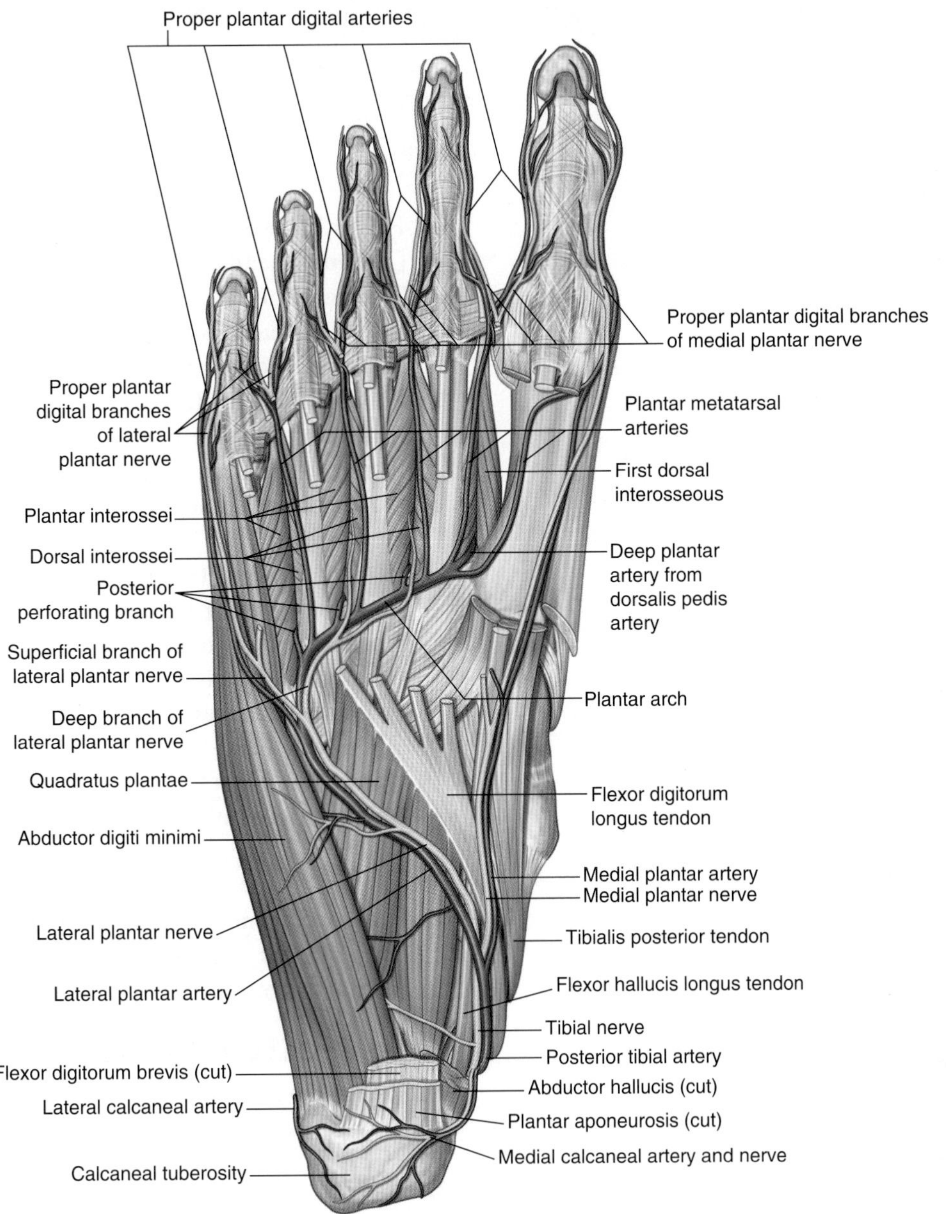

Plate 19.2 Arteries and nerves of the sole of the foot (deep). (From Drake RL et al. *Gray's Atlas of Anatomy*, 3rd edition, Philadelphia, Elsevier, 2021.)

LABORATORY IDENTIFICATION CHECKLIST

NERVES

- ☐ Medial plantar
  - ☐ Common plantar digital
  - ☐ Plantar digital
- ☐ Lateral plantar
  - ☐ Common plantar digital
  - ☐ Plantar digital
- ☐ Superficial fibular
  - ☐ Dorsal digital branches
- ☐ Deep fibular
  - ☐ Dorsal digital branches
- ☐ Medial calcaneal
- ☐ Lateral calcaneal

ARTERIES

- ☐ Dorsalis pedis
  - ☐ Lateral tarsal
  - ☐ Arcuate
  - ☐ Deep plantar
- ☐ Dorsal metatarsal
  - ☐ Dorsal digital
- ☐ Medial plantar
- ☐ Plantar metatarsal
  - ☐ Common plantar digital
  - ☐ Plantar digital
- ☐ Lateral plantar
- ☐ *Plantar arch*
  - ☐ Plantar metatarsal
  - ☐ Common plantar digital
  - ☐ Plantar digital

VEINS

- ☐ Dorsal venous arch

MUSCLES

- ☐ *Dorsal muscles and tendons*
  - ☐ Extensor hallucis brevis
  - ☐ Extensor digitorum brevis
  - ☐ Extensor hallucis longus tendon
  - ☐ Extensor digitorum longus tendons
  - ☐ Tibialis anterior tendon
- ☐ *Plantar muscles and leg muscle tendons*
- ☐ Abductor hallucis
- ☐ Flexor hallucis brevis
  - ☐ Medial head
  - ☐ Lateral head
- ☐ Flexor hallucis longus tendon
- ☐ Flexor digitorum brevis
- ☐ Flexor digiti minimi brevis
- ☐ Abductor digiti minimi
- ☐ Flexor digitorum longus tendons
- ☐ Quadratus plantae
- ☐ Lumbricals
- ☐ Fibularis longus tendon
- ☐ Tibialis posterior tendon
- ☐ Fibularis brevis tendon
- ☐ Adductor hallucis
  - ☐ Transverse head
  - ☐ Oblique head
- ☐ Plantar interossei
- ☐ Dorsal interossei

LIGAMENTS

- ☐ Plantar calcaneonavicular (spring) ligament
- ☐ Long plantar ligament
- ☐ Plantar calcaneocuboid (short plantar) ligament

CONNECTIVE TISSUE

- ☐ Plantar aponeurosis
- ☐ Inferior extensor retinaculum

BONES

- ☐ *Tarsal bones*
  - ☐ Calcaneus
  - ☐ Talus
  - ☐ Cuboid
  - ☐ Navicular
  - ☐ Medial cuneiform
  - ☐ Middle cuneiform
  - ☐ Lateral cuneiform
  - ☐ Metatarsals
  - ☐ Phalanges
    - ☐ Proximal
    - ☐ Middle
    - ☐ Distal

CLINICAL APPLICATIONS

TROCHANTERIC BURSITIS INJECTION

Clinical Application

Introduce local anesthetic using an intrabursal injection to relieve pain of inflamed trochanteric bursa.

Anatomical Landmarks (Figs. VII.1 and VII.2)

- **Skin**
- **Subcutaneous tissue**
- **Iliotibial tract**
- **Tensor fasciae latae**
- **Trochanteric bursa**
- **Greater trochanter**

PREPATELLAR BURSITIS ASPIRATION/INJECTION

Clinical Application

Introduce local anesthesia into the prepatellar bursa to withdraw fluid and relieve pain.

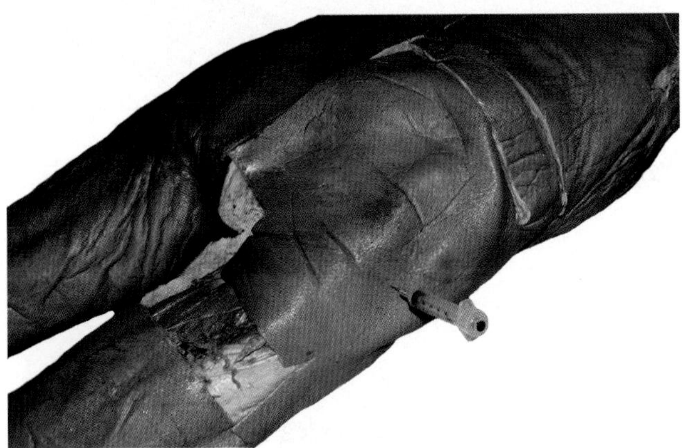

Fig. VII.1

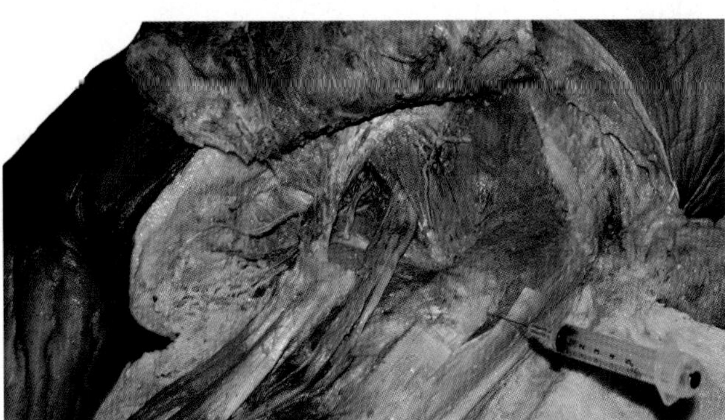

Fig. VII.2

Anatomical Landmarks (Fig. VII.3)

- **Skin**
- **Patella**
- **Subcutaneous tissue**
- **Prepatellar bursa**

SUPRAPATELLAR BURSITIS ASPIRATION/INJECTION

Clinical Application

Introduce local anesthesia into suprapatellar bursa to relieve pain from prepatellar bursa.

Anatomical Landmarks (Fig. VII.4)

- **Skin**
- **Subcutaneous tissue**
- **Suprapatellar bursa**

PLANTAR FASCIITIS INJECTION

Clinical Application

Injection of local anesthetic at the point of maximal tenderness within the plantar aponeurosis, often near its attachment to the medial process of the calcaneal tuberosity, to relieve pain caused by inflamed fascia.

Anatomical Landmarks (Figs. VII.5 and VII.6)

- **Skin**
- **Subcutaneous tissue/fat pad**
- **Plantar fascia/aponeurosis**
- **Calcaneal tuberosity**

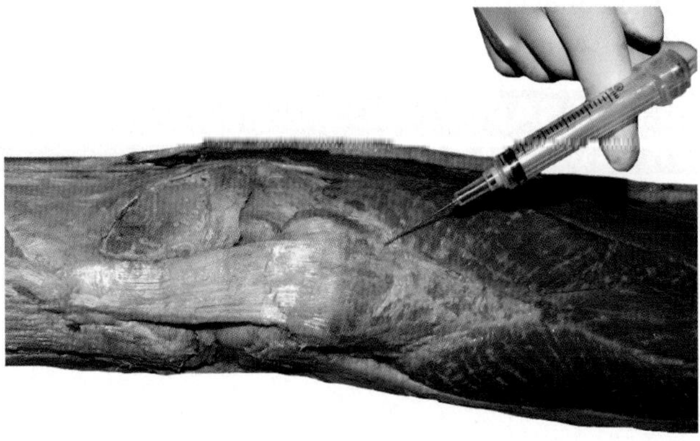

Fig. VII.3

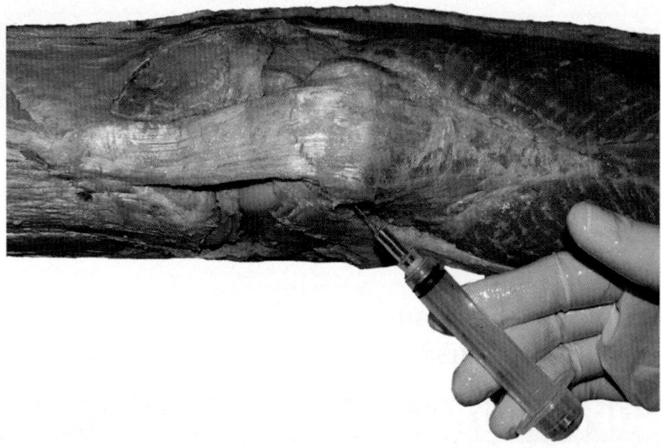

Fig. VII.4

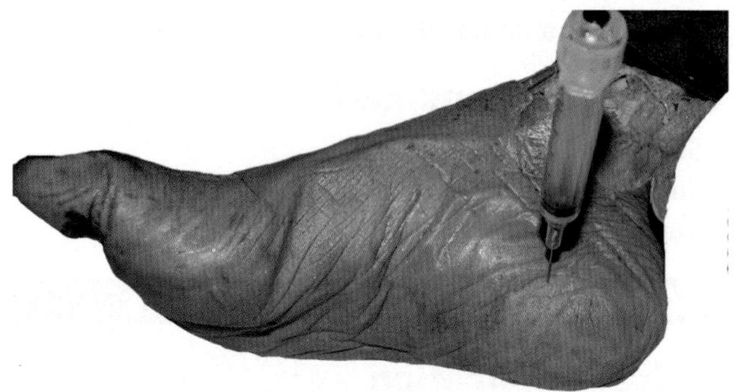

Fig. VII.5

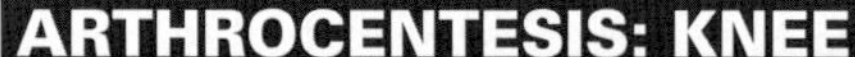

ARTHROCENTESIS: KNEE

Clinical Application

Introduce a needle into the knee joint to withdraw fluid and to inject medication.

Anatomical Landmarks

- **Skin**
- **Subcutaneous tissue**
- **Patella**
- **Intercondylar notch**
- **Joint cavity**

GREAT SAPHENOUS VEIN CUTDOWN OR CANNULATION

Clinical Application

Procedure to cannulate great saphenous vein for infusion of fluids.

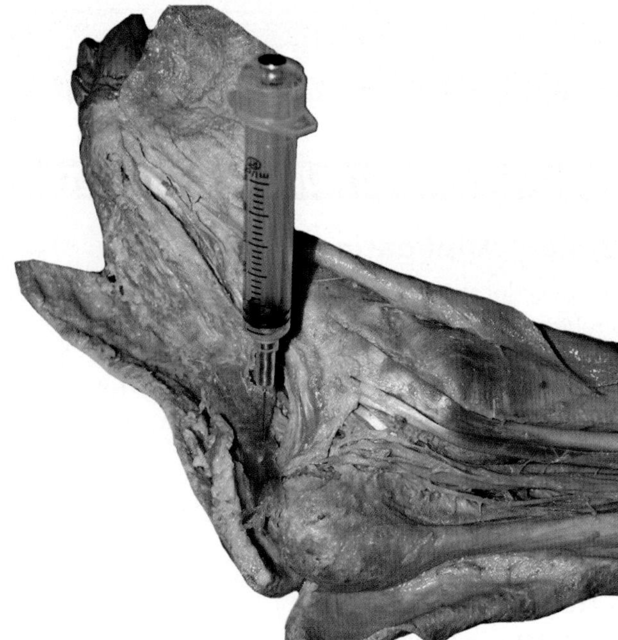

Fig. VII.6

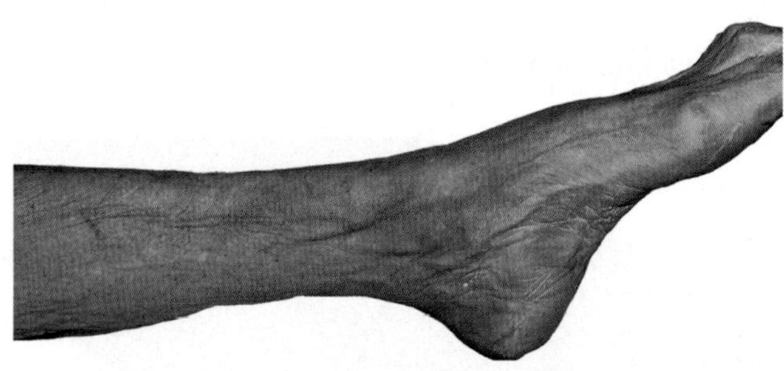

Fig. VII.7

Anatomical Landmarks (Figs. VII.7 and VII.8)

- **Medial malleolus**
- **Skin**
- **Subcutaneous tissue**
- **Great saphenous vein**
- **Saphenous nerve**

FEMUR AND KNEE REPLACEMENT

Fig. VII.9 depicts the head of a femur replacement. Fig. VII.10 depicts a knee replacement.

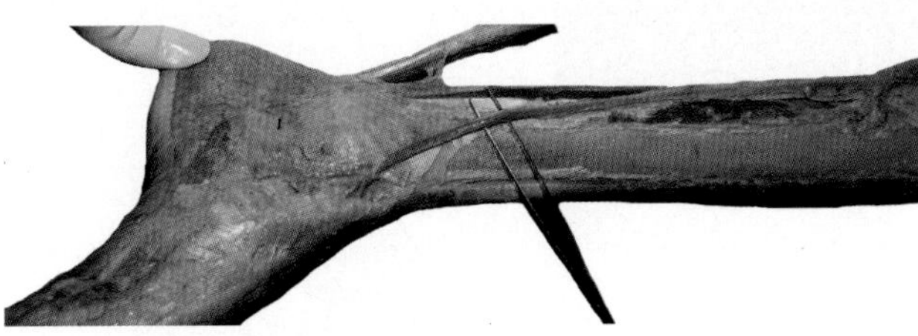

Fig. VII.8

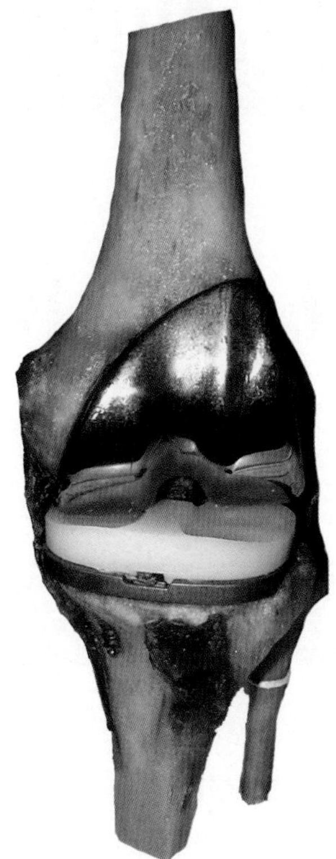

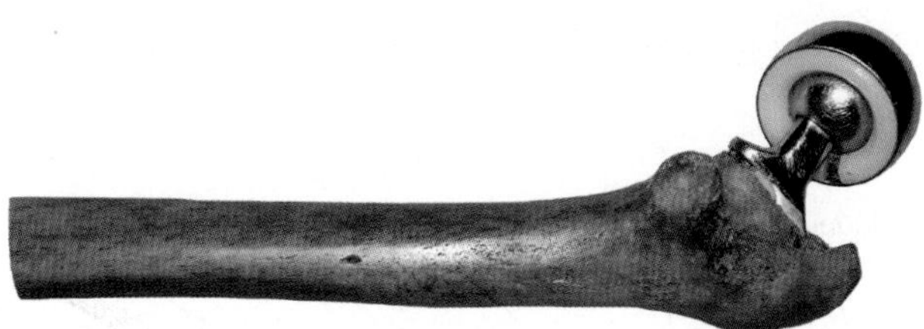

Fig. VII.9

Fig. VII.10

SECTION VIII

HEAD AND NECK

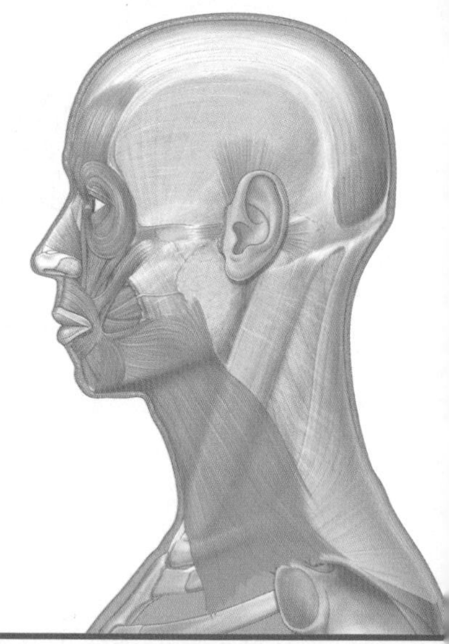

CHAPTER 20 NECK

BEFORE YOU BEGIN

Palpate the following landmarks on your neck or the cadaver:

- Mental protuberance
- Hyoid bone
- Laryngeal prominence
- Cricoid cartilage
- Jugular notch
- Thyroid gland

ANATOMIC TRIANGLES

ANATOMY NOTE

The neck may be divided into smaller topographic areas, the *triangles* of the neck. Specifically, the "carotid triangle" and the "root of the neck" are involved in many surgical procedures on the neck. There are two major triangles of the neck, the anterior and posterior cervical triangles (Fig. 20.1). The *anterior cervical triangle* is demarcated anteriorly by the midline of the neck; its base is the lower border of the mandible, and the posterior border is the anterior boundary of the sternocleidomastoid muscle. The *posterior cervical triangle* is bounded by the posterior border of the sternocleidomastoid muscle, the middle third of the clavicle, and the anterior border of the trapezius muscle. The cervical triangles may be subdivided as follows:

Anterior cervical triangle

1. Digastric triangle
2. Submental triangle
3. Carotid triangle
4. Muscular triangle

Posterior cervical triangle

5. Occipital triangle
6. Supraclavicular triangle

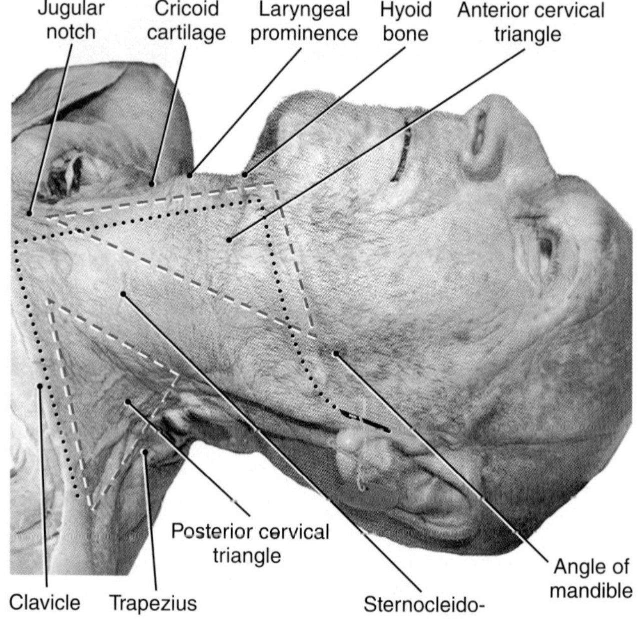

Fig. 20.1 Anterolateral view of surface anatomy of the neck, highlighting the hyoid bone, laryngeal prominence, jugular notch, angle of the mandible, sternocleidomastoid muscle, and anterior and posterior triangles of the neck.

NECK DISSECTION

- **Make a midline incision through the skin from the jugular notch to the mental protuberance.**
- **A second incision should be made from the jugular notch laterally, along the clavicle to the acromion.**
- **Make a final incision from the mental protuberance along the inferior border of the mandible, toward the earlobe (Fig. 20.2). Carefully reflect the skin over the neck.**

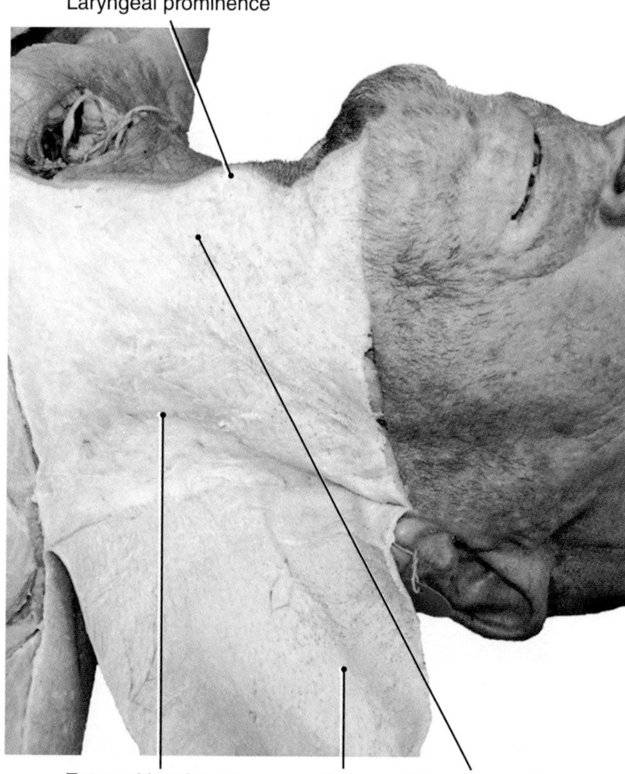

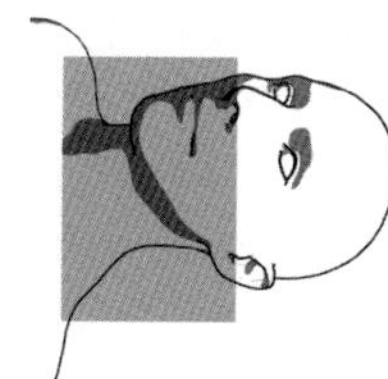

Fig. 20.2 Skin of the neck reflected laterally, revealing the subcutanous tissues (subcutaneous tissue), laryngeal prominence, superficial lobe of the submandibular gland, external jugular vein, and midline of the neck.

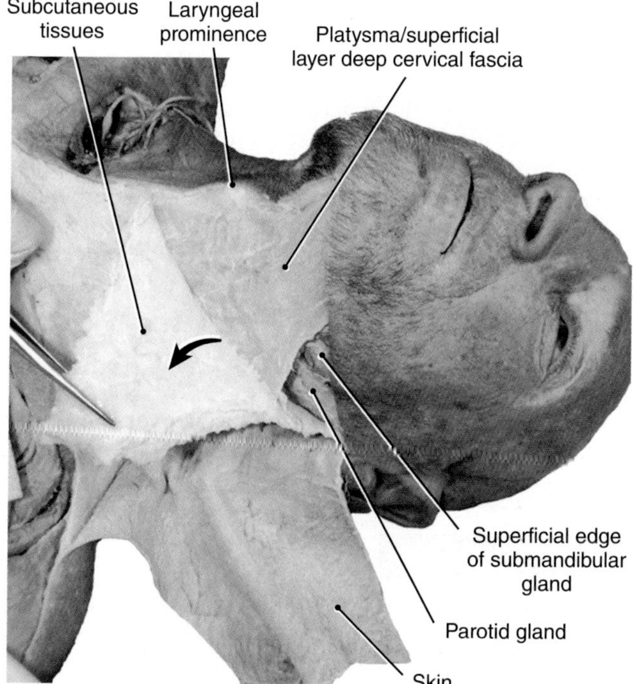

Fig. 20.3 Skin and subcutaneous tissues reflected laterally, revealing the platysma muscle, superficial layer of deep cervical fascia, superficial part of the submandibular gland, and sternocleidomastoid muscle.

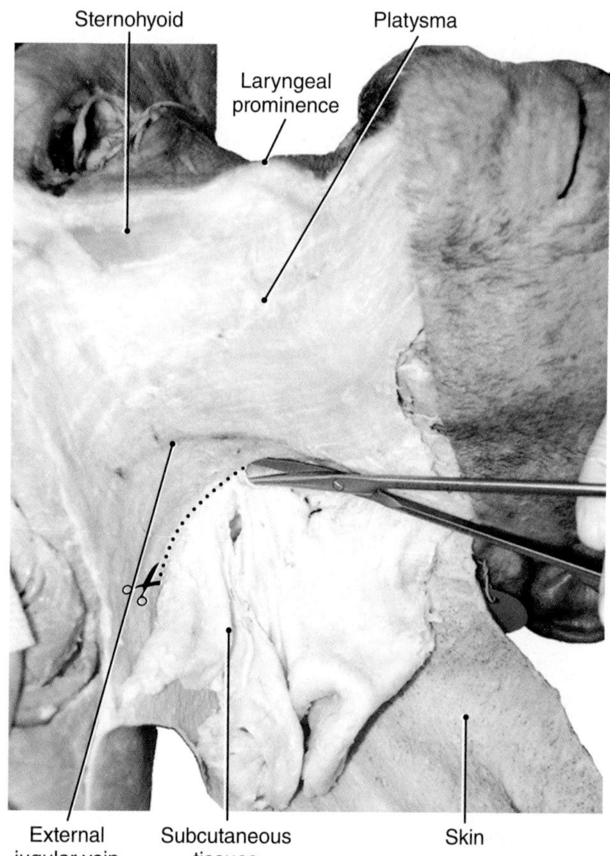

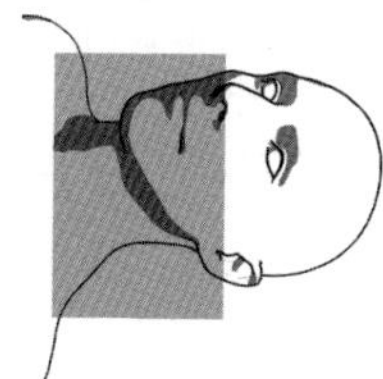

Fig. 20.4 Separation of lateral border of platysma muscle from the subcutaneous tissues.

DISSECTION TIP

The skin over the neck is thin. Pay special attention during its reflection for the subcutaneous tissue so that you do not reflect the platysma muscle with the skin.

- **Start the dissection by reflecting the subcutaneous tissue from the mental protuberance inferiorly and laterally toward the clavicles to expose the platysma muscle (Fig. 20.3).**
- **The platysma is pierced by the transverse cervical and supraclavicular nerves of the cervical plexus. Reflect the subcutaneous tissue over the platysma muscle (Fig. 20.4).**
- **Separate the lateral border of the platysma from the subcutaneous tissue. Identify the sternocleidomastoid muscle posterior to the platysma muscle.**
- **At the level of the clavicle, cut and reflect the platysma upward, toward the mandible (Figs. 20.5 and 20.6).**
- **Similarly, at the angle of the mandible, cut and reflect the platysma anteriorly (Fig. 20.7).**

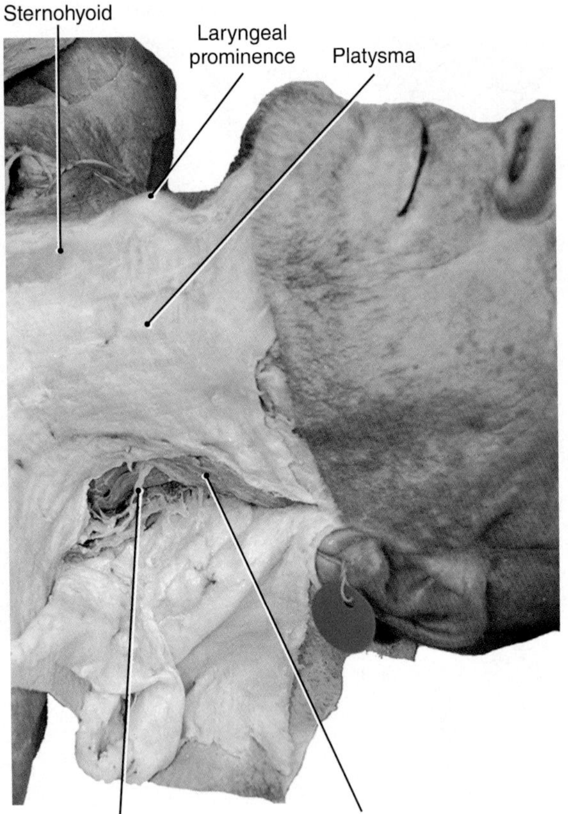

Fig. 20.5 Identification of the accessory nerve at the junction between the platysma, sternocleidomastoid, and trapezius muscles.

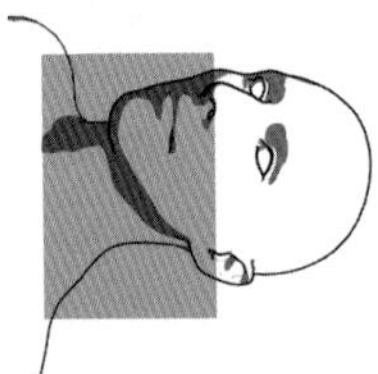

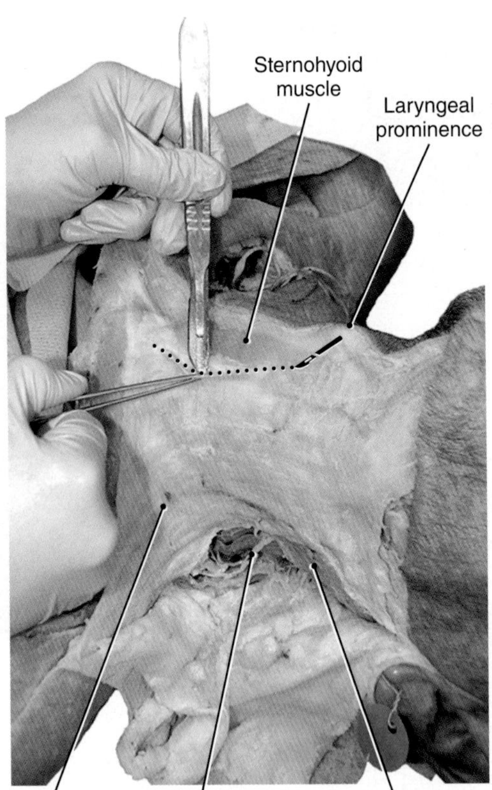

Fig. 20.6 Dissection of the medial border of the platysma muscle from underlying tissues.

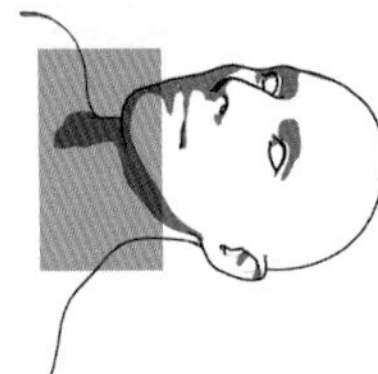

- **Preserve the attachment of the platysma muscle along the mandible (Fig. 20.8).**

DISSECTION **TIP**

At this stage, it is possible to identify the cervical branch of the facial nerve, which innervates the platysma muscle, coursing from the inferior border of the parotid gland toward the platysma.

- **About 1 cm inferior to the angle of the mandible, expose the marginal mandibular branch of the facial nerve.**

ANATOMY **NOTE**

The cervical branch of the facial nerve passes superficial to the facial vein and artery. The facial vein usually drains into the internal jugular vein through the retromandibular vein.

- **Notice the investing *cervical fascia* covering the sternocleidomastoid muscle (see Fig. 20.8). Observe the external jugular vein running lateral to the sternocleidomastoid muscle.**

ANATOMY **NOTE**

The investing cervical fascia encircles the trapezius and sternocleidomastoid muscles before reaching the midline of the neck. In the gap between these muscles, this fascia forms the "roof" of the posterior cervical triangle. The "floor" of the posterior cervical triangle is provided by another fascia, the *prevertebral fascia,* which covers the musculature of the lateral and anterior aspects of the vertebral column. Between these two fascial layers there is a potential space.

- **Clean the superficial investing fascia over the sternocleidomastoid muscle (Fig. 20.9 and Plate 20.1).**

DISSECTION **TIP**

Use care when you reflect the fascia so as not to sever any of the cutaneous nerves arising deep to the posterior edge of the sternocleidomastoid muscle.

- **Identify the external jugular vein running superficial to the sternocleidomastoid muscle, as well as the**

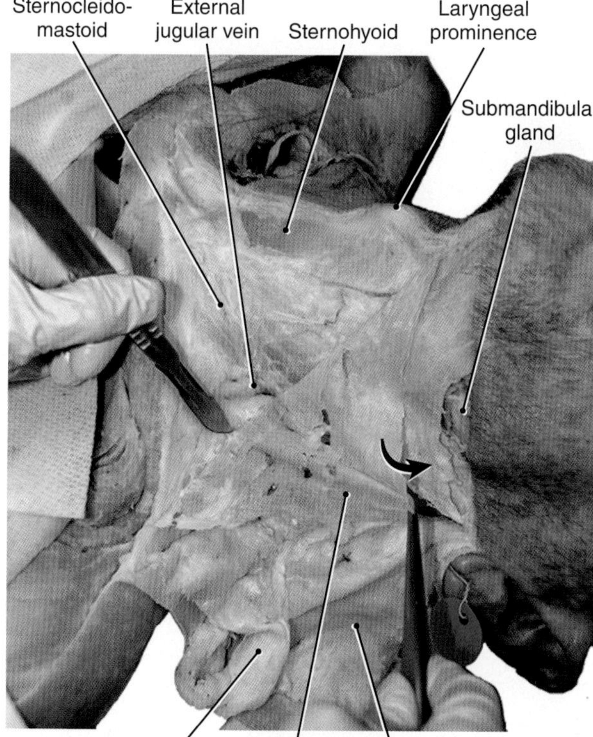

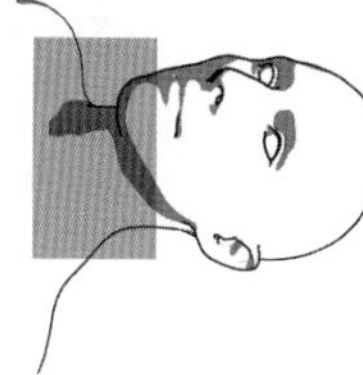

Fig. 20.7 Anterolateral view of neck with skin, subcutaneous tissues, and platysma reflected laterally, revealing the sternocleidomastoid muscle, external jugular vein, sternohyoid muscle, thyroid cartilage, and submandibular gland.

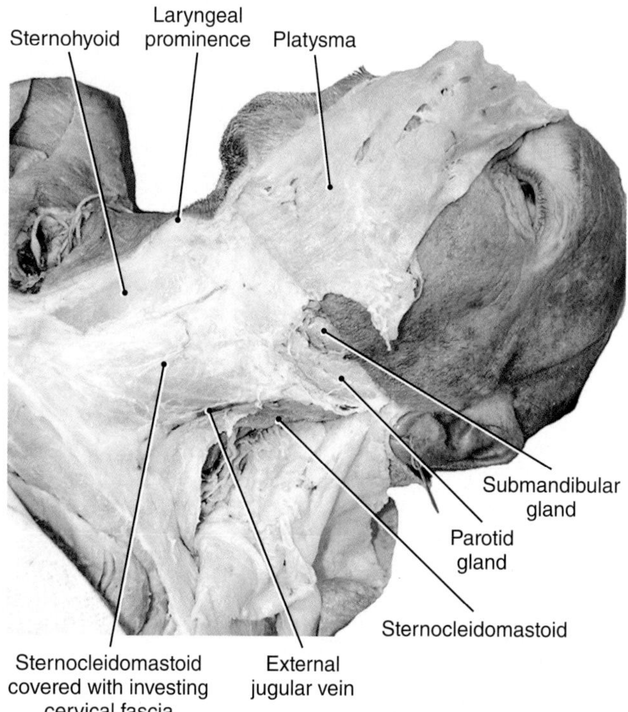

Fig. 20.8 Complete reflection of platysma muscle and exposure of underlying structures.

following cutaneous nerve branches of the cervical plexus:

- **Lesser occipital nerve (C2–C3)**
- **Great auricular nerve (C2–C3)**
- **Transverse cervical nerve (C2–C3)**
- **Supraclavicular nerves (C3–C4)**

- **These nerves emerge, from top to bottom, along the posterior border of the sternocleidomastoid muscle in the following order: the lesser occipital, great auricular, and transverse cervical nerves.**
- **Once you expose these nerves, look for the accessory nerve; it appears posterior to the sternocleidomastoid, about two-thirds the distance up its posterior edge, and then crosses the posterior triangle to reach the trapezius muscle.**

DISSECTION TIP

In many specimens the transverse cervical nerve, which is a cutaneous nerve, communicates with the cervical branch of the facial nerve, which is a motor nerve.

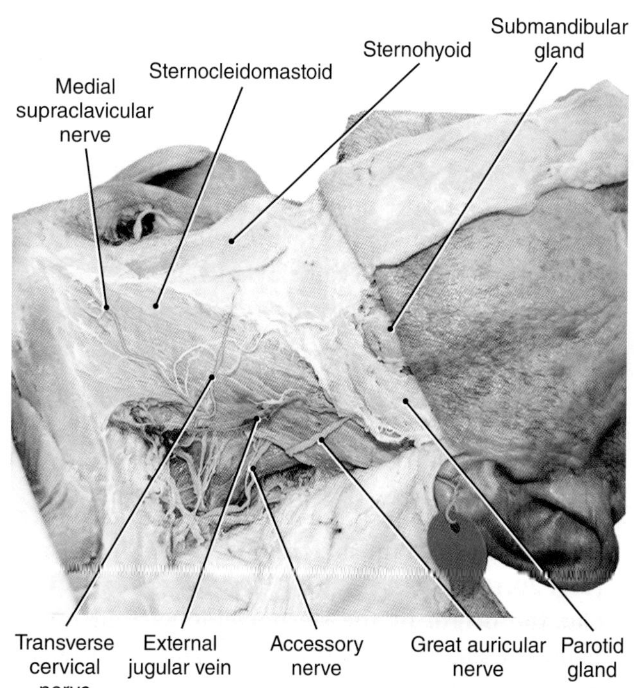

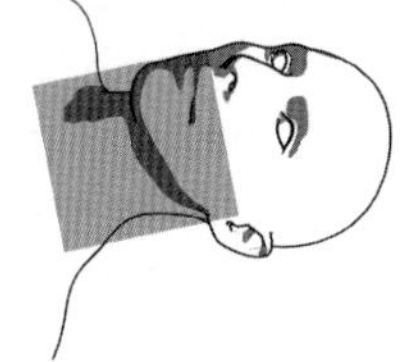

Fig. 20.9 Anterolateral view of the neck with skin and subcutaneous tissues reflected laterally and the platysma reflected superiorly.

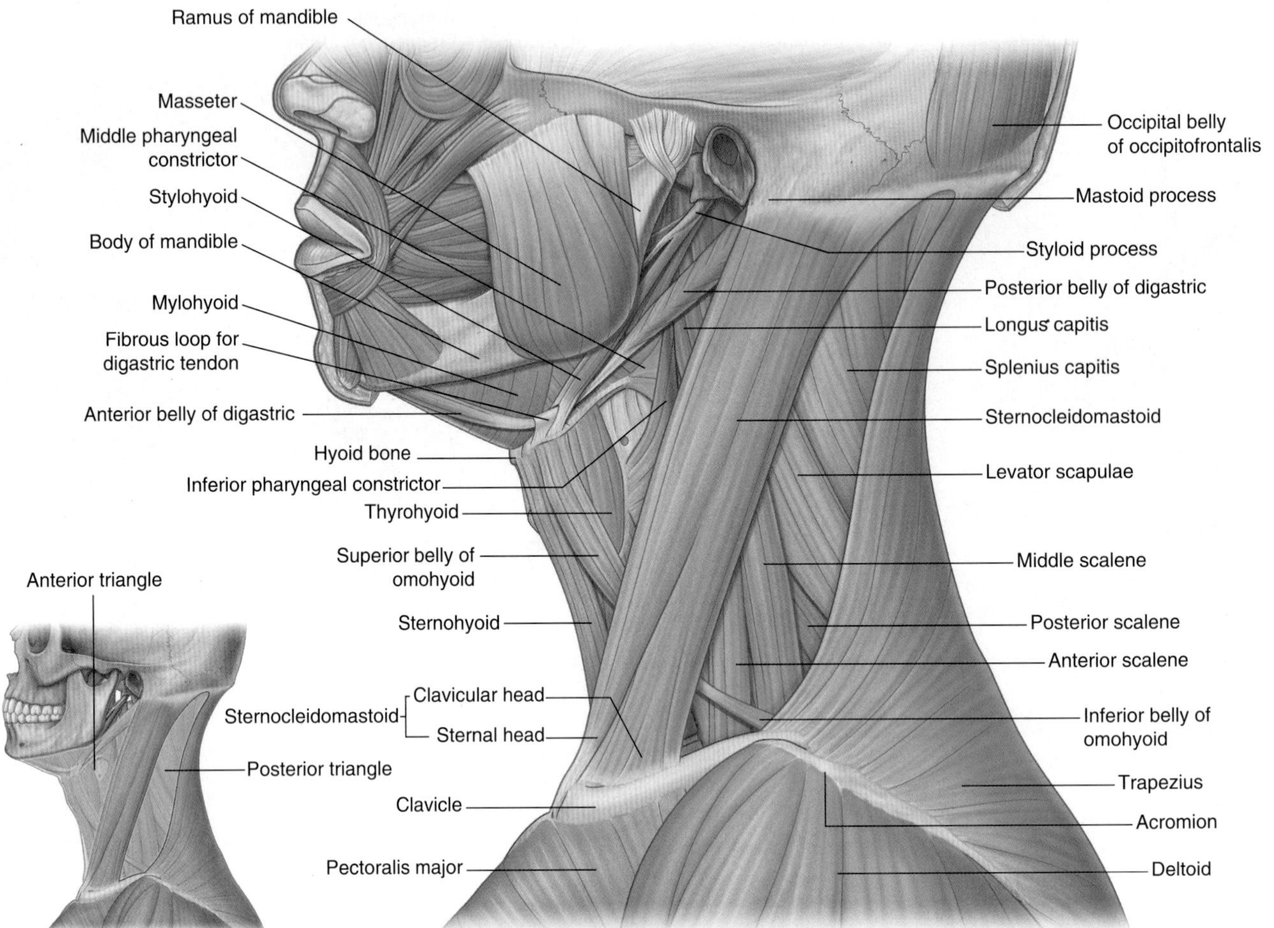

Plate 20.1 Lateral view of the muscles and triangle of the neck. (From Drake RL et al. *Gray's Atlas of Anatomy*, 3rd edition, Philadelphia, Elsevier, 2021.)

- **Identify the external jugular vein, which arises at the junction of the posterior auricular vein and the posterior division of the retromandibular vein. This vein terminates in the subclavian vein.**

DISSECTION **TIP**

The external jugular vein may be absent in the presence of a large anterior jugular vein.

- **With scissors, detach the medial border of the sternocleidomastoid muscle from its fascial investment (Fig. 20.10).**
- **Cut the origin of the sternocleidomastoid muscle from the clavicle and the manubrium of the sternum (Fig. 20.11).**
- **Reflect the sternocleidomastoid muscle upward, away from its fascia. Leave the posterior layer of the superficial cervical fascia intact.**
- **Trace the accessory nerve from the posterior aspect of the sternocleidomastoid muscle and preserve this nerve for later dissection.**
- **Dissect out the fascia and separate the parotid gland from the sternocleidomastoid muscle without damaging the great auricular and lesser occipital nerves.**

ANATOMY **NOTE**

In some specimens the accessory nerve will exhibit communications with C3 and C4 anterior rami. The accessory nerve in the posterior triangle is found between the superficial investing fascia and the prevertebral fascia.

DISSECTION **TIP**

In some cadavers the parotid gland may cover the most proximal portion of the sternocleidomastoid muscle (Fig. 20.12). It is important to separate the parotid gland from the sternocleidomastoid to reflect the muscle as laterally as possible. The more the sternocleidomastoid is reflected, the more space that will be available for later dissection.

- **Reflect the superficial layer of the investing fascia and note its contribution to the formation of the carotid sheath (Fig. 20.13).**

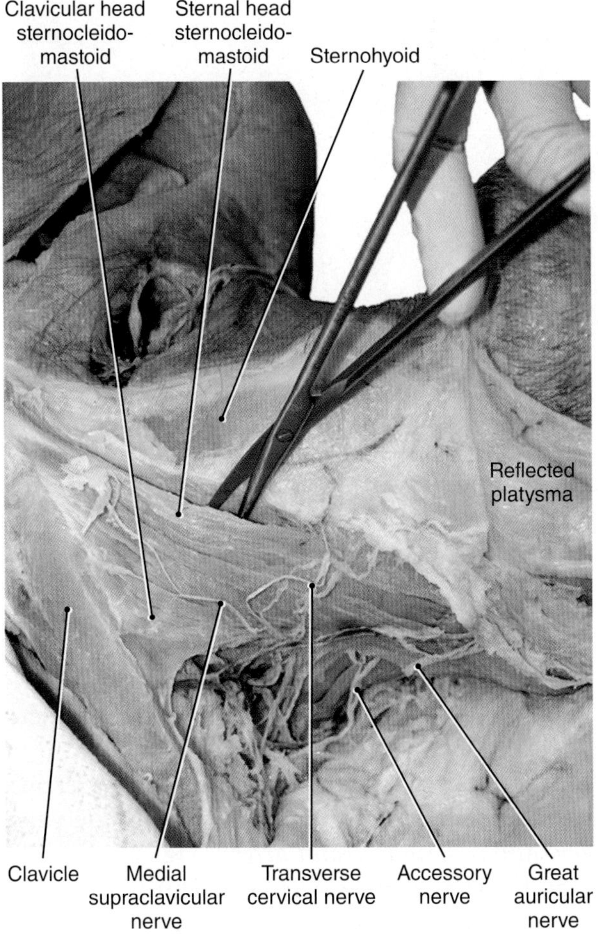

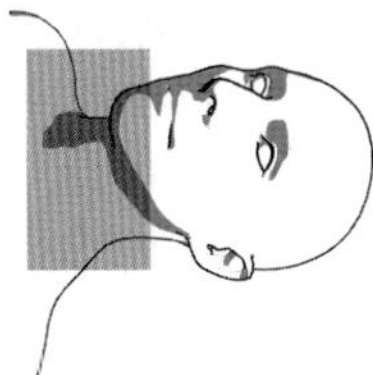

Fig. 20.10 Medial border of underlying tissues detached.

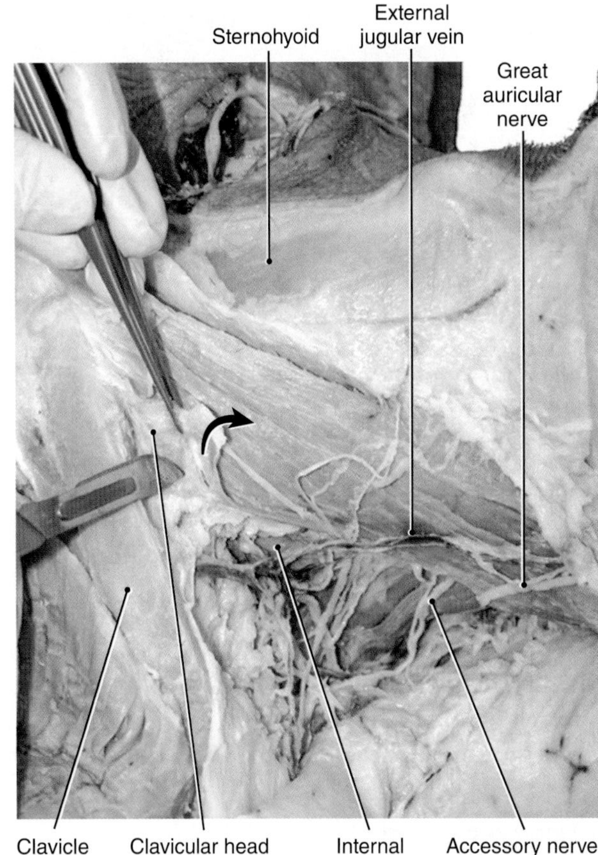

Fig. 20.11 Sternocleidomastoid muscle detached from clavicle.

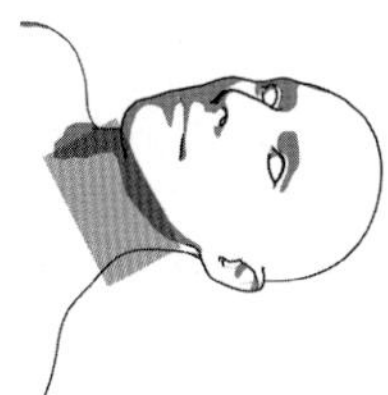

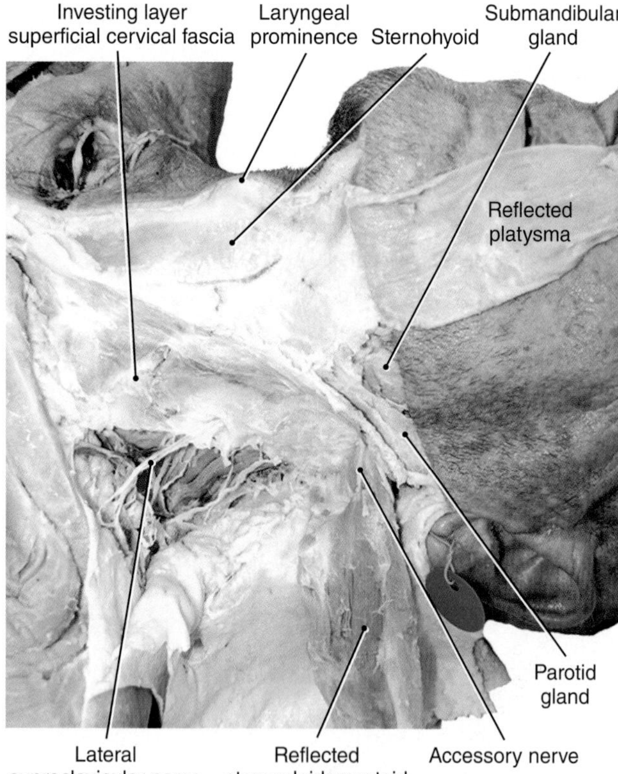

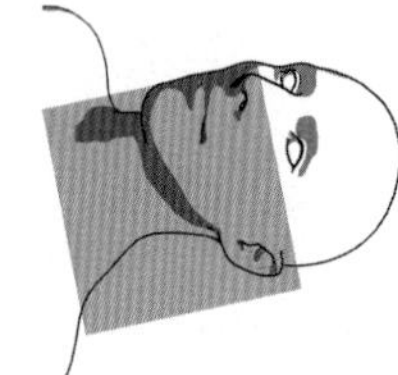

Fig. 20.12 Anterolateral view of the neck with skin, subcutaneous tissues, and sternocleidomastoid muscle reflected laterally and platysma reflected superiorly.

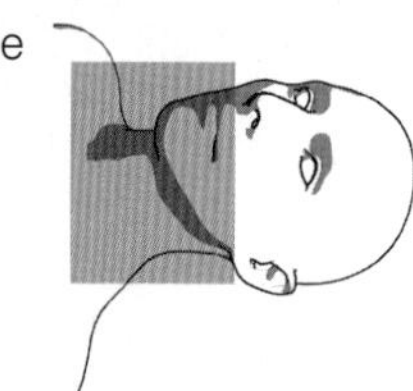

Fig. 20.13 Carotid sheath cleaned over the internal jugular vein.

- **Identify the carotid sheath, omohyoid muscle, and internal jugular vein.**
- **Clean the carotid sheath over the internal jugular vein.**

DISSECTION TIP

As you expose the internal jugular vein from the carotid sheath and superficial layer of the investing cervical fascia, look for the deep cervical lymph nodes. These lymph nodes are often prominent where the omohyoid crosses the internal jugular vein (jugulo-omohyoid node) and where the digastric muscle crosses the internal jugular vein (jugulodigastric node).

- **Identify the *ansa cervicalis.* The ansa cervicalis usually lies superficial to the internal jugular vein, outside the carotid sheath (Fig. 20.14). There are two techniques for the identification of the ansa cervicalis:**
  1. **Look superficial and lateral to the internal jugular vein in the lower part of the neck and identify the ansa cervicalis.**
  2. **Identify and clean the strap muscles. Follow their nerve supply backward and trace it to the ansa cervicalis. Specifically, identify the sternohyoid muscle and follow its small nerve branches proximally.**
- **Pull the internal jugular vein laterally and expose the other contents of the carotid sheath, the *vagus nerve* and *common carotid artery* (Fig. 20.15).**
- **Clean the connective tissue and identify the "strap muscles": the omohyoid (superior and inferior bellies), sternohyoid, sternothyroid, and thyrohyoid muscles (Fig. 20.16).**
- **Clear away the carotid sheath and fully expose the internal jugular vein, common carotid artery, and vagus nerve (Fig. 20.17).**

DISSECTION TIP

With scissors, pull the common carotid artery from the carotid sheath (see Fig. 20.17) to avoid severing important arteries and nerves.

- **Clean the connective tissue, fat, and carotid sheath and expose the cervical plexus (Fig. 20.18).**

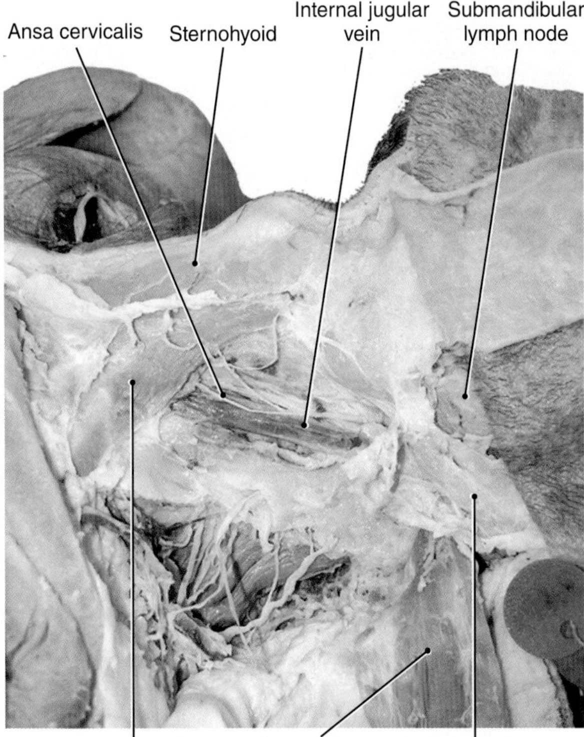

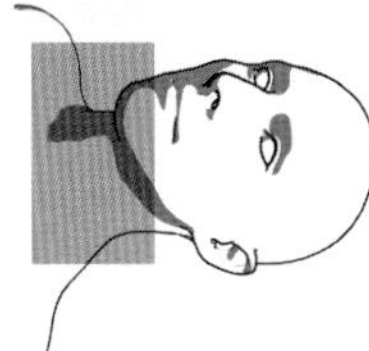

Fig. 20.14 Superior belly of omohyoid muscle exposed, revealing the ansa cervicalis superficial to the internal jugular vein.

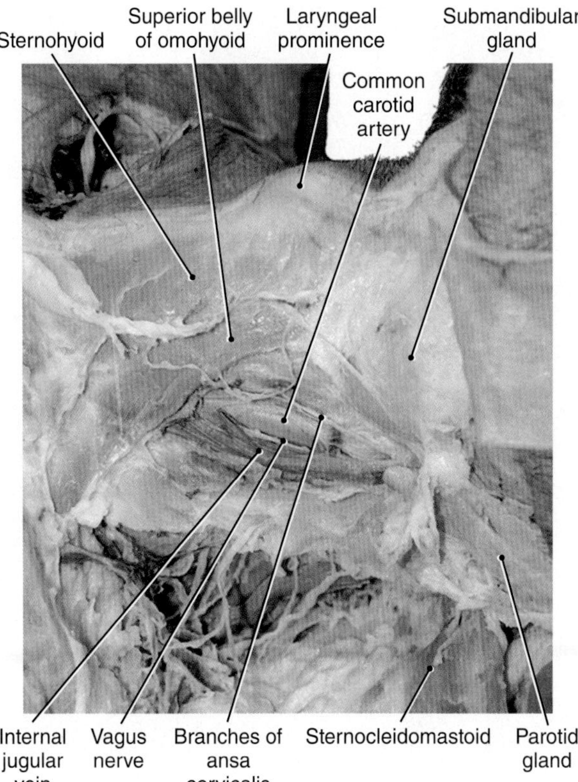

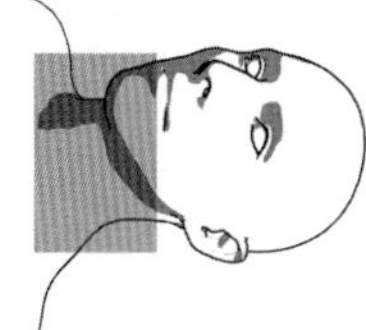

Fig. 20.15 Anterolateral view of the neck with the skin, subcutaneous tissues, and sternocleidomastoid muscle reflected laterally and the platysma muscle reflected superiorly. The internal jugular vein is pulled laterally to expose the other contents of the carotid sheath: vagus nerve and common carotid artery.

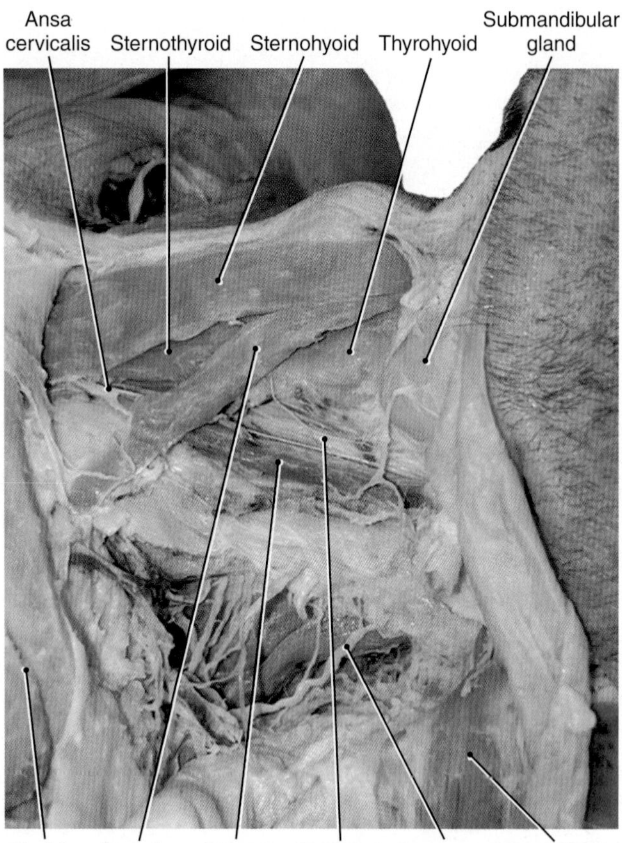

Fig. 20.16 Connective tissue cleaned, highlighting the strap muscles (omohyoid superior/inferior bellies, sternohyoid, sternothyroid, thyrohyoid).

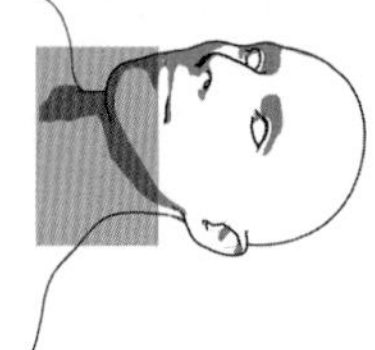

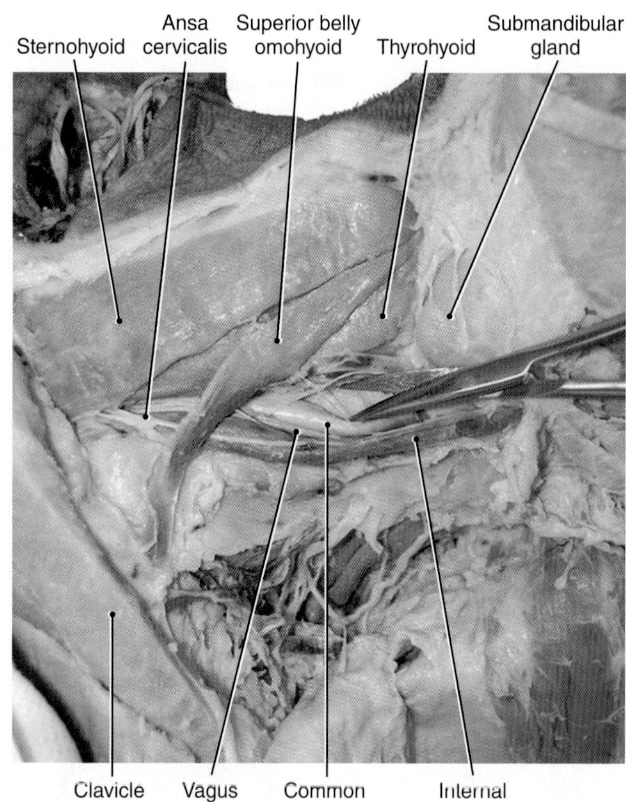

Fig. 20.17 Remaining carotid sheath cleaned, fully exposing the vagus nerve and the common carotid artery.

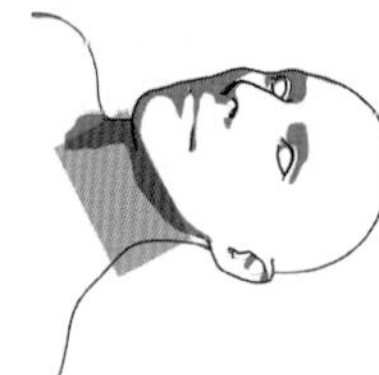

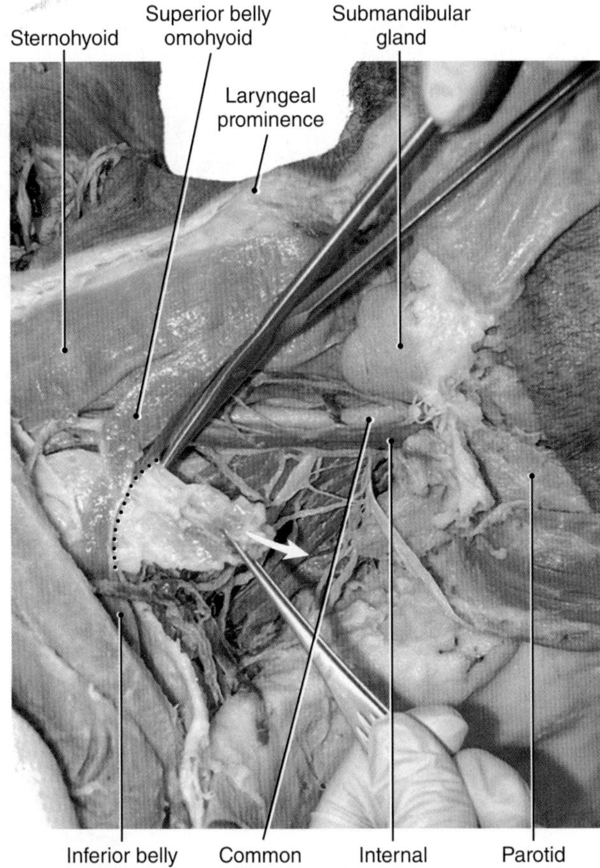

Fig. 20.18 Adipose tissue removed from the posterior cervical triangle, leaving intact the nerves and arteries.

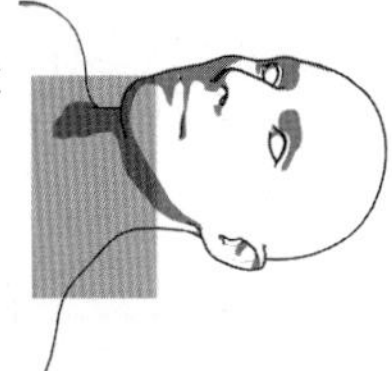

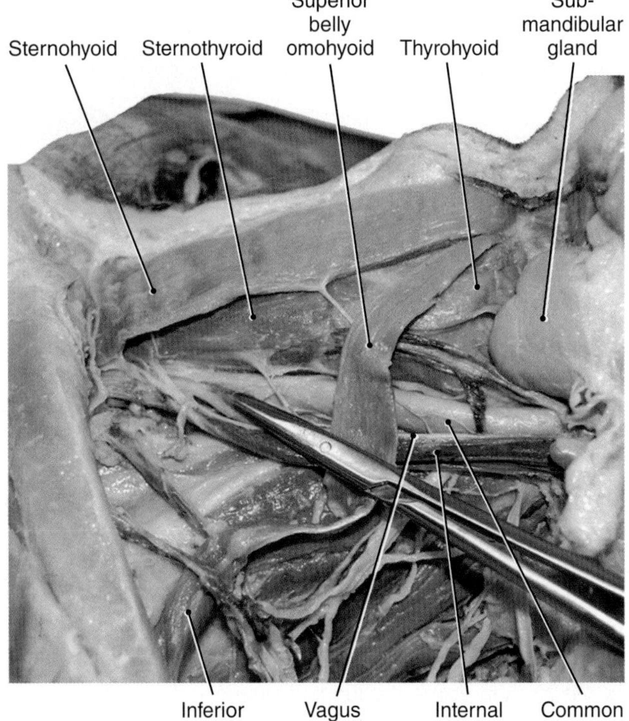

Fig. 20.19 Carotid sheath cleaned inferiorly, revealing the vagus nerve and carotid artery toward the root of neck.

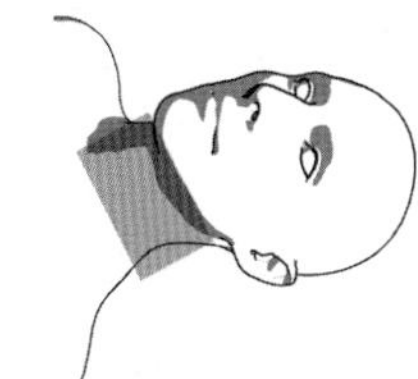

- **Continue the exposure of the contents of the carotid sheath toward the clavicle (Fig. 20.19).**
- **Identify the submandibular gland and pull it toward the midline.**
- **Clean the carotid sheath toward the angle of the mandible and identify (if prominent) the *jugulodigastric lymph nodes* (Fig. 20.20).**
- **Clean away fat and connective tissue around the common carotid artery and medial to the carotid sheath and identify the superior thyroid artery (Fig. 20.21). This artery runs between the thyrohyoid muscle and the carotid sheath. Do not try to identify the origin of this artery yet.**
- **Remove the jugulodigastric lymph nodes, and by pulling the parotid gland laterally, expose the posterior belly of the digastric muscle (Fig. 20.22).**
- **Expose the digastric muscle, with its posterior and anterior bellies, and the stylohyoid muscle.**
- **Observe the tendon insertion of the stylohyoid muscle onto the hyoid and its relationship with the posterior belly of the digastric muscle.**
- **Identify the hyoid bone and expose the mylohyoid muscle, which is partially hidden by the anterior belly of the digastric muscle (see Fig. 20.22).**
- **Expose the distal portion of the common carotid artery at its division into the internal and external carotid arteries (Fig. 20.23).**
- **Identify the origin of the *superior thyroid artery* from the external carotid artery and trace it to its termination in the thyroid gland.**

DISSECTION **TIP**

To create more space for exposing the branches of the external carotid artery, detach the submandibular gland from its base (Fig. 20.24) and mobilize it medially.

- **Dissect out the facial artery, which passes deep to the submandibular gland before emerging at the angle of the mandible (Fig. 20.25).**
- **Mobilize the submandibular gland medially and expose the stylohyoid muscle and the posterior belly of the digastric muscle. Identify the hypoglossal nerve running parallel to the posterior belly of the digastric muscle (Fig. 20.26).**

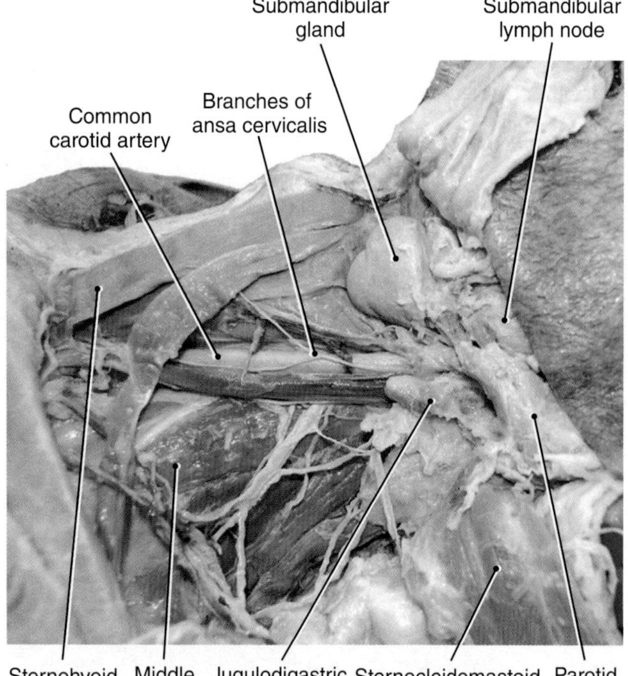

Fig. 20.20 Appreciate the jugulodigastric lymph nodes and parotid and submandibular glands.

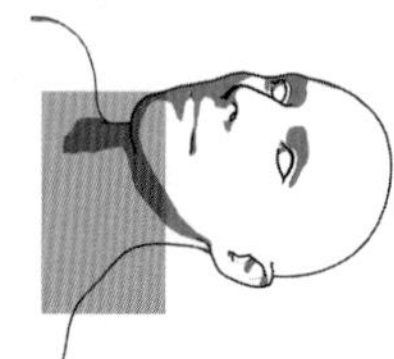

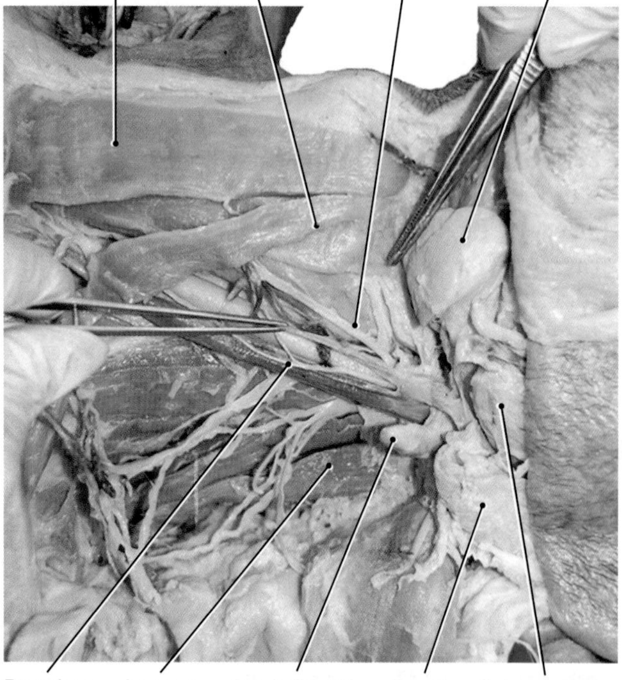

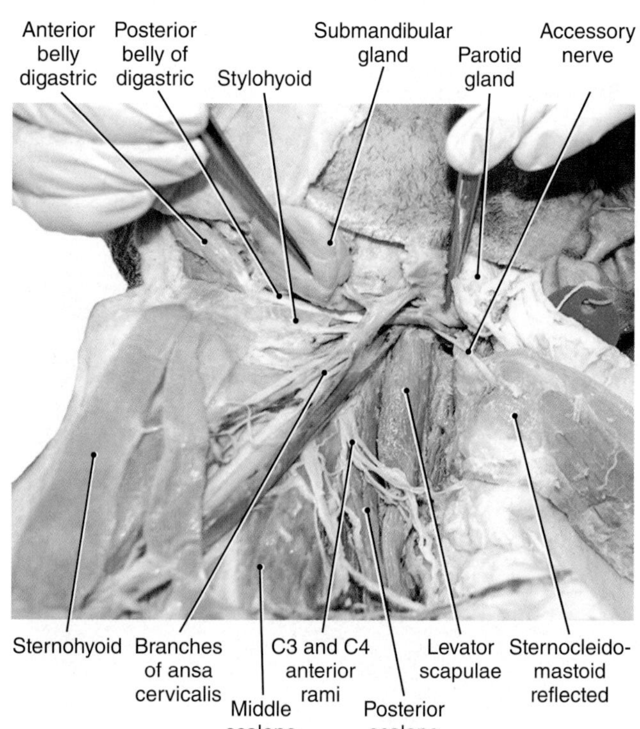

Fig. 20.22 Submandibular and parotid glands lifted to expose the external and internal carotid arteries.

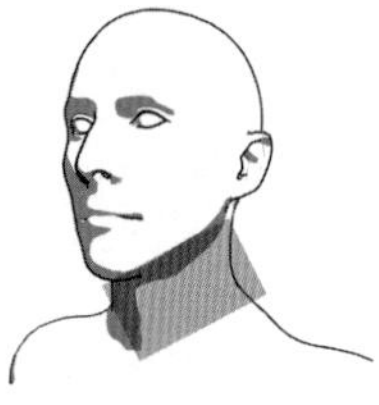

Fig. 20.21 Fat and connective tissue removed around the common carotid artery and medial to the carotid sheath to highlight the superior thyroid artery.

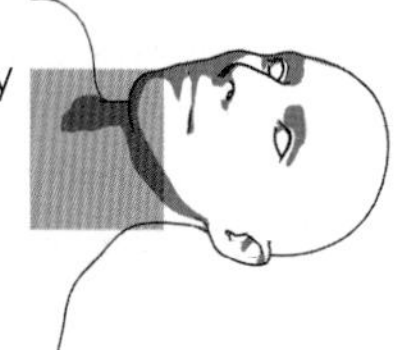

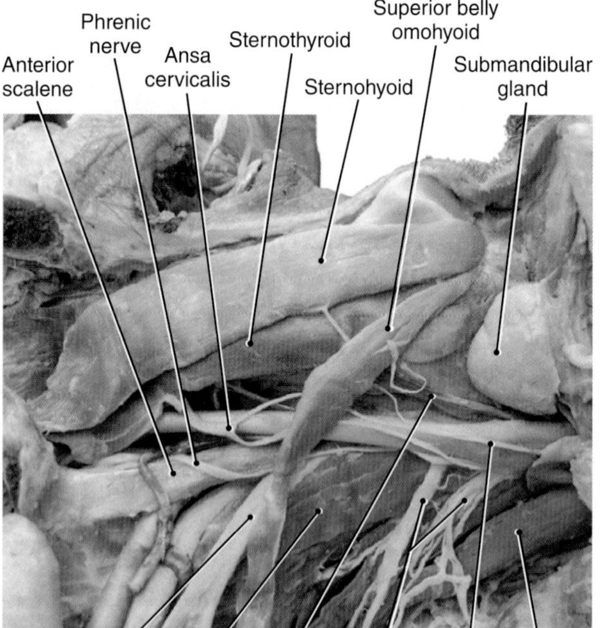

Fig. 20.23 Anterolateral view of neck revealing neurovascular structures of anterior and posterior cervical triangles.

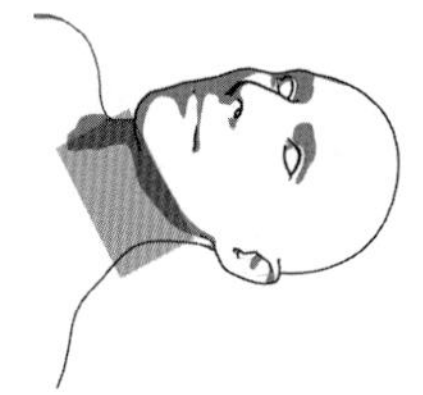

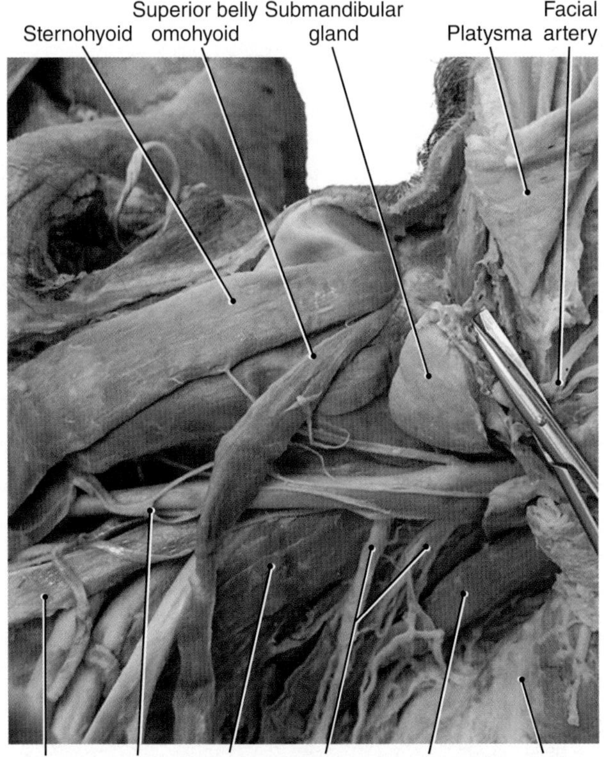

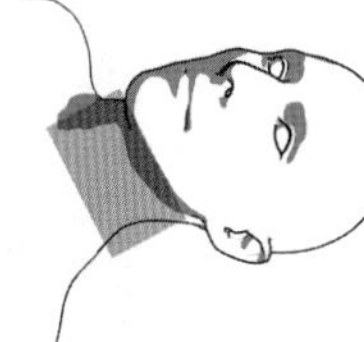

Fig. 20.24 Submandibular gland detached from the base to create more space for exposing branches of the external carotid artery.

- **Note the small branch of the superior thyroid artery, the *superior laryngeal artery*, which travels medially and penetrates the thyrohyoid membrane (Fig. 20.27).**

ANATOMY **NOTE**

The superior laryngeal artery has a variable origin. If it does not arise from the superior thyroid artery, the superior laryngeal may arise directly from the external carotid artery.

- **Parallel to the superior laryngeal artery, expose the internal branch of the superior laryngeal nerve, which also penetrates the thyrohyoid membrane.**
- **Observe the superior root of the ansa cervicalis all the way to the hypoglossal nerve. Note that the ansa cervicalis travels within the connective tissue sheath of the hypoglossal nerve.**
- **At the origin of the internal carotid artery, look for a dilation of its wall, the *carotid sinus* (Fig. 20.28).**

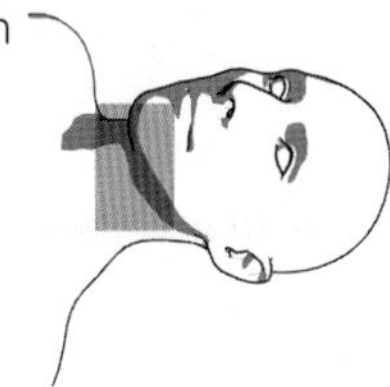

Fig. 20.25 Dissection of facial artery, which passes deep to submandibular gland before emerging at the angle of mandible.

ANATOMY **NOTE**

The carotid sinus contains nerve fibers responsible for detecting blood pressure changes at this location.

- **Using scissors, expose the division of the common carotid artery and identify the *carotid body* (Fig. 20.29), a small mass of specialized cells that act as chemoreceptors (Plate 20.2).**

ANATOMY **NOTE**

A branch of the glossopharyngeal nerve (carotid sinus nerve or Hering's nerve) is responsible for the nerve supply to the carotid body and sinus.

- **Pull the common carotid artery laterally (Fig. 20.30) and expose the *lingual artery*.**

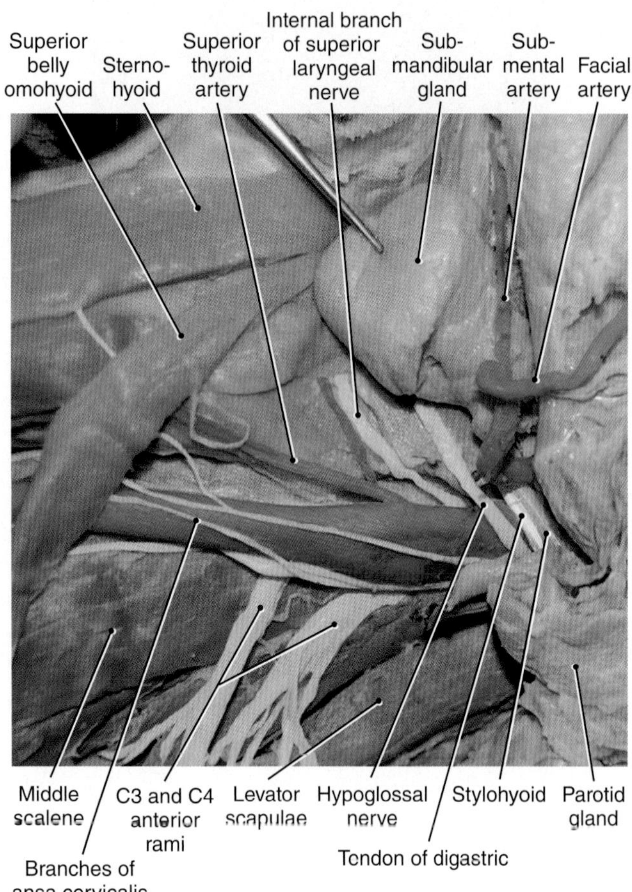

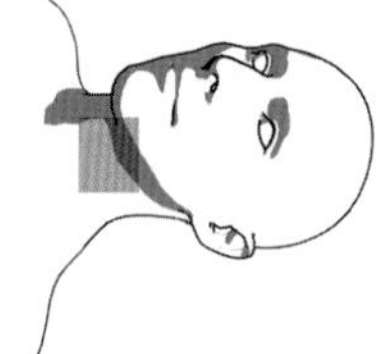

Fig. 20.26 Submandibular gland lifted to expose the internal laryngeal and hypoglossal nerves, posterior belly of the digastric muscle, and the facial artery.

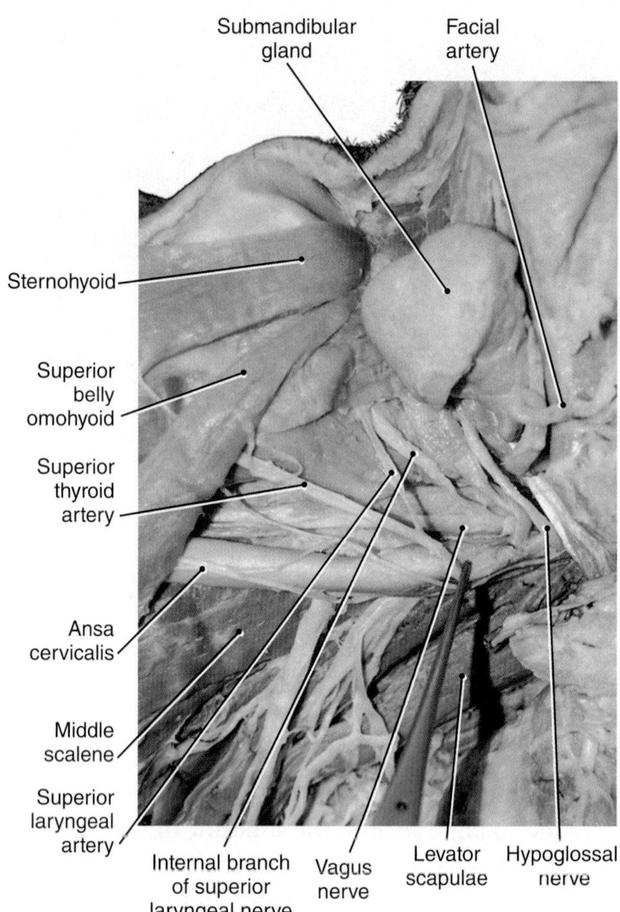

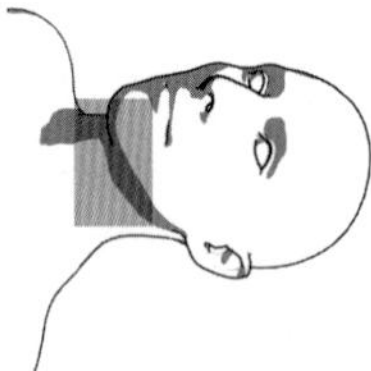

Fig. 20.27 Anterolateral view of the neck.

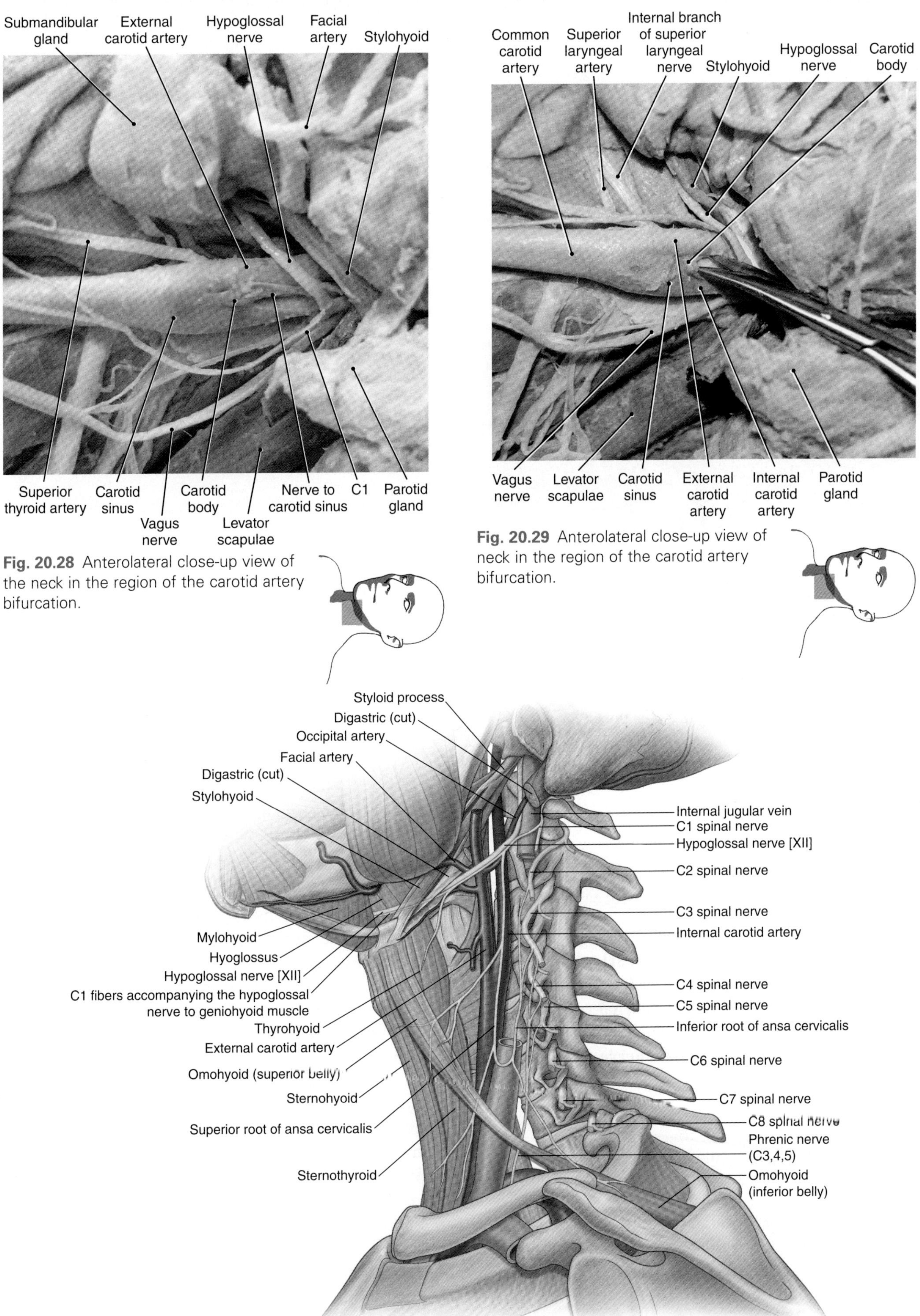

Fig. 20.28 Anterolateral close-up view of the neck in the region of the carotid artery bifurcation.

Fig. 20.29 Anterolateral close-up view of neck in the region of the carotid artery bifurcation.

Plate 20.2 Lateral view of the neck exposing cervical spinal nerves, ansa cervicalis, and hypoglossal nerve. (From Drake RL et al. *Gray's Atlas of Anatomy*, 3rd edition, Philadelphia, Elsevier, 2021.)

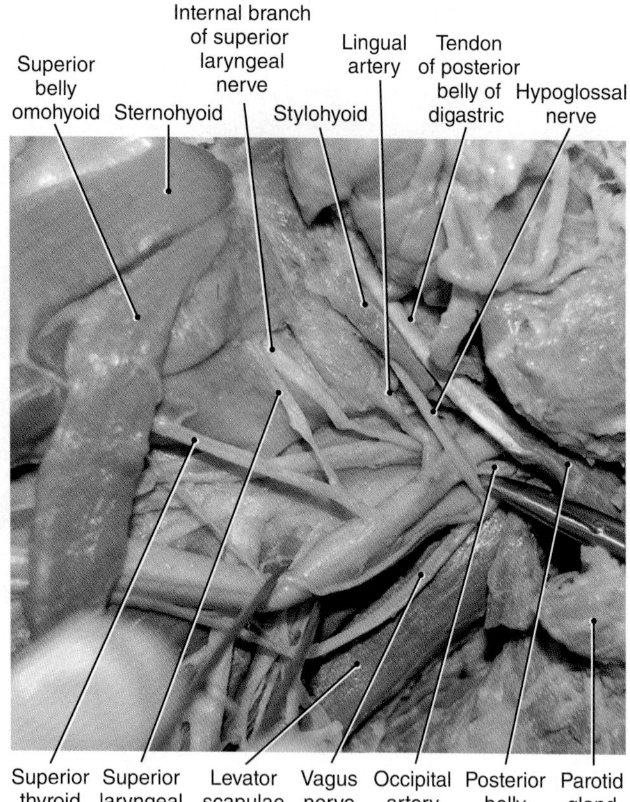

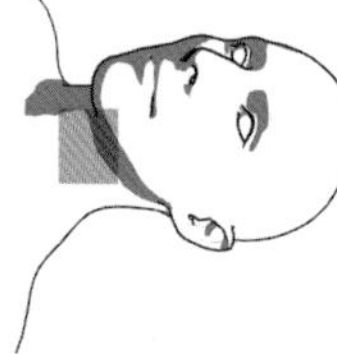

Fig. 20.30 Anterolateral view of the neck with the skin, subcutaneous tissues, sternocleidomastoid reflected laterally, and platysma reflected superiorly. The common carotid artery is pulled laterally to reveal the various nerves and arteries.

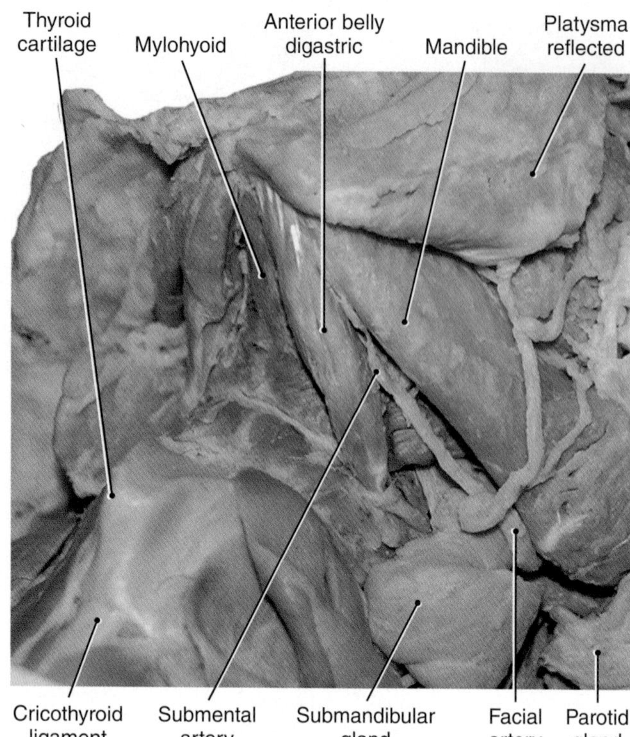

Fig. 20.31 Anteroinferior view of the midline of the neck with skin, subcutaneous tissues, and platysma reflected.

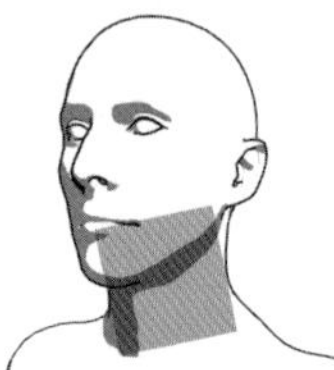

ANATOMY **NOTE**

The lingual artery is commonly the second branch of the external carotid artery in the majority of cases.

- **If time permits, trace the lingual artery to the point where it passes deep to the hyoglossus muscle.**
- **At the lateral border of the external carotid artery, expose the *occipital artery*, which passes posteriorly, crossing over the hypoglossal nerve (see Fig. 20.30 and Plate 20.2).**

ANATOMY **NOTE**

In the majority of cases, the occipital artery gives rise to the artery of the sternocleidomastoid muscle.

- **Opposite the occipital artery, at the medial border of the external carotid artery and superior to the lingual artery, identify the *facial artery*, and trace it to the submandibular gland at the angle of the mandible (Fig. 20.31).**

ANATOMY **NOTE**

In some cadavers the facial and lingual arteries may have a common origin, the *faciolingual trunk*. Similarly, the lingual and the superior thyroid arteries may originate as a common trunk.

- **Posterior to the origin of the external carotid artery, identify the ascending pharyngeal artery, which travels between the internal carotid artery and the lateral aspect of the pharynx.**
- **Clean any muscle attachments and connective tissue from the clavicle to expose the *brachial plexus* in the supraclavicular area (Fig. 20.32).**
- **Cover the neck and thorax with paper towels to protect the dissected structures from bone dust (Fig. 20.33).**
- **With an electric saw, cut the clavicle at the jugular notch and at its distal one-third (Fig. 20.34).**
- **With scissors, detach the clavicle from the underlying connective tissue and subclavius muscle (Figs. 20.35 and 20.36).**
- **Reflect the subclavius muscle laterally and expose the root of the neck and the brachial plexus (Fig. 20.37).**
- **Identify the anterior scalene muscle (Fig. 20.38), and on its surface identify the phrenic nerve (Fig. 20.39).**

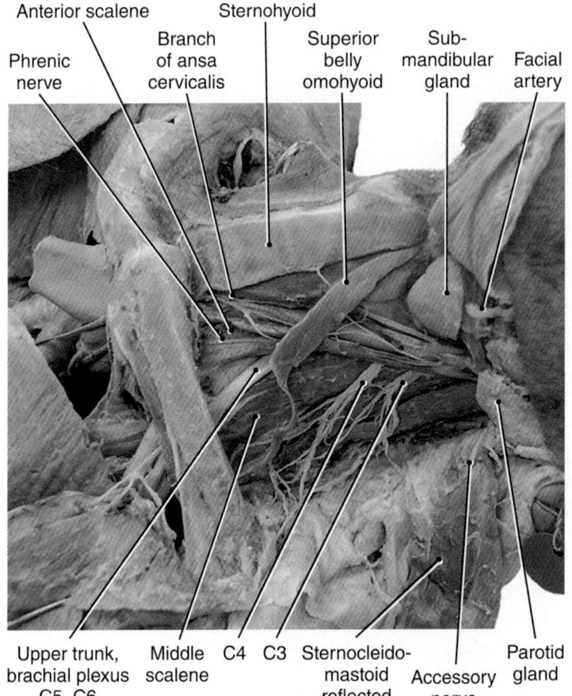

Fig. 20.32 Cleaned clavicle and adipose tissue removed, further revealing key neurovascular structures.

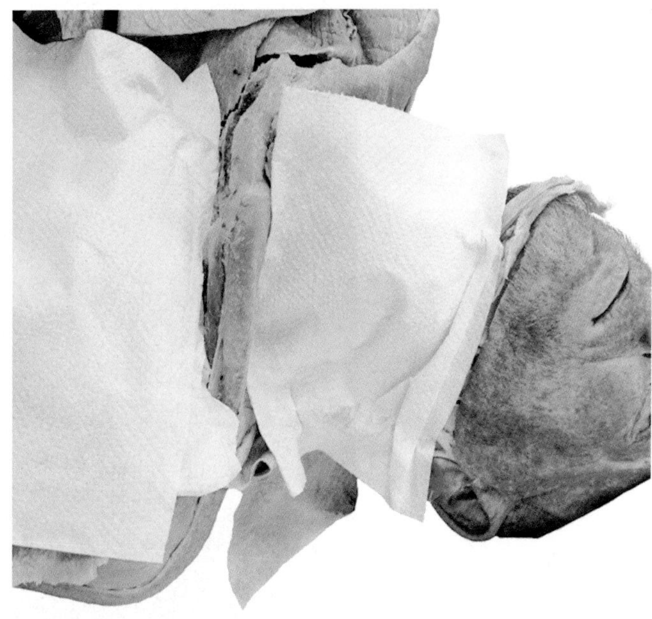

Fig. 20.33 Neck and thorax covered with paper towels to protect the dissected structures from bone dust when using a bone saw.

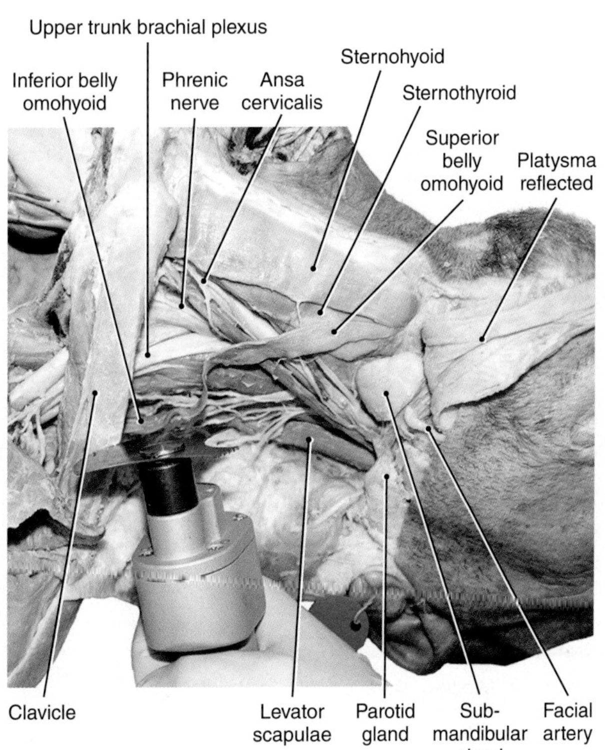

Fig. 20.34 Clavicle cut at jugular notch and at its distal one-third.

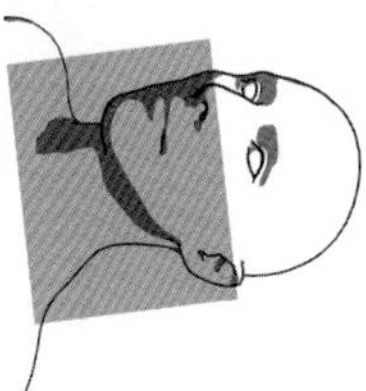

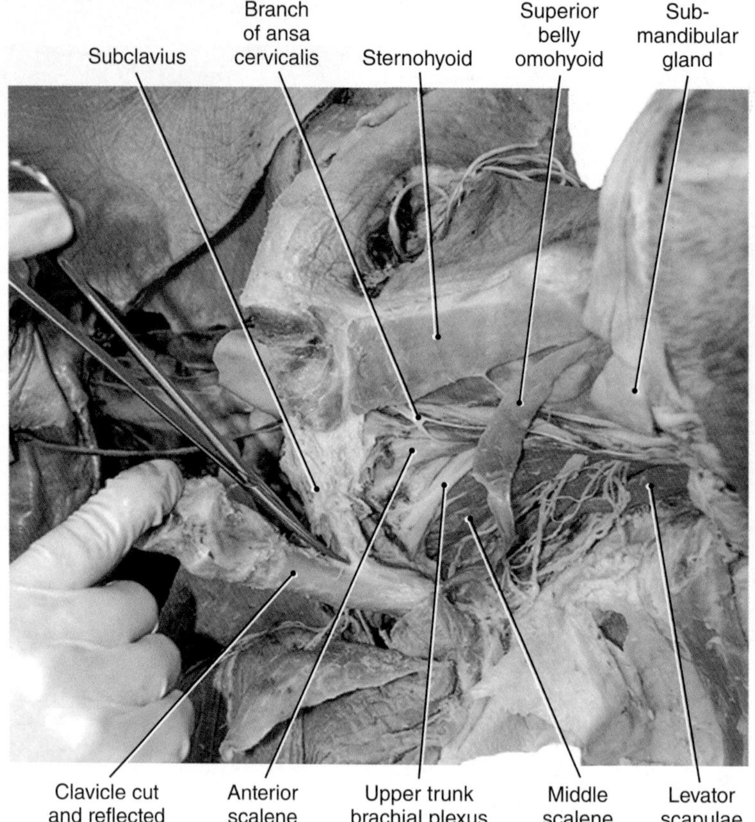

Fig. 20.35 Clavicle detached from underlying connective tissue and subclavius muscle.

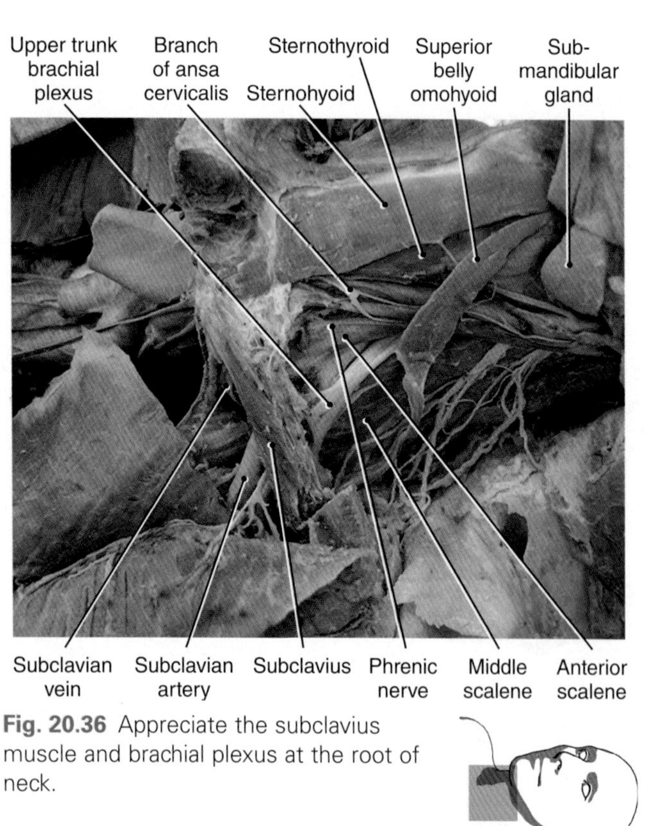

Fig. 20.36 Appreciate the subclavius muscle and brachial plexus at the root of neck.

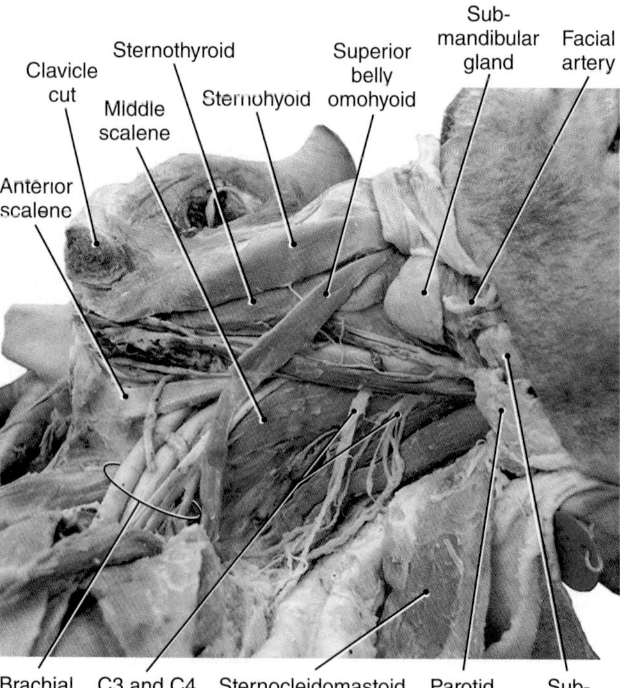

Fig. 20.37 Subclavius muscle reflected laterally to expose the root of neck.

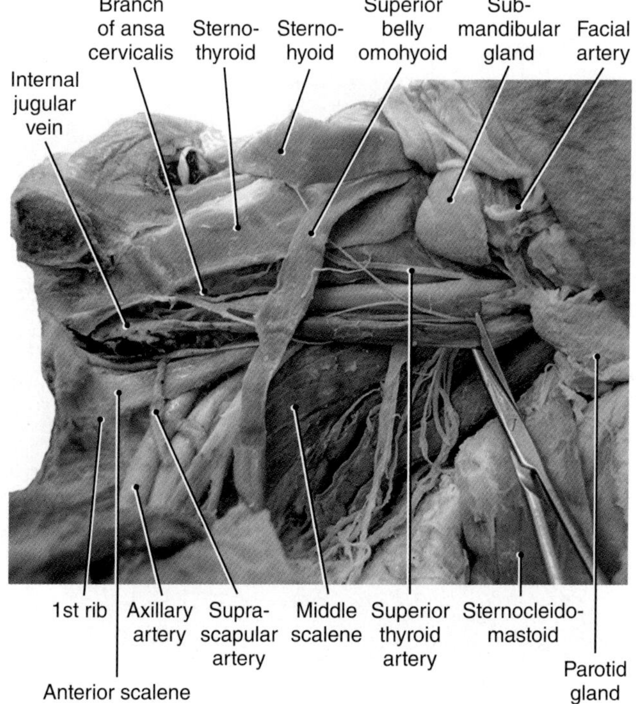

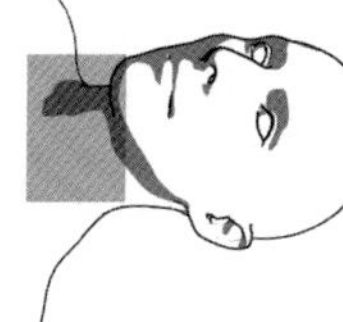

Fig. 20.38 Internal jugular vein incised at the level of the bifurcation of the common carotid artery and removed from the neck.

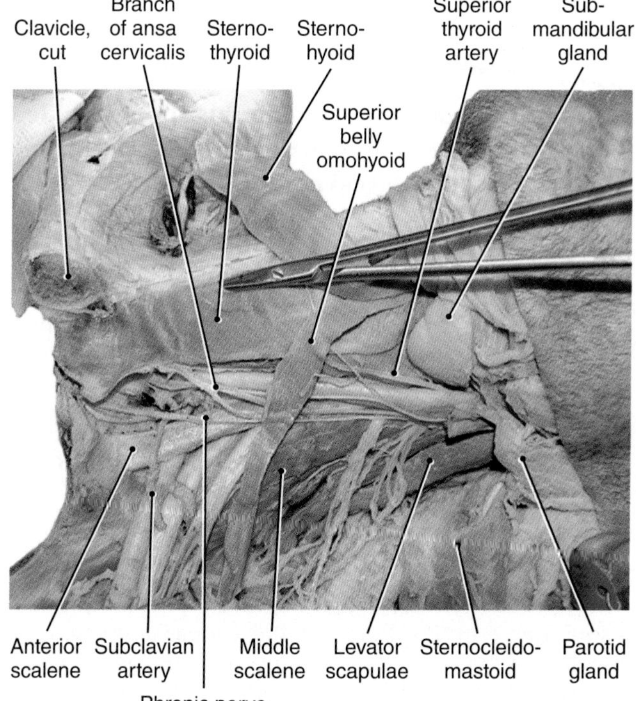

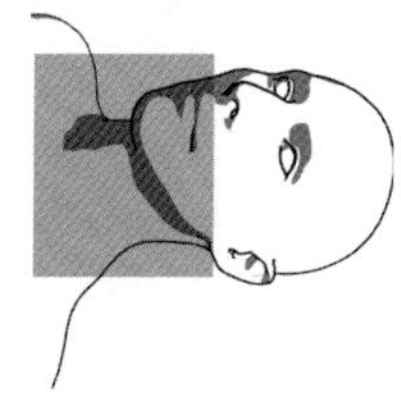

Fig. 20.39 Appreciate the course of the phrenic nerve in the neck.

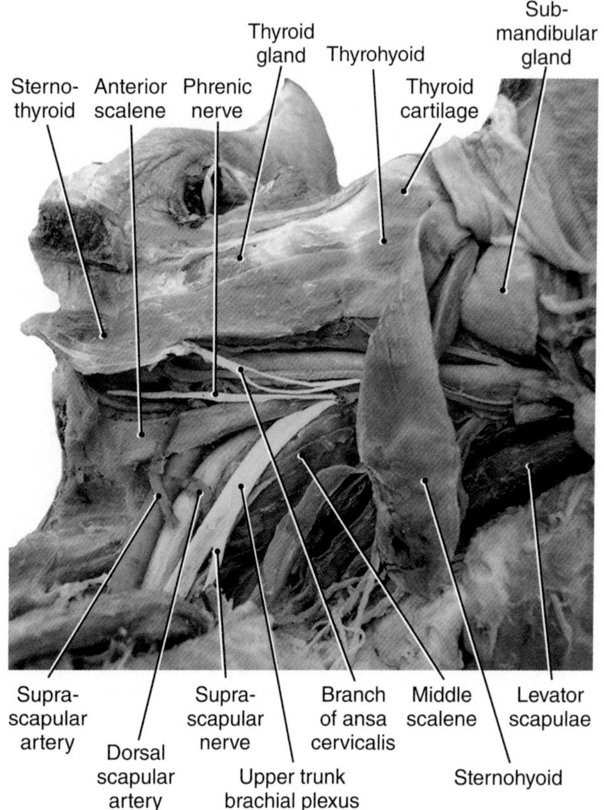

Fig. 20.40 Appreciate the supraclavicular nerves and phrenic nerve crossed by branches of the thyrocervical trunk.

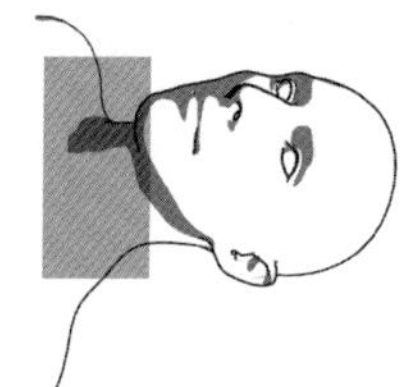

- **With scissors, cut the internal jugular vein at the level of the bifurcation of the common carotid artery and remove it from the neck.**
- **Trace the supraclavicular nerves, noting their origin from cervical nerves 3 and 4 (C3, C4) (see Fig. 20.39).**
- **On the anterior surface of the anterior scalene muscle, note the phrenic nerve is crossed by branches of the thyrocervical trunk, the transverse cervical and suprascapular arteries (Fig. 20.40).**
- **Cut the inferior attachments of the sternohyoid and sternothyroid muscles and reflect them upward to expose the *thyroid gland* (Figs. 20.41 and 20.42).**
- **Notice the branches from the ansa cervicalis innervating the strap muscles.**
- **Follow the superior thyroid artery medial to its termination into the thyroid gland. Identify the cricothyroid muscle superior to the thyroid gland (see Fig. 20.40).**
- **Note the two lobes of the thyroid gland connected by the isthmus.**

ANATOMY **NOTE**

A pyramidal lobe may be present, traveling from the thyroid gland toward the hyoid bone.

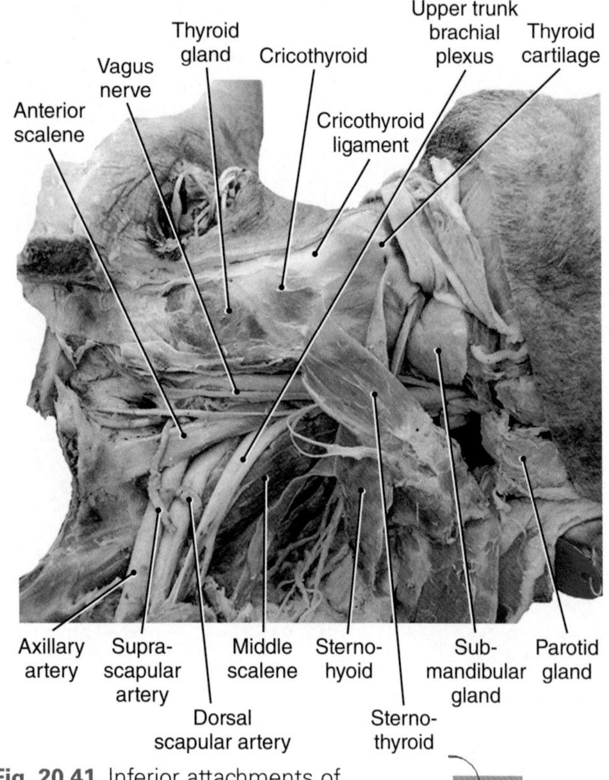

Fig. 20.41 Inferior attachments of sternohyoid and sternothyroid muscles reflected upward to expose thyroid gland.

Fig. 20.42 Thyroid gland and cricothyroid muscle exposed.

- If time permits, cut the isthmus of the thyroid gland and reflect the gland laterally from the trachea.
- Look on the posterior surface of the thyroid gland for the *parathyroid glands,* typically found close to the posterior branches of the superior and inferior thyroid arteries.
- If time permits, identify the superior and middle thyroid veins and trace them back to the internal jugular vein.
- Pull the common carotid artery laterally and trace the superior thyroid artery (Fig. 20.43).
- Locate the internal laryngeal branch of the superior laryngeal nerve and trace its origin back to the superior laryngeal nerve.
- Pull the internal laryngeal nerve away from its origin and identify the external laryngeal branch. Follow this nerve as it descends into the neck medial to the common carotid artery, running along the superior thyroid artery.
- Clean the superior thyroid artery and find the external laryngeal nerve piercing the cricothyroid muscle.
- Pull the common carotid artery laterally to expose the space between the anterior scalene muscle and trachea (Fig. 20.44).
- Clean the connective tissue in this space and identify the inferior thyroid artery, thyrocervical trunk, and recurrent laryngeal nerve (Fig. 20.45).

ANATOMY **NOTE**

The *inferior thyroid artery* is a branch of the thyrocervical trunk that supplies the inferior pole of the thyroid gland.

- Dissect the fat and connective tissue medial to the trachea (tracheoesophageal groove) and identify the *recurrent laryngeal nerve* (Fig. 20.46).

ANATOMY **NOTE**

The left recurrent laryngeal nerve arises from the left vagus nerve in the thorax as the vagus nerve crosses the arch of the aorta. The right recurrent laryngeal nerve arises from the right vagus nerve as it crosses the right subclavian artery.

ANATOMY **NOTE**

The *inferior thyroid artery* crosses the recurrent laryngeal nerve at the inferior pole of the thyroid artery (Fig. 20.47). This is an important surgical landmark.

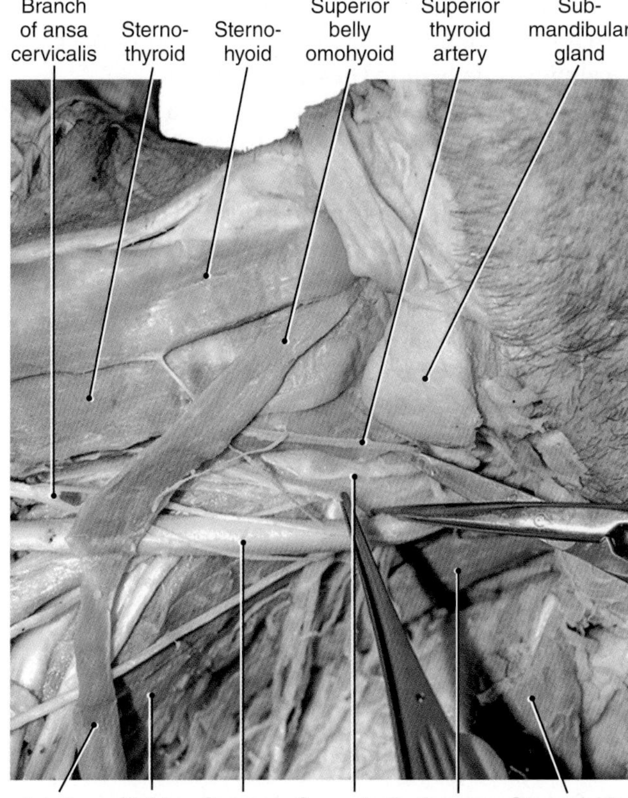

Fig. 20.43 Common carotid artery pulled laterally to trace the superior thyroid artery, internal laryngeal nerve, superior laryngeal artery, and external laryngeal nerve.

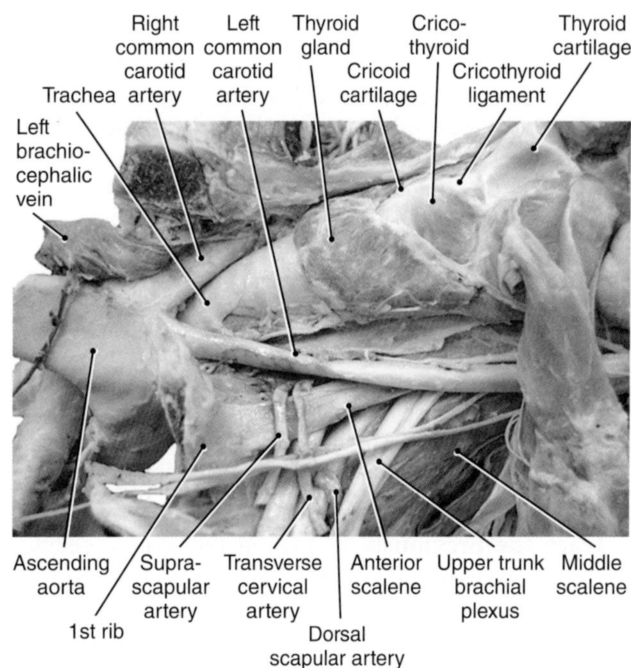

Fig. 20.44 Appreciate the common carotid artery in the tracheoesophageal region, with the recurrent laryngeal nerve traveling in the tracheoesophageal groove.

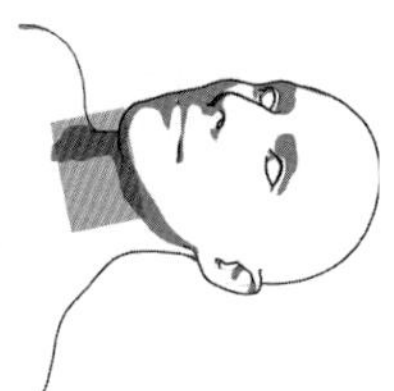

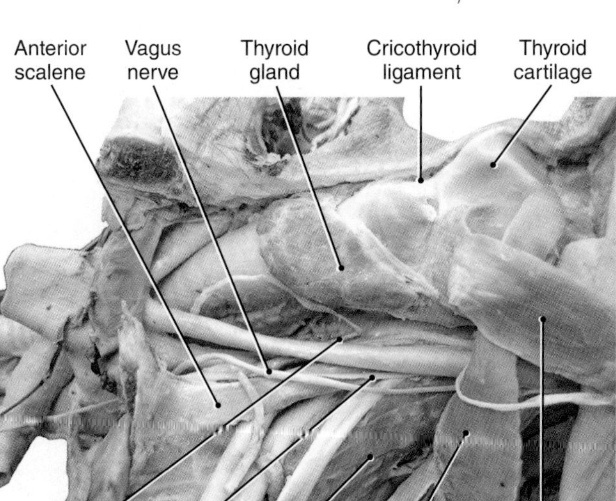

Fig. 20.45 Appreciate the inferior thyroid artery, a key surgical landmark.

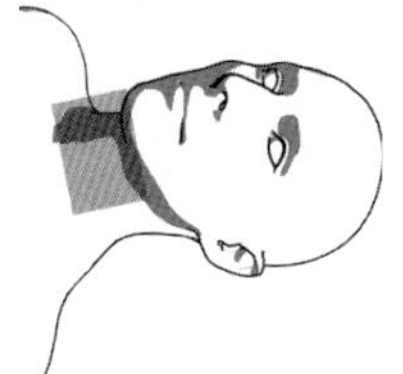

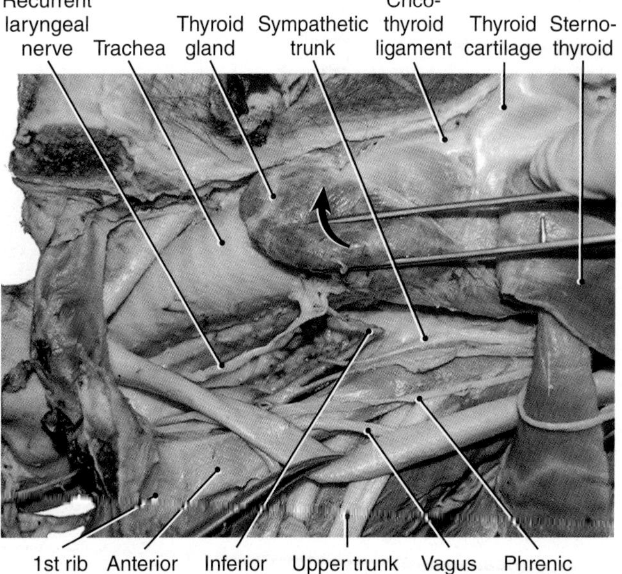

Fig. 20.46 Common carotid artery pulled laterally, revealing branches of the thyrocervical trunk. Note the relationship between the recurrent laryngeal nerve and inferior thyroid artery.

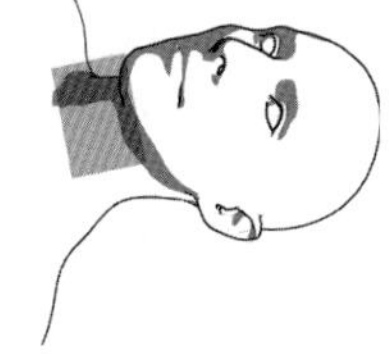

ANATOMY NOTE

When the inferior thyroid artery arises from the aortic arch, brachiocephalic trunk, or common carotid or vertebral artery, it is called the *thyroidea ima* (lowest thyroid) artery. This variation is present in approximately 5% of the population.

ANATOMY NOTE

In some specimens a nonrecurrent laryngeal nerve is present. This variation is caused by a delay in the development of the aortic arches, resulting in the right vagus nerve giving off a transversely oriented, nonrecurrent laryngeal nerve, which passes directly toward the larynx without reaching the thorax. This anatomic situation is usually associated with a retroesophageal right subclavian artery.

- **Trace the previously identified transverse cervical and suprascapular arteries deep to their origin from the thyrocervical trunk (see Fig. 20.47).**

ANATOMY NOTE

The transverse cervical or suprascapular arteries may be absent. In such cases the dorsal scapular artery may be large and may arise from the subclavian artery, crossing over the 1st rib.

- **Lift the contents of the carotid sheath (internal jugular vein, common carotid artery, vagus nerve), and look posterior for the cervical part of the sympathetic trunk, or sympathetic trunk (see Fig. 20.50). Note that the sympathetic trunk and the roots of the cervical plexus lie behind the carotid sheath.**
- **The sympathetic trunk lies within a dense fascial layer, the prevertebral fascia. Clean the prevertebral fascia (and remnants of the carotid sheath) posterior to the common carotid artery.**
- **Trace the sympathetic trunk inferiorly and identify the superior, middle, and inferior cervical ganglia (see Fig. 20.53).**

DISSECTION TIP

The middle cervical ganglion is variable in origin and is often not present. The superior cervical ganglion can be identified at the level of the angle of the mandible. However, during the retropharyngeal dissection, it will be fully exposed.

- **Once the thyrocervical trunk is identified and its branches exposed, pull it laterally and look for the *vertebral artery*, which ascends medial and deep to it (see Figs. 20.47 and 20.48).**
- **Near the origin of the vertebral artery, identify the inferior cervical ganglion and/or the stellate ganglion (Figs. 20.49 and 20.50).**
- **The inferior cervical ganglion is large and often fused with the first thoracic trunk ganglion, forming the stellate (cervicothoracic) ganglion (Fig. 20.51).**

Inferior thyroid artery
Recurrent laryngeal nerve
Thyroid gland
Anterior scalene
Cervical sympathetic trunk
1st rib
Thyrocervical trunk
Vagus nerve
Common carotid artery
Ascending cervical artery
Phrenic nerve

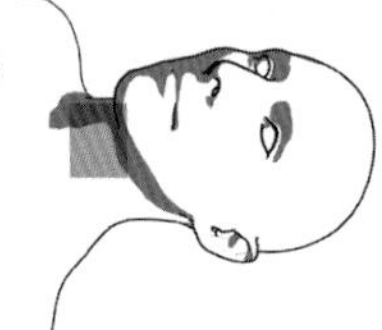

Fig. 20.47 Medial to the thyrocervical trunk, identify the vertebral artery arising as the first branch of the subclavian artery.

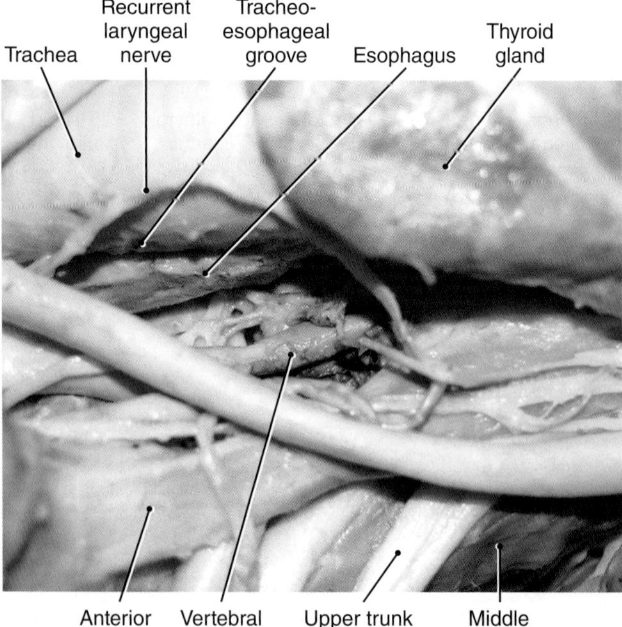

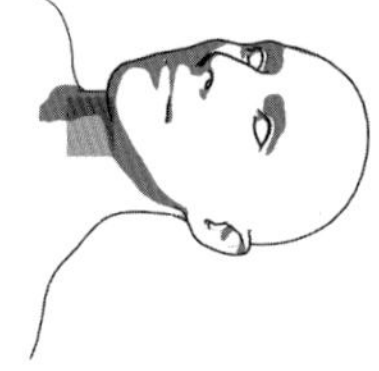

Fig. 20.48 Common carotid artery and thyrocervical trunk pulled laterally to identify the vertebral artery and sympathetic trunk.

- **After identifying the stellate ganglion or inferior cervical ganglion, remove 2 to 3 cm of the inferior portion of the common carotid artery (Fig. 20.52). Immediately beneath this artery, identify the *thoracic duct.***

Vertebral artery
Stellate ganglion
Trachea
Inferior thyroid artery
Thyroid gland
Cervical sympathetic trunk
Thyrocervical trunk
Ascending cervical artery
Common carotid artery
Internal jugular vein

Fig. 20.49 Retractors used (as necessary) to keep common the carotid artery and thyrocervical trunk reflected laterally, highlighting the sympathetic trunk with its stellate ganglion and vertebral artery.

ANATOMY **NOTE**

On the left side, the thoracic duct will empty into the junction between the internal jugular and subclavian veins. On the right side, the smaller right lymphatic duct will terminate at the junction of the right internal jugular and right subclavian veins.

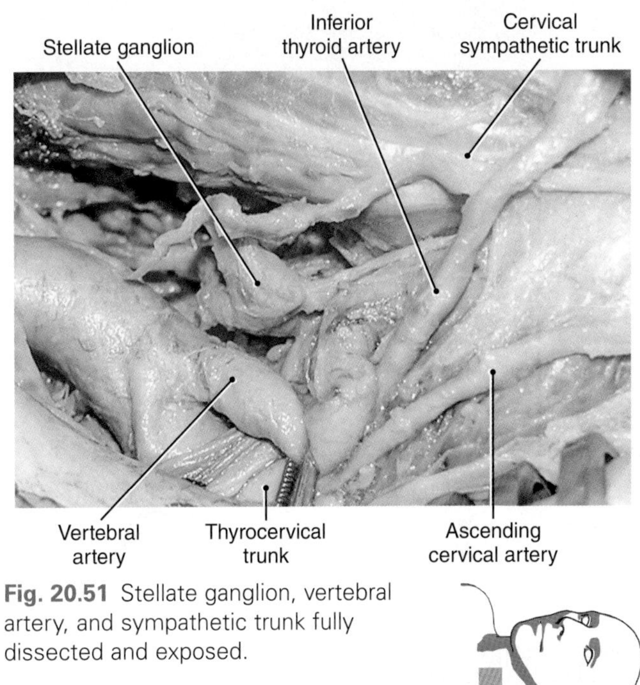

Fig. 20.51 Stellate ganglion, vertebral artery, and sympathetic trunk fully dissected and exposed.

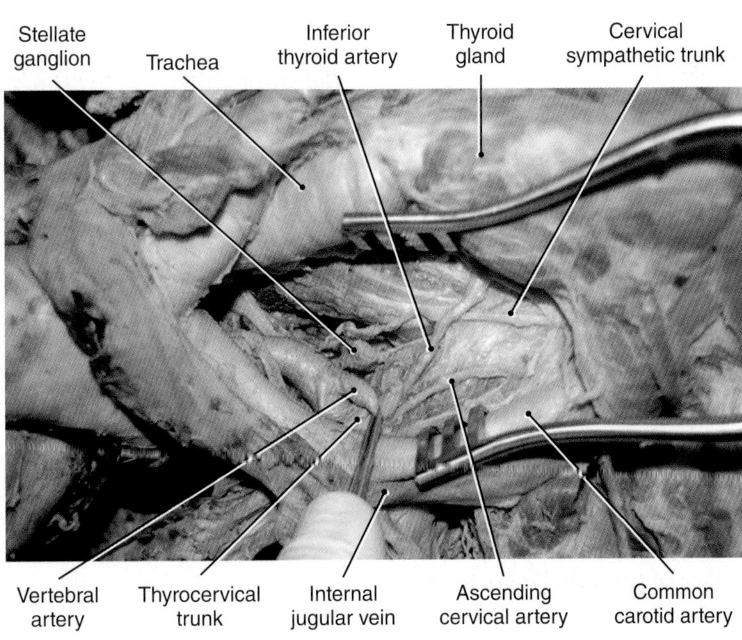

Fig. 20.50 Appreciate the stellate ganglion, vertebral artery, and sympathetic trunk fully exposed.

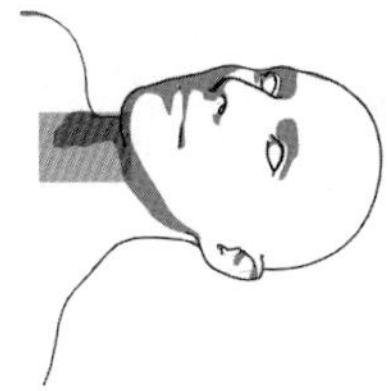

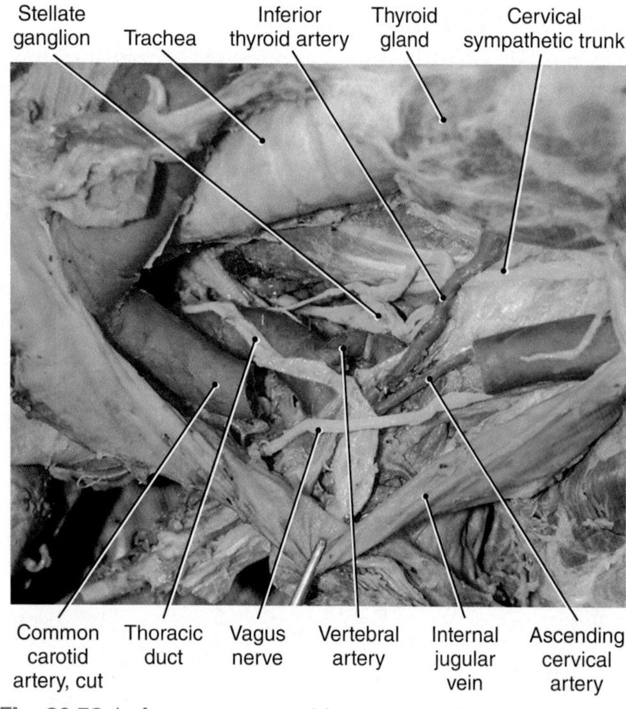

Fig. 20.52 Left common carotid artery cut, revealing the thoracic duct.

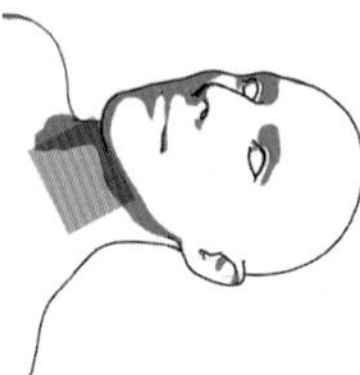

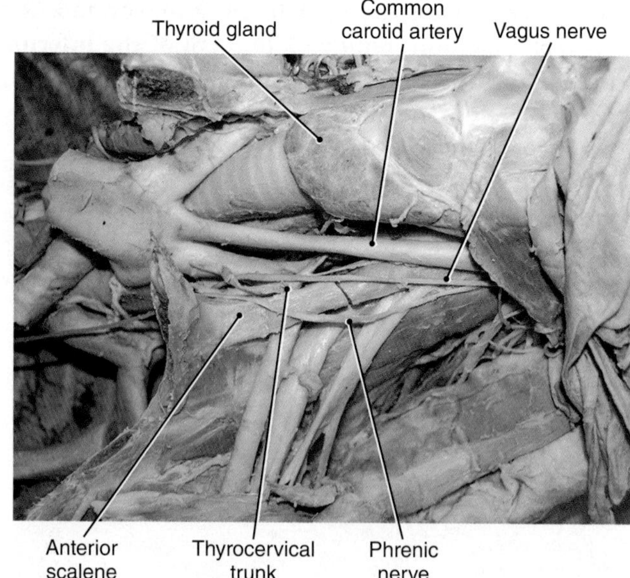

Fig. 20.53 Anterior scalene muscle cut midway from its attachment onto the 1st rib.

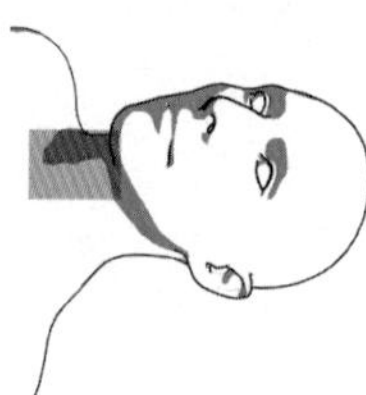

DISSECTION **TIP**

The thoracic duct is located close to the stellate or inferior cervical ganglion and can be severed during this dissection.

OPTIONAL DISSECTION

ANATOMY **NOTE**

The subclavian artery gives rise to the following branches:
1. Thyrocervical trunk
2. Vertebral artery
3. Internal thoracic artery
4. Costocervical trunk

- **The *costocervical trunk* is located on the deep surface of the subclavian artery posterior to the anterior scalene muscle. It usually gives off the highest intercostal artery, which supplies the upper two intercostal spaces.**
- **Cut the anterior scalene muscle midway from its attachment to the 1st rib (Fig. 20.53).**
- **Look at the posterior surface of the subclavian artery and identify the costocervical trunk (Fig. 20.54).**

DISSECTION **TIP**

This dissection can also take place from the internal surface of the already-dissected thorax.

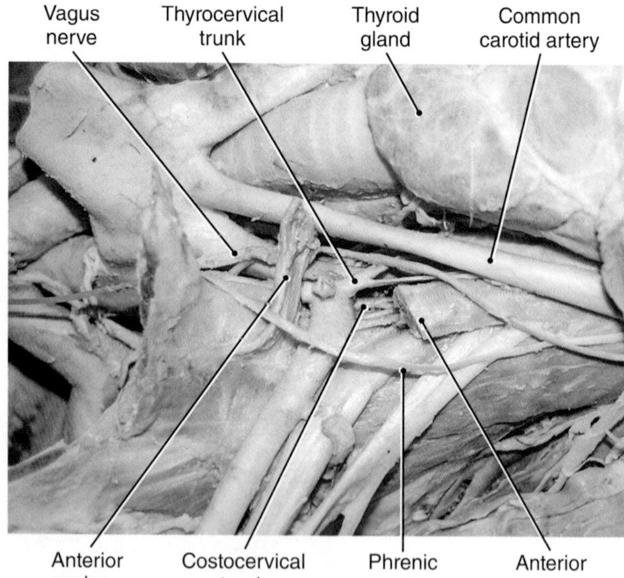

Fig. 20.54 Anterior scalene muscle and posterior surface of subclavian artery lifted, revealing the origin of the costocervical trunk.

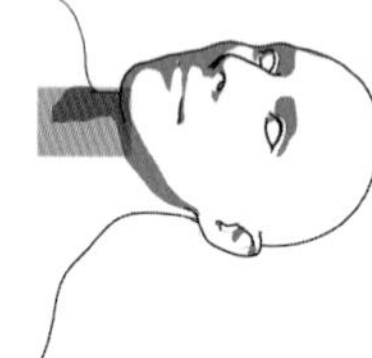

ANATOMY **NOTE**

The other branch of the costocervical trunk is the deep cervical artery, which ascends in the neck posterior to the transverse processes of the cervical vertebrae.

LABORATORY IDENTIFICATION CHECKLIST

NERVES

Cervical Plexus

- ☐ Great auricular
- ☐ Transverse cervical
- ☐ Supraclavicular
- ☐ Lesser occipital
- ☐ C1 fibers to thyrohyoid muscle
- ☐ Ansa cervicalis (C1–C3)
  - ☐ Superior root (C1)
  - ☐ Inferior root (C2 and C3)
- ☐ Phrenic (C3–C5)

Cranial Nerves (CN)

- ☐ Accessory (CN XI)
- ☐ Hypoglossal (CN XII)
- ☐ Vagus (CN X)
- ☐ Nerve to mylohyoid/anterior digastric muscle (CN V; from inferior alveolar nerve)
- ☐ Cervical branch from facial (CN VII)

Remaining Nerves

- ☐ Vagus
- ☐ Superior laryngeal
  - ☐ External laryngeal
  - ☐ Internal laryngeal
  - ☐ Recurrent laryngeal
  - ☐ Inferior laryngeal
- ☐ Cervical sympathetic trunk

Ganglia

- ☐ Superior cervical
- ☐ Middle cervical
- ☐ Cervicothoracic (stellate)

ARTERIES

- ☐ Common carotid
  - ☐ Internal carotid
  - ☐ External carotid
- ☐ Superior thyroid
  - ☐ Superior laryngeal
- ☐ Lingual
- ☐ Facial
- ☐ Occipital
- ☐ Ascending pharyngeal
- ☐ Subclavian
- ☐ Vertebral
- ☐ Thyrocervical trunk
  - ☐ Inferior thyroid
  - ☐ Transverse cervical
  - ☐ Suprascapular
- ☐ Dorsal scapular

VEINS

- ☐ External jugular
- ☐ Anterior jugular
- ☐ Internal jugular
  - ☐ Superior thyroid
  - ☐ Middle thyroid
- ☐ Subclavian
- ☐ Inferior thyroid

MUSCLES

- ☐ Platysma
- ☐ Sternocleidomastoid
  - ☐ Sternal head
  - ☐ Clavicular head
- ☐ Sternohyoid
- ☐ Omohyoid
- ☐ Sternothyroid
- ☐ Thyrohyoid
- ☐ Anterior belly of digastric
- ☐ Mylohyoid
- ☐ Posterior belly of digastric
- ☐ Stylohyoid
- ☐ Splenius capitis
- ☐ Levator scapulae
- ☐ Posterior scalene
- ☐ Middle scalene
- ☐ Anterior scalene
- ☐ Trapezius

FASCIA

- ☐ Subcutaneous tissues
- ☐ Deep fascia
  - ☐ Investing layer
  - ☐ Pretracheal layer
  - ☐ Prevertebral layer

BONES

- ☐ Mandible
- ☐ Hyoid
- ☐ Manubrium
- ☐ Clavicle
- ☐ Cervical vertebrae (C1–C7)
  - ☐ Atlas (C1)
  - ☐ Axis (C2)
- ☐ Occipital
- ☐ Temporal
  - ☐ Mastoid process
  - ☐ Styloid process

CONNECTIVE TISSUE

- ☐ Thyroid cartilage
- ☐ Cricoid cartilage
- ☐ Cricothyroid ligament
- ☐ Stylohyoid ligament
- ☐ Stylomandibular ligament
- ☐ Thyrohyoid membrane

GLANDS

- ☐ Submandibular
- ☐ Thyroid
  - ☐ Right lobe
  - ☐ Left lobe
  - ☐ Pyramidal lobe (variant)
- ☐ Parathyroid

BEFORE YOU BEGIN

Review the superficial anatomy of the face:

- Glabella
- Root of nose, dorsum of nose
- Tip of nose
- Ala
- Columella nasi
- Philtrum
- Mental protuberance
- Modiolus
- Vermillion border

Palpate the following facial landmarks on the cadaver:

- Jugular notch
- Mental protuberance
- Nasion
- Glabella
- Vertex
- External occipital protuberance (inion)
- Mastoid process
- Ramus, angle, and body of mandible
- Zygomatic arch
- Infraorbital margin
- Supraorbital margin
- Superciliary arch

SKIN AND SUPERFICIAL FASCIA

- **With a marker, outline the dissection for the cadaver as follows (Fig. 21.1):**
  1. **Make a line from the mental protuberance to the vertex. The line should encircle the lips, nostrils, and eyelids.**
  2. **Make a second line from the mental protuberance to the lobule of the ear.**
  3. **Make a third line from the vertex to the upper part of the helix of the ear.**
- **Identify the six major surface regions (temporal, frontal, zygomatic, maxillary, mandibular, mental).**
- **Based on the lines drawn, make an incision between the angle of the mandible and the mental protuberance (Fig. 21.2).**
- **Carefully reflect the flaps of skin (from medial to lateral) created by the incisions (Figs. 21.3 and 21.4).**

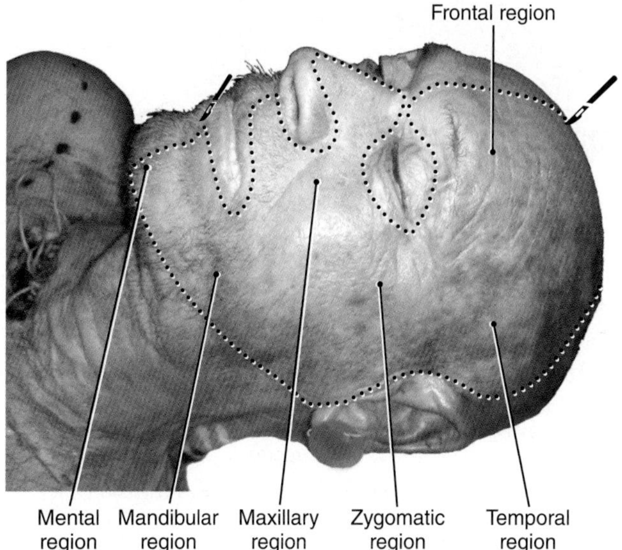

Fig. 21.1 Anterolateral view of the face with stippled lines for incisions, showing the six major surface regions.

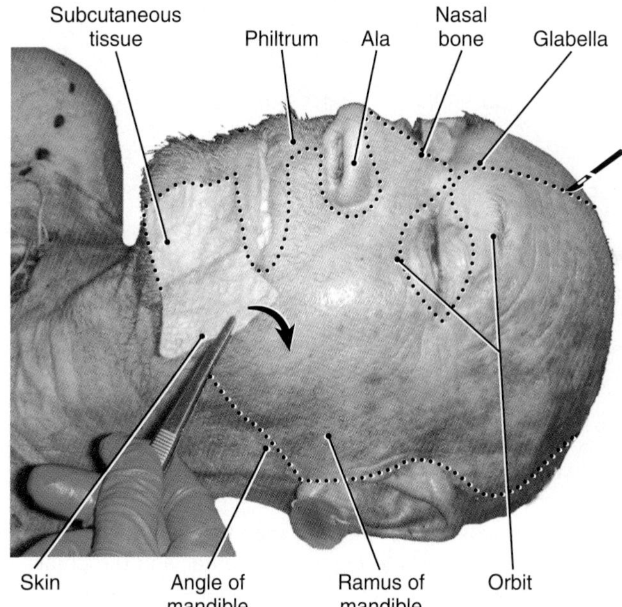

Fig. 21.2 Anterolateral view of the face with the skin reflected from the mental region.

ANATOMY **NOTE**

Beneath the skin, notice the surface of the face covered almost entirely with fat. This fibrofatty tissue is also known as the **superficial musculoaponeurotic space** or system (SMAS) (Fig. 21.5).

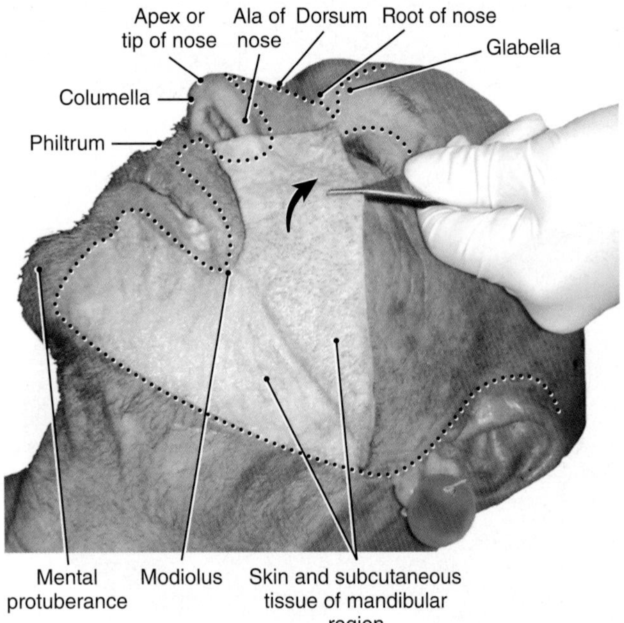

Fig. 21.3 Anterolateral view of the face with the skin reflected from the mandibular region.

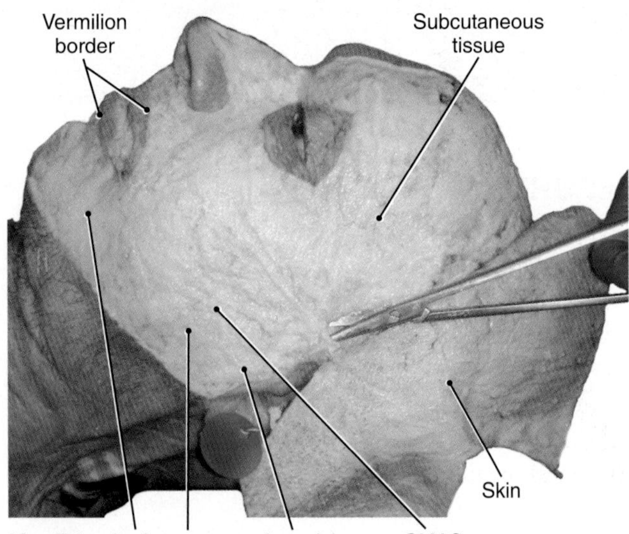

Fig. 21.5 Lateral view of the face with the skin reflected from mandibular, maxillary, zygomatic, frontal, and temporal regions. *SMAS,* Superficial musculoaponeurotic space.

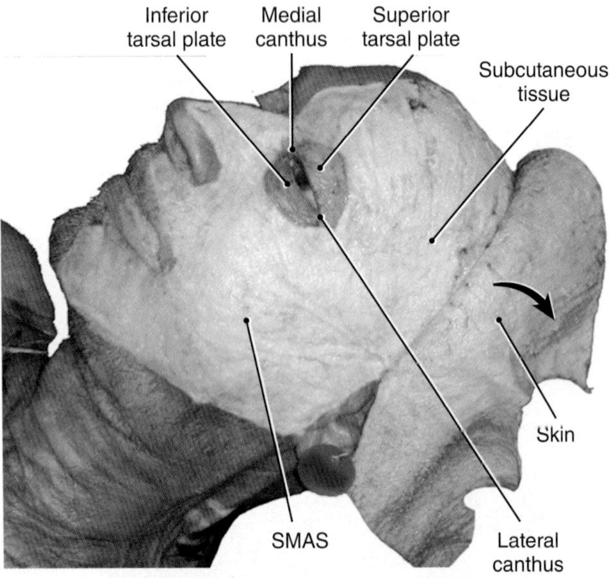

Fig. 21.4 Lateral view of the face with the skin reflected from the mandibular, maxillary, zygomatic, frontal, and temporal regions. *SMAS,* Superficial musculoaponeurotic space.

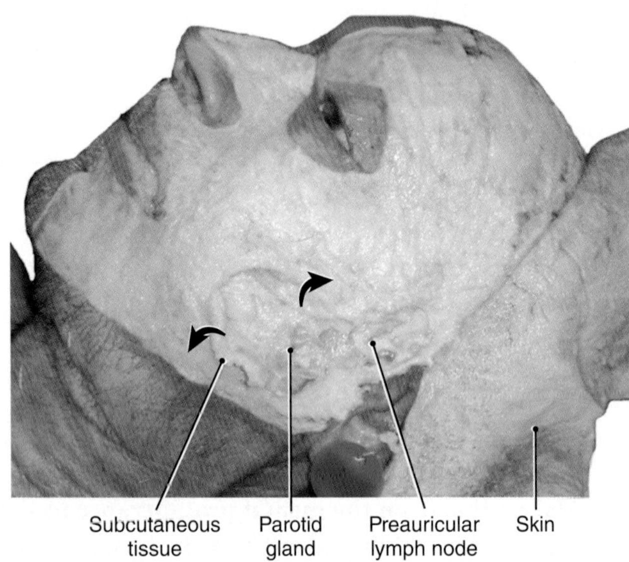

Fig. 21.6 Lateral view of the face with the skin reflected and the SMAS removed from the mandibular region. *SMAS,* Superficial musculoaponeurotic space.

DISSECTION **TIP**

The muscles of facial expression vary in thickness. Pay special attention when removing the skin and SMAS to avoid cutting any muscles, because many attach directly into the subcutaneous tissues.

PAROTID GLAND

- **Situated in front of the ear (auricle), the parotid gland is covered with variable amounts of fat. Using the separating technique with your scissors, reflect as much fat as possible.**
- **Identify the parotid gland, which typically extends into the space between the zygomatic arch and the angle of the mandible (Fig. 21.6).**

ANATOMY **NOTE**

The parotid gland is covered by a dense fibrous capsule, which sends septae into the gland, dividing it into lobules.

- **Begin to reflect the SMAS medially over the mandibular region to reveal the parotid gland (see Fig. 21.5).**
- **Continue to remove the SMAS from the mandibular region (Fig. 21.7).**

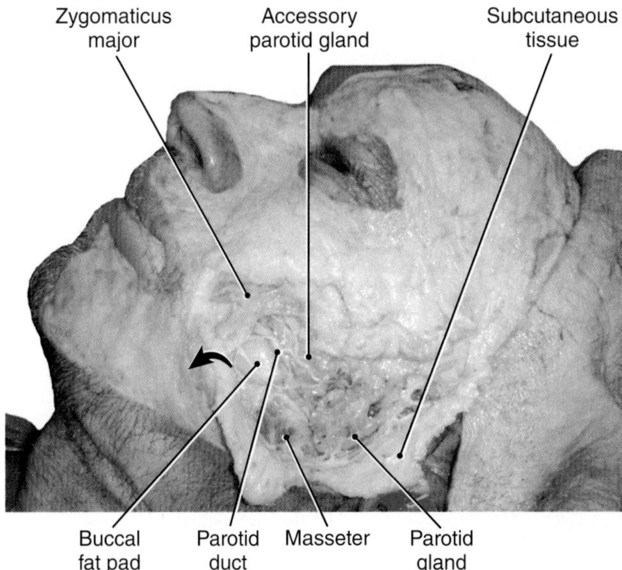

Fig. 21.7 Lateral view of the face with the skin reflected and the SMAS removed from the mandibular region. *SMAS,* Superficial musculoaponeurotic space.

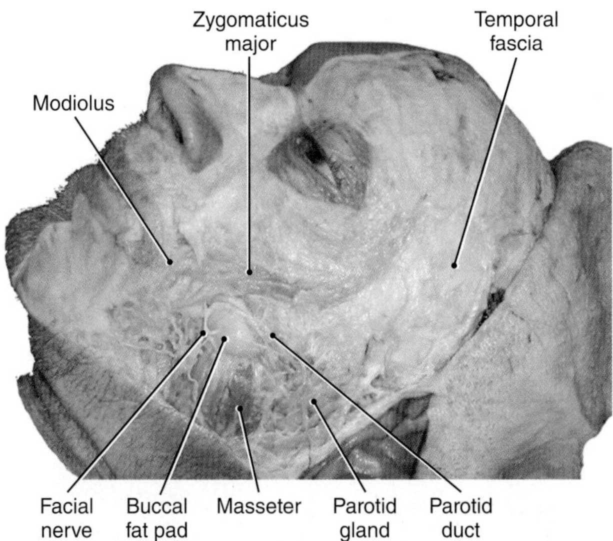

Fig. 21.8 Lateral view of the face with the skin reflected and the SMAS removed from mandibular, maxillary, and temporal regions. *SMAS,* Superficial musculoaponeurotic space.

- **Identify the parotid duct, usually found emerging from the anterior edge of the parotid gland, about 2.5 cm (1 inch) inferior to the zygomatic arch (Figs. 21.7 and 21.8).**

ANATOMY NOTE

From this point, the parotid duct passes horizontally across the masseter muscle, then turns around the anterior edge of the masseter and pierces the bucinator muscle (Fig. 21.9).

- **Remove the SMAS from the maxillary and temporal regions (see Fig. 21.8).**

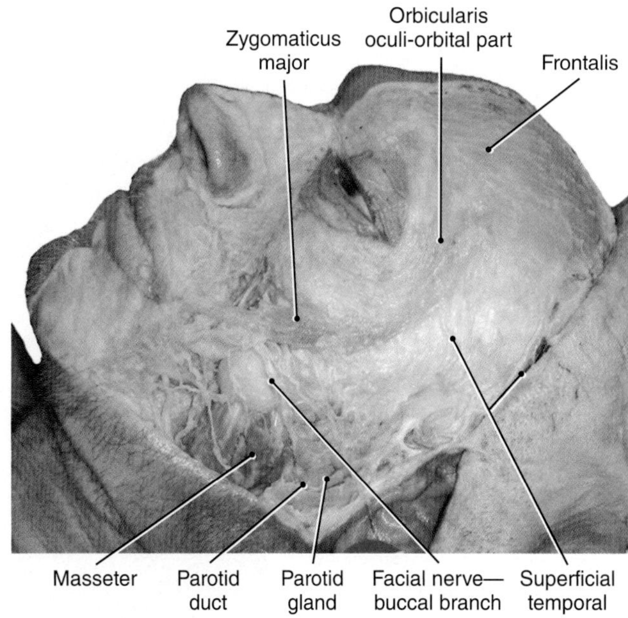

Fig. 21.9 Lateral view of the face with the skin and subcutaneous tissue removed from the mandibular, maxillary, and orbital regions.

- **Note the following structures: zygomaticus major muscle, masseter muscle, and temporal fascia (see Figs. 21.7 and 21.8).**
- **Identify the buccal fat pad.**

ANATOMY NOTE

The buccal fat pad is an encapsulated mass of adipose tissue, which lies between the masseter and bucinator muscles.

DISSECTION TIP

An accessory parotid gland can often be identified along the parotid duct in its course across the masseter muscle (see Figs. 21.7 and 21.8).

MIMETIC MUSCLES

- **Clean the mimetic muscles, taking care to preserve the branches of the facial nerve, which innervate them.**
- **Remove the SMAS from the orbital region and identify the frontalis and orbicularis oculi muscles (see Fig. 21.9 and Plate 21.1).**
- **Identify the parts of the orbicularis oculi muscles:**
  - **Orbital**
  - **Palpebral**
  - **Lacrimal**
- **Identify the superficial temporal artery just superior to the zygomatic arch in front of the external acoustic meatus (see Fig. 21.9).**

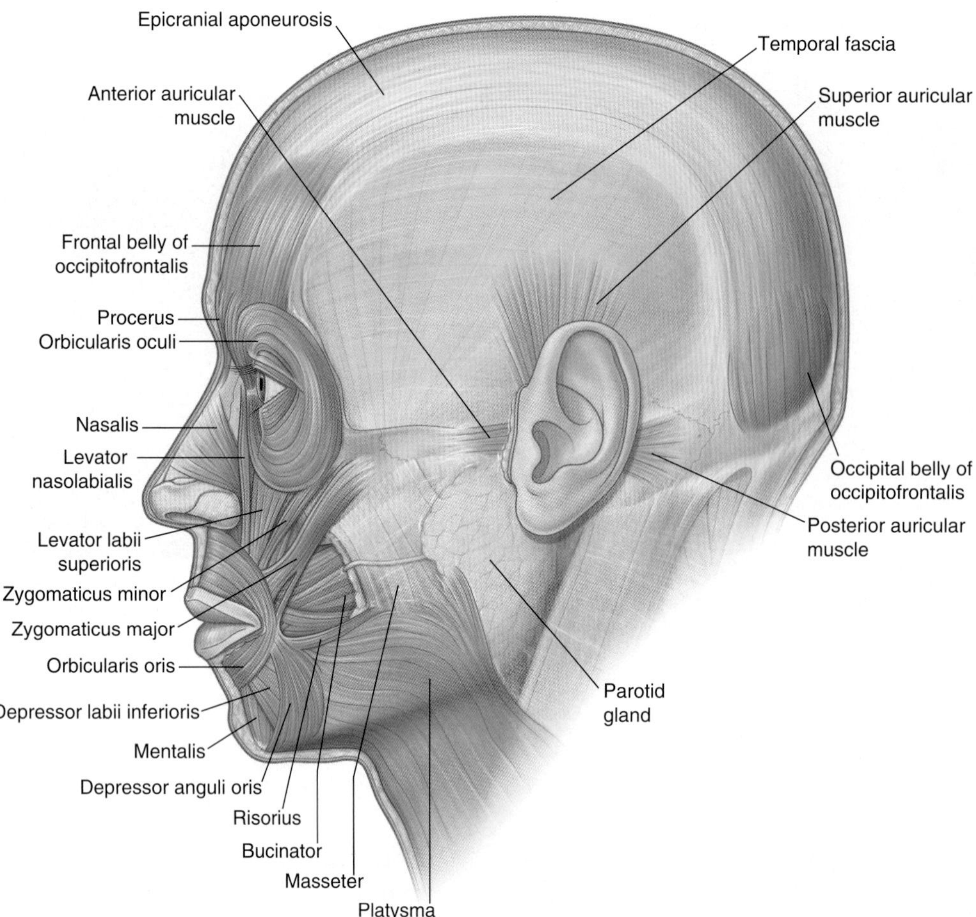

Plate 21.1 Lateral view of the muscles of the facial expression. (From Drake RL et al. *Gray's Atlas of Anatomy*, 3rd edition, Philadelphia, Elsevier, 2021.)

ANATOMY **NOTE**

The auriculotemporal nerve can be found just posterior to this artery.

DISSECTION **TIP**

The transverse facial artery runs superior to the parotid duct, but because of its small size, identifying this artery is often difficult.

- **Identify several of the mimetic muscles (Fig. 21.10).**
- **The muscle surrounding the lips is the *orbicularis oris*.**

DISSECTION **TIP**

Often you will need to remove additional skin from the margins of the lips to expose the orbicularis oris fully. Fibers from several other facial muscles merge with the orbicularis oris, including the bucinator and the elevators and depressors of the angles of the mouth.

- **Identify the zygomaticus major muscles.**
- **Identify the zygomaticus minor muscles.**
- **Identify the depressor anguli oris muscles.**
- **Identify the depressor labii inferioris muscles.**

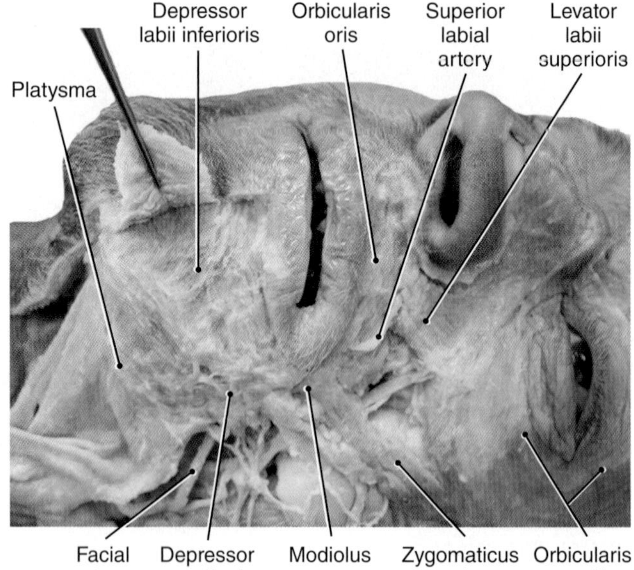

Fig. 21.10 Anterior view of the lower face with the skin removed, revealing various muscles.

- **Identify the levator nasolabialis muscles.**
- **Identify the bucinator muscle.**
- **The platysma muscle has been identified in the dissection of the neck (see Chapter 20).**

DISSECTION **TIP**

Some platysma fibers pass up over the lower border of the mandible and mingle with the depressor muscles of the lips and with the risorius muscle more laterally.

FACIAL NERVE

- **Identify the *buccal branch* of the facial nerve, which usually runs alongside the parotid duct (Fig. 21.11).**

DISSECTION **TIP**

Tracing the branches of the facial nerve can be challenging. In some specimens, some of the parotid nodes may be encountered as the gland is dissected.

- **After you have exposed the buccal branch of the facial nerve, carefully trace it into the substance of the parotid gland until you find its junction(s) with other branches.**
- **Dissect out the other branches of the facial nerve to their target muscles (Fig. 21.12). Landmarks for other branches of the facial nerve follow:**
  - ***Temporal* branch: Dissect near the posterior part of the zygomatic arch.**
  - ***Zygomatic* branch: Dissect around the zygomaticus major muscle at the base of the zygomatic bone.**
  - ***Buccal* branch: Runs parallel to the parotid duct and crosses the masseter muscle.**
  - ***Marginal mandibular* branch: Dissect at the posteroinferior margin of the mandible.**
  - ***Cervical* branch: Dissect deep to the platysma muscle, approximately one fingerbreadth posterior to the angle of the mandible.**

ANATOMY **NOTE**

The facial nerve typically bifurcates into temporofacial and cervicofacial divisions (see Fig. 21.12).

- **Identify the terminal branches of the facial nerve:**
  - Temporal
  - Zygomatic
  - Buccal
  - Marginal mandibular
  - Cervical

ANATOMY **NOTE**

The terminal branches of the facial nerve often connect to one another or with cutaneous (infraorbital) branches of the trigeminal nerve.

DISSECTION **TIP**

Several branches of the facial nerve are not identified with the cadaver in the supine position, including the posterior auricular nerve, which innervates musculature of the external ear and the occipitalis muscle, and the digastric branch, which supplies the posterior belly of the digastric muscle and the stylohyoid muscle.

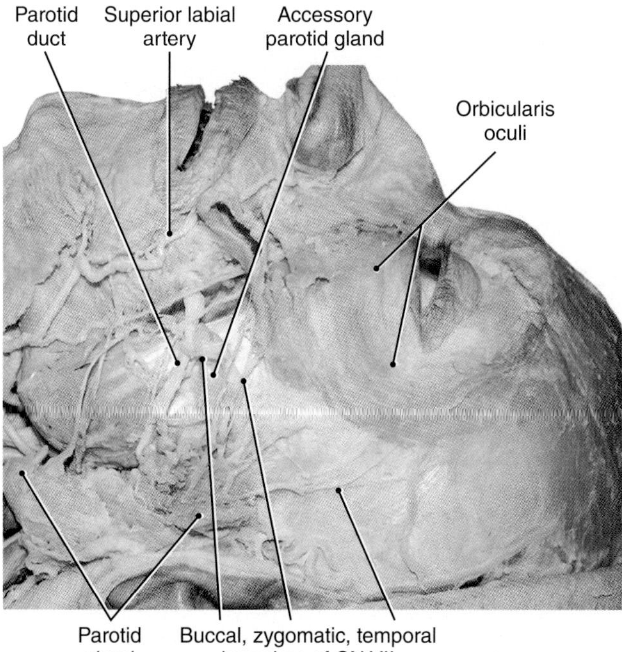

Fig. 21.11 Anterolateral view of the face with the skin and subcutaneous tissue removed.

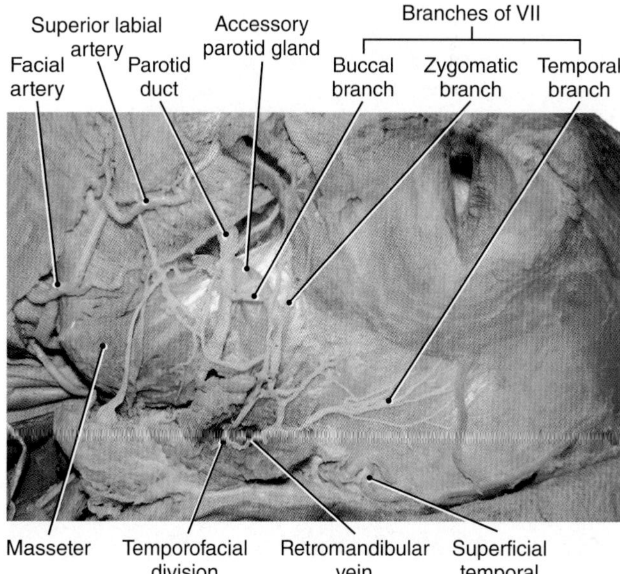

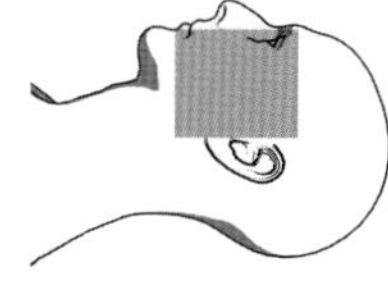

Fig. 21.12 Anterolateral view of the face with the skin and subcutaneous tissue removed.

BUCCAL FAT PAD

- After you expose all terminal branches of the facial nerve, identify and remove the *buccal fat pad*, an encapsulated mass of adipose tissue, which lies between the masseter and bucinator muscles (Figs. 21.13 and 21.14).
- Trace the parotid duct to its point of penetration into the bucinator muscle.
- Lift the buccal fat pad with forceps and use scissors to cut its attachments to nearby structures (Figs. 21.14 and 21.15).
- Pay special attention to preserve the neurovascular structures in the area as you remove the fat pad.

DISSECTION **TIP**

As you remove the buccal fat pad, you will probably notice branches of the buccal artery and nerve. The buccal nerve usually is located between the masseter and bucinator muscles and follows the anterior border of the temporalis muscle to its insertion onto the coronoid process of the mandible. Do not spend time completely exposing the temporalis now; this occurs during the infratemporal fossa dissection (see Chapter 22).

ARTERIES OF THE FACE

- Identify the superior labial artery within the substance of the orbicularis oris muscle.

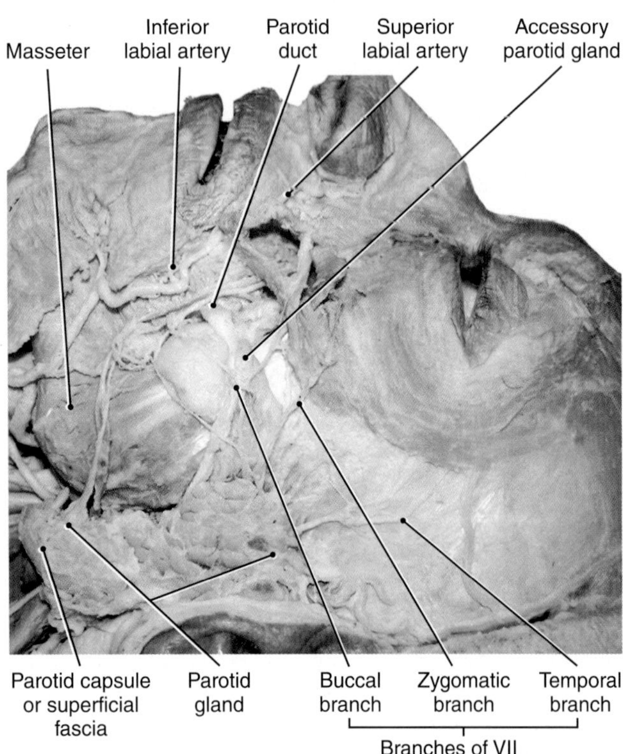

Fig. 21.13 Anterolateral view of the face with the skin and subcutaneous tissue removed, revealing temporofacial division of the facial nerve and its branches.

- Expose the *superior labial artery* and trace it backward toward the angle of the mandible (see Fig. 21.11).
- The *facial artery* is hidden along part of its course by the submandibular gland and by several mimetic muscles. Identify the facial artery as it becomes superficial at the inferior border of the mandible near its angle. It then crosses the cheek, passes near the

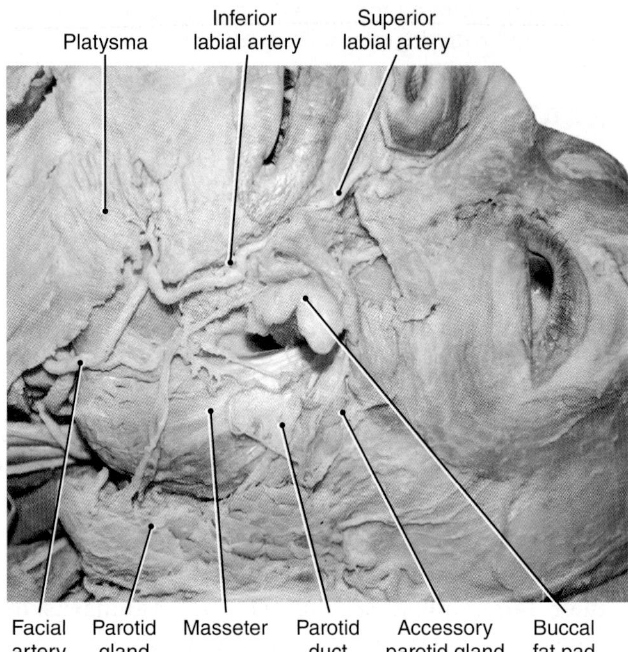

Fig. 21.14 Anterolateral view of the face with the skin and subcutaneous tissue removed.

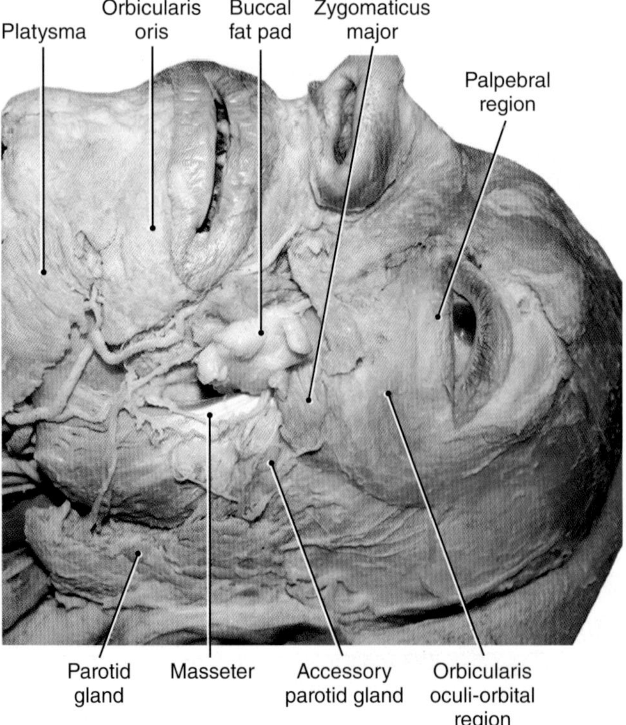

Fig. 21.15 Anterolateral view of the face with the skin and subcutaneous tissue removed.

angle of the mouth, and ends near the medial angle of the eye as the *angular artery* (Plate 21.2).

- Medially reflect any of the mimetic muscles covering the facial artery. Once the facial artery is exposed, continue exposing the terminal part, the angular artery.

DISSECTION **TIP**

The facial artery will terminate in approximately 50% of the specimens as the angular artery. The course of the facial artery is tortuous and in contact with the facial vein, which lies just posterior to it.

- With scissors, remove the platysma, depressor labii inferioris, and depressor anguli oris muscles medially over the periosteum of the mandible (see Fig. 21.17).

TRIGEMINAL NERVE

- Expose the fibers of the platysma muscle (Fig. 21.16).
- With scissors, remove the platysma, depressor labii inferioris, and depressor anguli oris muscles medially over the periosteum of the mandible (Fig. 21.17).
- Identify the mental foramen and the mental nerve (Fig. 21.18).

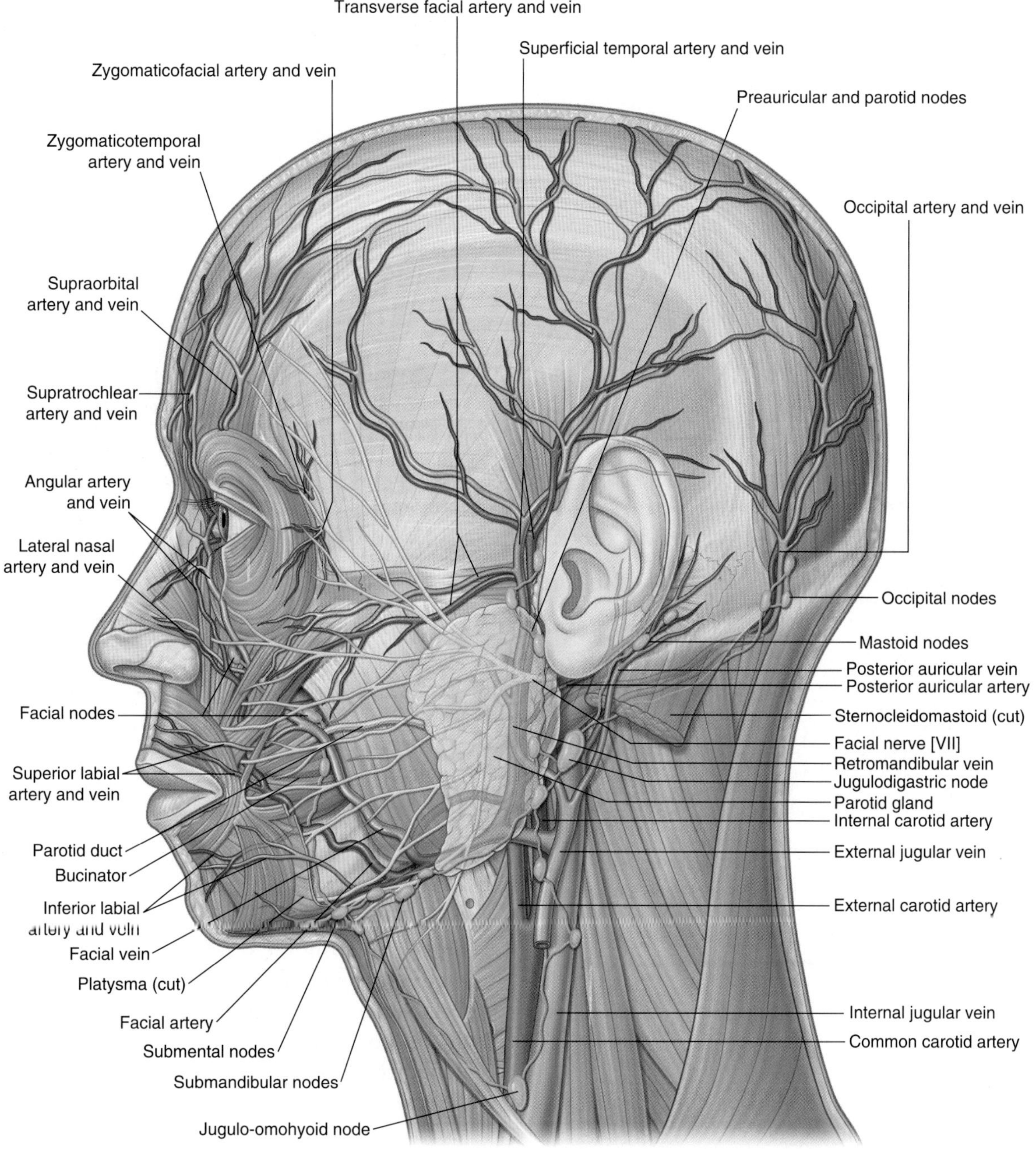

Plate 21.2 Lateral view of the muscles of the facial expression with accompanying nerves and arteries. (From Drake RL et al. *Gray's Atlas of Anatomy*, 3rd edition, Philadelphia, Elsevier, 2021.)

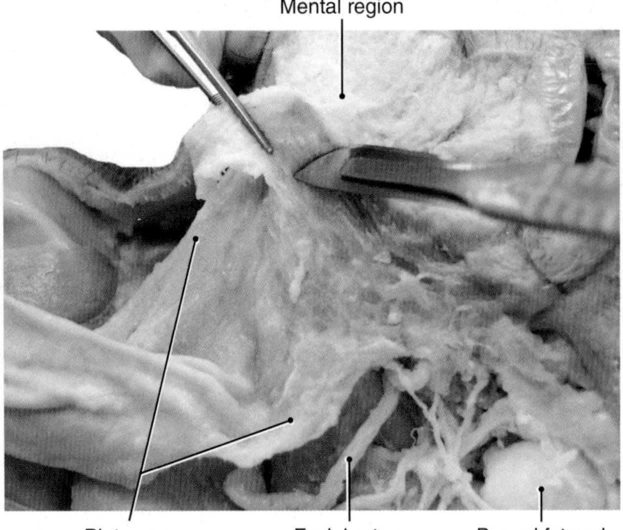

Fig. 21.16 Anterolateral view of the face and neck with the skin and subcutaneous tissue removed.

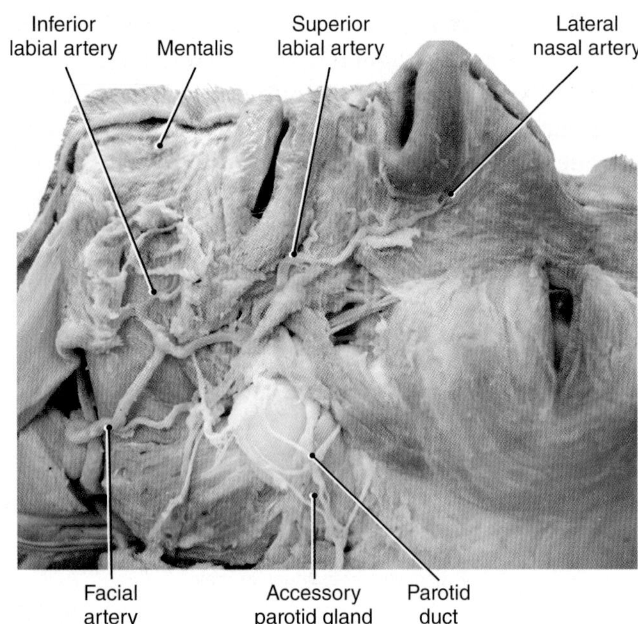

Fig. 21.18 Anterolateral view of the face and neck with the skin and subcutaneous tissue removed.

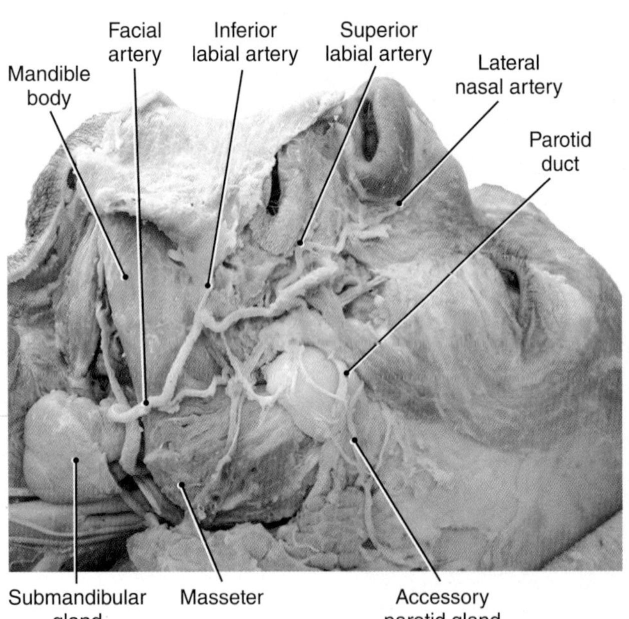

Fig. 21.17 Anterolateral view of the face and neck with the skin and subcutaneous tissue removed.

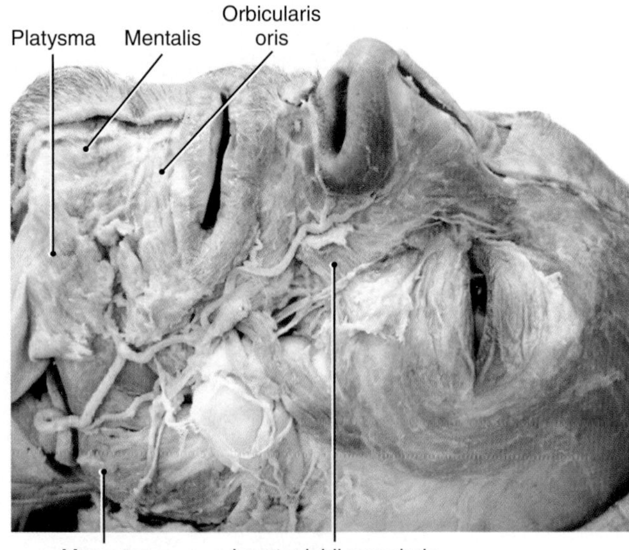

Fig. 21.19 Anterolateral view of the face and neck with the skin and subcutaneous tissue removed.

DISSECTION **TIP**

One way to identify the infraorbital and mental nerves is to draw an imaginary line from the supraorbital notch vertically to the mandible, which will pass over, or near, the infraorbital and mental foramina.

- **Detach the inferior part of the orbicularis oris superiorly from the inferior orbital rim (medial to zygomaticus major muscle) (Fig. 21.19).**
- **Detach the levator nasolabialis medially and identify the infraorbital nerve (Figs. 21.20–21.22).**
- **Reflect the superior part of the orbicularis oculi muscle and identify the superior tarsal plate (Figs. 21.23 and 21.24).**
- **Reflect the superior tarsal plate and notice the fascia of the levator palpebrae superioris muscle (Fig. 21.25).**

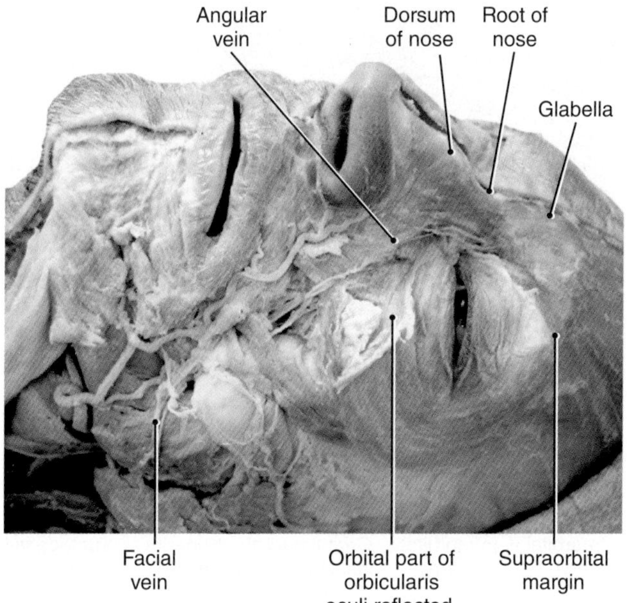

Fig. 21.20 Anterolateral view of the face and neck with the skin and subcutaneous tissue removed and orbital part of orbicularis oculi reflected.

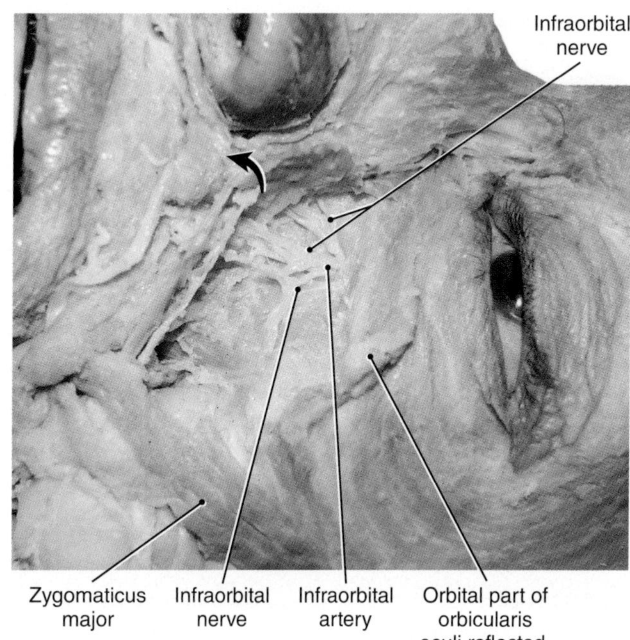

Fig. 21.22 Anteroinferior view of the orbital region with the skin and subcutaneous tissue removed and orbital part of orbicularis oculi reflected.

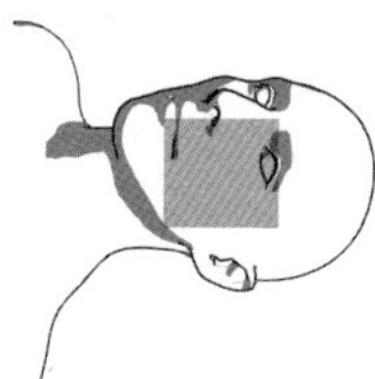

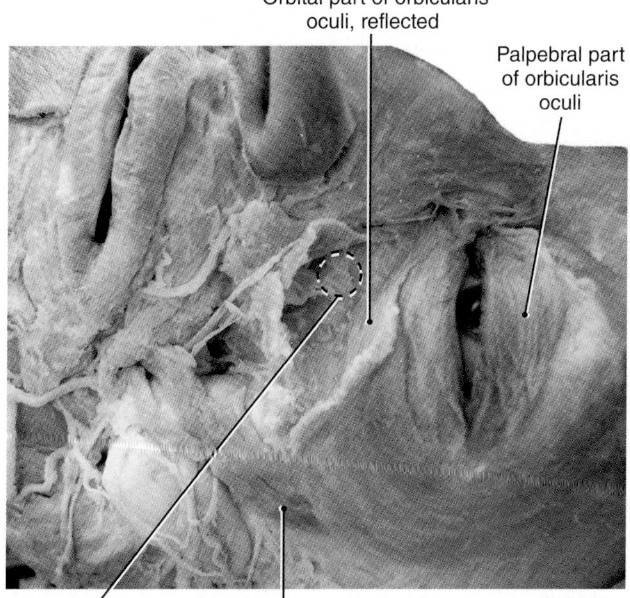

Fig. 21.21 Anteromedial view of the nasal, orbital, and maxillary regions with the skin and subcutaneous tissue removed.

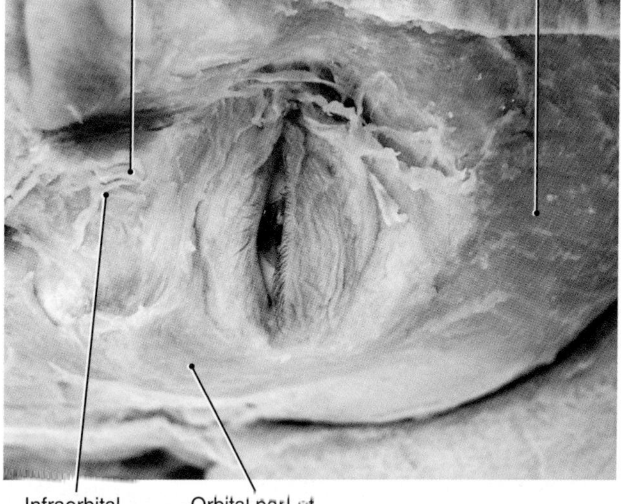

Fig. 21.23 Anteroinferior view of the orbital region with the skin and subcutaneous tissue removed.

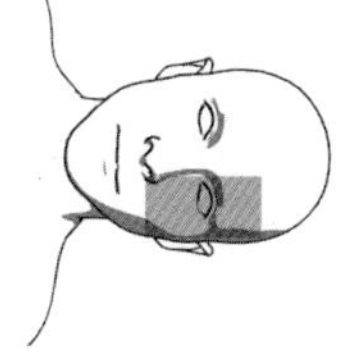

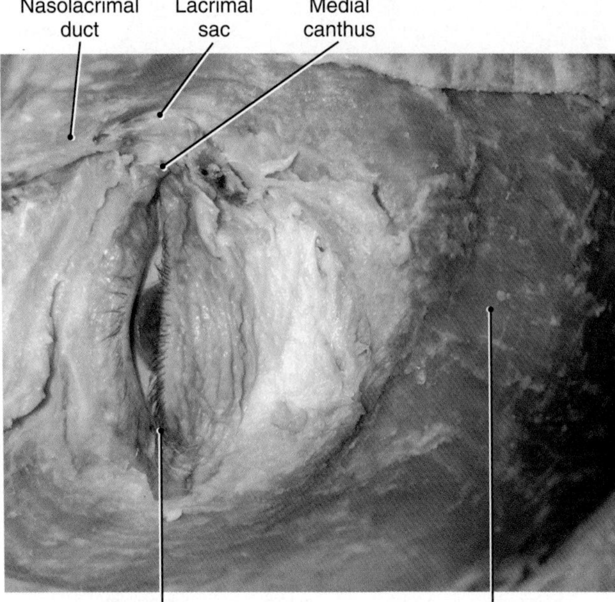

Fig. 21.24 Anterior view of the orbital region with the skin and subcutaneous tissue removed.

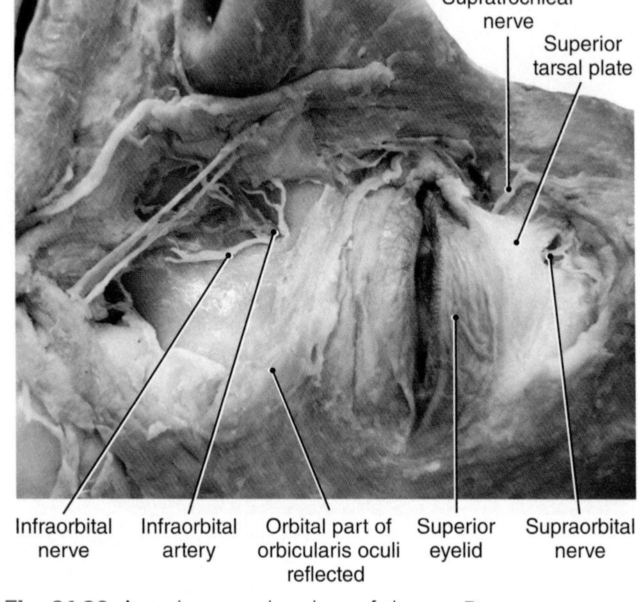

Fig. 21.26 Anterior superior view of the orbital region with the skin removed.

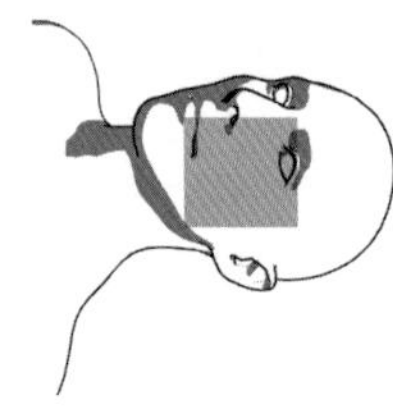

Lacrimal sac

Supraorbital notch

Fascia over levator palpebrae superioris

Frontalis

Fig. 21.25 Anterior view of the orbital region with the skin and subcutaneous tissue removed.

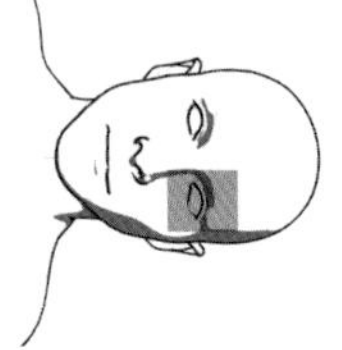

- **Palpate the supraorbital notch, and with scissors, separate the muscle fibers and the connective tissue superficial (inferior and superior) to the notch to expose the *supraorbital nerve* (Fig. 21.26).**
- **Identify the superficial temporal vein. This vein joins the maxillary vein to form the retromandibular vein.**

DISSECTION **TIP**

In most specimens the supraorbital nerve, artery, and vein emerge through the orbital septum and superior tarsal plate (see Fig. 21.26), whereas the supratrochlear nerve emerges medially (Fig. 21.27).

- **You may remove the parotid gland now (Fig. 21.28), or during the dissection of the infratemporal fossa (see Chapter 22).**

VEINS OF THE FACE

- **Identify the *retromandibular vein* deep to the facial nerve.**

ANATOMY **NOTE**

The retromandibular vein splits into anterior and posterior divisions; the posterior division joins the posterior auricular vein to form the external jugular vein, and the anterior division joins the facial vein to form the common facial vein.

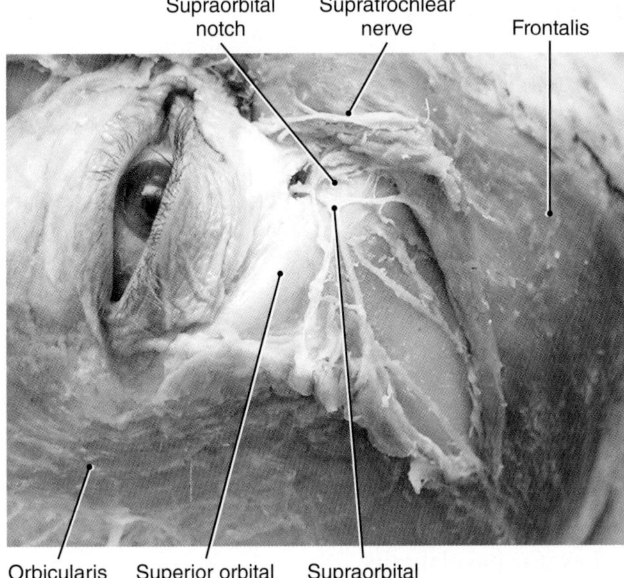

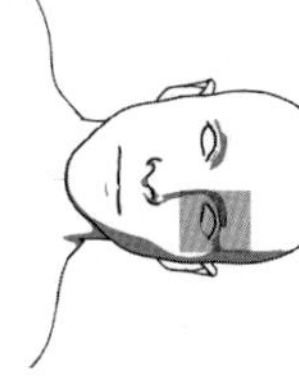

Fig. 21.27 Anterosuperior view of the orbital region with the skin and subcutaneous tissue removed.

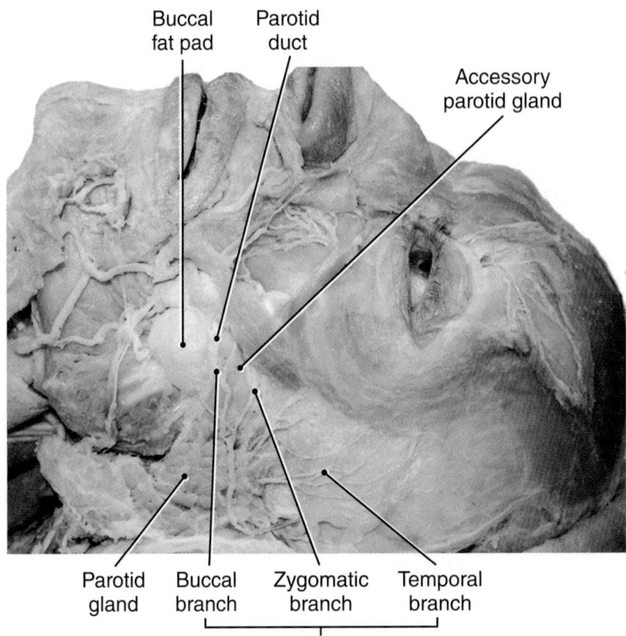

Fig. 21.28 Anterolateral view of the face with the skin and subcutaneous tissue removed.

- **Identify and trace the *facial vein* and look for its drainage into the common facial vein (Fig. 21.29).**
- **The facial vein begins at the medial orbit as the angular vein, then courses with the facial artery toward the angle of the mandible (see Fig. 21.20).**
- **Identify the junction of the posterior division of the retromandibular vein with the posterior auricular vein, forming the external jugular vein.**
- **Trace the facial vein's drainage into the anterior division of the retromandibular vein, forming the common facial vein, which drains into the internal jugular vein.**

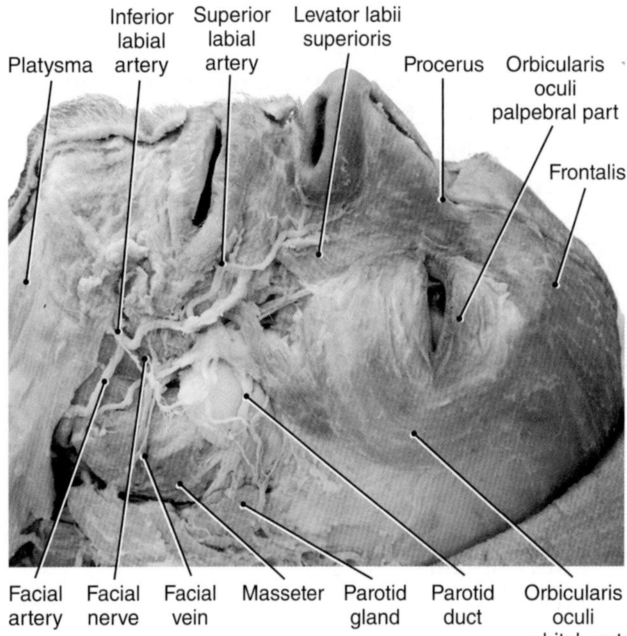

Fig. 21.29 Anterolateral view of the face and neck with the skin and subcutaneous tissue removed.

LABORATORY IDENTIFICATION CHECKLIST

NERVES

Trigeminal nerve branches (cutaneous)

- ☐ Supratrochlear
- ☐ Supraorbital
- ☐ Zygomaticotemporal
- ☐ Zygomaticofacial
- ☐ Auriculotemporal
- ☐ Infratrochlear
- ☐ Infraorbital
- ☐ Mental

Facial nerve branches (motor)

- ☐ Facial nerve trunk (deep within parotid gland)
- ☐ Temporal branches
- ☐ Zygomatic branches
- ☐ Buccal branches
- ☐ Marginal mandibular branches
- ☐ Cervical branches

ARTERIES

- ☐ External carotid (within parotid gland)
- ☐ Superficial temporal
- ☐ Maxillary
- ☐ Transverse facial
- ☐ Facial
  - ☐ Superior labial
  - ☐ Inferior labial
  - ☐ Angular

VEINS

- ☐ Facial
- ☐ Angular
- ☐ Retromandibular (within parotid gland)

MUSCLES

- ☐ Occipitofrontalis
  - ☐ Frontalis belly
  - ☐ Galea aponeurotica
  - ☐ Occipitalis belly
- ☐ Procerus
- ☐ Orbicularis oculi
  - ☐ Orbital part
  - ☐ Palpebral part
  - ☐ Lacrimal part
- ☐ Levator nasolabialis
- ☐ Levator labii superioris
- ☐ Levator anguli oris
- ☐ Risorius
- ☐ Zygomaticus major/minor
- ☐ Bucinator
- ☐ Orbicularis oris
- ☐ Depressor anguli oris
- ☐ Depressor labii inferioris
- ☐ Mentalis
- ☐ Platysma

BONES

- ☐ Frontal
- ☐ Zygomatic
- ☐ Temporal
- ☐ Maxillary
- ☐ Mandible

GLAND

- ☐ Parotid
  - ☐ Parotid duct (Stensen's duct)

BEFORE YOU BEGIN

- The infratemporal fossa dissection requires the use of an electric saw or a hammer and chisel. Make sure that you wear eye protection when you use these tools.
- Cut the terminal branches of the facial nerve and reflect the nerves posteriorly toward the parotid gland (Fig. 22.1).
- Similarly, cut the parotid duct as it penetrates the buccinator muscle (Fig. 22.2) and reflect it posteriorly toward the parotid gland (see Fig. 22.1).
- Palpate the zygomatic arch and expose it from the surrounding adipose tissue and temporal fascia (Fig. 22.3).

DISSECTION STEPS

- **Identify the temporalis muscle and trace its course medial to the zygomatic arch (Fig. 22.4).**

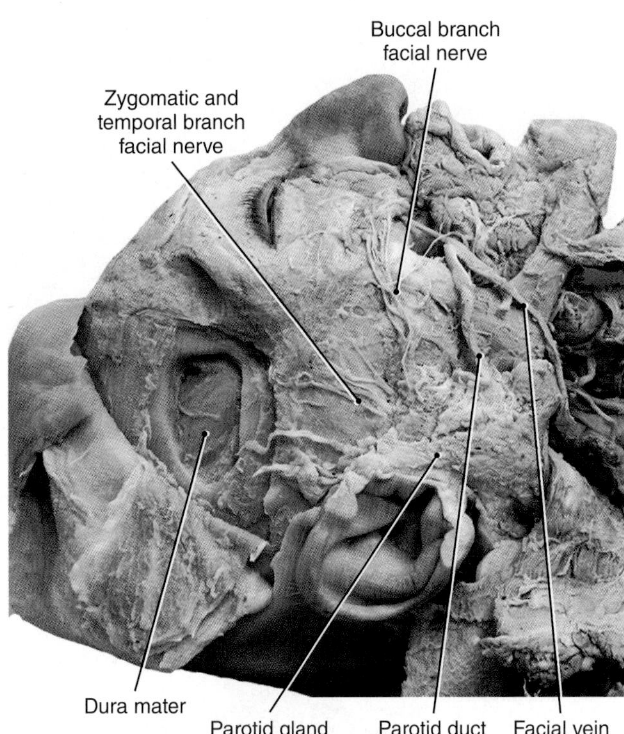

Fig. 22.2 Lateral view of the face with the skin reflected, revealing the superficial structures.

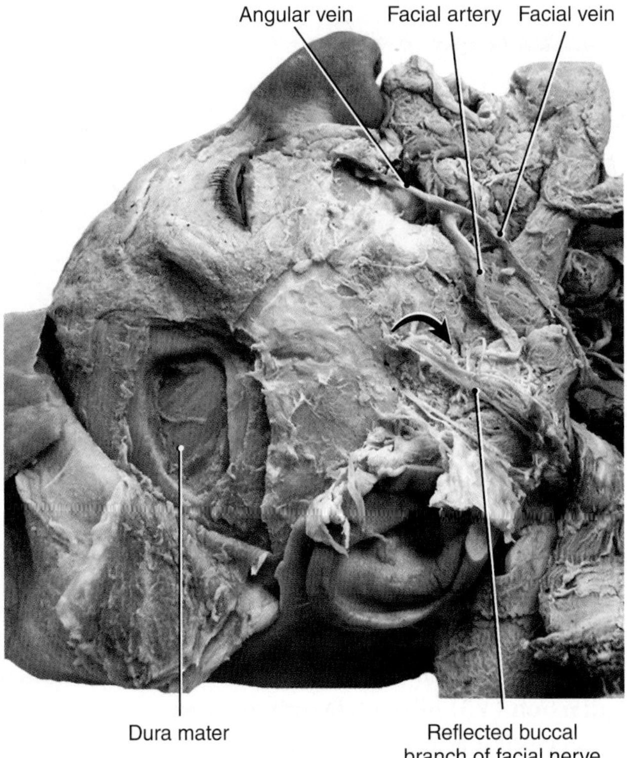

Fig. 22.1 Lateral view of the face, with the parotid duct and branches of facial nerve reflected.

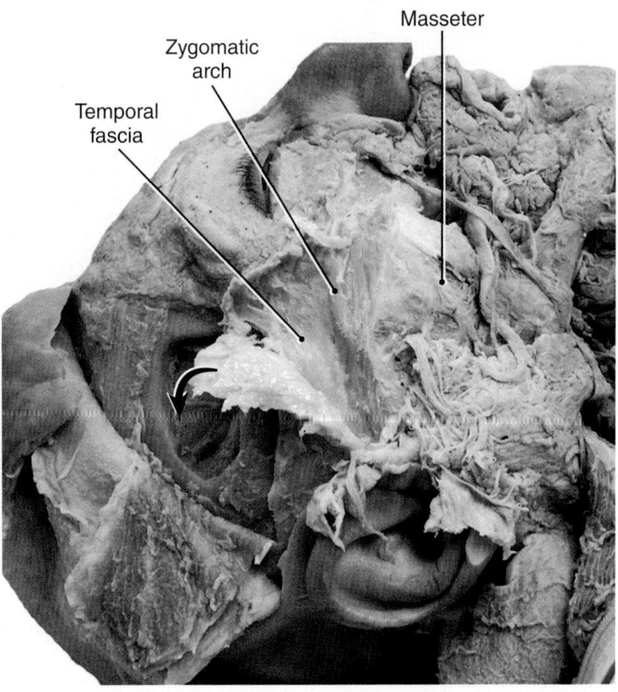

Fig. 22.3 Lateral view of the face, with the skin and the subcutaneous tissue removed and temporal fascia reflected.

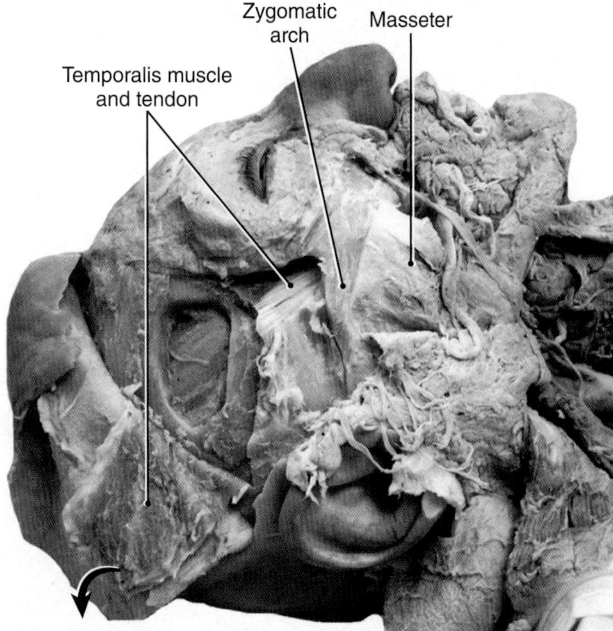

Fig. 22.4 Lateral view of the face, with the skin, subcutaneous tissue, and the temporal fascia removed.

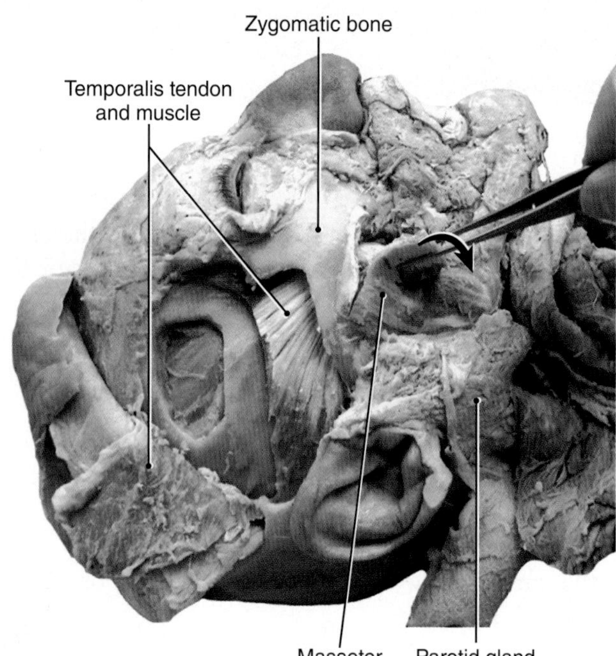

Fig. 22.6 Reflection of the masseter muscle from the inferior border of the zygomatic arch.

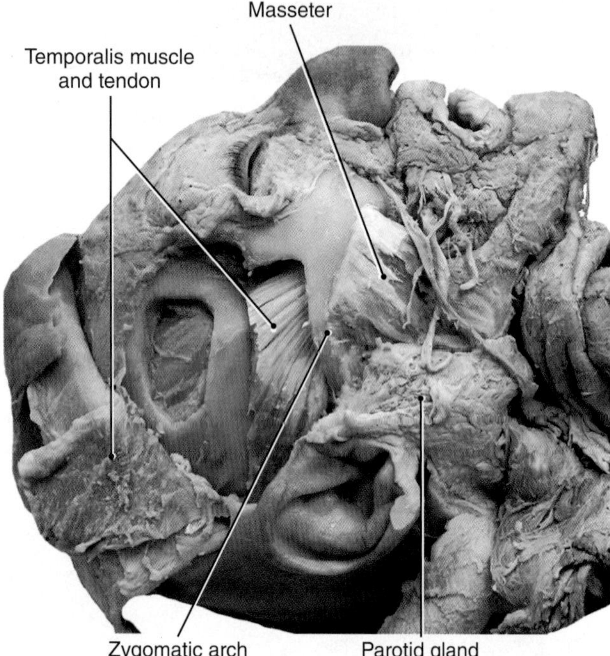

Fig. 22.5 Lateral view with the skin and subcutaneous tissue removed.

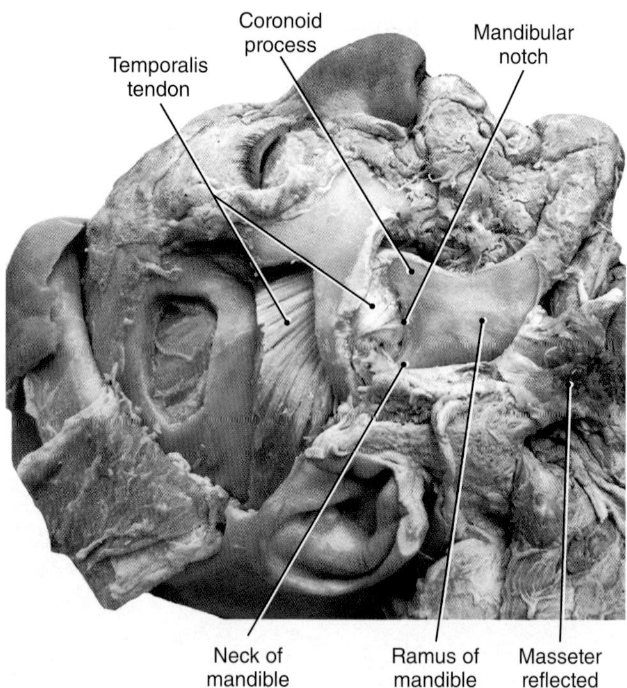

Fig. 22.7 Lateral view of the face with superficial skin and subcutaneous skin removed and the masseter muscle reflected.

- **Clean the lateral surface of the masseter muscle and expose its borders (Fig. 22.5).**
- **Detach the masseter muscle from the inferior border of the zygomatic arch (Fig. 22.6) and reflect it inferiorly toward the angle of the mandible.**
- **Clean the remaining soft tissues over the mandible and expose its surface (Fig. 22.7).**
- **Identify the temporal, zygomatic, and mandibular bony regions.**
- **Just deep to the anterior border of the ramus of the mandible, in the fat and connective tissue of the anterior edge of the temporalis muscle, identify and clean the *buccal nerve*, a branch of the mandibular division (V3) of the trigeminal nerve.**
- **Place scissors or a probe underneath the zygomatic arch.**
- **Using a saw, cut the zygomatic arch just anterior to the attachment of the masseter muscle (Fig. 22.8).**

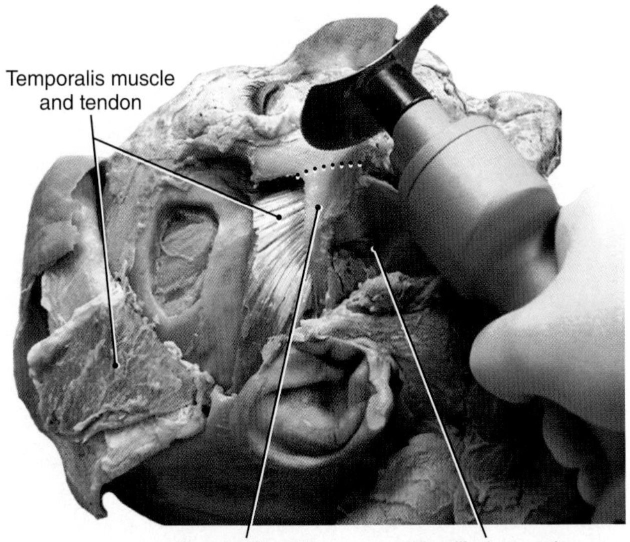

Fig. 22.8 Saw cut of the zygomatic arch just anterior to attachment of masseter muscle.

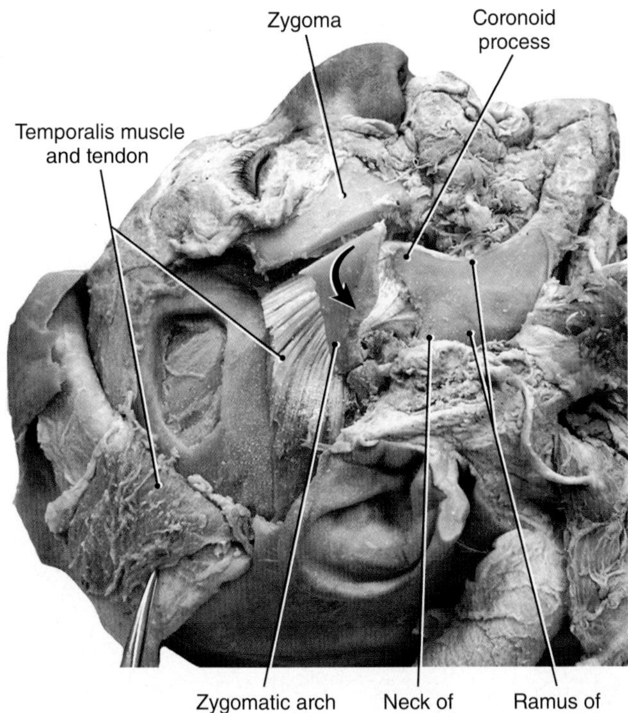

Fig. 22.9 Lateral view of the face, revealing the zygomatic arch osteotomy anterior to the masseter attachment, with a second cut anterior to the temporomandibular joint.

- **Make a second cut through the arch just posterior to the masseter and anterior to the temporomandibular joint (Fig. 22.9).**
- **Detach the cut piece of zygomatic bone (Fig. 22.10).**
- **With scissors, cut the *temporalis muscle* from the coronoid process and ramus of the mandible (Fig. 22.11).**
- **Reflect the temporalis upward and clean the soft tissues and fat over the mandibular notch (Fig. 22.12).**

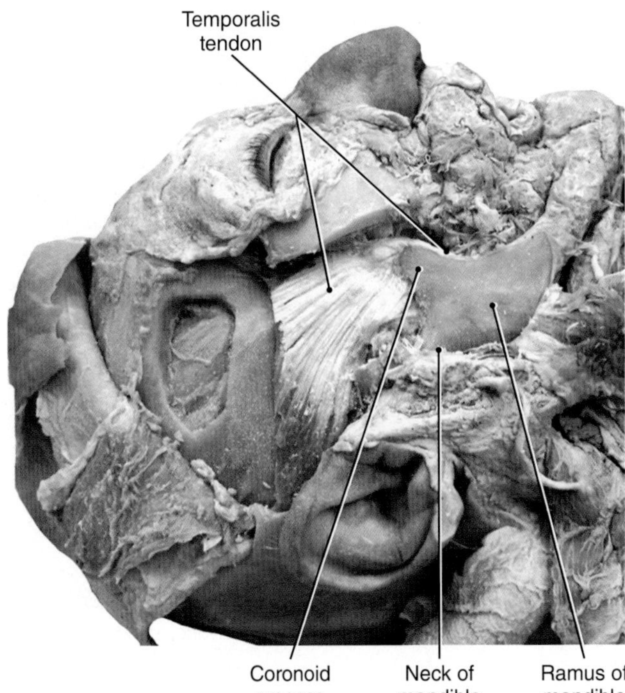

Fig. 22.10 Removal of the zygomatic arch, exposing attachments of the temporalis muscle and bony landmarks of the mandible.

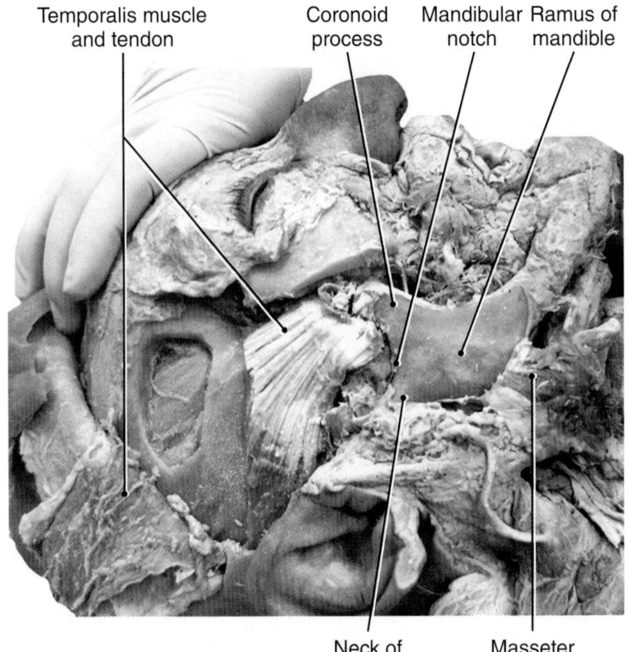

Fig. 22.11 Detachment of the temporalis muscle from the coronoid process and mandibular notch.

- **Place your scissors or a probe or scalpel handle immediately beneath the ramus of the mandible (Fig. 22.13).**
- **Push the soft tissues, musculature, and vessels inferiorly.**

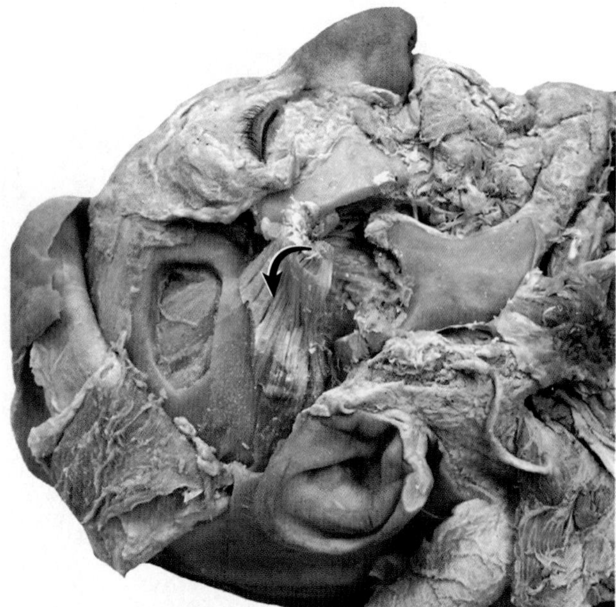

Fig. 22.12 Reflection of the temporalis muscle *(arrow)*.

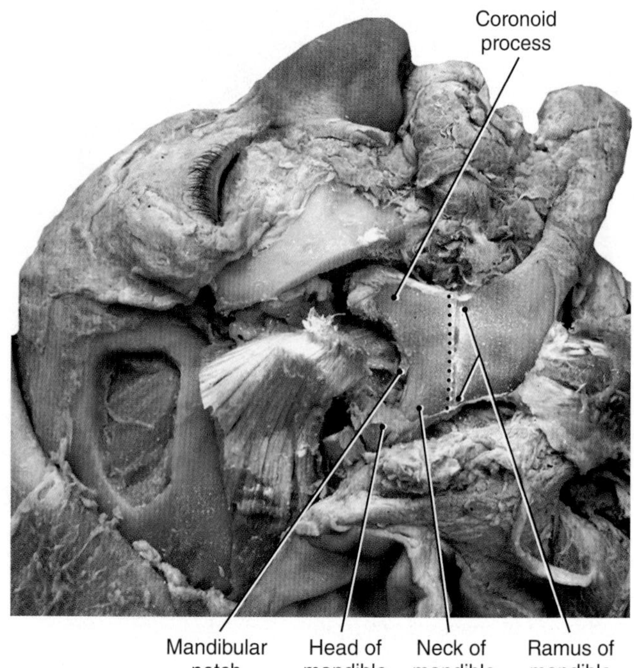

Fig. 22.14 Saw cut horizontally through the ramus of mandible below the coronoid process.

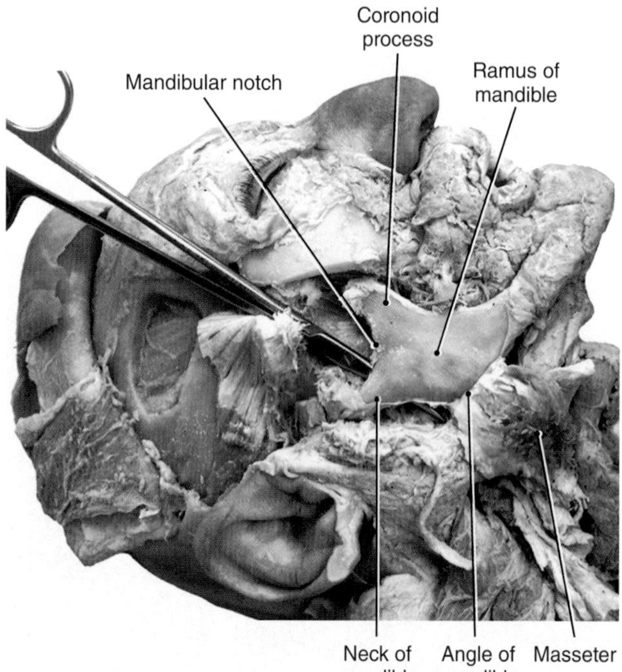

Fig. 22.13 Placing scissors underneath the ramus of the mandible and pushing the soft tissues, muscles, and vessels inferiorly preserves the underlying structure when the mandible is cut with an electric saw.

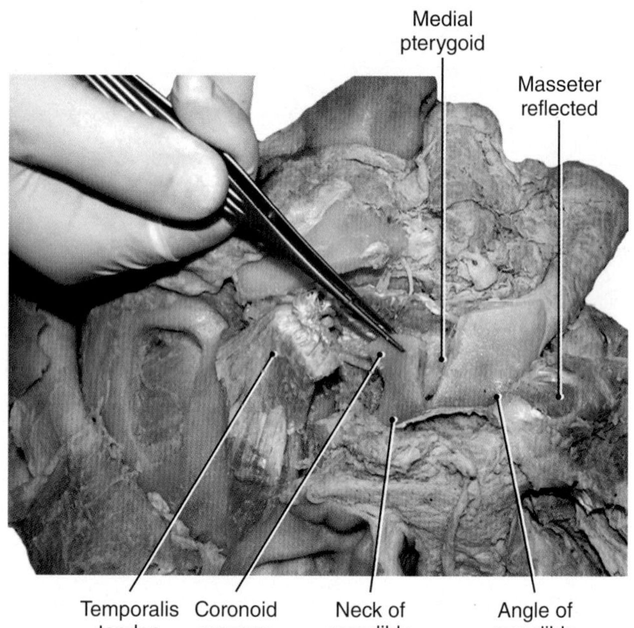

Fig. 22.15 Severed coronoid process and the temporalis muscle reflected superiorly.

DISSECTION **TIP**

This maneuver (see Fig. 22.13) is important for preserving underlying structures when the mandible is cut. You may leave the probe or scissors in place to protect the inferior alveolar neurovascular bundle and lingual nerve when you perform the cut (see next step).

- **With an electric saw, cut horizontally through the ramus of the mandible 2 to 3 inches (5–7.5 cm) below the coronoid process, leaving the articular process in place (Fig. 22.14).**
- **Reflect the severed coronoid process and the temporalis muscle superiorly (Figs. 22.15–22.17).**

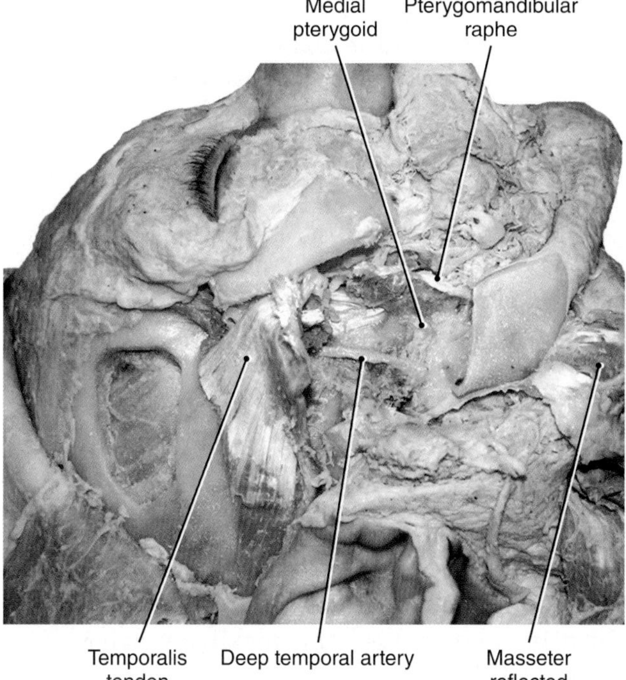

Fig. 22.16 Appreciate the medial pterygoid muscle with all soft tissues removed.

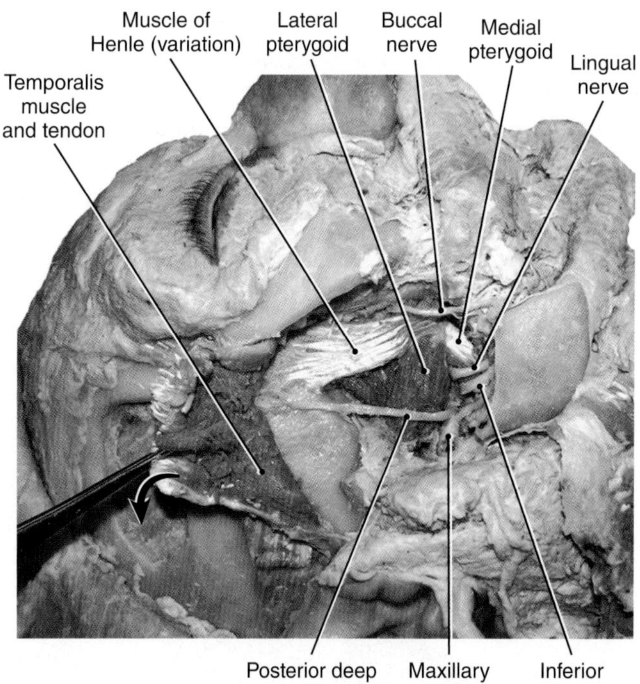

Fig. 22.18 Appreciate the medial and lateral pterygoid muscles. The maxillary artery is located deep to the lateral pterygoid in this specimen; also note the uncommon pterygoideus proprius (muscle of Henle).

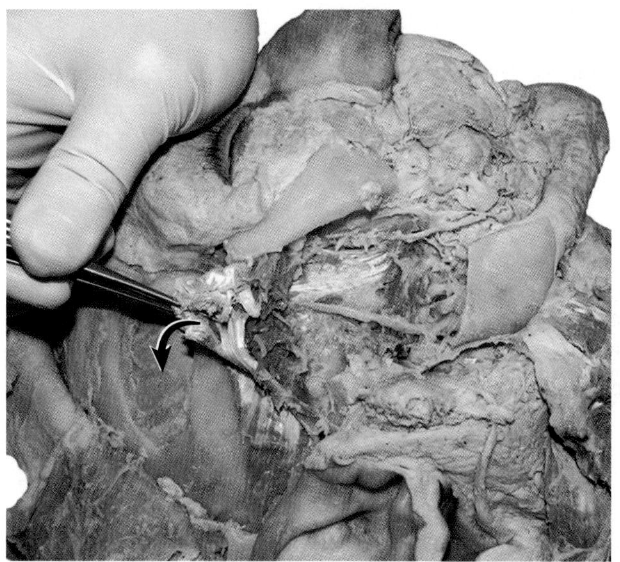

Fig. 22.17 Further reflection of the temporalis muscle to expose the contents of the infratemporal fossa.

DISSECTION **TIP**

Take special care when you reflect the coronoid process and the temporalis muscle so as not to injure the buccal nerve.

- **As the temporalis is reflected superiorly, observe the deep temporal arteries supplying this muscle.**

DISSECTION **TIP**

You can choose either to sever the arteries or to keep them. In this dissection, we choose to keep the deep temporal vessels (see Figs. 22.16 and 22.17).

- **Once temporalis has been reflected, identify the medial pterygoid muscle (see Figs. 22.15–22.17).**
- **Once the temporalis muscle is reflected and the soft tissues are cleaned, identify and expose the *lateral pterygoid muscle*, which lies just beneath the temporalis (Fig. 22.18).**

ANATOMY **NOTE**

The lateral pterygoid muscle arises from the lateral pterygoid plate and passes horizontally to insert onto the articular disc of the temporomandibular joint (see Fig. 22.18).

ANATOMY **NOTE**

In some cadavers, a variant muscle may be seen in the infratemporal fossa. In this specimen, a pterygoideus proprius was identified (muscle of Henle). This muscle originates from the anterior infratemporal crest, runs vertically downward to insert onto the lateral pterygoid plate, and crosses superficially to the lateral pterygoid muscle (see Fig. 22.18). Typically, the muscle of Henle has no functional significance, but it may compress the mandibular nerve, resulting in possible trigeminal neuralgia.

- Clean the soft tissues and fat at the inferior border of the lateral pterygoid muscle (Fig. 22.19 and Plate 22.1).
- Identify the *inferior alveolar nerve* and inferior alveolar artery superficial to the medial pterygoid muscle (see Figs. 22.18 and 22.19).
- Clean the inferior alveolar nerve and trace it to the inferior alveolar foramen.

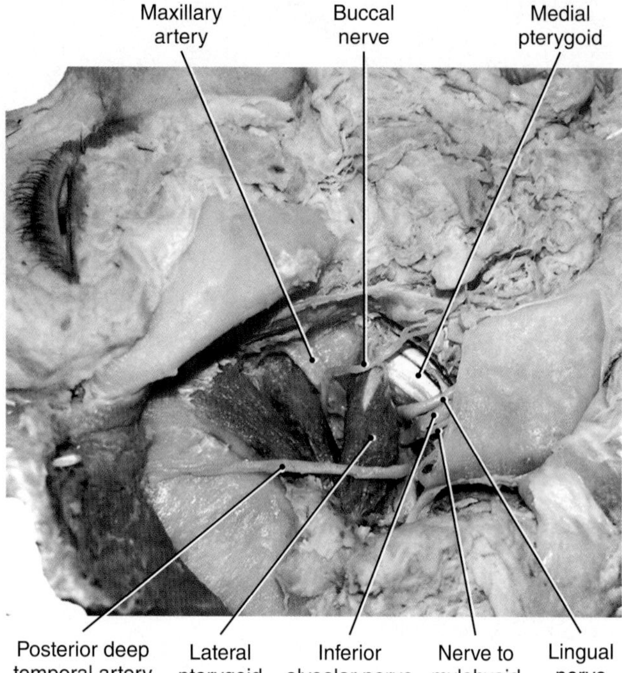

Fig. 22.19 Soft tissue in the space between the medial and lateral pterygoid muscles cleaned, exposing key structures.

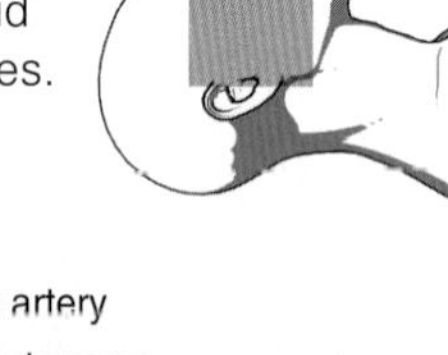

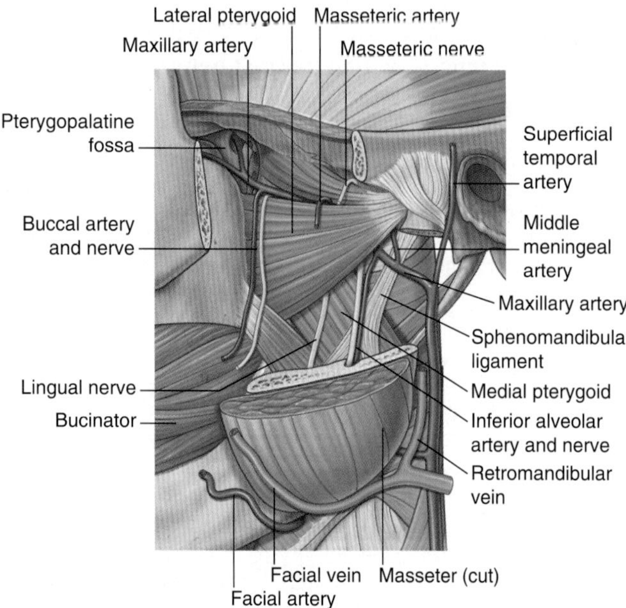

Plate 22.1 Nerves and vessels of the infratemporal fossa. (From Drake RL et al. *Gray's Atlas of Anatomy*, 3rd edition, Philadelphia, Elsevier, 2021.)

- Look at the lateral surface of the inferior alveolar nerve and note the small branch that runs parallel with it, the nerve to the mylohyoid muscle (see Fig. 22.19).

ANATOMY **NOTE**

The nerve to the mylohyoid arises just before the inferior alveolar nerve enters the inferior alveolar foramen. The nerve to the mylohyoid travels inferiorly, beneath the ramus and body of the mandible, to innervate the mylohyoid muscle and the anterior belly of the digastric muscle.

- Lateral to the inferior alveolar nerve, identify the *lingual nerve* (Figs. 22.20 and 22.21).
- Medial to the inferior alveolar nerve, identify the *buccal nerve.*
- Immediately underneath these nerves, observe the medial pterygoid muscle passing from the pterygoid plate to its insertion onto the inferior and posterior parts of the medial surface of the mandibular ramus.
- Identify and expose the maxillary artery (see Figs. 22.19–22.21 and 22.29).

ANATOMY **NOTE**

In the majority of cadavers, the lateral pterygoid muscle is crossed superficially by branches of the maxillary artery; in the remaining specimens, the artery travels deep to the muscle (see Fig. 22.21).

- Proceed by carefully detaching the lateral pterygoid muscle from its origin on the lateral pterygoid plate with scissors and forceps (Figs. 22.22–22.24).

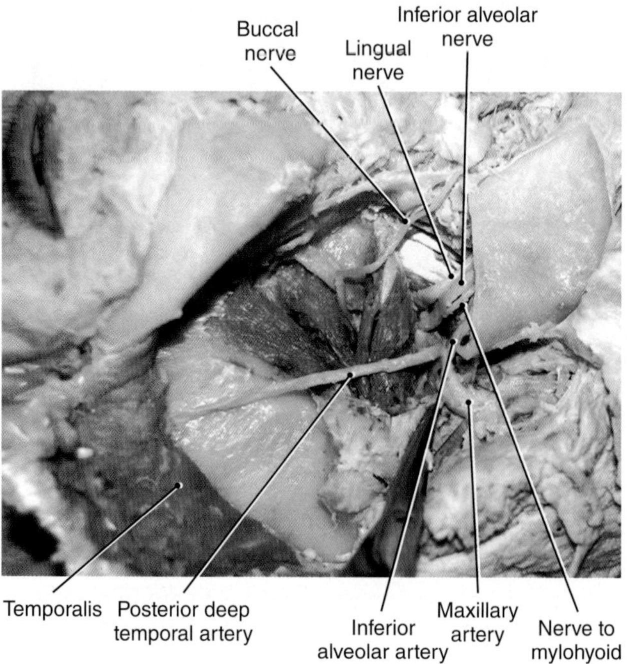

Fig. 22.20 The maxillary artery is exposed.

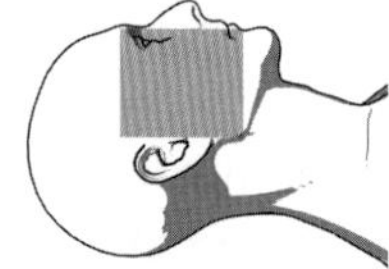

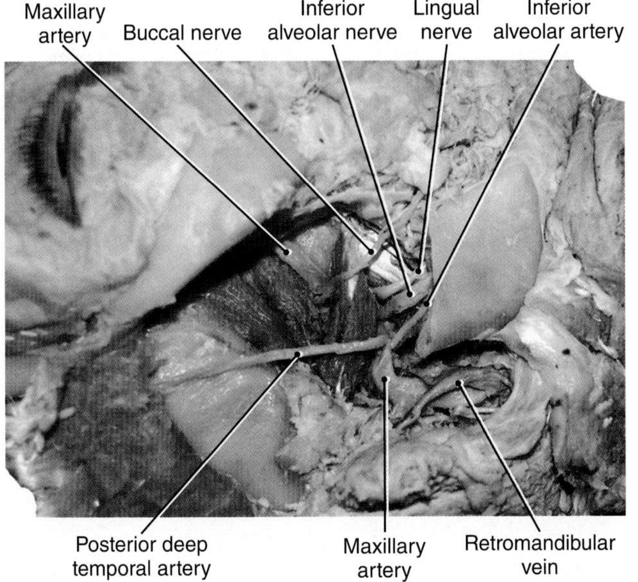

Fig. 22.21 Further exposure of the maxillary artery and accompanying maxillary and retromandibular veins.

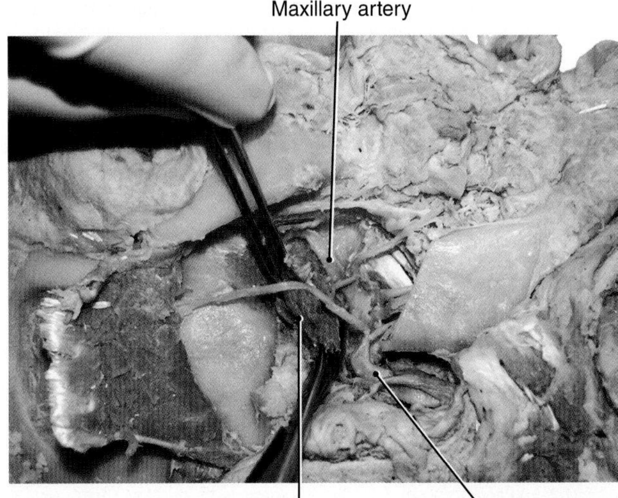

Fig. 22.22 Lateral pterygoid muscle removed with scissors and forceps.

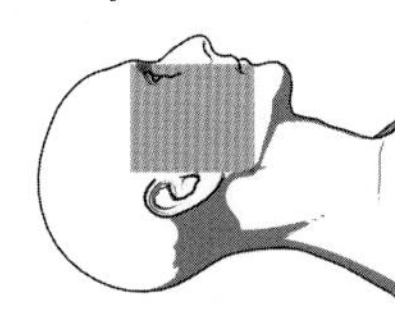

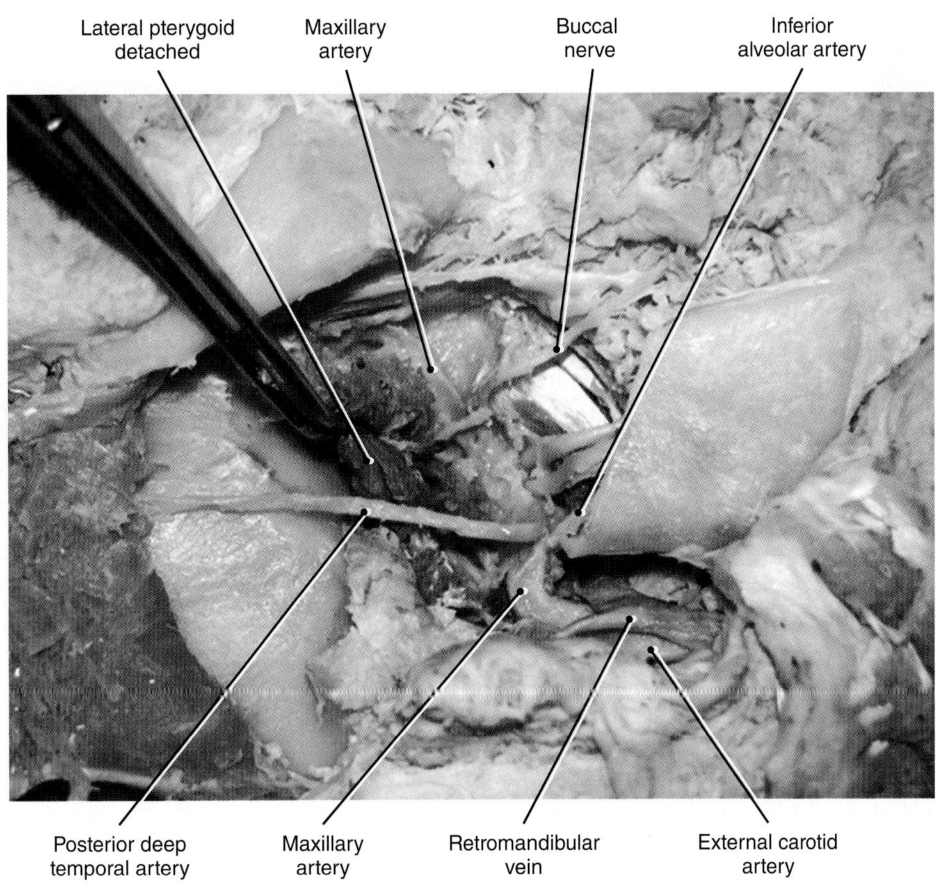

Fig. 22.23 Removal of remaining lateral pterygoid muscle fibers.

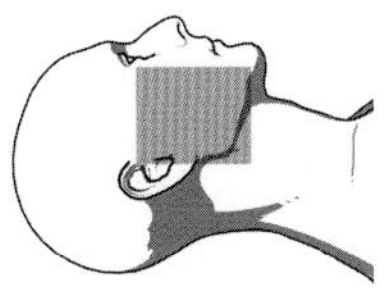

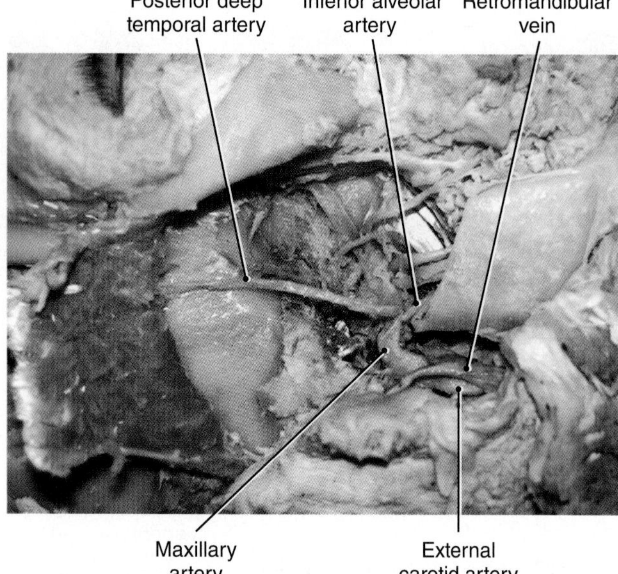

Fig. 22.24 Complete removal of lateral pterygoid muscle. Note the soft tissues around the maxillary artery; carefully remove all soft tissues.

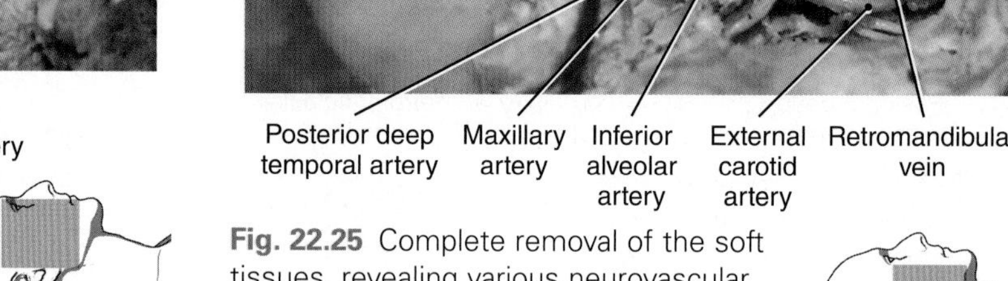

Fig. 22.25 Complete removal of the soft tissues, revealing various neurovascular structures.

DISSECTION TIP

Removing the lateral pterygoid muscle can be a challenge. Be patient, and detach its muscle fibers carefully, paying special attention to the branches of the maxillary artery deep to it (see Figs. 22.22–22.24).

- **Carefully remove all soft tissues around the maxillary artery.**
- **Posterior to the inferior alveolar artery and nerve and anterior to the medial pterygoid muscle, identify the sphenomandibular ligament.**

DISSECTION TIP

This ligament is thin and may resemble a nerve, and it is often confused with the inferior alveolar nerve.

- **Once the lateral pterygoid muscle is removed, expose the maxillary artery and its branches (Fig. 22.25).**
- **Note the retromandibular vein formed by the junction of the superficial temporal and maxillary veins (see Fig. 22.25).**
- **Identify the middle meningeal artery, which typically runs vertically toward the sphenoid bone, to enter the foramen spinosum (see Figs. 22.25 and 22.27).**
- **Identify the two roots of the auriculotemporal nerve, which, in the majority of cases, you will find encircling the middle meningeal artery (Figs. 22.26 and 22.27 and Plates 22.2 and 22.3).**
- **Lift the lingual nerve and trace it superiorly until you see it joined on its posterior surface by a small nerve, the *chorda tympani*, which is a branch of the**

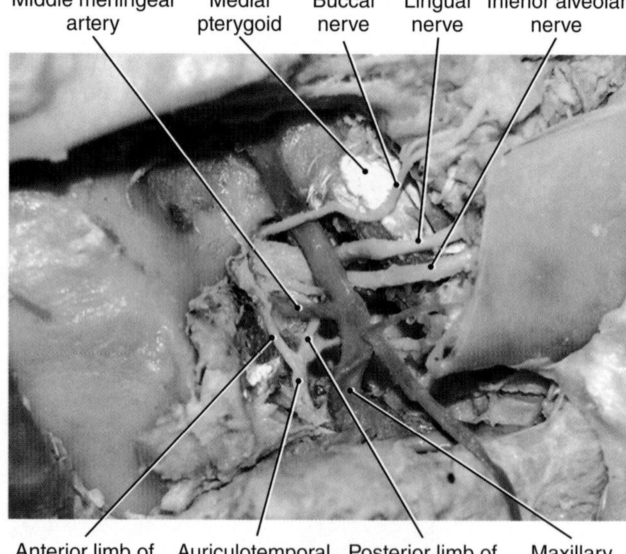

Fig. 22.26 Lateral view of infratemporal fossa, revealing the medial pterygoid muscle and neurovascular structures.

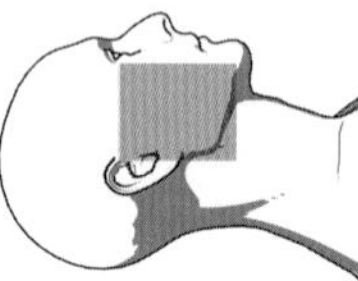

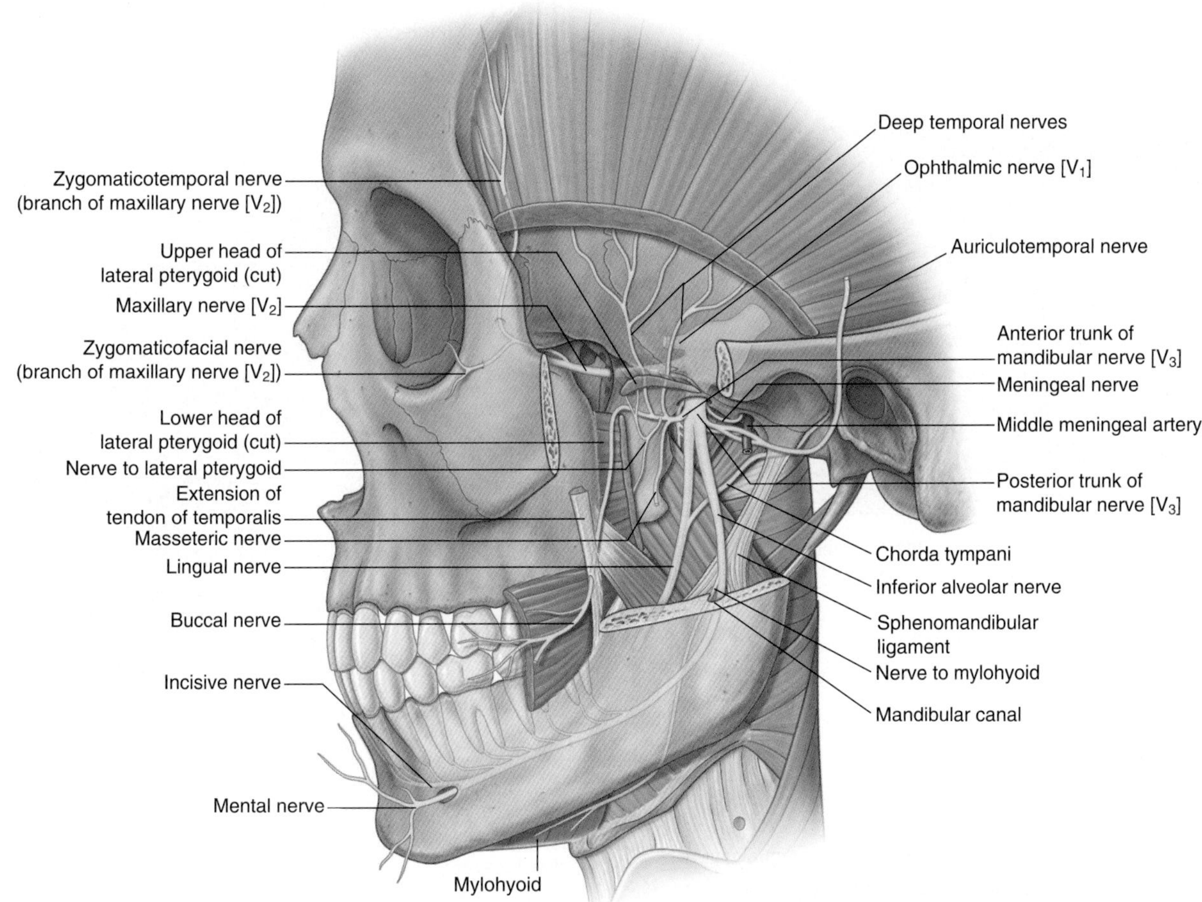

Plate 22.2 Nerves of the infratemporal fossa. (From Drake RL et al. *Gray's Atlas of Anatomy*, 3rd edition, Philadelphia, Elsevier, 2021.)

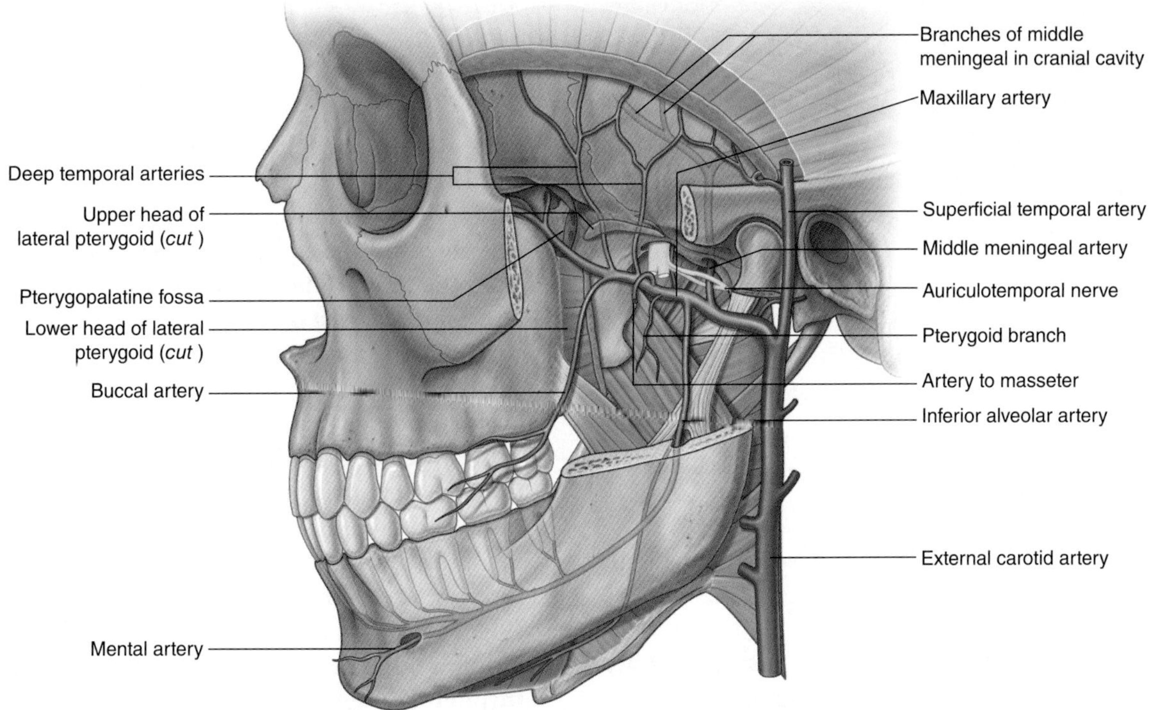

Plate 22.3 Arteries of the temporal and infratemporal fossae. (From Drake RL et al. *Gray's Atlas of Anatomy*, 3rd edition, Philadelphia, Elsevier, 2021.)

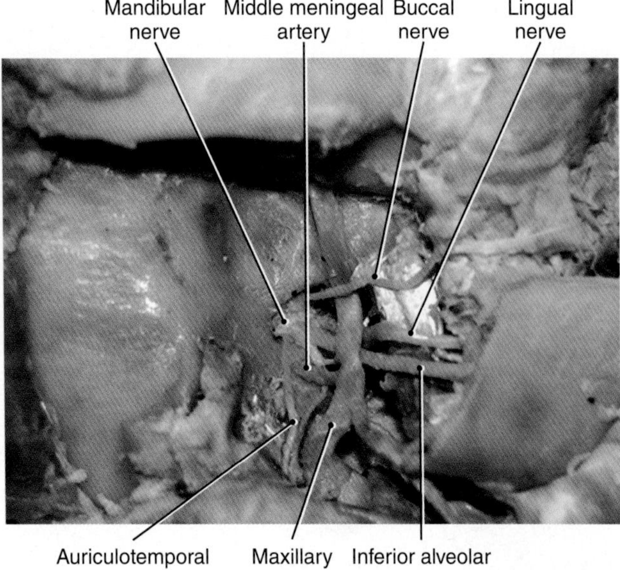

Fig. 22.27 Lateral view of the infratemporal fossa, revealing the medial pterygoid muscle and neurovascular structures.

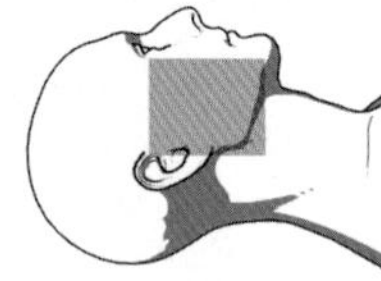

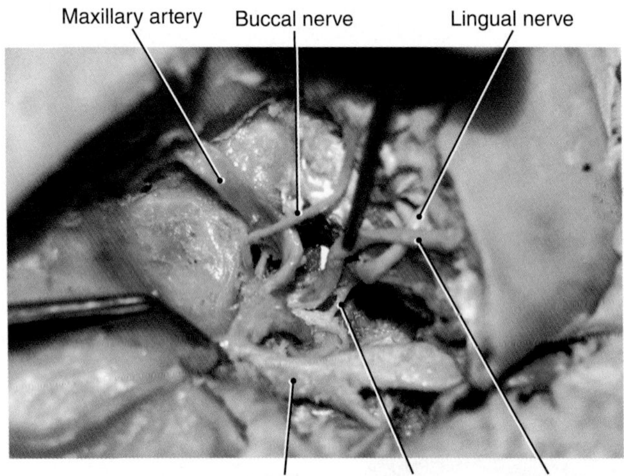

Fig. 22.28 Lingual nerve lifted and followed posteriorly to its connection with chorda tympani.

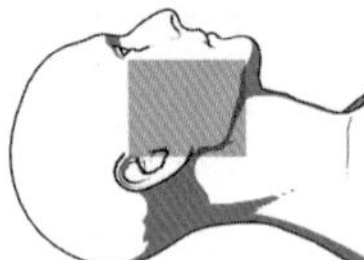

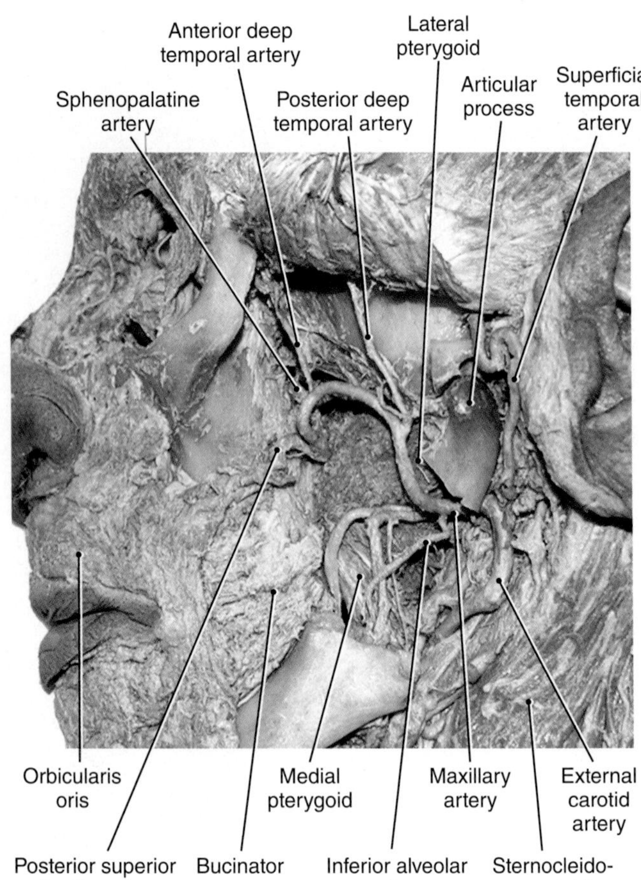

Fig. 22.29 A different specimen, with branches of the maxillary artery, exposed superficial to the lateral pterygoid muscle.

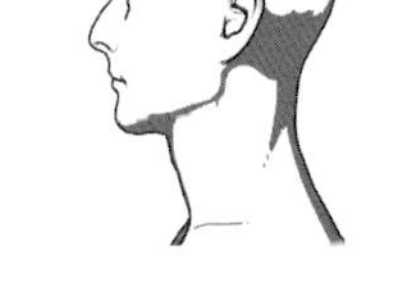

facial nerve (Fig. 22.28). If this nerve is not evident, clean the soft tissue around the lingual nerve more posteriorly.

- **Clean the lingual and inferior alveolar nerves and trace their passage deep to the medial pterygoid muscle.**
- **Deep to the infratemporal fossa, trace and follow the termination of the maxillary artery, the *sphenopalatine artery,* toward the sphenopalatine foramen (Figs. 22.29 and 22.30).**
- **Typically, two additional branches are easily identifiable. Identify the *infraorbital artery* as it ascends to enter the infraorbital canal, and the *posterior superior alveolar artery* as it descends to enter the infratemporal surface of the maxilla (see Fig. 22.30).**
- **Identify the mandibular canal and the inferior alveolar nerve (Figs. 22.31–22.33).**
- **With an electric drill, cut the mandible in a direction demarcating a line between the mandibular canal and mental foramen (see Fig. 22.32).**
- **With fine forceps, lift the small branches of the inferior alveolar nerve terminating on the teeth (Fig. 22.34).**
- **Using a bone saw, make a shallow parasagittal cut through the temporomandibular joint. Identify the articular disc, the two synovial cavities, and the articular capsule of that joint.**

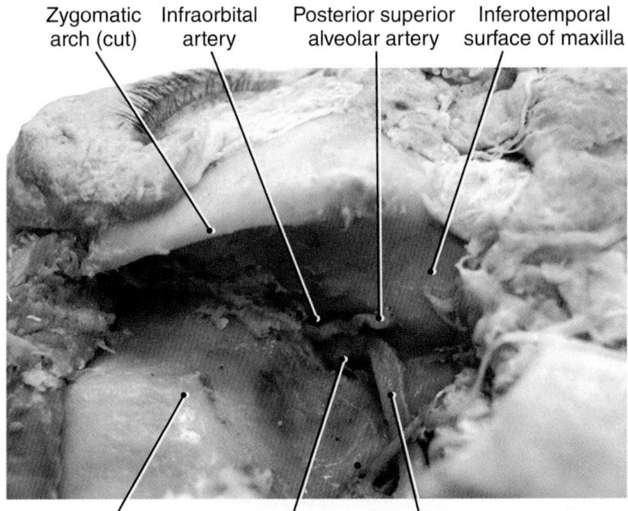

Fig. 22.30 Deep view of the infratemporal fossa, revealing the termination of the maxillary artery.

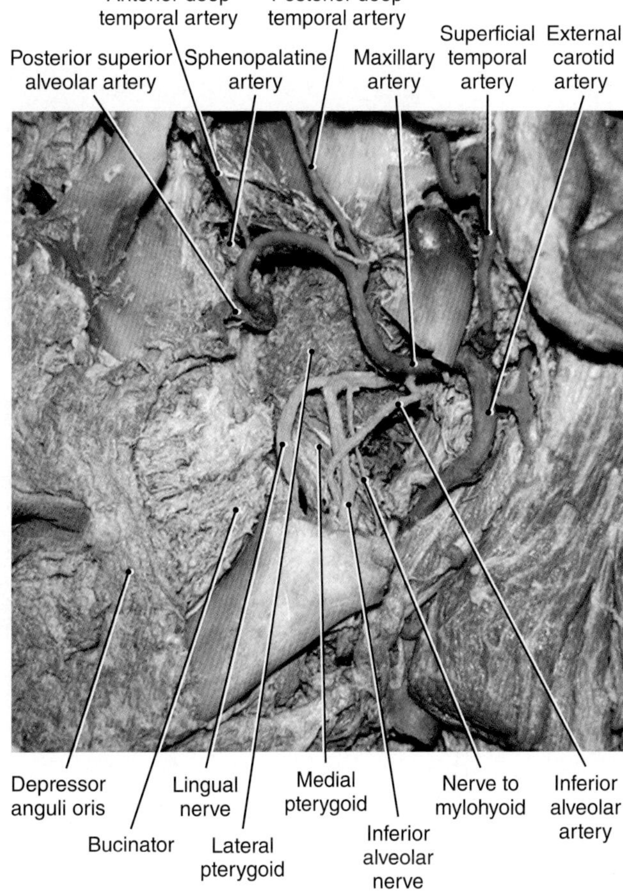

Fig. 22.31 Lateral view of the infratemporal fossa.

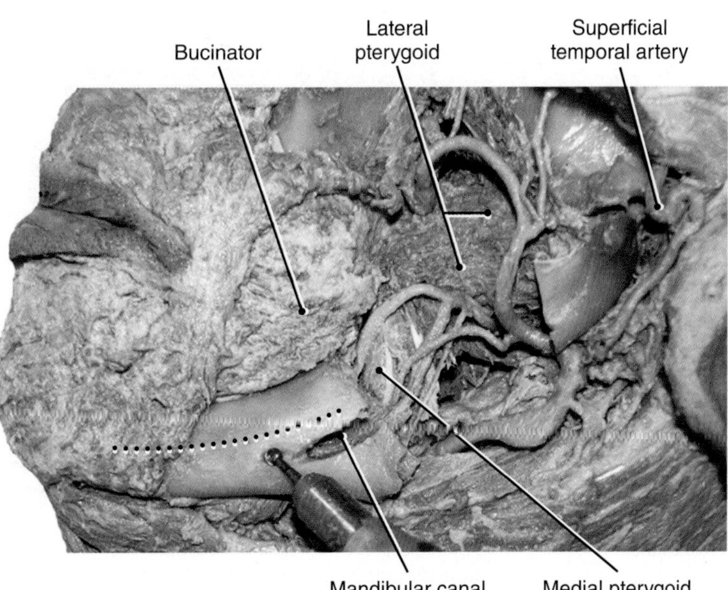

Fig. 22.32 Mandible drilled over the mandibular canal *(broken line)* between the inferior alveolar foramen and mental foramen.

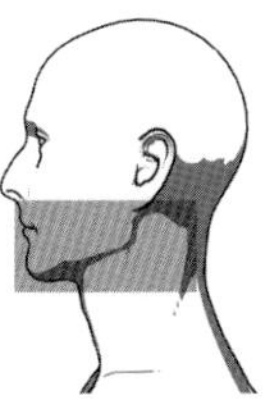

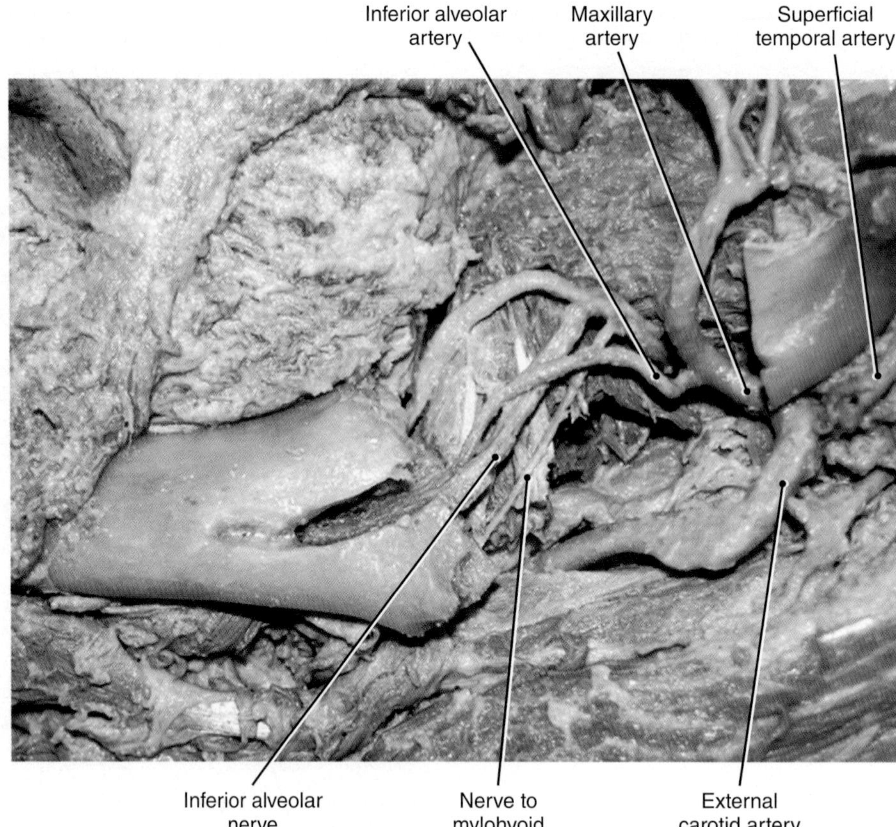

Fig. 22.33 Exposure of the contents of the mandibular canal.

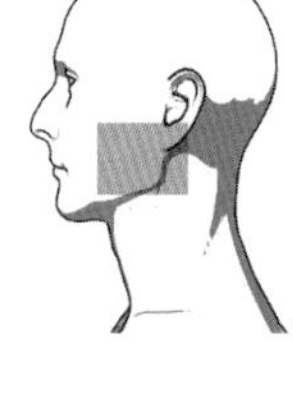

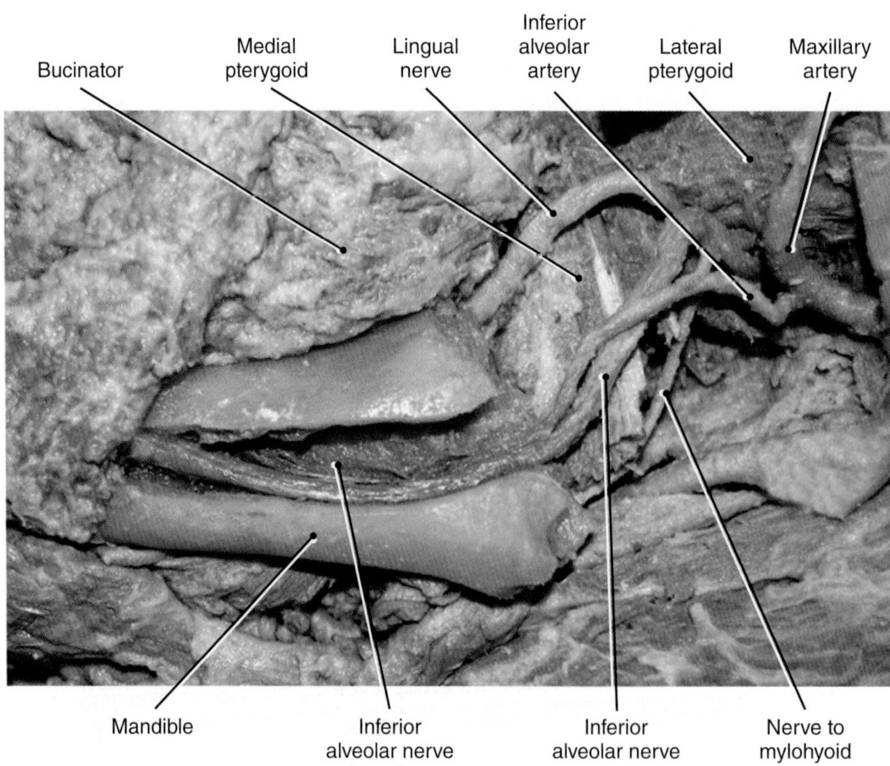

Fig. 22.34 Further exposure of the inferior alveolar nerve within the mandibular canal. Note the small branches to the teeth.

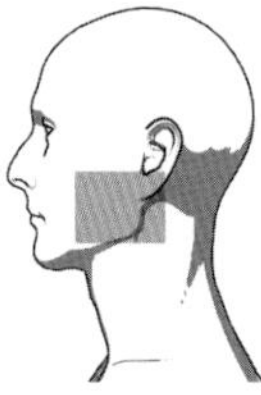

LABORATORY IDENTIFICATION CHECKLIST

NERVES

- ☐ Trigeminal, mandibular division (V3)
- ☐ Auriculotemporal
- ☐ Inferior alveolar
- ☐ Nerve to mylohyoid
- ☐ Lingual
- ☐ Chorda tympani
- ☐ Buccal

ARTERIES

- ☐ Maxillary
  - ☐ Middle meningeal
  - ☐ Inferior alveolar
  - ☐ Deep temporal arteries
  - ☐ Muscular branches
    - ☐ Masseteric artery
    - ☐ Artery to medial pterygoid
    - ☐ Artery to lateral pterygoid
- ☐ Sphenopalatine (terminal branch of maxillary artery)
- ☐ Posterior superior alveolar
- ☐ Infraorbital
- ☐ Buccal

VEINS

- ☐ Pterygoid venous plexus (often difficult to isolate in cadaveric tissue)

MUSCLES

- ☐ Masseter
- ☐ Temporalis
- ☐ Lateral pterygoid
- ☐ Medial pterygoid

BONES

- ☐ Temporal
- ☐ Sphenoid
- ☐ Mandible
  - ☐ Head
  - ☐ Coronoid process
  - ☐ Notch
  - ☐ Ramus
  - ☐ Angle
  - ☐ Neck

CONNECTIVE TISSUE

- ☐ Temporomandibular joint capsule
- ☐ Temporomandibular joint (articular) disc
- ☐ Stylomandibular ligament

BEFORE YOU BEGIN

The skin of the face has been previously removed (see Chapter 21).

DISSECTION STEPS

- **Continue the removal of the facial skin toward the occipital region and separate the skin from the subcutaneous tissue (Fig. 23.1).**
- **Identify and expose the superficial temporal artery and its branches (Fig. 23.2).**
- **Once the superficial temporal artery has been fully exposed, separate the subcutaneous tissue and fat from the underlying galea aponeurotica, or *epicranial aponeurosis* (see Fig. 23.2).**
- **This aponeurosis is a flattened tendon that connects the occipitalis and frontalis muscles, forming the occipitofrontalis muscle.**
- **Cut and detach the frontalis muscle from the frontal bone.**
- **With forceps, grasp the frontalis muscle and reflect it posteriorly (Fig. 23.3).**

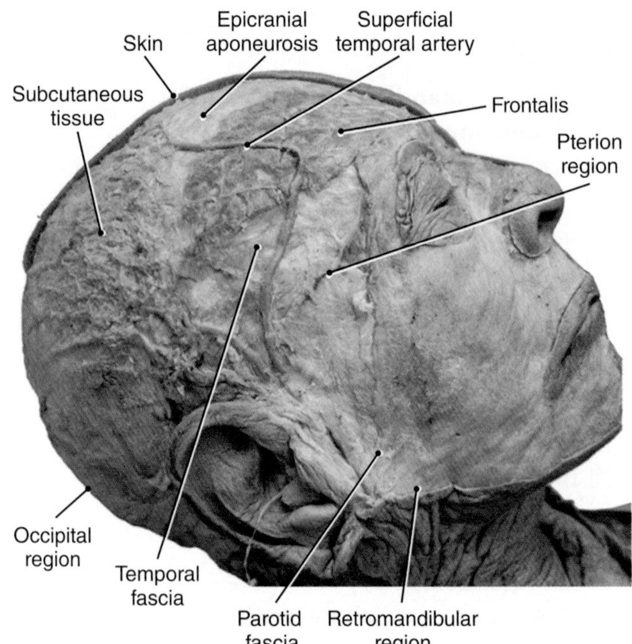

Fig. 23.2 Lateral view of the exposed superficial temporal artery and branches.

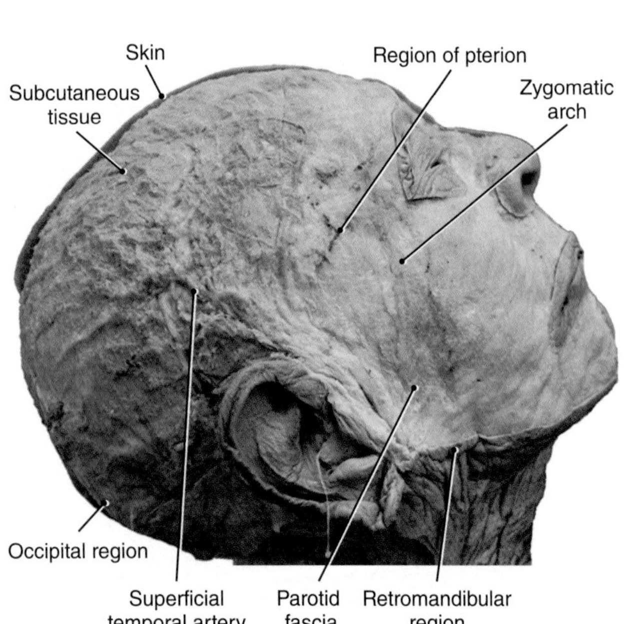

Fig. 23.1 Lateral view of the external cranium and face.

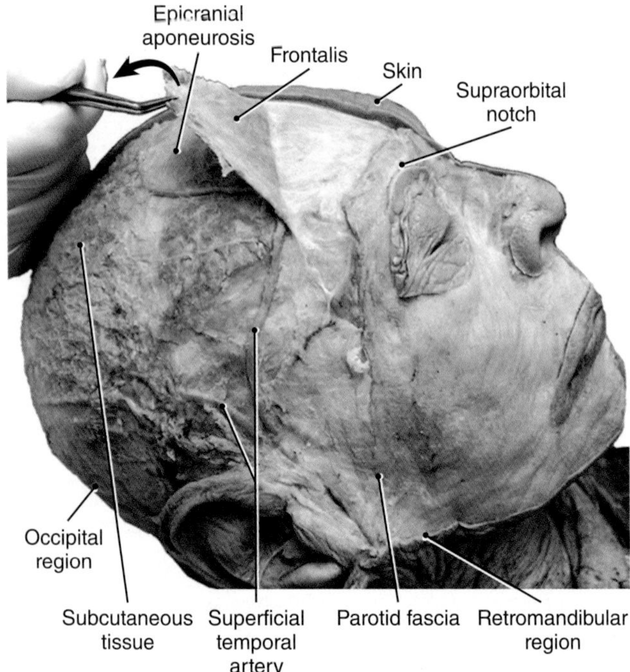

Fig. 23.3 Frontalis muscle detached from the frontal bone and reflected posteriorly.

- On the internal surface of the frontalis muscle, note the loose connective tissue, and on the surface of the cranium, note the *pericranium* (Fig. 23.4).
- At this part of the dissection, identify all the previously dissected layers of the *scalp* (Plate 23.1):
  - *Skin*
  - *Connective tissue (subcutaneous tissue)*
  - *Aponeurotic layer*
  - *Loose connective tissue*
  - *Pericranium*
- To expose the brain, the *calvaria*, or "skullcap," must be removed. The calvaria consists primarily of the parietal, frontal, and occipital bones. Dissect away the occipitofrontalis muscle and expose the pericranium, leaving the temporalis fascia intact (Fig. 23.5).
- With a scalpel, reflect the temporal fascia and expose the temporalis muscle (Fig. 23.6).

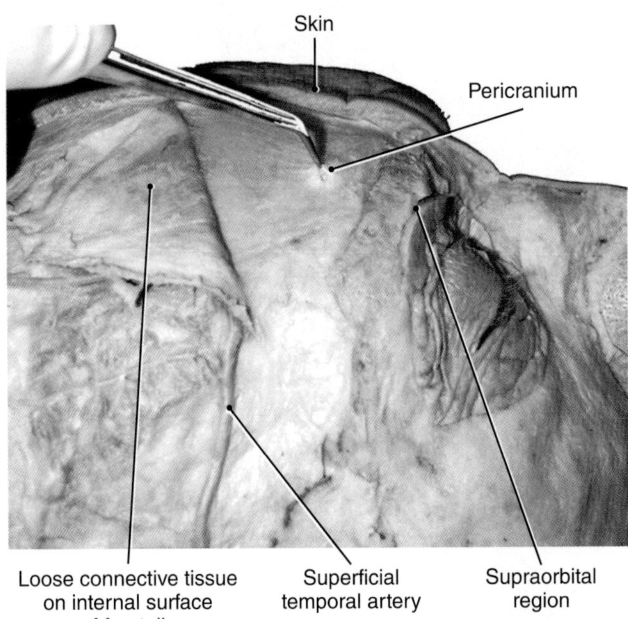

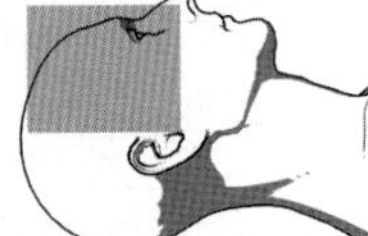

Fig. 23.4 Appreciate the loose connective tissue at the internal surface of the frontalis muscle and the pericranium on the cranial surface.

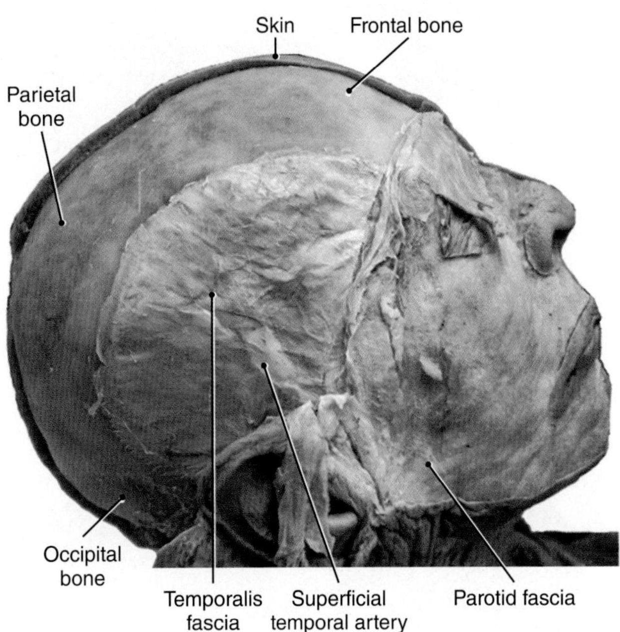

Fig. 23.5 Occipitofrontalis muscle removed, exposing pericranium and leaving the temporalis fascia intact.

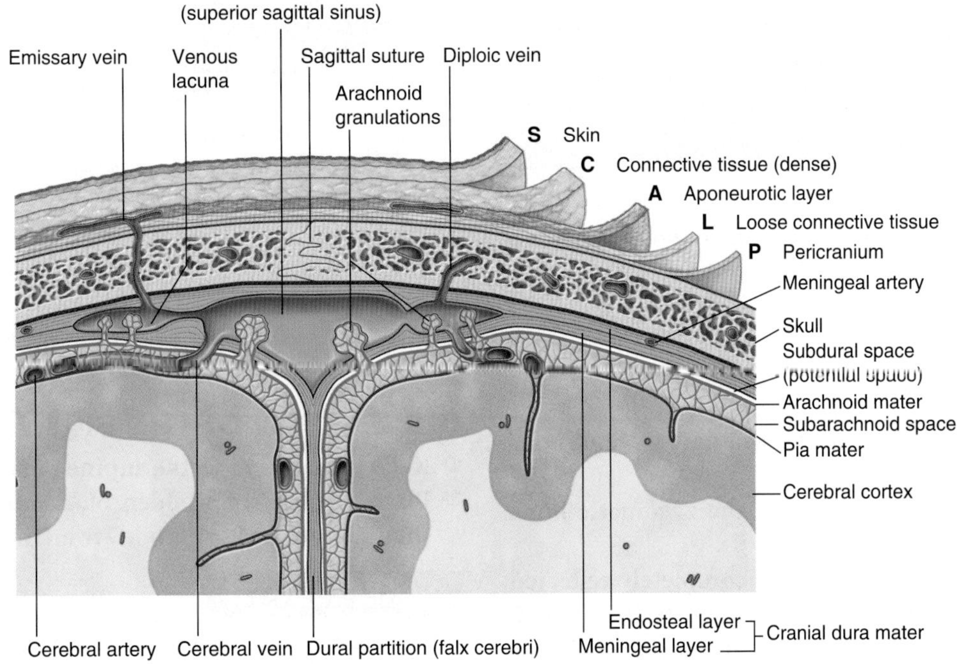

Plate 23.1 Scalp and cranial meninges. (From Drake RL et al. *Gray's Atlas of Anatomy*, 3rd edition, Philadelphia, Elsevier, 2021.)

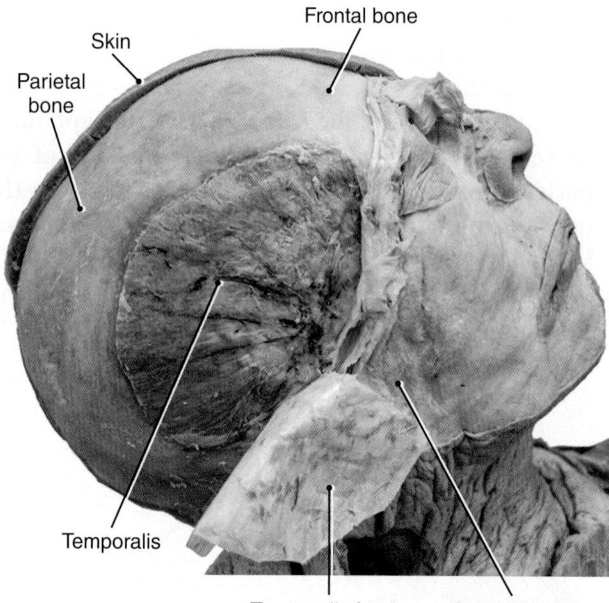

Fig. 23.6 Temporalis fascia reflected, exposing temporalis muscle.

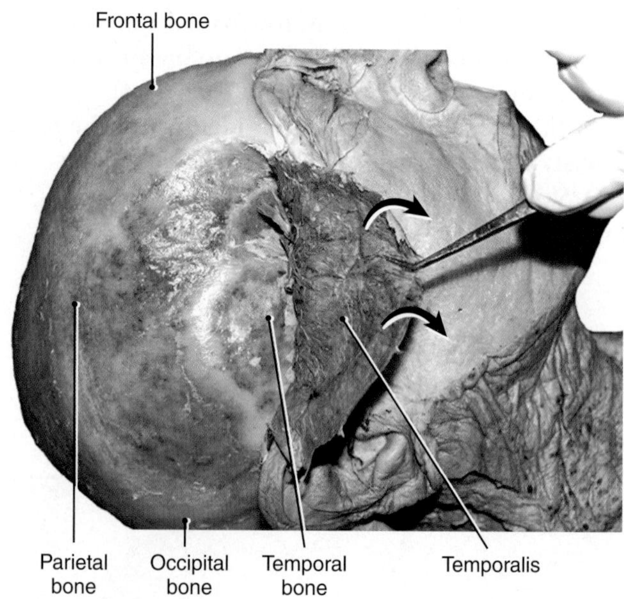

Fig. 23.8 Temporalis muscle reflected toward zygomatic bone, exposing pterion.

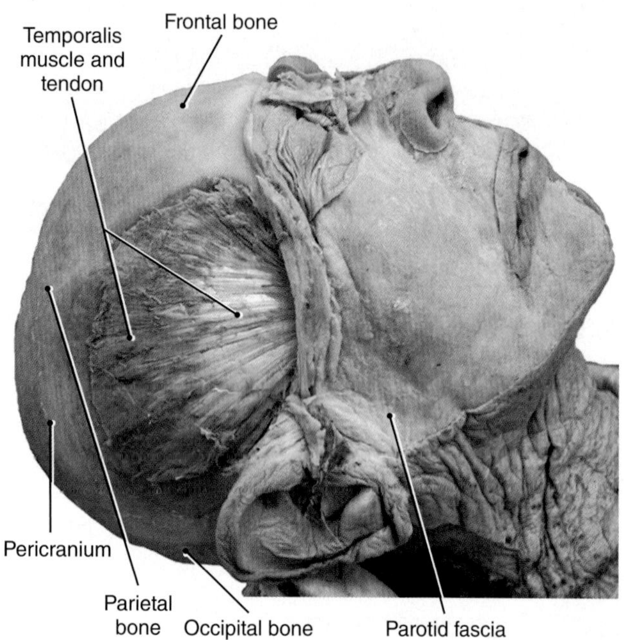

Fig. 23.7 Appreciate the temporalis muscle and its tendinous fibers.

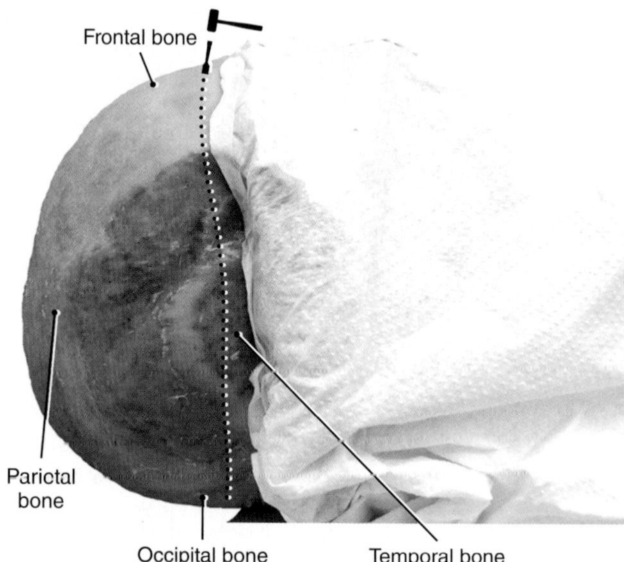

Fig. 23.9 Lateral view of the external cranium and face (covered).

- **Clean the temporalis muscle and note its tendinous fibers (Fig. 23.7).**
- **Reflect the temporalis toward the zygomatic bone and expose the *pterion* (Fig. 23.8).**
- **Once the temporalis muscle is completely reflected and the calvaria fully exposed, identify the frontal, parietal, temporal, and occipital bones, as well as the sagittal, coronal, and lambdoid sutures.**

DISSECTION OF THE SKULL

- **Keep the cadaver in the supine position.**
- **Place a plastic or wooden block under the head or shoulders to elevate the body from the dissection table.**

DISSECTION **TIP**

Place paper towels over the face and temporalis muscles to protect them from bone dust (Fig. 23.9).

- Two different techniques can be used to expose the contents of the skull.

Technique 1

- With a marker, draw a stippled midsagittal line from the nasion to the external occipital protuberance.
- Draw a second, circumferential line passing 1 to 2 cm above the superciliary arches and ears to reach 1 to 2 cm above the external occipital protuberance posteriorly (see Fig. 23.9).
- With an electric saw, make a cut 2 to 3 cm (~1 inch) lateral to the midline, on both sides. In this way, the superior sagittal sinus and the falx cerebri will remain intact (Fig. 23.10).

DISSECTION TIP

Caution! Use the electric saw carefully.

- Make a shallow, circumferential cut of approximately 1 cm in depth.

DISSECTION TIP

Do not place the saw too deeply, as you will cut the dura and the brain. To complete the cut toward the external occipital protuberance, it is necessary to rotate the cadaver.

Once the first cut is complete, use the chisel and mallet to break through the bone and detach the two bone flaps (Fig. 23.11).

DISSECTION TIP

Detaching the bone flap from the underlying dura mater can be challenging. Place the forceps or a chisel into the gap (created by the saw cut) between the two adjacent bones and use it to lift it up from the dura. If the dura is attached to the calvaria, use a probe to reflect the endosteal layer away from the calvaria, leaving the dura mater intact.

- After removal of the calvaria, examine the dura mater and identify the middle meningeal artery and its branches (see Figs. 23.11 and 23.12).
- Cut and reflect the dura and expose the subdural space (Fig. 23.13).
- Observe the arachnoid layer covering the brain and the cerebral veins penetrating the arachnoid mater (see Fig. 23.13).
- Place your hands on one of the cerebral hemispheres and retract it laterally (Fig. 23.14).
- Notice the midline connection between the two hemispheres, the corpus callosum (see Fig. 23.14).
- With a scalpel, make a midsagittal cut and reflect one of the brain hemispheres, leaving intact the dural venous sinuses (Fig. 23.15).
- Perform the same technique on the contralateral side and expose the sinuses bilaterally (Figs. 23.16 and 23.17).
- Identify the *falx cerebri,* a dural partition separating the right from the left cerebral hemispheres.

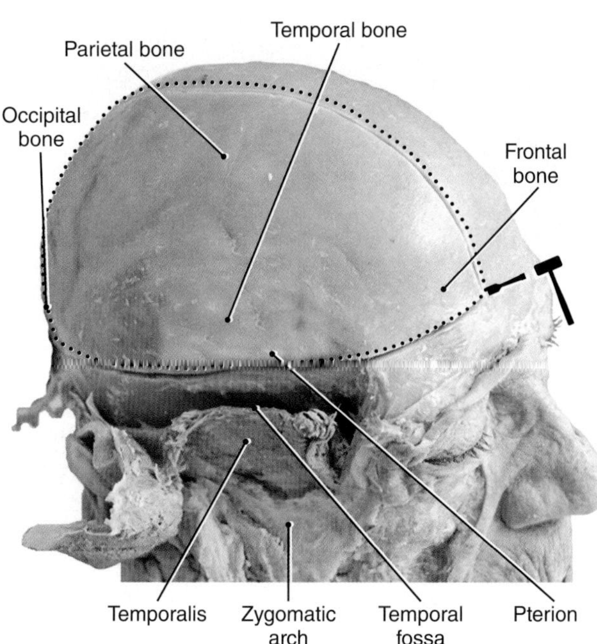

Fig. 23.10 Anterolateral view of the external cranium and face.

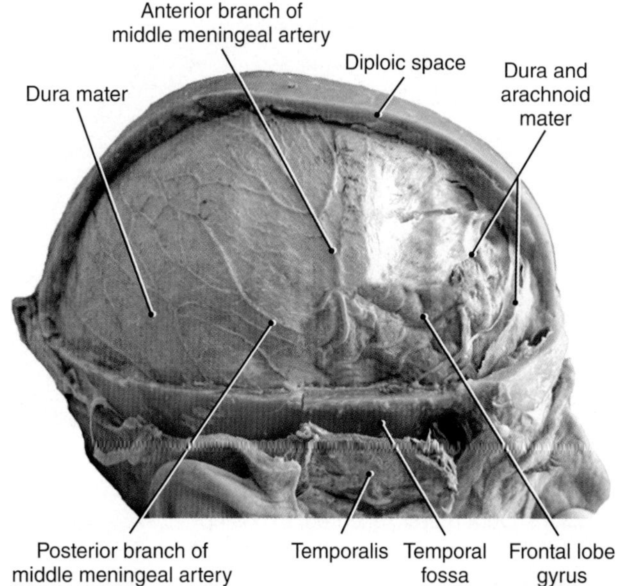

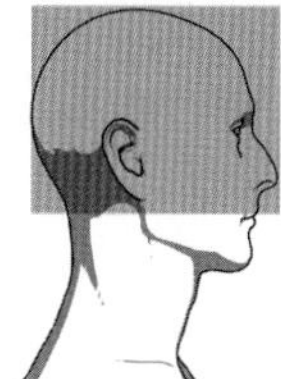

Fig. 23.11 Lateral view of the right hemisphere after craniotomy.

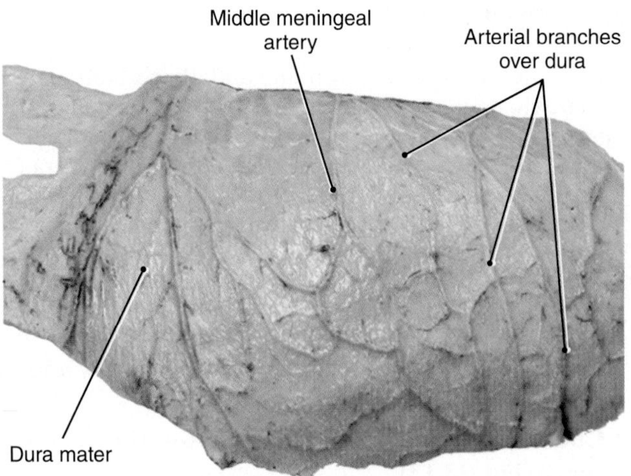

Fig. 23.12 External surface of removed dura mater, revealing the middle meningeal artery and arterial branches to dura mater.

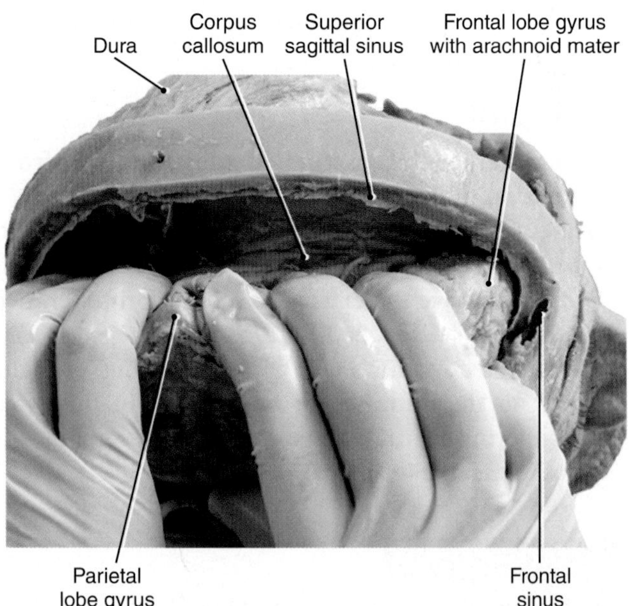

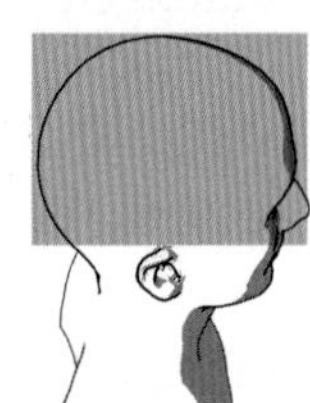

Fig. 23.14 Cerebral hemisphere retracted laterally; note the frontal and superior sagittal sinuses and corpus callosum. Appreciate the connection between the two hemispheres, the corpus callosum.

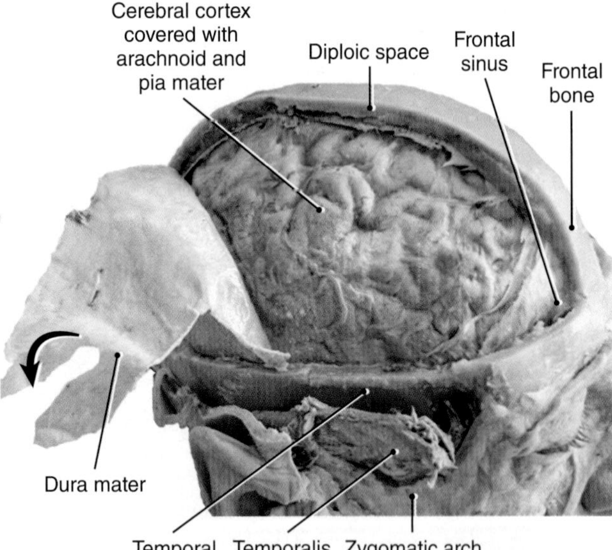

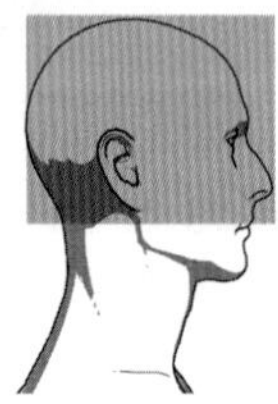

Fig. 23.13 Dura mater reflected, exposing the subdural space. Observe the arachnoid layer covering the brain and cerebral veins deep to it.

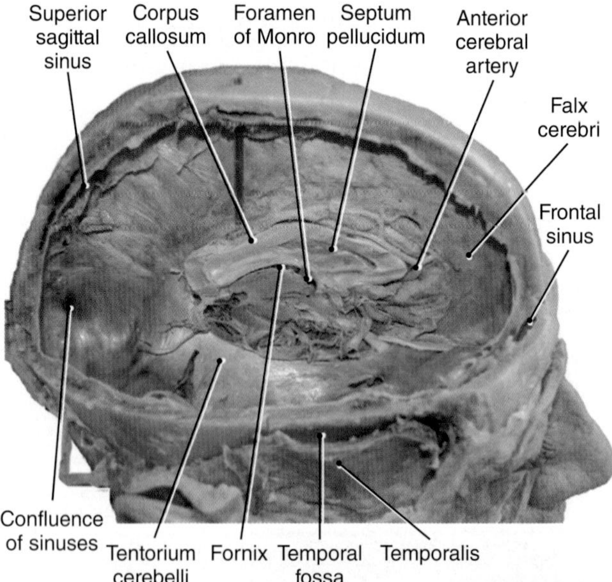

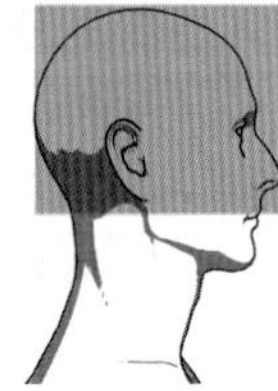

Fig. 23.15 With a midsagittal cut, the cerebral hemisphere is reflected, leaving the dural venous sinuses intact.

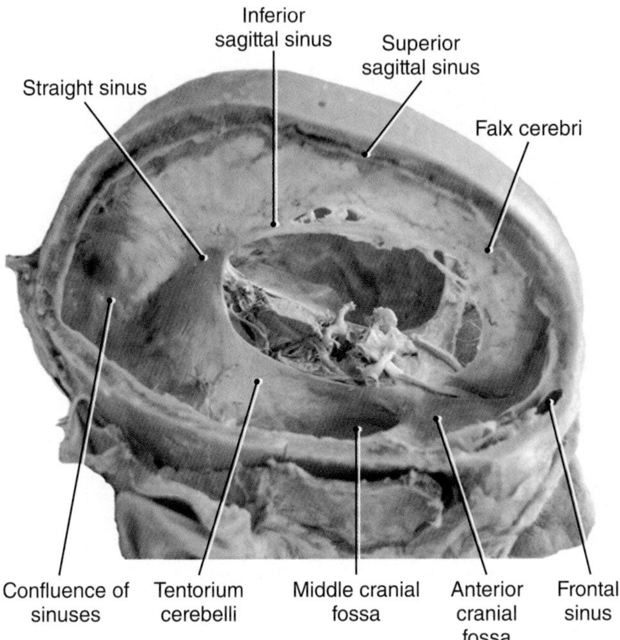

Fig. 23.16 Right-sided view of the craniotomy with the cerebral hemispheres removed.

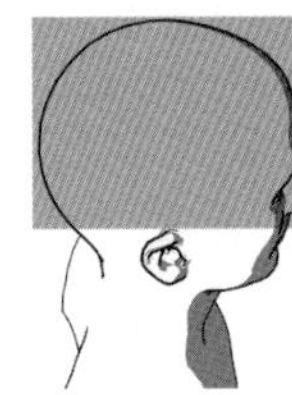

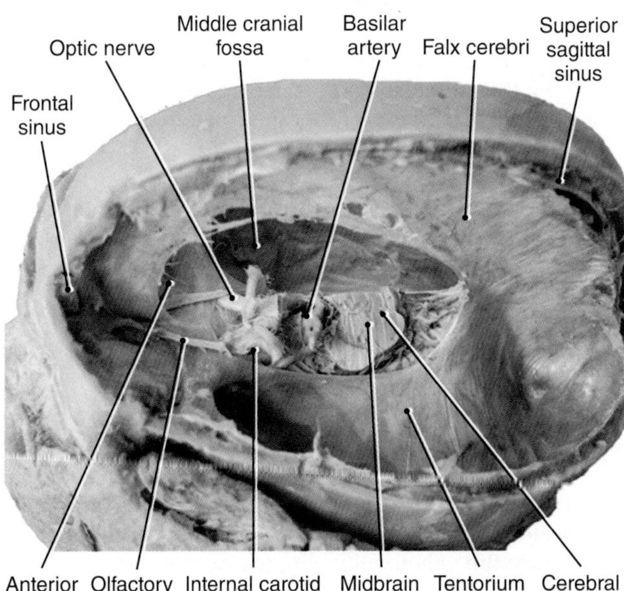

Fig. 23.17 Left-sided view of the craniotomy with the cerebral hemispheres removed.

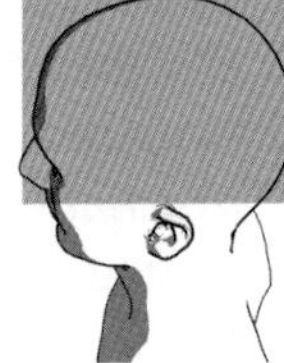

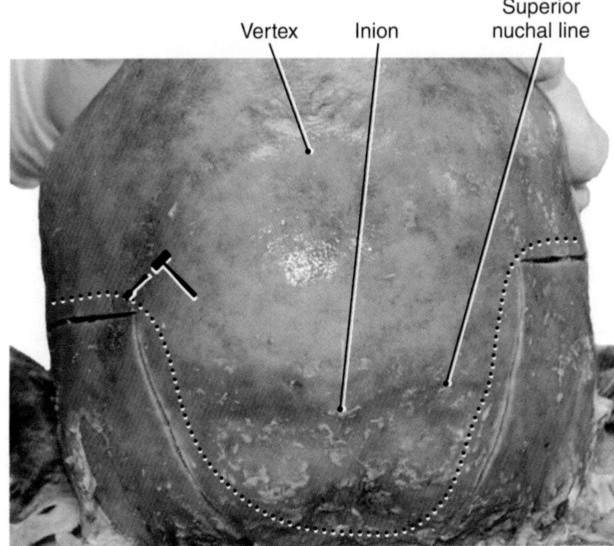

Fig. 23.18 Superoposterior view of the external cranium revealing the superior nuchal line, inion, posterior craniotomy *(dashed line)*, and vertex.

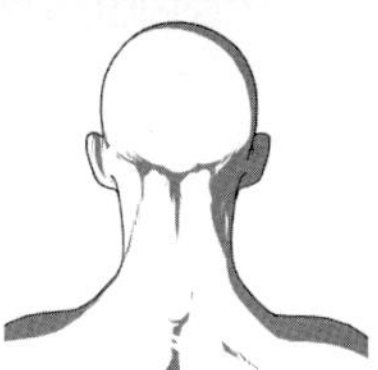

- **Superior to the falx cerebri, identify the *superior sagittal sinus*, which joins the two transverse sinuses at the confluence of sinuses ("torcular herophili," or wine-press of Herophilus).**
- **Inferolateral to the falx cerebri, look for the *tentorium cerebelli*, a large dural infolding separating the occipital lobes from the cerebellar hemispheres.**

DISSECTION **TIP**

If time permits, remove the midportion of the calvaria and expose the superior sagittal sinus. Incise the dura forming the sinus and notice its internal structure. In the majority of specimens the superior sagittal sinus will drain primarily into the right transverse sinus.

- **At this point, the dissection can continue as outlined later.**

Technique 2

- **With a pen, draw a circumferential line passing 1 to 2 cm above the superciliary ridges and ears to reach 1 to 2 cm above the external occipital protuberance posteriorly (Figs. 23.18 and 23.19).**
- **With an electric saw, make a shallow, circumferential cut of about 1 cm along this line (Fig. 23.20).**

DISSECTION **TIP**

Use the electric saw carefully. To complete the cut at the external occipital protuberance, the cadaver must be rotated. Do not insert the saw too deeply, or you may sever the dura mater and the brain (Fig. 23.21).

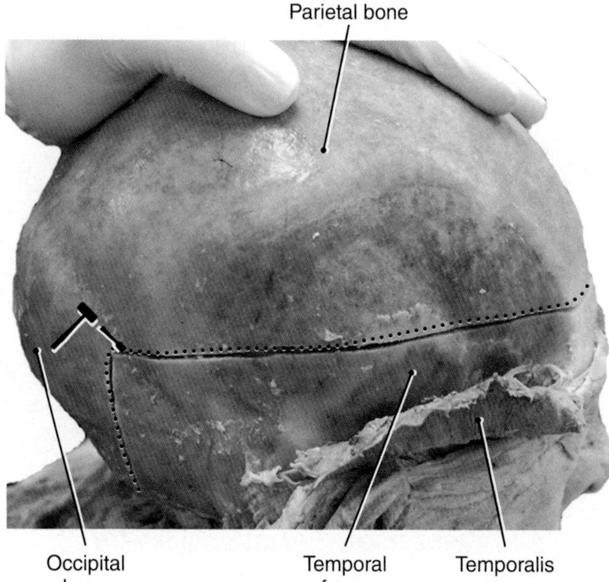

Fig. 23.19 Postcraniotomy lateral view of the external cranium, revealing the frontal bone, parietal bone, temporal bone/fossa, and temporalis muscle reflected inferiorly over the zygomatic arch.

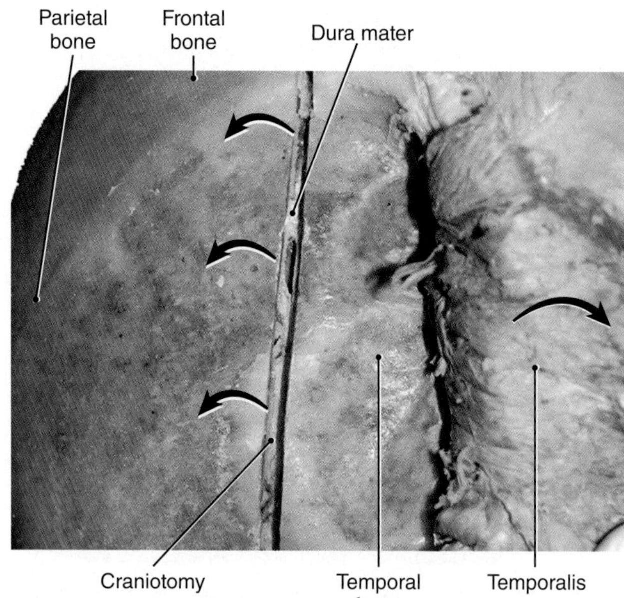

Fig. 23.21 Once the first cut is complete, use a chisel and mallet to break through the bone and detach it from the dura.

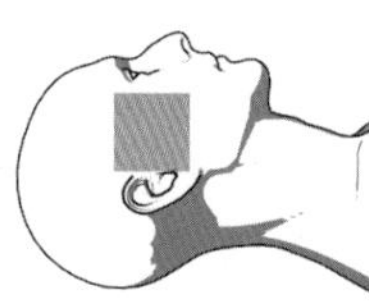

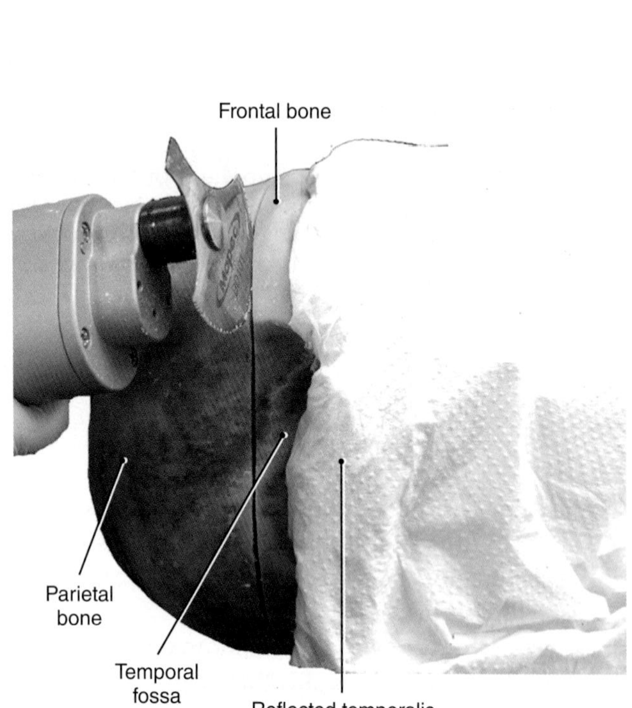

Fig. 23.20 Posterolateral view of the external cranium, revealing the wedge resection cut.

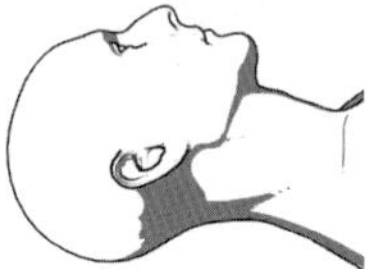

DISSECTION TIP

The bone cut can extend below the external occipital protuberance to the posterolateral aspects of the foramen magnum, including the posterior portions of the atlas and axis. With this extension, removal of the brain and spinal cord is easier. However, this extension will sever the muscles of the suboccipital triangle. If you want to preserve the suboccipital muscles, make the cut through the external occipital protuberance instead (Fig. 23.22).

- **Second, complete the bone removal with a chisel and mallet to break through the bone and detach it from the underlying dura mater (Fig. 23.23).**

DISSECTION TIP

Detaching the bone from the underlying dura can be challenging. Place the chisel in the gap (created by the saw cut) between the adjacent bones, slightly rotating it to lift the bone from the dura. If the dura is still connected to the calvaria, use a probe to reflect the endosteal layer from the calvaria, leaving the dura intact.

- **Inspect the internal surface of the calvaria and identify the small openings for emissary veins.**
- **Note the small pits (granular *fovea*) produced by the *arachnoid granulations* (large arachnoid *villi* that protrude into dural venous sinuses) (Fig. 23.24).**
- **Look for the frontal sinus extending into the calvaria.**

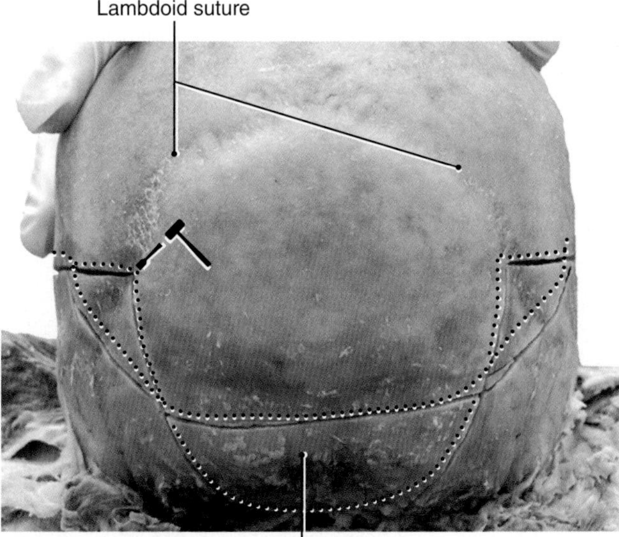

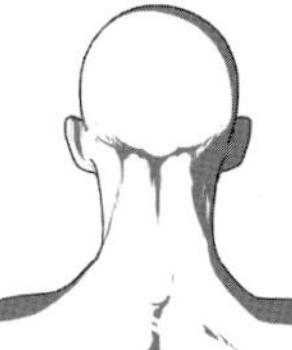

Fig. 23.22 Posterior view of the external cranium shows the cranium *(dashed line)*, lambdoid suture, and occipital bone, preserving the muscles of the suboccipital triangle.

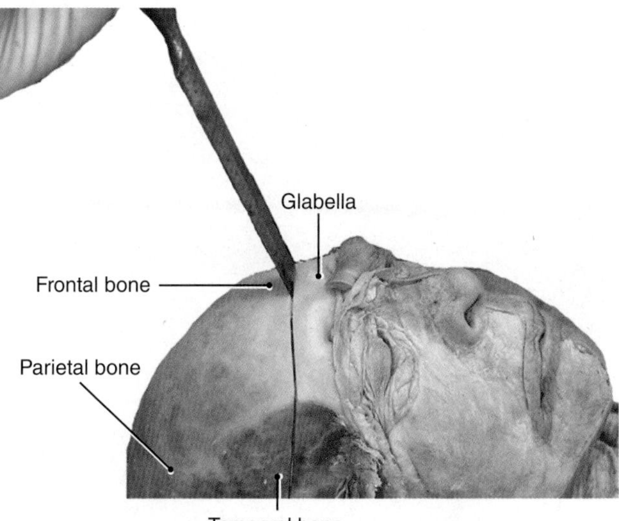

Fig. 23.23 Anterolateral view of the external cranium and face revealing sagittal suture line for craniotomy, with chisel inserted into scoring line and glabella.

- **Note the spongy bone occupying the space between the outer and inner compact bony layers (tables), the *diploic space.***
- **Identify the impressions made by the superior sagittal sinus and the middle meningeal arteries.**
- **Inspect the dura mater and identify the middle meningeal artery and its branches (Fig. 23.25).**
- **Identify the superior sagittal sinus and look for the *lateral lacunae* (Fig. 23.26). The lateral lacunae are lateral venous extensions of the superior sagittal sinus.**

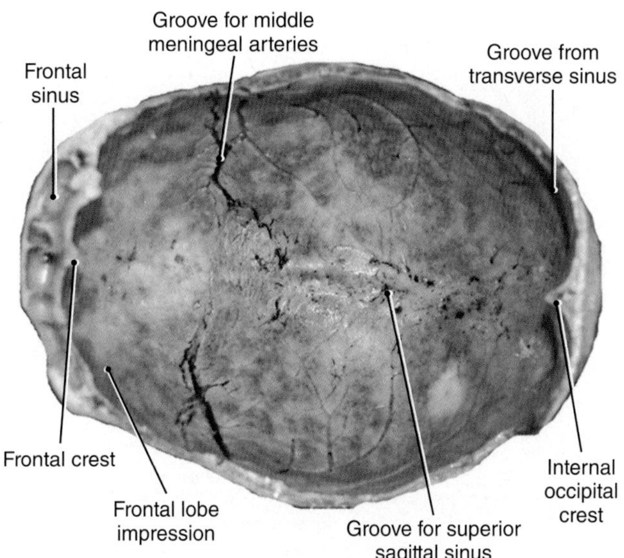

Fig. 23.24 Internal surface of the calvaria.

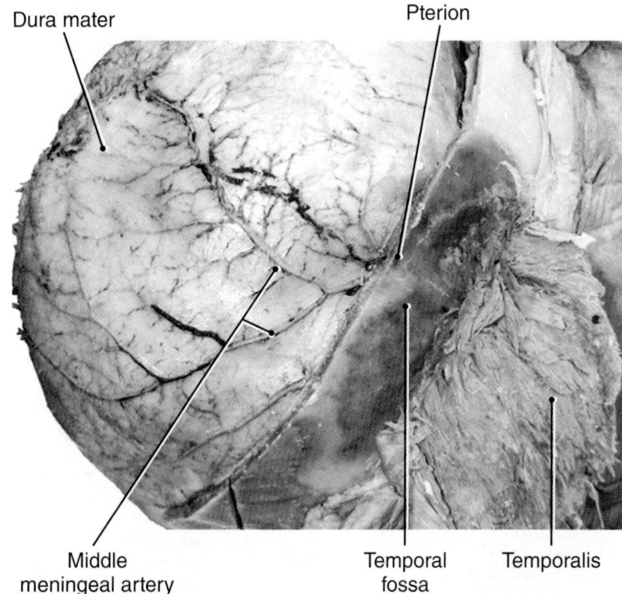

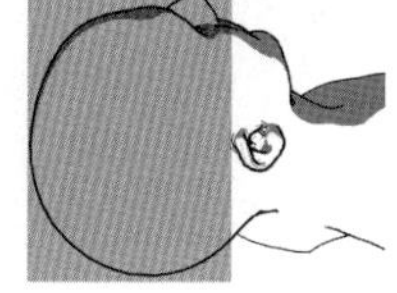

Fig. 23.25 Lateral view showing the dura mater, middle meningeal artery branches, pterion, temporal fossa, and temporalis muscle.

DISSECTION **TIP**

If time permits, with a scalpel, make an incision into the lateral lacunae and note their openings into the superior sagittal sinus.

- **Cut the dura 2 to 3 cm (Ĥ1 inch) lateral to the midline and reflect it inferiorly (Figs. 23.27 and 23.28).**
- **Inspect the subdural space and the arachnoid layer.**
- **Identify the arachnoid mater and make a small incision to expose the pia mater.**
- **Notice how the cerebral arteries and veins are covered with pia mater.**

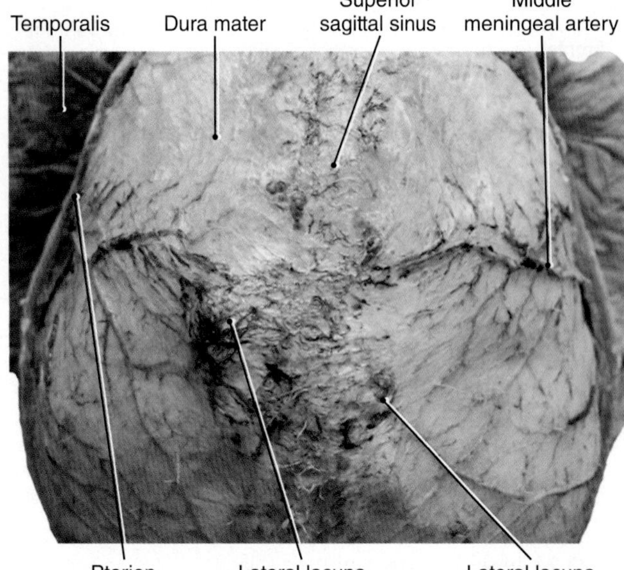

Fig. 23.26 Superior view, revealing the superior sagittal sinus, middle meningeal artery, lateral lacuna, dura mater, temporalis muscle, and pterion.

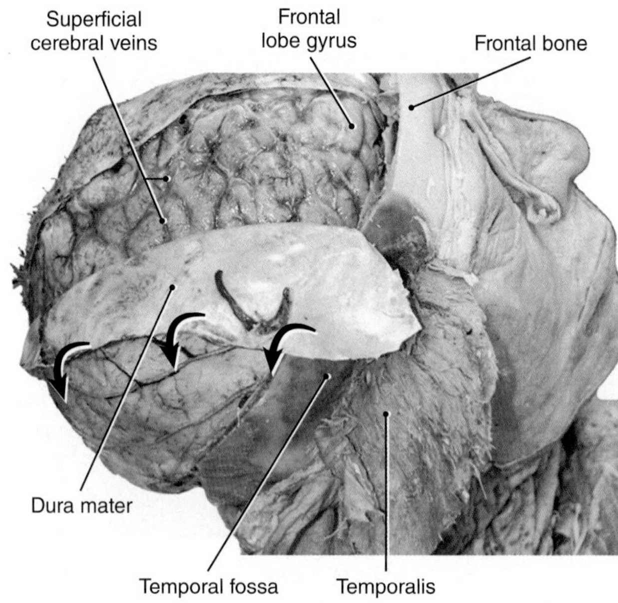

Fig. 23.28 Anterolateral view revealing the reflected dura mater, temporal bone, temporalis muscle, frontal bone, frontal lobe covered with arachnoid and pia mater, and superior cerebral veins of the parietal lobe.

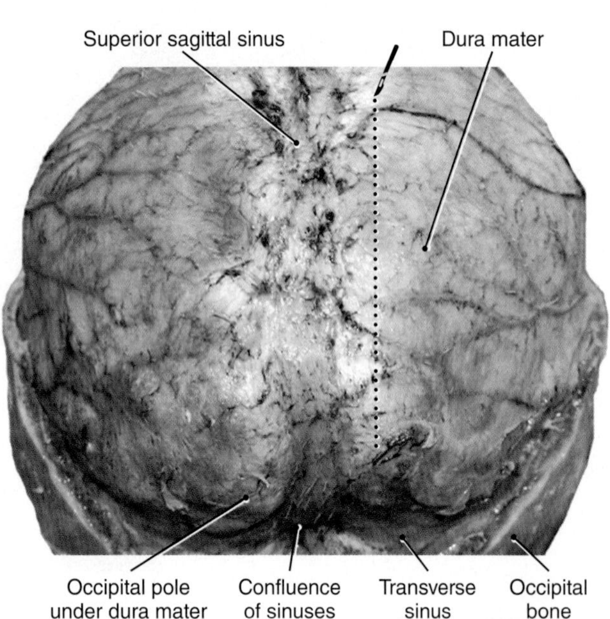

Fig. 23.27 Incision for cutting the dura mater laterally from midline *(dashed line)* and reflected inferiorly.

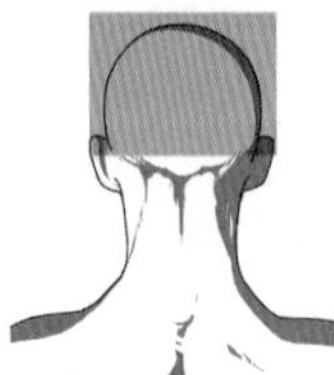

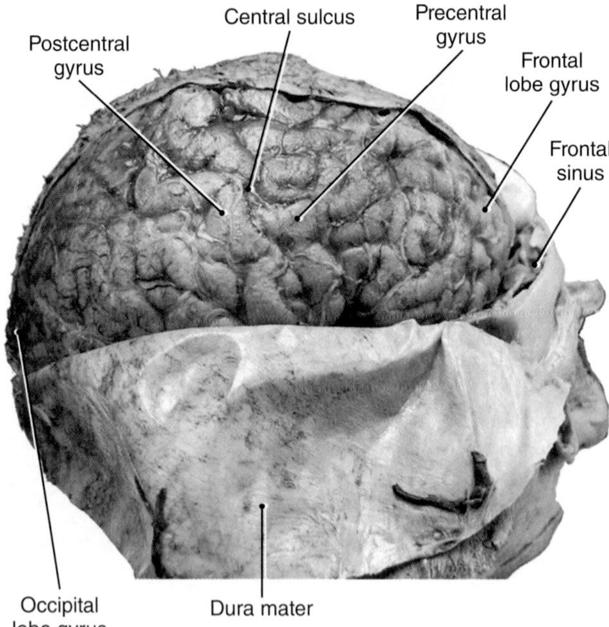

Fig. 23.29 Lateral view with the dura mater reflected laterally, revealing key gyri, the central sulcus, and the frontal sinus.

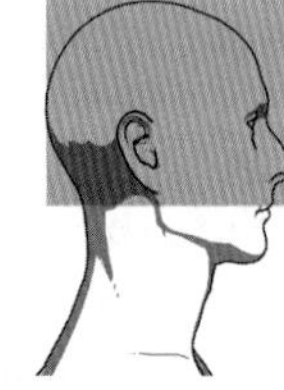

- **On the brain, identify the central sulcus, precentral gyrus, postcentral gyrus, and the frontal and occipital lobes (Fig. 23.29).**
- **On the other side of the brain, remove the arachnoid mater (Fig. 23.30).**
- **With forceps, pull the superior sagittal sinus and the falx cerebri laterally and observe the corpus callosum (Fig. 23.31).**
- **Observe the superior sagittal sinus and identify the lacunae joining it.**
- **Look for the tuft-like projections, the arachnoid granulations (Fig. 23.32).**

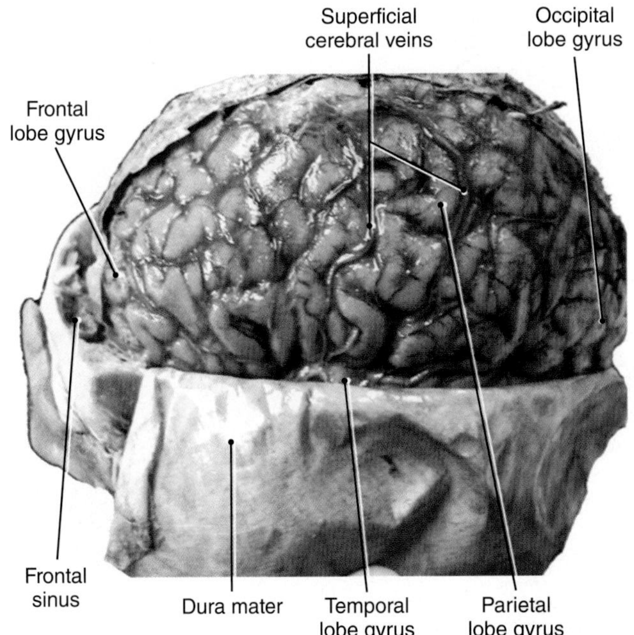

Fig. 23.30 Arachnoid mater removed from the brain.

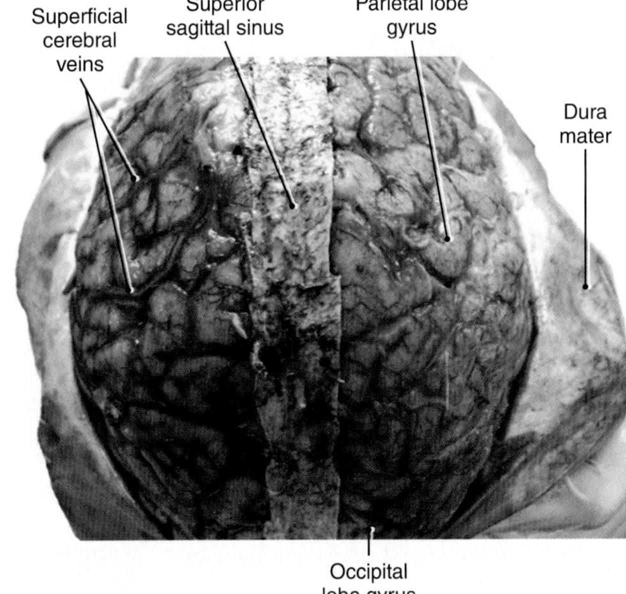

Fig. 23.32 Appreciate the superior sagittal sinus, lateral lacunae, and the tuft-like arachnoid granulations.

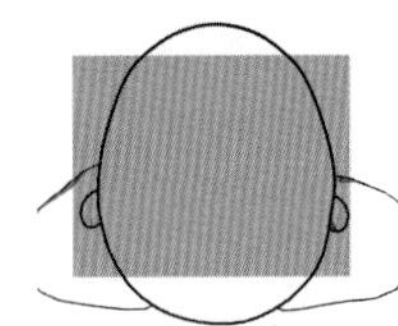

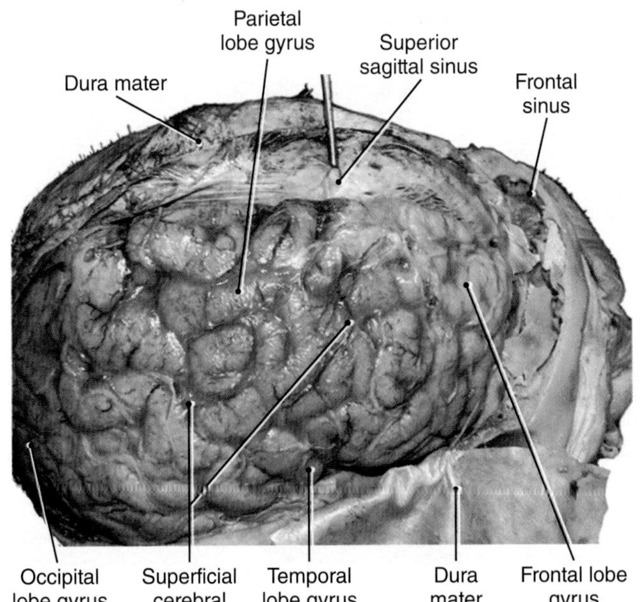

Fig. 23.31 Superior sagittal sinus and falx cerebri pulled laterally, revealing the corpus callosum.

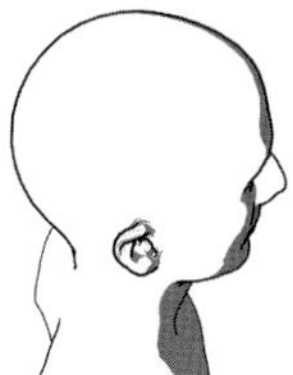

ANATOMY **NOTE**

Appreciate the relationships of the following:

- The *falx cerebri* separates the two cerebral hemispheres.
- The *falx cerebelli* separates the two cerebellar hemispheres.
- The *tentorium cerebelli* separates the cerebellum from the occipital lobes.

- **Gently lift the cerebral hemispheres.**
- **Inferior to the frontal lobes identify the attachment of the falx cerebri at the *crista galli.***
- **Cut this attachment from the crista galli and from the cerebral veins draining into the superior sagittal sinus.**
- **Pull the detached falx cerebri and superior sagittal sinus posteriorly (Fig. 23.33).**
- **Gently lift the cerebral hemispheres by placing your fingertips underneath the frontal lobes of the brain (Fig. 23.34).**
- **Look at the space between the cribriform plate of the ethmoid bone and the frontal lobes for the internal carotid artery, olfactory tracts, olfactory bulbs, optic nerve, optic chiasm, and anterior cerebral artery (Fig. 23.35).**

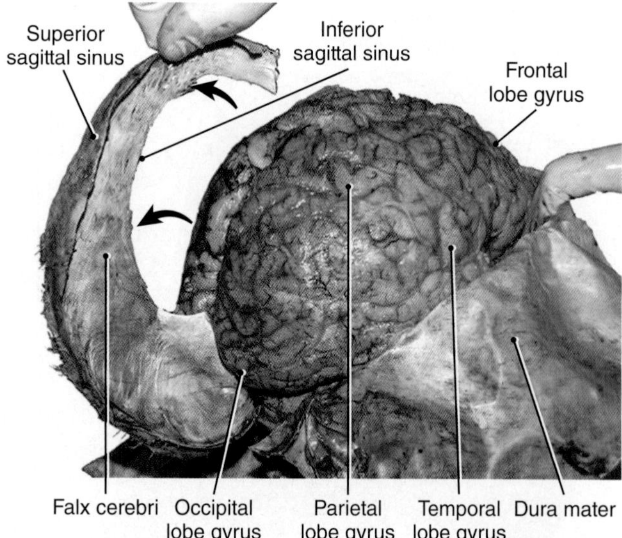

Fig. 23.33 Anterolateral view with the dura mater reflected laterally.

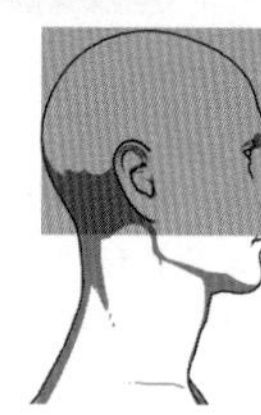

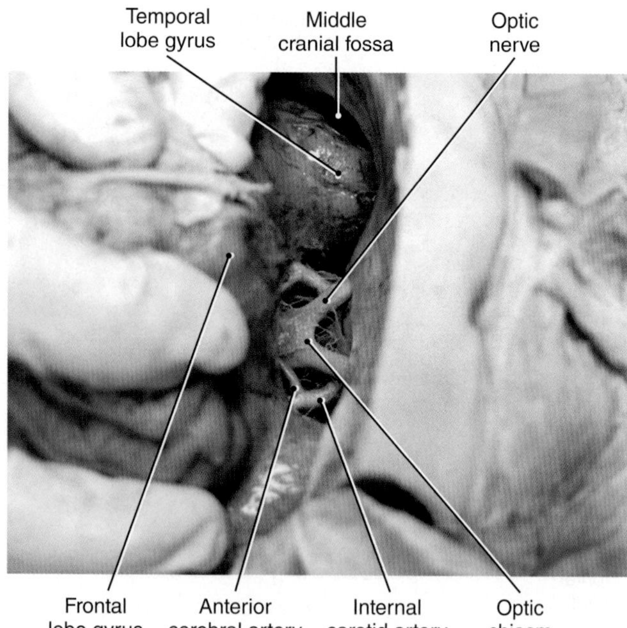

Fig. 23.35 In the space between the cribriform plate of the ethmoid bone and the frontal lobes, appreciate the internal carotid artery, olfactory tracts/bulbs, optic nerve/chiasm, and anterior cerebral artery.

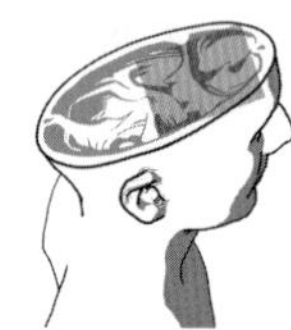

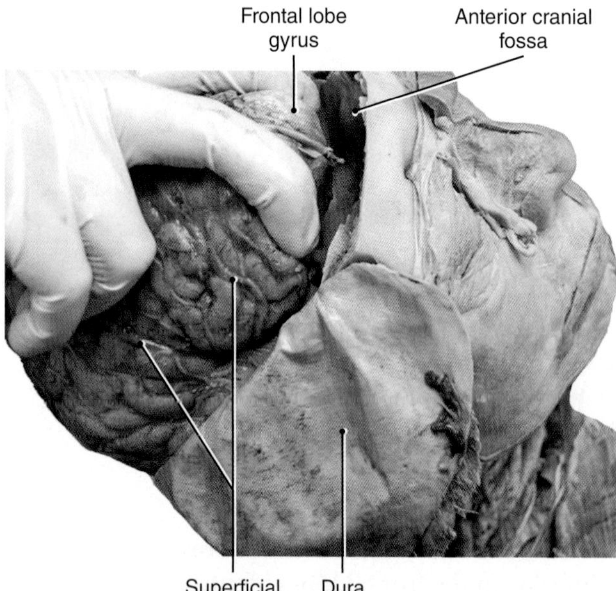

Fig. 23.34 Gently lift cerebral hemispheres by placing fingertips underneath frontal lobes.

- **With scissors, cut the aforementioned structures (Fig. 23.36).**
- **Gently keep lifting the frontal lobes upward and expose the brainstem and the basilar artery (Figs. 23.37 and 23.38).**
- **At this point, lift the occipital lobes of the cerebral hemisphere and appreciate the tentorium cerebelli and the straight sinus (Fig. 23.39).**
- **With a scalpel, carefully make a circumferential cut along the lateral attachment of the tentorium cerebelli.**

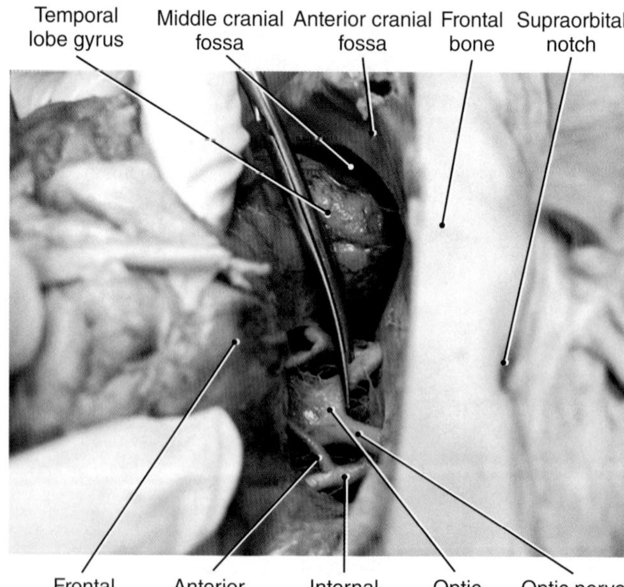

Fig. 23.36 Insert a pair of scissors and cut the optic nerve and internal carotid artery.

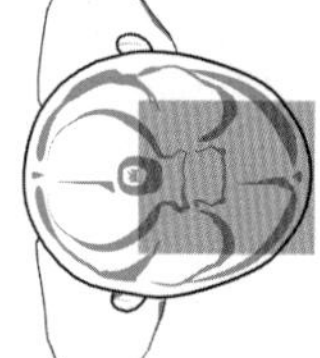

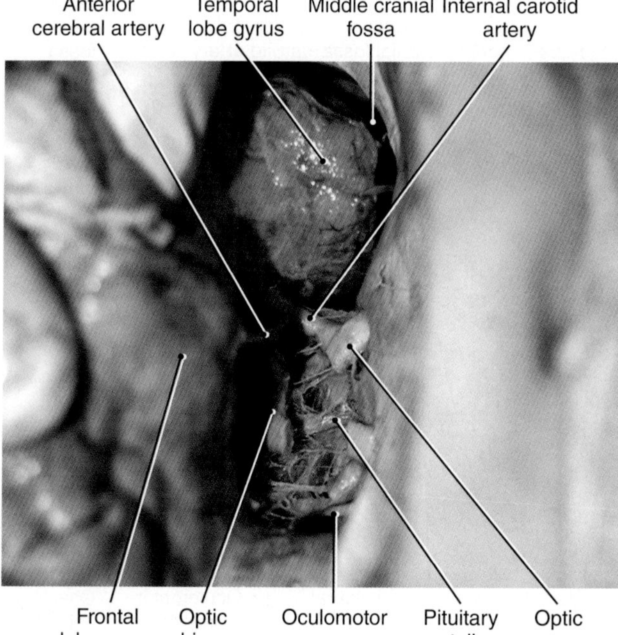

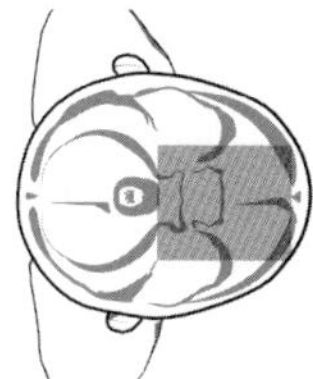

Fig. 23.37 View with the frontal lobes reflected superoposteriorly revealing the temporal lobe, middle cranial fossa, cut optic nerves, internal carotid artery, anterior cerebral artery, optic chiasm, oculomotor nerve, and pituitary stalk.

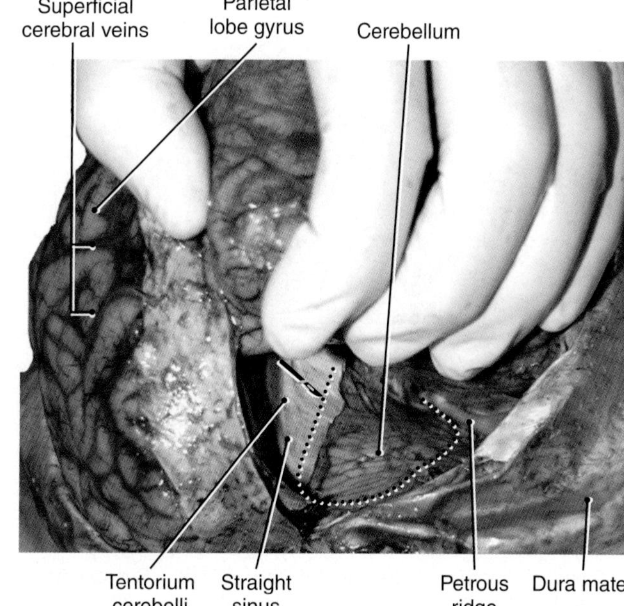

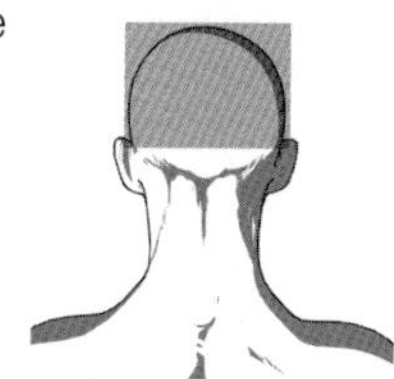

Fig. 23.39 Occipital lobes lifted to visualize the tentorium cerebelli and straight sinus; circumferential cut from the lateral attachment of the tentorium cerebelli alongside the transverse sinus toward the petrous ridge to the tentorial notch.

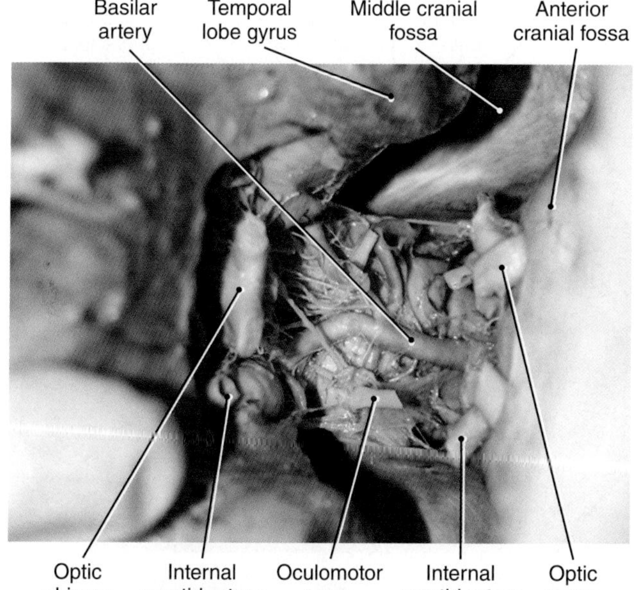

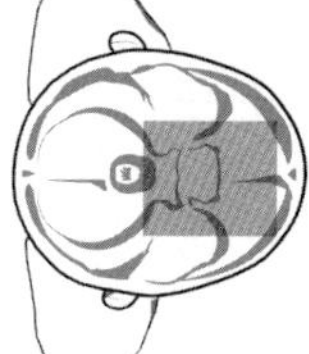

Fig. 23.38 Anterosuperior view of craniotomy with frontal lobes reflected superiorly and posteriorly, revealing anterior/middle cranial fossae, temporal lobe, optic nerve cut, internal carotid artery cut, basilar artery, optic chiasm cut, and oculomotor nerve.

- **Return to the frontal lobes and pull them upward (Fig. 23.40).**
- **Cut the facial, vestibulocochlear, trigeminal, abducens, and trochlear nerves.**
- **Because the tentorium cerebelli has been cut, pull the brain farther back and note the vertebral arteries forming the basilar artery (Fig. 23.41).**

DISSECTION **TIP**

The point at which you need to stop pulling the brain backward is when you visualize the junction where the vertebral arteries form the basilar artery.

- **Once you observe the vertebral arteries, cut the hypoglossal, accessory, glossopharyngeal, and vagus nerves.**
- **At this point, place a scalpel as deeply as possible within the foramen magnum and cut the spinal cord (Fig. 23.42).**
- **Retract the brain from the base of the skull, leaving intact the dural venous sinuses (Fig. 23.43).**
- **Once the brain is removed, identify the different dural venous sinuses: the superior sagittal sinus, inferior sagittal sinus, confluence of the sinuses, straight sinus, transverse sinus, sigmoid sinus, and the great vein of Galen (see Fig. 23.18).**

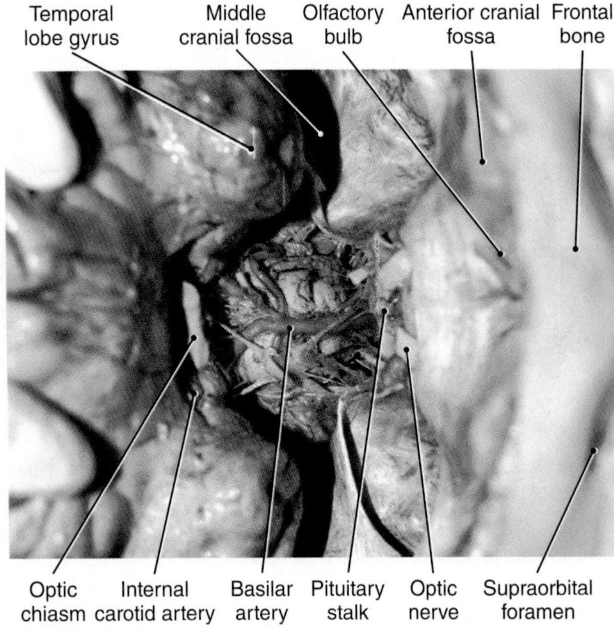

Fig. 23.40 Anterosuperior view of craniotomy with the frontal lobes reflected superiorly and posteriorly revealing the frontal bone, supraorbital foramen, anterior cranial fossa, olfactory tract (cut), optic nerve (cut), middle cranial fossa, temporal lobe, internal carotid artery (cut), optic nerves (cut), pituitary stalk (cut), and basilar artery.

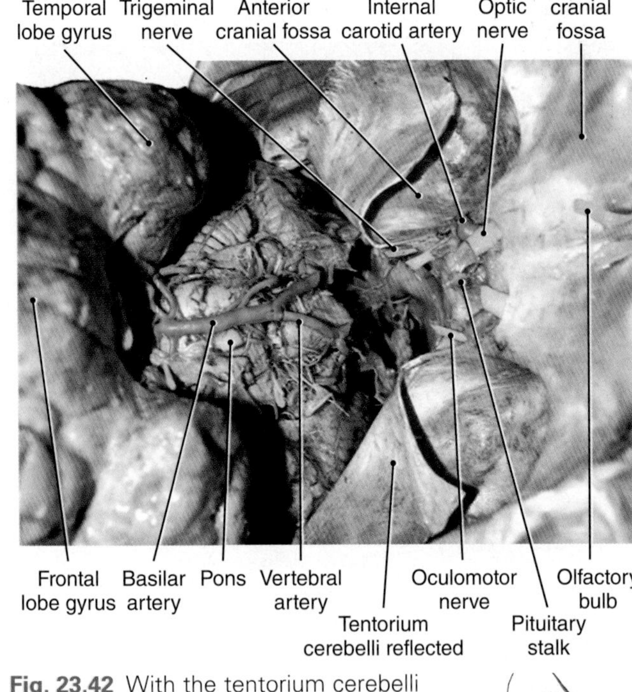

Fig. 23.42 With the tentorium cerebelli reflected, appreciate the hypoglossal, accessory, glossopharyngeal, and vagus nerves.

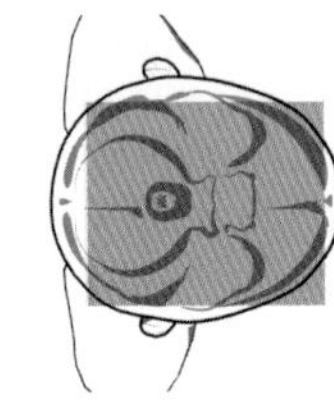

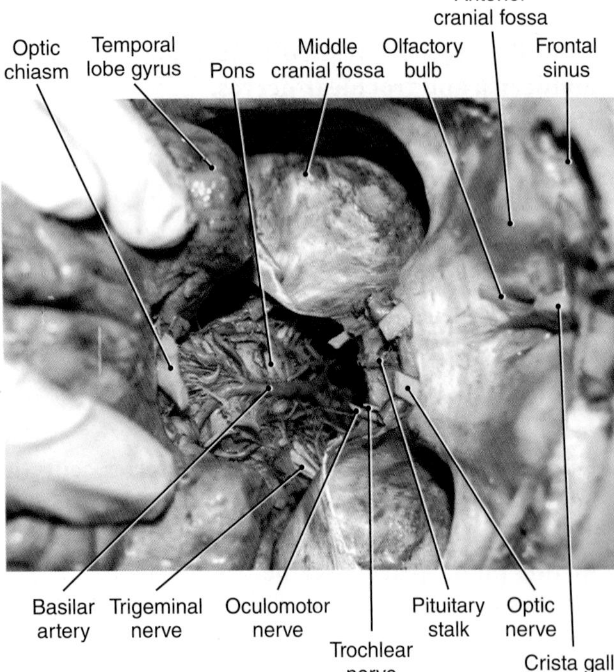

Fig. 23.41 Appreciate the facial, vestibulocochlear, trigeminal, abducens, and trochlear nerves; brain pulled farther back to visualize the vertebral arteries forming the basilar artery.

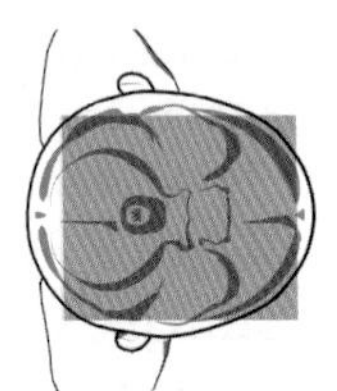

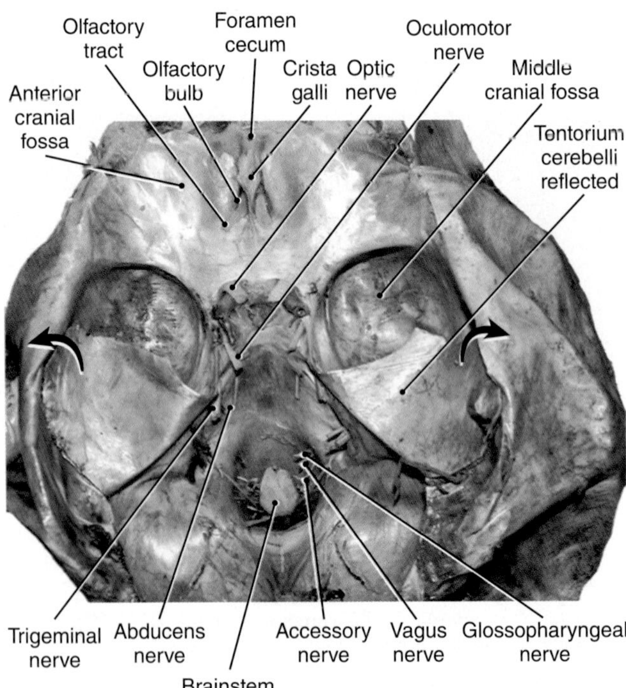

Fig. 23.43 Brain retracted from the base of the skull, leaving the dural venous sinuses intact.

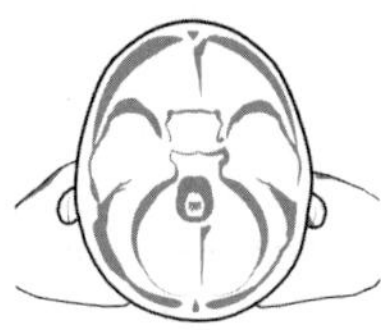

EXAMINATION OF THE BRAIN

- **Once the brain is removed, dissect away the arachnoid and pia mater from its ventral surface.**
- **Identify the cranial nerves on the brain (Figs. 23.44 and 23.45, Plate 23.2), as follows:**
  - **Cranial nerve I: The *olfactory bulbs and tracts* usually are found in contact with the frontal lobes of the brain.**
  - **Cranial nerve II: The *optic nerves* and the *optic chiasm* are usually well preserved in most cadavers. Posterior to the optic chiasm, identify the pituitary stalk.**
  - **Cranial nerve III: The *oculomotor nerve* passes between the posterior cerebral and superior cerebellar arteries, near the termination of the basilar artery.**
  - **Cranial nerve IV: The *trochlear nerve* is the smallest cranial nerve (less the olfactory nerves) and often is cut during brain removal. It passes anteriorly around the sides of the midbrain.**
  - **Cranial nerve V: The *trigeminal nerve* arises from the middle of the lateral aspect of the pons.**
  - **Cranial nerve VI: The *abducens nerve* arises from the inferior border of the pons, immediately superior to the medullary pyramids.**
  - **Cranial nerve VII: The *facial nerve* arises on the lateral aspect of the junction of the pons and the medulla oblongata, medial to the origin of cranial nerve VIII.**

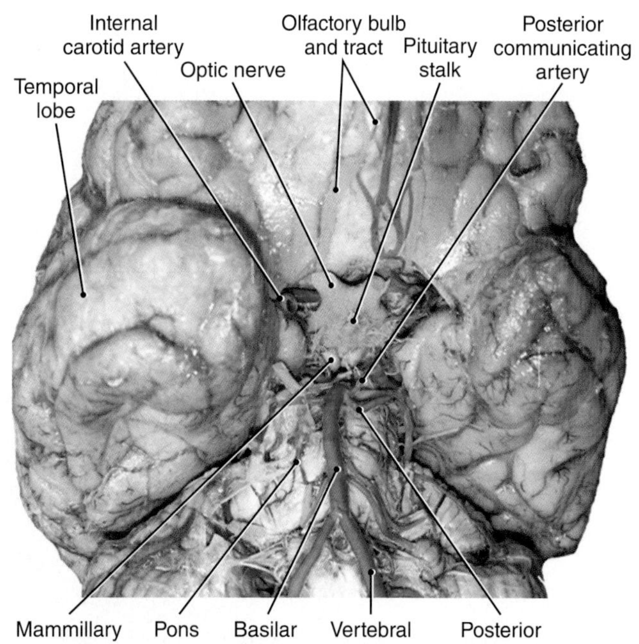

Fig. 23.44 Inferior aspect of the brain, revealing the olfactory bulb and tract, optic nerve, pituitary stalk, temporal lobe, mammillary bodies, and arteries (internal carotid, posterior communicating, basilar, vertebral, and posterior cerebral).

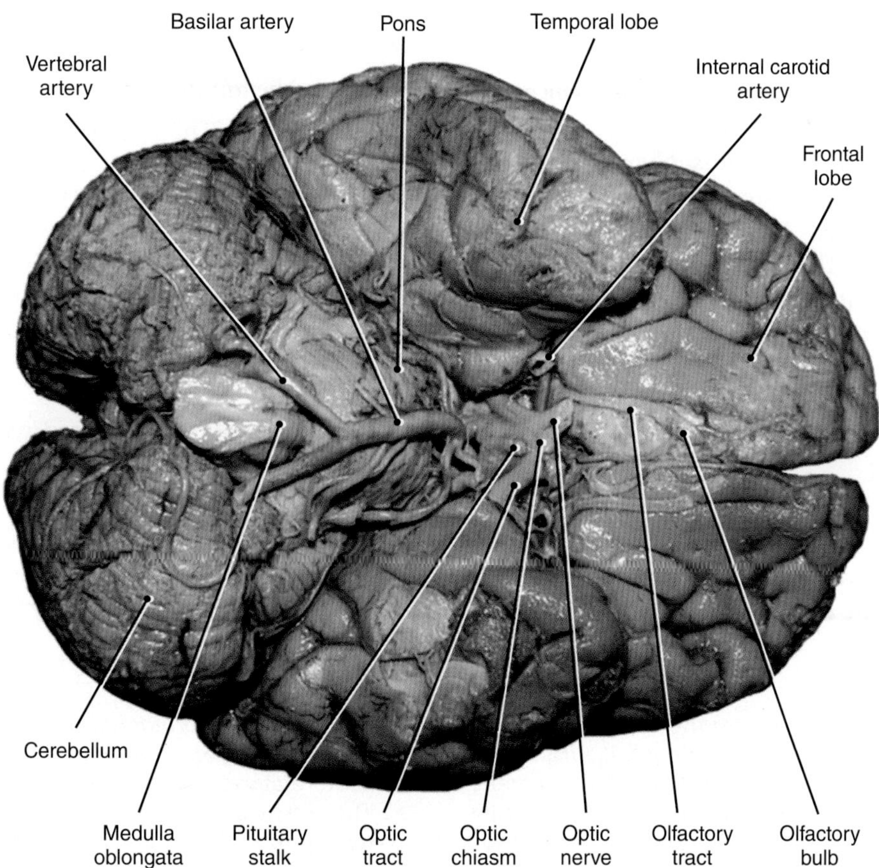

Fig. 23.45 Inferior aspect of the brain, revealing the olfactory bulb and tract, frontal lobe, optic chiasm, optic nerve, optic tract, internal carotid artery, pituitary stalk, temporal lobe, pons, medulla oblongata, basilar artery, vertebral artery, and cerebellum.

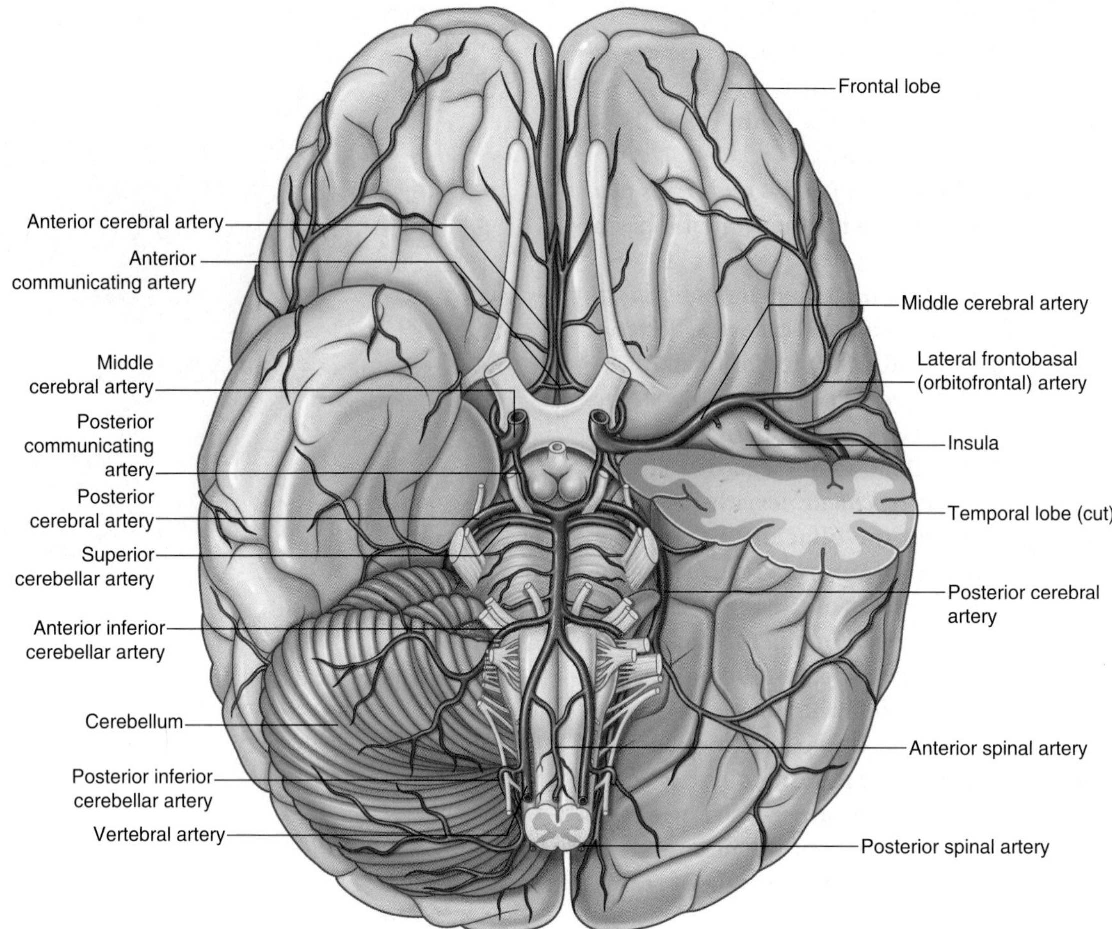

Plate 23.2 Arterial supply of the brain and cranial nerves. (From Drake RL et al. *Gray's Atlas of Anatomy*, 3rd edition, Philadelphia, Elsevier, 2021.)

- **Cranial nerve VIII: The *vestibulocochlear nerve* arises lateral to the facial nerve.**
- **Cranial nerve IX: The *glossopharyngeal nerve* arises at the groove posterior to the olive on the medulla oblongata.**
- **Cranial nerve X: The *vagus nerve* arises from the medulla oblongata by 8 to 10 rootlets between the olive and the inferior cerebellar peduncle.**
- **Cranial nerve XI: The *accessory nerve* arises from cranial rootlets from the medulla oblongata and from rootlets of the upper five cervical levels of the spinal cord.**
- **Cranial nerve XII: The *hypoglossal nerve* arises from a series of rootlets from the medulla oblongata on the ventrolateral sulcus between the pyramid and the olive.**

POINT OF **DEBATE**

Some anatomists do not consider the accessory nerve a "cranial nerve" because (1) it does not arise from the brain, and (2) it enters the skull through the foramen magnum. The definition of a cranial nerve states that it should arise from the brain and exit through one of the skull foramina.

- **Identify the following arteries contributing to the formation of the arterial circle of Willis (see Figs. 23.43 and 23.44, Plate 23.2):**
  - **The *anterior cerebral* arteries, connected by the anterior communicating artery**
  - **The *internal carotid* arteries, connected to the posterior cerebral arteries by posterior communicating arteries**

ANATOMY **NOTE**

Common variations encountered in the formation of the circle of Willis include the following:

- Absent anterior communicating artery
- Absent posterior communicating artery
- Large posterior communicating artery
- Posterior cerebral artery arising from the internal carotid (fetal posterior cerebral artery).

DISSECTION **TIP**

- The *anterior choroidal artery* arises near the origin of the posterior communicating artery and passes posterolaterally along the optic tract.
- The *trochlear nerve* and *oculomotor nerve* pass between the superior cerebellar and posterior cerebral arteries.

- Make a midsagittal incision through the brain, separating the right from the left hemisphere.
- Identify the thalamus, hypothalamus, and the three parts of the brainstem—midbrain, pons, and medulla oblongata (see Fig. 23.45).
- Identify the corpus callosum and fornix.
- Note the lateral ventricles, which open into the third ventricle through the foramen of Monro.
- Identify the foramen of Monro (Fig. 23.46).
- Note that the third ventricle is continuous inferiorly with the cerebral aqueduct, connecting the third with the fourth ventricles.

EXAMINATION OF THE CRANIAL BASE

- Identify the tentorium cerebelli and the anterior clinoid process.
- Visualize the dura covering the trigeminal nerve as it passes into the middle cranial fossa.
- With scissors, make a small cut in the dura covering the trigeminal nerve and pull it upward (Fig. 23.47 and Plate 23.3).
- Pull the dura covering the trigeminal nerve away from the middle cranial fossa and expose *Meckel's cave,* the area where the trigeminal (semilunar) ganglion resides (Fig. 23.48).
- Gently dissect out the soft tissues around Meckel's (trigeminal) cave and expose the trigeminal ganglion (Fig. 23.49).
- Continue the dissection to the trigeminal ganglion.
- Identify the ophthalmic (V1), maxillary (V2), and mandibular (V3) divisions of the trigeminal nerve entering into the superior orbital fissure, foramen

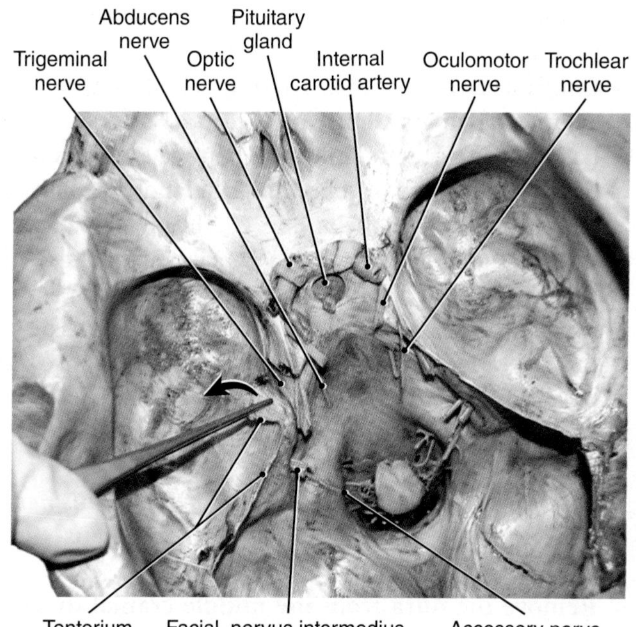

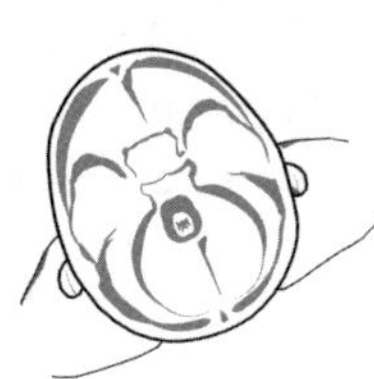

Fig. 23.47 Appreciate the tentorium cerebelli, anterior clinoid process, and dura mater covering the trigeminal nerve that is pulled upward.

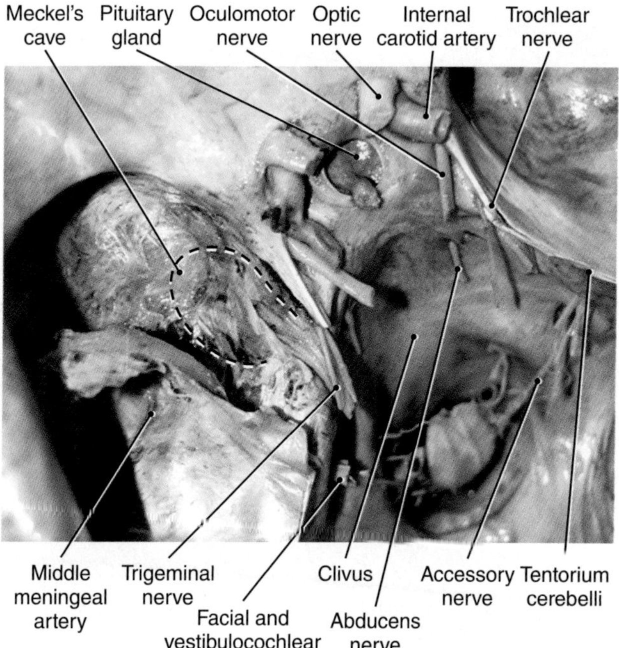

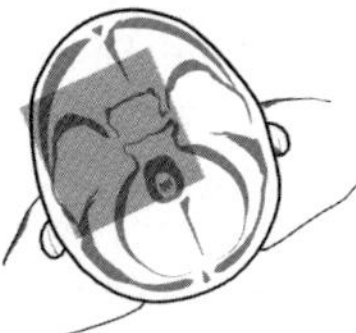

Fig. 23.48 Trigeminal nerve dura pulled from the middle cranial fossa, exposing the pituitary gland, Meckel's cave *(dashed arch),* and clivus (bony surface of posterior cranial fossa).

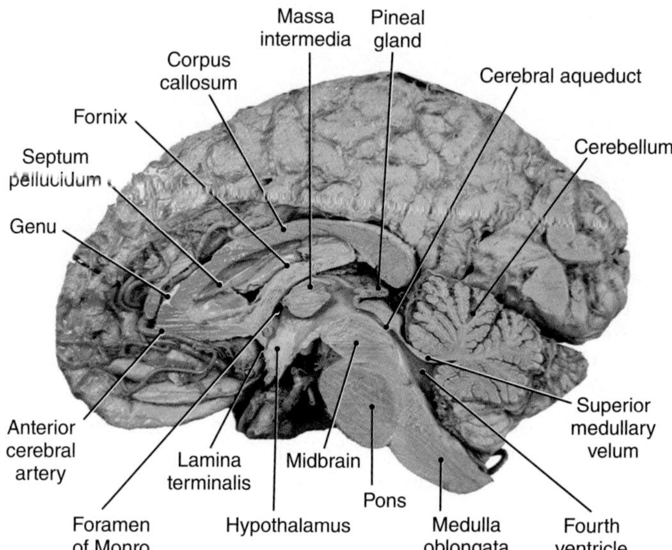

Fig. 23.46 Sagittal section of the cerebellum and brainstem.

rotundum, and foramen ovale, respectively (see Figs. 23.49 and 23.50).

- Continue laterally by identifying the internal carotid arteries passing underneath the optic nerves.
- Posterior to the optic chiasm and optic nerves, identify the infundibulum of the pituitary gland *(hypophysis)* and the diaphragma sella (Fig. 23.51 and Plate 23.3).
- Identify the cavernous sinus, appreciating that the walls of the cavernous sinuses are formed by dura mater.
- Identify the oculomotor nerve as it passes underneath the free edge of the tentorium cerebelli toward the posterior clinoid process.
- At the posterior clinoid process, identify the trochlear nerve.
- Inferior to the sella turcica, note the *abducens nerve* penetrating the dural wall of the cavernous sinus (Fig. 23.52).
- Remove the dura from the middle cranial fossa as well as from the medial side of the cavernous sinus (Fig. 23.53).
- Separate the soft tissue around the oculomotor nerve and internal carotid artery.

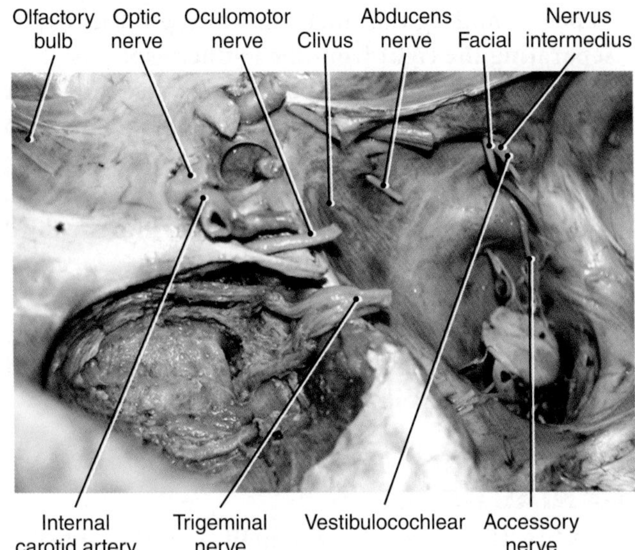

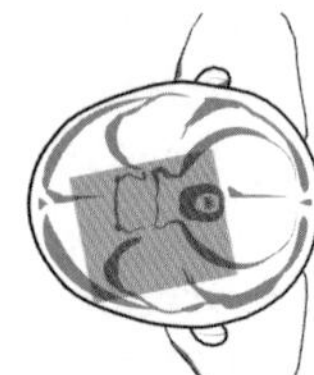

Fig. 23.50 Anterolateral view of the anterior, middle, and posterior cranial fossae.

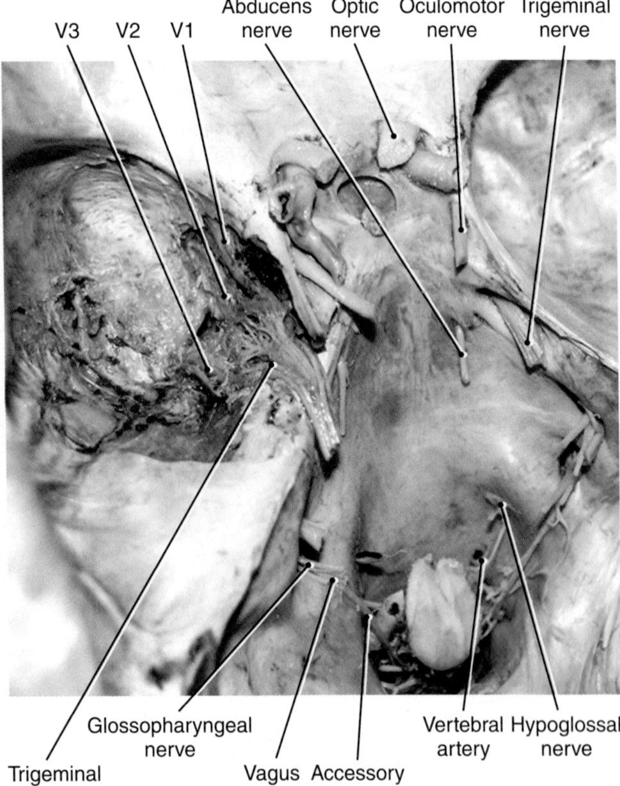

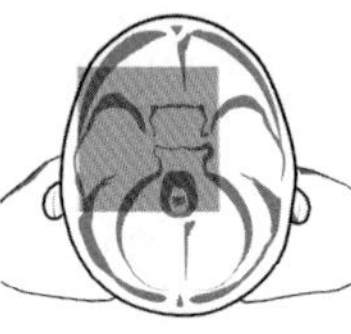

Fig. 23.49 Dissection continued anteriorly to the trigeminal ganglion revealing the ophthalmic *(V1)*, maxillary *(V2)*, and mandibular *(V3)* divisions of the trigeminal nerve and key neurovascular structures.

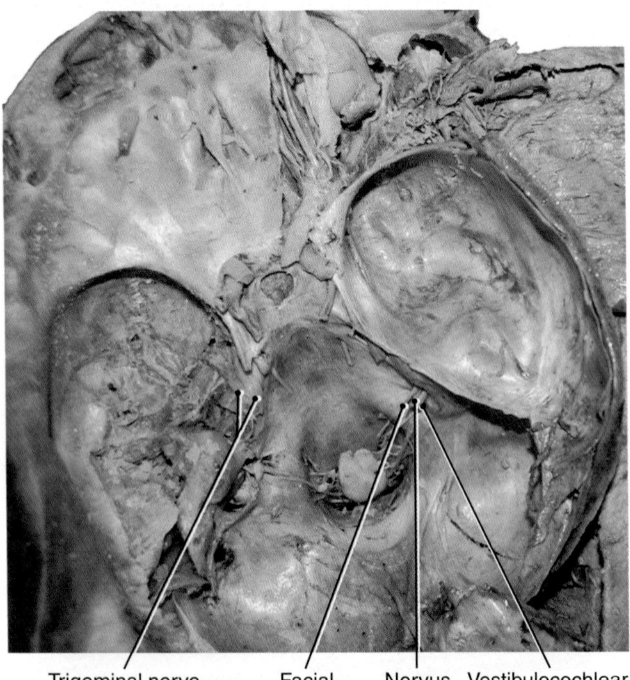

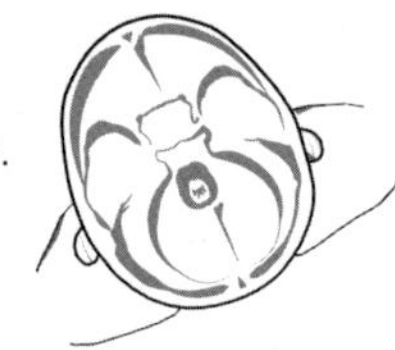

Fig. 23.51 Appreciate the foramina for the trigeminal nerve branches and facial, intermediate, and vestibulocochlear nerves.

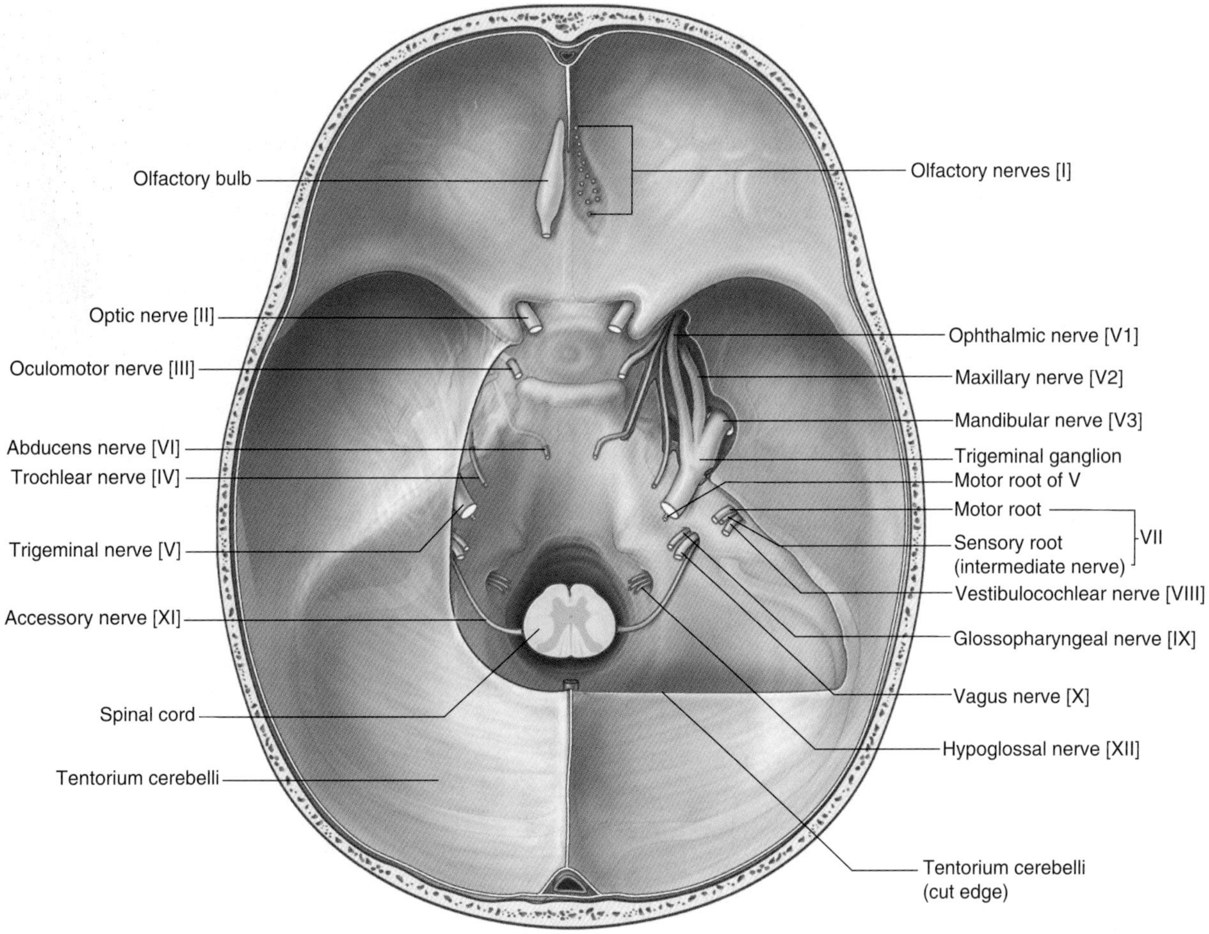

Olfactory bulb
Olfactory nerves [I]
Optic nerve [II]
Oculomotor nerve [III]
Abducens nerve [VI]
Trochlear nerve [IV]
Trigeminal nerve [V]
Accessory nerve [XI]
Spinal cord
Tentorium cerebelli
Ophthalmic nerve [V1]
Maxillary nerve [V2]
Mandibular nerve [V3]
Trigeminal ganglion
Motor root of V
Motor root
Sensory root
(intermediate nerve)
VII
Vestibulocochlear nerve [VIII]
Glossopharyngeal nerve [IX]
Vagus nerve [X]
Hypoglossal nerve [XII]
Tentorium cerebelli
(cut edge)

Plate 23.3 Cranial nerves as they traverse the cranium. (From Drake RL et al. *Gray's Anatomy for Students*, 5th edition, Philadelphia, Elsevier, 2024.)

Trigeminal nerve
Facial nerve
Nervus intermedius
Vestibulocochlear nerve

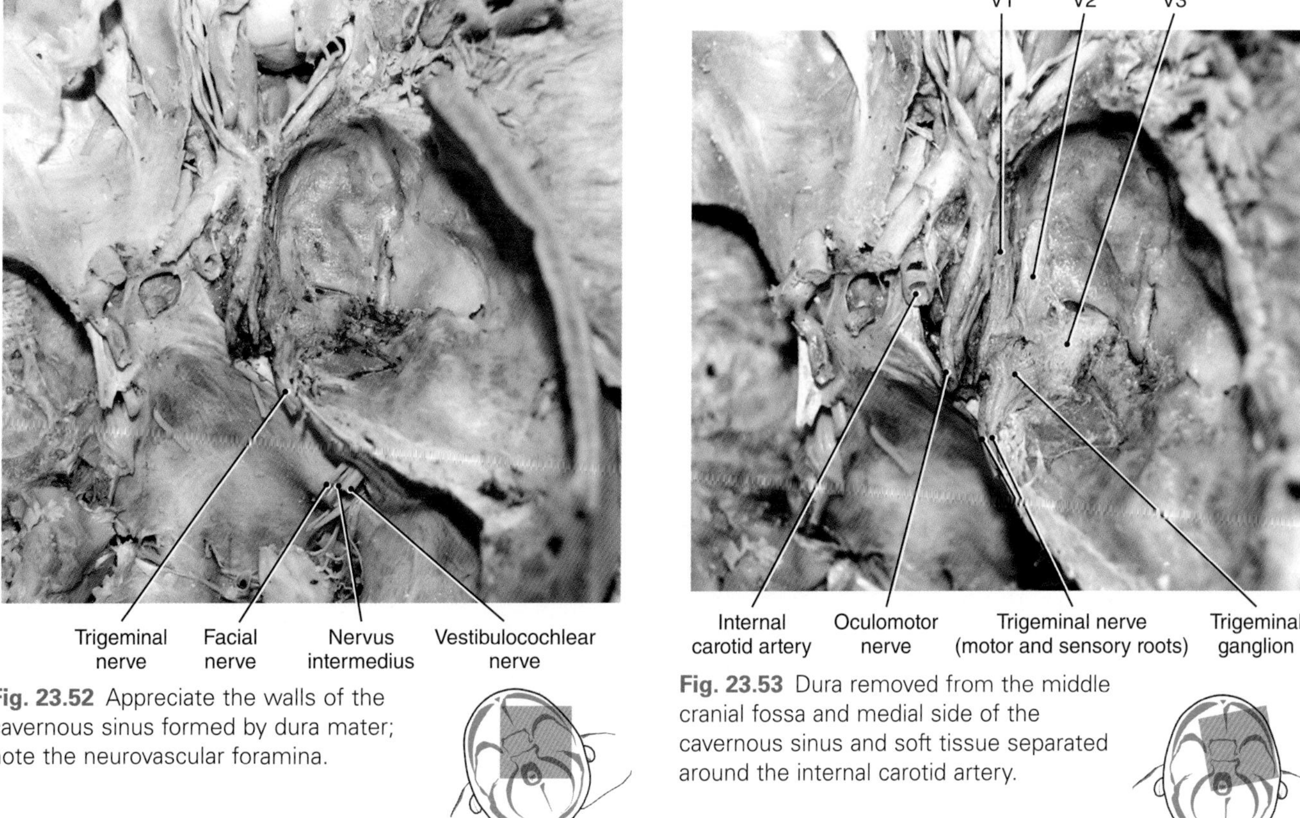

Fig. 23.52 Appreciate the walls of the cavernous sinus formed by dura mater; note the neurovascular foramina.

V1
V2
V3
Internal carotid artery
Oculomotor nerve
Trigeminal nerve (motor and sensory roots)
Trigeminal ganglion

Fig. 23.53 Dura removed from the middle cranial fossa and medial side of the cavernous sinus and soft tissue separated around the internal carotid artery.

- Notice the **S**-shaped course of the internal carotid artery (carotid siphon) within the cavernous sinus.
- Identify the abducens nerve running lateral to the internal carotid artery within the cavernous sinus.
- Incise the dura at the entrance of the abducens nerve and follow it into the cavernous sinus.

ANATOMY **NOTE**

The internal carotid artery and the abducens nerve are covered by a layer that separates them from the adjacent venous blood (Fig. 23.54).

- Identify the sigmoid sinus and cut the dura that forms it.
- Cut the dura off the superior and inferior petrosal sinuses.
- Identify the internal acoustic meatus and trace the facial and vestibulocochlear nerves as they enter this canal.
- Look inferior to the internal acoustic meatus for the jugular foramen and trace the glossopharyngeal, vagus, and accessory nerves (see Figs. 23.47 and 23.51).
- Note the upper cervical spinal fibers of the accessory nerve entering through the foramen magnum. Inferior to the jugular foramen and superior to the foramen magnum, identify the hypoglossal canal with the hypoglossal nerve (see Figs. 23.47 and 23.51).

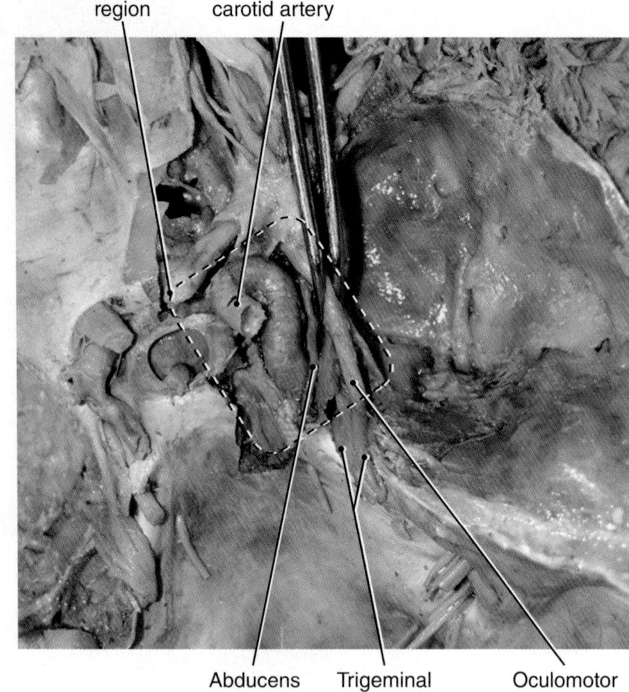

Fig. 23.54 *Dashed lines* indicate the cavernous sinus region with the abducens nerve running lateral to the internal carotid artery.

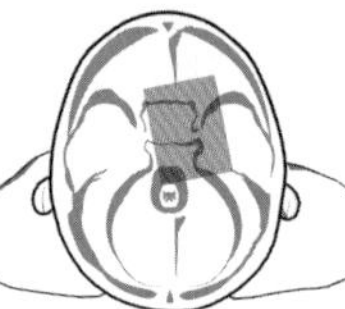

LABORATORY IDENTIFICATION CHECKLIST

BRAIN/BRAINSTEM

- ☐ Frontal lobe
  - ☐ Precentral gyrus
- ☐ Central sulcus
- ☐ Parietal lobe
  - ☐ Postcentral gyrus
- ☐ Occipital lobe
  - ☐ Occipital lobe gyri
- ☐ Temporal lobe
  - ☐ Temporal lobe gyri
- ☐ Corpus callosum
  - ☐ Genu
- ☐ Septum pellucidum
- ☐ Fornix
- ☐ Midbrain
- ☐ Hypothalamus
- ☐ Lamina terminalis
- ☐ Pineal gland
- ☐ Medulla oblongata
- ☐ Fourth ventricle
- ☐ Pons
- ☐ Mammillary body
- ☐ Foramen of Monro
- ☐ Cerebral aqueduct
- ☐ Pituitary stalk/gland
- ☐ Cerebellum

NERVES

- ☐ Olfactory bulb
- ☐ Olfactory tract
- ☐ Optic
- ☐ Optic chiasm
- ☐ Oculomotor
- ☐ Trochlear
- ☐ Trigeminal
  - ☐ V1 (ophthalmic) division
  - ☐ V2 (maxillary) division
  - ☐ V3 (mandibular) division
- ☐ Abducens
- ☐ Facial
- ☐ Nervus intermedius
- ☐ Vestibulocochlear
- ☐ Glossopharyngeal
- ☐ Vagus
- ☐ Accessory
- ☐ Hypoglossal

ARTERIES

- ☐ Internal carotid
- ☐ Basilar
- ☐ Middle meningeal
  - ☐ Anterior branch
  - ☐ Posterior branch
- ☐ Superficial temporal
- ☐ Anterior cerebral
- ☐ Middle cerebral
- ☐ Posterior cerebral
- ☐ Posterior communicating
- ☐ Vertebral

VEINS/SINUSES

- ☐ Confluence of sinuses
- ☐ Superior sagittal
- ☐ Inferior sagittal
- ☐ Transverse
- ☐ Straight
- ☐ Emissary veins
- ☐ Superficial cerebral veins
- ☐ Cavernous
- ☐ Superior petrosal
- ☐ Inferior petrosal
- ☐ Sigmoid

MUSCLE

- ☐ Temporalis

CONNECTIVE TISSUE

- ☐ Skin
- ☐ Subcutaneous tissue
- ☐ Epicranial aponeurosis
- ☐ Dura mater
- ☐ Lateral lacunae
- ☐ Falx cerebri
- ☐ Tentorium cerebelli
- ☐ Arachnoid mater
- ☐ Pia mater
- ☐ Temporalis fascia

BONES/FOSSAE/SINUSES

- ☐ Frontal bone
  - ☐ Frontal sinus
  - ☐ Supraorbital notch/foramen
  - ☐ Glabella

- ☐ Ethmoid bone
  - ☐ Crista galli
- ☐ Temporal bone
- ☐ Parietal bone
- ☐ Occipital bone
  - ☐ Internal occipital crest
  - ☐ Inion
  - ☐ Superior nuchal line
- ☐ Zygomatic arch
- ☐ Diploic space
- ☐ Pterion
- ☐ Sagittal suture
- ☐ Lambdoid suture
- ☐ Parietal foramen
- ☐ Temporal fossa
- ☐ Anterior cranial fossa
- ☐ Middle cranial fossa
- ☐ Posterior cranial fossa

BEFORE YOU BEGIN

Remove all soft tissues with a scalpel and expose the frontal and temporal bones. Reflect the temporalis muscle as laterally as possible.

OSTEOTOMY OF ORBITAL ROOF

- **With an electric saw or a mallet and chisel, make a second vertical cut through the frontal bone, lateral to the supraorbital notch (Fig. 24.1).**
- **Extend this cut posteriorly through the roof of the orbit between the optic nerve and ethmoidal cells (Fig. 24.2).**
- **With an electric saw or a mallet and chisel, make a second vertical cut through the squamous part of the temporal bone.**
- **Continue the cut horizontally toward the orbital process of the zygomatic bone at the infraorbital margin (see Fig. 24.2).**

> **DISSECTION TIP**
>
> Once all bones are cut, the orbital roof and the orbital process of the zygomatic bone can be reflected en bloc, while the periorbita (periosteal covering of orbital bones) is left intact (Fig. 24.3). This is referred to as an *orbitozygomatic approach.*

- **Complete the reflection of the orbital roof anteriorly but do not detach it from the orbit (Fig. 24.4).**

ORBIT

- **With sharp scissors, make a small cut in the periorbital fascia (Fig. 24.5).**
- **Identify the frontal nerve and its two branches, the supraorbital and supratrochlear nerves (Fig. 24.6).**
- **Clean and expose the frontal nerve and note the levator palpebrae superioris muscle lying underneath it (Fig. 24.7).**
- **Lateral and inferior to the levator palpebrae superioris, expose the superior rectus muscle (Fig. 24.8).**
- **Medial to the levator palpebrae superioris muscle, remove a small portion of the periorbital fat and identify the *nasociliary nerve* (Fig. 24.9 and Plate 24.1).**

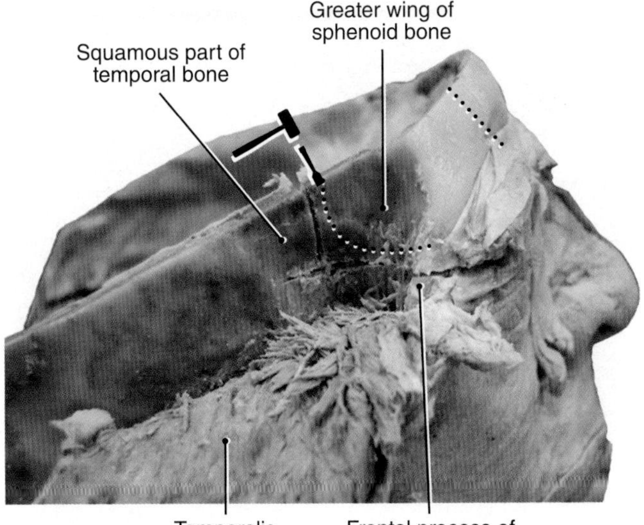

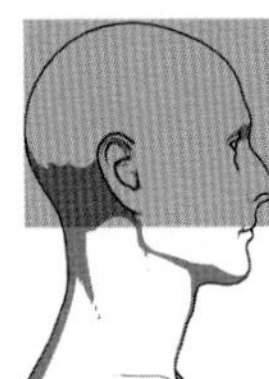

Fig. 24.1 Anterolateral view of the external orbit after craniotomy, with reflected temporalis muscle revealing bony landmarks; *dotted lines* indicate cuts through the frontal bone and orbital roof.

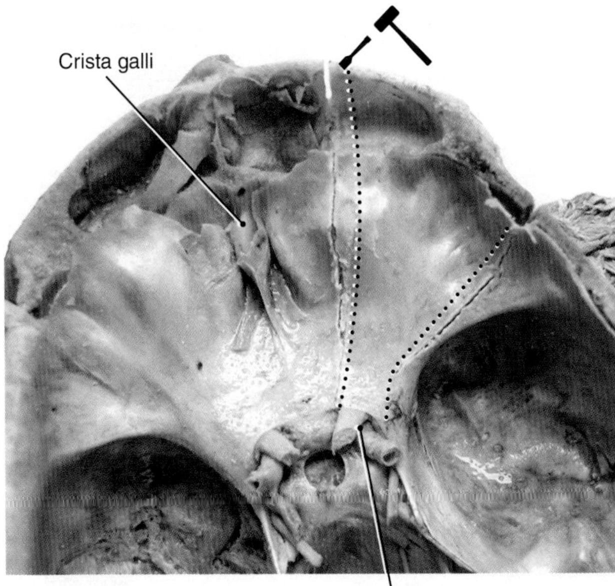

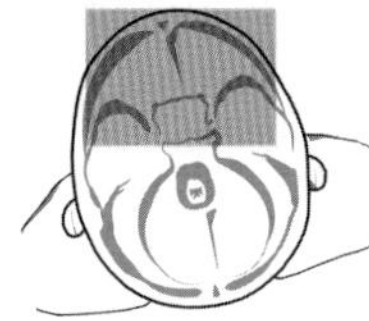

Fig. 24.2 View of the anterior cranial fossa, and roof of the orbit; *dotted lines* over dura represent the osteotomy cuts.

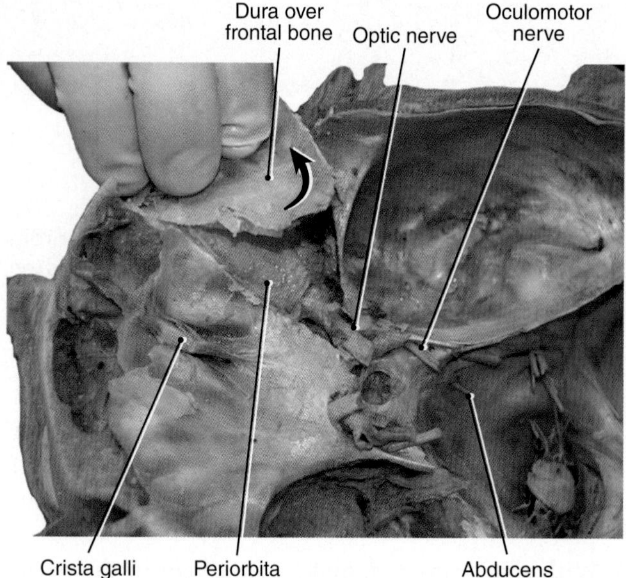

Fig. 24.3 Craniotomy view highlighting the anterior cranial fossa and dura mater, periorbita, crista galli, frontal bone, and nerves (optic, oculomotor, abducens).

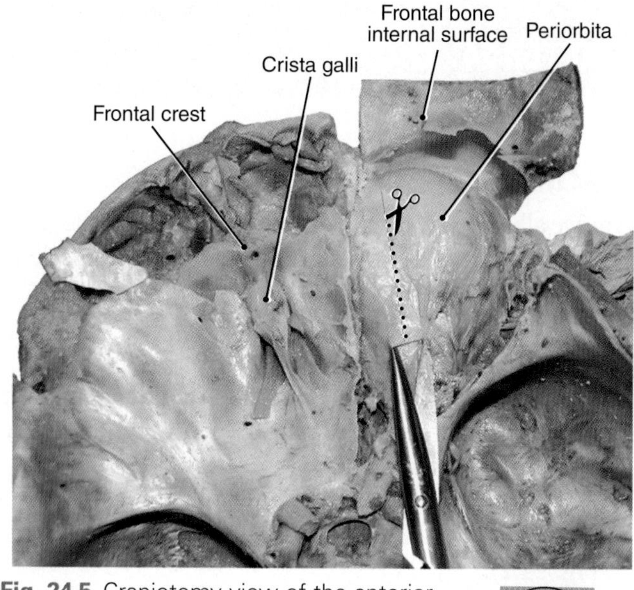

Fig. 24.5 Craniotomy view of the anterior cranial fossa with osteotomy of the roof of right orbit, revealing scissors cutting periorbita.

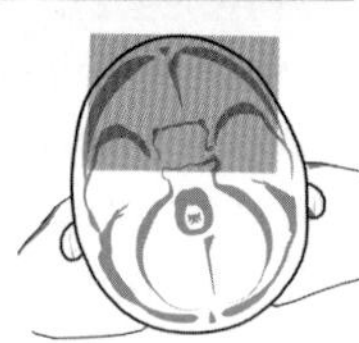

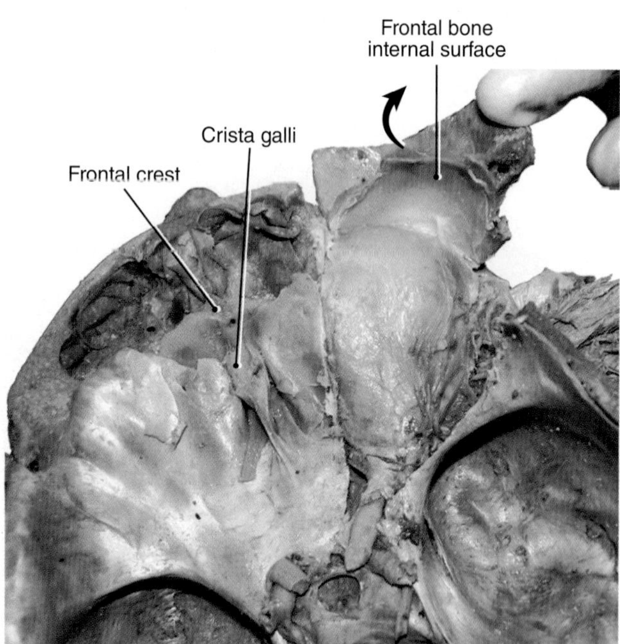

Fig. 24.4 Craniotomy view of the anterior cranial fossa with osteotomy performed to the roof of the right orbit.

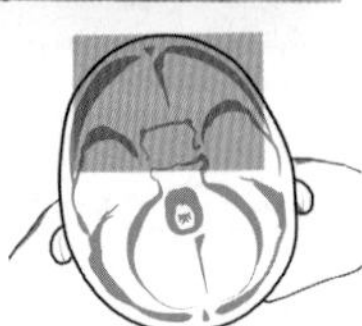

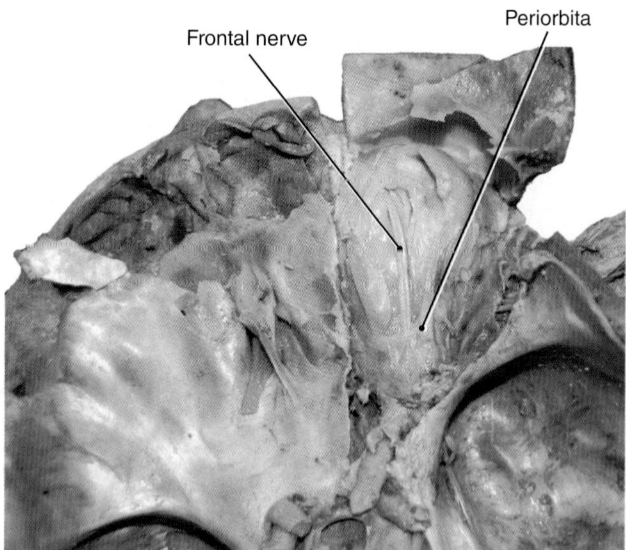

Fig. 24.6 Craniotomy view of the anterior cranial fossa with osteotomy to the orbital roof.

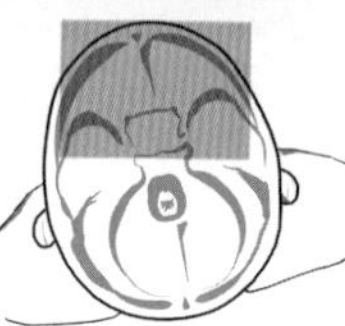

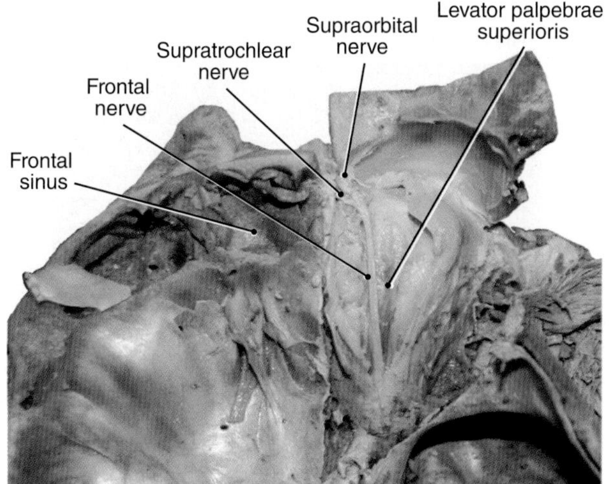

Fig. 24.7 Craniotomy view of the anterior cranial fossa with osteotomy to the roof of the orbit.

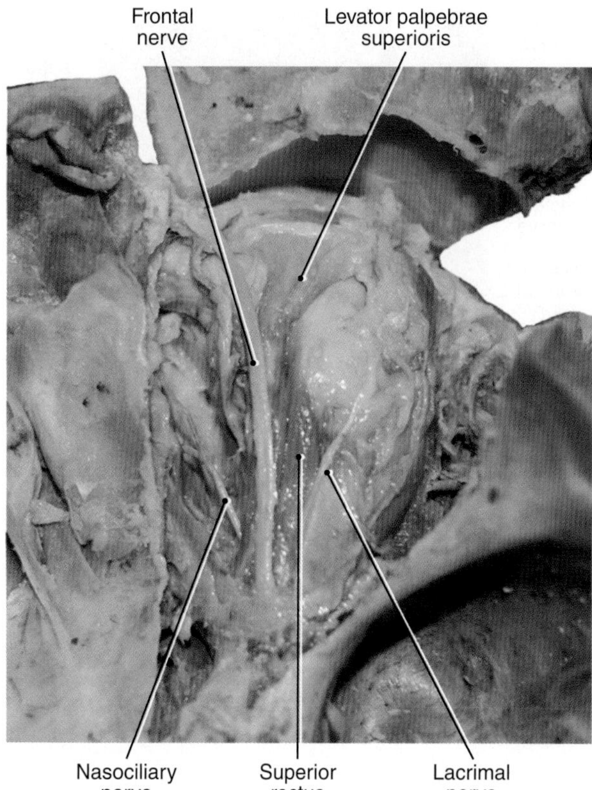

Fig. 24.8 Craniotomy view of the anterior cranial fossa with orbital roof osteotomy, revealing various nerves.

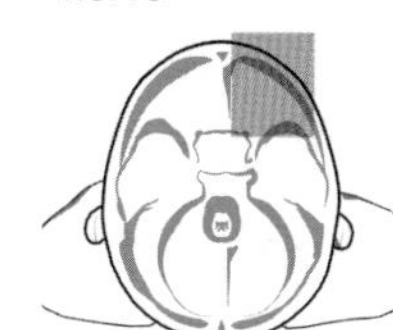

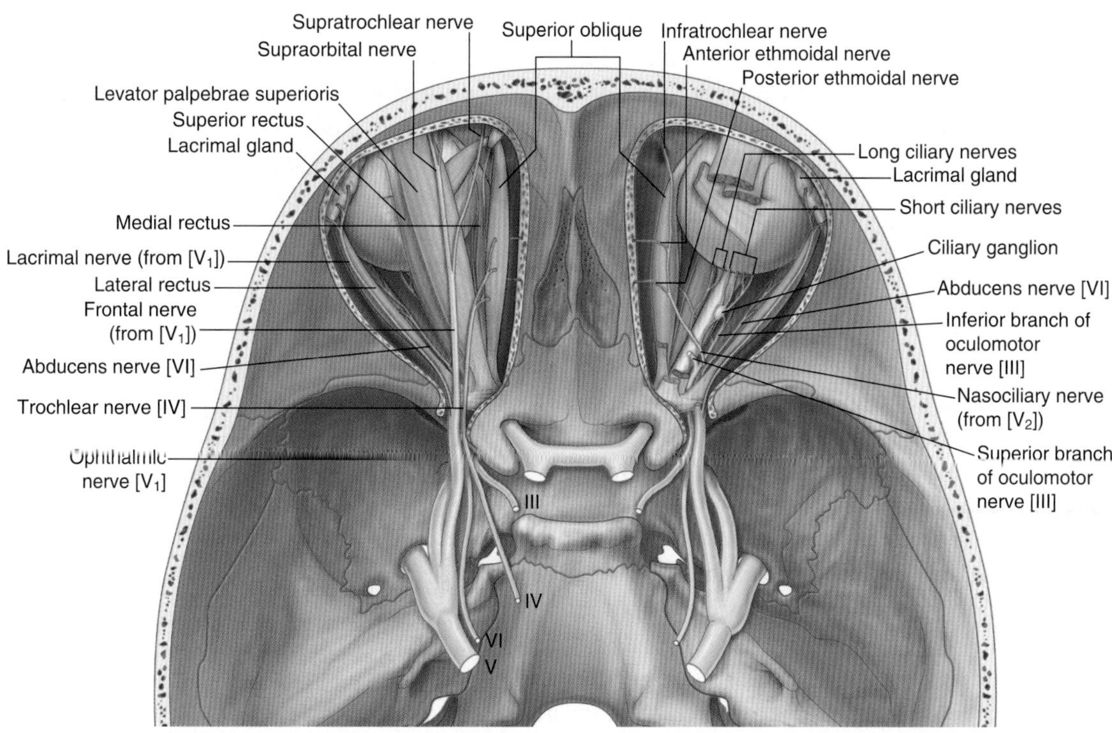

Plate 24.1 Superior view of the nerves and musculature of the orbit. (From Drake RL et al. *Gray's Atlas of Anatomy*, 3rd edition, Philadelphia, Elsevier, 2021.)

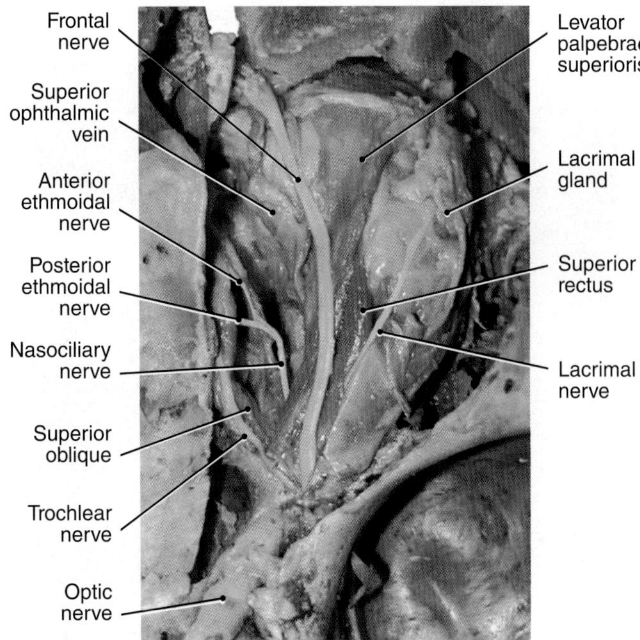

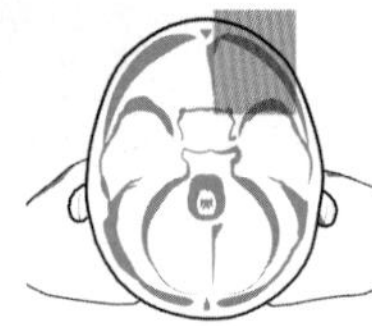

Fig. 24.9 Craniotomy view of the anterior cranial fossa with osteotomy to the roof of the orbit highlighting nerves and muscles.

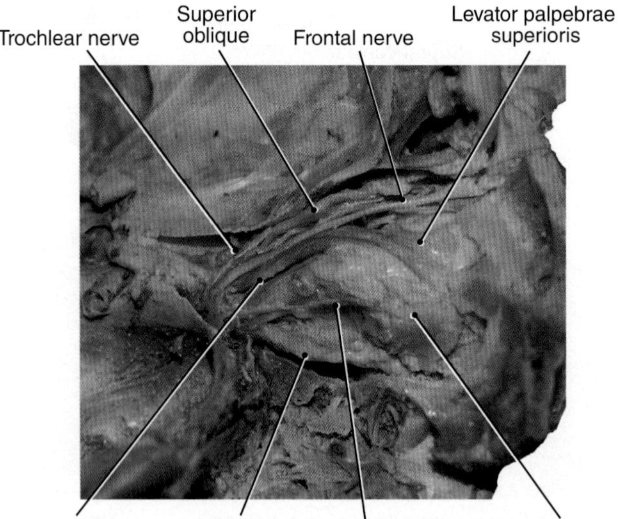

Fig. 24.10 Craniotomy view of the anterior cranial fossa with osteotomy to roof of orbit highlighting nerves and muscles.

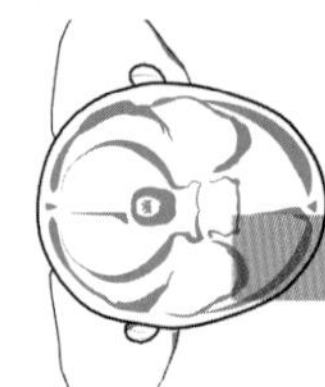

ANATOMY **NOTE**

The nasociliary nerve is located in the interval between the levator palpebrae superioris and the superior oblique muscles and crosses the optic nerve from lateral to medial (see Fig. 24.9).

- **Trace the terminal branches of the nasociliary nerve—the posterior ethmoidal, anterior ethmoidal, and infratrochlear nerves.**

DISSECTION **TIP**

The branches of the nasociliary nerve are small and delicate. The infratrochlear nerve is especially delicate and easily severed during dissection. The posterior ethmoidal nerve is often absent.

- **The superior oblique muscle is usually hidden medially under the orbital roof. Break away portions of the orbital roof to identify and clean the superior oblique muscle.**
- **Clean the periorbital fat away from the superior oblique muscle and note the *trochlear nerve* entering the superior surface of the muscle proximally (see Fig. 24.9).**
- **Distal to the interval between the superior oblique and levator palpebrae superioris muscles, look for a flat vessel, the superior ophthalmic vein.**
- **Remove all small tributaries of the ophthalmic veins (see Fig. 24.9).**
- **On the lateral surface of the superior rectus muscle, trace and expose the lacrimal nerve and lacrimal gland (see Fig. 24.9).**

DISSECTION **TIP**

The lacrimal gland is located distally and is often confused with periorbital fat. Lift and pull up on the lacrimal nerve to trace it to the lacrimal gland.

- **Deep to the lacrimal nerve, expose the lateral rectus muscle (Fig. 24.10).**
- **Pull the lateral rectus muscle laterally and expose the *abducens nerve* on its medial side (Fig. 24.11).**
- **Look for the *superior ophthalmic vein* in the space between the superior rectus and lateral rectus muscles (Fig. 24.12).**
- **After identifying the superior ophthalmic vein, remove the periorbital fat between the superior and lateral rectus muscles (Fig. 24.13).**
- **Observe the optic nerve, surrounded by short and long ciliary nerves (Fig. 24.14).**
- **Identify the *ciliary ganglion* on the lateral surface of the optic nerve and medial to the lateral rectus muscle (see Fig. 24.14).**

DISSECTION **TIP**

Another important landmark is the ciliary ganglion. It is connected by a small branch (motor root of ciliary ganglion) with the inferior division of the oculomotor nerve. The ganglion may be confused with periorbital fat.

- **In the interval between the optic nerve and the lateral rectus muscle, identify the *ophthalmic artery* (Fig. 24.15).**

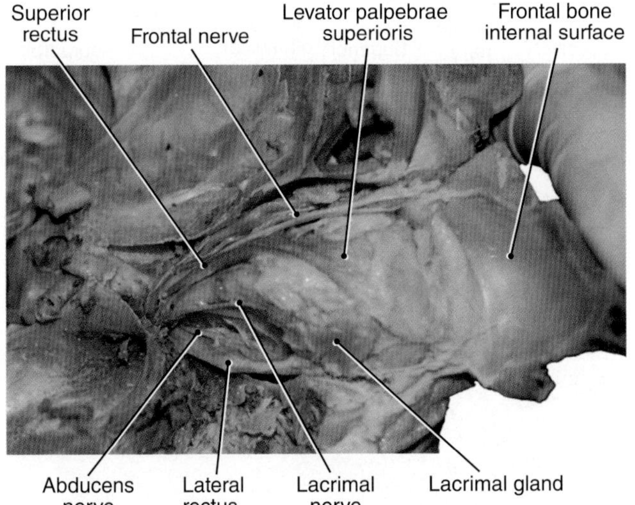

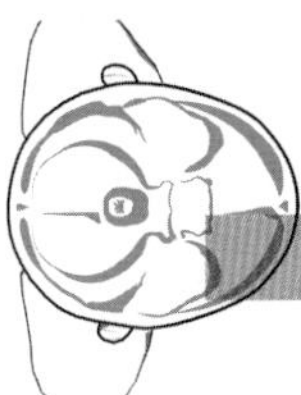

Fig. 24.11 Craniotomy view of the anterior cranial fossa with orbital osteotomy.

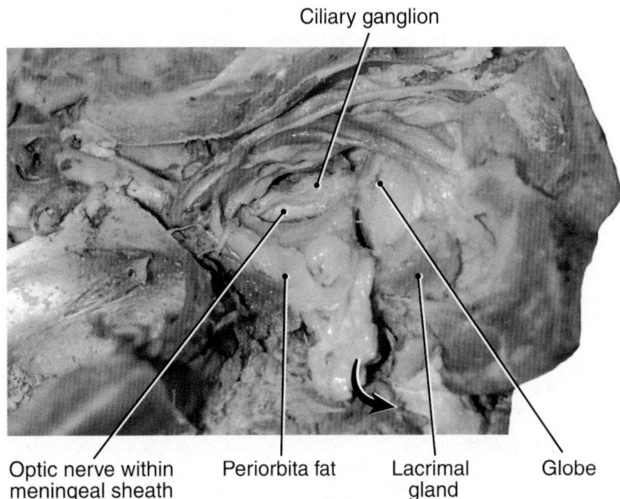

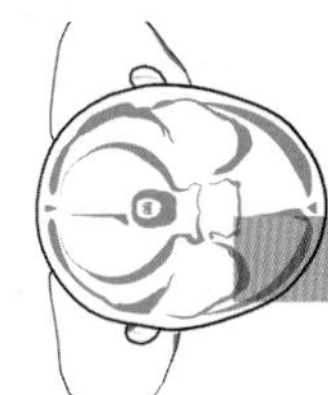

Fig. 24.13 Craniotomy view of the anterior cranial fossa following osteotomy to the roof of the orbit.

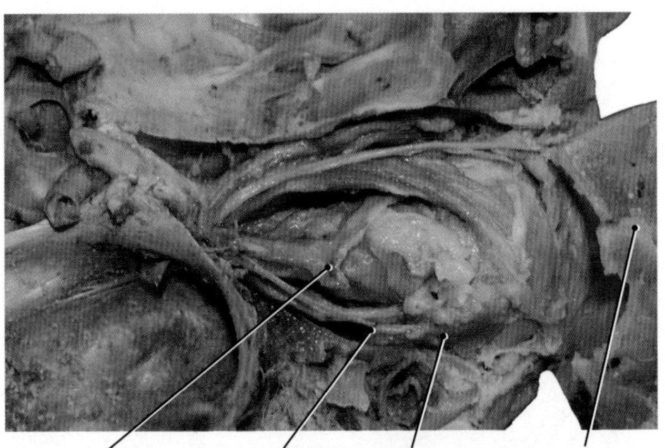

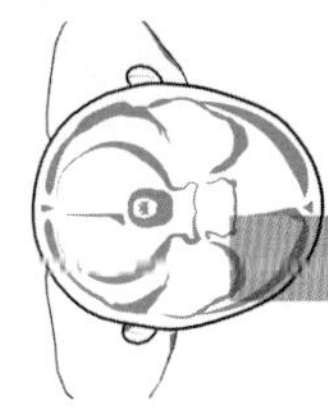

Fig. 24.12 Craniotomy view of the anterior cranial fossa with osteotomy to orbital roof, highlighting the superior ophthalmic vein.

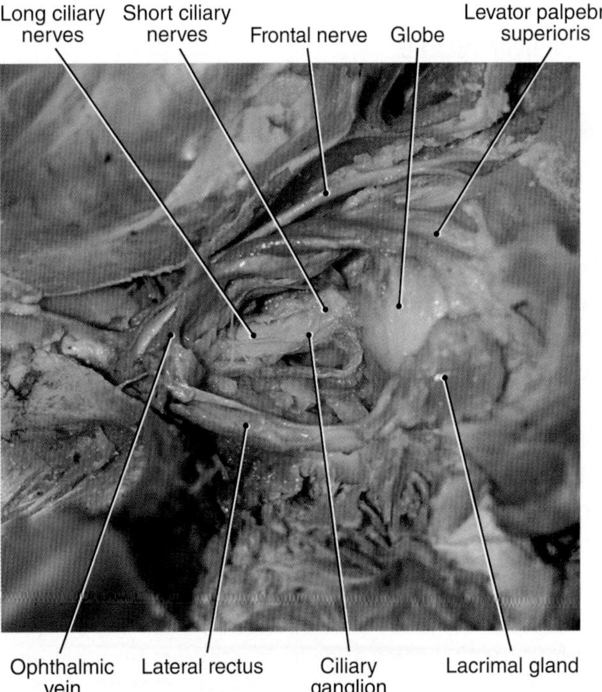

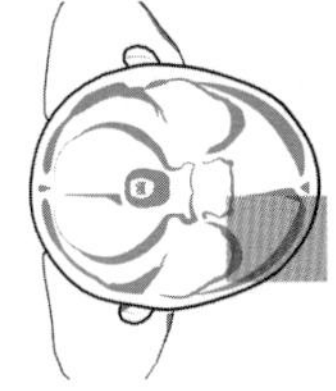

Fig. 24.14 Craniotomy view of the anterior cranial fossa with osteotomy to the orbital roof, revealing frontal nerve, reflected levator palpebrae superioris muscle, and highlighting the long and short ciliary nerves and the ciliary ganglion.

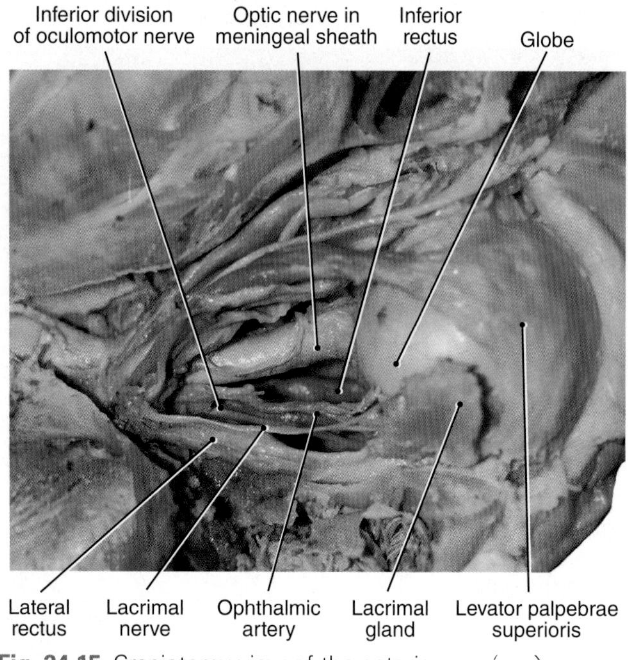

Fig. 24.15 Craniotomy view of the anterior cranial fossa with an osteotomy.

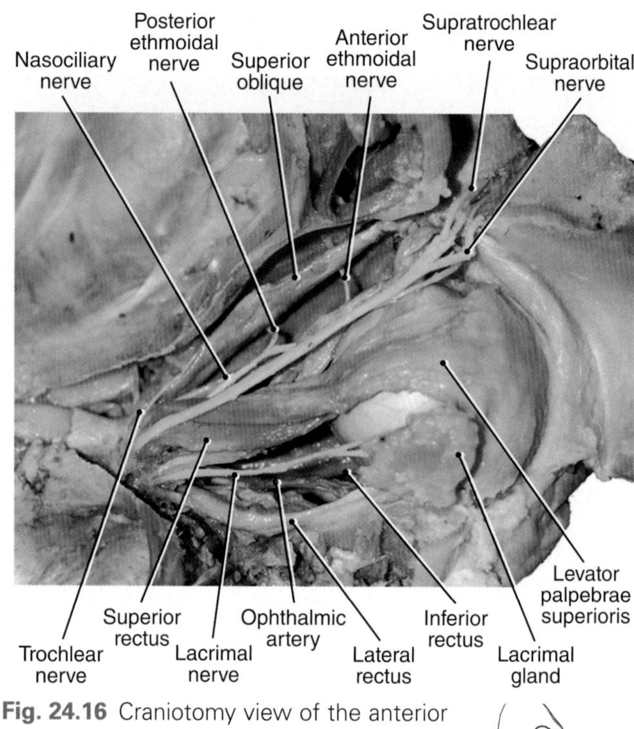

Fig. 24.16 Craniotomy view of the anterior cranial fossa with an osteotomy to the orbital roof.

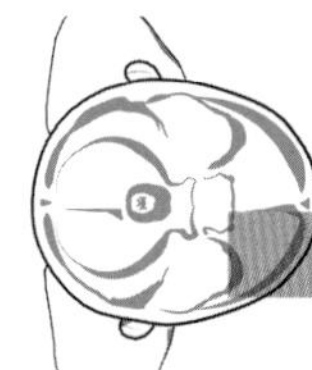

ANATOMY **NOTE**

After entering the orbit, the ophthalmic artery gives off a central retinal branch to the optic nerve and usually crosses over the nerve and passes toward the medial wall of the orbit.

- **Inferior to the optic nerve, remove the periorbital fat and identify the inferior division of the oculomotor nerve, which runs parallel to the inferior rectus muscle (see Fig. 24.15).**
- **Clean the periorbital fat inferior to the superior oblique muscle.**
- **Trace the anterior and posterior ethmoidal nerves to their entrance into the anterior and posterior ethmoidal foramina, respectively (Fig. 24.16 and Plate 24.2).**

ANATOMY **NOTE**

The four recti muscles arise from a fibrous ring that encircles the optic foramen and a portion of the superior orbital fissure. The superior oblique and levator palpebrae muscles arise from points superior and medial to this anulus (anulus of Zinn) (Fig. 24.17).

- **Reflect the nasociliary nerve and ophthalmic artery posteriorly and expose the medial rectus muscle (Fig. 24.18).**

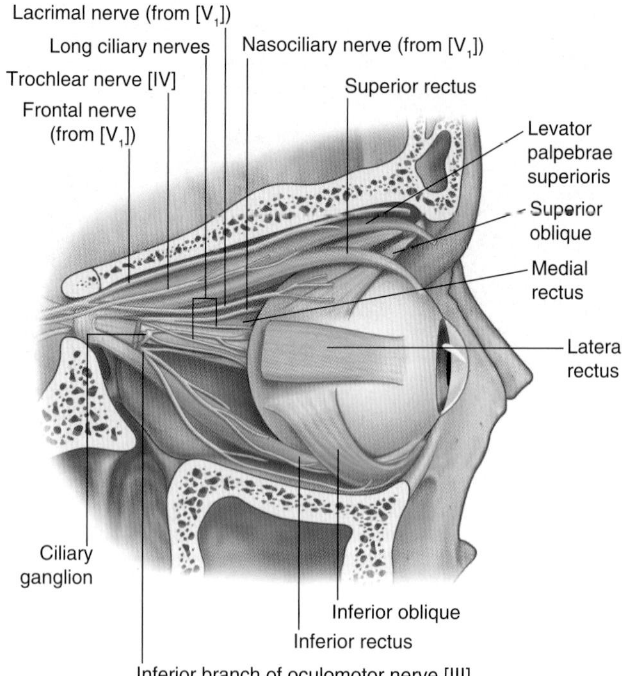

Plate 24.2 Lateral view of the nerves and musculature of the orbit. (From Drake RL et al. *Gray's Atlas of Anatomy*, 3rd edition, Philadelphia, Elsevier, 2021.)

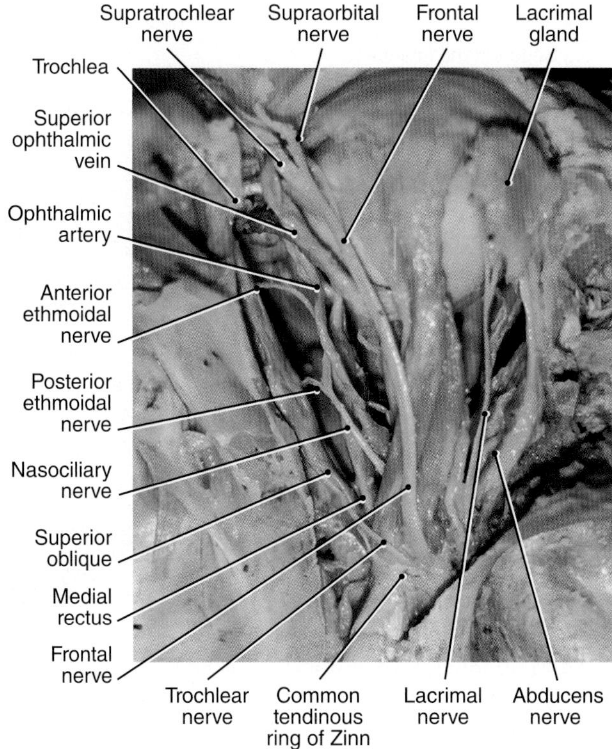

Fig. 24.17 Craniotomy view of the anterior cranial fossa with an osteotomy to the roof of the orbit.

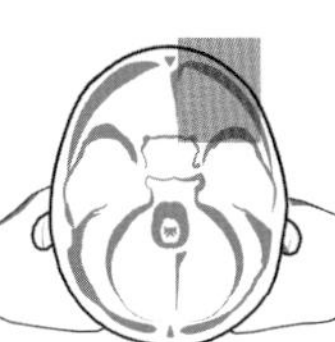

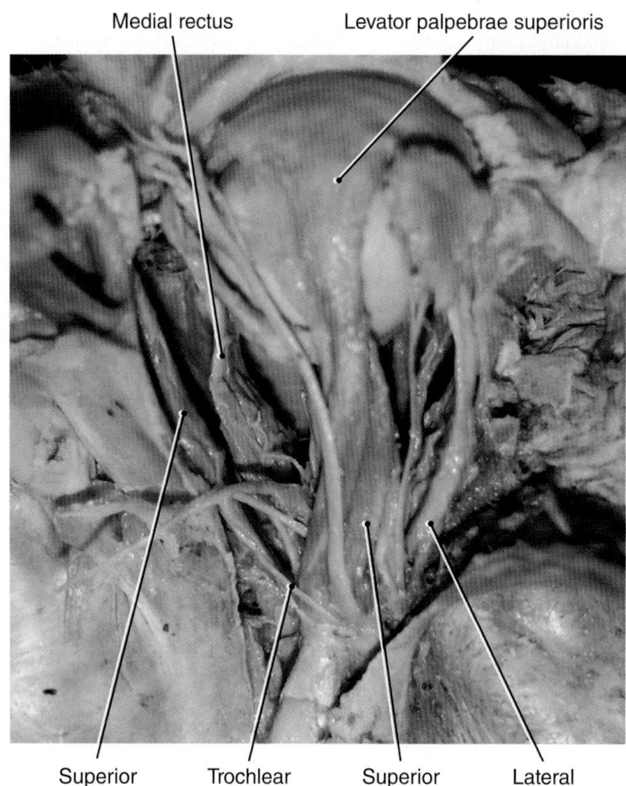

Fig. 24.18 Craniotomy view revealing the trochlear nerve and key muscles.

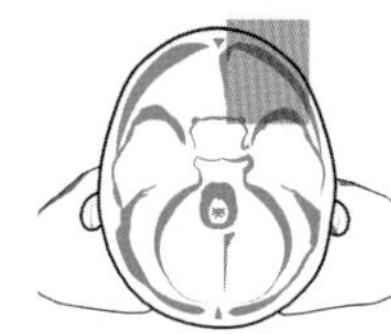

- **Pull the lateral rectus muscle laterally and the optic nerve medially and expose the inferior rectus muscle (Fig. 24.19 and Plate 24.3).**

DISSECTION **TIP**

To trace the inferior oblique muscle, the inferior rectus muscle, and the nerve to the inferior oblique muscle, you need to dissect inferior to the globe.

INFRAORBITAL APPROACH

- **Detach the orbital septum from the infraorbital margin.**
- **Lift the orbit and periorbital fat superiorly (Fig. 24.20).**
- **Clean away the periorbital fat and expose the inferior oblique muscle running obliquely from lateral to medial (Fig. 24.21).**
- **Remove all periorbital fat and identify the inferior rectus muscle and the nerve to the inferior oblique muscle (Fig. 24.22).**
- **Lift the orbicularis oculi muscle and identify the medial palpebral ligament (Fig. 24.23).**
- **Reflect all musculature from the frontal process of the maxilla (Fig. 24.24).**

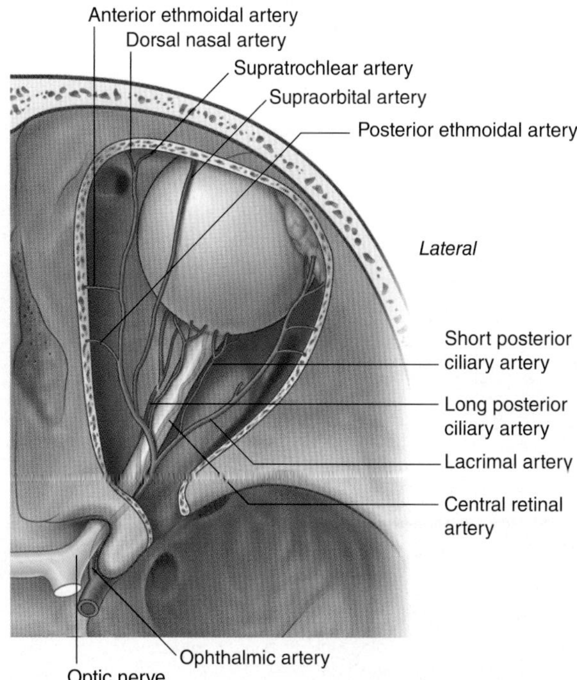

Plate 24.3 Superior view of the arteries of the orbit. (From Drake RL et al. *Gray's Anatomy for Students*, 5th edition, Philadelphia, Elsevier, 2024.)

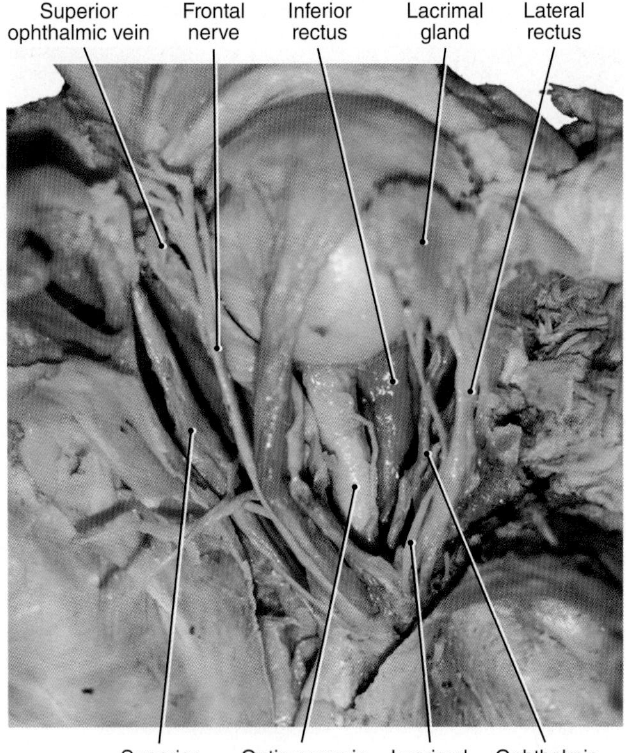

Fig. 24.19 Craniotomy view of the anterior cranial fossa with an osteotomy to the roof of the orbit revealing the frontal nerve, superior ophthalmic vein, optic nerve, lacrimal nerve, and lacrimal gland.

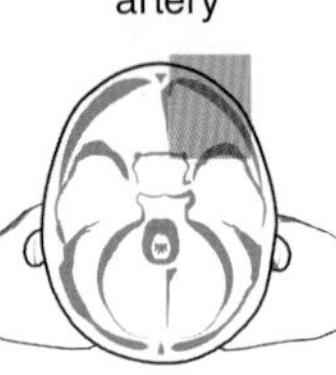

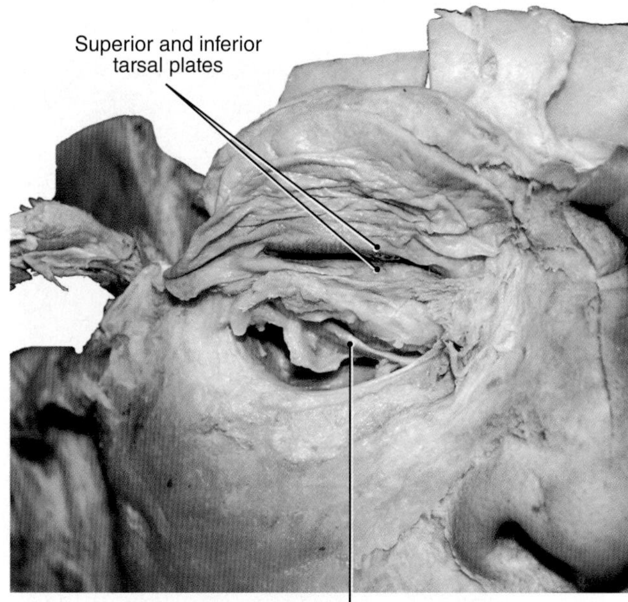

Fig. 24.21 Anterior view of the external orbit with craniotomy showing an infraorbital approach and highlighting the tarsal plates.

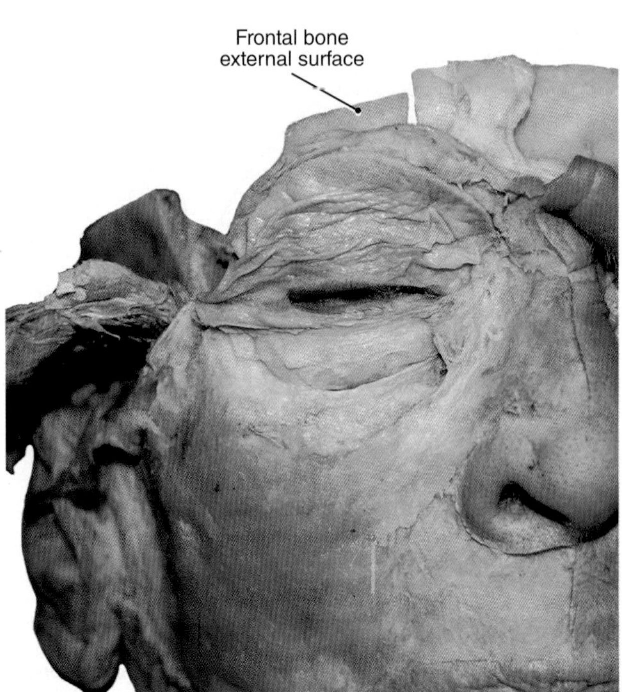

Fig. 24.20 Anterior view of the external orbit with craniotomy and vertical frontal bone osteotomy.

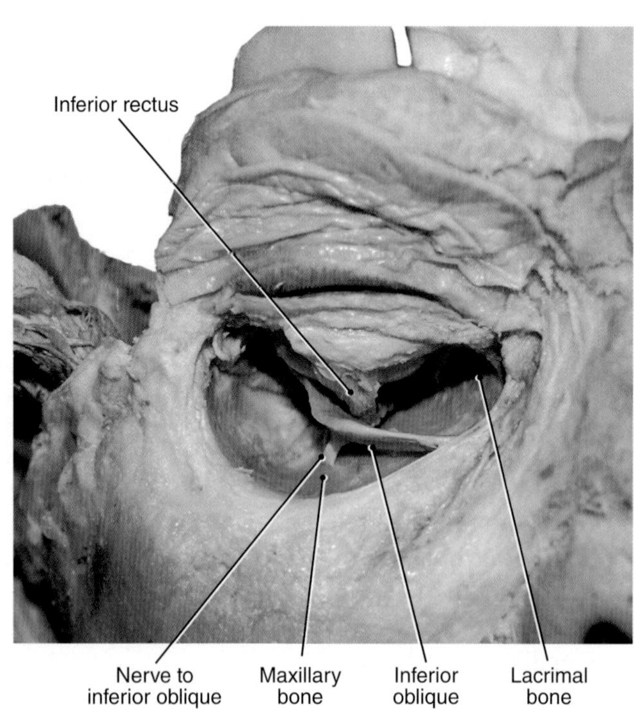

Fig. 24.22 Anterior view of the orbit with the eyeball removed.

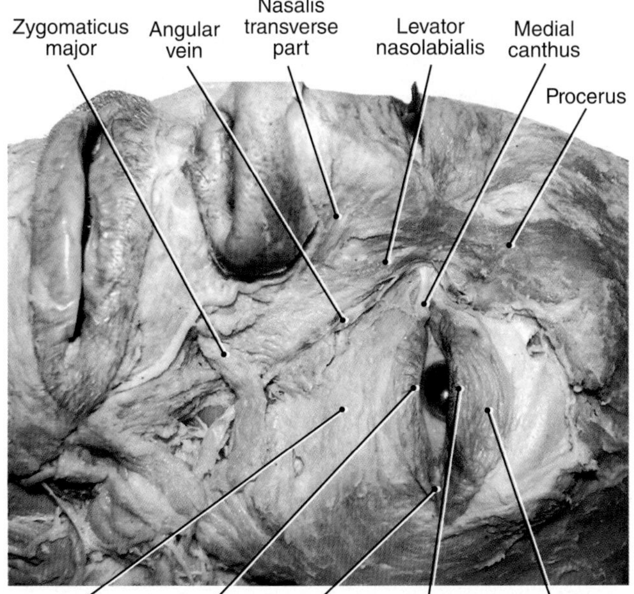

Fig. 24.23 Anterior view of the external orbit with the skin reflected superiorly, revealing canthi, tarsal plates, angular vein, and key muscles.

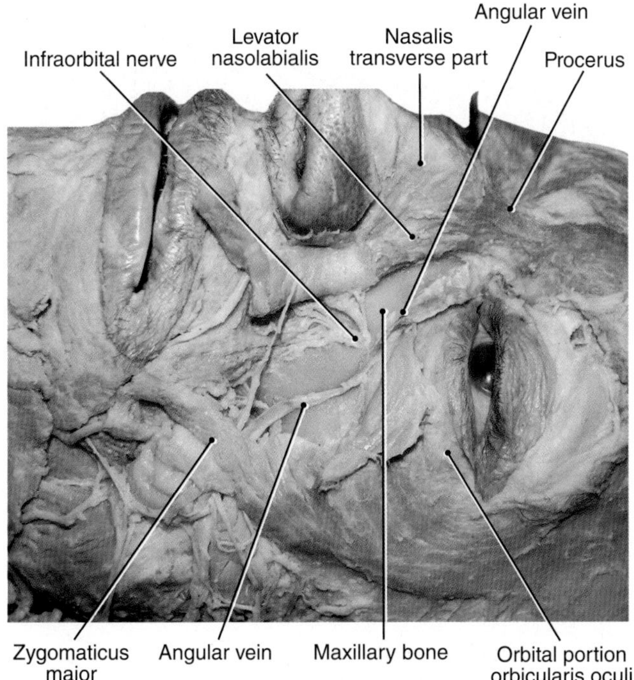

Fig. 24.24 Anterior view of the external orbit, nose, and maxilla.

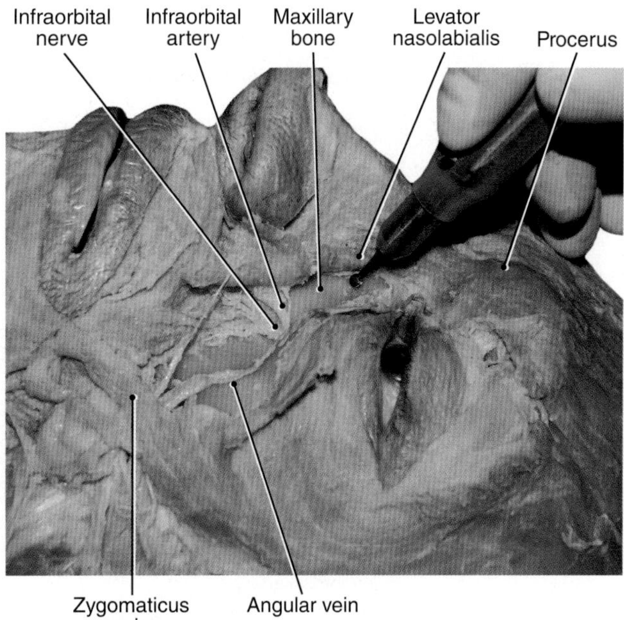

Fig. 24.25 Anterolateral view of the orbit with the skin and subcutaneous tissues removed and the orbital part of orbicularis oculi muscle reflected.

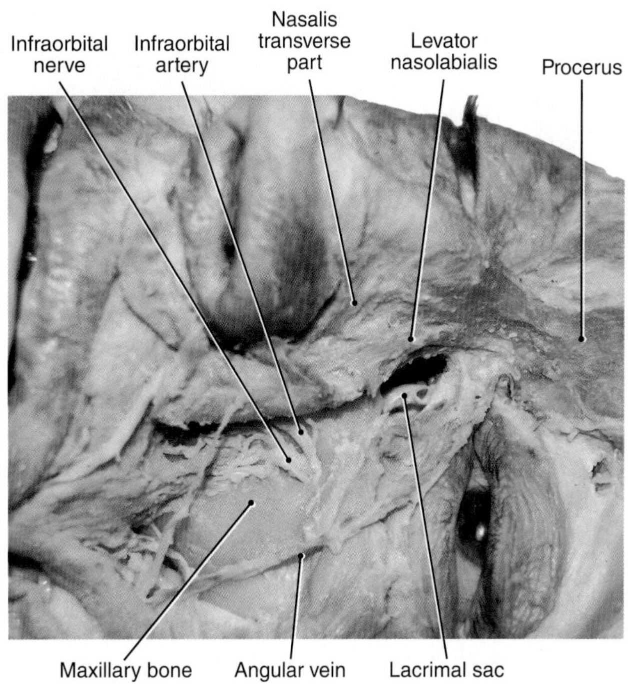

Fig. 24.26 Anterior view of the external orbit, highlighting the medial region with the skin and subcutaneous tissues removed.

- **With an electric saw, cut the area inferior to the medial canthus and the inferomedial portion of the infraorbital margin (Fig. 24.25).**
- **Identify the nasolacrimal duct within the lacrimal canal (Fig. 24.26 and Plate 24.4).**

ANATOMY **NOTE**

Excess lacrimal fluid is drained by the *puncta* into *canaliculi*, which drain the fluid to the lacrimal sac. From this sac, the nasolacrimal duct passes into the nasal cavity.

- **If time permits, remove the eyeball en bloc with the surrounding extraocular muscles (Fig. 24.27).**

DISSECTION **TIP**

The sclera is usually compressed and distorted. To restore its original shape, inject water into the eyeball with a hypodermic needle attached to a syringe (Fig. 24.28). Once the shape of the *sclera* has been restored, observe the extraocular muscle attachments (Fig. 24.29).

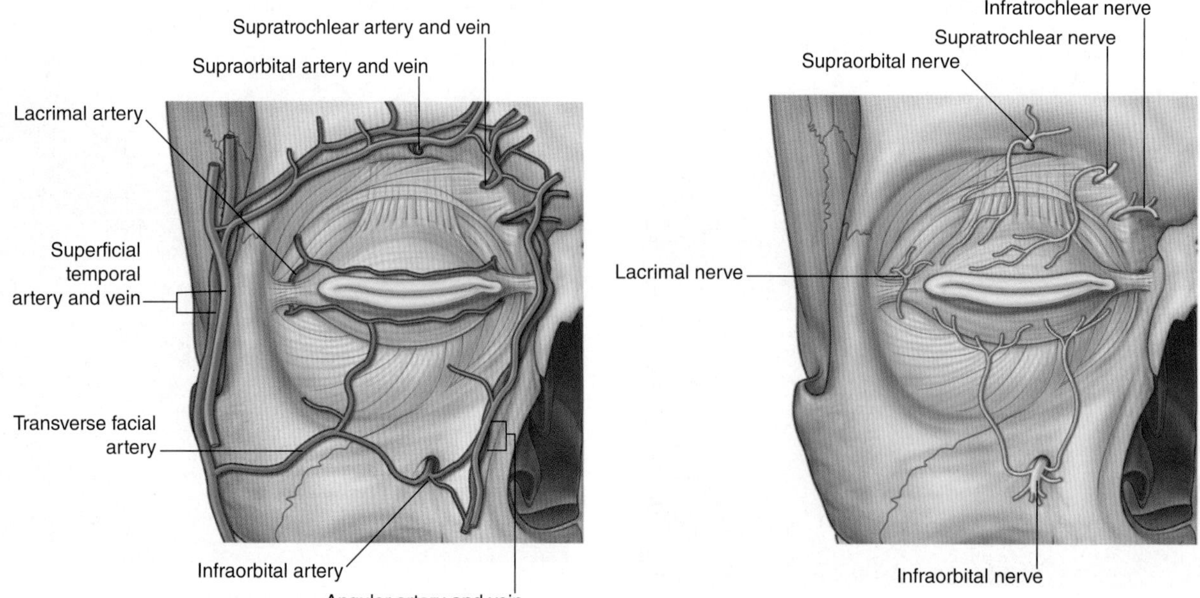

Plate 24.4 Anterior view of the vessels around the eye. (From Drake RL et al. *Gray's Anatomy for Students*, 5th edition, Philadelphia, Elsevier, 2024.)

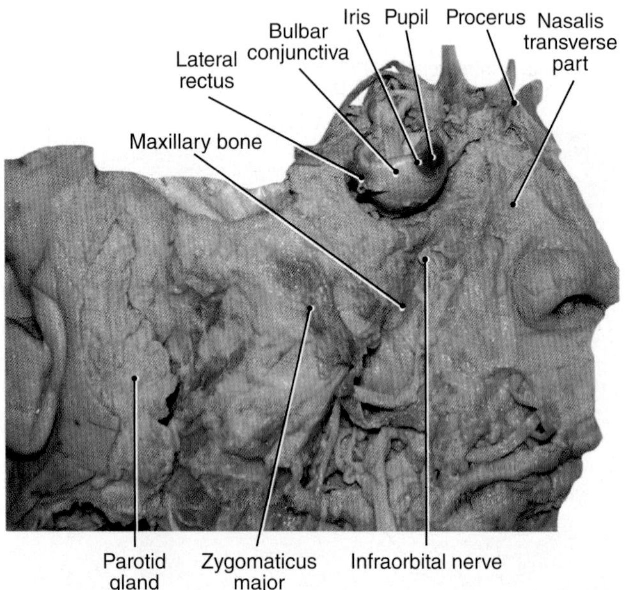

Fig. 24.27 Lateral craniotomy view of the orbit with the skin and subcutaneous tissue removed and an osteotomy to the zygomatic bone, revealing the eyeball, musculature, and parotid gland.

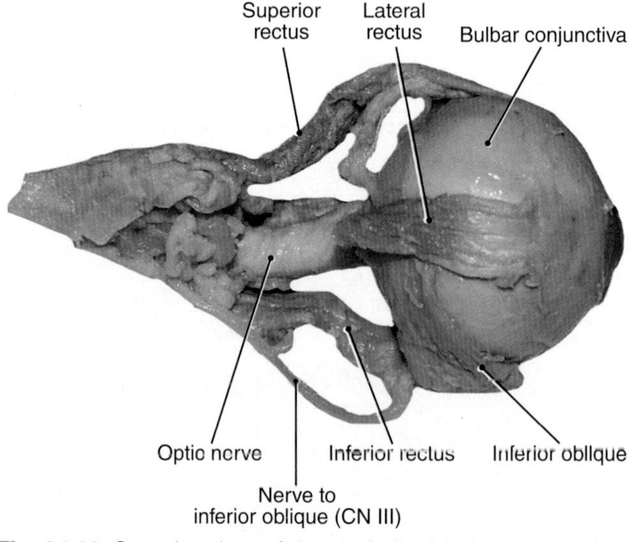

Fig. 24.29 Superior view of the eyeball with the extraocular muscles removed from the orbit.

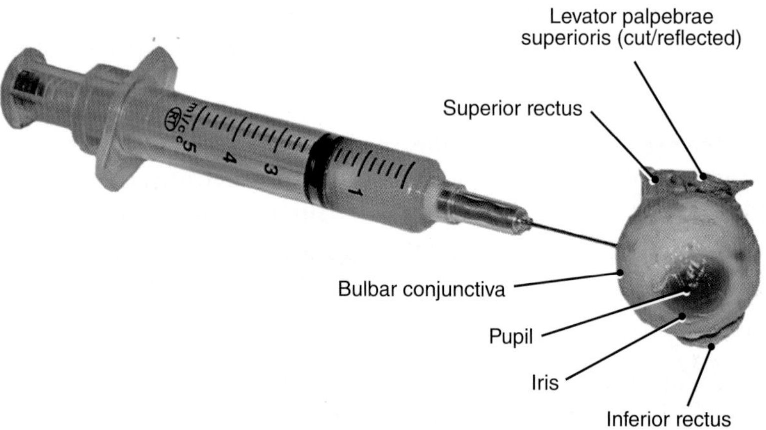

Fig. 24.28 Anterosuperior view of the eyeball removed from the orbit, with fluid injected to maintain its morphologic shape.

- **With a scalpel, cut the *optic nerve* and note the thick dura mater encircling it.**
- **At the middle of the cross-section of the optic nerve, observe the small lumen that represents the central retinal artery (Fig. 24.30).**
- **Have a classmate hold the sclera firmly with their fingers (Fig. 24.31).**
- **Carefully incise the sclera with a scalpel (Fig. 24.32).**
- **On the hemisected orbit, identify the *limbus*, which is the junction of the cornea and the sclera (Fig. 24.33).**
- **The space between the iris and cornea is the anterior chamber. This is usually filled with the aqueous humor, but in the cadaver it will be empty (Fig. 24.34).**

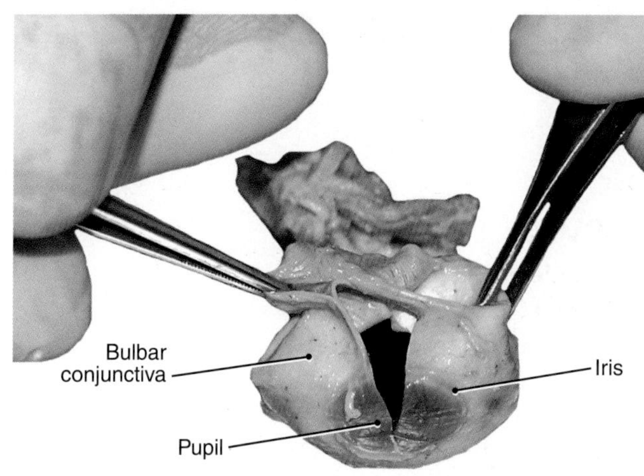

Fig. 24.32 Anterosuperior view of the eyeball removed from the orbit.

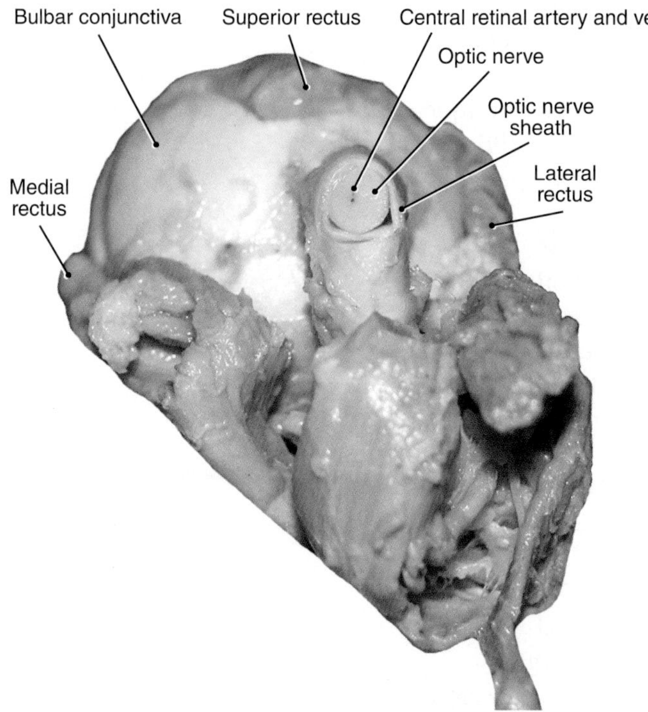

Fig. 24.30 Posterior view of the eyeball with the extraocular muscles removed from orbit.

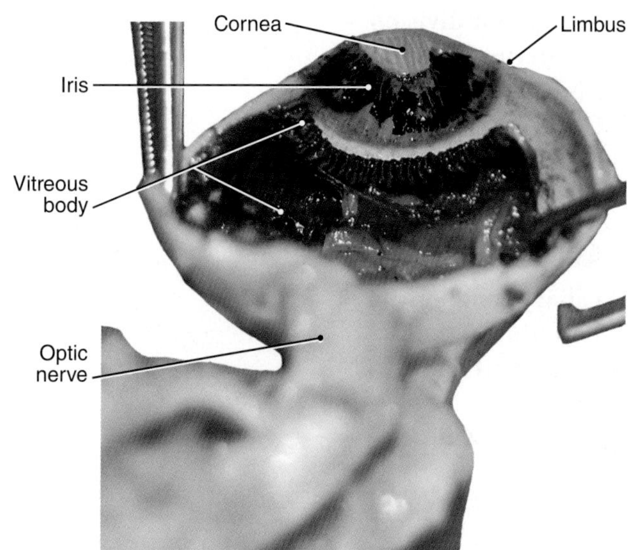

Fig. 24.33 Sagittal section of the eyeball with vitreous humor removed.

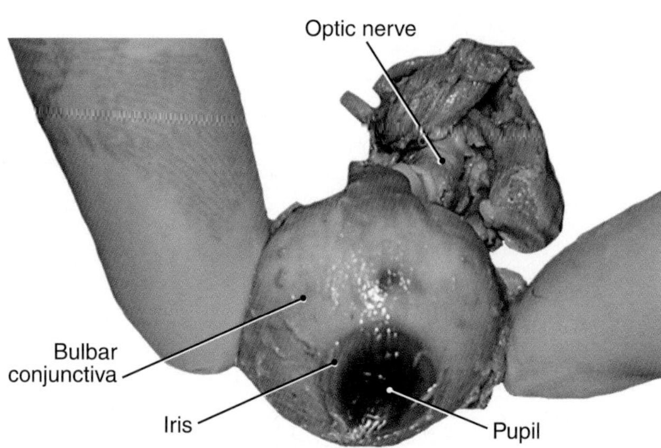

Fig. 24.31 Anterosuperior view of the eyeball with the extraocular muscles cut and reflected.

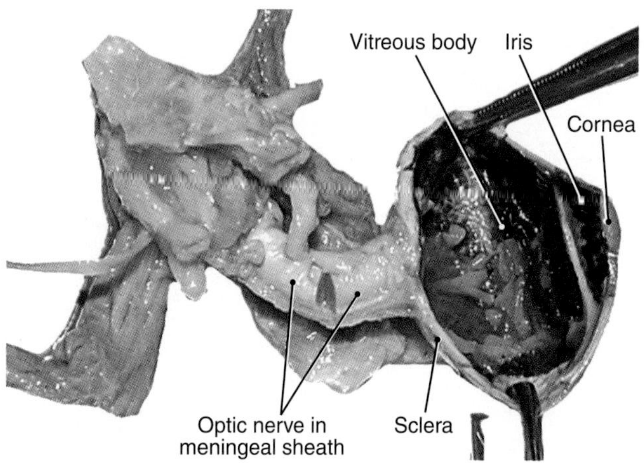

Fig. 24.34 Sagittal section of the eyeball removed from the orbit.

LABORATORY IDENTIFICATION CHECKLIST

NERVES

- ☐ Trochlear
- ☐ Frontal
  - ☐ Supratrochlear
  - ☐ Supraorbital
- ☐ Lacrimal
- ☐ Nasociliary
  - ☐ Posterior ethmoidal (inconstant)
  - ☐ Anterior ethmoidal
  - ☐ Infratrochlear
  - ☐ Long ciliary
- ☐ Oculomotor
  - ☐ Superior division
  - ☐ Inferior division
- ☐ Abducens
- ☐ Optic
- ☐ Short ciliary (8–10)
- ☐ Infraorbital

GANGLION/FASCIA/FAT

- ☐ Ciliary ganglion
- ☐ Periorbita
- ☐ Periorbital fat
- ☐ Trochlea
- ☐ Anulus of Zinn

ARTERIES

- ☐ Ophthalmic
  - ☐ Anterior ethmoidal
  - ☐ Posterior ethmoidal
  - ☐ Central retinal
  - ☐ Lacrimal

VEINS

- ☐ Superior ophthalmic
- ☐ Inferior ophthalmic

MUSCLES

- ☐ Procerus

Recti

- ☐ Superior rectus
- ☐ Inferior rectus
- ☐ Medial rectus
- ☐ Lateral rectus

Obliques

- ☐ Superior oblique
- ☐ Inferior oblique
- ☐ Levator palpebrae superioris

BONES

- ☐ Frontal
- ☐ Lacrimal
- ☐ Maxilla
- ☐ Ethmoid
- ☐ Zygomatic

GLAND

- ☐ Lacrimal

SINUSES

- ☐ Frontal
- ☐ Ethmoidal
  - ☐ Anterior cells
  - ☐ Middle cells
  - ☐ Posterior cells

BEFORE YOU BEGIN

Identify the following bones in your atlas, text, and on a skull:

- Petrous part of temporal bone
- Squamous part of temporal bone
- Petrosquamous fissure (at junction of petrous and squamous parts of the temporal bone)
- Arcuate eminence (overlies anterior semicircular canal)
- Internal acoustic meatus
- Hiatus of facial canal (greater petrosal nerve exits temporal bone from here)
- Groove for superior petrosal sinus
- Tegmen tympani (roof of middle ear between petrosquamous fissure and hiatus of facial canal)
- Jugular foramen
- Tympanic part of temporal bone (provides much of bony wall of external acoustic meatus)
- Mandibular fossa
- Petrotympanic fissure (for passage of chorda tympani)
- Styloid process and stylomastoid foramen

External Ear

The ear is subdivided into external, middle, and internal parts.

On the external ear of a classmate, identify the following structures (Fig. 25.1):

- Helix
- Antihelix and crura of antihelix
- Triangular fossa
- Concha
- Lobule
- Tragus
- Antitragus
- Intertragic notch
- External acoustic meatus

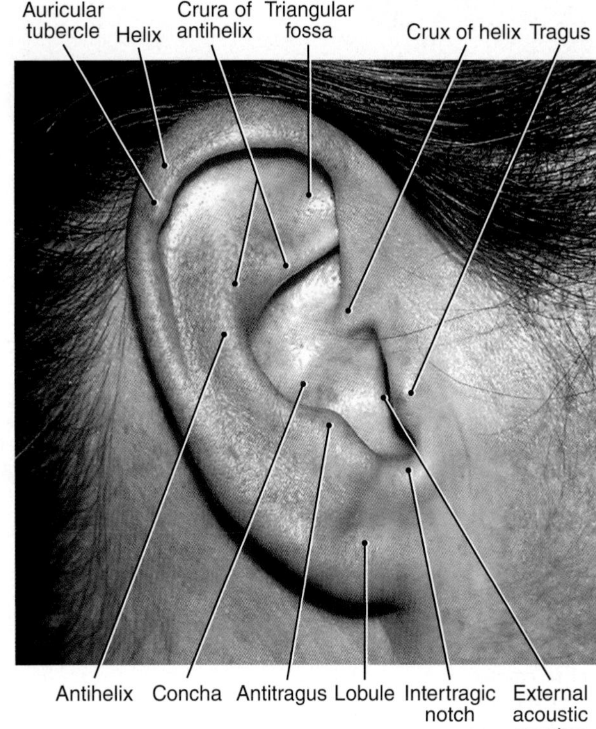

Fig. 25.1 External view of the external ear with various surface features.

OPTIONAL DISSECTION (MIDDLE EAR)

- **Students in most anatomy courses do not dissect the ear because it is a time-consuming dissection. This chapter presents a new, time-efficient method for exposing the structures of the middle ear.**
- **If time permits, create a skin flap from the helix to expose the part of the elastic fibrocartilage.**
- **Create a second skin flap at the lobule and note the dense, fibrous connective tissue.**
- **With your scalpel, make an incision posterior to the auricle toward the neck.**
- **Dissect away most of the soft tissue and the external acoustic meatus (Fig. 25.2).**
- **Remove any debris present in the remaining part of the external meatus.**

DISSECTION TIP

With the aid of an otoscope, attempt to inspect the tympanic membrane. Remove any wax (cerumen) that may obstruct your view.

- **Draw a line along the bony roof of the middle ear, the *tegmen tympani*, demarcating the length of the canal from the external acoustic meatus to the tympanic membrane.**
- **Draw two dashed lines at the outer borders of the meatus (Fig. 25.3).**

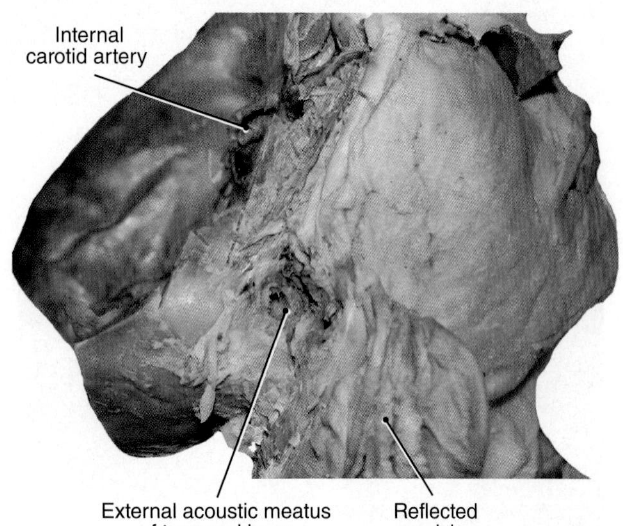

Fig. 25.2 Postcraniotomy reveals a lateral view of the middle cranial fossa with external ear reflected, highlighting the external acoustic meatus of temporal bone.

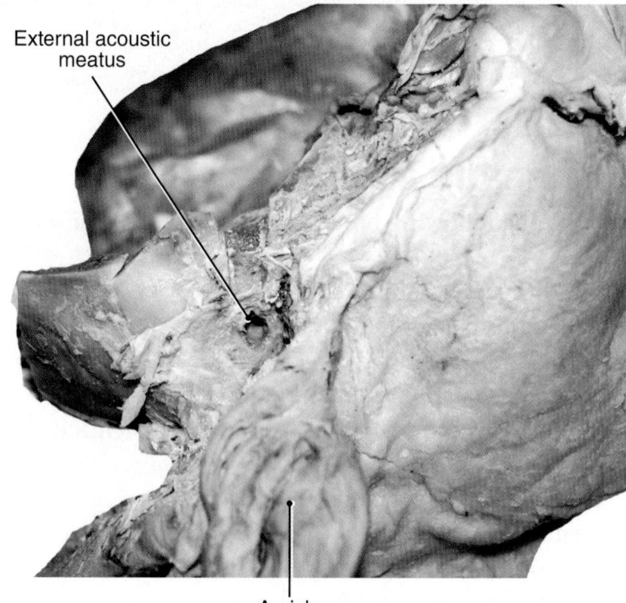

Fig. 25.4 Postcraniotomy view reveals the middle cranial fossa with the external ear reflected.

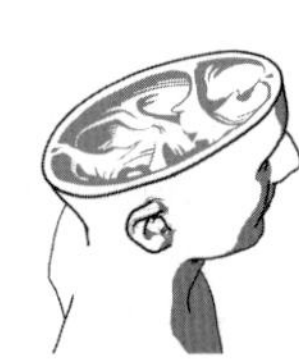

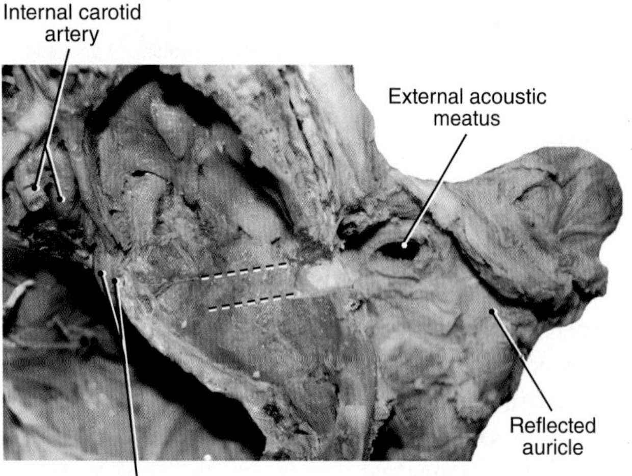

Fig. 25.3 Middle cranial fossa with external ear reflected, highlighting the external acoustic meatus, trigeminal nerve, and internal carotid artery. *Dashed lines* demarcate the lateral borders of the external acoustic meatus on tegmen tympani (roof of middle ear).

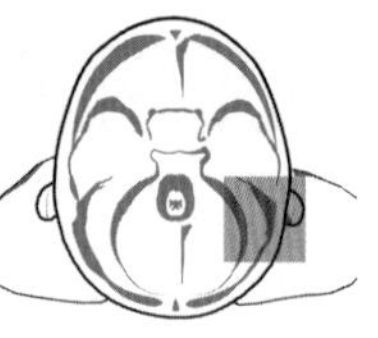

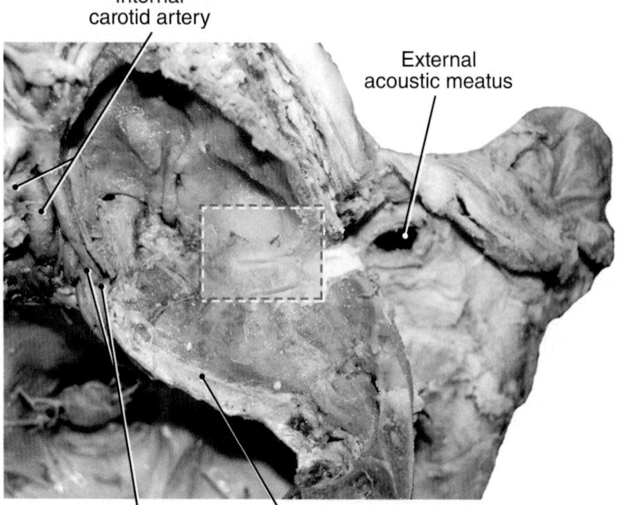

Fig. 25.5 Middle cranial fossa with external ear reflected; highlighted over tegmen tympani, *chisel marks* and *square* in center indicate lateral borders of external acoustic meatus.

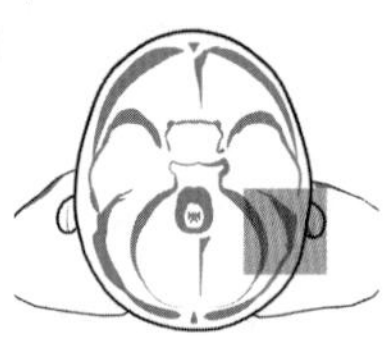

- **With a chisel and a mallet, remove a small piece of bone and expose the outer portion of the canal for inspection (Fig. 25.4).**
- **With a cotton swab or forceps, clean the acoustic meatus of debris and cerumen (Fig. 25.5).**

DISSECTION TIP

Do not place the swab or forceps too deeply into the canal to prevent damage to the tympanic membrane.

- **Continue the removal of bone with the chisel and the mallet on the surface of the tegmen tympani (see Fig. 25.5). The external acoustic meatus is about 3 to 4 cm**

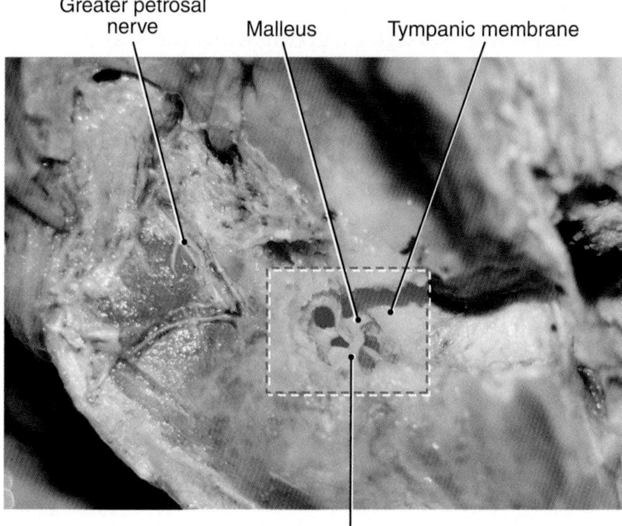

Fig. 25.6 The tegmen tympani over the middle ear is removed, exposing tympanic membrane and two auditory ossicles.

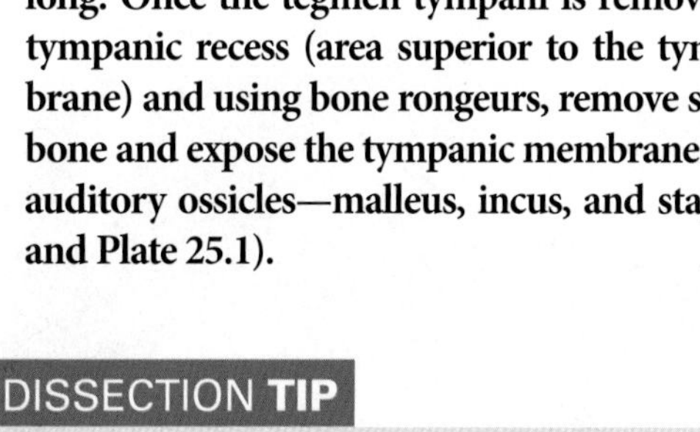

long. Once the tegmen tympani is removed to the epitympanic recess (area superior to the tympanic membrane) and using bone rongeurs, remove small pieces of bone and expose the tympanic membrane and the three auditory ossicles—malleus, incus, and stapes (Fig. 25.6 and Plate 25.1).

DISSECTION **TIP**

When exposing the tegmen tympani to reveal the malleus, incus, and stapes, grasp the outer part of the tympanic membrane and pull it gently upward to maintain the position of the ossicles.

- **At the final stage of dissection, cut the connective tissue layer covering the external acoustic meatus and appreciate the orientation of the tympanic membrane (see Fig. 25.6).**
- **The membrane is positioned obliquely in the external acoustic meatus at an angle of about 55 degrees (Fig. 25.7).**

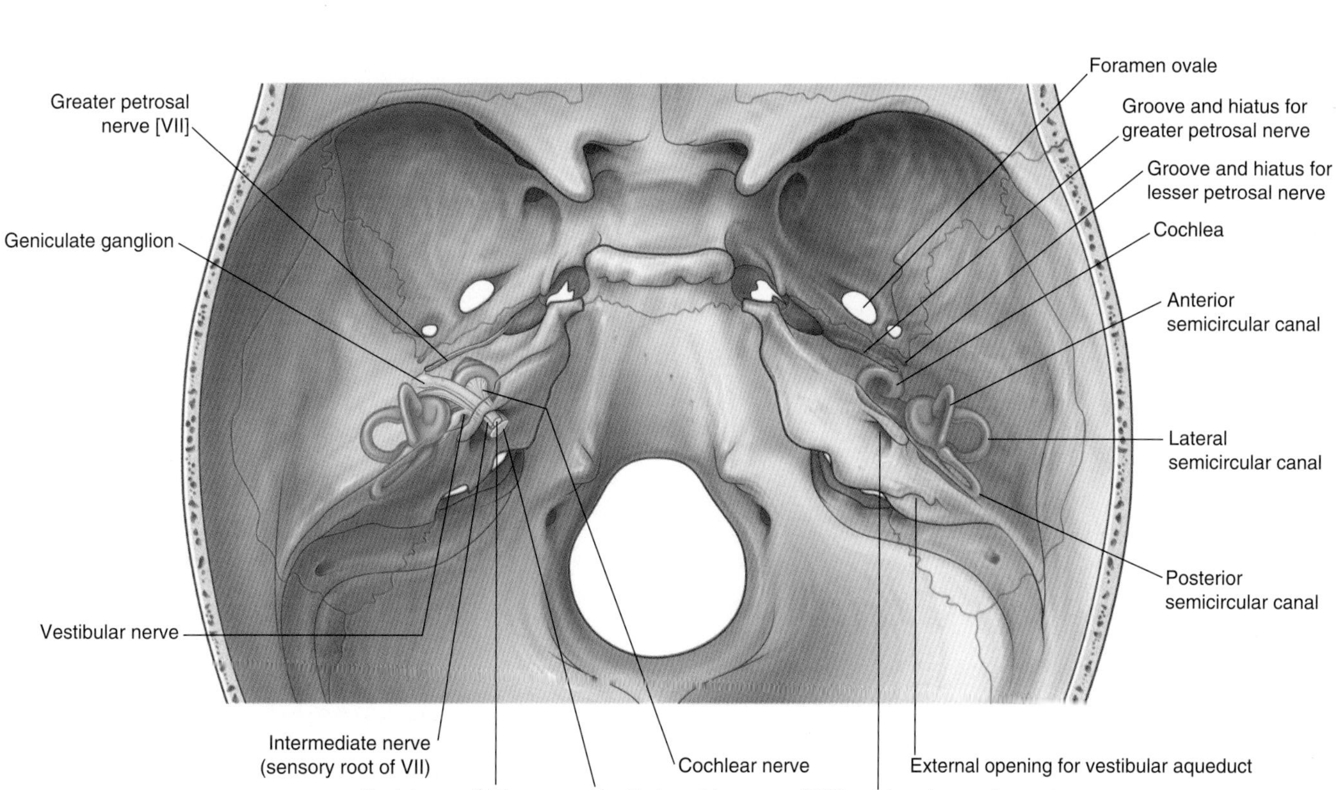

Plate 25.1 Superior projection of the internal ear in the temporal bone. (From Drake RL et al. *Gray's Atlas of Anatomy*, 3rd edition, Philadelphia, Elsevier, 2021.)

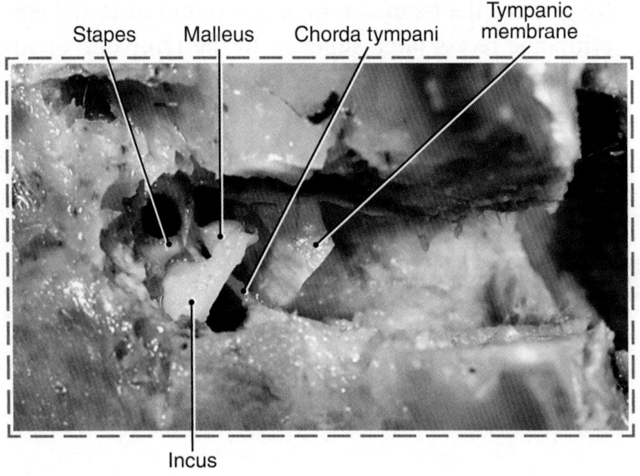

Fig. 25.7 Magnified view of the external acoustic meatus and middle ear, revealing the tympanic membrane, auditory ossicles (malleus, incus, stapes), and chorda tympani.

- **Note the following relationships:**
  - **Stapedius muscle inserting onto the stapes.**
  - **Tendon of the tensor tympani muscle inserting onto the malleus.**
  - **Malleus attached to the tympanic membrane.**

DISSECTION **TIP**

Dissecting the internal ear cavity is time-consuming; more importantly, however, inspection requires a dissecting microscope to identify the structures clearly.

LABORATORY IDENTIFICATION CHECKLIST

NERVES

- ☐ Trigeminal
  - ☐ Mandibular (V3)
- ☐ Nervus intermedius
- ☐ Greater petrosal
- ☐ Facial
- ☐ Chorda tympani
- ☐ Vestibulocochlear
- ☐ Vagus

GANGLIA

- ☐ Trigeminal
- ☐ Geniculate

ARTERY

- ☐ Internal carotid

MUSCLES

- ☐ Tensor tympani
- ☐ Stapedius
- ☐ Auricularis

BONES

- ☐ Petrous part of temporal bone
- ☐ Tegmen tympani
- ☐ Auditory ossicles
  - ☐ Malleus
  - ☐ Incus
  - ☐ Stapes

OTHER STRUCTURES

- ☐ External acoustic meatus
- ☐ Tympanic membrane
- ☐ Oval window

CARTILAGE

- ☐ Helix
- ☐ Antihelix
- ☐ Tragus
- ☐ Antitragus
- ☐ Auricular tubercle (of Darwin)

DISSECTION STEPS

- **Exposure of the contents of the nasal cavity requires a midsagittal transection through the head (Fig. 26.1).**

DISSECTION TIP

Electric saws are usually too small for transection of the head. Make sure that one of your classmates holds the cadaver head firmly as you cut with the saw.

- **Place the saw as close as possible to the midline. Begin the cut externally from the face toward the midportion of the head (Fig. 26.2).**
- **Split the head in half and choose one of the two halves to decapitate (Figs. 26.3 and 26.4).**
- **Clean away soft tissues or any bony fragments after the hemisection (compare Fig. 26.4 with Fig. 26.5).**
- **Identify several landmarks as indicated on the dissection photographs of the hemisected head.**
- **The nasal cavities extend from the nares anteriorly to the choanae posteriorly, constituting the *nasal cavity proper*. Identify the superior, middle, and inferior**

Frontal bone
Nasal bone
Ala
Nares
Philtrum

Fig. 26.2 Anterolateral view of the face with previous craniotomy, demonstrating a sagittal cut of the head.

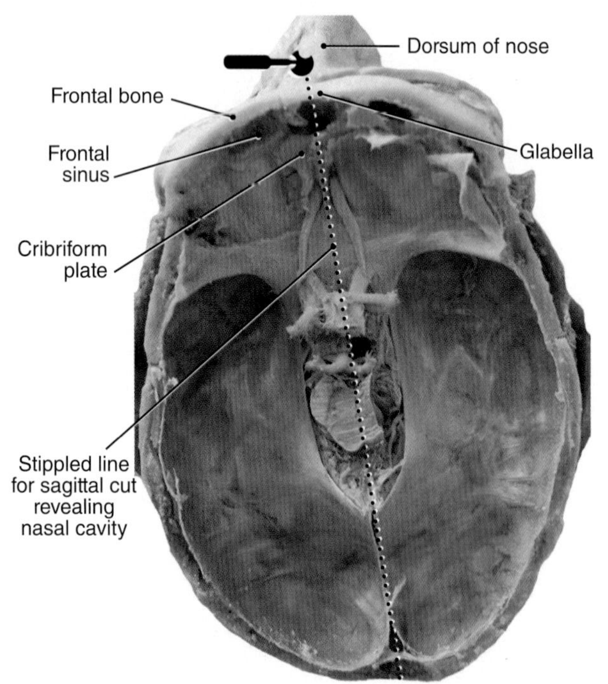

Fig. 26.1 Craniotomy view with *dashed line* for sagittal section.

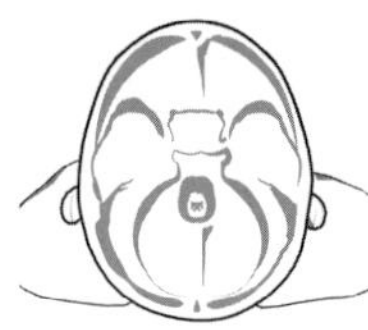

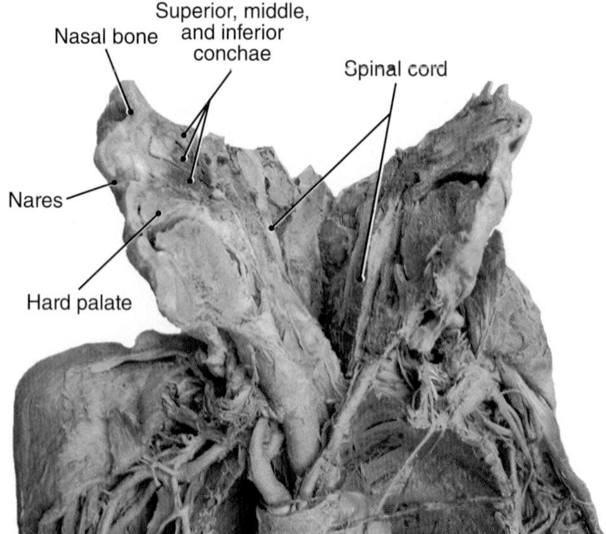

Fig. 26.3 Anterior view of the sagittal cut; revealing the nasal septum on the left and section through the conchae on the right.

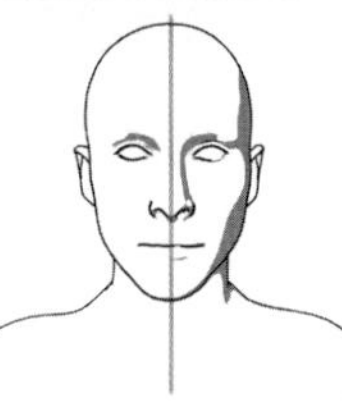

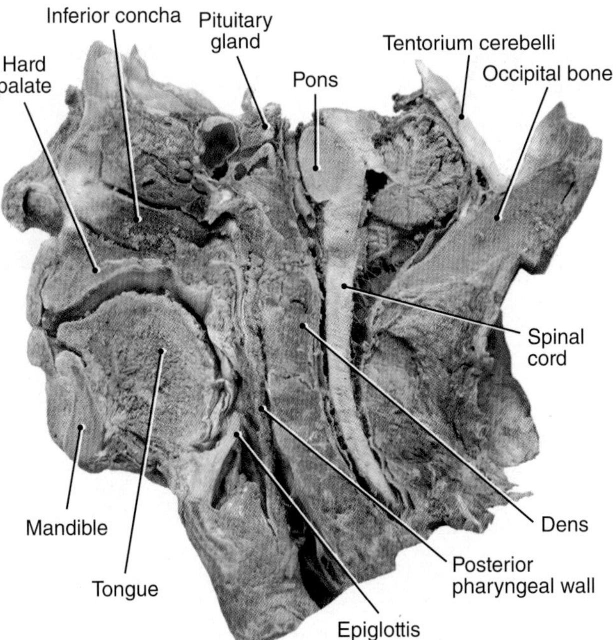

Fig. 26.4 Sagittal view of the nasal and oral cavities revealing the nasal bone, cartilage, concha, and openings. Structures of the mouth and pharynx include the hard palate, soft palate, tongue, mandible, epiglottis, and posterior pharyngeal wall.

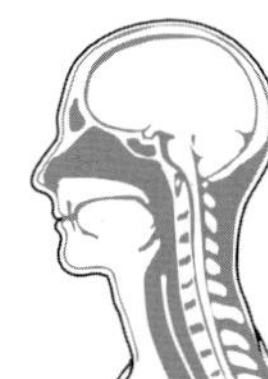

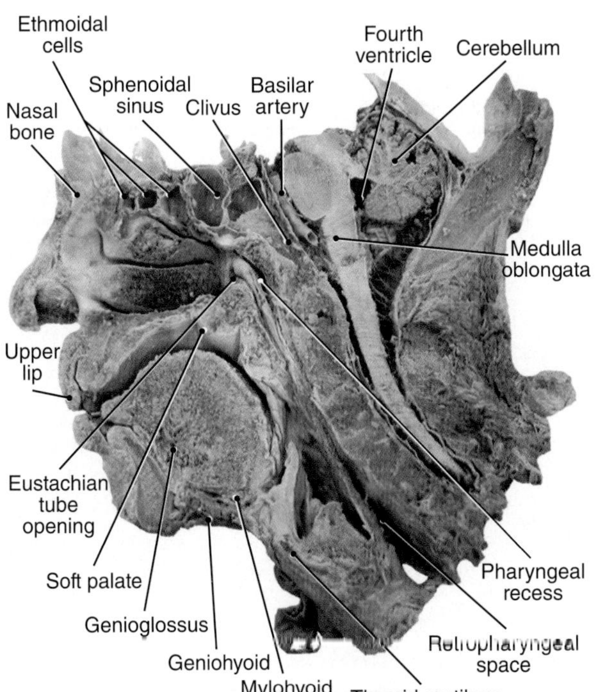

Fig. 26.5 Sagittal view of the nasal and oral regions. Nasal region structures include the sphenoidal sinus, ethmoidal sinus (anterior, middle, and posterior cells), nasal conchae, and eustachian tube opening. Oral structures include the lips, hard and soft palate, tongue, oral floor muscles (genioglossus, geniohyoid, mylohyoid), epiglottis, pharyngeal recess, and retropharyngeal space.

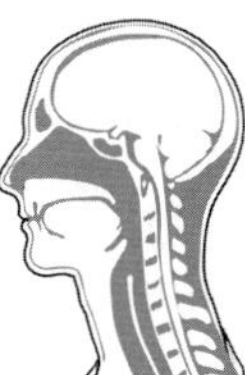

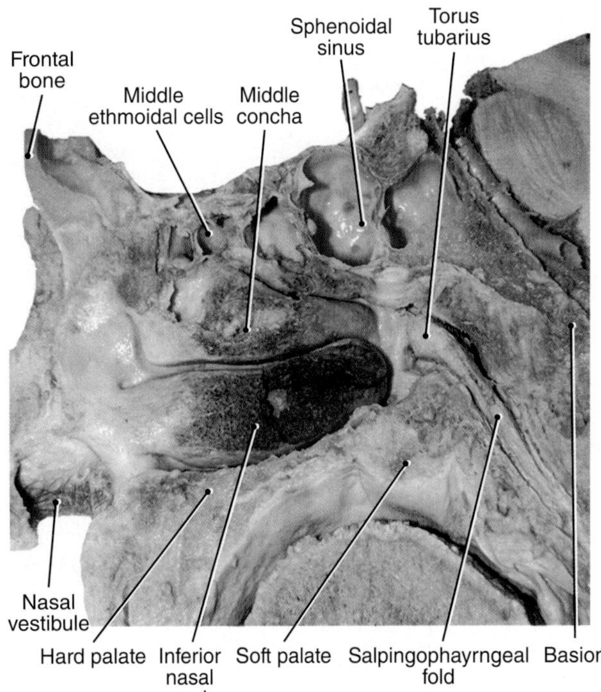

Fig. 26.6 Sagittal view of the nasal cavity revealing sphenoidal, ethmoidal, and frontal sinuses; concha; nasal bone; torus tubarius; and salpingopharyngeal fold.

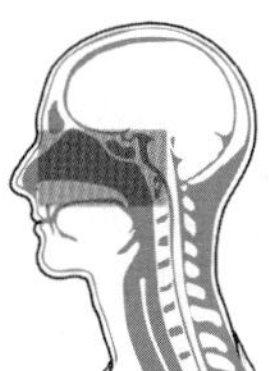

nasal *conchae*, which are located within the nasal cavity proper (Figs. 26.6 and 26.7).

- **Identify the *superior meatus*, the space between the superior and middle conchae.**
- **Continue inferiorly and identify the space between the middle and inferior conchae, the *middle meatus*.**
- **Finally, identify the space between the inferior concha and the hard palate, the *inferior meatus* (see Figs. 26.6 and 26.7).**
- **Posterior to the superior concha is a space referred to as the *sphenoethmoidal recess*. Identify the opening for the sphenoidal sinus into this recess (see Figs. 26.6 and 26.7).**

DISSECTION TIP

Some specimens have an increased thickness of the nasal mucosa (see Figs. 26.6 and 26.7).

DISSECTION TIP

In most cadavers it is necessary to break away part of the thin, medial wall of the sphenoidal sinus to gain access to its interior. Some specimens may also have a "supreme" concha.

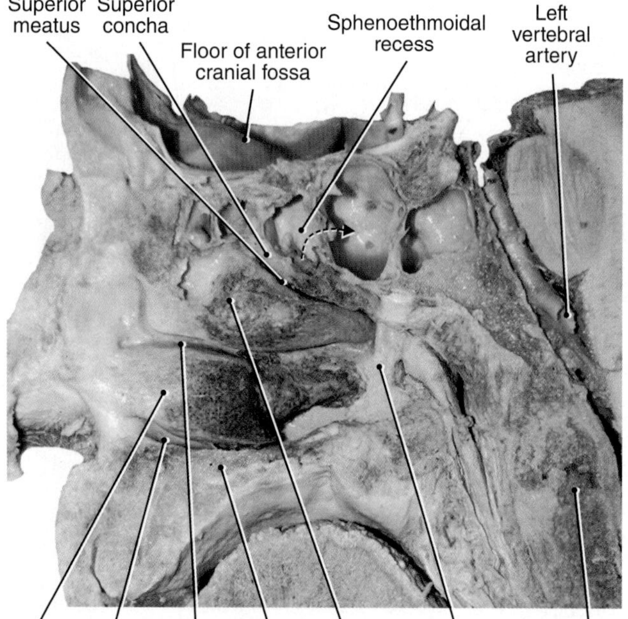

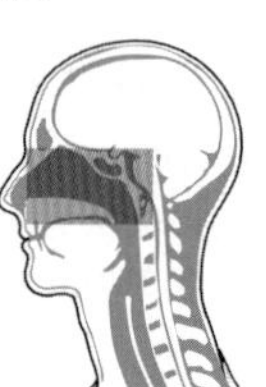

Fig. 26.7 Sagittal view of the nasal cavity revealing the sphenoidal and ethmoid sinuses and nasal concha highlighting drainage pathways that include sphenoethmoidal recess and meatus associated with superior, middle, and inferior conchae.

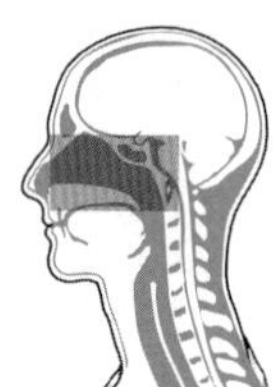

Fig. 26.8 Sagittal view of the nasal cavity with the middle concha reflected, revealing opening of ethmoidal cells, ethmoidal bulla, semilunar hiatus, and maxillary sinus opening.

- **With forceps, lift the middle nasal meatus upward and identify the ethmoidal bulla.**

ANATOMY **NOTE**

The ethmoidal bulla can be oversized from hypertrophy of the ethmoidal cells.

- **Locate the opening of the ethmoidal infundibulum into the semilunar hiatus (Fig. 26.8).**
- **With scissors or a scalpel, cut the middle nasal concha away from its junction with the lateral wall of the nasal cavity and completely expose the middle meatus (Fig. 26.9).**
- **Identify the anterior, middle, and posterior *ethmoidal cells.* In the superior nasal meatus, find the ostia of the posterior ethmoidal cells (see Fig. 26.9 and Plate 26.1).**

ANATOMY **NOTE**

The *hiatus semilunaris* is the long, semicircular groove into which the frontonasal duct drains (drainage of frontal sinus through the infundibulum), as well as the anterior ethmoidal cells.

- **Identify the opening of the maxillary sinus. Pass a probe into this opening.**

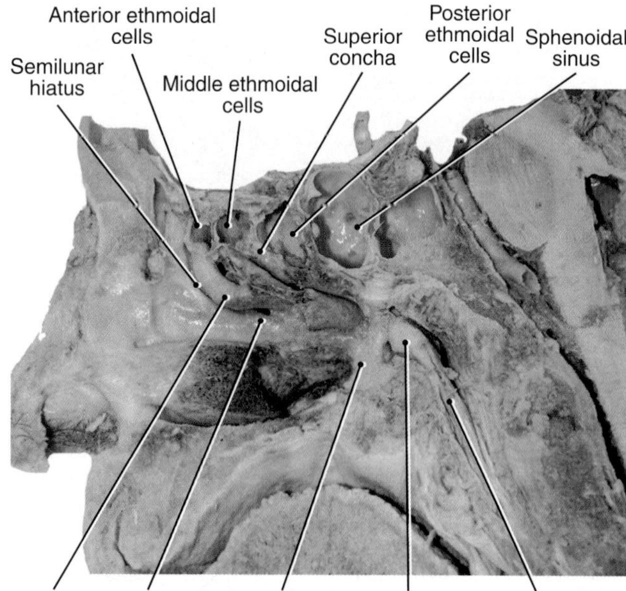

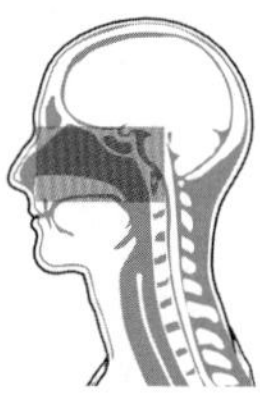

Fig. 26.9 Sagittal view of the nasal cavity with the superior concha cut and the middle concha removed revealing the sphenoidal sinus and posterior, middle, and anterior ethmoidal cells. Middle concha removed, highlighting the ethmoidal bulla, semilunar hiatus, and maxillary sinus opening.

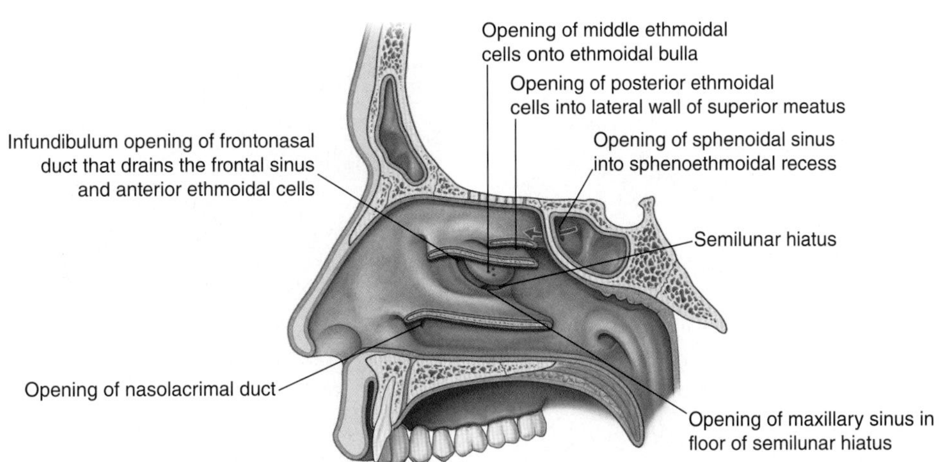

Plate 26.1 A lateral view of the structures of the nasal cavity, with conchae cut away. (From Drake RL et al. *Gray's Anatomy for Students*, 5th edition, Philadelphia, Elsevier, 2024.)

DISSECTION **TIP**

Inspect the area of the middle meatus to determine whether there may be accessory openings for the maxillary sinus.

- **The *ethmoidal bulla* is formed by the bulging of ethmoidal cells into the middle meatus (see Fig. 26.9).**
- **Remove the anterior half of the inferior nasal concha and identify the opening of the nasolacrimal duct (Fig. 26.10).**
- **Place a probe in the nasolacrimal duct.**
- **Before dissection of the pterygopalatine fossa, identify the opening to the auditory or pharyngotympanic tube *(eustachian tube)* and place a probe into it (see Fig. 26.10).**
- **Identify the elevation of the auditory tube and its muscular ridge, the *salpingopharyngeal fold.* At the opening of the eustachian tube, dissect away the mucous membrane (Fig. 26.11).**
- **Identify the *levator* veli palatini muscle (Fig. 26.12).**
- **Anterior to the levator veli palatini, dissect out fat and other connective tissues (Fig. 26.13).**
- **Identify the *tensor* veli palatini muscle (see Fig. 26.13).**

DISSECTION **TIP**

The tensor veli palatini and levator veli palatini muscles are easy to distinguish because of the white, *tendinous* fibers of the *tensor* veli palatini (see Fig. 26.13).

- **Lift the soft tissues and mucous membranes at the space posterior to the nasal conchae and the tensor veli palatini (in essence, the posterior plate of the pterygoid process of the sphenoid bone) (Fig. 26.14).**
- **Cut the posterior one-third of the middle and superior conchae and remove the mucosa and soft tissues to expose the palatine bone (Fig. 26.15).**

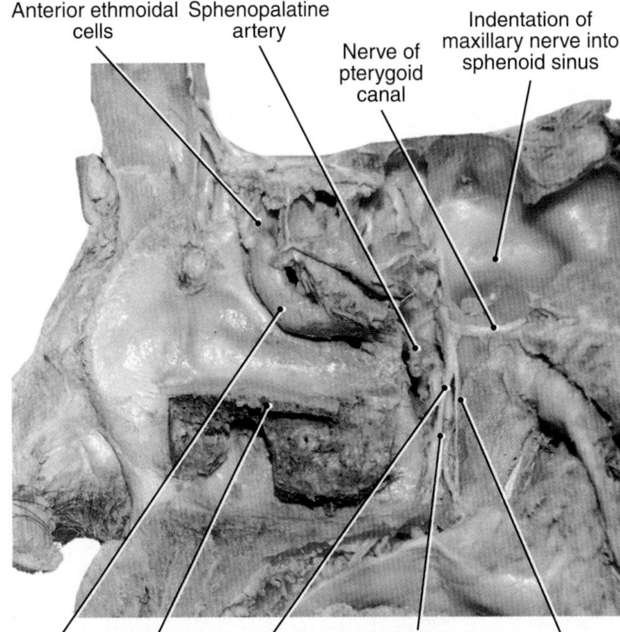

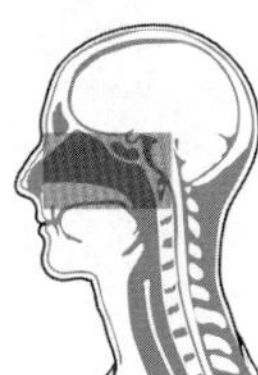

Fig. 26.10 Sagittal view of the nasal cavity with the middle concha removed and the inferior concha cut and partially removed, revealing drainage pathway of nasolacrimal duct and osteotomy into the pterygopalatine fossa. The pterygopalatine fossa includes the pterygopalatine ganglion, nerve of pterygoid canal, greater and lesser palatine nerves, and the sphenopalatine and descending palatine arteries.

DISSECTION **TIP**

The palatine bone is thin, and you can identify the course of the greater and lesser palatine nerves and vessels before removing it.

- **With a small electric drill, cut away the palatine bone, making a vertical cut from the sphenoidal sinus to**

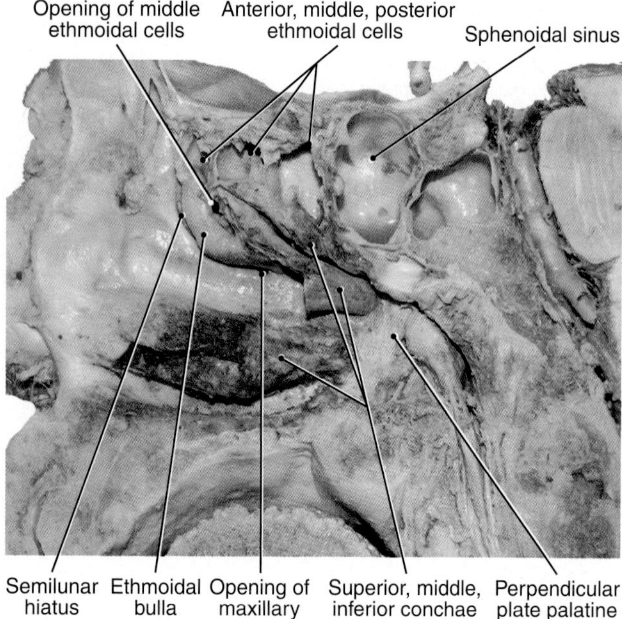

Fig. 26.11 Sagittal view of the nasal cavity revealing sphenoidal, posterior middle, and anterior ethmoidal cells. Middle concha removed, revealing the semilunar hiatus, ethmoid bulla, maxillary sinus opening, and superior, middle, and inferior conchae, as well as the perpendicular plate of the palatine bone.

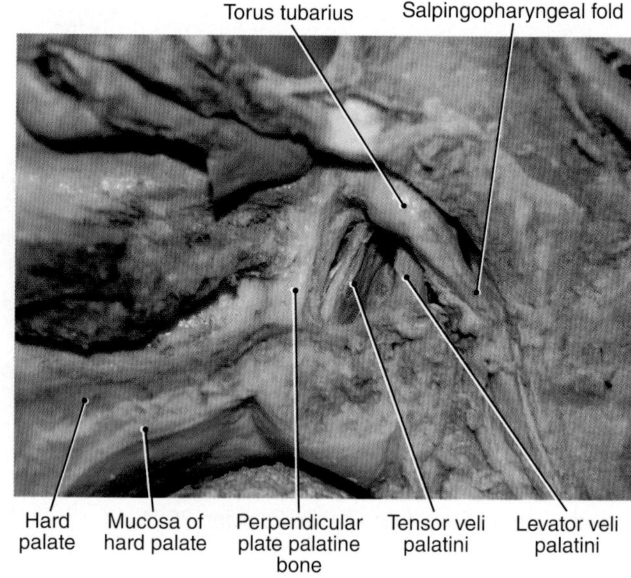

Fig. 26.13 Sagittal view of the nasal cavity highlighting the hard palate and revealing the tensor and levator veli palatini muscles, torus tubarius, and salpingopharyngeal fold.

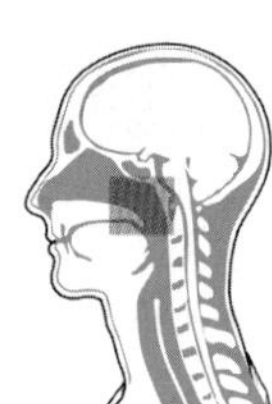

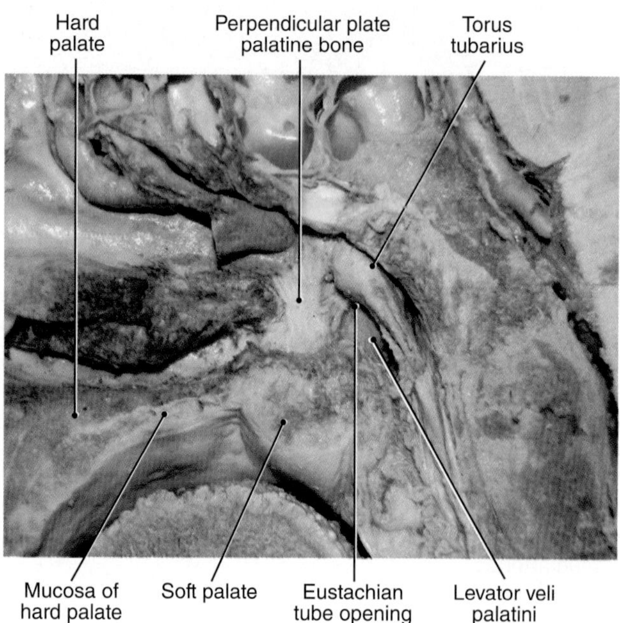

Fig. 26.12 Sagittal view of the nasal cavity revealing the hard and soft palate, torus tubarius, salpingopharyngeal fold, opening of the eustachian tube, and the levator veli palatini muscle.

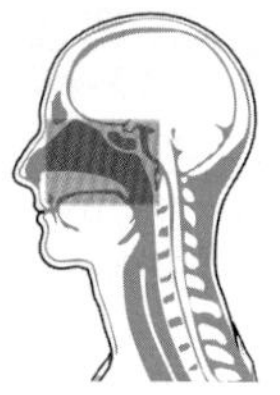

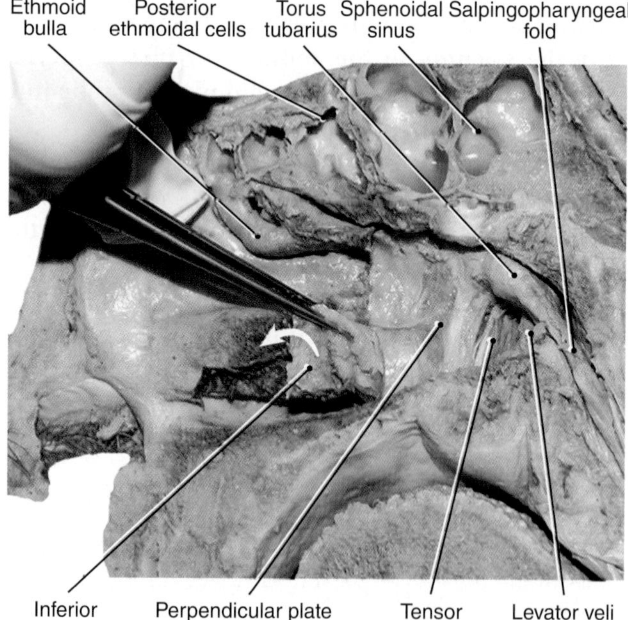

Fig. 26.14 Sagittal view of the nasal cavity with superior, middle, and inferior concha cut, revealing perpendicular plate of palatine bone, tensor and levator veli palatini, torus tubarius, and salpingopharyngeal fold.

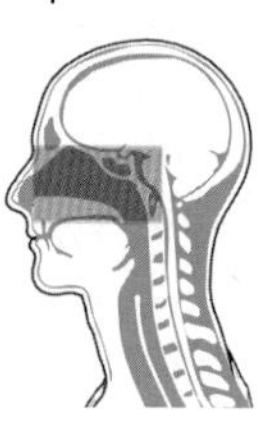

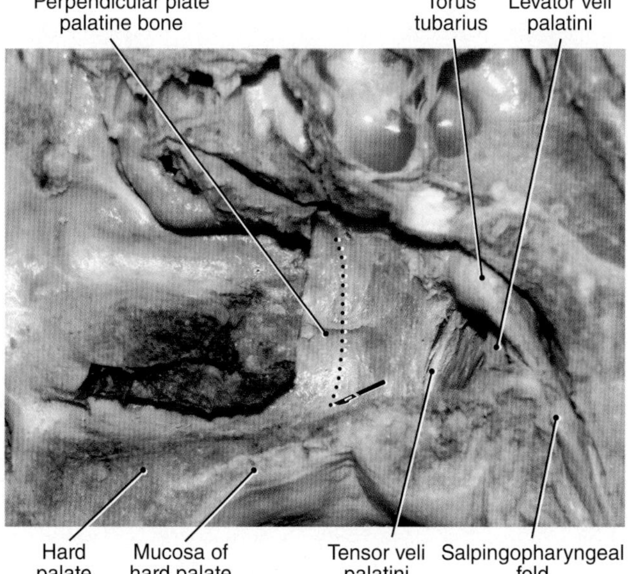

Fig. 26.15 Sagittal view of the nasal cavity highlighting the perpendicular plate of palatine bone, tensor and levator veli palatini muscles, torus tubarius, and mucosa of hard palate.

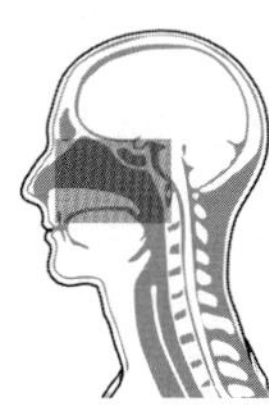

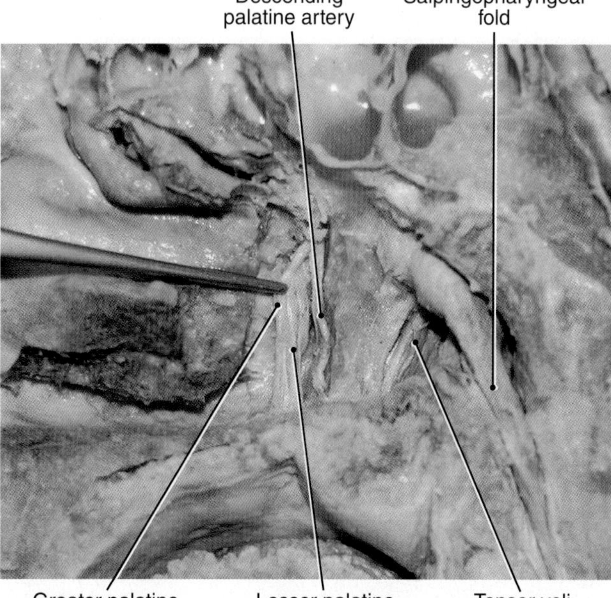

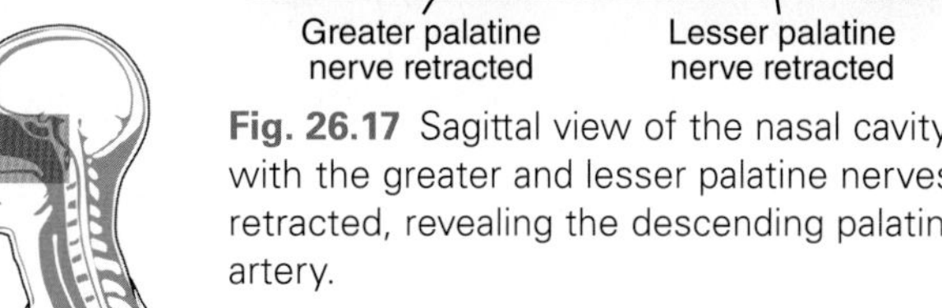

Fig. 26.17 Sagittal view of the nasal cavity with the greater and lesser palatine nerves retracted, revealing the descending palatine artery.

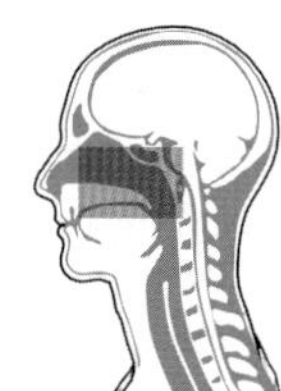

Fig. 26.16 Sagittal view of the nasal cavity highlighting the middle and superior conchae cut and perpendicular plate of palatine bone with small osteotomy to reveal pterygopalatine fossa structures.

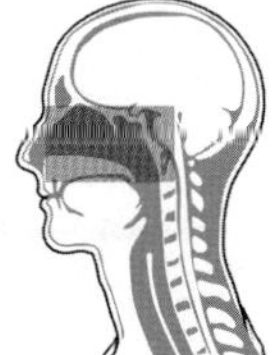

the hard palate and posteriorly to the middle concha (see Figs. 26.15 and 26.16).

- **First, expose the greater and lesser palatine nerves, as well as the descending palatine artery and the greater and lesser palatine arteries (Figs. 26.17 and 26.18).**
- **Continue drilling upward to the sphenoidal sinus. Identify the sphenopalatine artery and the pterygopalatine ganglion (Fig. 26.19 and Plate 26.2).**

DISSECTION **TIP**

In this part of dissection, use fine forceps and scissors to separate the delicate nerves and arteries.

- **Continue drilling posteriorly to the pterygopalatine ganglion and inferior to the sphenoidal sinus. Expose the *vidian nerve* (nerve to pterygoid canal) (Fig. 26.20).**

ANATOMY **NOTE**

The greater and deep petrosal nerves unite and form the nerve of the pterygoid canal. This nerve passes through the pterygoid canal of the sphenoid bone and then into the pterygopalatine fossa.

- **If time permits, drill away the sphenoidal sinus and expose the connection of the pterygopalatine ganglion with the maxillary nerve (Fig. 26.21).**
- **With scissors, reflect the oral mucosa from the hard palate and identify the distribution of the greater and lesser palatine nerves (Fig. 26.22).**
- **The lateral wall of the nasal cavity is dissected on one side of the head, as well as the pterygopalatine fossa. Dissect the nasal septum on the opposite side, i.e., the other hemisected part of the head (Fig. 26.23).**

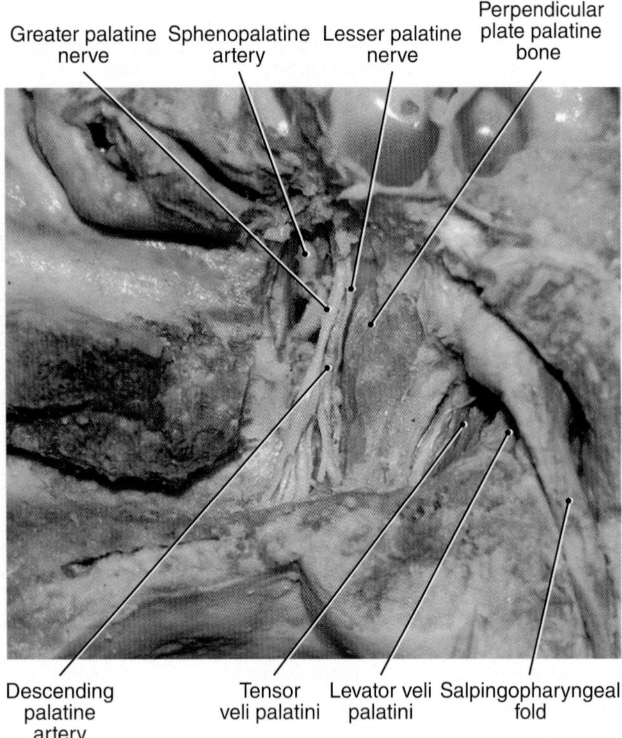

Fig. 26.18 Sagittal view of the nasal cavity following osteotomy of the perpendicular plate of the palatine bone revealing the sphenopalatine artery, greater and lesser palatine nerves, and descending palatine artery.

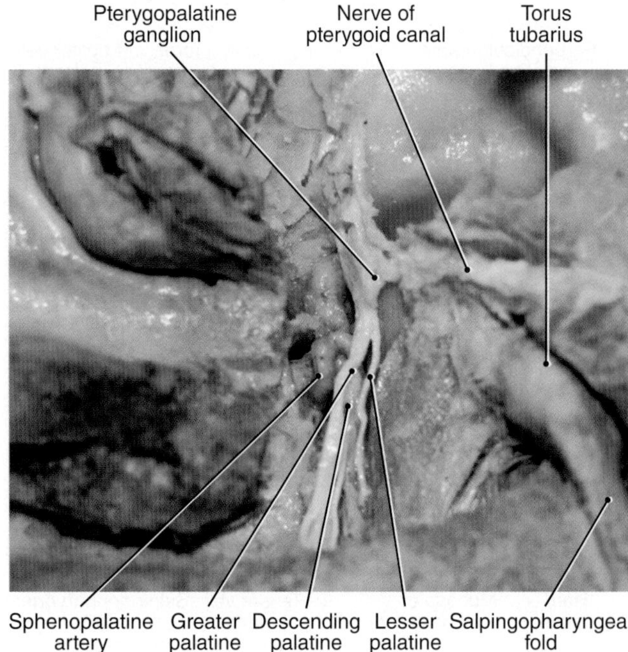

Fig. 26.19 Sagittal view of the nasal cavity following osteotomy of the perpendicular plate of the palatine bone revealing the sphenopalatine artery, pterygopalatine ganglion, nerve of pterygoid canal, greater and lesser palatine nerves, and descending palatine artery.

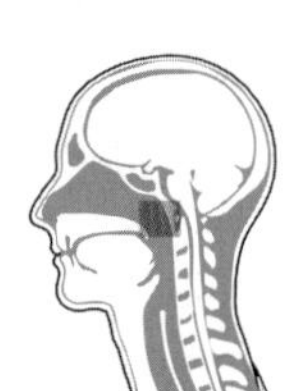

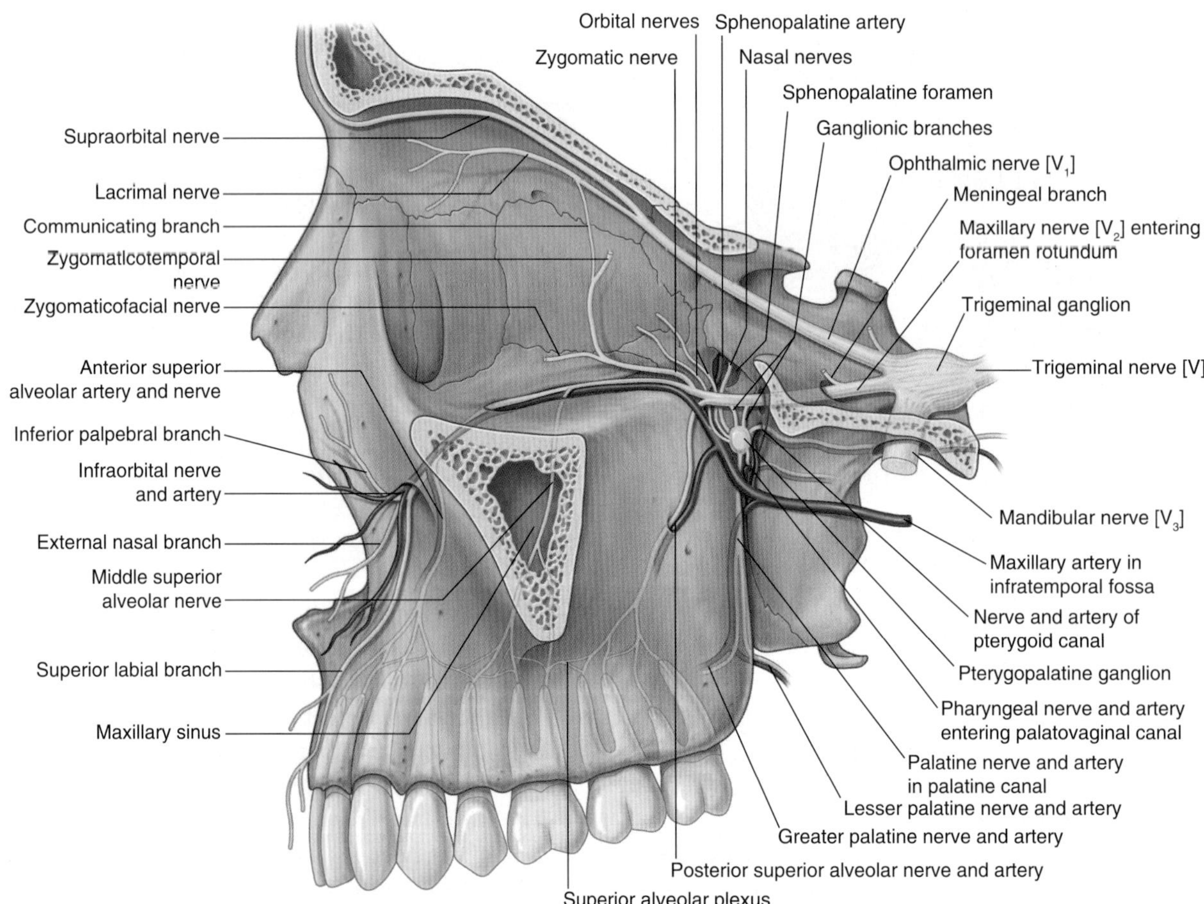

Plate 26.2 Nerves and arteries of the pterygopalatine fossa. (From Drake RL et al. *Gray's Atlas of Anatomy*, 3rd edition, Philadelphia, Elsevier, 2021.)

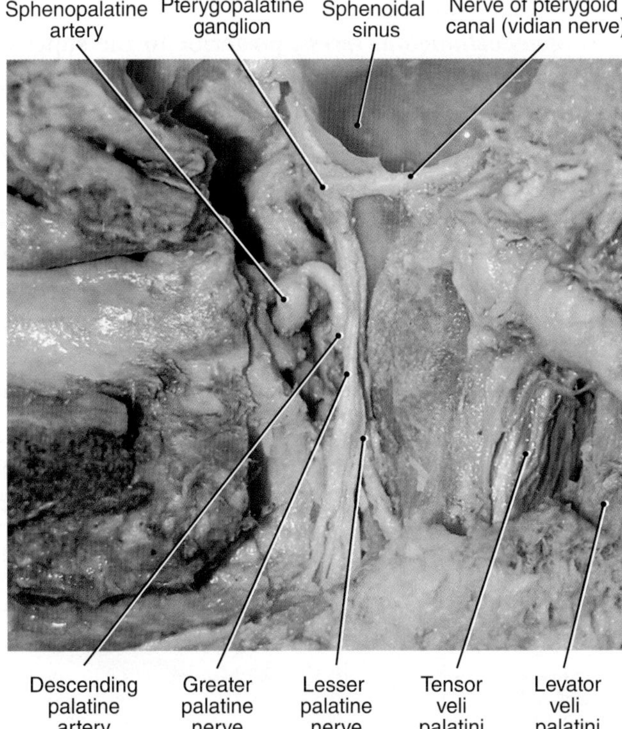

Fig. 26.20 Sagittal view of the nasal cavity with osteotomy of the perpendicular plate of the palatine bone, revealing the pterygopalatine ganglion, nerve of pterygoid canal, greater and lesser palatine nerves, and descending palatine artery.

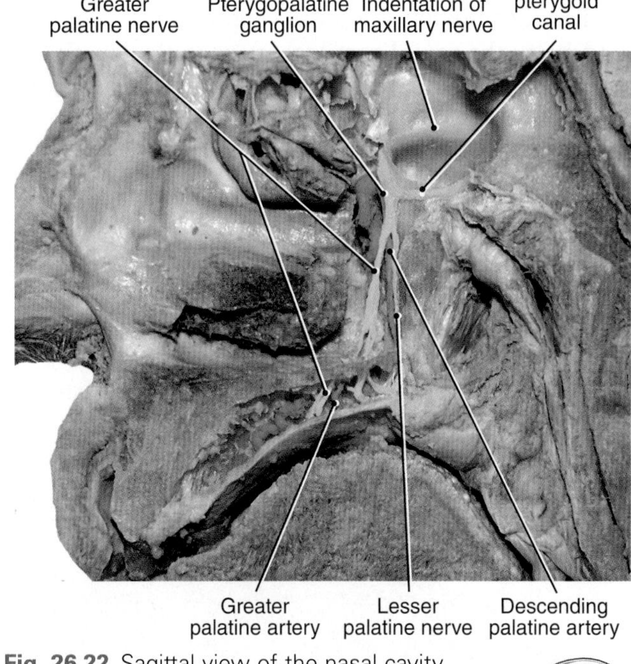

Fig. 26.22 Sagittal view of the nasal cavity highlighting the perpendicular plate of the palatine bone, showing pterygopalatine fossa with pterygopalatine ganglion, nerve of pterygoid canal, greater and lesser palatine nerves and arteries, and descending palatine artery.

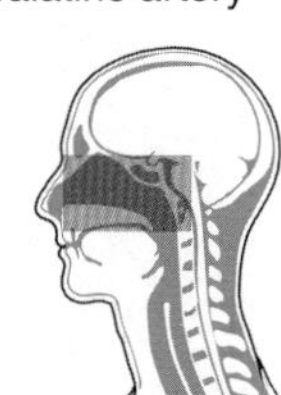

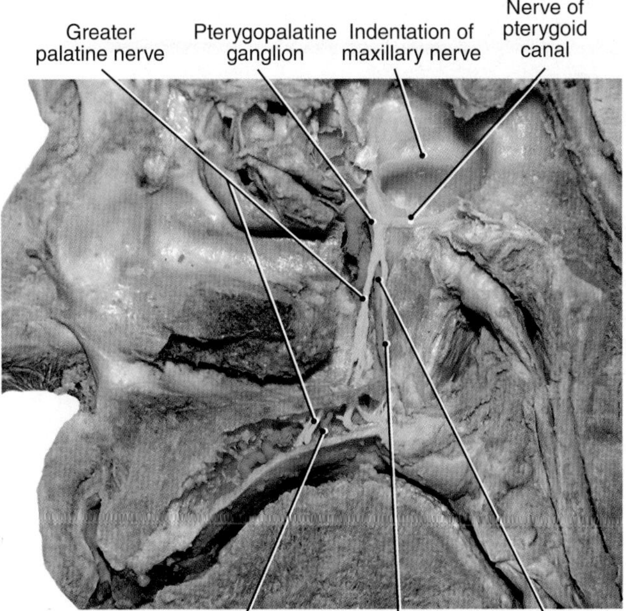

Fig. 26.21 Sagittal view of the nasal cavity highlighting the perpendicular plate of the palatine bone and the sphenoidal sinus and revealing pterygopalatine fossa with pterygopalatine ganglion, nerve of pterygoid canal, greater palatine nerve, descending palatine artery, and maxillary nerve.

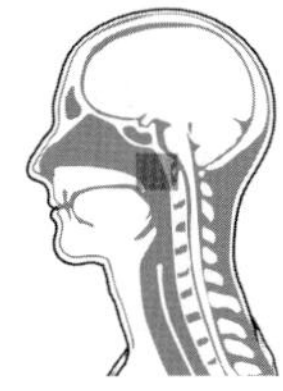

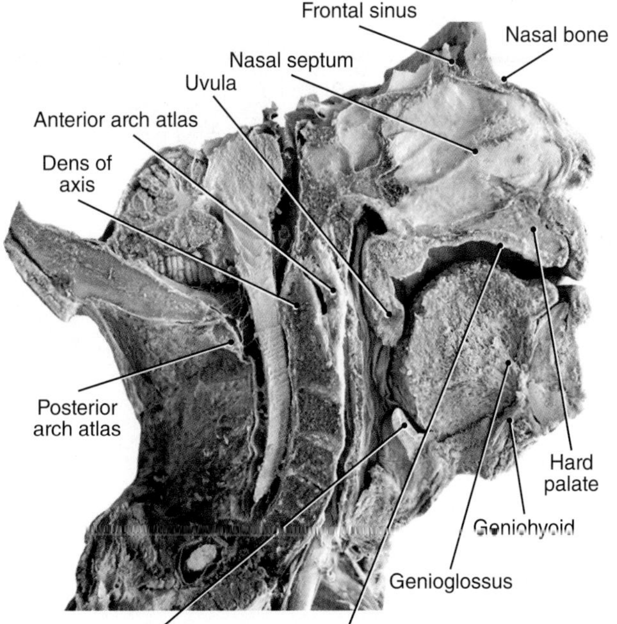

Fig. 26.23 Sagittal view of the nasal and oral cavities revealing the nasal septum and sphenoidal/frontal sinuses. The hard palate, soft palate, uvula, pharynx, floor of tongue muscles (genioglossus, geniohyoid), and epiglottis are seen.

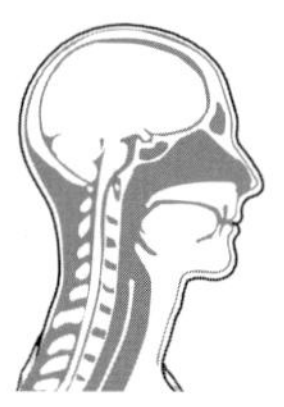

- Remove the mucous membranes from the exposed surface of the nasal septum (Fig. 26.24).
- Identify the septal cartilage, perpendicular plate of the ethmoid bone, and the vomer bone (Fig. 26.25).

DISSECTION TIP

Usually, it is difficult and time-consuming to find any of the nerves or vessels in the nasal mucosa, because of drying and shrinkage from fixation.

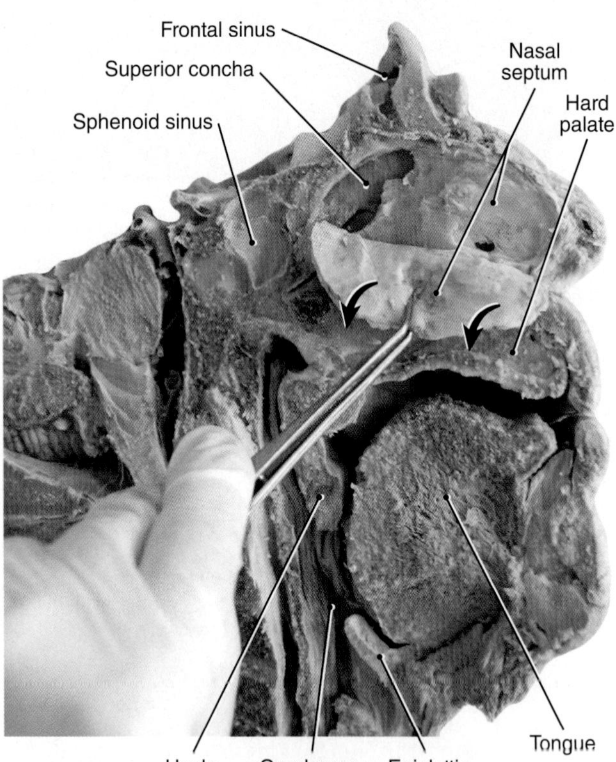

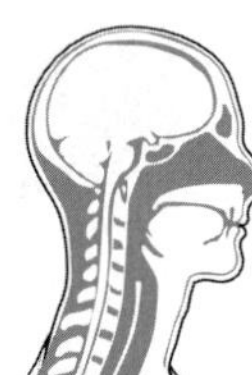

Fig. 26.24 Sagittal view of the nasal and oral cavities with the nasal septum reflected revealing the superior concha, vomer, sphenoidal sinus, and frontal sinus. Uvula, epiglottis, and pharynx are seen.

Identify the following:

- **1. *Sphenoethmoidal recess*, posterior to the superior concha, the location of the opening for the sphenoidal sinus**
- **2. *Superior nasal meatus*, beneath the superior concha, the opening for the posterior ethmoidal cells**
- **3. *Middle nasal meatus*, the ethmoidal bulla, with openings for the middle ethmoid cells and the maxillary sinus**
- **4. *Inferior nasal meatus*, the opening of the nasolacrimal duct**
- **5. *Ethmoidal infundibulum*, for the opening of the frontonasal duct from the frontal sinus**
- **6. *Hiatus semilunaris*, the semilunar hiatus, the long, crescent-shaped opening for the anterior ethmoidal cells**

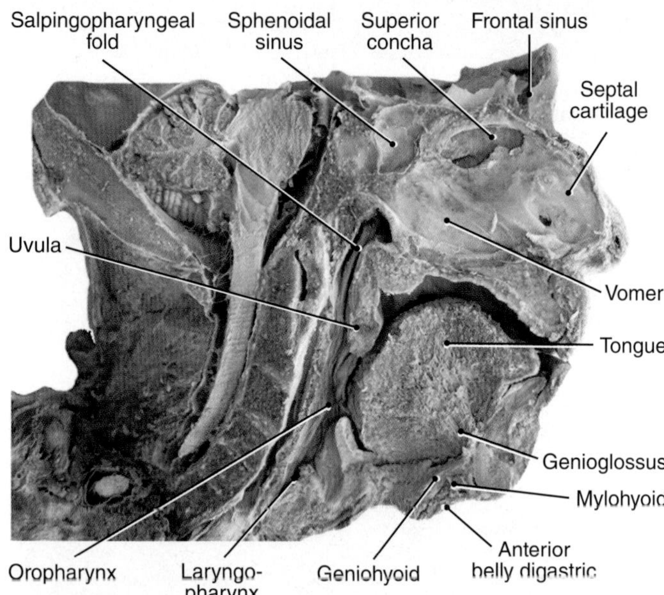

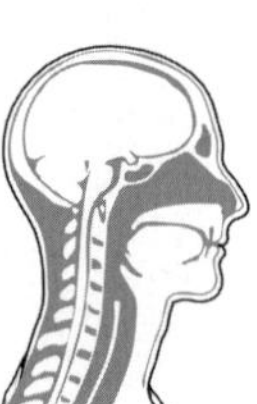

Fig. 26.25 Sagittal view of the nasal and oral cavities revealing sphenoidal and frontal sinuses, septal cartilage, vomer, superior concha, and nasal pharynx. Uvula, tongue, genioglossus, geniohyoid, mylohyoid, and anterior belly of digastric muscles are seen.

LABORATORY IDENTIFICATION CHECKLIST

NERVES

- ☐ Nerve of pterygoid canal
- ☐ Greater palatine
- ☐ Lesser palatine
- ☐ Maxillary

ARTERIES

- ☐ Sphenopalatine
  - ☐ Descending palatine
    - ☐ Greater palatine
    - ☐ Lesser palatine

MUSCLES

- ☐ Tensor veli palatini
- ☐ Levator veli palatini
- ☐ Salpingopharyngeus

BONES

- ☐ Nasal
- ☐ Frontal
- ☐ Ethmoid
  - ☐ Cribriform plate
  - ☐ Perpendicular plate
- ☐ Sphenoid
- ☐ Palatine
  - ☐ Horizontal plate
  - ☐ Perpendicular plate
- ☐ Palatine process of maxilla
- ☐ Vomer
- ☐ Conchae
  - ☐ Superior
  - ☐ Middle
  - ☐ Inferior

SINUSES

- ☐ Sphenoidal
- ☐ Ethmoidal
  - ☐ Posterior cells
  - ☐ Middle cells
  - ☐ Anterior cells
- ☐ Frontal
- ☐ Maxillary

DRAINAGE PATHWAYS

- ☐ Sphenoethmoidal recess
- ☐ Superior meatus
- ☐ Middle meatus
- ☐ Inferior meatus
- ☐ Ethmoidal bulla
- ☐ Semilunar hiatus
- ☐ Nasolacrimal duct
- ☐ Sphenopalatine foramen
- ☐ Maxillary sinus ostium
- ☐ Nares (nostrils)
  - ☐ Choanae
  - ☐ Vestibule

GANGLION

- ☐ Pterygopalatine

OTHER STRUCTURES

- ☐ Basion
- ☐ Clivus
- ☐ Dens
- ☐ Epiglottis
- ☐ Torus tubarius
- ☐ Uvula
- ☐ Septal cartilage

DISSECTION STEPS

- Identify the borders of the nasopharynx, oropharynx, and laryngopharynx on the cadaver (Fig. 27.1).
- The tensor veli palatini and the levator veli palatini muscles have been identified during the dissection of the pterygopalatine fossa (see Fig. 27.1 and Chapter 26).
- Identify the *torus tubarius*, a cartilaginous elevation of the auditory tube (see Figs. 27.1 and 27.4), and locate the pharyngeal tonsil superior to it.
- Extending inferiorly from the torus tubarius is the *salpingopharyngeal fold*, formed by the underlying salpingopharyngeus muscle (see Fig. 27.3 and Plate 27.1).
- Locate the borders of the tonsillar fossa in the oropharynx and identify the palatine tonsil bounded by two arches. Anteriorly, observe the *palatoglossal arch*, a mucosal fold formed by the palatoglossus muscle (see Fig. 27.1).
- Posteriorly, a second arch, the *palatopharyngeal arch*, is formed by a mucosal fold from the underlying palatopharyngeus muscle (see Fig. 27.1).
- In the tonsillar fossa, use your forceps to lift the mucous membrane and pull it off the underlying musculature (Fig. 27.2).
- Similarly, remove the mucous membrane and expose the palatopharyngeus muscle (see Fig. 27.2).

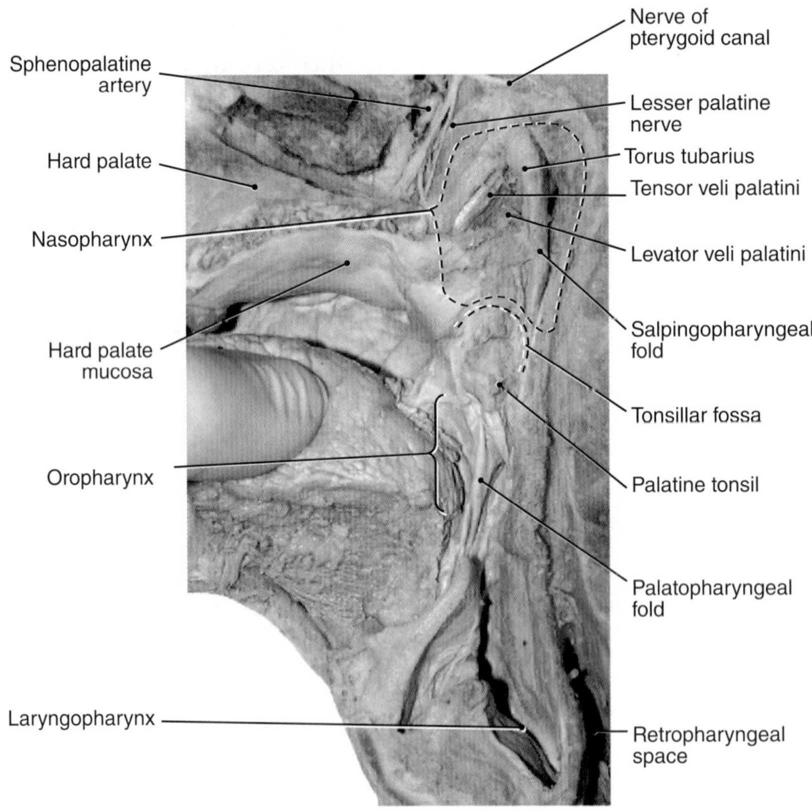

Fig. 27.1 Sagittal view of the oral cavity, nasal and pharyngeal regions, revealing the hard palate, nasopharynx, hard palate mucosa, oral pharynx, laryngopharynx, retropharyngeal space, and salpingopharyngeal fold.

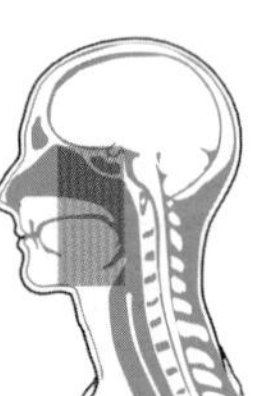

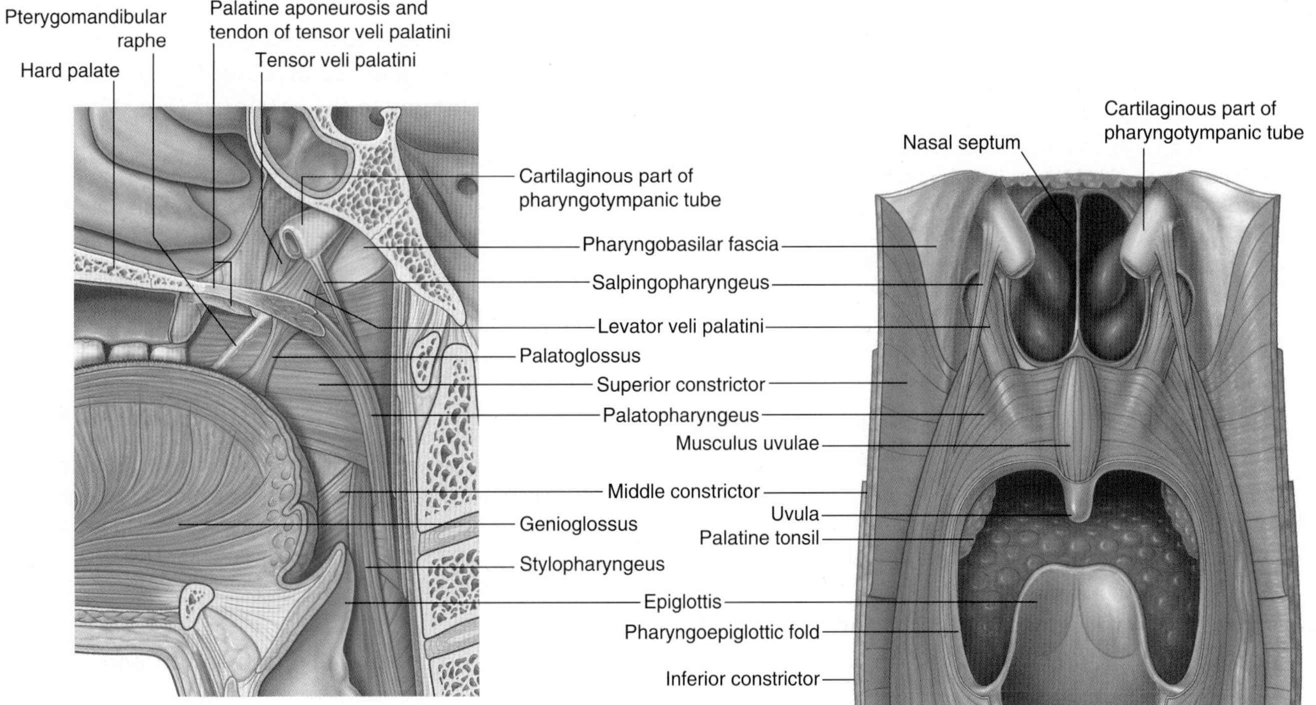

Plate 27.1 Muscles of soft palate, sagittal and posterior views. (From Drake RL et al. *Gray's Atlas of Anatomy*, 3rd edition, Philadelphia, Elsevier, 2021.)

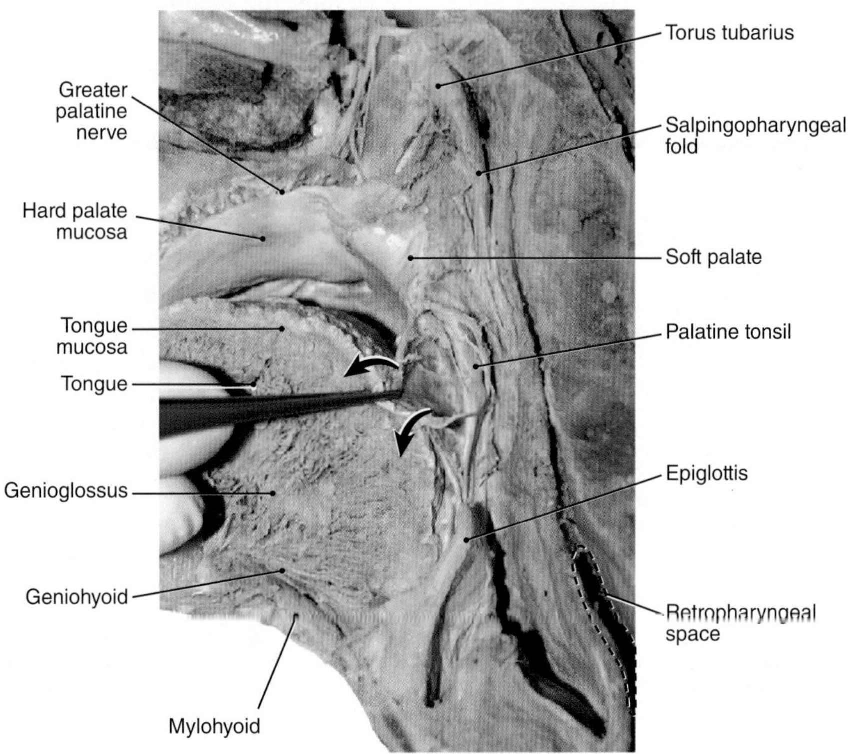

Fig. 27.2 Removal of mucous membranes and exposure of underlying musculature.

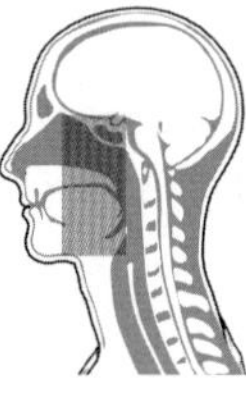

DISSECTION TIP

In the laryngopharynx, at the level of the epiglottis, the palatopharyngeus, salpingopharyngeus, and stylopharyngeus muscles give the impression that they blend and fuse with the posterior pharyngeal constrictor muscles (see Fig. 27.2). However, the posterior pharyngeal constrictors are separated from these muscles by a thin fascia, the *buccopharyngeal fascia*. In some specimens, this fascia may appear as a white vertical line.

- **Pull the palatine tonsil forward and expose the palatopharyngeus muscle (Fig. 27.3).**
- **Continue the dissection by removing the mucous membranes from the palatoglossal arch and expose the palatoglossus muscle (Fig. 27.4).**
- **Because this muscle is located deep and lateral to the tongue, pull the tongue forward and the palatine tonsil backward to expose it fully.**
- **Divide the palatoglossus muscle and identify the glossopharyngeal nerve (Fig. 27.5).**
- **At the base of the tongue, identify the *lingual tonsil.***

DISSECTION TIP

To find the glossopharyngeal nerve, place your thumb at the lateral border of the epiglottis, between the palatine tonsil and the epiglottis. Split the palatoglossus muscle lateral to your thumb (see Fig. 27.5).

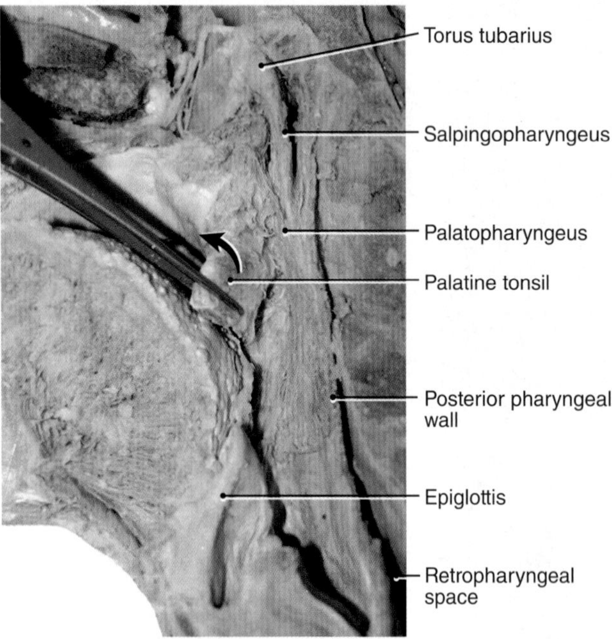

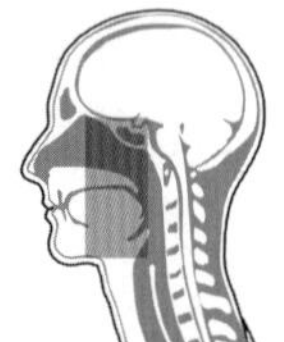

Fig. 27.3 Palatine tonsil reflected anteriorly, exposing the salpingopharyngeus, palatopharyngeus, and posterior pharyngeal wall.

- **Identify the space between the epiglottis and the tongue. Look for a membranous ridge, the *median glossoepiglottic fold,* connecting the posterior surface of the tongue to the epiglottis (Fig. 27.6).**

ANATOMY NOTE

This fold divides the area between the epiglottis and the tongue into two spaces, the *valleculae* (see Fig. 27.6).

INSPECTION

ANATOMY NOTE

The oral cavity occupies the space between the lips anteriorly and the palatoglossal folds posteriorly. For descriptive purposes, the oral cavity is also divided into the vestibule and the oral cavity proper. The *vestibule* includes the area between the external surfaces of the teeth and the internal surface of cheeks. The *oral cavity proper* is the space filled by the tongue.

- **Pull the tongue toward the midline and note the *vestibule.***
- **Identify the mucous membrane, the *frenulum,* between the inferior aspect of the tongue and the floor of the mouth (Fig. 27.7).**
- **Lateral to the frenulum, identify multiple tributaries of the lingual veins and orifices of the submandibular glands, the *sublingual* papilla (sublingual *caruncle*).**
- **Continue the inspection of the anterior surface of the tongue and identify the *filiform* papillae.**
- **Appreciate the much larger and sometimes reddish *fungiform* papillae.**

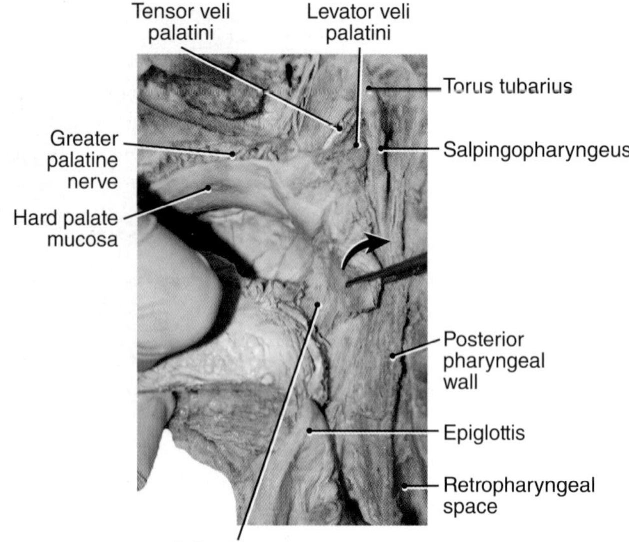

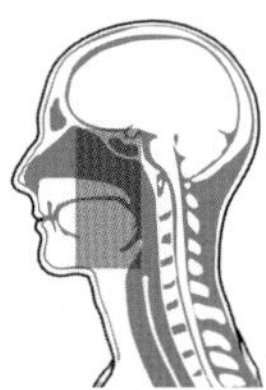

Fig. 27.4 Soft palate reflected posteriorly, exposing the palatoglossal fold and palatoglossus muscle.

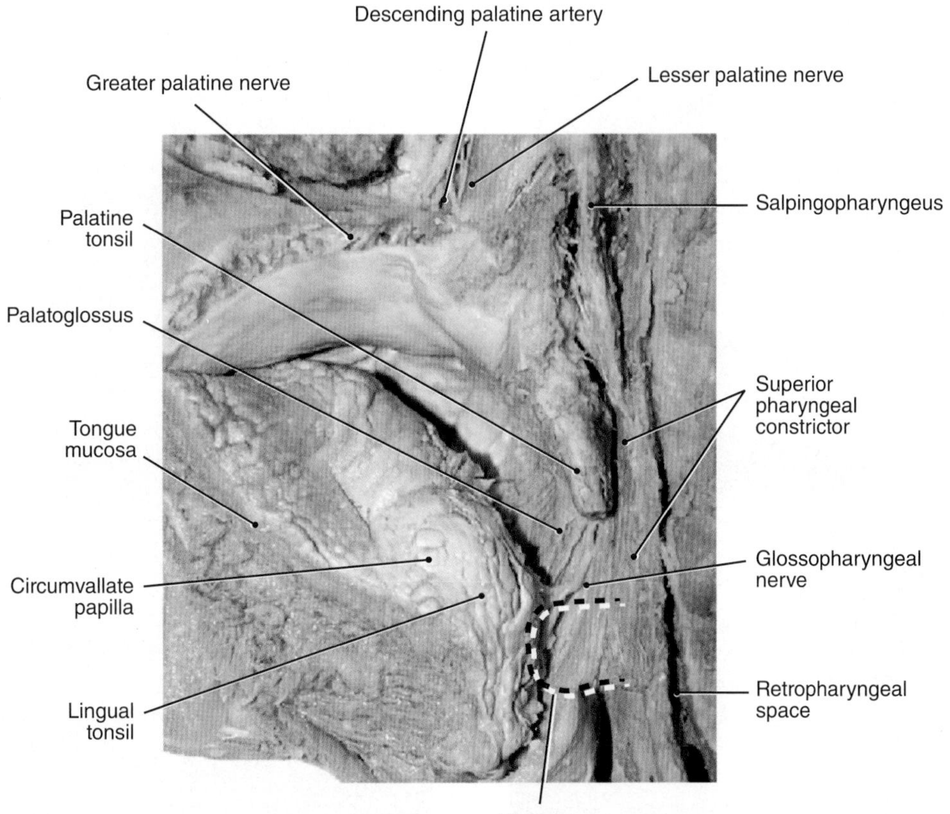

Fig. 27.5 To find the glossopharyngeal nerve, the thumb is placed *(dashed area)* lateral to the epiglottis between it and the palatine tonsil.

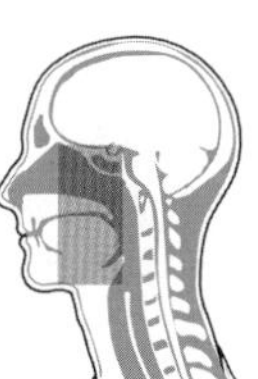

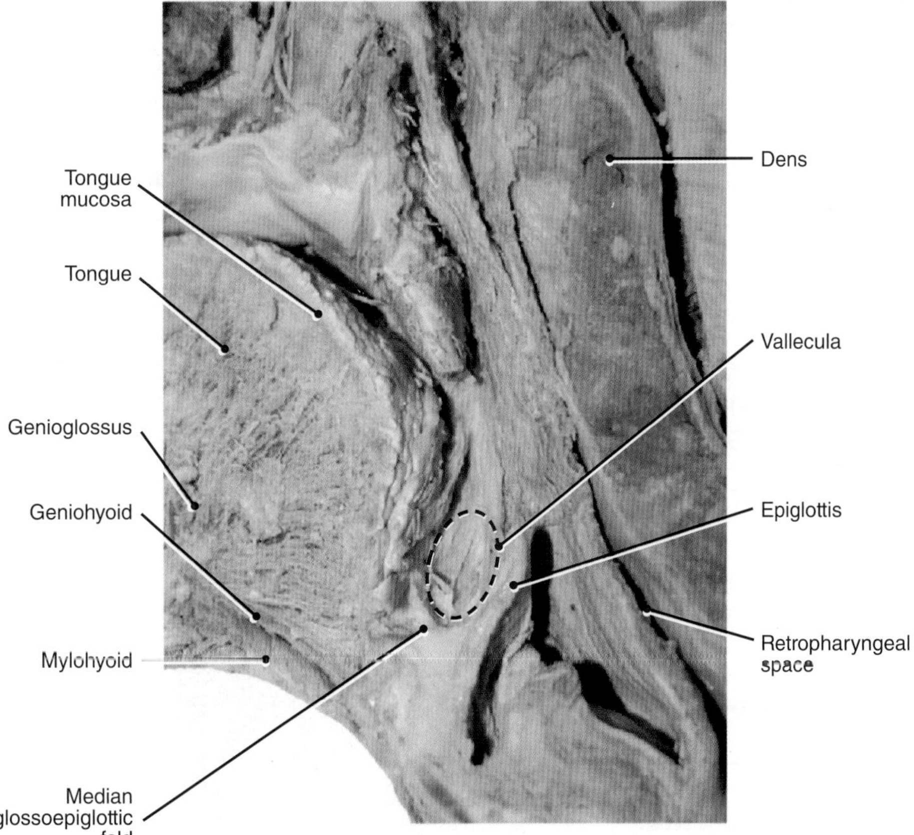

Fig. 27.6 Appreciate the connection between the tongue and epiglottis, the median glossoepiglottic fold, and spaces lateral to it (valleculae).

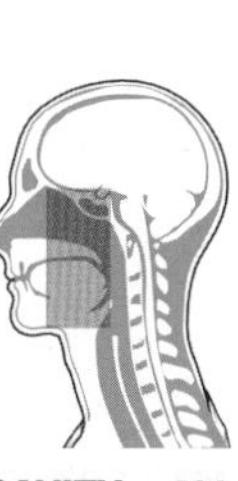

- At the posterior surface of the tongue, identify the sulcus terminalis and *vallate* papillae.
- At the midpoint of the sulcus terminalis, attempt to visualize the *foramen cecum* (Fig. 27.8 and Plate 27.2).
- Pull the tongue medially and make a shallow incision through the mucous membranes lateral to the tongue alongside the mandible (Fig. 27.9).

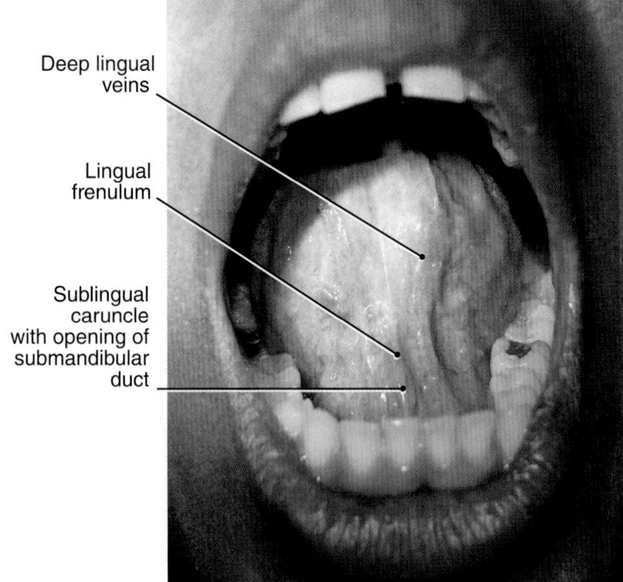

Fig. 27.7 Appreciate the lingual frenulum, deep lingual vein, and submandibular duct.

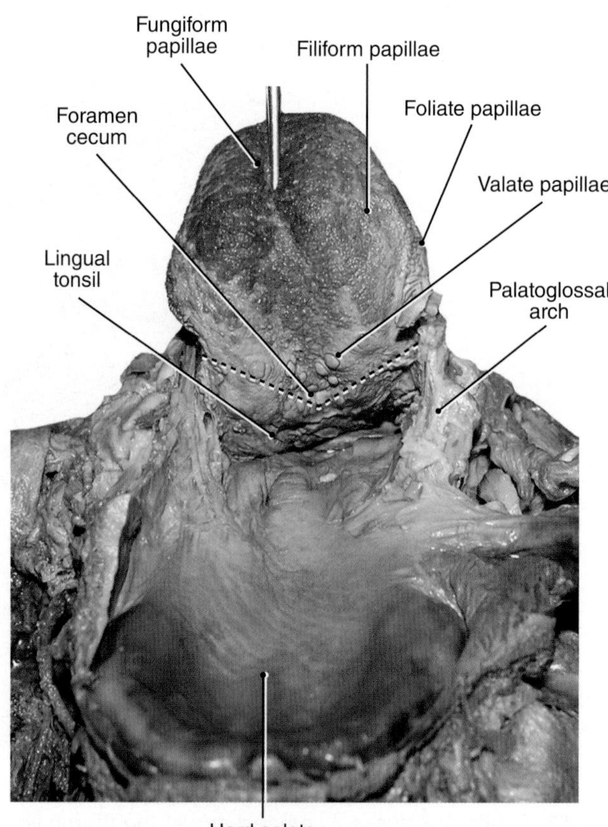

Fig. 27.8 Hard palate reflected posteriorly with view from above revealing the filiform, fungiform, and foliate papillae, and at the posterior third of the tongue, the sulcus terminalis *(dashed line)* and 10 to 12 vallate papillae.

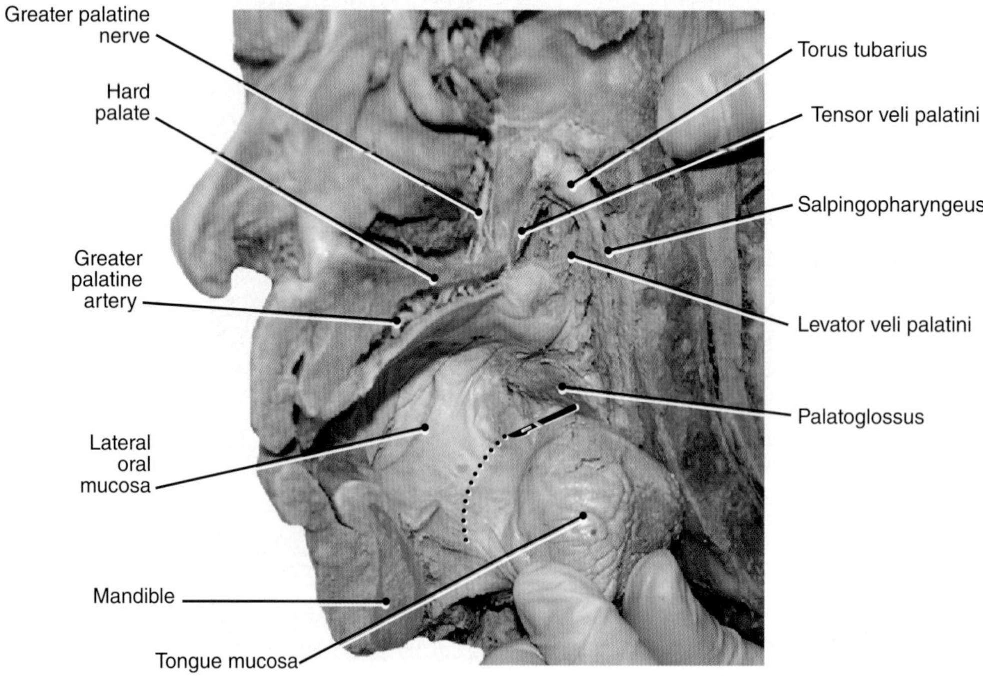

Fig. 27.9 Tongue pulled medially with shallow incision *(dotted line)* through the mucous membranes lateral to the tongue alongside mandible.

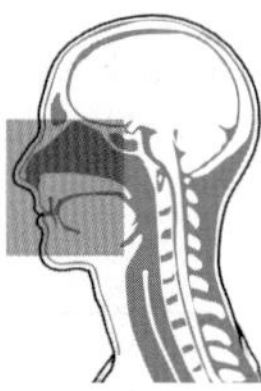

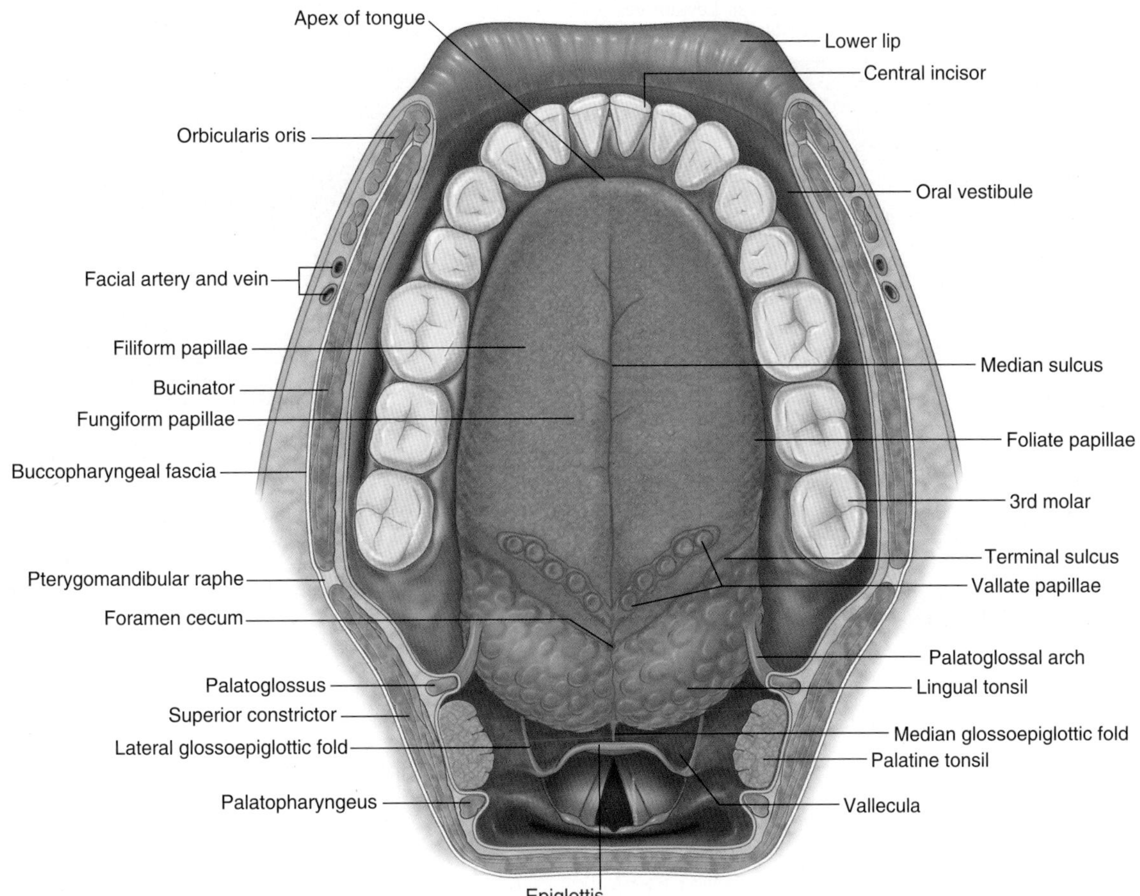

Plate 27.2 Horizontal section showing superior view of the tongue. (From Drake RL et al. *Gray's Atlas of Anatomy*, 3rd edition, Philadelphia, Elsevier, 2021.)

- **Extend the incision toward the palatoglossus but do not sever this muscle (Fig. 27.10).**
- **Lift the mucous membranes of the vestibule and expose the mylohyoid muscle (Fig. 27.11).**
- **Appreciate neuromuscular structures with the mylohyoid muscle exposed.**
- **In the space between the palatoglossus and mylohyoid muscles, identify the *lingual nerve* descending from the infratemporal fossa into the floor of the mouth (Figs. 27.12 and 27.13). Clean the soft tissues and mucous membranes around the lingual nerve.**

DISSECTION TIP

The dissection of the lingual nerve also continues from the floor of the mouth. Therefore do not attempt to dissect the nerve too deeply.

- **Make an incision through the mucous membrane of the floor of the mouth between the geniohyoid and mylohyoid muscles (Figs. 27.14 and 27.15) and identify the *lingual artery* (Fig. 27.16).**
- **As the mucous membranes are reflected laterally from the midline, identify the *submandibular duct* (Wharton's duct) and the *sublingual gland.***
- **Expose the submandibular duct posteriorly to its origin from the submandibular gland, around the posterior edge of the mylohyoid muscle (Fig. 27.17).**
- **Distal to the tortuous lingual artery, identify the lingual nerve.**

ANATOMY NOTE

The lingual nerve passes medially toward the tongue as it crosses over the submandibular duct (Fig. 27.18).

- **Posterior to the tongue, expose the hypoglossal nerve.**
- **Pull the tongue posteriorly and expose the mylohyoid muscle (Fig. 27.19).**
- **Trace the lingual nerve as it descends from the infratemporal fossa between the palatoglossus and mylohyoid muscles. Note the submandibular duct crossing the lingual nerve (Fig. 27.20).**

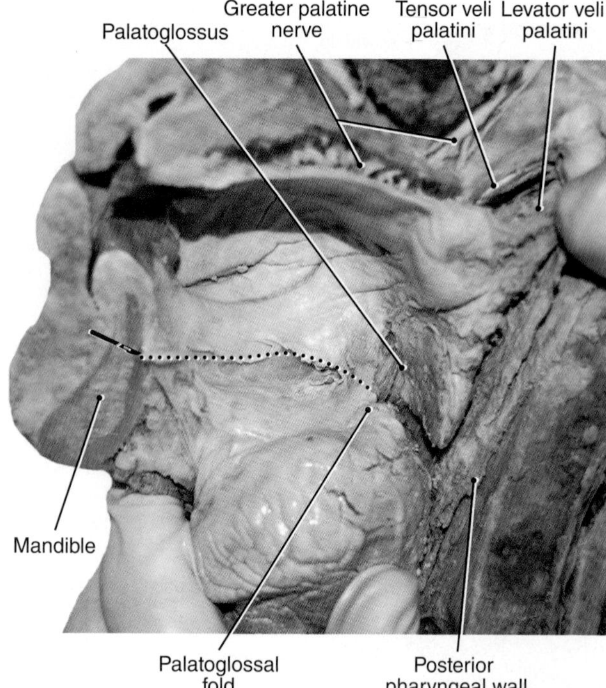

Fig. 27.10 Incision extended toward the palatoglossus muscle.

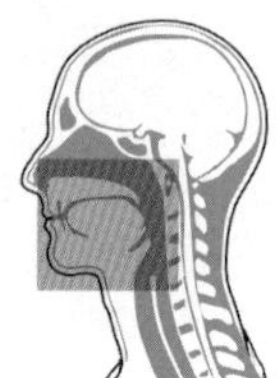

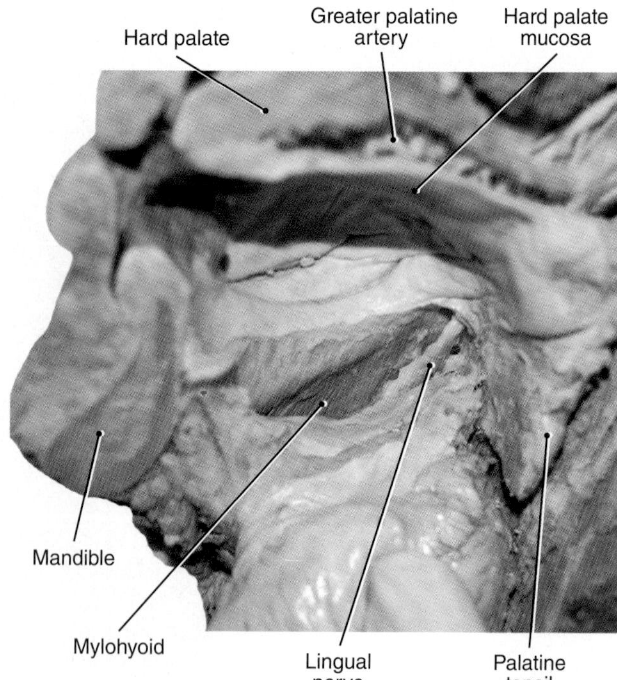

Fig. 27.12 Appreciate the lingual nerve descending from the infratemporal fossa into the floor of the mouth, between the palatoglossus and mylohyoid muscles.

Hard palate mucosa
Soft palate
Levator veli palatini
Tensor veli palatini
Mylohyoid
Palatoglossus
Palatine tonsil
Posterior pharyngeal wall

Fig. 27.11 Mucous membranes of the vestibule lifted, exposing the mylohyoid muscle.

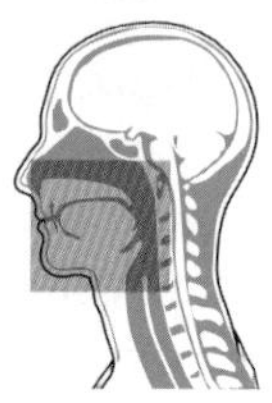

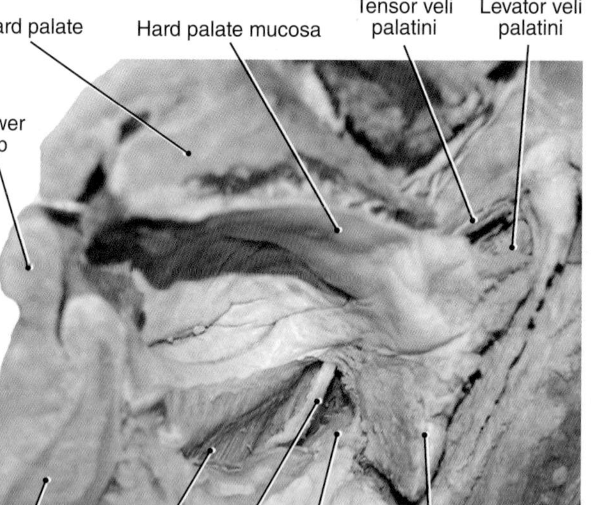

Fig. 27.13 Soft tissues and mucous membranes cleaned around the lingual nerve.

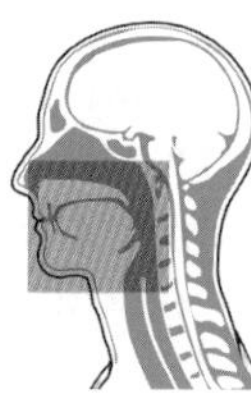

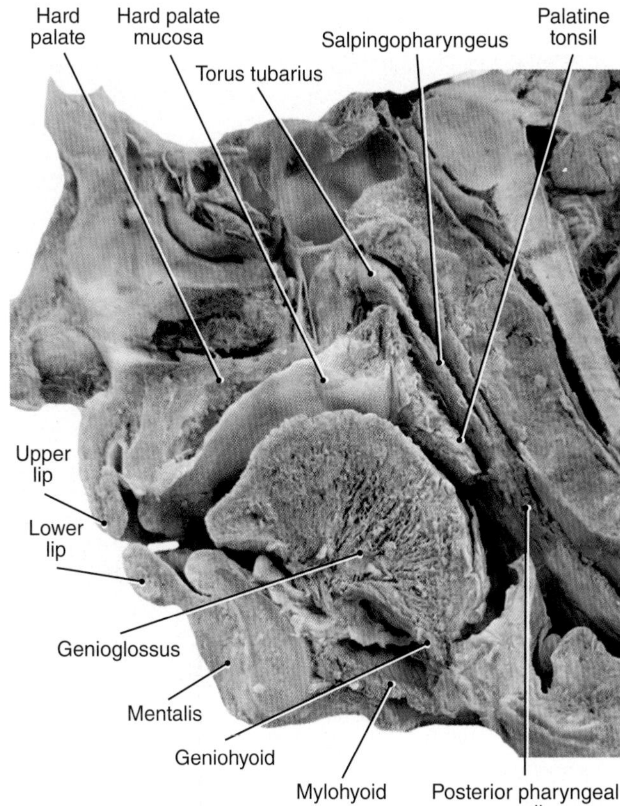

Fig. 27.14 Sagittal view of the oral cavity, including the nasal and pharyngeal regions, revealing the hard palate mucosa, upper/lower lips, uvula, and mentalis, genioglossus, geniohyoid, mylohyoid, and salpingopharyngeus muscles.

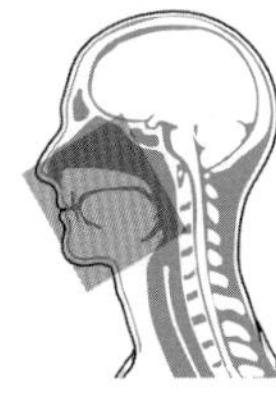

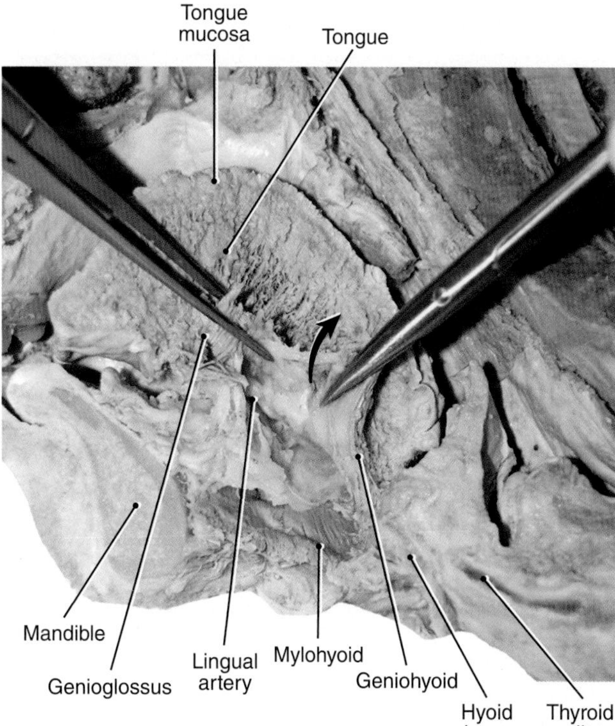

Fig. 27.15 Geniohyoid muscle lifted upward to clean the soft tissues underneath.

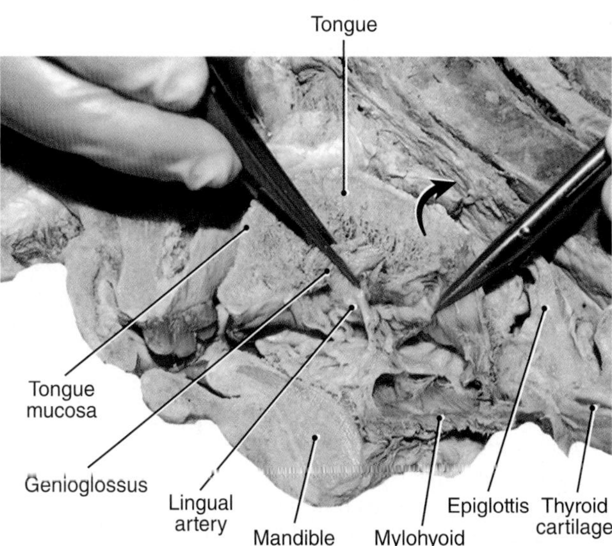

Fig. 27.16 Sagittal view of the oral cavity revealing the mucosa of the tongue, genioglossus muscle, lingual artery, mandible, mylohyoid muscle, hyoid bone, and epiglottis.

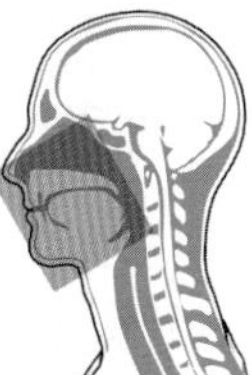

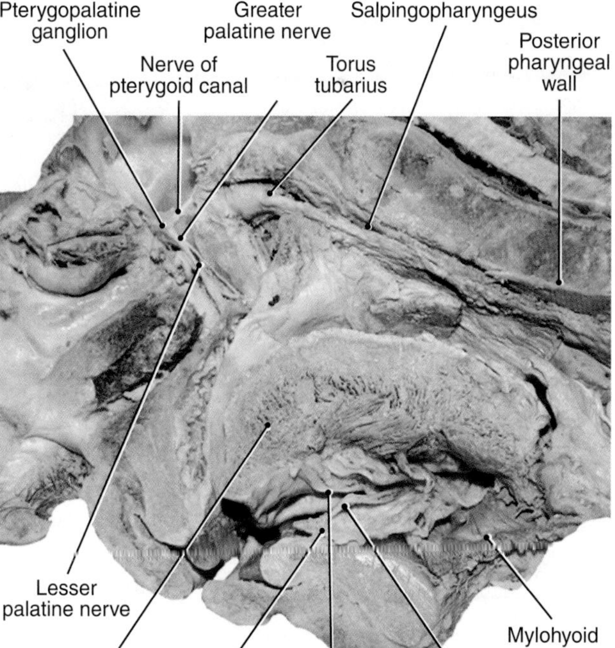

Fig. 27.17 Submandibular duct exposed posteriorly from its origin at the submandibular gland around the posterior edge of the mylohyoid muscle.

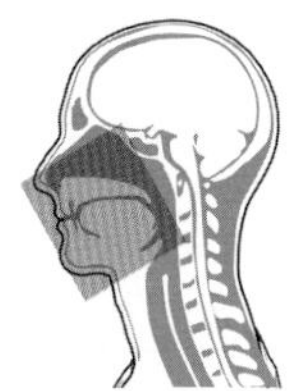

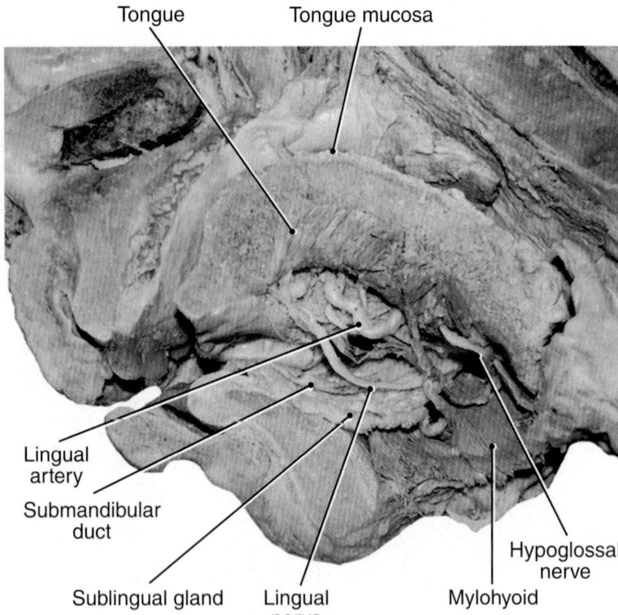

Fig. 27.18 Appreciate the lingual nerve distal to tortuous lingual artery, passing medially toward the tongue and crossing over the submandibular duct, and hypoglossal nerve posteriorly.

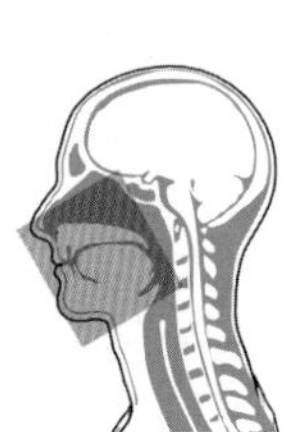

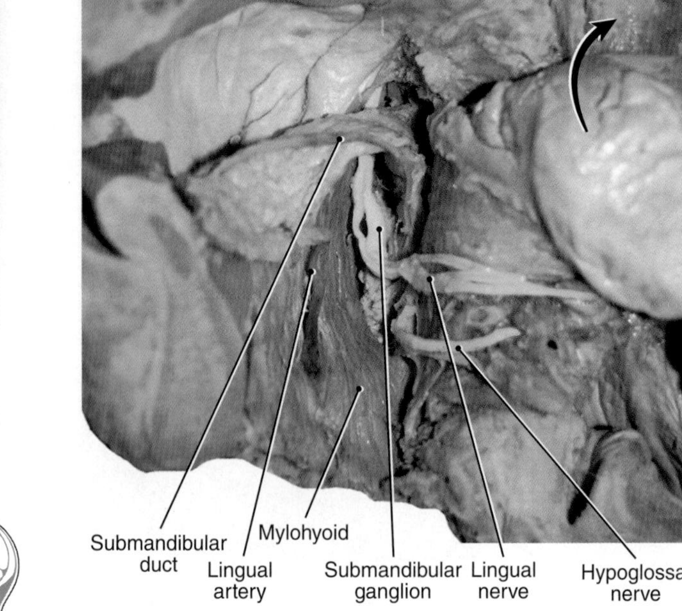

Fig. 27.20 Appreciate the lingual nerve descending from the infratemporal fossa and submandibular duct crossing over it.

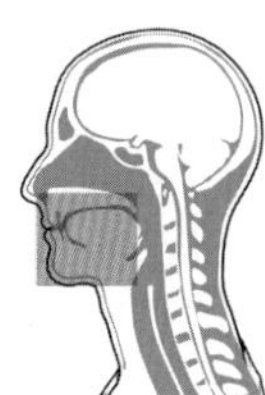

Tensor veli palatini
Levator veli palatini
Hard palate mucosa
Lingual nerve
Mylohyoid
Submandibular duct
Sublingual gland
Lingual artery

Fig. 27.19 Tongue pulled posteriorly, exposing the mylohyoid muscle.

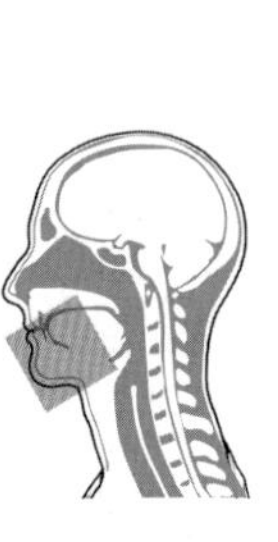

- **With the tongue pulled posteriorly, dissect between the lingual nerve and submandibular gland and expose the *submandibular ganglion* (see Fig. 27.20).**

DISSECTION **TIP**

The following landmarks help to identify the different structures in the floor of the mouth (Figs. 27.21 and 27.22):

- The *lingual artery* passes deep to the hyoglossus muscle and is often tortuous.
- The *hypoglossal nerve* passes superficial to the hyoglossus muscle and is seen at the posterior part of the tongue.
- Seen from the midline with the tongue in situ, the *lingual nerve* passes medially toward the tongue as it crosses over the submandibular duct (see Fig. 27.18).

With the tongue reflected posteriorly, note the *submandibular duct* crossing over the lingual nerve (see Figs. 27.19 and 27.20 and Plate 27.3).

- **If time permits, separate and expose the hyoglossus, genioglossus, geniohyoid, styloglossus, and mylohyoid muscles.**

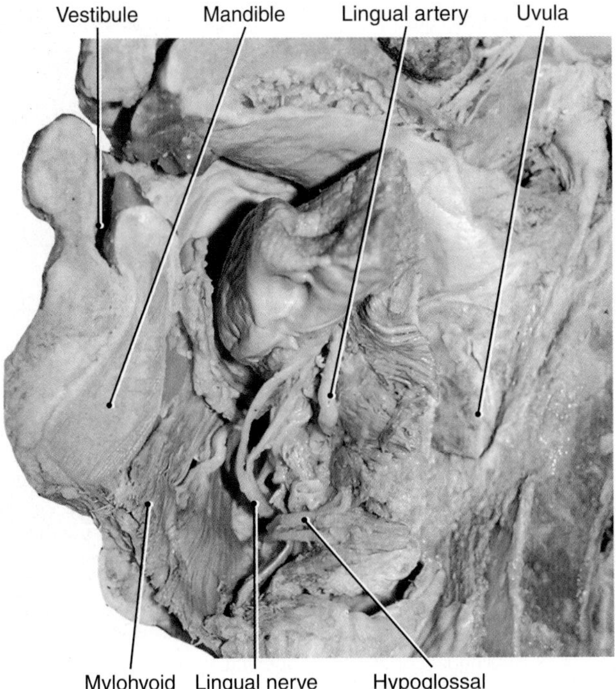

Fig. 27.21 Sagittal view of the oral cavity, including the nasal and pharyngeal regions, revealing vestibule, lingual artery, hypoglossal nerve, lingual nerve, mylohyoid muscle, uvula, and hyoid bone.

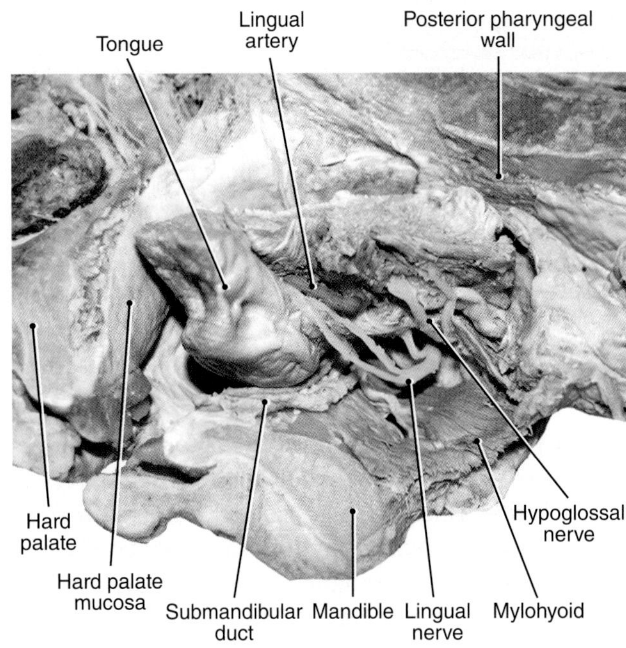

Fig. 27.22 Sagittal view of the oral cavity, highlighting the hard palate and mucosa, tongue, hypoglossal nerve, lingual artery and nerve, mylohyoid muscle, and posterior pharyngeal wall.

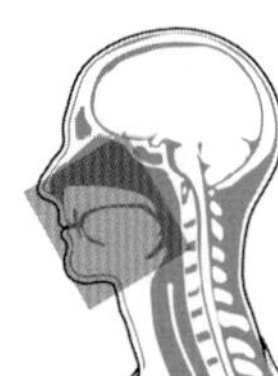

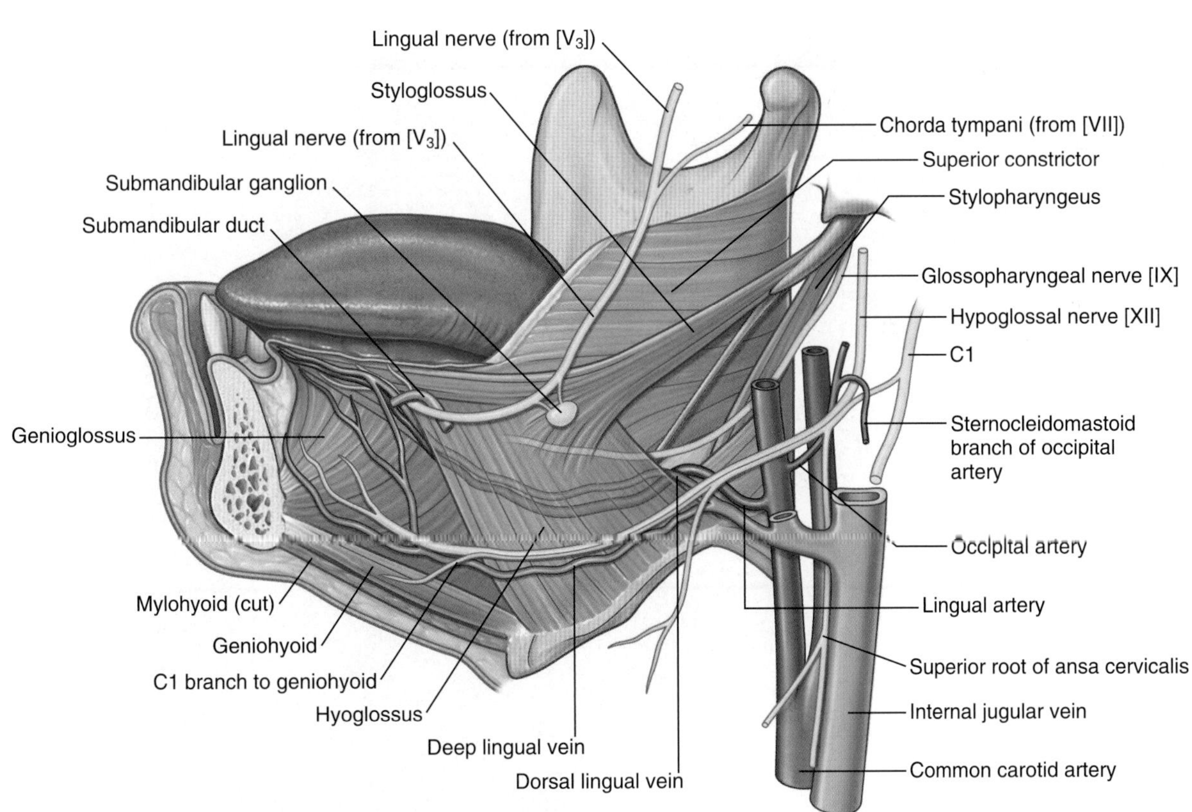

Plate 27.3 Arteries, veins, and nerves around the tongue. (From Drake RL et al. *Gray's Atlas of Anatomy*, 3rd edition, Philadelphia, Elsevier, 2021.)

DISSECTION TIP

To identify the following muscles, note their course:

- The *genioglossus* muscle runs from the mandible to the tongue.
- The *geniohyoid* runs from the mandible to the hyoid bone.
- The *hyoglossus* runs from the tongue to the hyoid bone.
- The *styloglossus* arises from the styloid process and enters the tongue posteriorly and passes under the palatoglossus to fuse with the hyoglossus muscle.

- ○ **After you identify these muscles, make a small vertical cut near the tip of the tongue and expose the vertical muscle fibers and intrinsic transverse muscle fibers.**
- ○ **Make another incision in the superficial tissue from the dorsum of the tongue and expose the intrinsic longitudinal fibers (Fig. 27.23).**

ANATOMY NOTE

In some cadavers, you may find some bony outgrowths in the oral cavity, the torus palatinus and torus mandibularis. The *torus palatinus* and *torus mandibularis* are variant benign excrescences of the hard palate and mandible, respectively (Fig. 27.24).

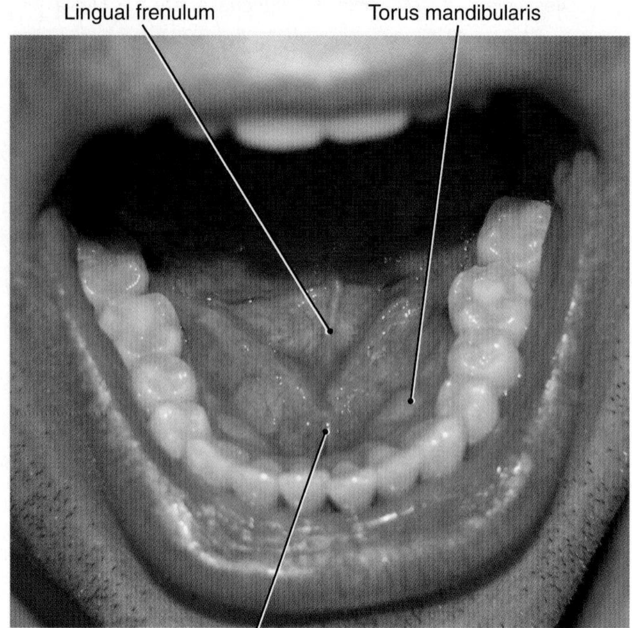

Fig. 27.24 The torus mandibularis is a benign, bony outgrowth of the mandible.

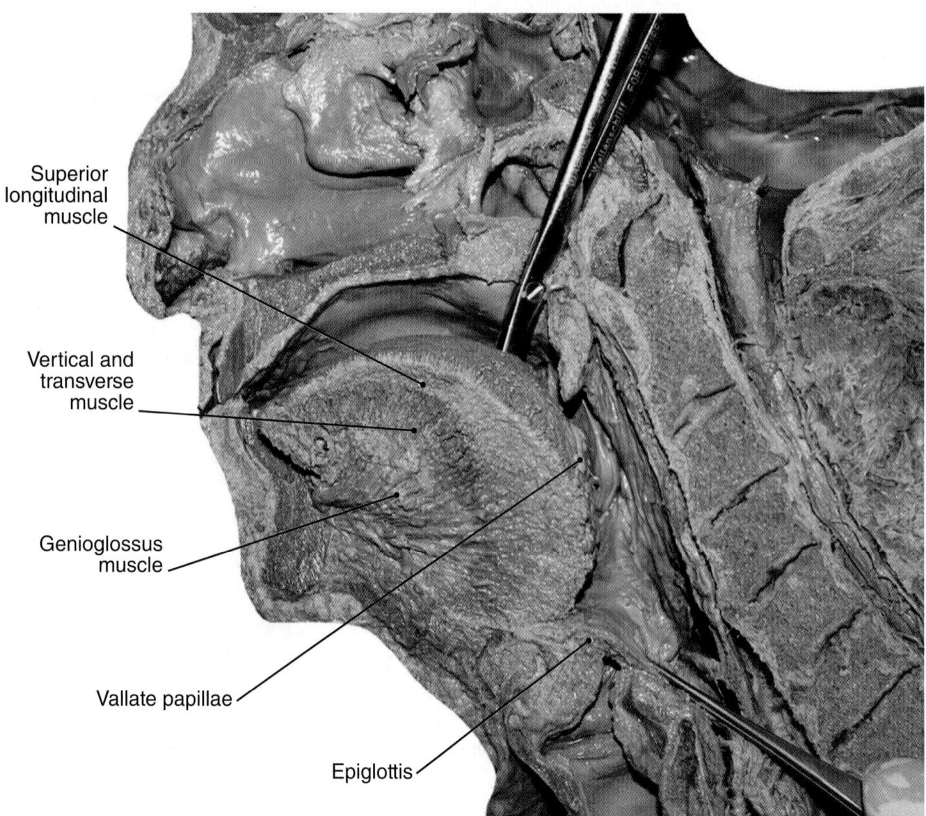

Fig. 27.23 Midsagittal section of the cadaveric head reveals the intrinsic muscle of tongue.

LABORATORY IDENTIFICATION CHECKLIST

NERVES

- ☐ Lingual
- ☐ Hypoglossal
- ☐ Nerve to mylohyoid
- ☐ Glossopharyngeal

GANGLION

- ☐ Submandibular

ARTERY

- ☐ Lingual

VEIN

- ☐ Lingual

MUSCLES

- ☐ Digastric
  - ☐ Anterior belly
  - ☐ Posterior belly
- ☐ Mylohyoid
- ☐ Geniohyoid
- ☐ Genioglossus
- ☐ Tongue
  - ☐ Superior longitudinal fibers
  - ☐ Inferior longitudinal fibers
  - ☐ Horizontal fibers
  - ☐ Vertical fibers
  - ☐ Hyoglossus
  - ☐ Styloglossus

BONES

- ☐ Mandible
- ☐ Hyoid
- ☐ Temporal
  - ☐ Styloid process
  - ☐ Mastoid process

SALIVARY GLANDS

- ☐ Submandibular
  - ☐ Superficial and deep parts
  - ☐ Submandibular duct (Wharton's duct)
- ☐ Sublingual

CHAPTER 28 LARYNX

BEFORE YOU BEGIN

The larynx occupies the space between the epiglottis superiorly and the inferior border of the cricoid cartilage.

INSPECTION

Technique 1

- **The inspection begins by examining the larynx in a hemisected head.**
- **In a hemisected specimen, identify the epiglottis, laryngopharynx, thyroid cartilage, vallecula, uvula, posterior pharyngeal wall, cervical vertebrae, and trachea (Fig. 28.1 and Plate 28.1).**
- **If the thyroid and cricoid cartilages are not hemisected, complete the hemisection and expose the contents of the larynx using scissors.**

DISSECTION **TIP**

Do not cut directly in the midline of the cricoid and thyroid cartilages. Try to perform the cut as laterally as possible.

- **With your fingertips, keep the larynx open and identify the supraglottic space, or *vestibule,* extending from the epiglottis to the vestibular folds (Fig. 28.2).**
- **The *ventricle* is the space between the vestibular (false vocal) folds and the vocal (true vocal) folds (Plate 28.2).**
- **Note the space between the vocal folds, the *rima glottidis* (Fig. 28.3).**
- **Identify the infraglottic space between the vocal fold and the first tracheal ring.**
- **Identify the *aryepiglottic fold,* the mucous membrane stretched between the epiglottis to the apex of the arytenoid cartilages.**
- **With scissors, cut the remaining part of the larynx in the midsagittal plane (see Fig. 28.3).**
- **Identify the epiglottis and the thyroid and cricoid cartilages (Fig. 28.4).**

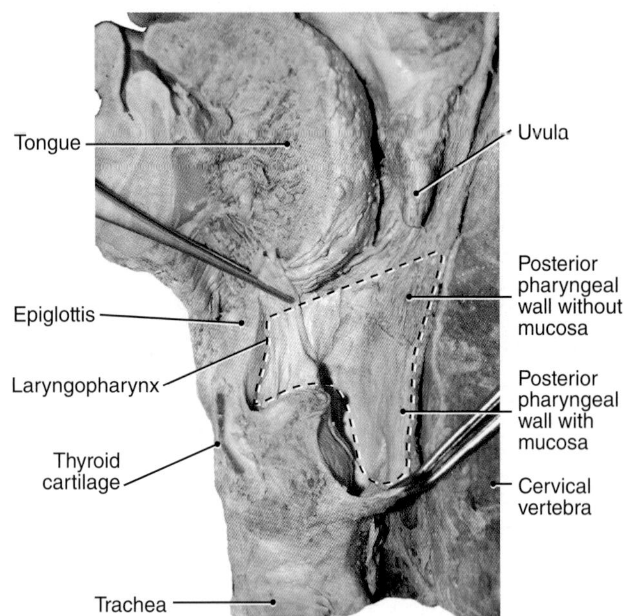

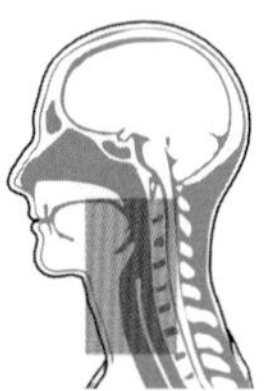

Fig. 28.1 Sagittal view of the mouth and larynx, revealing the tongue, epiglottis, laryngopharynx, thyroid cartilage, vallecula, uvula, posterior pharyngeal wall, cervical vertebrae, and trachea.

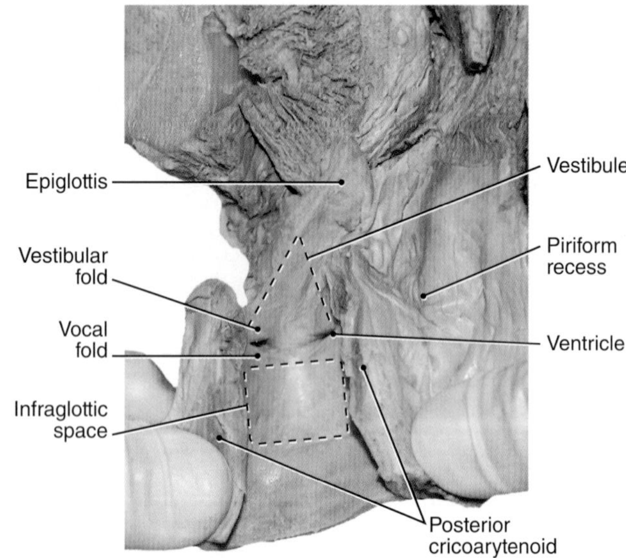

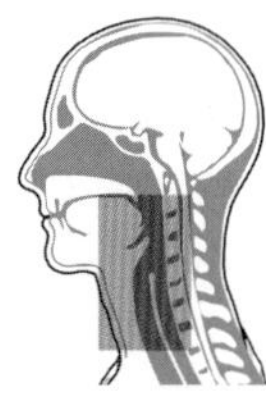

Fig. 28.2 Sagittal view of the mouth with open posterior view of the larynx, highlighting the epiglottis, vestibule/laryngeal inlet, vocal fold, vestibular fold, ventricle, posterior cricoarytenoid muscle, and piriform recess.

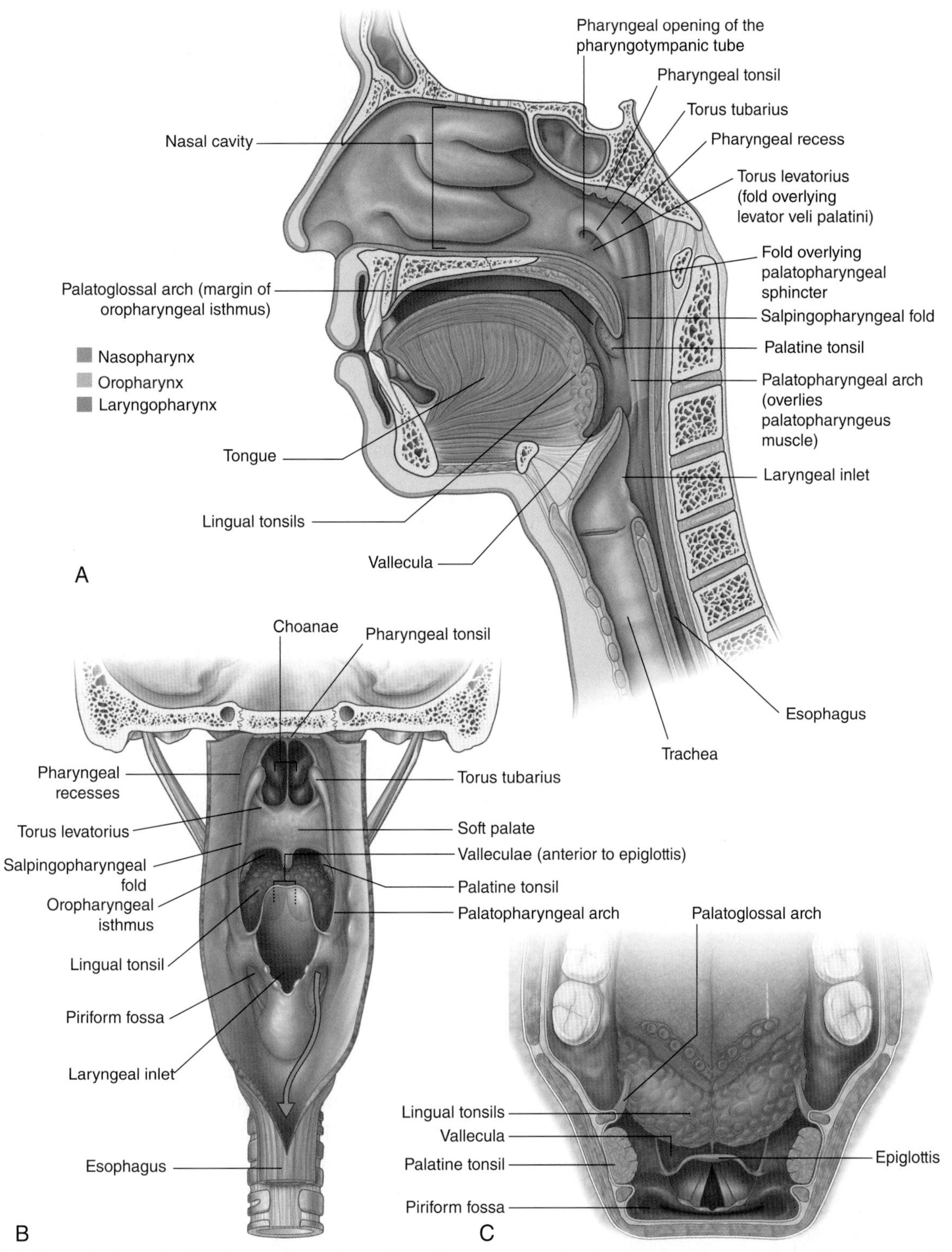

Plate 28.1 A, Lateral view of a hemisected specimen featuring structures in the nasal cavity, oral cavity, larynx, and pharynx. B, Posterior view of the pharynx. C, Superior view of the oropharynx and larynx. (From Drake RL et al. *Gray's Atlas of Anatomy*, 3rd edition, Philadelphia, Elsevier, 2021.)

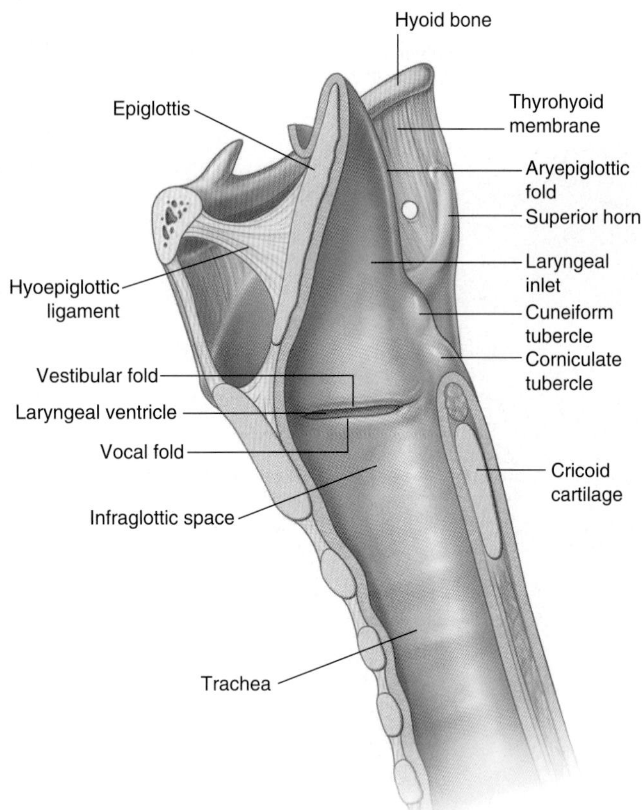

Plate 28.2 A sagittal section through the laryngeal cavity showing the vocal and vestibular folds. (From Drake RL et al. *Gray's Atlas of Anatomy*, 3rd edition, Philadelphia, Elsevier, 2021.)

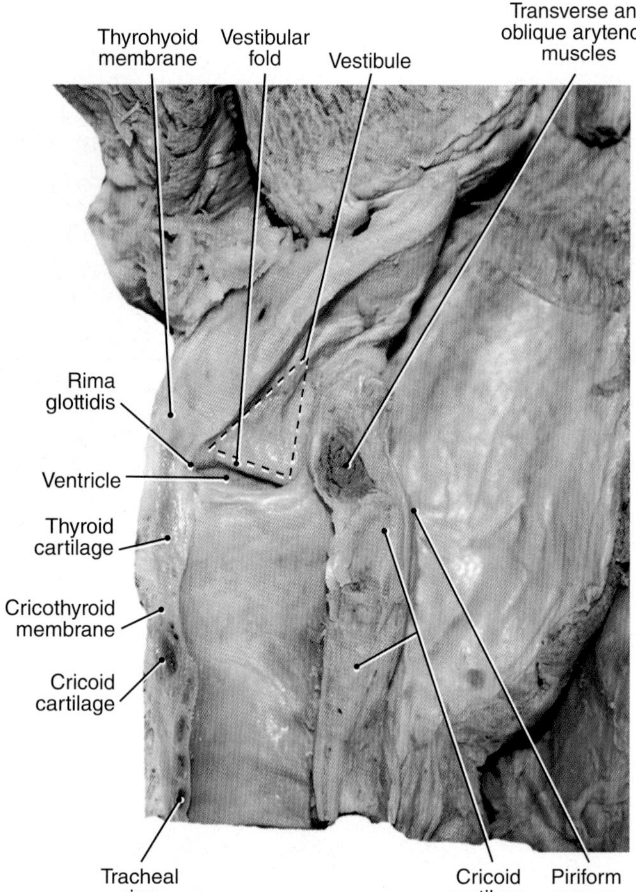

Fig. 28.4 Sagittal view with vestibule/laryngeal inlet, vestibular fold, vocal fold, ventricle, thyroid and cricoid cartilages, tracheal ring, transverse arytenoid muscle, and piriform recess.

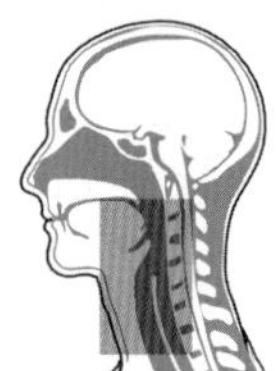

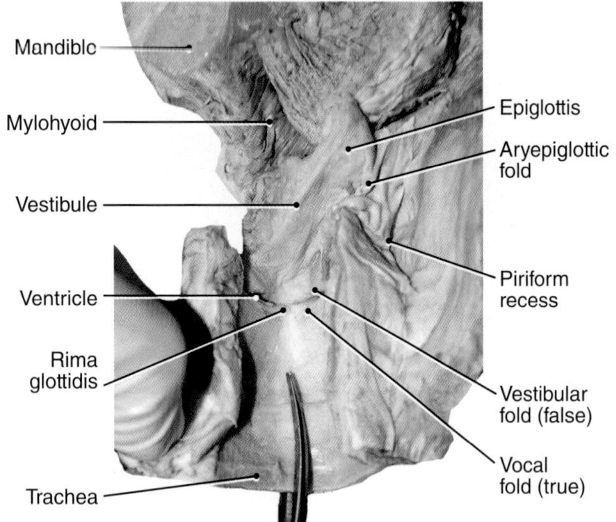

Fig. 28.3 Posterior view, revealing the mandible, mylohyoid muscle, epiglottis, vestibule/laryngeal inlet, piriform recess, vestibular fold, vocal fold, ventricle, and trachea.

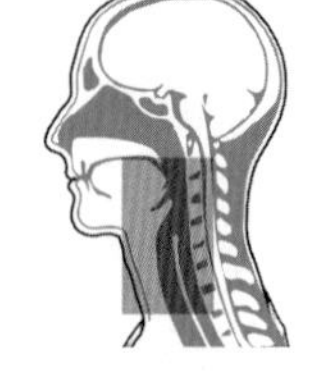

- **Note the thyroid cartilage and its attachment to the hyoid bone through the thyrohyoid membrane.**
- **Identify the attachment of the thyroid cartilage to the cricoid cartilage by the cricothyroid membrane.**
- **Palpate the arytenoid cartilages (Fig. 28.5) and at their free edge in the aryepiglottic fold, feel for the corniculate and cuneiform cartilages.**
- **Palpate the cricoid cartilage and make a midline incision along its posterior surface through the mucous membrane exposing the posterior cricoarytenoid muscle (see Fig. 28.5).**
- **Superior to the posterior cricoarytenoid muscle, identify the transverse and oblique arytenoid muscles (Figs. 28.6 and 28.7).**
- **Reflect the mucous membrane over the aryepiglottic fold and expose the corniculate and cuneiform cartilages (see Fig. 28.7).**

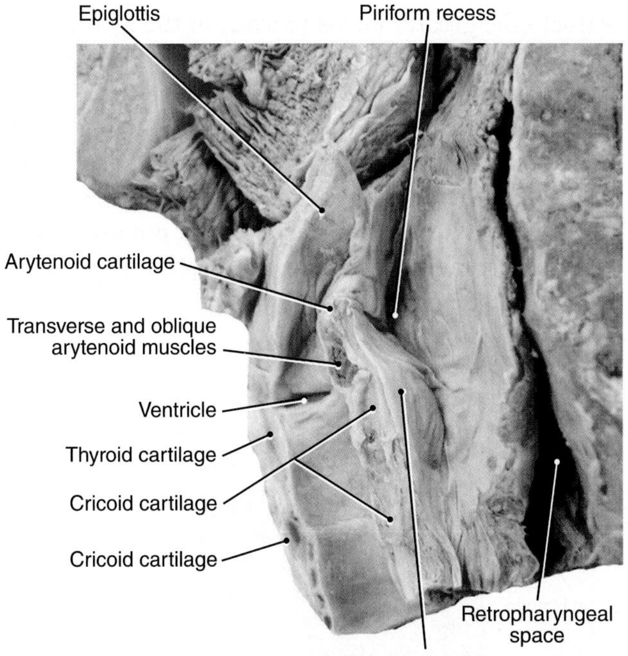

Fig. 28.5 Sagittal view of the mouth and larynx with the posterior wall of the pharynx reflected from the cervical vertebrae, revealing the epiglottis, transverse arytenoid muscle, ventricle, thyroid cartilage, anterior and posterior regions of cricoid cartilage, posterior cricoarytenoid mucosa, retropharyngeal space, and piriform recess.

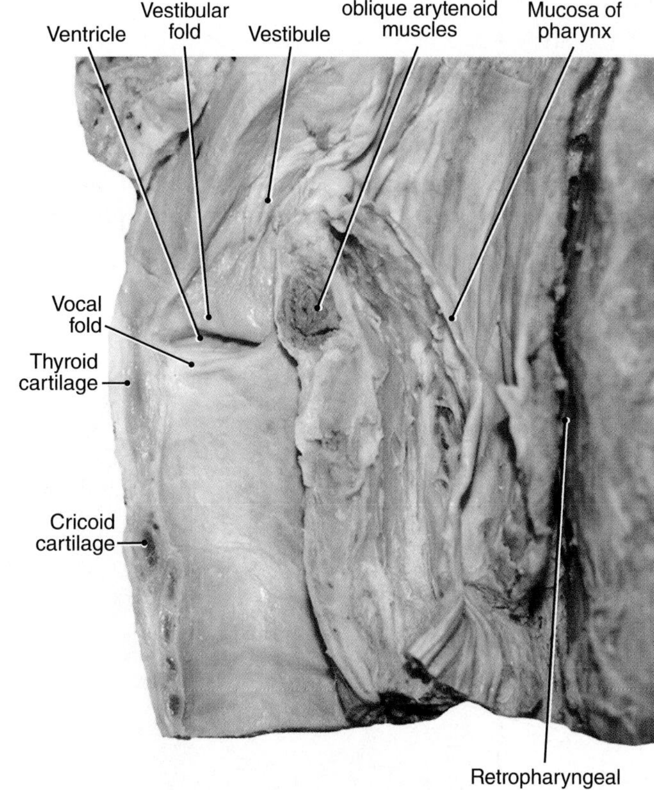

Fig. 28.6 Sagittal view of the laryngeal region, revealing the vestibule/laryngeal inlet, arytenoid muscle, vestibular fold, vocal fold, ventricle, cricoid cartilage, thyroid cartilage, mucosa of the pharynx, and retropharyngeal space.

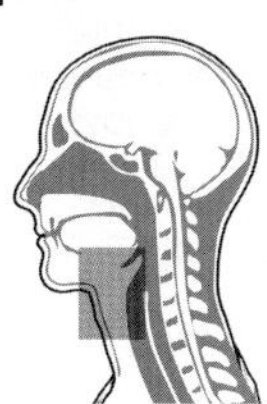

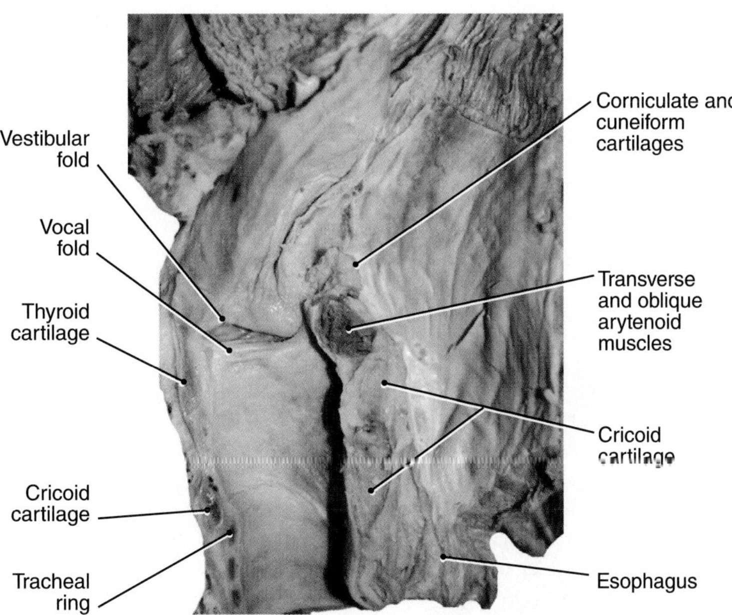

Fig. 28.7 Sagittal view of the laryngeal region, highlighting corniculate and cuneiform cartilages, pharyngeal mucosa, and esophagus.

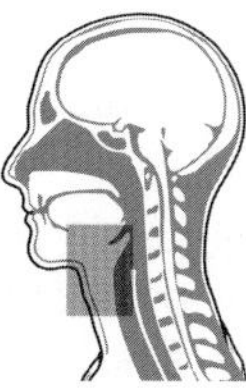

INSPECTION
Technique 2

- **Another technique for exposing the structures of the larynx is to remove the laryngopharynx and larynx en bloc from the cadaver and examine it.**
- **Remove the laryngopharynx en bloc from the cadaver and identify the aryepiglottic fold, piriform recess, and epiglottis (Fig. 28.8).**
- **Palpate the greater horns (cornu) of the hyoid bone and thyroid cartilage and remove the soft tissues around the larynx (Fig. 28.9).**
- **Just inferior to the greater cornu of the hyoid bone, notice the internal branch of superior laryngeal nerve penetrating the thyrohyoid membrane (Fig. 28.10).**
- **Reflect the mucosa over the posterior portion of the cricoid cartilage and expose the posterior cricoarytenoid muscle (Fig. 28.11).**

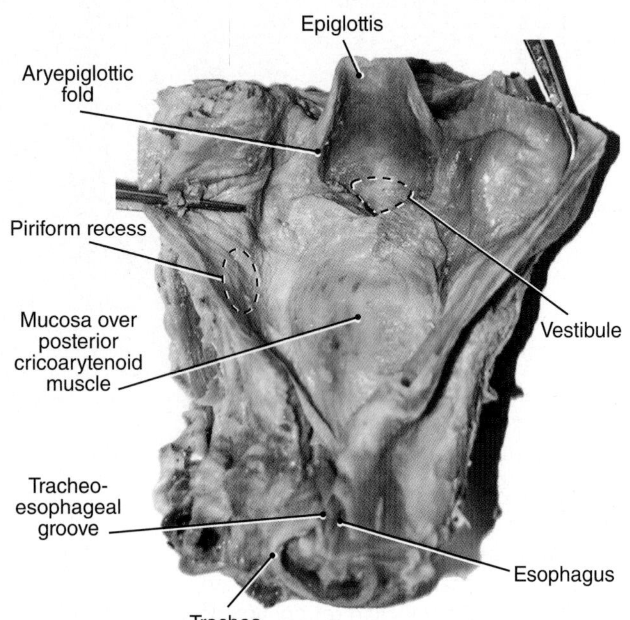

Fig. 28.8 Posterior view of the larynx with the posterior pharyngeal wall reflected from the midline, revealing the epiglottis, aryepiglottic fold, vestibule/laryngeal inlet, piriform recess, and tracheoesophageal groove.

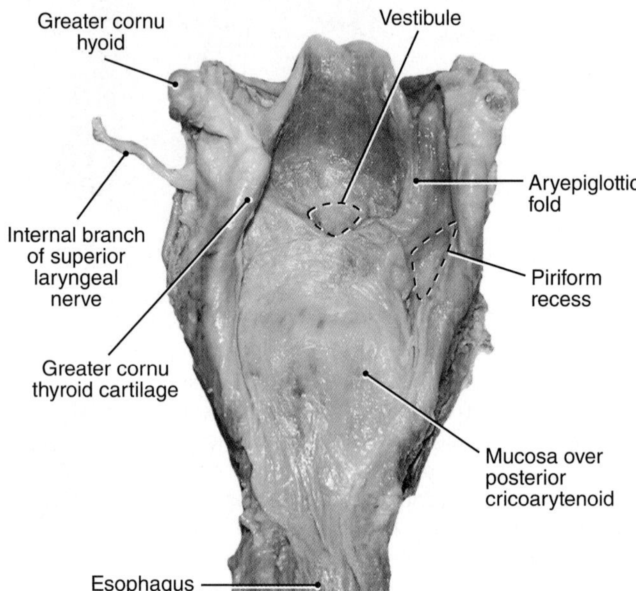

Fig. 28.10 Posterior view of the larynx with the posterior pharyngeal wall reflected, revealing vestibule/laryngeal inlet, greater cornu of the hyoid and thyroid cartilage, and internal branch of the superior laryngeal nerve.

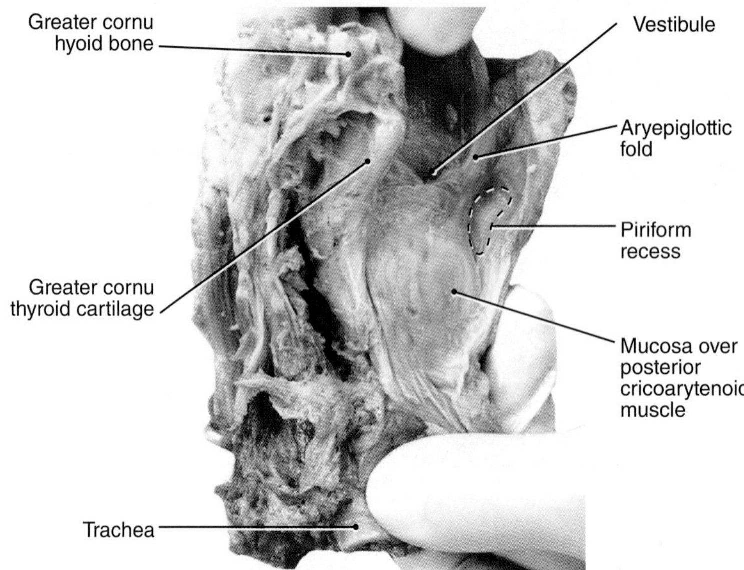

Fig. 28.9 Posterior view of the larynx with the posterior pharyngeal wall reflected from the midline, highlighting the horns (cornua) of the hyoid and thyroid cartilages, mucosa over the posterior cricoarytenoid muscle, aryepiglottic fold, and piriform recess.

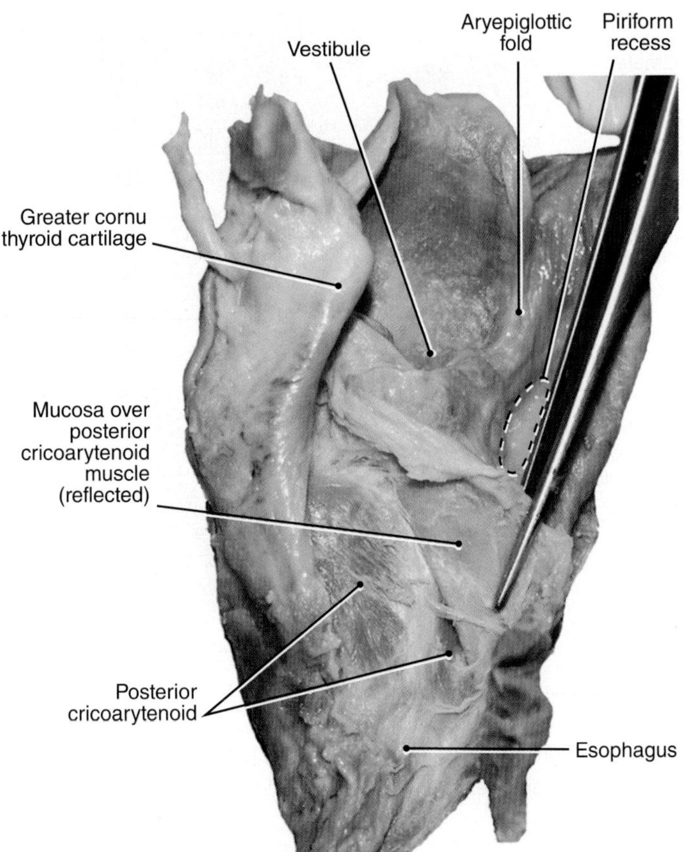

Fig. 28.11 Posterior view of the larynx with pharyngeal wall cut from the midline, revealing the vestibule/laryngeal inlet, greater cornu of the thyroid cartilage, posterior cricoarytenoid, esophagus, mucosa over the posterior cricoarytenoid muscle, aryepiglottic fold, and piriform recess.

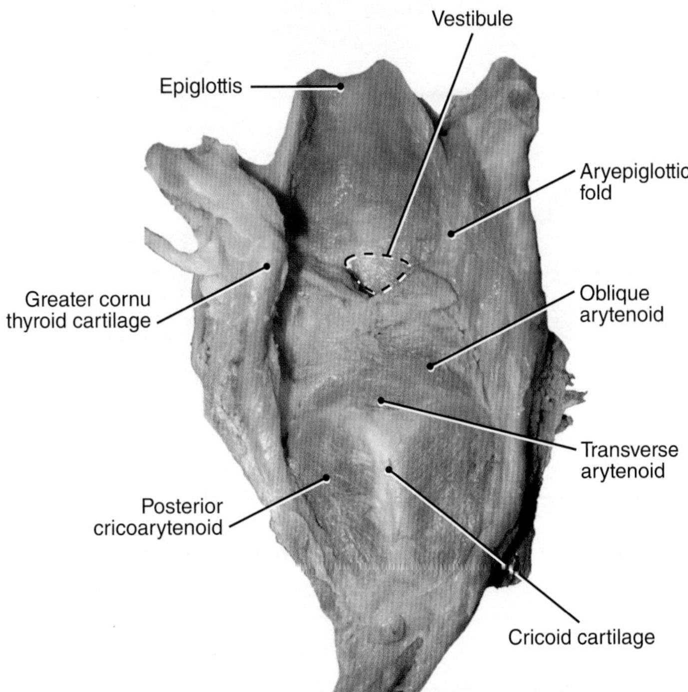

Fig. 28.12 Posterior view of the larynx with the posterior pharyngeal wall reflected, revealing the epiglottis, vestibule/laryngeal inlet, posterior cricoarytenoid muscle, posterior cricoid cartilage, transverse and oblique arytenoids, and aryepiglottic fold.

- **Identify the posterior cricoarytenoid and transverse and oblique arytenoid muscles (Fig. 28.12).**
- **Make a midline incision through the cricoid cartilage and identify the vocal and vestibular folds (Fig. 28.13).**
- **Pull the lateral edges of the cartilages open to fully expose the space between the vocal folds (Fig. 28.14).**
- **Turn the specimen anteriorly and identify the *crico-thyroid muscle.***

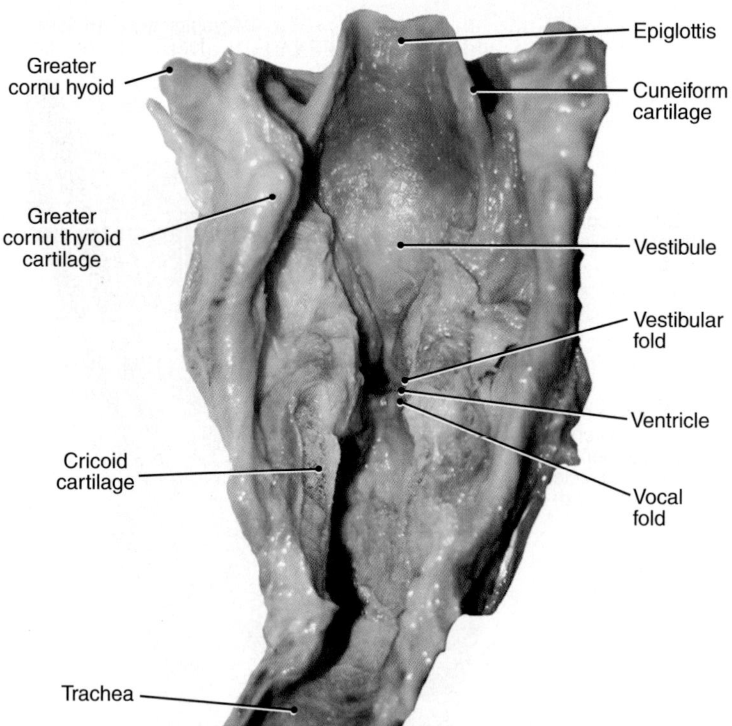

Fig. 28.13 Posterior midline view of the larynx with the cricoid cartilage reflected from the midline, highlighting the epiglottis, greater cornu (hyoid, thyroid cartilage), vocal and vestibular folds, cuneiform cartilage, ventricle, posterior region of cricoid cartilage, and trachea.

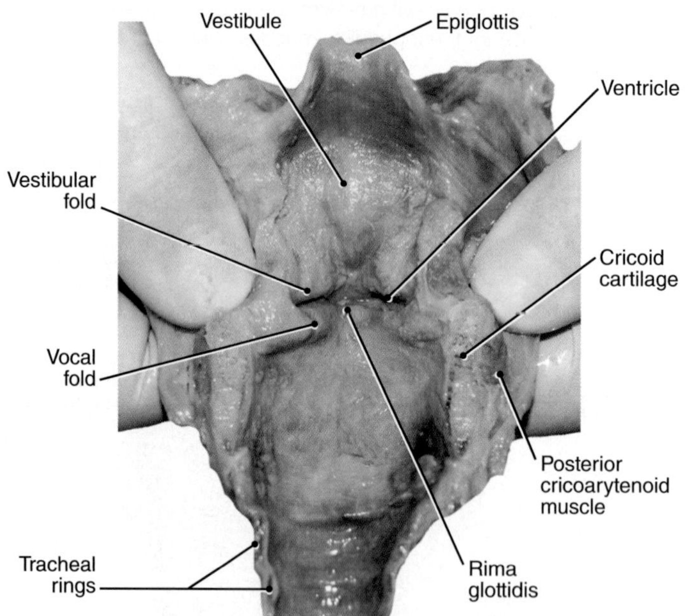

Fig. 28.14 Posterior view of the larynx with the cricoid cartilage reflected from the midline, revealing the epiglottis, vestibule/laryngeal inlet, vestibular fold, vocal fold, ventricle, posterior region of cricoid cartilage, posterior cricoarytenoid muscle, and tracheal rings.

- **Reflect the cricothyroid muscle anteriorly from the cricoid cartilage and identify the median cricothyroid ligament in the midline between the thyroid and cricoid cartilages.**
- **Identify the *thyroarytenoid muscle* lateral to the transverse and oblique arytenoids, ascending posteriorly from the midline to the arytenoid cartilage.**
- **Inferior to the thyroarytenoid muscle, a small muscle, the *lateral cricoarytenoid muscle,* runs obliquely superior to the arytenoid cartilage.**

DISSECTION TIP

If time permits, reflect the thyrohyoid membrane and trace the course of the internal branch of the superior laryngeal nerve to the piriform recess.

LABORATORY IDENTIFICATION CHECKLIST

NERVES

- ☐ Superior laryngeal
- ☐ External branch of superior laryngeal
- ☐ Internal branch of superior laryngeal
- ☐ Recurrent laryngeal
- ☐ Inferior laryngeal

ARTERIES

- ☐ Superior laryngeal

MUSCLES

- ☐ Uvula
- ☐ Cricothyroid
- ☐ Posterior cricoarytenoid
- ☐ Transverse arytenoid
- ☐ Oblique arytenoid
- ☐ Vocalis
- ☐ Lateral cricoarytenoid
- ☐ Thyroarytenoid

BONES

- ☐ Hyoid
    - ☐ Greater cornu

CARTILAGES

- ☐ Epiglottis
- ☐ Thyroid
    - ☐ Greater cornu
- ☐ Cricoid
- ☐ Arytenoid
- ☐ Corniculate
- ☐ Cuneiform
- ☐ Tracheal rings

MEMBRANES

- ☐ Thyrohyoid
- ☐ Cricothyroid

LIGAMENT

- ☐ Cricothyroid

SPACES/RECESS/FOLDS

- ☐ Piriform recess
- ☐ Vestibule
- ☐ Vocal folds
- ☐ Ventricle
- ☐ Vestibular folds
- ☐ Aryepiglottic folds
- ☐ Laryngopharynx

BEFORE YOU BEGIN

Place the cadaver in the supine position and identify the following landmarks in the postcraniotomy skull (Fig. 29.1):

- Anterior, middle, and posterior cranial fossae
- Transverse and sigmoid sinuses
- Confluence of sinuses

DISSECTION STEPS

- **With toothed forceps and a scalpel, remove the dura mater from the posterior cranial fossa.**
- **With a mallet and chisel, make an inverted V-shaped cut (*dashed line* in Fig. 29.2) in the posterior cranial fossa (Plate 29.1).**
- **Place the chisel 1 to 2 cm in the front of the foramen magnum at the midportion of the clivus and make a deep cut.**
- **Continue this cut laterally and posteriorly between the jugular foramen and the hypoglossal canal toward the edge of the occipital bone (Fig. 29.3).**
- **Once the incisions are complete, pull the occipital bone backward to separate it from the skull base.**
- **Use a scalpel to cut the soft tissues between the bone fragments.**
- **Have a laboratory partner keep the head stable by holding it as shown in Fig. 29.4.**

DISSECTION TIP

Be careful in making the separation in the region posterior to the jugular foramen. This is where the carotid sheath emerges, and aggressive dissection can damage its contents. As you pull the posterior cranial fossa backward (Fig. 29.5), place your finger in the opening you created at the clivus and pull backward (Fig. 29.6).

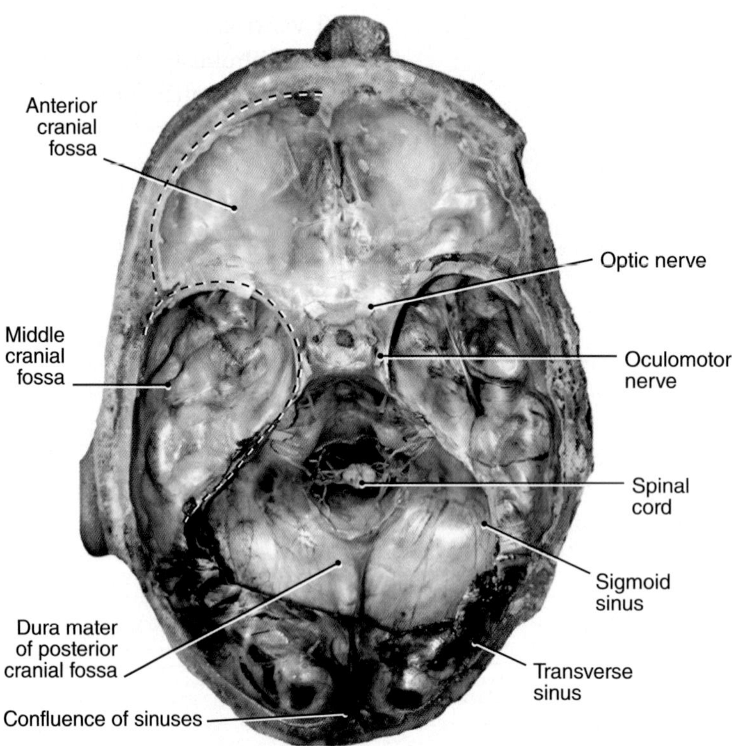

Fig. 29.1 View of the anterior, middle, and posterior cranial fossae, dura mater, dural venous sinuses (transverse, sigmoid, confluence), spinal cord, and cranial nerves (optic, oculomotor).

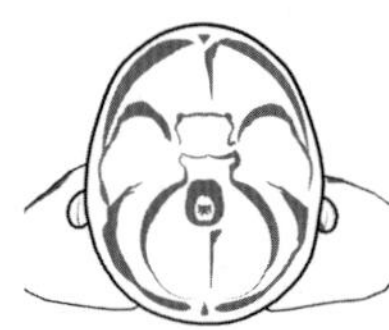

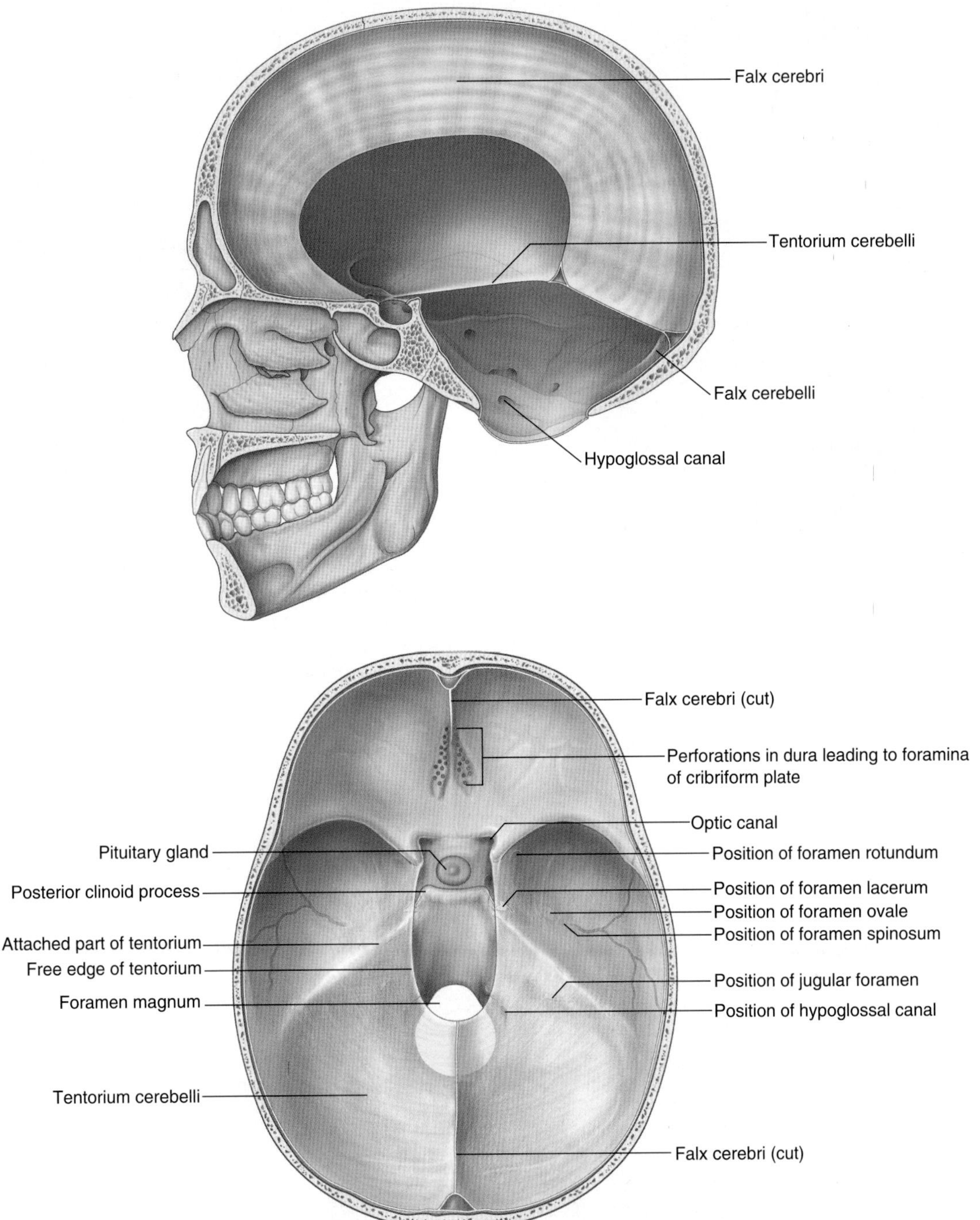

Plate 29.1 Depiction of the cranial fossae, dura mater, and venous sinuses. (From Drake RL et al. *Gray's Atlas of Anatomy*, 3rd edition, Philadelphia, Elsevier, 2021.)

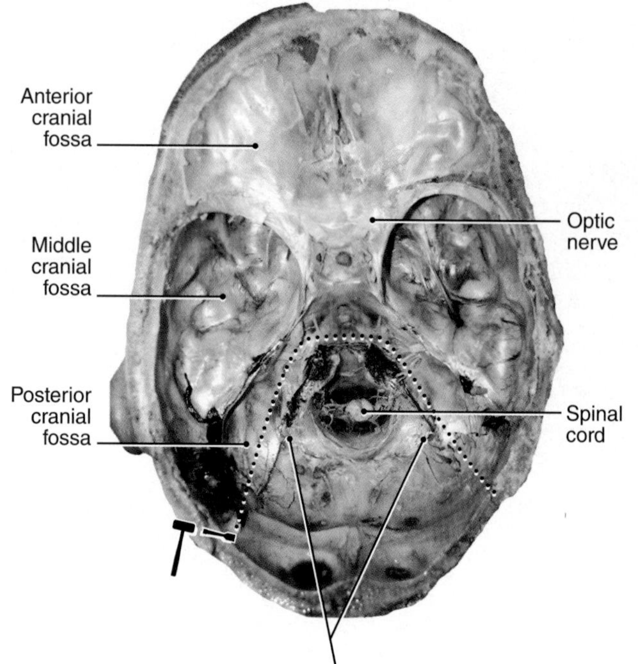

Fig. 29.2 Postcraniotomy horizontal section reveals the anterior, middle, and posterior cranial fossae, with inverted V-shaped section of dura mater removed from the posterior cranial fossa, highlighting dural venous sinuses, spinal cord, and cranial nerves.

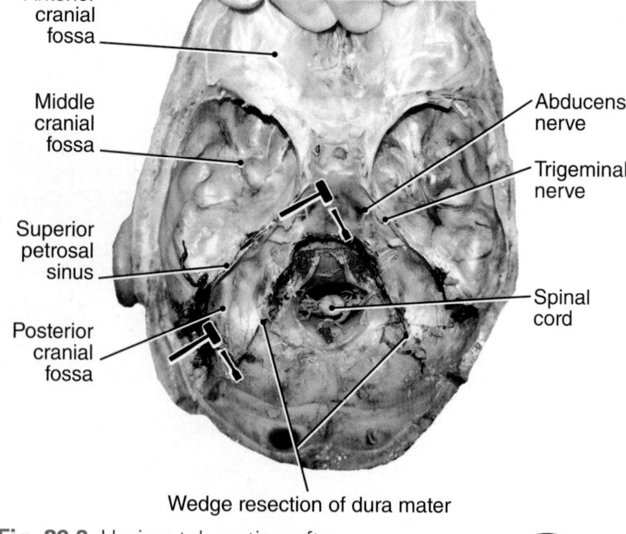

Fig. 29.3 Horizontal section after craniotomy reveals the anterior, middle, and posterior cranial fossae, with removal of dura mater from posterior cranial fossae, highlighting dura mater, dural venous sinuses (superior petrosal), spinal cord, and cranial nerves (abducens, trigeminal).

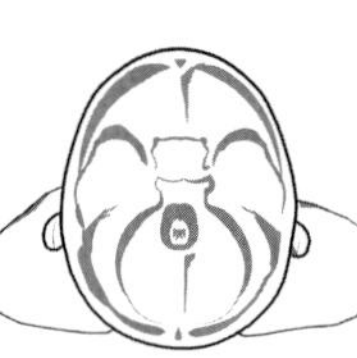

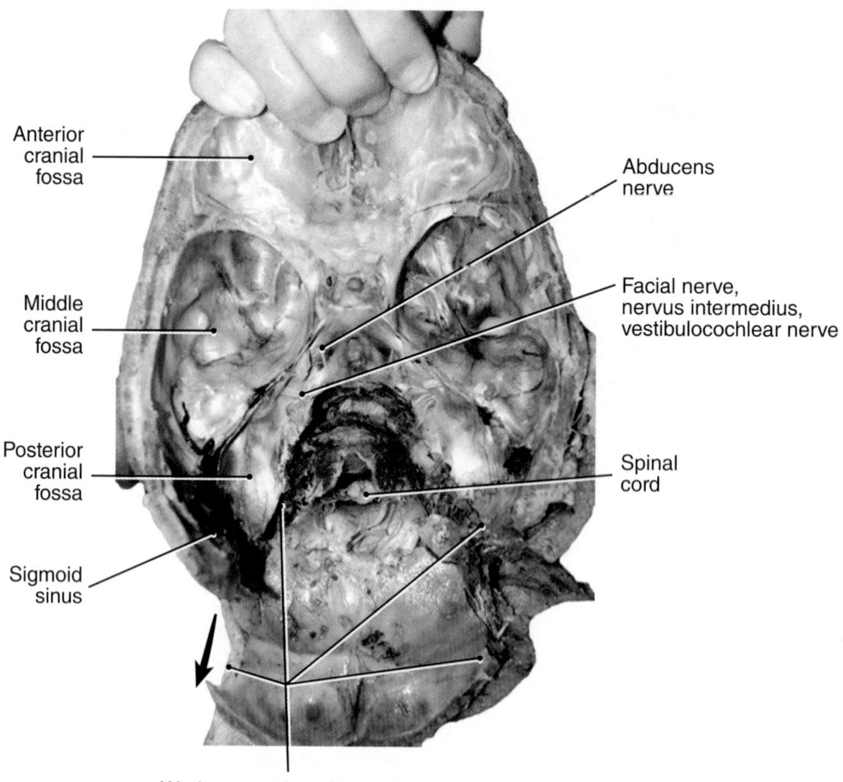

Fig. 29.4 Postcraniotomy horizontal section reveals the anterior, middle, and posterior cranial fossae, with wedge resection from the posterior cranial fossa reflected, highlighting the dural venous sinuses (sigmoid sinus), spinal cord, and cranial nerves (abducens, facial, nervus intermedius, and vestibulocochlear).

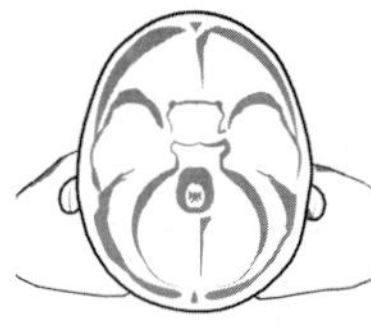

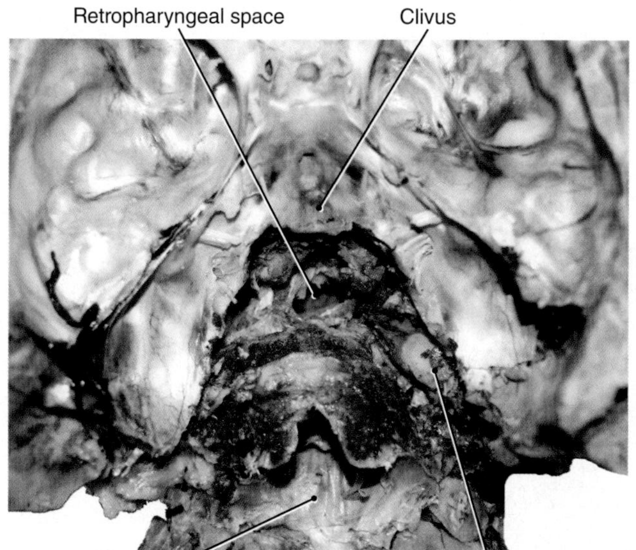

Fig. 29.5 Horizontal section after craniotomy, magnifying the clival region of the posterior cranial fossa and revealing a small opening in the retropharyngeal space.

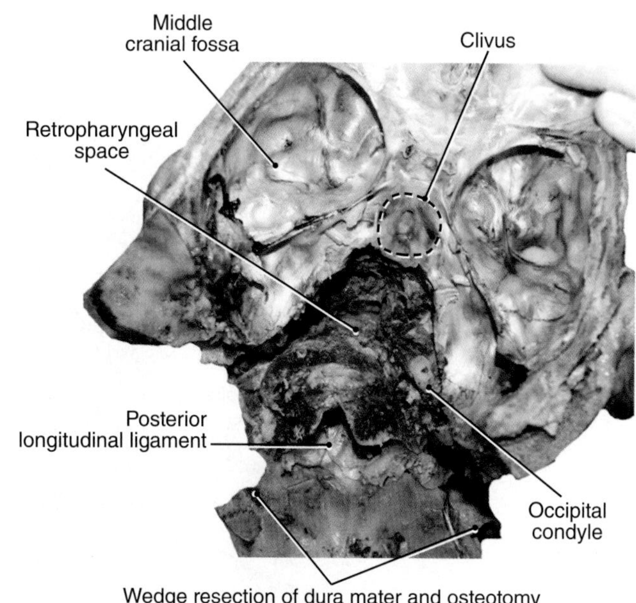

Fig. 29.7 Horizontal section after craniotomy of the middle and posterior cranial fossae, with wedge osteotomy resection of posterior cranial fossa, revealing a large opening, the *retropharyngeal space*.

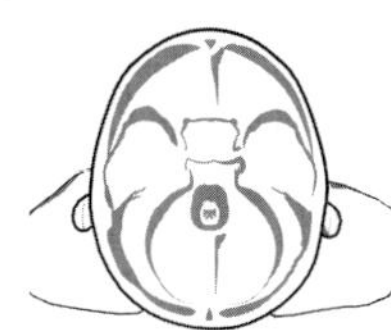

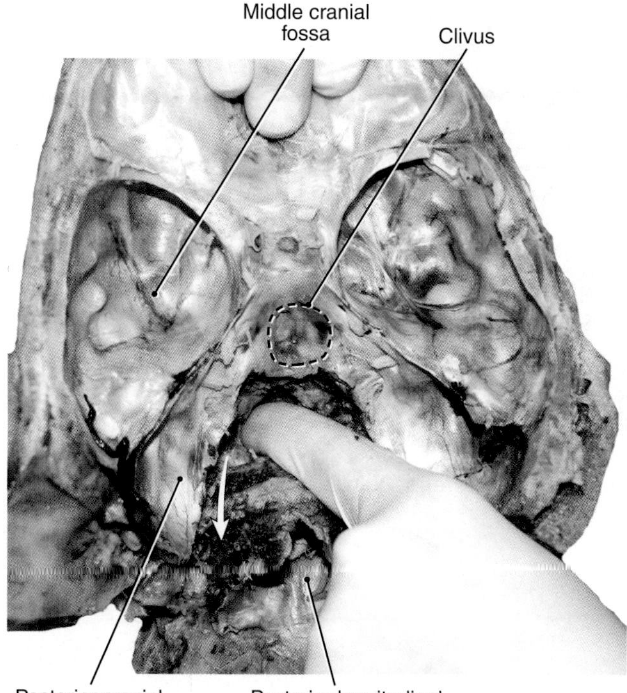

Fig. 29.6 Postcraniotomy horizontal section highlighting the anterior, middle, and posterior cranial fossae, with wedge osteotomy resection of the posterior cranial fossa and finger in the retropharyngeal space, pulling the cranial fossa posteriorly.

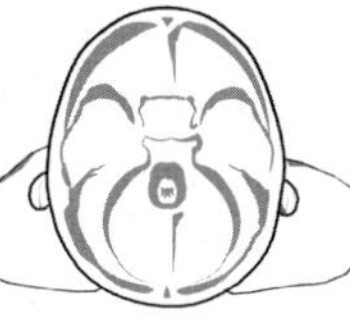

- **Complete the separation of the posterior cranial fossa and musculature from the retropharyngeal space. Carefully cut any soft tissues obstructing the separation (Fig. 29.7).**
- **Once the separation is complete, stabilize the head in the upright position and fully expose the retropharyngeal space (Fig. 29.8).**
- **Palpate the *pharyngeal tubercle*, which provides attachment to the fibrous raphe (seam) of the pharynx and is the point of attachment for the superior pharyngeal constrictor muscle (Fig. 29.9 and Plate 29.2).**
- **Identify the sternocleidomastoid muscle laterally.**
- **Beneath the tubercle, the *buccopharyngeal fascia* invests the constrictor muscles of the pharynx.**
- **Lateral to this fascia, note a thickened, whitish condensed fascia, the *carotid sheath*.**
- **With forceps, lift up the carotid sheath and expose its contents (Figs. 29.10 and 29.11).**
- **Identify and clean the internal jugular vein, common carotid artery, superior cervical ganglion, and vagus nerve (Fig. 29.12).**
- **Dissect the internal jugular vein and identify the accessory nerve at its entrance into the sternocleidomastoid muscle (Fig. 29.13).**

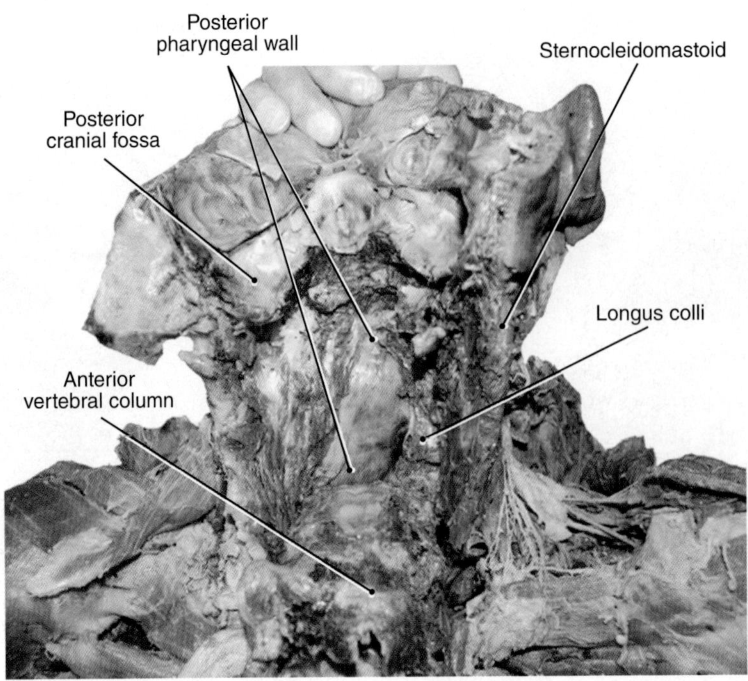

Fig. 29.8 Posterior view of the pharynx after retropharyngeal dissection. Anterior view of the vertebral column reveals fascia, sternocleidomastoid, longus colli muscles, and the posterior cranial fossa.

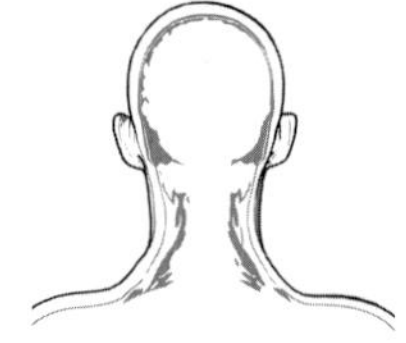

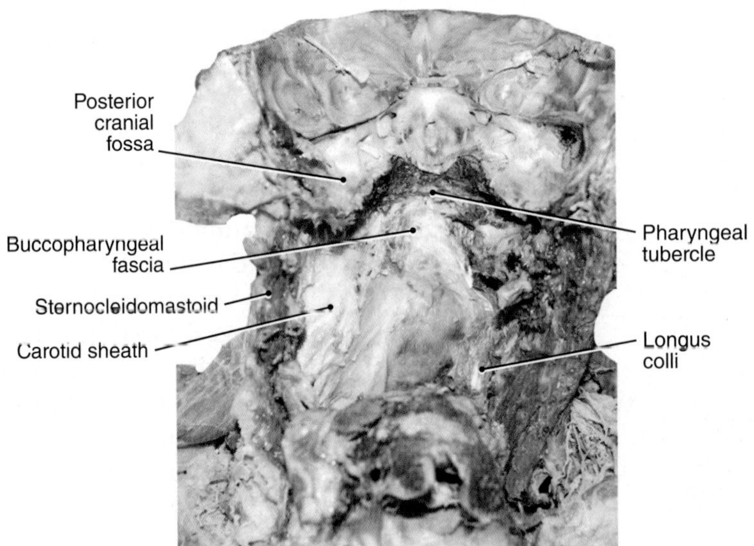

Fig. 29.9 Posterior view of the pharynx with wedge osteotomy resection of the posterior cranial fossa, highlighting the buccopharyngeal fascia and pharyngeal tubercle.

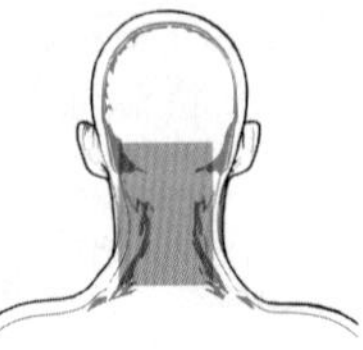

- **Continue cleaning the carotid sheath and the buccopharyngeal fascia inferiorly (Fig. 29.14) and fully expose its contents (Fig. 29.15).**
- **Identify the superior laryngeal nerve from its origin from the vagus nerve.**
- **Trace the hypoglossal nerve from its emergence from the hypoglossal canal (Fig. 29.16). The *hypoglossal nerve* passes lateral to the internal carotid artery.**
- **Medial to the internal carotid artery, identify the superior laryngeal nerve. Its internal branch travels near**

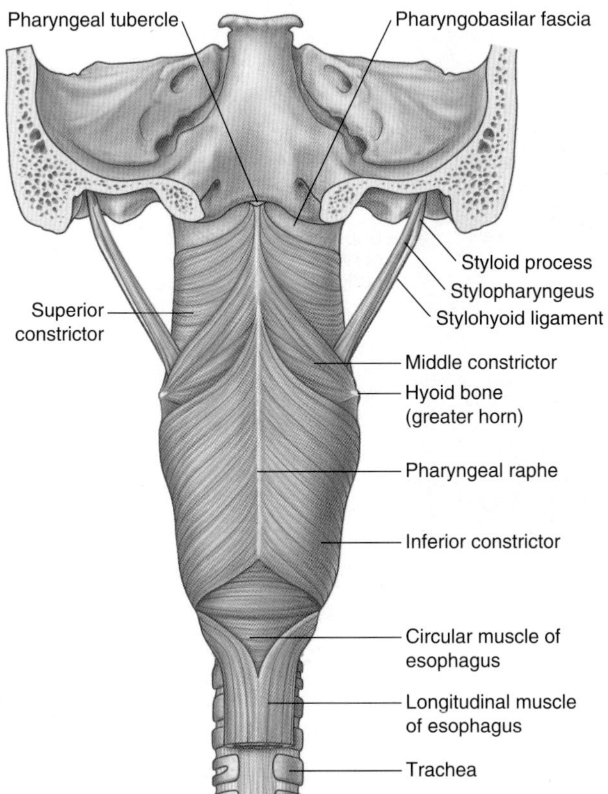

Plate 29.2 Depiction of the pharyngeal tubercle and the superior, middle, and inferior constrictors (posterior view). (From Drake RL et al. *Gray's Atlas of Anatomy*, 3rd edition, Philadelphia, Elsevier, 2021.)

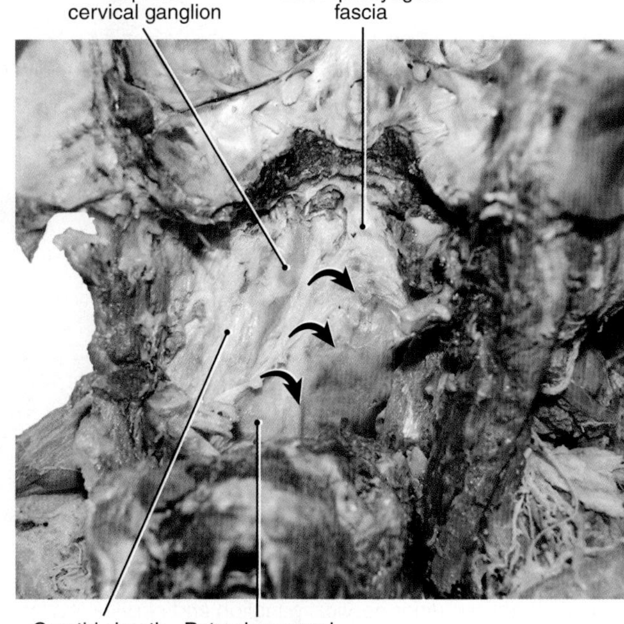

Fig. 29.10 Posterior view of the pharynx with the wedge osteotomy resection of the posterior cranial fossa, revealing the buccopharyngeal fascia, sternocleidomastoid muscle, and base of the skull.

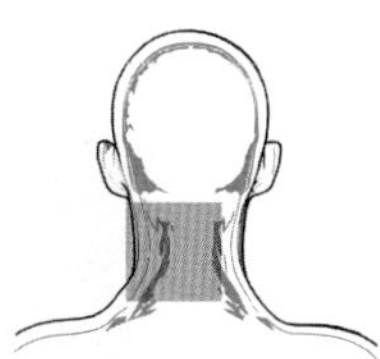

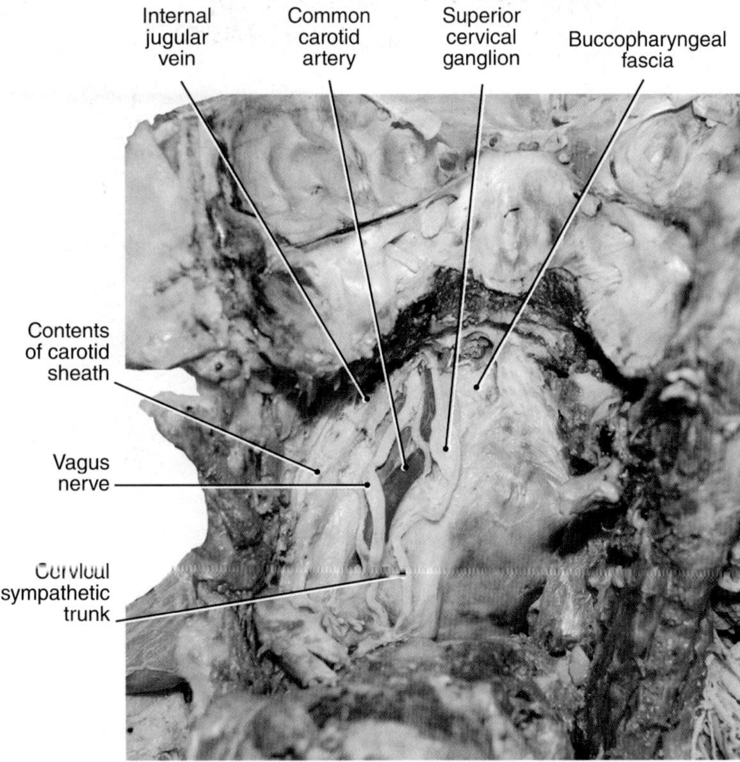

Fig. 29.11 Posterior view of the pharynx with wedge osteotomy resection of the posterior cranial fossa, revealing the buccopharyngeal fascia, cervical sympathetic trunk, superior cervical ganglion, common carotid artery, internal jugular vein, and vagus nerve.

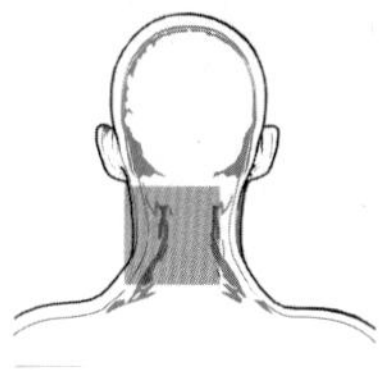

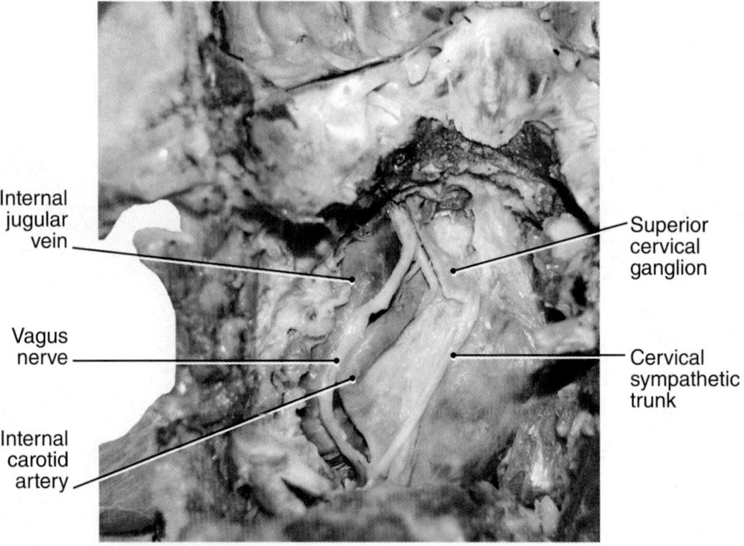

Fig. 29.12 Posterior view of the pharynx with wedge osteotomy resection of the posterior cranial fossa, highlighting contents of the carotid sheath (internal jugular vein, common carotid artery, and vagus nerve), as well as the superior cervical ganglion and cervical sympathetic trunk.

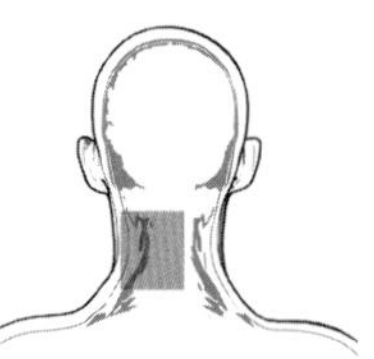

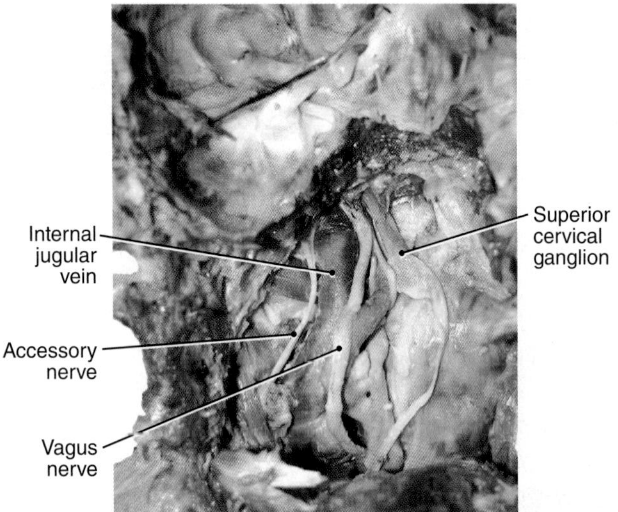

Fig. 29.13 Posterior view of the pharynx with wedge osteotomy resection of posterior cranial fossa, revealing the internal jugular vein, common carotid artery, inferior vagal ganglion (nodose ganglion), vagus nerve, superior cervical ganglion, and cervical sympathetic trunk.

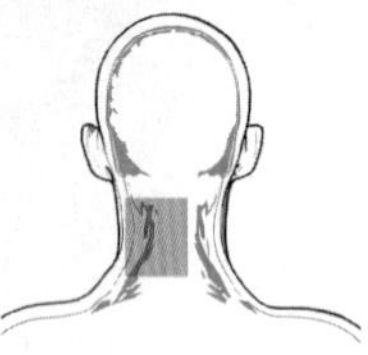

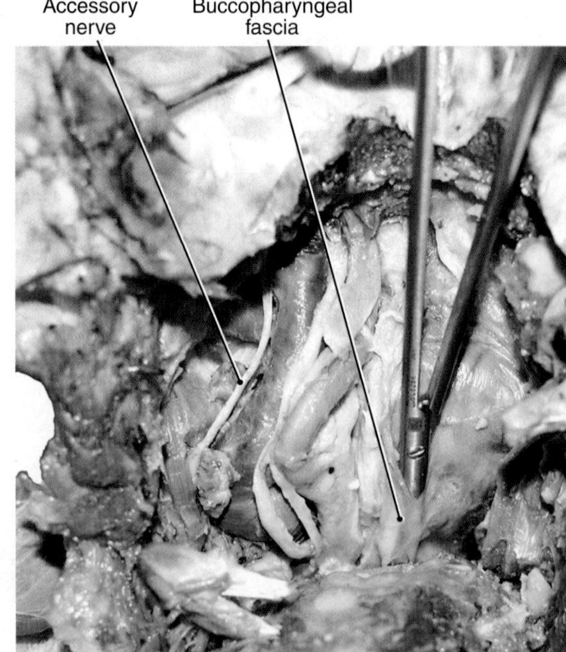

Fig. 29.14 Scissors removing remnants of the carotid sheath and buccopharyngeal fascia, further exposing neurovascular structures and the superior, middle, and inferior pharyngeal muscles.

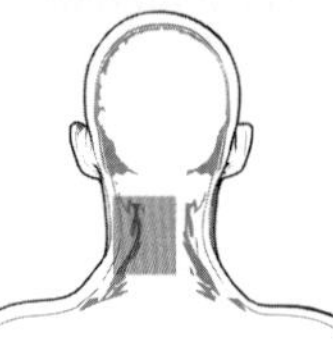

the gap between the middle and inferior constrictor muscles of the pharynx or the space between the external carotid artery and cornua of the hyoid bone.

DISSECTION **TIP**

You may encounter multiple lymph nodes around the internal jugular vein. After you identify these, remove them from the field of dissection (Fig. 29.17).

- **Lift the internal carotid artery to trace the pathway of the internal laryngeal artery and its division into internal and external branches (see Fig. 29.17).**
- **Identify the superior, middle, and inferior pharyngeal constrictor muscles and carefully clean the buccopharyngeal fascia and adipose tissue (see Fig. 29.17).**

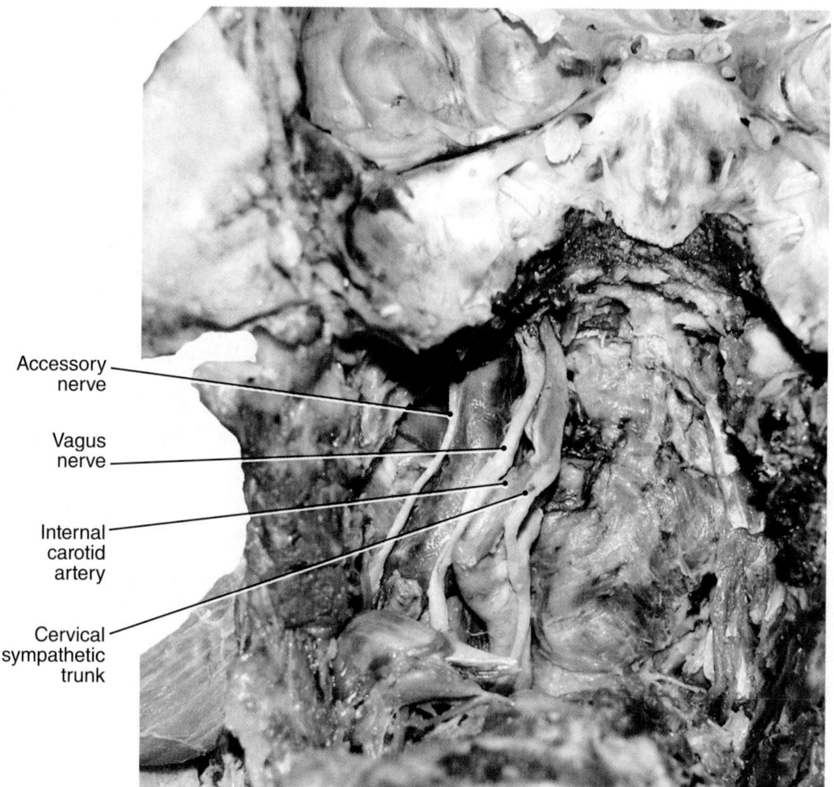

Fig. 29.15 Posterior view of the pharynx with wedge osteotomy resection of the posterior cranial fossa, highlighting the accessory and vagus nerves and cervical sympathetic trunk, as well as internal jugular vein, common carotid artery, inferior (nodose) ganglion, vagus nerve, and superior cervical ganglion.

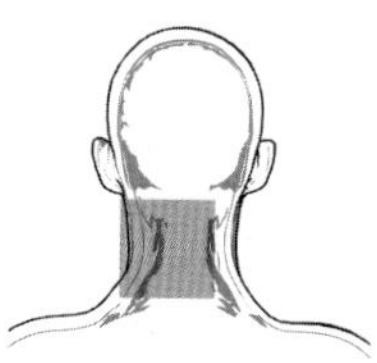

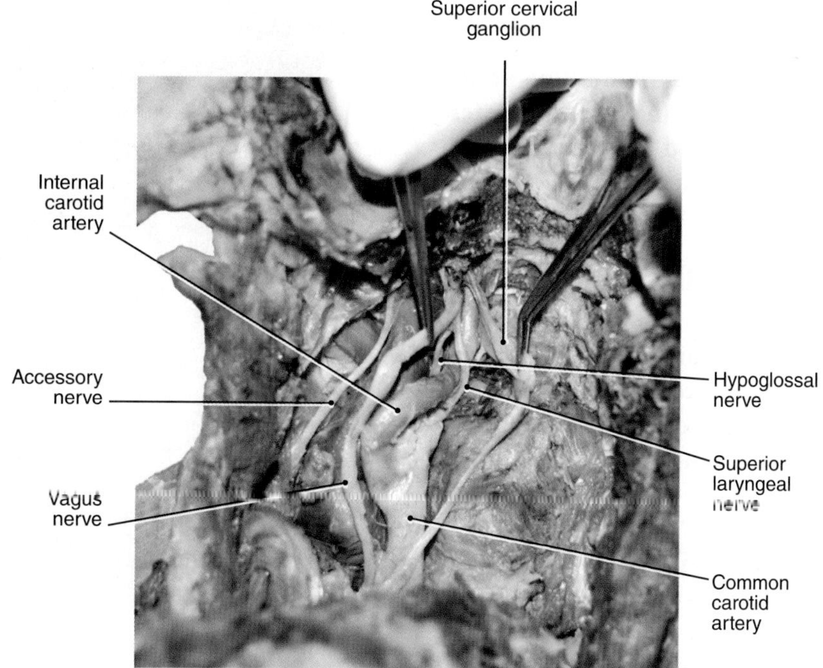

Fig. 29.16 Forceps retracting the superior cervical ganglion medially, further exposing the internal jugular vein, common carotid artery, inferior (nodose) ganglion, vagus nerve, superior laryngeal nerve, and hypoglossal nerve.

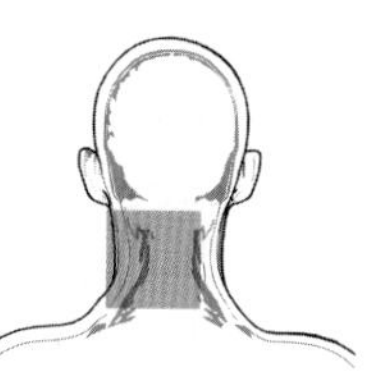

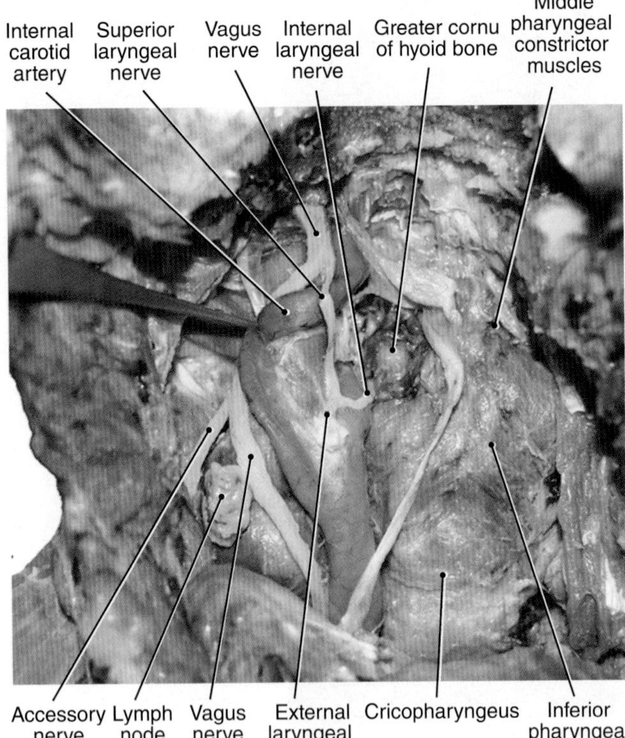

Fig. 29.17 Posterior view of the pharynx with wedge osteotomy resection of the posterior cranial fossa revealing the inferior pharyngeal constrictor (cricopharyngeus). Forceps retracting the internal carotid artery laterally, further exposing the division of the superior laryngeal nerve into the internal and external branches.

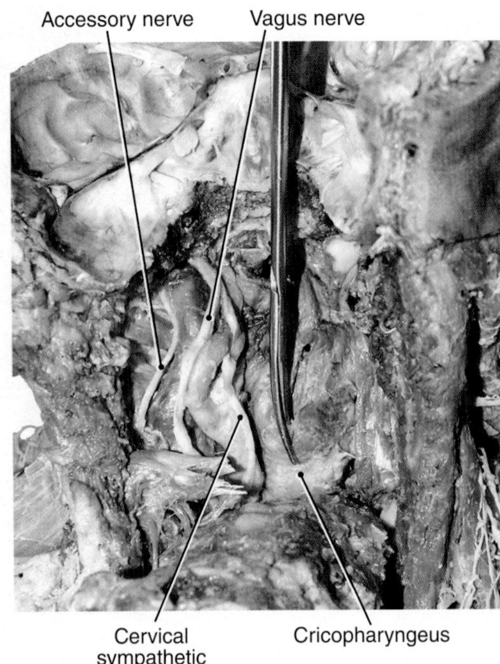

Fig. 29.18 Midsagittal incision at the midline of the superior middle and inferior pharyngeal constrictors, exposing the internal aspect of pharynx.

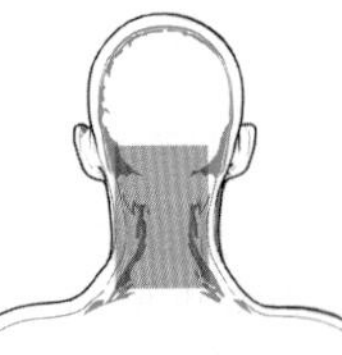

- **Make a midsagittal incision at the midline of the pharyngeal constrictor muscles to expose the internal aspect of the pharynx and to visualize such structures as the cervical sympathetic trunk and the epiglottis (Figs. 29.18 and 29.19).**

DISSECTION OF UNDIVIDED SPECIMEN

- **A different method of dissection of the retropharyngeal space is through the suboccipital region. In this approach, all the musculature of the back, as well as the cervical vertebrae and spinal cord, is removed, exposing the retropharyngeal space (Fig. 29.20 and Plates 29.3 and 29.4).**
- **The pharyngeal constrictor muscles are especially useful landmarks that can be identified with both dissecting methods as follows:**
  - ***Superior pharyngeal constrictor:* Identify the gap between the upper border of the superior pharyngeal constrictor muscle and the base of the skull. Clean the pharyngobasilar fascia that occupies this space and expose the levator veli palatini muscle, auditory tube, and ascending palatine artery (Fig. 29.21).**

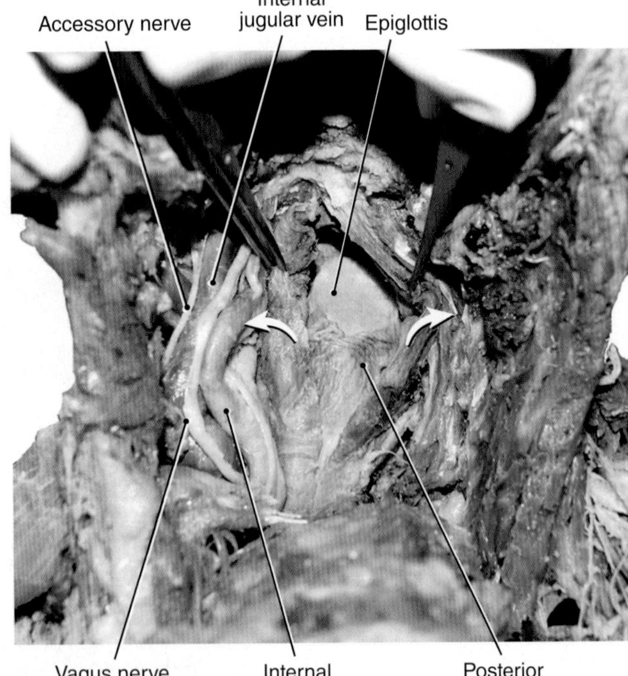

Fig. 29.19 Vertical incision of the pharynx with the pharyngeal wall reflected, revealing the epiglottis and posterior cricoarytenoid muscle.

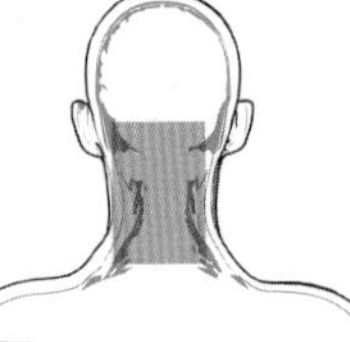

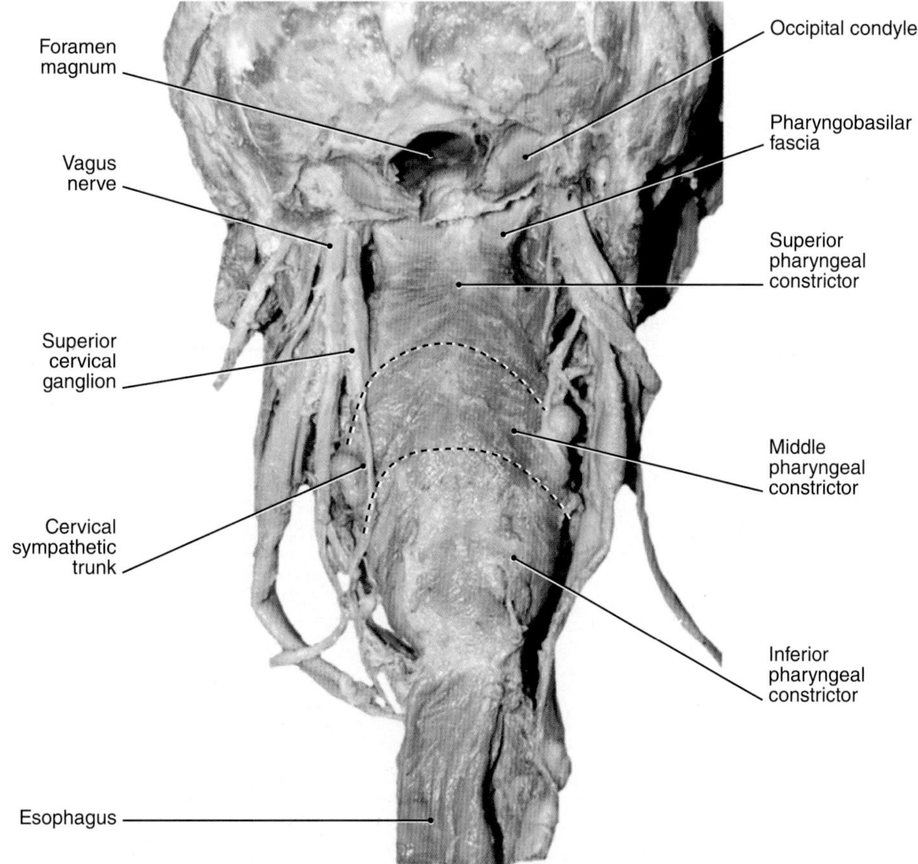

Fig. 29.20 Posterior view of the pharynx and base of the skull, revealing the foramen magnum, occipital condyle, pharyngobasilar fascia, and superior, middle, and inferior pharyngeal constrictors, as well as the superior cervical ganglion and cervical sympathetic trunk.

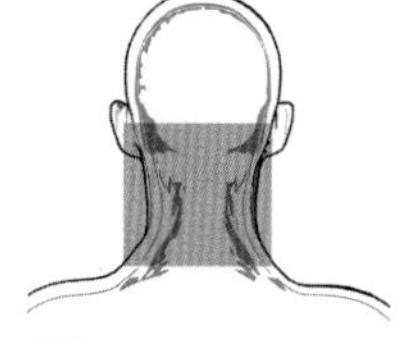

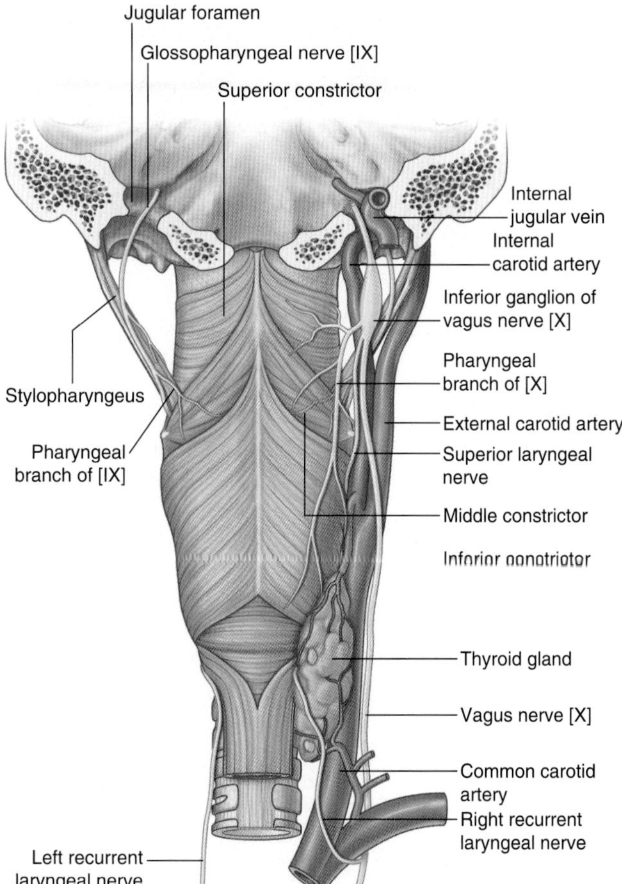

Plate 29.3 Posterior view of the retropharyngeal space, with several neurovascular structures and muscles exposed. (From Drake RL et al. *Gray's Atlas of Anatomy*, 3rd edition, Philadelphia, Elsevier, 2021.)

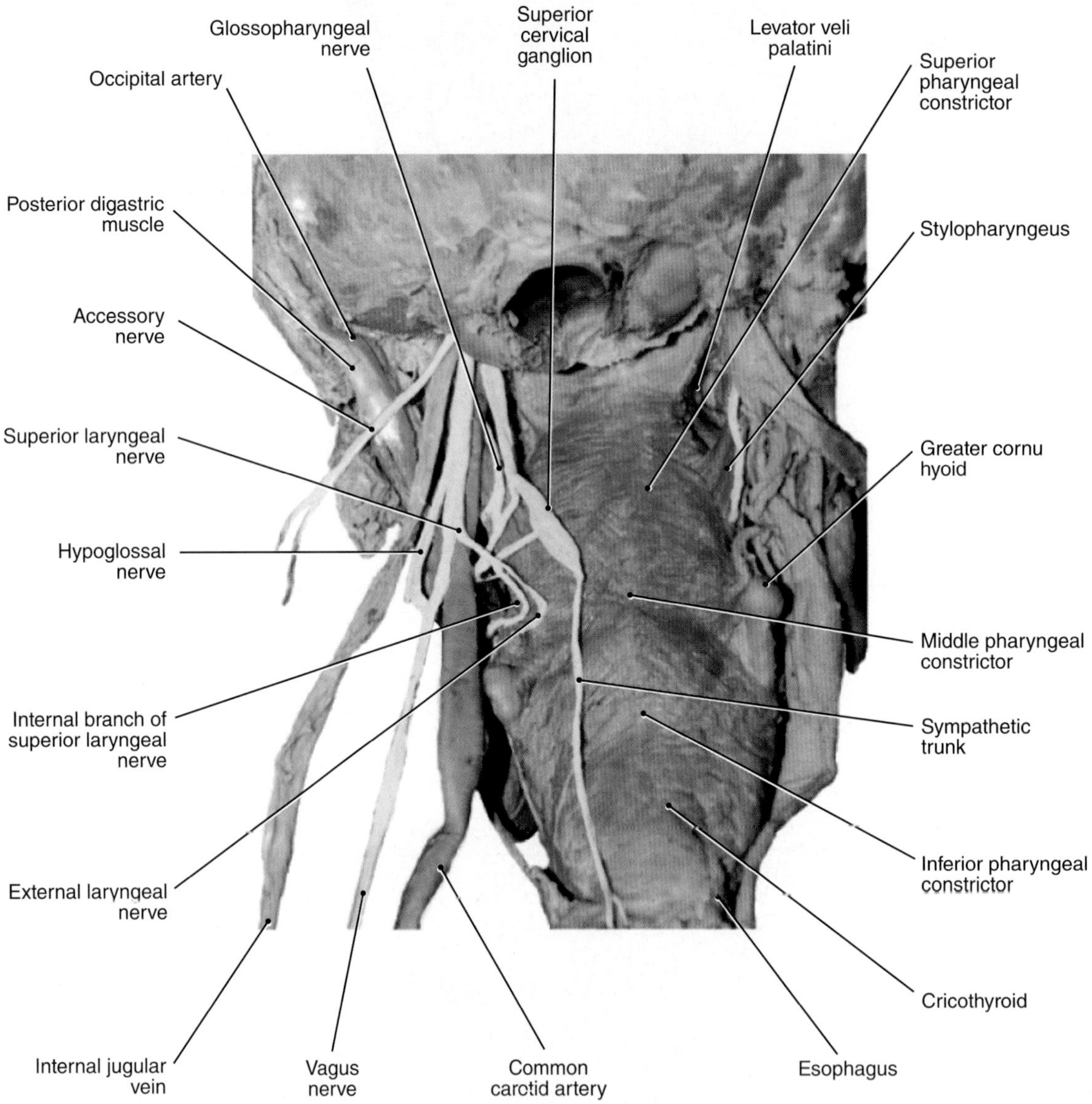

Glossopharyngeal nerve

Superior cervical ganglion

Levator veli palatini

Occipital artery

Superior pharyngeal constrictor

Posterior digastric muscle

Stylopharyngeus

Accessory nerve

Superior laryngeal nerve

Greater cornu hyoid

Hypoglossal nerve

Middle pharyngeal constrictor

Internal branch of superior laryngeal nerve

Sympathetic trunk

Inferior pharyngeal constrictor

External laryngeal nerve

Cricothyroid

Internal jugular vein

Vagus nerve

Common carotid artery

Esophagus

Fig. 29.21 View of the retropharyngeal space, with several neurovascular structures and muscles exposed.

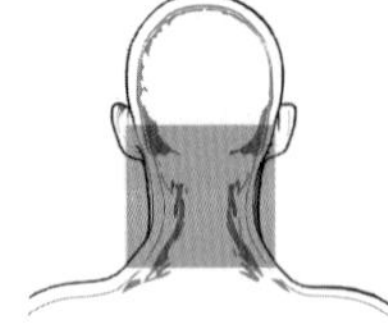

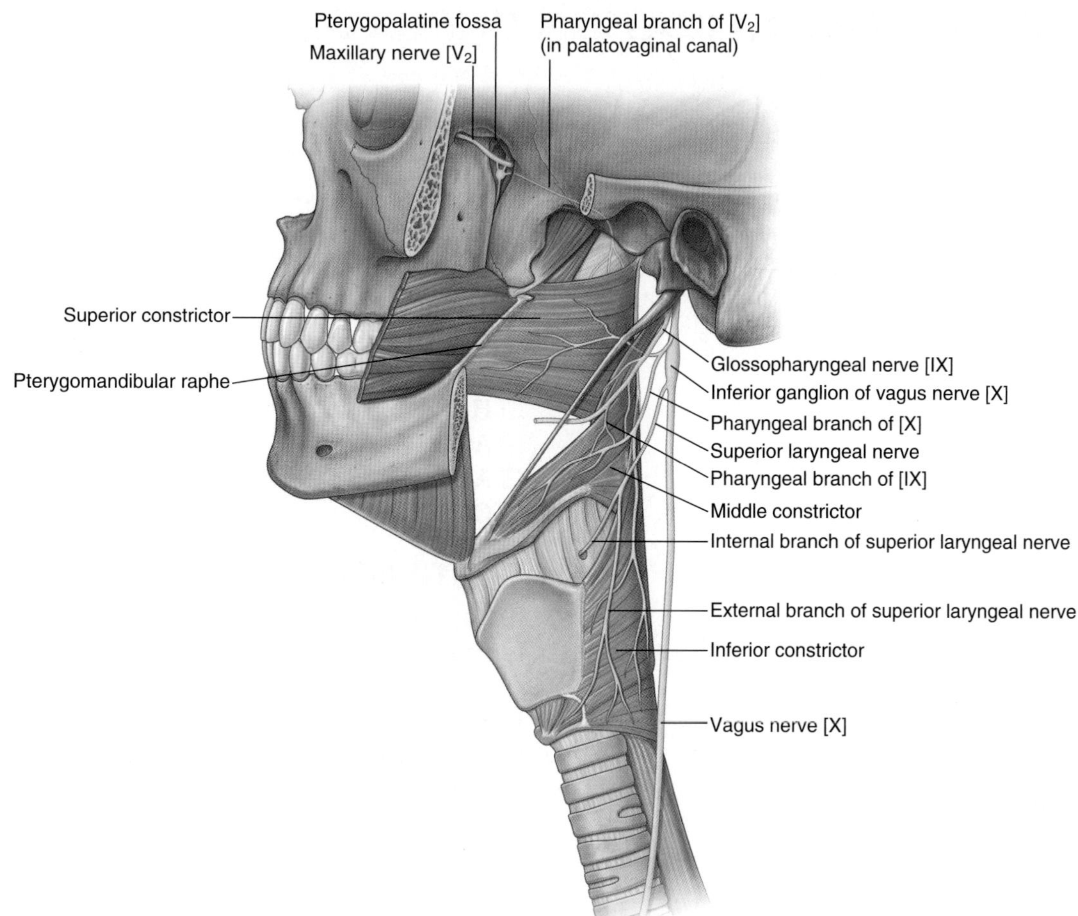

Plate 29.4 Lateral view of the retropharyngeal space, illustrating regional nerves and muscles. (From Drake RL et al. *Gray's Atlas of Anatomy*, 3rd edition, Philadelphia, Elsevier, 2021.)

- ***Middle pharyngeal constrictor:*** **This muscle attaches to the greater cornu of the hyoid bone. At the junction of the superior and middle pharyngeal constrictors, identify the stylopharyngeus muscle and the glossopharyngeal nerve (see Fig. 29.21).**
- ***Inferior pharyngeal constrictor:*** **This muscle arises from the sides of the thyroid and cricoid cartilages. At the junction of the middle and inferior pharyngeal constrictors, identify the internal laryngeal nerve and the superior laryngeal artery (see Fig. 29.21). The inferior part of the inferior constrictor is also known as the cricopharyngeus muscle.**

LABORATORY IDENTIFICATION CHECKLIST

NERVES

- ☐ Sympathetic trunk
- ☐ Vagus
  - ☐ Recurrent laryngeal
  - ☐ Inferior laryngeal
- ☐ Accessory
- ☐ Hypoglossal
- ☐ Glossopharyngeal

GANGLIA

- ☐ Superior cervical
- ☐ Middle cervical

ARTERIES

- ☐ Common carotid
- ☐ Internal carotid
- ☐ External carotid
- ☐ Vertebral

VEIN

- ☐ Internal jugular

MUSCLES

- ☐ Sternocleidomastoid
- ☐ Stylopharyngeus
- ☐ Superior constrictor
- ☐ Middle constrictor
- ☐ Inferior constrictor
- ☐ Longus colli

BONES

- ☐ Occipital
- ☐ Temporal
  - ☐ Mastoid process
  - ☐ Styloid process
- ☐ Hyoid
- ☐ Atlas (C1)
- ☐ Axis (C2)
- ☐ C3 to C7

CARTILAGES

- ☐ Thyroid
- ☐ Cricoid

LIGAMENTS

- ☐ Transverse, of atlas
- ☐ Alar

GLANDS

- ☐ Thyroid
- ☐ Parathyroid

FASCIAE

- ☐ Buccopharyngeal
- ☐ Retropharyngeal
- ☐ Prevertebral

CLINICAL APPLICATIONS

CRICOTHYROTOMY

Clinical Application

Procedure creates an emergent airway through the cricothyroid membrane.

Anatomical Landmarks (Figs. VIII.1 and VIII.2)

Palpation of midline structures

- **Hyoid cartilage**
- **Thyroid cartilage**
- **Cricoid cartilage**

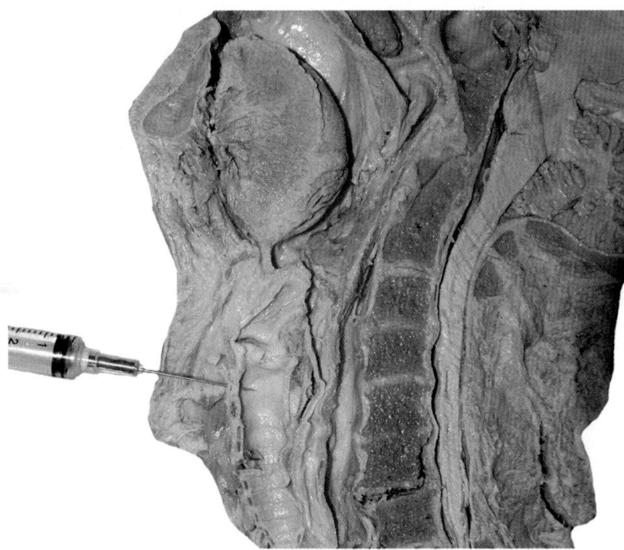

Fig. VIII.1

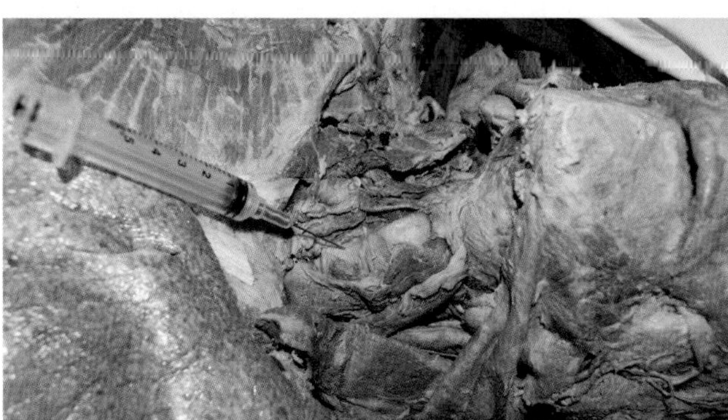

Fig. VIII.2

Skin/subcutaneous tissue

- **Cricothyroid arteries and small veins (may traverse the cricothyroid membrane)**
- **Cricothyroid membrane**

TRACHEAL INTUBATION

Clinical Application

Procedure maintains and controls definitive airway by introducing a tube orally that passes through the larynx between the vocal cords, stopping before the tracheal bifurcation.

Anatomical Landmarks (Fig. VIII.3)

- **Mouth**
  Incisor teeth
  Anterior arch: palatoglossus muscle
  Palatine tonsil
  Posterior arch: palatopharyngeus muscle
- **Oral pharynx**
- **Epiglottis**
- **Vallecula**
- **Piriform recess**
- **Vocal cords**
- **Trachea**

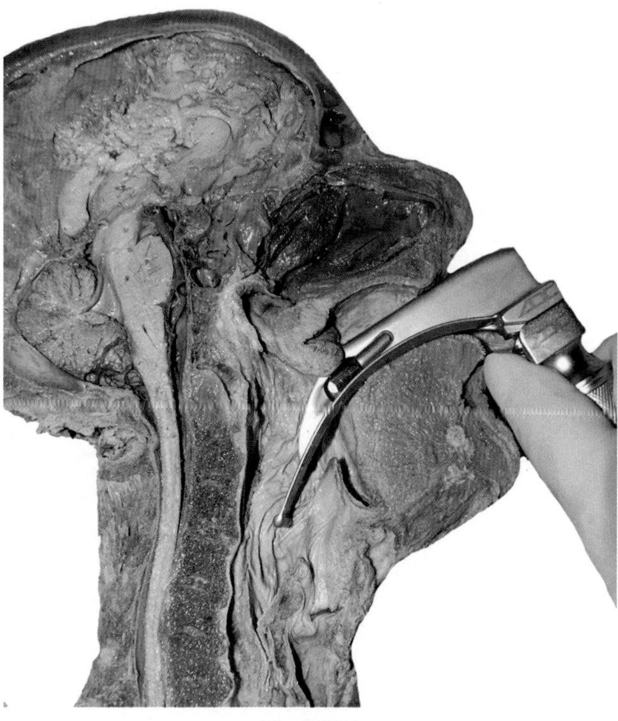

Fig. VIII.3

NASOTRACHEAL INTUBATION

Clinical Application

Procedure maintains and controls the airway by introducing a tube nasally that passes through the oral pharynx and larynx between the vocal cords, stopping short of the tracheal bifurcation.

Anatomical Landmarks

- **Right or left nostril**
- **Conchae**
- **Nasopharynx**
- **Oropharynx**
- **Laryngopharynx**
- **Trachea**

BURR HOLES FOR CRANIOTOMY

Clinical Application

Procedure creates an opening in the skull to evacuate blood from an epidural or subdural hemorrhage.

Anatomical Landmarks

- **Scalp**
- **Skin**
- **Connective tissue**
- **Aponeurosis**
- **Loose connective tissue**
- **Periosteum**
- **Bones of the calvaria**
- **Dura mater**

AKINOSI TECHNIQUE: TRIGEMINAL-MANDIBULAR NERVE BLOCK

Clinical Application

Procedure allows a local anesthetic to be deposited near the mandibular division of the trigeminal nerve when opening the mouth is prohibited.

Anatomical Landmarks

- **Oral vestibule**
- **Mucosa medial to ramus**
- **Maxillary bone and mucosa**
- **Trigeminal nerve–mandibular nerve branches**

Page numbers followed by "*f*" indicate figures, and "*b*" indicate boxes.

A

B

C

D

E

J

K

L

P

Q

R

S

T